Brief Contents

1 Introduction to Health Care, 1
2 The Person's Rights, 10
3 The Nursing Assistant, 18
4 Ethics and Laws, 30
5 Student and Work Ethics, 42
6 Communicating With the Person, 53
7 Health Team Communications, 64
8 Medical Terminology, 78
9 Body Structure and Function, 89
10 The Older Person, 108
11 Safety Needs, 117
12 Preventing Falls, 133
13 Restraint Alternatives and Restraints, 144
14 Preventing Infection, 159
15 Isolation Precautions, 175
16 Body Mechanics, 189
17 Moving the Person, 199
18 Transferring the Person, 214
19 The Person's Unit, 232
20 Bedmaking, 244
21 Oral Hygiene, 261
22 Daily Hygiene and Bathing, 271
23 Grooming, 291
24 Dressing and Undressing, 304
25 Urinary Needs, 316
26 Urinary Catheters, 333
27 Bowel Needs, 344
28 Nutrition, 355

29 Meeting Nutrition Needs, 365
30 Fluid Needs, 377
31 Measurements, 388
32 Exercise and Activity Needs, 412
33 Comfort and Rest Needs, 425
34 Collecting Specimens, 434
35 Wound Care, 446
36 Pressure Injuries, 464
37 Oxygen Needs, 475
38 Rehabilitation Needs, 486
39 Hearing, Speech, and Vision Problems, 493
40 Common Health Problems, 503
41 Mental Health Disorders, 529
42 Confusion and Dementia, 539
43 Emergency Care, 555
44 End-of-Life Care, 569
45 Getting a Job, 578

Review Question Answers, 587

Appendices, 590

A The Patient Care Partnership—Understanding Expectations, Rights, and Responsibilities (A Summary), 590
B National Nurse Aide Assessment Program (NNAAP®) Written Examination Content Outline and Skills Evaluation, 591
C Minimum Data Set: Selected Pages, 592

Glossary, 594

Key Abbreviations, 602

Index, 604

7TH EDITION

MOSBY'S®
ESSENTIALS
FOR *Nursing Assistants*

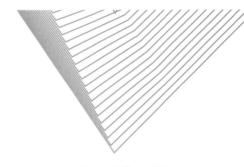

LEIGHANN N. REMMERT, MS, RN
SHEILA A. SORRENTINO, PhD, RN

ELSEVIER

Elsevier
3251 Riverport Lane
St. Louis, Missouri 63043

MOSBY'S® ESSENTIALS FOR NURSING ASSISTANTS, SEVENTH EDITION   ISBN: 978-0-323-79631-6
Copyright © 2023 by Elsevier, Inc. All rights reserved.

Notice

Practitioners and researchers must always rely on their own experience and knowledge in evaluating and using any information, methods, compounds or experiments described herein. Because of rapid advances in the medical sciences, in particular, independent verification of diagnoses and drug dosages should be made. To the fullest extent of the law, no responsibility is assumed by Elsevier, authors, editors or contributors for any injury and/or damage to persons or property as a matter of products liability, negligence or otherwise, or from any use or operation of any methods, products, instructions, or ideas contained in the material herein.

Previous editions copyrighted 2019, 2014, 2010, 2006, 2001, and 1997.

International Standard Book Number: 978-0-323-79631-6

Executive Content Strategists: Nancy O'Brien, Kelly Skelton, and Sonya Seigafuse
Senior Content Development Specialists: Melissa Rawe, Laura Klein, and Kathleen Nahm
Publishing Services Manager: Catherine Jackson
Health Content Management Specialist: Kristine Feeherty
Design Direction: Brian Salisbury

Printed in Canada

Last digit is the print number: 9   8   7   6   5   4   3   2

Working together
to grow libraries in
developing countries

www.elsevier.com • www.bookaid.org

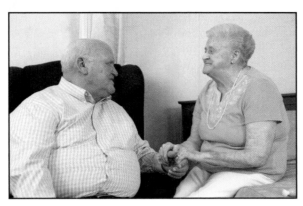

In memory of my grandfather and friend,
Roger ("Curly") Dennison, Sr.
In honor of 65 years of marriage and a lifetime of cherished moments.

With love,
"Annie" (Leighann)

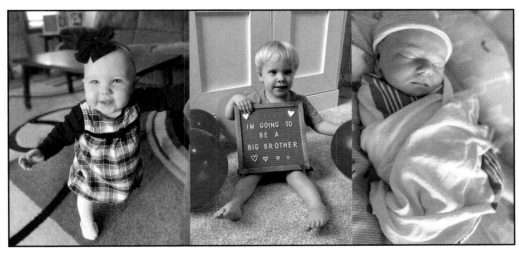

To the newest members of our family…
My brother's granddaughters…
Ava Loraine and Mason's baby sister, Makenzie Grace.
Wishing them a lifetime of health, happiness, and love.

With much love,
Aunt Sheila

About the Authors

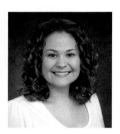

Leighann N. Remmert is a registered nurse and nursing assistant instructor. She has taught in high school, vocational, and community college nursing assistant programs in central Illinois.

Ms. Remmert has a Bachelor of Science degree in nursing from Bradley University (Peoria, Illinois) and a Master of Science degree in nursing education from Southern Illinois University Edwardsville (Edwardsville, Illinois).

Nursing practice for Ms. Remmert began at St. John's Hospital (Springfield, Illinois) as a nursing assistant/technician. As a registered nurse, Ms. Remmert concentrated in the area of emergency nursing at Memorial Medical Center (Springfield, Illinois). There, her roles included staff nurse, charge nurse, nurse preceptor, and trauma nurse specialist. As a clinical nursing instructor at Capital Area School of Practical Nursing (Springfield, Illinois), Ms. Remmert supervised, instructed, and evaluated student learning in various long-term care and acute care settings.

In her current focus on nursing assistant education, Ms. Remmert emphasizes the importance of professionalism and work ethics, safety, teamwork, communication, and accountability. Valuing the role of the nursing assistant and treating the person with dignity, care, and respect are integral to her instruction.

Ms. Remmert is co-author of *Mosby's® Textbook for Nursing Assistants* (ed 8–10), *Mosby's® Essentials for Nursing Assistants* (ed 4–7), and *Mosby's® Textbook for Medication Assistants* (ed 1). She was a consultant on *Mosby's® Textbook for Long-Term Care Nursing Assistants* (ed 6) and served as a content adviser for *Mosby's® Nursing Assistant Video Skills* (version 4.0).

Ms. Remmert is a Basic Life Support instructor. She is a member of Sigma Theta Tau International, the Honor Society of Nursing, and the Certified Nursing Assistant Educator's Association (Illinois, Central Region).

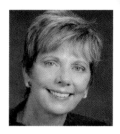

Sheila A. Sorrentino was instrumental in the development and approval of CNA-PN-ADN career-ladder programs in the Illinois community college system and has taught at various levels of nursing education—nursing assistant, practical nursing, associate degree nursing, and baccalaureate and higher degree programs. Her career includes experiences in nursing practice and higher education—nursing assistant, staff nurse, charge and head nurse, nursing faculty, program director, assistant dean, and dean.

A Mosby author and co-author of several nursing assistant titles since 1982, Dr. Sorrentino's titles include:
- *Mosby's® Textbook for Nursing Assistants*
- *Mosby's® Essentials for Nursing Assistants*
- *Mosby's® Textbook for Long-Term Care Nursing Assistants*
- *Mosby's® Textbook for Nursing Assistive Personnel*
- *Mosby's® Basic Skills for Nursing Assistants*
- *Mosby's® Textbook for Medication Assistants*

She was also involved in the development of an early version of *Mosby's® Nursing Assistant Video Skills* and *Mosby's® Nursing Video Skills*, winner of an AJN Book of the Year Award (electronic media).

Dr. Sorrentino has a Bachelor of Science degree in nursing, a Master of Arts degree in education, a Master of Science degree in nursing, and a PhD in higher education administration. She is a member of Sigma Theta Tau International, the Honor Society of Nursing. Her past community activities include the Rotary Club of Anthem (Anthem, Arizona), the Provena Senior Services Board of Directors (Mokena, Illinois), the Central Illinois Higher Education Health Care Task Force, the Iowa-Illinois Safety Council Board of Directors, and the Board of Directors of Our Lady of Victory Nursing Center (Bourbonnais, Illinois).

She received an alumni achievement award from Lewis University for outstanding leadership and dedication in nursing education. She is also a member of the Illinois State University College of Education Hall of Fame.

Acknowledgments

Many individuals help to develop an accurate, up-to-date, and timely publication. With gratitude and appreciation, we acknowledge:

- The staff of The Christian Village (Lincoln, Illinois). Many of the new photos were shot in this location.
- MPS North America, LLC, for their talented artistry and prompt revisions.
- The reviewers who made comments and offered suggestions to improve the text. See "Reviewers" on p. viii.
- Anne Skowronski, PT, for her feedback and professional insight to questions regarding positioning devices.
- Susan Broadhurst for her role as copyeditor and her attention to detail.
- Graphic World for their proofreading efforts.
- And finally, the Elsevier staff involved:
  - Nancy O'Brien, Kelly Skelton, and Sonya Seigafuse, Content Strategists
  - Melissa Rawe, Laura Klein, and Kathleen Nahm, Senior Content Development Specialists
  - Kristine Feeherty, Health Content Management Specialist
  - Brian Salisbury, Designer

To all of the individuals who contributed to this effort in any way, we are sincerely grateful.

Leighann N. Remmert and Sheila A. Sorrentino

Reviewers

Monica Asare-Boadu, BSN, RN-BC
Program Director/Director of Nursing
Serenity Nurse Aide Academy/Serenity Nursing Services
Charlotte, North Carolina

Mary Barr, RN
Health Sciences
Lancaster County Career & Technology Center
Willow Street, Pennsylvania

Nicole Bartreau, MSN, APRN, FNP-C, IBCLC, CVT
Residential Faculty
Nursing/Nurse Assisting
Mesa Community College
Mesa, Arizona

Demy Blake, RN, MSN
Nurse Educator
South Dade Technical College
Homestead, Florida

Rebecca Deibwert, RN, MSN
Nurse Educator
Cochise College
Sierra Vista, Arizona

Abimbola Farinde, PhD, PharmD
Licensed Pharmacist, Licensed Professional Counselor
Certified Geriatric Pharmacist
Professor
Columbia Southern University
Phoenix, Arizona

Marie Furtado, MBBS, MPH
Doctor, Workforce Solution Group – Health Care
St. Louis Community College
Bridgeton, Missouri

Sara Hansen, M.Ed
State Licensed and Nationally Certified Athletic Trainer,
    Health Science Instructor
Career & Technology
Humble Independent School District
Humble, Texas

Daphene L. Kimball, RN, PCM, CLC, SANE
Community Health Instructor
District 6 Health Department MRC
Augusta, Georgia

Ali Morton, LPN
Nursing Assistant Instructor
Career Technical Training
Whitney M. Young Job Corps Center
Simpsonville, Kentucky

Laura Oldaker
Certified Dementia Trainer, First Aid/CPR Certified
    Instructor
Nursing Assistant Program Administrator
Administration
Academy for Caregiving Excellence
Tucson, Arizona

Suzanne Pinos, RN, MSN
Professor I
Department of Nursing
Palm Beach State College
Lake Worth, Florida

Caron Que, MHA, BSN, RN
Registered Nurse/Certified Teacher
Career and Technology Education (CTE)
Centennial High School
Burleson, Texas

Fatima Demonteverde Reyes, RN, MS, CCRN
Program Coordinator
Avid CNA School
Streamwood, Illinois

Darlene Seay, RN, BSN, MSEd
RN Health and Medical Sciences Instructor
Career and Technology Education (CTE)
Nelson County Public Schools
Lovingston, Virginia

Cassellen J. Springer
Registered Dental Assistant
Certified Professional Coder – Apprentice
MBA with Healthcare Management
Allied Health Director
Allied Health
Emergency Medical Training Professionals
Lexington, Kentucky

The seventh edition of *Mosby's® Essentials for Nursing Assistants* serves several purposes.

- Prepares students to function as nursing assistants in nursing centers and hospitals.
- Assists faculty in meeting educational goals.
- Serves as a resource when preparing for the competency evaluation.
- Serves as a resource for nursing assistants wanting to review or learn new information for safe care.

The following foundational principles and values are presented in specific chapters and integrated in content and key features (pp. xiv-xix) throughout the book.

- Patients and residents are *persons* with dignity having a past, a present, and a future. Such persons are physical, social, psychological, and spiritual beings with basic needs and protected rights.
- Nursing assistant roles, functions, and limitations are described in federal and state laws with dependence on effective delegation and good work ethics.
- Body structure and function, body mechanics, preventing infection, and safety and comfort measures form an essential knowledge base.
- Communication skills enhance relationships with the nursing and health teams, patients and residents, and families and visitors.
- The nursing assistant has a key role in the nursing process.

Content Issues

Content decisions are based on changes in laws or in guidelines and standards issued by federal and state governments, accrediting agencies, and national organizations. So are changes to state curricula and competency evaluations.

Student learning needs and abilities, instructor desires, work-related issues, course/program and book length, and student cost also are among the many factors considered.

New Content

Chapter 1: Introduction to Health Care

- Purposes
- Types of Agencies
- Staffing
- Safety and Quality
- Box 1-1 HHS Agencies
- Policies and Procedures

Chapter 2: The Person's Rights

- Protecting Rights

Chapter 3: The Nursing Assistant

- FOCUS ON COMMUNICATION: Follow-Up and Feedback

Chapter 5: Student and Work Ethics

- Attention
- FOCUS ON COMMUNICATION: Planning Your Work
- Burnout
- Box 5-3 Burnout—Causes, Signs, and Symptoms

Chapter 6: Communicating With the Person

- CARING ABOUT CULTURE: Culture and Religion
- Health Care Beliefs and Practices
- CARING ABOUT CULTURE: Listening
- FOCUS ON OLDER PERSONS: Behavior

Chapter 7: Health Team Communications

- Table 7-1 Parts of a Medical Record
- FOCUS ON COMMUNICATION: Assessment

Chapter 8: Medical Terminology *(new)*

- Learning Word Elements
- Abdominal Quadrants
- Positional Terms
- Common Terms and Phrases
- Table 8-6 Common Health Care Terms and Phrases

Chapter 10: The Older Person

- Table 10-1 The Aging Process—Physical Changes and Care Measures (Immune System)

Chapter 11: Safety Needs

- Pandemics

Chapter 12: Preventing Falls

- PROMOTING SAFETY AND COMFORT: Using Position Change Alarms
- Moving the Person From the Floor

Chapter 13: Restraint Alternatives and Restraints

- FOCUS ON OLDER PERSONS: Restraint Types

Chapter 14: Preventing Infection

- Moments for Hand Hygiene
- Box 14-3 WHO's 5 Moments for Hand Hygiene
- Antiseptics
- Biohazardous Waste

Chapter 15: Isolation Precautions *(new)*

Chapter 16: Body Mechanics
- Box 16-2 Musculo-Skeletal Disorders—Risk Factors for Nursing Assistants
- Safe Handling Programs
- PROMOTING SAFETY AND COMFORT: Safe Handling Programs

Chapter 17: Moving the Person
- DELEGATION GUIDELINES: Moving the Person

Chapter 18: Transferring the Person
- Lateral Transfers
- PROMOTING SAFETY AND COMFORT: Lateral Transfers

Chapter 19: The Person's Unit
- Personal Care Items

Chapter 20: Bedmaking *(new)*
- Box 20-1 Guidelines for Handling Used Linens

Chapter 21: Oral Hygiene *(new)*
- Structure and Function of Teeth
- Equipment
- Reporting and Recording

Chapter 22: Daily Hygiene and Bathing *(new)*
- Reporting and Recording
- Box 22-4 Daily Hygiene and Bathing Observations

Chapter 23: Grooming *(new)*
- FOCUS ON OLDER PERSONS: Nail and Foot Care

Chapter 24 Dressing and Undressing *(new)*
- Garments
- FOCUS ON COMMUNICATION: Garments
- PROMOTING SAFETY AND COMFORT: Changing Garments

Chapter 25: Urinary Needs
- Voiding Equipment
- PROMOTING SAFETY AND COMFORT: Voiding Equipment

Chapter 27: Bowel Needs
- FOCUS ON COMMUNICATION: Normal Bowel Elimination
- Emptying Ostomy Pouches

Chapter 28: Nutrition
- Dietary and Activity Guidelines
- Food Labels
- FOCUS ON MATH: Food Labels

Chapter 29: Meeting Nutrition Needs *(new)*

Chapter 31: Measurements
- PROCEDURE: Measuring Blood Pressure With an Electronic Manometer

Chapter 32: Exercise and Activity Needs
- Preventing Complications
- PROMOTING SAFETY AND COMFORT: Preventing Complications
- PROMOTING SAFETY AND COMFORT: Canes

Chapter 33: Comfort and Rest Needs
- Comfort
- FOCUS ON COMMUNICATION: Comfort
- Rest
- Promoting Sleep

Chapter 34: Collecting Specimens
- Urinary Catheter Specimens
- Blood Glucose Testing Equipment

Chapter 36: Pressure Injuries
- Observations

Chapter 37: Oxygen Needs
- Devices for Sleep Apnea

Chapter 38: Rehabilitation Needs
- Economic Aspects

Chapter 40: Common Health Problems
- Cancer Signs and Symptoms

Chapter 41: Mental Health Disorders
- FOCUS ON COMMUNICATION: Panic Disorder
- Psychotic Disorders
- Mood Disorders

Chapter 42: Confusion and Dementia
- FOCUS ON OLDER PERSONS: Delirium
- Risk Factors

Chapter 43: Emergency Care
- CPR Skills Testing
- Box 43-3 Stroke Emergency Care—FAST
- Box 43-4 Seizures—Activating EMS

New Key Terms
- Abbreviation (Chapter 8)
- Accountable (Chapter 3)
- Acute pain (Chapter 33)
- Advocate (Chapter 2)
- Afebrile (Chapter 31)
- Affected side (Chapter 24)

- Assessment (Chapter 7)
- Bath blanket (Chapters 20 and 22)
- Bed rest (Chapter 32)
- Bloodborne pathogens (Chapter 14)
- Bradycardia (Chapter 31)
- Burnout (Chapter 5)
- Cardiopulmonary resuscitation (Chapter 43)
- Cholesterol (Chapter 28)
- Chronic pain (Chapter 33)
- Comfort (Chapter 33)
- Coping (Chapter 41)
- Deconditioning (Chapter 32)
- Delegation (Chapter 3)
- Discharge (Chapter 1)
- Drawsheet (Chapter 20)
- Esteem (Chapter 6)
- Evaluation (Chapter 7)
- Febrile (Chapter 31)
- Garment (Chapter 24)
- Gender identity (Chapter 6)
- Glucometer (Chapter 34)
- Hazard (Chapter 11)
- Hygiene (Chapter 21)
- Hyperglycemia (Chapter 40)
- Hypoglycemia (Chapter 40)
- Immobility (Chapter 32)
- Implementation (Chapter 7)
- Incident (Chapter 11)
- Lateral transfer (Chapter 18)
- Left semi-prone position (Chapter 16)
- Melena (Chapter 34)
- Mobility (Chapter 32)
- Normal flora (Chapter 14)
- Nursing intervention (Chapter 7)
- Occupied (Chapter 20)
- Paraphrasing (Chapter 6)
- Personality (Chapter 41)
- Person's unit (Chapter 19)
- Position change alarm (Chapter 12)
- Prefix (Chapter 8)
- Reflex (Chapter 9)
- Regulations (Chapter 1)
- Rest (Chapter 33)
- Risk factor (Chapter 6)
- Root (Chapter 8)
- Self-esteem (Chapter 6)
- Sleep apnea (Chapter 33)
- Standard of care (Chapter 4)
- Sterile technique (Chapter 14)
- Stimulus (Chapter 9)
- Stressor (Chapter 41)
- Suffix (Chapter 8)
- Surgical asepsis (Chapter 14)
- Survey (Chapter 1)
- Tachycardia (Chapter 31)
- Unaffected side (Chapter 24)
- Unconscious (Chapter 11)
- Under-garment (Chapter 24)
- Waterproof under-pad (Chapter 20)
- Word element (Chapter 8)

New Key Abbreviations

AFO	Ankle-foot orthosis
ANA	American Nurses Association
APRN	Advanced practice registered nurse
BON	Board of nursing
CAUTI	Catheter-associated urinary tract infection
CKD	Chronic kidney disease
CPAP	Continuous positive airway pressure
ESRD	End-stage renal disease
GAD	Generalized anxiety disorder
HHS	U.S. Department of Health & Human Services
STI	Sexually transmitted infection
UI	Urinary incontinence
WHO	World Health Organization

New Figures

Figure 5-3	A watch with a second (sweep) hand.
Figure 7-6	24-hour time. **A,** In 24-hour time, there are 4 digits. The first 2 digits are for the hours. The last 2 digits are for minutes. A colon and AM and PM are not used.
Figure 7-7	From 1:00 PM to 11:00 PM, add 12 to the hours digit(s) to change from conventional time to 24-hour time. Remove the colon and PM.
Figure 8-1	Prefixes, roots, and suffixes are combined to form medical terms.
Figure 8-2	A prefix is at the beginning of the word. Changing the prefix changes the meaning of the word.
Figure 8-3	A root contains the basic meaning of the word. A word can have more than 1 root.
Figure 8-4	A suffix is at the end of the word.
Figure 8-5	The 4 abdominal quadrants.
Figure 9-10	The nervous system is divided into the central nervous system and the peripheral nervous system.
Figure 12-13	Moving the person from the floor using a mechanical lift.
Figure 14-13	WHO's 5 Moments for Hand Hygiene.
Figure 14-16	**B,** Sharps containers.
Figure 15-1	Personal protective equipment is in a cabinet outside the person's room.
Figure 15-2	Sample sign for contact precautions.
Figure 15-3	A respirator.
Figure 15-4	Applying (donning) gloves.
Figure 17-4	A trapeze.
Figure 17-5	Turning the person to position a friction-reducing device.
Figure 17-9	**C,** Positioning on the side with pillows for support.
Figure 18-2	Removing wheelchair front rigging.

Figure 18-11   A slide sheet is used to transfer a person from a bed to a stretcher.

Figure 18-13   **A,** A stand-assist mechanical lift supports the upper body.

Figure 18-15   A full sling.

Figure 19-4   **C,** Bed controls on the outer part of a bed rail.

Figure 19-7   Over-bed table.

Figure 20-10   A hamper for used linens.

Figure 20-23   Occupied bed. **A,** The person is turned to the other side. Used linens are removed. (Gloves are removed and hand hygiene is performed before touching clean linens.) **B,** The clean bottom linens are pulled through and tucked in.

Figure 20-24   Making a toe pleat.

Figure 21-5   **A,** Oral sponge swabs. **B,** Bite block.

Figure 22-2   Moisture can collect between skin folds, causing irritation. Dry between skin folds thoroughly.

Figure 22-15   A shower bench.

Figure 24-5   Applying a shirt that opens in the front with the person lying down.

Figure 25-6   **B,** Urinal designed for females.

Figure 25-7   Using the male urinal. **A,** Standing. **B,** In bed.

Figure 26-5   Catheter securing devices. **A,** Tube holder. **B,** Leg band.

Figure 27-9   A clamp is used to close the ostomy pouch.

Figure 29-2   **A,** Nectar-thick liquid. **B,** Honey-thick liquid. **C,** Pudding-thick (spoon-thick) liquid.

Figure 30-1   Edema in the lower leg. The nurse applies pressure to the body part to check for edema.

Figure 30-8   Electronic IV pump.

Figure 31-1   **D,** Non-contact infrared thermometer.

Figure 31-19   Using a watch with a second (sweep) hand to count for 30 seconds.

Figure 31-25   A standing scale.

Figure 31-26   A wheelchair scale.

Figure 34-3   Collecting a specimen from a urinary catheter. A syringe is connected to the port on the drainage tubing.

Figure 35-2   **C,** Diabetic foot ulcers.

Figure 37-13   A continuous positive airway pressure (CPAP) device used for sleep apnea.

Figure 38-2   **E,** Shoehorn.

Figure 39-2   **B,** A behind-the-ear hearing aid.

Figure 40-20   Myocardial infarction. Blood flow to part of the heart muscle is blocked, causing death of heart tissue.

Figure 40-21   COPD. Emphysema damages the inner walls of alveoli. Chronic bronchitis causes inflammation and mucus in the airways.

Figure 43-8   A bag valve mask.

Figure 43-9   Sequence of adult CPR.

Review Questions

- True/False sections have been removed. Replacement questions are multiple choice.
- Questions have been added that evaluate the student's ability to apply knowledge.

Features and Design

For features and design elements, see "Student Preface" on page xiii.

May this book serve you and your students well. We aim to provide current information for teaching and learning safe and effective care during a time of dynamic change in health care.

Leighann N. Remmert, BSN, MS, RN
Sheila A. Sorrentino, BSN, MA, MSN, PhD, RN

This book with special features (pp. xiv-xix) was designed to help you learn. This preface gives study guidelines to help you use the book. To study effectively, use a study system with these steps.

- Preview or survey
- Question
- Read and record
- Recite and review

Preview or Survey

Preview or survey the reading assignment for a few minutes. This gives an idea of what the assignment covers. It also helps you to recall what you know about the subject. Carefully look over the assignment. Preview the chapter title, objectives, key terms and abbreviations, headings, subheadings, and key ideas in italics. Also survey the boxes and chapter review questions.

Question

Questioning sets a purpose for reading. Form questions to answer while reading. Questions should relate to how the information applies to care or possible test questions. Use the headings and subheadings to form questions. *What*, *why*, or *how* questions are helpful. Avoid questions with 1-word answers. If a question does not help you study, change the question.

Read and Record

You read to:

- Gain new information.
- Connect new information to what you already know.
- Find answers to your questions.

Break the assignment into small parts. Then answer your questions as you read each part. Underline or highlight important information. This reminds you of what you need to learn. Review the marked parts later. Make notes by writing down important information in the margins or in a notebook. Use words and statements to prompt your memory about the material.

To remember what you read, organize information into a study guide. Create diagrams or charts to show relationships or steps in a process. Note taking in an outline also is very useful. For example:

1 Main heading
  A Second level
  B Second level
    (1) Third level
    (2) Third level

Recite and Review

Finally, recite and review. Use your notes and study guides. Answer your questions and others from reading and answering chapter "Review Questions." Answer all questions out loud (recite).

Reviewing is more about *when* to study rather than *what* to study. You decided *what* to study during your preview, question, and reading steps. It is best to review right after the first study session, 1 week later, and before a quiz or test.

We hope you enjoy learning and your work. You and your work are important. You and the care you give make a difference in the person's life!

Leighann N. Remmert
Sheila A. Sorrentino

SPECIAL FEATURES

Chapter Openers
Chapter openers contain a list of Objectives, Key Terms, and Key Abbreviations.
- *Objectives* are goals to accomplish while studying. The Objectives section lists what is presented in the chapter.
- *Key Terms* are important words and phrases used in the chapter. Each word or phrase is defined in the Key Terms section. In text, terms and definitions are identified with *magenta and italic* treatment. The term is **bold**.
- *Key Abbreviations* are important abbreviations used in the chapter.

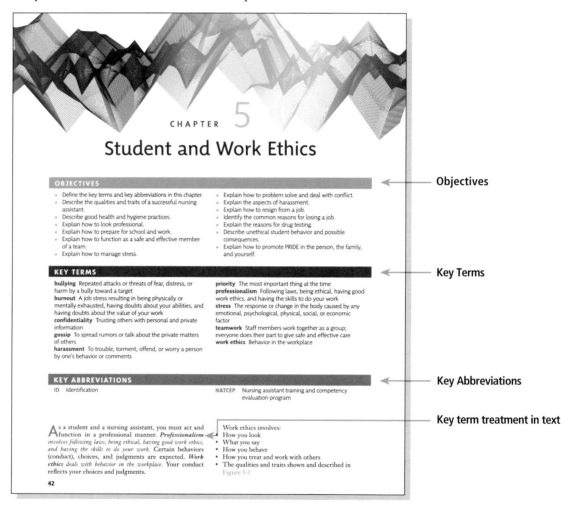

Focus Boxes
The following boxes highlight a certain part of the nursing assistant role. Callouts for these boxes are in *blue font and italics.*
- *Focus on Communication* boxes suggest what to say and questions to ask when interacting with patients, residents, visitors, and the nursing team.
- *Caring About Culture* boxes describe various cultural beliefs and practices that relate to health care.
- *Focus on Older Persons* boxes identify needs and considerations of older persons, especially persons with Alzheimer's disease and other dementias.
- *Focus on Surveys* boxes list questions that surveyors may ask you or tasks they may observe you doing.
- *Delegation Guidelines* boxes list information needed from the nurse and the care plan to perform a procedure. They also list the observations to report and record.
- *Promoting Safety and Comfort* boxes identify safety and comfort measures to consider when giving care.
- *Focus on Math* boxes explain math skills involved in various care measures and procedures.

FOCUS ON **COMMUNICATION**
The Training Program

Student clinical experiences involve giving care to patients or residents. The patient or resident has the right to know who you are. Introduce yourself. Tell the person you are a student. For example:

> *Hello. My name is Jesse Smith. I am a nursing assistant student. I will be working with your nurse today.*

CARING ABOUT CULTURE
Listening

Communicating respect is important in all cultural groups. This can be shown in how you listen. Giving the person your attention and showing kindness and interest communicate respect. In some cultures, eye contact communicates listening. In others, the listener turns an ear to listen.

Modified from Giger JN: *Transcultural nursing: assessment and intervention*, ed 7, St Louis, 2017, Mosby.

FOCUS ON **OLDER PERSONS**
Behavior

Changes in the brain with Alzheimer's disease and other forms of dementia can affect communication and judgment. Unable to communicate needs as usual, the brain uses other methods. Caregivers and staff must remember that behaviors communicate needs. For example, a person is hot. Instead of saying "I am hot," the person begins taking off clothes in the dining room. You will learn about behavior changes and how to provide for the person's needs in Chapter 42.

FOCUS ON **SURVEYS**
Grooming

Grooming promotes self-esteem. Therefore surveyors will observe if patients and residents:
- Are groomed according to their wishes.
- Have hair combed and styled.
- Have beards shaved or trimmed.
- Can reach grooming supplies.

DELEGATION GUIDELINES
Changing Garments

To assist with dressing and undressing, you need this information from the nurse and the care plan.
- How much help the person needs
- If the person can sit up and lean forward
- If the person can raise the hips to lift the buttocks off of the bed
- If the person has an affected side (weak side)
- If the person has limited range of motion in any joints
- If certain garments are needed
- What observations to report and record:
  - How much help was given
  - How the person tolerated the procedure
  - Complaints by the person
  - Changes in the person's behavior
- When to report observations
- What patient or resident concerns to report at once

PROMOTING SAFETY AND COMFORT
Bed Rails

Safety
You raise the bed to give care. Follow these safety measures to prevent falling.
- *For a person who uses bed rails:* Always raise the far bed rail(s) if you are working alone. Raise bed rails on both sides and lower the bed if you need to leave the bedside.
- *For a person who does not use bed rails:* Ask a co-worker to help you. The co-worker stands on the far side of the bed to protect the person from falling.
- Never leave the person alone when the bed is raised.
- Lower the bed to a comfortable and safe level for the person after giving care. Follow the care plan.

Comfort
The person has to reach over raised bed rails for items on the bedside stand and over-bed table (Chapter 19). That is unsafe. Adjust the over-bed table so needed items (water mug, tissues, phone, TV and light controls) are within reach. Ask what other items to place nearby. Always make sure needed items, including the call light, are within reach.

FOCUS ON **MATH**
Measuring Blood Pressure

Aneroid manometers have long and short lines (Fig. 31-22).
- Long lines mark 10 mm Hg values.
- Short lines mark 2 mm Hg values (2, 4, 6, and 8).

Read the manometer as the cuff deflates. The needle is dropping.
- If the needle is at a long line, note this value. Long line values end in 0. For example: 70, 80, 90, 100, 110, 120, and so on.
- If the needle is between 2 long lines:
  - Note the value of the long line below the needle.
  - Note the short line. Count up from the long line below by even numbers. Short line values end with 2, 4, 6, or 8. See Figure 31-22.

For example: *The needle is at the 3rd short line between 90 and 100. Count up by even numbers from 90. Line 1 is 92. Line 2 is 94. Line 3 is 96. The value is 96.*

If needed, round up to the nearest 2 mm Hg. When you *round up, you choose the higher value. For example: The needle is between 82 and 80. Report and record the value as 82 mm Hg.*

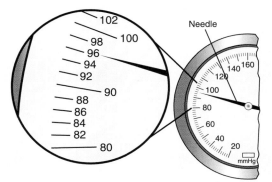

FIGURE 31-22 Reading the aneroid manometer. Long lines mark 10 mm Hg values. Short lines mark 2 mm Hg values.

Boxes, Tables, and Figures
- *Boxes and tables* list rules, principles, guidelines, signs and symptoms, nursing measures, and other information useful for study.
- *Figures* include color illustrations (drawings) and photographs. They visually present key ideas, concepts, and procedure steps.
- Callouts for boxes, tables, and figures are in blue font.

Callouts in blue font

Box

Figure

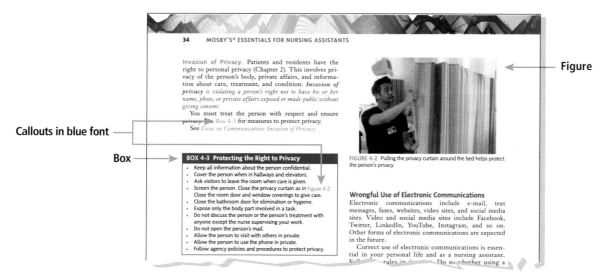

Table

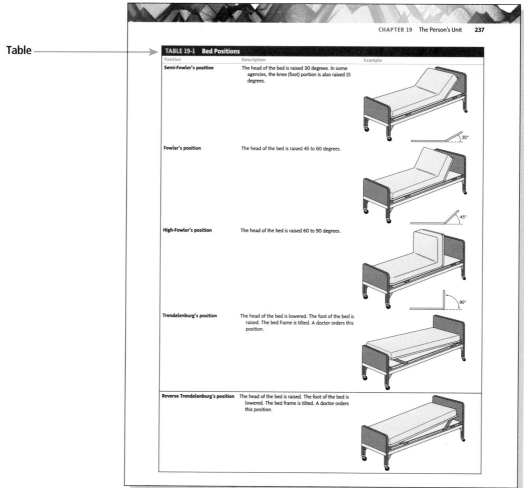

Procedures

Procedures are skills to perform. Heading icons and procedure callouts alert that a procedure will follow. Procedure callouts are in *blue font and italics.* Procedures include the following features.

- Title bar icons:
  - *NATCEP icon*—the skill may be part of a state's competency evaluation.
  - *Video Clip icon*—the skill has a video clip available on-line on *Evolve Student Learning Resources.*
  - *Video icon*—the skill has a procedure included in *Mosby's® Nursing Assistant Video Skills 4.0.*
- Procedures are divided into *Quality of Life, Pre-Procedure, Procedure,* and *Post-Procedure* sections. The *Quality of Life* section lists 6 simple courtesies that show respect for the person.

Heading icon ———→

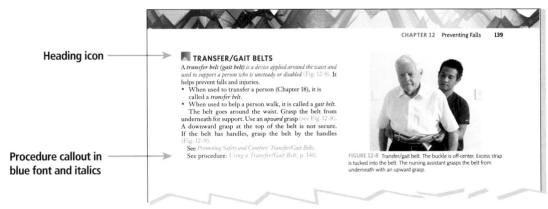

Procedure callout in blue font and italics ———→

Title bar icons:
- *NATCEP*
- *Video Clip*
- *Video*

Procedure sections:
- *Quality of Life*
- *Pre-Procedure*
- *Procedure*
- *Post-Procedure*

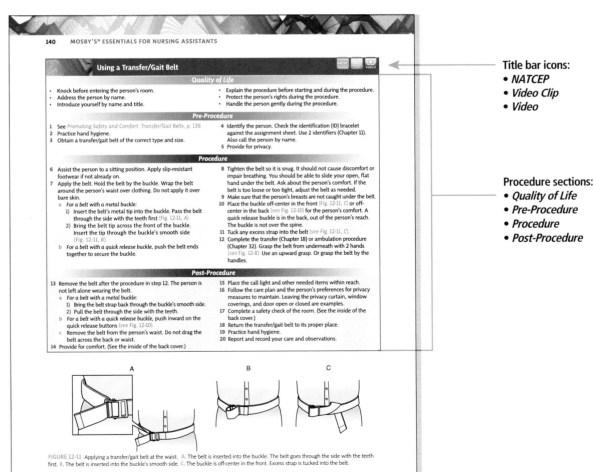

Focus on PRIDE: The Person, Family, and Yourself

This feature builds on chapter content to promote *pride* in the person, family, and yourself. The first letter of each section spells *PRIDE*.

- *Personal and Professional Responsibility*—how to have pride in yourself through personal and professional behaviors and development.
- *Rights and Respect*—how to promote the rights of others and respect them as persons with dignity and value.
- *Independence and Social Interaction*—ways to help the person remain or attain independence and interact socially with others.
- *Delegation and Teamwork*—how to work efficiently with and help nursing team members.
- *Ethics and Laws*—laws affecting nursing care and doing the right thing when dealing with patients, residents, and co-workers.

Each box ends with a *Focus on PRIDE: Application* section. Questions are intended for personal thought or classroom discussion. They relate to how you will apply the information in Focus on PRIDE.

Focus on PRIDE →

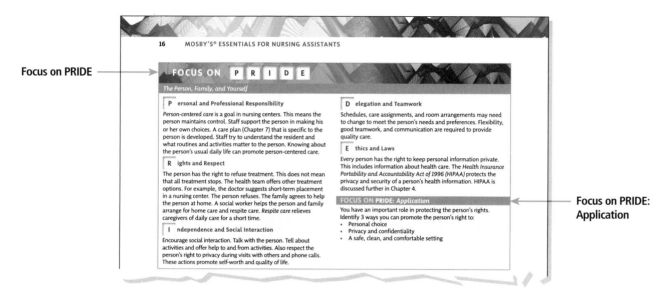

Focus on PRIDE: Application

16   MOSBY'S® ESSENTIALS FOR NURSING ASSISTANTS

FOCUS ON P R I D E
The Person, Family, and Yourself

P ersonal and Professional Responsibility

Person-centered care is a goal in nursing centers. This means the person maintains control. Staff support the person in making his or her own choices. A care plan (Chapter 7) that is specific to the person is developed. Staff try to understand the resident and what routines and activities matter to the person. Knowing about the person's usual daily life can promote person-centered care.

R ights and Respect

The person has the right to refuse treatment. This does not mean that all treatment stops. The health team offers other treatment options. For example, the doctor suggests short-term placement in a nursing center. The person refuses. The family agrees to help the person at home. A social worker helps the person and family arrange for home care and respite care. *Respite care* relieves caregivers of daily care for a short time.

I ndependence and Social Interaction

Encourage social interaction. Talk with the person. Tell about activities and offer help to and from activities. Also respect the person's right to privacy during visits with others and phone calls. These actions promote self-worth and quality of life.

D elegation and Teamwork

Schedules, care assignments, and room arrangements may need to change to meet the person's needs and preferences. Flexibility, good teamwork, and communication are required to provide quality care.

E thics and Laws

Every person has the right to keep personal information private. This includes information about health care. The *Health Insurance Portability and Accountability Act of 1996 (HIPAA)* protects the privacy and security of a person's health information. HIPAA is discussed further in Chapter 4.

FOCUS ON PRIDE: *Application*

You have an important role in protecting the person's rights. Identify 3 ways you can promote the person's right to:
- Personal choice
- Privacy and confidentiality
- A safe, clean, and comfortable setting

Review Questions

Review Questions are multiple-choice questions at the end of every chapter. They are useful as study guides to review what you have learned. Use them to study for a test or for the competency evaluation. Answers are at the back of the book. See p. 587.

Each chapter ends with a *Focus on Practice: Problem Solving* scenario. A situation is presented that you may encounter as a student or in the work setting. For classroom discussion or self-study, questions relate to what you should do, how you should act, or how you can improve the situation.

Review Questions →

Focus on Practice: Problem Solving

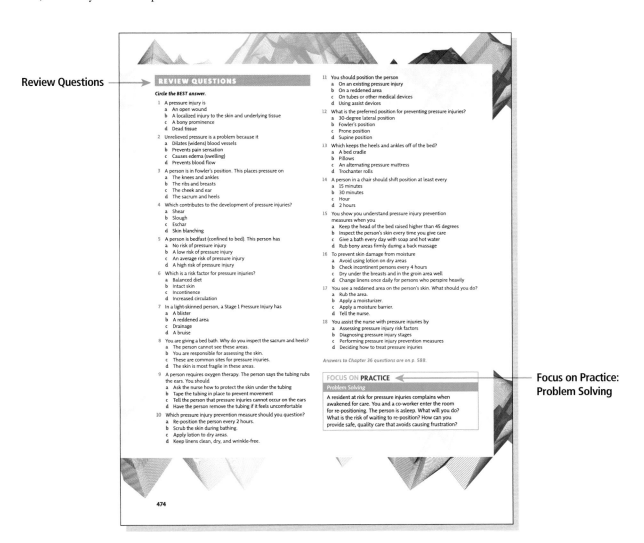

REVIEW QUESTIONS

Circle the BEST answer.

1 A pressure injury is
   a An open wound
   b A localized injury to the skin and underlying tissue
   c A bony prominence
   d Dead tissue

2 Unrelieved pressure is a problem because it
   a Dilates (widens) blood vessels
   b Prevents pain sensation
   c Causes edema (swelling)
   d Prevents blood flow

3 A person is in Fowler's position. This places pressure on
   a The knees and ankles
   b The ribs and breasts
   c The cheek and ear
   d The sacrum and heels

4 Which contributes to the development of pressure injuries?
   a Shear
   b Slough
   c Eschar
   d Skin blanching

5 A person is bedfast (confined to bed). This person has
   a No risk of pressure injury
   b A low risk of pressure injury
   c An average risk of pressure injury
   d A high risk of pressure injury

6 Which is a risk factor for pressure injuries?
   a Balanced diet
   b Intact skin
   c Incontinence
   d Increased circulation

7 In a light-skinned person, a Stage 1 Pressure Injury has
   a A blister
   b A reddened area
   c Drainage
   d A bruise

8 You are giving a bed bath. Why do you inspect the sacrum and heels?
   a The person cannot see these areas.
   b You are responsible for assessing the skin.
   c These are common sites for pressure injuries.
   d The skin is most fragile in these areas.

9 A person requires oxygen therapy. The person says the tubing rubs the ears. You should
   a Ask the nurse how to protect the skin under the tubing
   b Tape the tubing in place to prevent movement
   c Tell the person that pressure injuries cannot occur on the ears
   d Have the person remove the tubing if it feels uncomfortable

10 Which pressure injury prevention measure should you question?
   a Re-position the person every 2 hours.
   b Scrub the skin during bathing.
   c Apply lotion to dry areas.
   d Keep linens clean, dry, and wrinkle-free.

11 You should position the person
   a On an existing pressure injury
   b On a reddened area
   c On tubes or other medical devices
   d Using assist devices

12 What is the preferred position for preventing pressure injuries?
   a 30-degree lateral position
   b Fowler's position
   c Prone position
   d Supine position

13 Which keeps the heels and ankles off of the bed?
   a A bed cradle
   b Pillows
   c An alternating pressure mattress
   d Trochanter rolls

14 A person in a chair should shift position at least every
   a 15 minutes
   b 30 minutes
   c Hour
   d 2 hours

15 You show you understand pressure injury prevention measures when you
   a Keep the head of the bed raised higher than 45 degrees
   b Inspect the person's skin every time you give care
   c Give a bath every day with soap and hot water
   d Rub bony areas firmly during a back massage

16 To prevent skin damage from moisture
   a Avoid using lotion on dry areas
   b Check incontinent persons every 4 hours
   c Dry under the breasts and in the groin area well
   d Change linens once daily for persons who perspire heavily

17 You see a reddened area on the person's skin. What should you do?
   a Rub the area.
   b Apply a moisturizer.
   c Apply a moisture barrier.
   d Tell the nurse.

18 You assist the nurse with pressure injuries by
   a Assessing pressure injury risk factors
   b Diagnosing pressure injury stages
   c Performing pressure injury prevention measures
   d Deciding how to treat pressure injuries

Answers to Chapter 36 questions are on p. 588.

FOCUS ON PRACTICE

Problem Solving

A resident at risk for pressure injuries complains when awakened for care. You and a co-worker enter the room for re-positioning. The person is asleep. What will you do? What is the risk of waiting to re-position? How can you provide safe, quality care that avoids causing frustration?

474

Contents

1 Introduction to Health Care, *1*
Purposes, *2*
Types of Agencies, *2*
Organization, *3*
The Nursing Team, *5*
Staffing, *5*
Nursing Care Patterns, *6*
Paying for Health Care, *6*
Safety and Quality, *7*

2 The Person's Rights, *10*
Patient Rights, *10*
Resident Rights, *10*
Protecting Rights, *15*

3 The Nursing Assistant, *18*
Nurse Practice Acts, *19*
The Omnibus Budget Reconciliation Act
   of 1987, *19*
Working in Another State, *21*
Roles and Responsibilities, *21*
Delegation Guidelines, *25*

4 Ethics and Laws, *30*
Ethical Aspects, *31*
Legal Aspects, *33*
Reporting Abuse, *35*
Other Laws, *39*

5 Student and Work Ethics, *42*
Health, Hygiene, and Appearance, *43*
Preparing for School or Work, *45*
Teamwork, *45*
Stress, *48*
Harassment, *50*
Resigning From a Job, *50*
Losing a Job, *51*
Drug Testing, *51*
Unethical Student Behavior, *51*

6 Communicating With the Person, *53*
The Whole Person, *53*
Basic Needs, *54*
Culture and Religion, *55*
Health Care Beliefs and Practices, *55*
Effective Communication, *56*
Behavior, *60*
Persons With Special Needs, *61*
Family and Friends, *62*

7 Health Team Communications, *64*
The Medical Record, *65*
The Nursing Process, *67*
Reporting and Recording, *71*
Electronic Devices, *75*
Phone Communications, *75*

8 Medical Terminology, *78*
Medical Terms, *78*
Abdominal Quadrants, *83*
Directional Terms, *84*
Positional Terms, *84*
Abbreviations, *84*
Common Terms and Phrases, *86*

9 Body Structure and Function, *89*
Organization of the Body, *90*
The Integumentary System, *92*
The Musculo-Skeletal System, *92*
The Nervous System, *95*
The Circulatory System, *98*
The Lymphatic System, *100*
The Respiratory System, *100*
The Digestive System, *101*
The Urinary System, *102*
The Reproductive System, *102*
The Immune System, *104*
The Endocrine System, *105*

10 The Older Person, *108*
Growth and Development, *108*
Psychological and Social Changes, *110*
Physical Changes, *110*
Nursing Center Care, *113*
Sexuality, *114*

11 Safety Needs, *117*
Accident Risk Factors, *118*
Identifying the Person, *119*
Preventing Burns, *120*
Preventing Poisoning, *120*
Preventing Suffocation, *121*
PROCEDURE: Relieving Choking—Adult or Child
   (Over *1* Year of Age), *122*
Preventing Equipment Accidents, *124*
Hazardous Chemicals, *125*
Disasters, *126*
PROCEDURE: Using a Fire Extinguisher, *127*
Workplace Violence, *128*
Risk Management, *129*

12 Preventing Falls, *133*
Causes and Risk Factors for Falls, *134*
Fall Prevention Programs, *134*
Transfer/Gait Belts, *139*
PROCEDURE: Using a Transfer/Gait Belt, *140*
The Falling Person, *141*
PROCEDURE: Helping the Falling Person, *141*
Moving the Person From the Floor, *142*

13 Restraint Alternatives and Restraints, *144*
Terms, *144*
History of Restraint Use, *145*
Restraint Alternatives, *145*
Restraint Types, *146*
Risks From Restraint Use, *147*
Laws, Rules, and Guidelines, *148*
Restraints, *152*
Applying Restraints, *154*
PROCEDURE: Applying Restraints, *155*
Reporting and Recording, *156*

14 Preventing Infection, *159*
Microorganisms, *160*
Infection, *160*
Asepsis, *162*
PROCEDURE: Hand-Washing, *166*
PROCEDURE: Using an Alcohol-Based Hand Sanitizer, *167*
Bloodborne Pathogen Standard, *170*

15 Isolation Precautions, *175*
Standard Precautions, *175*
Transmission-Based Precautions, *177*
Personal Protective Equipment, *180*
PROCEDURE: Donning and Removing Personal
    Protective Equipment, *185*
Used Laundry, *186*
Used Supplies and Equipment, *186*
Collecting Specimens, *186*
Transporting Persons, *187*

16 Body Mechanics, *189*
Principles of Body Mechanics, *189*
Work-Related Injuries, *191*
Positioning the Person, *193*

17 Moving the Person, *199*
Planning a Safe Move, *200*
Protecting the Skin, *201*
Moving Persons in Bed, *202*
PROCEDURE: Moving the Person Up in Bed With a
    Friction-Reducing Device, *204*
PROCEDURE: Moving the Person to the Side
    of the Bed, *205*
Turning Persons, *206*
PROCEDURE: Turning and Positioning the Person
    on the Side, *207*
PROCEDURE: Logrolling the Person, *208*
Sitting on the Side of the Bed (Dangling), *209*
PROCEDURE: Sitting on the Side of the Bed
    (Dangling), *210*
Re-Positioning in a Chair or Wheelchair, *211*

18 Transferring the Person, *214*
Wheelchair and Stretcher Safety, *215*
Stand and Pivot Transfers, *217*
PROCEDURE: Transferring the Person to a Chair or
    Wheelchair, *218*
PROCEDURE: Transferring the Person From a Chair or
    Wheelchair to Bed, *221*
PROCEDURE: Transferring the Person To and From the
    Toilet, *222*
Lateral Transfers, *223*
Mechanical Lifts, *224*
PROCEDURE: Transferring the Person Using a
    Stand-Assist Mechanical Lift, *226*
PROCEDURE: Transferring the Person Using a Full-Sling
    Mechanical Lift, *228*

19 The Person's Unit, *232*
Comfort, *234*
Room Furniture and Equipment, *235*

20 Bedmaking, *244*
Types of Beds, *244*
Linens, *245*
Making Beds, *248*
PROCEDURE: Making a Closed Bed, *249*
PROCEDURE: Making an Occupied Bed, *254*
PROCEDURE: Making a Surgical Bed, *258*

21 **Oral Hygiene,** 261
Structure and Function of Teeth, 261
Purpose of Oral Hygiene, 262
Flossing, 262
Equipment, 262
Brushing and Flossing Teeth, 262
PROCEDURE: Brushing and Flossing the Person's
    Teeth, 263
PROCEDURE: Providing Mouth Care for the Unconscious
    Person, 266
Dentures, 267
PROCEDURE: Providing Denture Care, 268
Reporting and Recording, 269

22 **Daily Hygiene and Bathing,** 271
Daily Care, 272
Bathing, 272
PROCEDURE: Giving a Complete Bed Bath, 276
PROCEDURE: Assisting With the Partial Bath, 279
PROCEDURE: Assisting With a Tub Bath or Shower,
    283
Perineal Care, 284
PROCEDURE: Giving Female Perineal Care, 286
PROCEDURE: Giving Male Perineal Care, 288
Reporting and Recording, 289

23 **Grooming,** 291
Hair Care, 292
PROCEDURE: Brushing and Combing Hair, 294
PROCEDURE: Shampooing the Person's Hair in Bed, 296
Shaving, 297
PROCEDURE: Shaving the Person's Face With a Safety
    Razor, 299
Nail and Foot Care, 300
PROCEDURE: Giving Nail and Foot Care, 301

24 **Dressing and Undressing,** 304
Garments, 304
PROCEDURE: Undressing the Person, 307
PROCEDURE: Dressing the Person, 309
Changing Patient Gowns, 312
PROCEDURE: Changing a Standard Patient Gown on a
    Person With an IV, 314

25 **Urinary Needs,** 316
Normal Urination, 317
Voiding Equipment, 318
PROCEDURE: Giving the Bedpan, 319
PROCEDURE: Giving the Male Urinal, 322
PROCEDURE: Helping the Person to the Commode, 324
Urinary Incontinence, 325
PROCEDURE: Applying an Incontinence Brief, 328
Bladder Training, 331

26 **Urinary Catheters,** 333
Catheters, 334
Catheter Care, 335
PROCEDURE: Giving Catheter Care, 337
Urine Drainage Systems, 338
PROCEDURE: Emptying a Urine Drainage
    Bag, 339
PROCEDURE: Applying a Condom Catheter, 341

27 **Bowel Needs,** 344
Normal Bowel Elimination, 345
Factors Affecting BMs, 346
Common Problems, 347
Bowel Training, 348
Enemas, 349
PROCEDURE: Giving a Small-Volume
    Enema, 350
The Person With an Ostomy, 351

28 **Nutrition,** 355
Basic Nutrition, 355
Special Diets, 359
Food Intake, 362

29 **Meeting Nutrition Needs,** 365
Factors Affecting Eating and Nutrition, 366
Dysphagia, 367
Nutrition and Food Requirements, 368
Preparing for Meals, 368
PROCEDURE: Preparing the Person for a Meal, 369
Serving Meals, 369
PROCEDURE: Serving Meal Trays, 370
Feeding the Person, 371
PROCEDURE: Feeding the Person, 372
Assisting With Special Needs, 373

30 **Fluid Needs,** 377
Fluid Balance, 378
Special Fluid Orders, 378
Intake and Output, 379
PROCEDURE: Measuring Intake and
    Output, 382
Providing Drinking Water, 383
PROCEDURE: Providing Drinking Water, 383
IV Therapy, 384

31 **Measurements,** 388
Vital Signs, 389
PROCEDURE: Taking a Temperature With an Electronic
   Thermometer, 393
PROCEDURE: Taking a Radial Pulse, 399
PROCEDURE: Taking an Apical Pulse, 399
PROCEDURE: Counting Respirations, 401
PROCEDURE: Measuring Blood Pressure With an Aneroid
   Manometer, 404
PROCEDURE: Measuring Blood Pressure With an
   Electronic Manometer, 406
Pulse Oximetry, 406
Pain, 406
Weight and Height, 406
PROCEDURE: Measuring Weight and Height With a
   Standing Scale, 409

32 **Exercise and Activity Needs,** 412
Mobility and Immobility, 413
Range-of-Motion Exercises, 414
PROCEDURE: Performing Range-of-Motion
   Exercises, 415
Positioning Devices, 418
Walking Aids, 420
Ambulation, 421
PROCEDURE: Assisting With Ambulation, 422

33 **Comfort and Rest Needs,** 425
Comfort, 425
PROCEDURE: Giving a Back Massage, 429
Rest, 430
Sleep, 430

34 **Collecting Specimens,** 434
Urine Specimens, 435
PROCEDURE: Collecting a Random Urine Specimen, 436
PROCEDURE: Collecting a Midstream Specimen, 437
PROCEDURE: Testing Urine With Reagent Strips, 440
Stool Specimens, 440
PROCEDURE: Collecting a Stool Specimen, 441
Sputum Specimens, 442
PROCEDURE: Collecting a Sputum Specimen, 443
Blood Glucose Testing, 444

35 **Wound Care,** 446
Skin Tears, 447
Circulatory Ulcers, 448
PROCEDURE: Applying Elastic Stockings, 451
PROCEDURE: Applying an Elastic Bandage, 453
Dressings, 453
PROCEDURE: Applying a Dry, Non-Sterile
   Dressing, 455
Binders and Compression Garments, 456
Heat and Cold Applications, 457
PROCEDURE: Applying Heat and Cold
   Applications, 461

36 **Pressure Injuries,** 464
Risk Factors, 466
Persons at Risk, 466
Pressure Injury Sites, 467
Pressure Injury Stages, 467
Prevention and Treatment, 470
Complications, 473

37 **Oxygen Needs,** 475
Altered Respiratory Function, 476
Respiratory Tests, 477
PROCEDURE: Using a Pulse Oximeter, 478
Meeting Oxygen Needs, 478
PROCEDURE: Assisting With Deep-Breathing and
   Coughing Exercises, 479
Assisting With Oxygen Therapy, 481
Devices for Sleep Apnea, 483

38 **Rehabilitation Needs,** 486
Restorative Nursing, 487
The Whole Person, 487
The Person's Setting, 490
The Rehabilitation Team, 490
Rehabilitation Programs, 490
Quality of Life, 491

39 **Hearing, Speech, and Vision Problems,** 493
Hearing Disorders, 493
Speech Disorders, 496
Eye Disorders, 496
PROCEDURE: Caring for Eyeglasses, 500

40 **Common Health Problems,** 503
Cancer, 504
Musculo-Skeletal Disorders, 506
Nervous System Disorders, 511
Cardiovascular Disorders, 514
Respiratory Disorders, 517
Digestive Disorders, 519
Urinary System Disorders, 521
Reproductive Disorders, 523
Endocrine Disorders, 523
Immune System Disorders, 524
Skin Disorders, 526

41 **Mental Health Disorders,** 529
Anxiety Disorders, 530
Psychotic Disorders, 532
Mood Disorders, 533
Personality Disorders, 534
Substance Use Disorder, 534
Eating Disorders, 536
Suicide, 536
Care and Treatment, 537

42 Confusion and Dementia, *539*
Confusion, *539*
Dementia, *541*
Alzheimer's Disease, *541*
Care of Persons With AD and Other Dementias, *547*

43 Emergency Care, *555*
Emergency Care, *556*
Sudden Cardiac Arrest, *557*
CPR, *557*
Choking, *562*
Respiratory Arrest, *562*
Poisoning, *563*
Heart Attack, *563*
Hemorrhage, *563*
Fainting, *564*
Shock, *564*
Stroke, *565*
Seizures, *565*
Concussions, *566*
Burns, *566*

44 End-of-Life Care, *569*
Terminal Illness, *569*
Attitudes About Death, *570*
The Stages of Dying, *571*
Comfort Needs, *571*
The Family, *573*
Legal Issues, *573*
Signs of Death, *573*
Care of the Body After Death, *574*
PROCEDURE: Assisting With Post-Mortem Care, *574*

45 Getting a Job, *578*
Sources of Jobs, *578*
What Employers Look For, *579*
Job Applications, *579*
The Job Interview, *582*
Accepting or Declining a Job Offer, *585*
Drug Testing, *585*

Review Question Answers, *587*

Appendices, *590*

A   The Patient Care Partnership—Understanding Expectations, Rights, and Responsibilities (A Summary), *590*

B   National Nurse Aide Assessment Program (NNAAP®) Written Examination Content Outline and Skills Evaluation, *591*

C   Minimum Data Set: Selected Pages, *592*

Glossary, *594*

Key Abbreviations, *602*

Index, *604*

CHAPTER 1

Introduction to Health Care

OBJECTIVES

- Define the key terms and key abbreviations in this chapter.
- Describe the purposes and types of health care agencies.
- Describe the persons cared for in nursing centers.
- Describe the health team and nursing team members.
- Describe 5 nursing care patterns.

- Describe the programs that pay for health care.
- Explain how government agencies and health care agencies ensure safe, quality care.
- Explain your role in meeting standards.
- Explain how to promote PRIDE in the person, the family, and yourself.

KEY TERMS

acute illness An illness of rapid onset and short duration; the person is expected to recover

admission The official entry of a person into a health care setting

assisted living residence (ALR) Provides housing, personal care, support services, health care, and social activities in a home-like setting to persons needing some help with daily activities

chronic illness A long-term health condition that may not have a cure; it can be controlled and complications prevented with proper treatment

discharge The official departure of a person from a health care setting

health team The many health care workers whose skills and knowledge focus on the person's total care; interdisciplinary health care team

hospice A health care agency or program that promotes comfort and quality of life for the dying person and the person's family

licensed practical nurse (LPN) A nurse who has completed a practical nursing program and has passed a licensing test; called *licensed vocational nurse (LVN)* in California and Texas

licensed vocational nurse (LVN) See "licensed practical nurse (LPN)"

nursing assistant A person who has passed a nursing assistant training and competency evaluation program (NATCEP); performs delegated nursing tasks under the supervision of a licensed nurse

nursing team Those who provide nursing care—RNs, LPNs/LVNs, and nursing assistants

registered nurse (RN) A nurse who has completed a 2-, 3-, or 4-year nursing program and has passed a licensing test

regulations Rules made by government agencies

survey The formal review of an agency through the collection of facts and observations

surveyor A person who collects information by observing and asking questions

terminal illness An illness or injury from which the person will not likely recover

KEY ABBREVIATIONS

ALR	Assisted living residence	LPN	Licensed practical nurse
APRN	Advanced practice registered nurse	LVN	Licensed vocational nurse
DON	Director of nursing	RN	Registered nurse
HHS	U.S. Department of Health & Human Services	SNF	Skilled nursing facility

The health care industry is one of the largest providers of jobs in the United States. Working in health care offers many opportunities. Nursing assistants are a valuable part of the health care team.

Persons of all ages need health care. The setting and reason for care vary. The *person* is always the focus of care.

PURPOSES

The purposes of health care are:
- *Health promotion and disease prevention.* The goal is to reduce the risk of illness. People learn about healthy living.
- *Detection and treatment of disease.* Physical exams and diagnostic tests are done. Treatment may involve life-style changes, drugs, surgeries, or other therapies.
- *Rehabilitation and restorative care.* This involves returning persons to their highest possible level of physical and mental function and to independence. *Independence* means *not relying on or needing care from others.*

Some health care agencies have a narrow focus. A certain health problem or age-group is the focus of care. Or a certain service is provided. Other agencies have many purposes and services.

TYPES OF AGENCIES

Health care agencies vary in size, services, and staff. Nursing assistants work in many settings.

Acute care agencies treat serious and urgent injuries and illnesses. A high level of medical and nursing care and close observation are needed. Care is costly. The length of stay is usually short. Acute care is needed until the person can be safely treated in another setting. A hospital is an example of an acute care setting. See "Hospitals."

Rehabilitation and sub-acute care agencies offer complex medical care or rehabilitation when hospital care is no longer needed. Care needs fall between acute care and long-term care. Some hospitals and long-term care centers have rehabilitation and sub-acute care units. Others are separate agencies. Some persons return home. Others need long-term care.

Long-term care settings are for persons who cannot care for themselves at home but do not need hospital care. See "Long-Term Care Centers."

Doctors' offices and clinics are used for routine appointments, preventive care, treatment of minor injuries and illnesses, and management of chronic illnesses.

Home care agencies provide services to persons living at home. Health teaching, nursing care, physical therapy, and rehabilitation services are examples of care provided.

Hospitals

Hospitals provide emergency care, surgery, nursing care, x-ray procedures and treatments, and laboratory testing. Respiratory, physical, occupational, speech, and other therapies are provided.

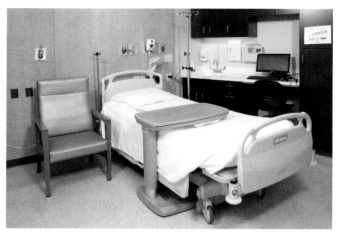

FIGURE 1-1 A hospital room.

Persons cared for in hospitals are called *patients.* Hospital care is either in-patient or out-patient.
- *In-patient care* is health care a person receives when admitted to an agency. **Admission** *is the official entry of a person into a health care setting.* At least 1 over-night stay is involved. See Figure 1-1.
- *Out-patient (ambulatory) care* includes medical or surgical care received when a person is not admitted to an agency. The person does not stay over-night.

People of all ages need hospital care. They have babies, surgery, physical and mental health disorders, and broken bones. Some are dying.

Hospitals are commonly divided into *units.* Each unit has a different focus. Surgical, medical, intensive (critical) care, pediatric, and mental health units are examples. Operating and recovery areas, emergency room, and maternity department are others. Some hospitals only treat certain illnesses, injuries, or age-groups.

Hospital patients have acute, chronic, or terminal illnesses.
- *Acute illness* *is an illness of rapid onset and short duration. The person is expected to recover.* A heart attack is an example.
- *Chronic illness* *is a long-term health condition that may not have a cure. The illness can be controlled and complications prevented with proper treatment.* Arthritis is an example.
- *Terminal illness* *is an illness or injury from which the person will not likely recover.* The person will die (Chapter 44). Cancers not responding to treatment are examples.

Discharge *is the official departure of a person from a health care setting.* The person returns home or goes to another agency after hospital care.

Long-Term Care Centers

Hospital patients are often discharged while still recovering from illness or surgery. Some need home care. Others need care until able to go home. Long-term care centers offer options for such persons. Some need care until death.

Persons in long-term care centers are called *residents.* They are not *patients.* The center is their short- or long-term home.

Nursing Centers. A *nursing center (nursing facility, nursing home)* provides medical, nursing, dietary, recreation, and social services. Rehabilitation services (physical, occupational, speech-language) are also available. Care needs range from simple to complex.

Skilled care refers to nursing or rehabilitation services that must be provided by licensed nurses and therapists. Wound care, intravenous (IV) therapy, urinary catheter care, and physical therapy are examples. A *skilled nursing facility (SNF)* provides skilled care.

See *Focus on Older Persons: Nursing Centers.*

Memory Care Units. A memory care unit is designed for persons with Alzheimer's disease and other dementias (Chapter 42). Such persons suffer increasing memory loss and confusion. Over time, they cannot tend to simple personal needs. Wandering is common. The unit is usually closed off from other parts of the center. The closed unit provides a safe setting where residents can wander freely.

Assisted Living Residences. An *assisted living residence (ALR) provides housing, personal care, support services, health care, and social activities in a home-like setting to persons needing some help with daily activities.* Some ALRs are part of nursing centers or retirement communities.

ALR residents may need help with 1 or more of the following.
- Personal care—bathing, dressing, grooming, elimination
- Meals—cooking, eating
- Taking drugs
- Housekeeping
- Personal safety
- Transportation

Mobility is often a requirement. The person walks or uses a wheelchair or motor scooter. The person can leave the building in an emergency. The person has stable health or needs limited health care or treatment.

The person has a room, an apartment, or a cottage. Three meals a day and 24-hour supervision are provided. So are housekeeping, laundry, social, recreational, transportation, and some health care services.

Home Care Agencies

Health care services are provided to people where they live. Nursing care, rehabilitation, and food services are common. People of all ages need home health care. Some persons need end-of-life care at home.

Hospices

A *hospice is a health care agency or program that promotes comfort and quality of life for the dying person and the person's family.* Hospice patients no longer respond to treatments aimed at cures. Usually they have less than 6 months to live.

The physical, emotional, social, and spiritual needs of the person and family are met. The focus is on comfort, not cure.

Hospice care is provided by hospitals, nursing centers, and home care and hospice agencies.

FOCUS ON **OLDER PERSONS**

Nursing Centers

Most nursing center residents are older. Many have chronic diseases, poor nutrition, memory problems, or poor health. Not all residents are old. Some are disabled from birth defects, accidents, or disease.

Health problems and care needs vary. Nursing center staff often care for:
- *Alert and oriented persons. Alert* describes a person's normal level of consciousness. *Oriented* relates to a person's awareness of his or her name, the time, and the location. Such persons know who they are and where they are. Care needs depend on their physical problems.
- *Confused and disoriented persons.* These persons are mildly to severely confused and disoriented. This may be a short-term or long-term problem. See Chapter 42.
- *Persons needing complete (total) care.* These persons cannot meet their own needs. Daily care needs must be met by staff. Some cannot understand or say what they need or want.
- *Short-term residents.* These people are recovering from fractures or other injuries, acute illness, or surgery. Some may need tube feedings, wound care, or other treatments. The goal is optimal level of function and to return home.
- *Persons needing respite care. Respite* means *rest* or *relief.* The person living at home goes to a nursing center for a short stay. The person's caregiver gets relief for a trip, business, or rest.
- *Life-long residents.* Such persons may have disabilities from birth defects or childhood or adult diseases or injuries. There may be physical impairments, intellectual impairments, or both. Life-long assistance, support, and special devices are needed.
- *Persons with mental health disorders.* Behavior and function are affected. Self-care and independent living may be impaired. Some persons have both physical and mental health disorders.
- *Persons who are terminally ill.* Terminally ill persons are dying. The goal is quality end-of-life care (Chapter 44).

ORGANIZATION

An agency has a governing body called the *board of trustees* or *board of directors.* The board makes policies. The focus is safe care at the lowest possible cost. Local, state, and federal laws are followed.

An administrator or chief executive officer (CEO) manages the agency. This person reports directly to the board. Directors or department heads manage certain areas (departments). For example, a director of nursing (DON) manages the nursing department (p. 5). Department directors report to the administrator or CEO.

Departments in a hospital setting often include:
- *Business*—human resources and payroll, admitting, billing, public relations and marketing, medical records
- *Facility services*—housekeeping, maintenance, food service, laundry, security, information technology (IT)
- *Ancillary services*—x-ray, laboratory, respiratory therapy, physical and occupational therapy, social services, speech therapy, pharmacy, dietary, spiritual care
- *Nursing*—see "Nursing Service" on p. 5
- *Medical staff*—doctors

Nursing centers have nursing, therapy, and food service departments. They also have housekeeping, maintenance, laundry, social service, activity, and other departments.

The Health Team

The **health team** *(interdisciplinary health care team) involves the many health care workers whose skills and knowledge focus on the person's total care.* Many team members may be involved in the care of each person. See Table 1-1.

Coordinated care is needed. This means the team communicates and works together well. There is a common focus and goal. The person is the focus of care. The goal is to provide quality care.

See *Focus on Communication: The Health Team.*

TABLE 1-1   Health Team Members

Title	Description
Activities director/recreational therapist	Plans and directs recreation treatment programs to help maintain or improve a person's physical, social, and emotional well-being.
Audiologist	Treats hearing, balance, and ear problems.
Cleric (clergyman; clergywoman)	Assists with spiritual needs.
Clinical nurse specialist (CNS)	Advanced practice registered nurse (APRN) who consults in a specialty. Geriatrics, critical care, diabetes, rehabilitation, and wound care are examples. Can prescribe drugs in some states.
Dietitian and nutritionist	Assesses and plans for nutritional needs to promote health and manage disease. Teaches about diet and healthy eating.
Licensed practical/vocational nurse (LPN/LVN)	Provides nursing care and gives drugs under the direction of RNs and doctors.
Medical or clinical laboratory technician	Collects specimens. Performs tests on blood, urine, and other body fluids.
Medication assistant-certified (MA-C)	Gives drugs as allowed by state law under the supervision of a licensed nurse.
Nurse practitioner (NP)	An APRN with specialized graduate education who diagnoses and treats common health problems. May prescribe some drugs and treatments.
Nursing assistant	Assists nurses and gives care. Supervised by a licensed nurse.
Occupational therapist (OT)	Assists persons to learn or retain skills needed for daily living and working.
Pharmacist	Fills drug orders and advises about safe prescription use. Consults with doctors and nurses about drug actions and interactions.
Physical therapist (PT)	Assists ill and injured persons with movement, pain management, and rehabilitation.
Physician (doctor)	Diagnoses and treats diseases and injuries.
Podiatrist	Prevents, diagnoses, and treats foot, ankle, and lower leg problems.
Radiographer/radiologic technologist	Takes images using x-rays and other equipment.
Registered nurse (RN)	Assesses, makes nursing diagnoses, plans, implements, and evaluates nursing care. Supervises LPNs/LVNs and nursing assistants.
Respiratory therapist (RT)	Assists in treating lung and heart disorders. Gives respiratory treatments and therapies.
Social worker	Deals with social, emotional, and environmental issues affecting illness and recovery. Coordinates community agencies to assist the person and family.
Speech-language pathologist/speech therapist	Diagnoses and treats communication and swallowing disorders.

Modified from Bureau of Labor Statistics, U.S. Department of Labor: *Occupational outlook handbook*, September 8, 2021.

Nursing Service

Nursing service is a large department (Fig. 1-2). The director of nursing (DON) is a registered nurse (RN). (*Director of nursing services, chief nurse executive,* and *vice president of nursing* are other titles.) Usually a bachelor's or higher degree is required. The DON is responsible for the entire nursing staff and the nursing care given.

Nursing supervisors and nurse managers (usually RNs) over-see a work shift, nursing unit, or certain nursing function. They are responsible for all nursing care and the actions of nursing staff in their areas.

Nursing units usually have RN *charge nurses* for each shift. LPNs/LVNs can be charge nurses in some states. The charge nurse is responsible for all nursing care and nursing staff actions during that shift. Staff RNs report to the charge nurse. LPNs/LVNs report to staff RNs or to the charge nurse. You report to the nurse supervising your work.

Nursing education (staff development) is part of nursing service. Nursing education staff:

- Plan and present educational programs (in-service programs). This includes programs that meet federal and state educational requirements.
- Provide new and changing information.
- Show how to use new equipment and supplies.
- Review policies and procedures on a regular basis.
- Educate and train nursing assistants.
- Conduct new employee orientation programs.

THE NURSING TEAM

The ***nursing team*** *involves those who provide nursing care—RNs, LPNs/LVNs, and nursing assistants.* All focus on the physical, social, emotional, and spiritual needs of the person and family.

Registered Nurses

A ***registered nurse (RN)*** *has completed a 2-, 3-, or 4-year nursing program and has passed a licensing test.*

- Community college programs—2 years
- Hospital-based diploma programs—2 or 3 years
- College or university programs—4 years

Graduates take a licensing test offered by their state board of nursing. They receive a license and become *registered* after passing the test. RNs must have a license recognized by the state in which they work.

RNs assess, make nursing diagnoses, plan, implement, and evaluate nursing care (Chapter 7). They provide care and delegate (Chapter 3) nursing care and tasks to the nursing team. They evaluate how nursing care affects each person. RNs teach the person and family how to improve health and independence.

RNs receive and carry out (implement) the doctor's orders. They may delegate care to other nursing team members. RNs do not prescribe treatments or drugs. However, RNs can become *clinical nurse specialists* or *nurse practitioners.* Depending on state law, these RNs have limited diagnosing and prescribing functions.

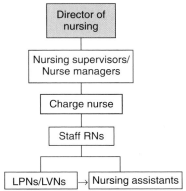

FIGURE 1-2 Sample organizational chart of the nursing department. (*LPN*—licensed practical nurse; *LVN*—licensed vocational nurse; *RN*—registered nurse.)

Licensed Practical Nurses and Licensed Vocational Nurses

A ***licensed practical nurse (LPN)*** *has completed a practical nursing program and has passed a licensing test.* Hospitals, community colleges, vocational schools, and technical schools offer programs. Programs are 10, 12, or 18 months long. Some high schools offer 2-year programs.

Graduates take a licensing test for practical nursing. After passing the test, they have a license to practice and the title of *licensed practical nurse.* ***Licensed vocational nurse (LVN)*** *is used in California and Texas.* LPNs/LVNs must have a license recognized by the state where they work.

LPNs/LVNs are supervised by RNs and doctors. They have fewer responsibilities and functions than RNs do. They need less supervision when the person's condition is stable and care is simple. They assist RNs with acutely ill persons and complex procedures.

Nursing Assistants

A ***nursing assistant*** *has passed a nursing assistant training and competency evaluation program (NATCEP). Nursing assistants perform delegated nursing tasks under the supervision of a licensed nurse.* Nursing assistants are discussed in Chapter 3.

STAFFING

Agencies must provide enough nursing staff to safely provide care. *Nurse staffing* describes the number and type of nursing team members assigned to care for a group of patients or residents for a certain amount of time (work shift). Work shifts vary—8-, 10-, and 12-hour shifts are common. The DON and nursing supervisors (nurse managers) are responsible for ensuring safe staffing.

Agencies use different methods to plan nurse staffing. Decisions are usually based on the number of patients or residents needing care and the care needs or *acuity levels* of the persons needing care. *Acuity* relates to the severity of illness and the level of care required. Education and experience of staff, safety and quality goals, and cost are other factors.

NURSING CARE PATTERNS

The *nursing care pattern* used depends on how many persons need care, the staff, and the cost. See Figure 1-3.

- *Functional nursing* focuses on tasks and jobs. Each nursing team member has certain tasks and jobs to do. For example, 1 nurse gives all drugs. Another gives all treatments. Nursing assistants give baths, make beds, and serve meals.
- *Team nursing* involves a team of nursing staff led by an RN "team leader." The team leader delegates care to other nurses and nursing assistants. (See "Delegation" in Chapter 3.) Decisions about care depend on the person's needs and team member abilities. Team members report observations and the care given to the team leader.
- *Primary nursing* involves total care. The primary nurse (an RN) is responsible for the person's total care. The nursing team assists as needed. The RN gives nursing care and makes discharge plans. The RN teaches and counsels the person and family.
- *Case management.* A nursing case manager coordinates the care of specific groups of patients from admission through discharge and into the home or long-term care setting. Case managers communicate with the health team, insurance companies, and community agencies. They work with certain doctors, certain age-groups, or persons with certain health problems. Heart disease, diabetes, and cancer are examples.
- *Patient-focused care* is when services are moved from departments to the bedside. Besides nursing care, the nursing team performs basic skills usually done by other health team members. For example, an RN draws a blood sample. This reduces the number of staff involved and the care costs.

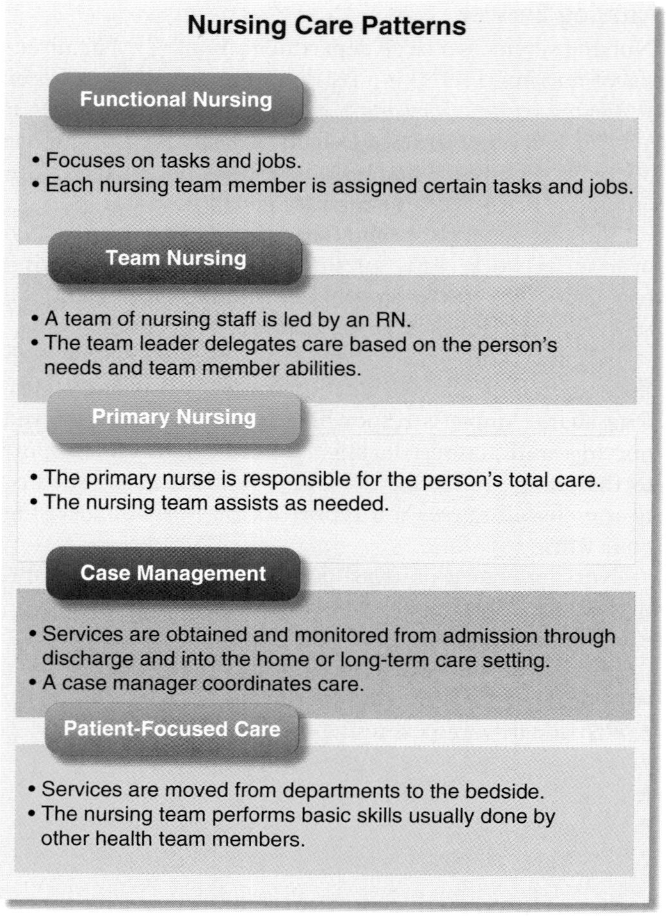

PAYING FOR HEALTH CARE

Health care is costly. Some people avoid health care because they cannot pay. Others pay doctor bills but go without food or drugs. Health insurance covers some costs. Rarely are all costs covered.

These programs help pay for health care.
- *Private insurance* is bought by individuals and families.
- *Group insurance* is bought by groups or organizations for individuals. This is often an employee benefit.
- *Medicare* is a federal program for persons 65 years of age or older. Some younger people with certain disabilities qualify. Persons of any age with end-stage renal disease (kidney failure) also qualify (Chapter 40). Part A is for hospital, SNF, hospice, and home care costs. Part B is for doctors' services, preventive care, ambulance services, medical supplies, mental health care, and some drugs. Part B is voluntary. The person pays a monthly premium.

Nursing Care Patterns

Functional Nursing
- Focuses on tasks and jobs.
- Each nursing team member is assigned certain tasks and jobs.

Team Nursing
- A team of nursing staff is led by an RN.
- The team leader delegates care based on the person's needs and team member abilities.

Primary Nursing
- The primary nurse is responsible for the person's total care.
- The nursing team assists as needed.

Case Management
- Services are obtained and monitored from admission through discharge and into the home or long-term care setting.
- A case manager coordinates care.

Patient-Focused Care
- Services are moved from departments to the bedside.
- The nursing team performs basic skills usually done by other health team members.

FIGURE 1-3 Nursing care patterns.

- *Medicaid* is jointly funded by the federal government and the states. People and families with low incomes usually qualify. It covers children and older, blind, and disabled persons.
- *Health Insurance Marketplace®* is a service that helps people shop for and enroll in affordable health insurance. The "Marketplace" or "exchange" began as part of the *Patient Protection and Affordable Care Act of 2010*. This act is commonly called the *Affordable Care Act (ACA)* or "Obamacare," after President Barack Obama. The federal government operates the Marketplace for most states. Some states run their own Marketplaces.

See *Promoting Safety and Comfort: Paying for Health Care.*

PROMOTING SAFETY AND COMFORT

Paying for Health Care

Safety

Some conditions can be prevented with proper care. Medicare pays a lower rate for such conditions if they are acquired during a hospital stay. Pressure injuries (Chapter 36) and certain types of falls, trauma, and infections are examples. You must help prevent such conditions.

Prospective Payment Systems

Prospective payment systems limit the amount paid by insurers, Medicare, and Medicaid. *Prospective* means *before*. The amount paid for services is determined before giving care. If costs are less than the amount paid, the agency keeps the extra money. If costs are greater, the agency takes the loss.

SAFETY AND QUALITY

The *U.S. Department of Health & Human Services (HHS)* is the government agency responsible for protecting the health and well-being of Americans. HHS has different divisions (agencies) that focus on certain areas of health care safety and quality. Box 1-1 lists some of the HHS agencies that over-see health care in the United States.

Regulations are rules made by government agencies. Regulations are based on standards that must be met. Health care agencies must meet the standards set by federal and state governments for:

- *Licensure.* A state license is required to operate and provide care.
- *Certification.* This is required to receive Medicare and Medicaid funds.

Accrediting agencies also have standards. *Accreditation* is voluntary. It signals quality and excellence. *The Joint Commission* is an example of an accrediting agency. The agency helps improve performance.

Policies and Procedures

Policies are guides for staff conduct and daily operation. *Procedures* explain how to perform certain tasks or skills. Policies and procedures communicate what the health care agency expects. They promote compliance with regulations and accreditation requirements. *Compliance* means the agency is meeting the standards.

BOX 1-1 HHS Agencies

- *Agency for Healthcare Research and Quality (AHRQ)*—focuses on information (evidence) that promotes safety, quality, and reduced health care costs. The AHRQ gathers information, monitors outcomes, and provides resources to improve practice. This agency works with other HHS agencies to make sure information is understood and used.
- *Centers for Disease Control and Prevention (CDC)*—provides leadership and direction on the prevention and control of diseases. This agency responds to public health emergencies.
- *Centers for Medicare & Medicaid Services (CMS)*—over-sees government-funded insurance programs such as Medicare, the federal part of the Medicaid program, and the Health Insurance Marketplace®.
- *Food and Drug Administration (FDA)*—regulates the safety of foods, drugs and vaccines (Chapter 14), medical devices, electronics that give off radiation, cosmetics, and tobacco products.
- *National Institutes of Health (NIH)*—conducts and supports medical research. The goal is to gain knowledge that helps prevent, detect, diagnose, and treat diseases and disabilities. The National Cancer Institute (NCI), National Institute on Aging (NIA), and the National Institute of Mental Health (NIMH) are examples of NIH institutes.

Modified from U.S. Department of Health & Human Services: *HHS agencies & offices,* January 5, 2022.

The Survey Process

Surveys are done to see if standards are met. A *survey is the formal review of an agency through the collection of facts and observations.* Survey teams are made up of surveyors. A *surveyor is a person who collects information by observing and asking questions.*

A survey team will:

- Review policies, procedures, and medical records.
- Interview staff, patients and residents, and families.
- Observe how care is given.
- Observe if dignity and privacy are promoted.
- Check for cleanliness and safety.
- Make sure staff meet state requirements. (Are doctors and nurses licensed? Are nursing assistants on the state registry?)

If standards are met, the agency receives a license, certification, or accreditation. Sometimes problems (*deficiencies*) are found. The agency usually has 60 days or less to correct the problem. The agency can be fined for uncorrected or serious deficiencies. Or it can lose its license, certification, or accreditation.

Your Role

You have an important role in meeting standards and in the survey process. You must:
- Provide quality care.
- Protect the person's rights.
- Provide for the person's and your own safety.
- Help keep the agency clean and safe.
- Act in a professional manner.
- Have good work ethics.
- Follow agency policies and procedures.
- Answer questions honestly and completely. See *Focus on Surveys: Your Role.*

FOCUS ON SURVEYS

Your Role

A surveyor may ask you questions. If so, be polite. Answer questions honestly and completely. If you do not understand a question, ask that it be re-phrased. Do not guess. Tell the surveyor where you can find the answer. You can say: "I will ask the nurse."

For example, a surveyor approaches you.

Surveyor: "May I ask you some questions?"

You: "Yes. I am happy to answer your questions."

Surveyor: "Thank you. First, what do you use for hand hygiene during routine patient care?"

You: "I use the hand sanitizer in the person's room."

Surveyor: "Thank you. Next, what are 2 appropriate patient identifiers?"

You: "I don't understand. Can you re-phrase the question?"

Surveyor: "Yes. Name 2 things you can use to identify a patient."

You: "Okay. Thank you. I can use the patient's full name and date of birth. I cannot use the room number."

Surveyor: "I have 1 last question. In a disaster, where would you find the Emergency Preparedness Plan?"

You: "I'm not sure. I will ask the charge nurse where to find it."

FOCUS ON P R I D E

The Person, Family, and Yourself

P ersonal and Professional Responsibility

Working in health care is rewarding. You provide care for a *person.* Your work affects the person's quality of care. Value the work that you do.

Focus on PRIDE is at the end of every chapter. The feature will help you promote pride in the person, the family, and yourself. Building on chapter content, it focuses on:
- *Personal and Professional Responsibility*—how personal and professional behaviors and development affect yourself and others.
- *Rights and Respect*—how to promote the rights of others and how to respect them as persons with dignity and value.
- *Independence and Social Interaction*—how to promote independence and positive interactions.
- *Delegation and Teamwork*—how to practice safe delegation (Chapter 3) and work well with and help other team members.
- *Ethics and Laws*—how to do the right thing when dealing with patients, residents, and co-workers. Laws affecting nursing care are also presented.

For discussion purposes, each chapter ends with a *Focus on PRIDE: Application* section. The questions challenge you to think about your role and how you will value the person, family, or yourself.

R ights and Respect

Why do you want to work in health care? Maybe you want to help people. Maybe a health team member inspired you. Or you may have a job opportunity or career goal in mind. Think about your reasons.

Consider what type of agency would suit you. One person may prefer working in long-term care while another prefers a hospital setting. Careful career planning shows respect for employers, patients and residents, and yourself.

I ndependence and Social Interaction

You will interact with patients and residents, nursing staff, health team members, surveyors, and families. How you interact with others affects quality of care and job satisfaction.

D elegation and Teamwork

Health team members must work together to provide quality care. Offer to help others when you can. Helping others shows you value teamwork.

E thics and Laws

Professional conduct is valued in all health care agencies. You will learn about ethical and legal aspects of care (Chapter 4) and student and work ethics (Chapter 5). As you study, consider how you will apply professional qualities as a student and in the workplace.

FOCUS ON PRIDE: Application

Why do you want to work in health care? Where do you want to work? What are your career goals?

Circle the BEST answer.

1 The purpose of rehabilitation is to
   a Prevent chronic illnesses
   b Detect terminal illnesses
   c Restore function and independence
   d Treat urgent illnesses

2 A person is admitted to a hospital. Which is *true*?
   a The person is called a resident.
   b Chronic illnesses are not treated.
   c The person cannot leave.
   d The person receives in-patient care.

3 A patient is ready for discharge from the hospital. The person needs more care before going home. Which is *best*?
   a Stay in the hospital for as long as possible.
   b Do short-term rehabilitation in a nursing center before going home.
   c Discharge from the hospital to home as soon as possible.
   d Avoid nursing center care.

4 You work in an assisted living residence. You
   a Give care in the person's home
   b Care for patients recovering from surgery
   c Help persons with their daily activities
   d Care for persons with acute illnesses

5 A person needs end-of-life care. Which can promote comfort and quality of life?
   a Hospice
   b Rehabilitation
   c Restorative care
   d Memory care

6 Who controls policy in a health care agency?
   a The survey team
   b The board of directors
   c The health team
   d Medicare and Medicaid

7 Who is responsible for the entire nursing staff and safe nursing care?
   a The case manager
   b The director of nursing
   c The charge nurse
   d The RN

8 Which health team member helps the person retain skills needed for daily living and work?
   a Occupational therapist
   b Social worker
   c Respiratory therapist
   d Pharmacist

9 The nursing team includes
   a Doctors
   b Pharmacists
   c Physical and occupational therapists
   d RNs, LPNs/LVNs, and nursing assistants

10 Which member of the nursing team requires the *most* education?
   a Licensed vocational nurse
   b Licensed practical nurse
   c Registered nurse
   d Nursing assistant

11 Nursing assistants are supervised by
   a Licensed nurses
   b Other nursing assistants
   c The health team
   d The medical director

12 Your hospital unit uses a team nursing care pattern. Your role is to
   a Ask which task you are assigned for your work shift
   b Report observations and the care you give to the nurse
   c Perform tasks that are usually done by other departments
   d Coordinate care with the case manager

13 Medicare is for persons who
   a Are 65 years of age or older
   b Need nursing center care
   c Have group insurance
   d Have low incomes

14 Which government agency over-sees government-funded insurance programs?
   a Food and Drug Administration (FDA)
   b Centers for Disease Control and Prevention (CDC)
   c National Institutes of Health (NIH)
   d Centers for Medicare & Medicaid Services (CMS)

15 Which is required for an agency to operate and provide care?
   a Accreditation
   b Certification
   c A license
   d A survey

16 Which is voluntary for health care agencies?
   a Licensure
   b Certification
   c Accreditation
   d Surveys

17 Surveys are done to
   a Reduce health care costs
   b See if agencies meet set standards
   c Educate the nursing team
   d Determine the amount paid by insurers

18 A surveyor asks you some questions. You should
   a Refer all questions to the nurse
   b Answer as the DON tells you to
   c Give as little information as possible
   d Give honest and complete answers

Answers to Chapter 1 questions are on p. 587.

FOCUS ON **PRACTICE**

Problem Solving

The nurse supervising you has not returned from a meal break. You have a question about a patient's care. Your nursing department is organized as shown in Figure 1-2. What will you do?

CHAPTER 2

The Person's Rights

OBJECTIVES

- Define the key terms and key abbreviation in this chapter.
- Explain the purpose of *The Patient Care Partnership: Understanding Expectations, Rights, and Responsibilities.*
- Describe the purposes and requirements of the *Omnibus Budget Reconciliation Act of 1987 (OBRA).*
- Identify the person's rights under OBRA.
- Explain how to protect the person's rights.
- Explain the ombudsman role.
- Explain how to promote PRIDE in the person, the family, and yourself.

KEY TERMS

advocate Someone who acts or speaks on behalf of another person

involuntary seclusion Separating a person from others against the person's will, keeping the person to a certain area, or keeping the person away from his or her room without consent

ombudsman Someone who supports or promotes the needs and interests of another person

representative Someone with the legal right to act on the patient's or resident's behalf when the person cannot do so alone

treatment The care provided to maintain or restore health, improve function, or relieve symptoms

KEY ABBREVIATION

OBRA Omnibus Budget Reconciliation Act of 1987

People want to know about their health problems and treatment. They want to understand and take part in treatment decisions. As patients and residents, they have certain rights.

PATIENT RIGHTS

The Patient Care Partnership: Understanding Expectations, Rights, and Responsibilities is from the American Hospital Association. The document explains the person's rights and expectations during hospital stays. The relationship between the doctor, health team, and patient is stressed. See Appendix A, p. 590.

RESIDENT RIGHTS

The *Omnibus Budget Reconciliation Act of 1987 (OBRA)* is a federal law. It applies to all 50 states. The law set minimum standards for quality of care in nursing centers. The Centers for Medicare & Medicaid Services (CMS) enforces OBRA through the survey process (Chapter 1).

OBRA requires that nursing centers provide care in a manner and in a setting that maintains or improves each person's quality of life, health, and safety. Nursing assistant training and competency evaluation are part of OBRA (Chapter 3). Resident rights are a major part of OBRA.

Residents have rights as United States citizens. For example, they have the right to vote. They also have rights relating to their every-day lives and care in a nursing center. These rights are protected by federal and state laws.

Nursing centers must protect and promote the person's rights. The center cannot interfere with a resident's rights. Some residents cannot exercise their rights.

A representative (spouse, partner, adult child, court-appointed guardian) does so for them. A *representative is someone with the legal right to act on the patient's or resident's behalf when the person cannot do so alone.*

Nursing centers must inform residents of their rights—orally and in writing. Residents are also informed of the rules about their conduct and responsibilities in the center. Information is given before or during admission to the center, as needed during the person's stay, and when laws or center rules change.

Resident rights and other information are given in the language the person uses and understands. An interpreter is used if the person speaks and understands a foreign language or communicates by sign language.

Resident rights (Box 2-1) also are posted throughout the center. Those affecting your role are described in this chapter.

See *Focus on Surveys: Resident Rights.*

FOCUS ON SURVEYS

Resident Rights

Resident rights are a major focus of surveys. Surveyors observe staff behaviors and actions. They listen to staff comments and remarks. Always assume they are doing so. What you say and do must promote quality of life, health, and safety. For example, a surveyor may observe:
- How you prevent exposure of the person's body
- How you help a person dress for the season and time of day
- How you label clothing
- If you knock on a person's door before entering the room
- If you change a person's music or TV without permission
- If you move personal items without permission
- How you address and speak to a person

You will learn how to protect the person's rights as you study this and other chapters. Always act and speak in a professional manner.

BOX 2-1   Resident Rights

- To be treated with dignity and respect. And to receive quality care.
- To exercise rights as a center resident and as a United States citizen.
- To be informed orally and in writing of rights and center rules. This is done in a language the person understands.
- To access all of his or her records.
- To obtain copies of his or her records. This is at the resident's expense.
- To refuse treatment.
- To refuse to take part in experimental research. This is the development and testing of new treatments and drugs.
- To make advance directives (Chapter 44).
- To be informed of Medicare benefits and services. This includes costs covered and not covered.
- To be informed of center services and service charges.
- To choose a doctor.
- To know the doctor's name, specialty, and contact information.
- To be informed of his or her health status and medical condition. Information is given in a language that the person understands. That language is used during care planning (Chapter 7).
- To be informed of:
  - Any accident or injury that may need medical attention.
  - A change in physical, mental, or psycho-social status.
  - The need to stop, change, or add a treatment.
  - A decision to transfer or discharge the person. *Transfer* means to move to a different setting. *Discharge* is when the person officially departs from the agency.
  - A room or roommate change.
  - A change in rights under federal or state law.
- To manage personal and financial affairs.
- To be informed in advance about care and treatment. This includes changes in care and treatment.
- To have privacy and confidentiality:
  - Of personal and medical records
  - Of treatment and care
  - Of written and phone communications
  - During visits with family and friends
  - When meeting with resident groups
- To voice grievances and have them solved promptly.
- To see the results of federal and state surveys and plans to correct problems or areas of weakness.
- To perform or refuse to perform services for the center.
- To send and receive un-opened mail. To buy supplies to send mail.
- To receive information about protecting persons with intellectual and developmental disabilities and mental health disorders.
- To have and use personal items and clothing.
- To take his or her drugs without help if able.
- To refuse to change to a different room.
- To be free from restraints (Chapter 13).
- To be free from abuse (verbal, sexual, physical), bodily punishment, involuntary seclusion, and other abuse or mistreatment (Chapter 4).
- To file complaints with the appropriate state agency about abuse, neglect, and the mis-use of property.
- To be cared for in a manner and setting that maintains or enhances quality of life.
- To choose activities, schedules, and health care that meet his or her interests and needs.
- To interact with community members inside and outside the center.
- To make choices about his or her life in the center.
- To organize and take part in resident groups.
- To take part in social, religious, and community activities.
- To have a setting and services that consider his or her needs and choices.
- To a clean, comfortable, and home-like setting. This includes temperature, lighting, and sound levels.
- To attain or maintain his or her highest level of function.
- To have closet space.
- To visit with a spouse or partner, family, and friends at any reasonable hour.

Information

The *right to information* means access to all records about the person. Medical records, contracts, incident reports, and financial records are included. The request can be oral or written.

The person has the right to be fully informed of his or her health condition. The person must also have information about his or her doctor. This includes the doctor's name, specialty, and contact information.

Report any information request to the nurse. *You do not give the information described above to the person or family* (Chapter 3).

See *Focus on Communication: Information.*

FOCUS ON COMMUNICATION

Information

You may be asked about a person's care. You must not give out information. This is the nurse's responsibility. You can say:

I am sorry. I am not allowed to give that information. I will report your request to the nurse.

Communicate the request promptly. You can tell the person:

I told the nurse about your question. The nurse will speak with you soon.

Refusing Treatment

The person has the *right to refuse treatment*. **Treatment** *means the care provided to maintain or restore health, improve function, or relieve symptoms.* A person cannot be treated without consent (Chapter 4).

The center must:
- Find out what the person is refusing and why.
- Explain the problems that can result from the refusal.
- Offer other treatment options.
- Continue to provide all other services.

Advance directives are part of the right to refuse treatment (Chapter 44). They include living wills and instructions about life support. *Advance directives* are written instructions about health care when the person is not able to make such decisions.

Report any treatment refusal to the nurse. The nurse may change the person's care plan (Chapter 7).

Privacy and Confidentiality

Residents have the *right to personal privacy*. Staff must maintain privacy of the person's body. Expose the person's body only as necessary. Only staff directly involved in care and treatment are present. Consent is needed for others to be present. For example, consent is needed for a student to observe a treatment.

Privacy is maintained for all personal care measures. Bathing, dressing, and elimination are examples. To protect privacy:
- Close privacy curtains, doors, and window coverings.
- Remove residents from public view.
- Provide clothes or drape the person to prevent unnecessary exposure of body parts.
- Practice the measures listed in Chapter 4.

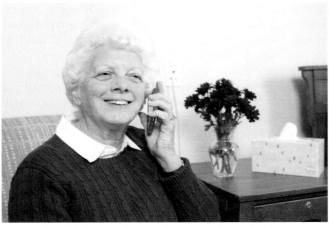

FIGURE 2-1 A resident is talking privately on the phone.

Leaving the person without a gown, clothing, or bed covers violates the right to privacy. So does an open door when the person uses the bathroom, commode, urinal, or bedpan.

Residents have the right to visit with others in private—where others cannot see or hear them. This includes phone calls (Fig. 2-1). Calls must not be over-heard. Privacy is provided for phone calls in offices or at the nurses' station. Phones are at the correct height for use by persons in wheelchairs. Phones for hard of hearing persons are also available. Some residents use their own phones.

The right to privacy also involves mail. No one can open mail the person sends or receives without the person's consent.

Information about the person's care, treatment, and condition is kept confidential. So are medical and financial records. Consent is needed for their release to other agencies or persons.

Privacy and confidentiality are discussed in Chapters 4 and 5.

Personal Choice

Residents have the *right to make their own choices*. This includes:
- Choosing doctors
- Choosing friends and visitors
- Helping to plan care and treatment
- Choosing activities, schedules, and care:
  - When to go to bed and when to get up
  - What to wear (Fig. 2-2)
  - How to spend time
  - What to eat

Personal choice promotes quality of life, dignity, and self-respect. Allow personal choice whenever safely possible.

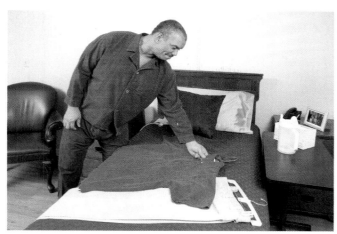

FIGURE 2-2 A resident is choosing what clothing to wear.

Grievances

Residents have the *right to voice concerns, questions, and complaints about treatment and care.* The problem may involve another person. It may be about care that was given or not given. The center must promptly try to correct the matter. No one can punish the person in any way for voicing a grievance.

Work

The person does not work for care, care items or other things, or privileges. The person is not required to perform services for the center.

However, the person has the *right to work or perform services if he or she desires.* Some people like to garden, repair or build things, clean, sew, mend, or cook. Other persons need work for rehabilitation or activity reasons. The care plan reflects the person's desire or need to work. Residents volunteer or are paid for their services.

Resident Groups

The person has the *right to form and take part in resident groups.* Families can meet with other families. These groups can plan activities, discuss concerns, take part in educational events, and suggest center improvements. They can support and comfort group members.

Residents have the right to take part in social, cultural, religious, and community events. They have the right to help in getting to and from such events.

Personal Items

Residents have the *right to keep and use personal items.* This includes clothing and some furnishings. The items allowed depend on space needs and the health and safety of others.

Treat the person's property with care and respect. The items may lack value to you but have meaning to the person. They also relate to personal choice, dignity, a home-like setting, and quality of life.

The person's property is protected. Items are labeled with the person's name. The center must investigate reports of lost, stolen, or damaged items. Sometimes the police help. The person and family are advised to keep jewelry and costly items at home.

Protect yourself and the center from being accused of stealing. Do not go through a closet, drawers, purse, or other space without the person's knowledge and consent. A nurse may ask you to inspect closets and drawers. Center policy should require that a co-worker and the person or legal representative be present. They witness your actions.

Freedom From Abuse, Mistreatment, and Neglect

Residents have the *right to be free from verbal, sexual, physical, and mental abuse. No one can abuse, neglect, or mistreat a resident. Abuse* and *neglect* are discussed in Chapter 4.

Residents also have the right to be free from *involuntary seclusion.*

- *Separating a person from others against the person's will*
- *Keeping the person to a certain area*
- *Keeping the person away from his or her room without consent*

No one can mistreat a resident. This includes center staff, volunteers, and staff from other agencies or groups. It also includes other residents, family members, visitors, and legal representatives. Centers must investigate suspected or reported cases of abuse, neglect, or mistreatment. The person must be protected from harm during an investigation. A center cannot employ a person who:

- Has been found guilty of abusing, neglecting, or mistreating others by a court of law.
- Has a finding entered into a state's nursing assistant registry (Chapter 3) about abuse, neglect, mistreatment, or wrongful acts involving a person's money or property. A *finding* means that a state determined that the employee abused, neglected, mistreated, or wrongfully used the person's money or property.

Freedom From Restraint

Residents have the *right not to have body movements restricted.* Restraints and certain drugs can restrict body movements. Some drugs are restraints because they affect mood, behavior, and mental function. Sometimes residents are restrained to protect them from harming themselves or others. A doctor's order is needed for restraint use. Restraints are not used for staff convenience or to discipline a person. They are used only if required to treat medical symptoms. Restraints are discussed in Chapter 13.

Quality of Life

Residents have the *right to quality of life.* They must be cared for in a manner and in a setting that promotes dignity and respect for self. Staff must provide care in a manner that maintains or enhances self-esteem and feelings of self-worth. Care must promote physical, mental, and social well-being. Protecting resident rights promotes quality of life. It shows respect for the person.

Be polite and courteous. Good, honest, and thoughtful care enhances quality of life. Box 2-2 lists OBRA-required actions that promote dignity and privacy.

See *Focus on Communication: Quality of Life.*

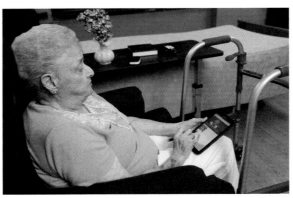

FIGURE 2-3 This resident's setting is safe, clean, and comfortable. Personal items are part of a home-like setting.

Environment. Residents have the *right to a safe, clean, comfortable, and home-like setting.* The person can have and use personal items to the extent possible. Doing so promotes personal choice and a home-like setting. See Figure 2-3.

FOCUS ON COMMUNICATION

Quality of Life

Every person deserves to be addressed in a manner that shows dignity and respect. Address the person by title and last name. For example: Mr. Baker, Mrs. Harty, or Dr. Collins. Do not use a person's first name or another name unless the person requests it. Avoid using terms like *sweetheart, honey, grandpa,* and *dear.*

BOX 2-2 OBRA-Required Actions to Promote Dignity and Privacy

Courteous and Dignified Interactions
- Use the right tone of voice.
- Use good eye contact.
- Stand or sit close enough as needed. Position yourself at the person's eye level. For example, sit to speak to a person who is seated.
- Use the person's proper name and title. For example: "Mrs. Crane." Or use the name the person prefers.
- Gain the person's attention before interacting with him or her.
- Explain the care you provide.
- Use touch if the person approves.
- Respect the person's social status.
- Listen with interest to what the person is saying.
- Do not yell at, scold, or embarrass the person.

Privacy and Self-Determination
- Knock on the door before entering. Wait to be asked in.
- Drape properly during care and procedures to avoid exposure and embarrassment.
- Use privacy curtains or screens during care and procedures.
- Close the room door during care and procedures. Also close window coverings.
- Close the bathroom door when the person uses the bathroom.
- Drape properly in a chair.

Personal Choice and Independence
- Person smokes in allowed areas.
- Person takes part in activities of interest.
- Person takes part in scheduling activities and care.
- Person gives input into the care plan about preferences and independence.
- Person is involved in a room or roommate change.
- The person's items are moved or inspected only with the person's consent.

Courteous and Dignified Care
- Respond to requests for help in a timely manner.
- Assist with dressing in the right clothing for time of day and personal choice. The person wears his or her own clothing.
- Promote independence and dignity in dining.
- Respect private space and property. For example, change music or TV stations only with the person's consent.
- Assist with walking and transfers. Do not interfere with independence.
- Assist with hygiene and grooming preferences. Do not interfere with independence.
  - Appearance is neat and clean.
  - Hair is styled as the person prefers.
  - The person is clean shaven or has a groomed beard and mustache.
  - Nails are trimmed and clean.
  - Dentures, hearing aids, eyeglasses, and other devices are used correctly.
  - Clothing is clean.
  - Clothing fits and is properly fastened.
  - Shoes, hose, and socks are on properly and fastened.
  - Extra clothing is worn for warmth as needed. Sweaters and lap blankets are examples.

Activities. Residents have the *right to activities that enhance each person's physical, mental, and psycho-social well-being.* The center provides religious services for spiritual health.

Activities are meaningful when they:

- Reflect the person's needs, interests, culture, background, and life-style.
- Are enjoyed by the person.
- Help the person feel useful or produce something useful.
- Provide a sense of belonging.

Activities involve large groups (bingo), small groups (a card game), or 2 people. The person may do something alone. Letter writing and computer games are examples.

You assist residents to and from activity programs of their choice. You may need to help them with activities (Fig. 2-4).

See *Focus on Communication: Activities.*

See *Focus on Surveys: Activities.*

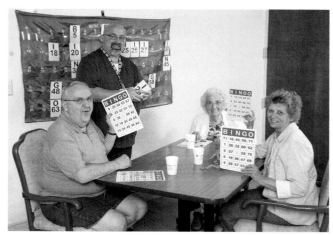

FIGURE 2-4   A nursing assistant is helping residents with an activity.

FOCUS ON **COMMUNICATION**

Activities

You may need help assisting residents to and from activity programs. Politely ask a co-worker to help you. Share the following with your co-worker.

- What time you need help.
- How much of the co-worker's time you need.
- The residents you need help with.
- If the person walks or uses a wheelchair.
- What adaptive (assistive) devices are used. Eyeglasses, hearing aids, canes, and walkers are examples.

Always say "please" when asking for help. And thank the person for helping you. For example:

Alex, can you please help me assist 2 residents to the concert? It starts at 2:00, so I'll need your help at 1:45. Mr. Harris needs his glasses, hearing aid, and walker. Mrs. Janz uses a wheelchair. She needs her glasses. The blanket for her lap is in the wheelchair. The concert is over at 3:00. Can you help me then, too? Thanks so much for helping me.

FOCUS ON **SURVEYS**

Activities

Surveyors may ask you about:

- Your role in getting residents ready for a group activity.
  - How do you make sure the person is dressed and ready for an activity?
  - How do you provide needed transportation?
- Your role in helping with activities of daily living during an activity. For example, does the person need to use the bathroom? Does the person need help eating?
- Your role in helping a person with an individual activity. For example, you play cards with a person. Do you have needed supplies? Is the person properly positioned? Do you provide good lighting?
- How are activities provided when the activities staff members are not available?

PROTECTING RIGHTS

An **advocate** *is someone who acts or speaks on behalf of another person.* Nurses act as advocates for their patients or residents. You also act as an advocate when you:

- Respect and protect the person's rights.
- Respect the person's decisions and choices.
- Treat the person with dignity.
- Are attentive to the person's needs, concerns, and requests.
- Promote a safe setting for the person.
- Tell the nurse about concerns.

Ombudsmen

The *Older Americans Act* is a federal law. It requires a long-term care ombudsman program in every state. An **ombudsman** *supports or promotes the needs and interests of another person.*

Ombudsmen are advocates for residents. They protect a person's health, safety, welfare, and rights. They:

- Investigate and resolve complaints.
- Provide services to assist the person.
- Assist with hospital access or discharge concerns.
- Provide information about long-term care services.
- Monitor nursing care and conditions.
- Provide support to resident and family groups.
- Help the person and family resolve family conflicts.
- Help the center manage difficult problems.

Nursing centers must post contact information for local and state ombudsmen. A resident or family may share a concern with you. Follow center policies and procedures for contacting an ombudsman. Ombudsman services are useful when:

- There is a concern about a person's care or treatment.
- Someone interferes with a person's rights, health, safety, or welfare.

FOCUS ON P R I D E
The Person, Family, and Yourself

P ersonal and Professional Responsibility

Person-centered care is a goal in nursing centers. This means the person maintains control. Staff support the person in making his or her own choices. A care plan (Chapter 7) that is specific to the person is developed. Staff try to understand the resident and what routines and activities matter to the person. Knowing about the person's usual daily life can promote person-centered care.

R ights and Respect

The person has the right to refuse treatment. This does not mean that all treatment stops. The health team offers other treatment options. For example, the doctor suggests short-term placement in a nursing center. The person refuses. The family agrees to help the person at home. A social worker helps the person and family arrange for home care and respite care. *Respite care* relieves caregivers of daily care for a short time.

I ndependence and Social Interaction

Encourage social interaction. Talk with the person. Tell about activities and offer help to and from activities. Also respect the person's right to privacy during visits with others and phone calls. These actions promote self-worth and quality of life.

D elegation and Teamwork

Schedules, care assignments, and room arrangements may need to change to meet the person's needs and preferences. Flexibility, good teamwork, and communication are required to provide quality care.

E thics and Laws

Every person has the right to keep personal information private. This includes information about health care. The *Health Insurance Portability and Accountability Act of 1996 (HIPAA)* protects the privacy and security of a person's health information. HIPAA is discussed further in Chapter 4.

FOCUS ON PRIDE: *Application*

You have an important role in protecting the person's rights. Identify 3 ways you can promote the person's right to:
- Personal choice
- Privacy and confidentiality
- A safe, clean, and comfortable setting

REVIEW QUESTIONS

Circle the BEST answer.

1 *The Patient Care Partnership: Understanding Expectations, Rights, and Responsibilities* is concerned with
   a Hospital care
   b Home care
   c Long-term care
   d All health care agencies and settings

2 The Omnibus Budget Reconciliation Act of 1987 (OBRA) is a federal law that
   a Requires health care agencies to limit treatment costs
   b Sets standards for quality of nursing center care
   c Restricts nursing center residents' rights
   d Provides affordable health insurance options

3 A son has the legal right to act on his mother's behalf. The son is his mother's legal
   a Ombudsman
   b Representative
   c Caregiver
   d Health care provider

4 Residents must be
   a Involved in resident groups
   b Able to provide some type of work for the center
   c Informed of rights orally and in writing
   d Willing to accept treatments ordered by their doctors

5 A resident says he does not want a shower. Which response is *best*?
   a "You smell badly and need a shower."
   b "You cannot refuse a shower."
   c "Why are you being difficult?"
   d "Why do you not want a shower?"

6 A daughter wants to read her father's medical record. What should you do?
   a Give her the medical record.
   b Ask the resident if she can read the record.
   c Tell the nurse.
   d Tell her that she cannot do so.

7 A resident asks about another resident's health.
   Which response is *best*?
   a "Mind your own business."
   b "The nurse can tell you."
   c "He had a heart attack."
   d "I cannot give information about another resident."

8 Which violates the person's right to privacy?
   a Closing the bathroom door when the bathroom is used
   b Opening window blinds when assisting with bathing
   c Covering the person for personal care
   d Asking the person's permission to observe a treatment

9 A resident has a phone and wants to make a call.
   What should you do?
   a Leave the room.
   b Tell the nurse.
   c Have the person use the phone at the nurses' station.
   d Close the privacy curtain so you can finish your tasks in the room.

10 Who decides how to style a person's hair?
   a The person
   b The nurse
   c You
   d The ombudsman

11 A resident would like to sleep later in the morning. You should
   a Explain why the agency has a set schedule
   b Tell the nurse why this is not convenient for you
   c Allow the person to sleep until the preferred time
   d Wake the person at a time best for you

12 Residents have the right to
   a Bring weapons into the center
   b Mistreat other residents
   c Use other residents' personal items
   d Voice complaints about care

13 Residents have the right to be free from
   a Disease
   b Grievances
   c Involuntary seclusion
   d Rules

14 A resident brought some items from home. They are
   a Kept at the nurses' station
   b Labeled with the person's name
   c Arranged as you prefer
   d Shared with the person's roommate

15 A resident carries a baby doll most of the day. You should
   a Ask the family to take the doll home
   b Remind the person that the doll is not allowed in the dining room
   c Threaten to take the doll away if the resident refuses care
   d Treat the doll with care and respect

16 A person found guilty of abuse
   a Cannot work in a nursing center
   b Can work in a nursing center with supervision
   c Can work as a nurse in a nursing center
   d Can work as a nursing assistant in a nursing center

17 Which is the correct way to address a person?
   a "Hello, sweetie."
   b "Hello."
   c "Hello, Mrs. Smith."
   d "Hello, grandpa."

18 Which action promotes dignity?
   a Restraining the person
   b Making clothing choices for the person
   c Scolding the person
   d Listening to the person

19 Which promotes privacy?
   a Entering a person's room without knocking
   b Closing the privacy curtain for a procedure
   c Leaving the door open during personal care
   d Looking through the person's belongings

20 Who selects activities for a resident?
   a The nurse
   b You
   c The person's representative
   d The person

21 A nursing center must provide
   a A safe, clean, and comfortable setting
   b An indoor smoking area
   c A bed near a window
   d A noise-free setting

22 A long-term care ombudsman
   a Is employed by the nursing center
   b Investigates resident complaints
   c Grants a nursing center a license or certification
   d Can prevent a resident from leaving the center

Answers to Chapter 2 questions are on p. 587.

FOCUS ON PRACTICE

Problem Solving

A resident is crying. She tells you a co-worker is rough when moving her and insults her. She says the co-worker threatens to "tie her down" if she tries to get up alone. What will you do? What is the nursing center's responsibility?

CHAPTER 3

The Nursing Assistant

OBJECTIVES

- Define the key terms and key abbreviations in this chapter.
- Describe the training and competency evaluation requirements for nursing assistants.
- Identify the information in the nursing assistant registry.
- List the reasons for denying, suspending, or revoking a nursing assistant's certification, license, or registration.
- Explain how to obtain certification, a license, or registration in another state.

- Describe what nursing assistants can do and their role limits.
- Describe the standards for nursing assistants developed by the National Council of State Boards of Nursing.
- Explain why a job description is important.
- Describe the delegation process and your role.
- Explain how to accept or refuse a delegated task.
- Explain how to promote PRIDE in the person, the family, and yourself.

KEY TERMS

accountable To answer to one's self and others about one's choices, decisions, and actions
certification Official recognition by a state that standards or requirements have been met
delegate To authorize or direct a nursing assistant to perform a nursing task
delegation The process a nurse uses to direct a nursing assistant to perform a nursing task; allowing a nursing assistant to perform a nursing task that is beyond the nursing assistant's usual role and not routinely done by the nursing assistant

endorsement A state recognizes the certificate, license, or registration issued by another state; reciprocity or equivalency
equivalency See "endorsement"
job description A document that describes what the agency expects you to do
nursing task Nursing care or a nursing function, procedure, skill, or activity
reciprocity See "endorsement"

KEY ABBREVIATIONS

ANA	American Nurses Association	NATCEP	Nursing assistant training and competency evaluation program
APRN	Advanced practice registered nurse		
BON	Board of nursing	NCSBN	National Council of State Boards of Nursing
LPN	Licensed practical nurse	OBRA	Omnibus Budget Reconciliation Act of 1987
LVN	Licensed vocational nurse	RN	Registered nurse

Federal and state laws and agency policies combine to define your roles and functions. To give safe care, you need to know:

- What you can and cannot do
- Rules and standards of conduct affecting your work
- Your role limits

Laws, job descriptions, and the person's condition shape your work. So does the amount of supervision you need.

NURSE PRACTICE ACTS

Each state has a nurse practice act. A nurse practice act:

- Defines the different nursing levels and their scope of practice.
  - Advanced practice registered nurse (APRN)
  - Registered nurse (RN)
  - Licensed practical nurse/licensed vocational nurse (LPN/LVN)
- Describes APRN, RN, and LPN/LVN education and licensing requirements.
- Protects the public from persons practicing nursing without a license. Persons who do not meet the state's requirements cannot perform nursing functions.

A nurse practice act is enforced by the state's board of nursing (BON). The BON can deny, revoke, or suspend a nurse's license. The intent is to protect the public from unsafe nurses. Reasons include:

- Selling or distributing drugs
- Using a person's drugs for oneself
- Placing a person in danger from the over-use of alcohol or drugs
- Being convicted of abusing or neglecting children or older persons
- Demonstrating incompetent behaviors

Nursing Assistants

Nurse practice acts are used to decide what nursing assistants can do. Some also regulate nursing assistant roles, functions, education, and certification requirements. Other states have separate laws for nursing assistants.

If you do something beyond the legal limits of your role, you could be practicing nursing without a license. This means serious legal problems for you, your supervisor, and the agency. Like nurses, you can have your certification (license, registration) denied, revoked, or suspended. (See "Certification" on p. 20.)

THE OMNIBUS BUDGET RECONCILIATION ACT OF 1987

The *Omnibus Budget Reconciliation Act of 1987 (OBRA)* is a federal law. It applies to all 50 states.

OBRA sets minimum requirements for nursing assistant training and evaluation. Each state must have a nursing assistant training and competency evaluation program (NATCEP). A nursing assistant must successfully

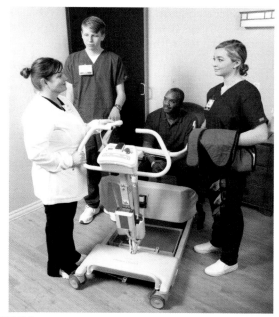

FIGURE 3-1 Nursing assistant training program. An instructor demonstrates a skill to students.

complete a NATCEP to work in a nursing center, hospital long-term care unit, or home care agency receiving Medicare funds.

The Training Program

OBRA requires at least 75 hours of instruction. Some states require more hours. Classroom and at least 16 hours of supervised practical training are required (Fig. 3-1). Practical training (clinical practicum or clinical experience) occurs in a laboratory or clinical setting. Students perform nursing tasks on another person. A nurse supervises this training.

See *Focus on Communication: The Training Program.*

FOCUS ON COMMUNICATION

The Training Program

Student clinical experiences involve giving care to patients or residents. The patient or resident has the right to know who you are. Introduce yourself. Tell the person you are a student. For example:

Hello. My name is Jesse Smith. I am a nursing assistant student. I will be working with your nurse today.

Competency Evaluation

The competency evaluation has a written test and a skills test (Appendix B, p. 591).

- The written test has multiple-choice questions. Each has 4 choices. Only 1 answer is correct.
- For the skills test, you perform certain skills learned in your training program.

You take the competency evaluation after your training program. Your instructor knows the testing service used in your state and how to schedule the evaluation and pay the required fee. If working in a nursing center, the employer pays the fee. Otherwise you pay the fee.

Your training prepares you for the competency evaluation. If you listen, study hard, and practice safe care, you should do well. If the first attempt was not successful, you can re-test. OBRA allows at least 3 attempts to successfully complete the evaluation.

Each testing service has a candidate handbook. Review the handbook carefully as you prepare for the competency evaluation.

Nursing Assistant Registry

OBRA requires a nursing assistant registry in each state. It is the official record or listing of persons who have successfully completed that state's approved NATCEP. The registry has information about each nursing assistant.

- Full name, including maiden name and any married names.
- Identifying information.
- Date the competency evaluation was passed.
- Information about findings of abuse, neglect, or dishonest use of property. The nature of the offense and supporting evidence are documented. If a hearing was held, the date and its outcome are included. The person has the right to include a statement disputing the finding. All information stays in the registry unless the finding was made in error, the person is found not guilty, or the state is notified of the registrant's death.

OBRA requires removing registry entries for persons who have not worked as nursing assistants for 24 consecutive (back-to-back) months. Entries remain for findings of abuse, neglect, or dishonest use of property.

Any health care agency can access registry information. You also receive a copy of your registry information. The copy is sent when the first entry is made and when information is changed or added. You can correct wrong information.

Certification

Certification is the official recognition by a state that standards or requirements have been met. After successfully completing your state's NATCEP, you have the title used in your state. Titles include:

- Certified nursing assistant (CNA) or certified nurse aide (CNA). CNA is used in most states.
- Licensed nursing assistant (LNA).
- Registered nurse aide (RNA).
- State registered nurse aide (SRNA).
- State tested nurse aide (STNA).

Nursing assistants can have their certifications (licenses, registrations) disciplined for actions that are harmful or dangerous to the public or a person's health. A state may deny, revoke, or suspend a certification (license, registration). See Box 3-1.

See *Promoting Safety and Comfort: Certification.*

BOX 3-1 Discipline Reasons

- Violating professional boundaries with a patient, resident, or family member. See "Professional Boundaries" in Chapter 4.
- Engaging in sexual conduct with a patient, resident, or family member.
- Leaving an assignment or abandoning a person. The nursing assistant left without notifying the nurse.
- Failing to accurately record the care given.
- Making a false or incorrect entry in a person's health record.
- Failing to follow agency policies and procedures for patient or resident safety.
- Failing to protect a person's safety or welfare.
- Failing to report observations to the nurse in a timely manner. See Chapter 7.
- Violating a person's rights or dignity.
- Violating a person's privacy by sharing the person's information.
- Neglecting or abusing a person. The abuse can be physical, verbal, emotional, or financial.
- Asking for or borrowing money or property from a patient, resident, or family member.
- Taking money, property, or personal items without permission.
- Requesting payment for services not performed from a person or the agency.
- Using or being under the influence of alcohol, a drug, or other substance that may impair judgment and safe care while on duty.
- Accepting or performing a task or function that the nursing assistant was not trained to perform.
- Removing drugs, supplies, equipment, or health records from the agency.
- Obtaining, possessing, using, or selling any narcotic, controlled substance, or illegal drug. Doing so violates agency policy or any federal or state law.
- Allowing or helping another person use the nursing assistant's certificate (license, registration) or identity.
- Making false or misleading advertisements about his or her practice as a nursing assistant.
- Offering or providing paid nursing assistant services without a nurse supervisor.
- Threatening, harassing, or exploiting a person. To *exploit* means *to use or take advantage of another person.*
- Using violent or abusive behavior in the work setting.
- Failing to cooperate with the BON during an investigation.
- Making a false or inaccurate statement to the BON or the BON's representative during an investigation.
- Engaging in fraud or deceit about the competency evaluation or an application for certification (license, registration) renewal.
- Making a false or misleading statement on an employment application about previous employment, work experience, education, or qualifications.
- Failing to notify the BON of any criminal conviction, plea arrangement, or deferred judgment.
- Practicing in any manner that gives the BON reasonable cause to believe a person or the public may be harmed.

Modified from National Council of State Boards of Nursing, Inc.: *NCSBN model rules*, Chicago, 2017, Author.

PROMOTING SAFETY AND COMFORT

Certification

Safety

OBRA and other federal and state laws require background checks on individuals with direct patient or resident contact in long-term care agencies. This may include FBI (Federal Bureau of Investigation) fingerprint checks. Long-term care agencies include:

- Nursing centers and skilled nursing facilities
- Home care agencies
- Hospices
- Long-term care hospitals
- Assisted living residences
- Adult day-care centers
- Centers for persons with developmental or intellectual disabilities

Findings of abuse, neglect, mistreatment, or misappropriation of property (Chapter 4) may affect your certification (license, registration) status. Also, OBRA does not allow persons convicted of such crimes to be employed in long-term care agencies.

Your NATCEP may require a background check before enrolling in the program or before clinical experiences begin. Clinical sites have the right to deny a student's participation depending on the student's criminal record. Satisfactory completion of your clinical experience is a NATCEP requirement. Follow your NATCEP's guidelines.

Maintaining Competence

OBRA requires that agencies provide 12 hours of education to nursing assistants every year. Performance reviews also are required. That is, your work is evaluated. These requirements help ensure that you have the current knowledge and skills to give safe, effective care.

OBRA has requirements to ensure the competence of nursing assistants who have not worked for 24 months. It does not matter how long you worked as a nursing assistant before. What matters is how long you did *not* work. States can require:

- A new competency evaluation
- Both re-training and a new competency evaluation
  See *Focus on Surveys: Maintaining Competence.*

FOCUS ON SURVEYS

Maintaining Competence

Surveyors must make sure that nursing assistants are competent to give safe care. They will:

- Check if nursing assistants have completed a NATCEP.
- Ask nursing assistants:
  - Where they received their training
  - The length of their training
  - How long they have worked in the agency
- Observe if nursing assistants:
  - Maintain or improve the person's independent functioning.
  - Perform range-of-motion exercises (Chapter 32).
  - Transfer the person from bed to a wheelchair safely (Chapter 18).
  - Observe, describe, and report the person's behavior and condition to the nurse (Chapter 7).
  - Follow instructions.
  - Practice infection control (Chapters 14 and 15) and safety measures (Chapters 11 and 12).

WORKING IN ANOTHER STATE

To work in another state, you must meet that state's NATCEP requirements. First, contact the state agency responsible for NATCEPs and the nursing assistant registry. To find that agency, do 1 of the following.

- Contact your current nursing assistant registry.
- Search on-line to locate the state agency.

Then apply to the desired state agency for endorsement (reciprocity, equivalency) as a CNA (LNA, RNA, SRNA, STNA). *Endorsement (reciprocity, equivalency) means that a state recognizes the certificate, license, or registration issued by another state.* This means that your application is reviewed to see if you meet the state's requirements.

The application review results in 1 or more of the following.

- Being granted or denied certification (a license, registration).
- Having to take a NATCEP competency test. This may be the written test, the skills test, or both.
- Having to take the entire NATCEP in that state (training program and competency test).

ROLES AND RESPONSIBILITIES

OBRA, nurse practice acts and other state laws, and legal and advisory opinions direct what you can do. To protect persons from harm, you must understand what you can do, what you cannot do, and the legal limits of your role. This is called *scope of practice* or *range of functions*.

Licensed nurses supervise your work. You perform nursing tasks related to the person's care. A *nursing task is nursing care or a nursing function, procedure, skill, or activity.* Often you function without a nurse in the room. At other times you help nurses give care. The rules in Box 3-2 will help you understand your role.

The range of functions for nursing assistants varies among states and agencies. Before performing a nursing task make sure that:

- Your state allows nursing assistants to do so.
- It is in your job description.
- You have the education and training to do so.
- A nurse is available to answer questions and to guide and assist you as needed.

BOX 3-2 Rules for Nursing Assistants

- You are an assistant to the nurse.
- A nurse assigns and supervises your work.
- You report observations about the person's physical and mental status to the nurse (Chapter 7). Report changes in the person's condition or behavior at once.
- The nurse decides what is done or not done for a person. You do not make these decisions.
- Review directions and the care plan (Chapter 7) with the nurse before going to the person.
- Perform only the nursing tasks that you are trained to do.
- Ask a nurse to guide and assist you if you are not comfortable performing a nursing task.
- Perform only the nursing tasks that your state and job description allow.

You perform nursing tasks to meet the person's hygiene, safety, comfort, nutrition, exercise, and elimination needs. You move and transfer persons and make observations. You measure temperatures, pulses, respirations, and blood pressures. And you help promote the person's mental comfort.

Box 3-3 describes the limits of your role—tasks that you should never do. State laws differ. Know what you can do in the state in which you are working.

Your job description reflects your state's laws and rules. An agency can further limit what you can do. So can a nurse based on the person's needs. However, no agency or nurse can expand your range of functions beyond what your state's laws and rules allow.

Nursing Assistant Standards

All NATCEPs include the range of functions required by OBRA. Some states allow other functions. NATCEPs also prepare nursing assistants to meet the standards listed in Box 3-4.

Job Description

The *job description is a document that describes what the agency expects you to do* (Fig. 3-2). It also states educational requirements and your job title.

Always obtain a written job description when you apply for a job. Ask questions about it during your job interview (Chapter 45). Before accepting a job, tell the employer about:
- Functions you did not learn
- Functions you cannot do for moral or religious reasons

Clearly understand what is expected before taking a job. Do not take a job that requires you to:
- Act beyond the legal limits of your role.
- Function beyond your training limits.
- Perform acts that are against your morals or religion.

No one can force you to do something beyond the legal limits of your role. You must understand:
- Your roles and responsibilities
- What you can safely do
- The things you should never do
- Your job description
- The ethical and legal aspects of your role (Chapter 4)

See *Focus on Communication: Job Description.*

FOCUS ON **COMMUNICATION**
Job Description

Your training prepares you for certain nursing tasks. The agency may not let you do everything you learned. Other agencies may want you to do things not learned. Use your job description to discuss these issues with the nurse.

For example, a job description includes changing a dressing (Chapter 35). You did not learn this skill in your training program. You can say:

I see changing dressings in my job description. I did not learn to do that. Will I be trained to perform this skill?

Carefully review your job description. Know what you can and cannot do. Ask if you have questions.

BOX 3-3 Role Limits

- ***Never give drugs.*** Nurses give drugs. Many states allow nursing assistants to give some drugs after completing a state-approved medication assistant training program.
- ***Never insert tubes or objects into body openings. Do not remove them from the body.*** Exceptions to this rule are the procedures you will study during your training. Giving enemas is an example.
- ***Never take oral or phone orders from doctors.*** Politely give your name and title, and ask the doctor to wait for a nurse. Promptly find a nurse to speak with the doctor.
- ***Never tell the person or family the person's diagnosis or medical or surgical treatment plans.*** This is the doctor's responsibility. Nurses may clarify what the doctor has said.
- ***Never diagnose or prescribe treatments or drugs for anyone.*** Doctors and some advanced practice nurses diagnose and prescribe.
- ***Never supervise others, including other nursing assistants.*** This is a nurse's responsibility. You will not be trained to supervise others. Supervising others can have serious legal problems.
- ***Never ignore an order or request to do something.*** This includes nursing tasks that you can do, those you cannot do, and those beyond your legal limits. Promptly and politely explain to the nurse why you cannot carry out the order or request. The nurse assumes you are doing what you were told to do unless you explain otherwise. You cannot neglect the person's care.

BOX 3-4 Nursing Assistant Standards

The nursing assistant:
- Performs nursing tasks within the range of functions allowed by the state's nurse practice act and its rules.
- Is honest and shows integrity. (*Integrity* involves following a code of ethics. See Chapter 4.)
- Accepts or refuses nursing tasks based on education, training, and the nurse's directions. See "Your Role in Delegation" on p. 27.
- Is accountable for personal behavior and actions while assisting the nurse and helping patients and residents. *Accountable means to answer to one's self and others about one's choices, decisions, and actions.*
- Assists the nurse in observing patients and residents. Also assists in identifying their needs.
- Communicates:
  - Progress toward completing nursing tasks
  - Problems in completing nursing tasks
  - Changes in the person's status
- Asks the nurse to clarify what is expected when unsure.
- Uses educational and training opportunities as available.
- Practices safety measures to protect the person, others, and self.
- Respects the person's rights, concerns, decisions, and dignity.
- Functions as a member of the health team. Helps implement the care plan (Chapter 7).
- Respects the person's property and the property of others.
- Protects confidential information unless required by law to share the information.

Modified from National Council of State Boards of Nursing, Inc.: *NCSBN model rules,* Chicago, 2017, Author.

POSITION DESCRIPTION / PERFORMANCE EVALUATION

Job Title: LTC Certified Nursing Assistant (CNA)   Supervised by: CNA Coordinator, Charge Nurse
Prepared by: _____   Approved by: _____
Date: _____   Date: _____

Job Summary: Provides direct and indirect resident care activities under the direction of an RN or LPN/LVN. Assists residents with activities of daily living, provides for personal care, comfort and assists in the maintenance of a safe and clean environment for an assigned group or residents.

DUTIES AND RESPONSIBILITIES:

3 = Exceeds Performance   2 = Expected Performance   1 = Needs Improvement

<u>Demonstrates Competency in the Following Areas:</u>

Assists in the preparation for admission of residents.	3	2	1
Assists in and accompanies residents in the admission, transfer and discharge procedures.	3	2	1
Provides morning care, which may include bed bath, shower or whirlpool, oral hygiene, combing hair, back care, dressing residents, changing bed linen, cleaning overbed table and bedside stand, straightening room and other general care as necessary throughout the day.	3	2	1
Provides evening care which includes hands/face washing as needed, oral hygiene, back rubs, peri-care, freshening linen, cleaning overbed tables, straightening room and other general care as needed.	3	2	1
Notifies appropriate licensed staff when resident complains of pain.	3	2	1
Provides postmortem care and assists in transporting bodies to the morgue.	3	2	1
Assists LPN/LVN in treatment procedures.	3	2	1
Provides general nursing care, such as positioning residents, lifting and turning residents, applying/utilizing special equipment, assisting in use of bedpan or commode and ambulating the residents.	3	2	1
Performs all aspects of resident care in an environment that optimizes resident safety and reduces the likelihood of medical/health care errors.	3	2	1
Supports and maintains a culture of safety and quality.	3	2	1
Takes and records temperature, pulse, respiration, weight, blood pressure and intake-output.	3	2	1
Makes rounds with outgoing shift; knows whereabouts of assigned residents.	3	2	1
Makes rounds with oncoming shift to ensure the unit is left in good condition.	3	2	1
Adheres to policies and procedures of the facility and the Nursing Department.	3	2	1
Participates in socialization activities on the unit.	3	2	1
Turns and positions residents as ordered and/or as needed, making sure no rough surfaces are in direct contact with the body. Lifts and turns with proper and safe body mechanics and with available resources.	3	2	1
Checks for reddened areas or skin breakdown and reports to RN or LPN/LVN.	3	2	1
Ensures residents are dressed properly and assists, as necessary. Ensures that used clothing is properly stored in bedside stand or on hangers in closet. Ensures that all residents are clean and dry at all times.	3	2	1
Checks unit for adequate linen. Folds neatly and arranges linen in linen closet. Cleans linen cart. Provides clean linen and clothing. Makes beds.	3	2	1
Treats residents and their families with respect and dignity.			
Restrains residents properly, when ordered.	3	2	1
Accompanies residents to appointments, as directed.	3	2	1
Provides reality orientation in daily care.	3	2	1
Prepares residents for meals; serves and removes food trays and assists with meals or feeds residents, if necessary.	3	2	1
Distributes drinking water and other nourishments to residents.	3	2	1
Performs general care activities for residents in isolation.	3	2	1
Answers residents' call lights, anticipates residents' needs and makes rounds to assigned residents.	3	2	1
Assists residents with handling and care of clothing and other personal property (including dentures, glasses, contact lenses, hearing aids and prosthetic devices).	3	2	1
Transports residents to and from various departments, as requested.	3	2	1
Reports and, when appropriate, records any changes observed in condition or behavior of residents and unusual incidents.	3	2	1
Participates in and contributes to interdisciplinary care conferences.	3	2	1
Must be able to follow directions, both oral and written, and work cooperatively with other staff members.	3	2	1
Must have the ability to acquire knowledge of and develop skills in basic nursing procedures and simple documenting.	3	2	1
Establishes and maintains interpersonal relationship with residents, family members and other facility staff while assuring confidentiality of resident information.	3	2	1
Attends inservice education programs, as assigned, to learn new treatments, procedures, developmental skills, etc.	3	2	1
Practices careful, efficient and nonwasteful use of supplies and linen and follows established charge procedure for resident charge items.	3	2	1
Maintains personal health in order to prevent absence from work due to health problems.	3	2	1
Possesses a genuine interest and concern for geriatric and disabled persons.	3	2	1

FIGURE 3-2 Portions of a sample job description. Note that the job description is also a performance evaluation tool. (Modified from Medical Consultants Network, Inc., Englewood, Colo.)

Continued

Professional Requirements:

Adheres to dress code, appearance is neat and clean.	3	2	1
Completes annual education requirements.	3	2	1
Maintains regulatory requirements.	3	2	1
Maintains resident confidentiality at all times.	3	2	1
Reports to work on time and as scheduled, completes work within designated time.	3	2	1
Wears identification while on duty, uses computerized punch time system correctly.	3	2	1
Completes inservices and returns in a timely fashion.	3	2	1
Attends annual review and department inservices, as scheduled.	3	2	1
Attends at least ____ staff meetings annually, reads and returns all monthly staff meeting minutes.	3	2	1
Represents the organization in a positive and professional manner.	3	2	1
Actively participates in performance improvement and continuous quality improvement (CQI) activities.	3	2	1
Complies with all organizational policies regarding ethical business practices.	3	2	1
Communicates the mission, ethics and goals of the facility.	3	2	1
Total Points	___	___	___

Regulatory Requirements:

- High School graduate or equivalent.

- Current Certified Nursing Assistant (CNA) certification in State of _____ for Long Term Care Facilities.

- Current Basic Cardiac Life Support certification within three (3) months of hire date.

Language Skills:

- Able to communicate effectively in English, both verbally and in writing.

- Additional languages preferred.

Skills:

- Basic computer knowledge.

Physical Demands:

- For physical demands of position, including vision, hearing, repetitive motion and environment, see following description.

  Reasonable accommodations may be made to enable individuals with disabilities to perform the essential functions of the position without compromising resident care.

===

I have received, read and understand the Position Description/Performance Evaluation above.

_____   _____
Name/Signature   Date Signed

FIGURE 3-2, cont'd

DELEGATION GUIDELINES

Nursing assistants function under the supervision of licensed nurses. Nurse practice acts give nurses the right to *assign* or *delegate* nursing tasks to nursing assistants. Definitions vary among state nurse practice acts, agency job descriptions, and national nursing organizations. (The *National Council of State Boards of Nursing [NCSBN]* and the *American Nurses Association [ANA]* are examples.) You need to know the definitions used in your state. The following definitions are used in this textbook.

- *Delegate—to authorize or direct a nursing assistant to perform a nursing task*
- *Delegation:*
  - *The process a nurse uses to direct a nursing assistant to perform a nursing task*
  - *Allowing a nursing assistant to perform a nursing task that is beyond the nursing assistant's usual role and not routinely done by the nursing assistant*

Some tasks are part of the nursing assistant's routine work. The tasks are commonly assigned to nursing assistants. You will learn these *routine nursing tasks* in your NATCEP. Moving and transfer procedures, hygiene and grooming measures, and how to measure weight and height are examples. Such tasks will be part of your usual work assignment.

Some states and agencies allow nurses to delegate tasks that are not routinely done by nursing assistants—*delegated nursing responsibilities.* The following guidelines outlined by the NCSBN and ANA are used for safe delegation of such tasks.

- The person delegating has the authority to do so. See "Who Can Delegate."
- The task is within the delegating nurse's scope of practice.
- The task is within the nursing assistant's range of functions and job description.
- The nursing assistant has the education and training to perform the task.
- The nursing assistant has shown competence in performing the task. *Competence* means *having the ability to do something successfully.*
- The task *does not* involve nursing judgment or critical decision making. Such tasks cannot be delegated.

Communication is an important part of the delegation process (p. 26). Before performing any task, you need information. *Delegation Guidelines* boxes accompany the procedures in this book. The guidelines list the information you need from the nurse and care plan before performing a task. They also list the observations to record and report to the nurse.

Who Can Delegate

Licensed nurses can delegate.

- An APRN can delegate to RNs, LPNs/LVNs, and nursing assistants.
- An RN can delegate to LPNs/LVNs and nursing assistants.
- An LPN/LVN can delegate to nursing assistants if allowed by the state's nurse practice act.

A nurse's delegation decisions must result in the best care for the person. Otherwise the person's health and safety are at risk. The delegating nurse is accountable for safe delegation decisions. The nurse must make sure the task was completed safely and correctly. You are responsible for completing tasks safely. See "Your Role in Delegation" on p. 27.

Nursing assistants cannot delegate. You cannot assign or delegate any task to other nursing assistants or to any other worker. You can ask someone to help you. For example, you ask a co-worker to help you move a person in bed. *But you cannot ask or tell someone to do your work.* If you are unable to complete a task or need guidance, tell the delegating nurse. The nurse decides whether to re-assign or re-delegate the task.

See *Promoting Safety and Comfort: Who Can Delegate.*

PROMOTING SAFETY AND COMFORT

Who Can Delegate

Safety

Delegation decisions require a nurse's knowledge and judgment. The nurse must understand the state's rules and the agency's policies and procedures on delegation. Delegated tasks must be:

- Within the nurse's scope of practice
- Within the nursing assistant range of functions allowed by the state
- Listed in the nursing assistant's job description
  Many other factors are involved. For example, the nurse must know:
- The person's individual needs
- The person's condition—stable (not likely to change) or unstable (likely to change)
- If the outcome is predictable or not
- The nursing assistant's competence and comfort level
- How much supervision will be needed
  Each situation is different. The nurse may decide not to assign or delegate a task in a certain situation.

Delegation Process

For safe delegation, the person's needs, the nursing task, and the staff member doing the task must fit (Fig. 3-3). The nurse decides if the task is safe for you to do. The person's needs and the task may require a nurse's knowledge, judgment, and skill. You may be asked to assist.

Delegation is a process involving:
- Assessment of needs
- Communication
- Guidance and assistance
- Follow-up and feedback

Assessment of Needs. The nurse needs to understand the person's needs. And the nurse needs to know your knowledge, skills, and job description.

To assess the person's needs, the nurse answers these questions.
- What are the person's needs? How complex and urgent are they? How can they vary?
- What are the most important long-term and short-term needs?
- How much judgment is needed to meet the person's needs and give care?
- How predictable is the person's health status? How does the person respond to health care?
- What problems might arise from the task? How severe might they be?
- What actions are needed if a problem occurs? How complex are the needed actions?
- What emergencies might arise? How likely might they occur?
- How involved is the person and family in health care decisions?
- How will delegating the task help the person? What are the risks?

To assess your knowledge and skills, the nurse answers these questions.
- What knowledge and skills are needed to safely perform the task?
- What is in your job description?
- What are the conditions affecting the task?
- What is expected from the task?
- What problems might the person develop during the task?
- What problems can arise from the task?

The nurse decides if you can safely perform the task. It must be safe for the person and you. If unsafe, the nurse stops the delegation process. If safe for the person and you, the nurse continues the delegation process.

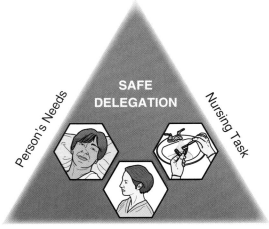

Nursing Team Member
(APRN, RN, LPN/LVN, Nursing Assistant)

FIGURE 3-3 The nurse considers the person's needs, the task, and the staff member's abilities when making delegation decisions.

Communication. This step involves the nurse and you. The nurse must give you clear and complete directions about:
- How to perform and complete the task
- What observations to report and record
- When to report observations
- What patient or resident concerns to report at once
- Priorities for tasks
- What to do if the person's condition changes or needs change

The nurse asks questions to make sure you understand. The nurse may ask you to explain what you will do. Do not be insulted by such questions. The intent is to protect the person and you.

Before performing a delegated task, discuss the task with the nurse. Make sure that you:
- Ask questions about the task and what you are expected to do.
- Tell the nurse if you have not done the task before or not often.
- Ask for needed training or supervision.
- Re-state what is expected of you.
- Re-state what patient or resident concerns to report to the nurse.
- Explain how and when you will report progress in completing the task.
- Know how to call the nurse for an emergency.
- Know what to do during an emergency.

After completing a task, report and record the care given. Also report and record your observations. See "Reporting and Recording" in Chapter 7.

Guidance and Assistance. The nurse supervises your work. The nurse must be available to guide and assist you as needed. The nurse:

* Observes the care you give as needed.
* Makes sure that you complete the task correctly.
* Observes the person's condition and response to care. The frequency of the nurse's observations depends on:
  * The person's health status and needs
  * If the person's condition is stable or unstable
  * If the nurse can predict the person's responses and risks to care
  * The setting where the task occurs
  * The resources and support available
  * If the task is simple or complex

The nurse follows up on problems or concerns. For example, the nurse takes action if:

* You did not complete the task in a timely manner.
* The task did not meet expectations.
* There is a change in the person's condition.

The nurse is alert for possible changes in the person's condition. With your help, the nurse can act before the person's condition changes.

Depending on the person's needs, the nurse might need to assist you with the task. Or the nurse can decide to perform the task.

After you complete the task, the nurse may review and discuss what happened with you. This helps you learn. If something similar happens again, you have ideas about how to adjust.

Follow-Up and Feedback. *Follow-up* means *to review and take needed action.* The nurse decides if the delegation was successful. The nurse answers these questions.

* Was the task done correctly?
* Did the person respond as expected?
* Was the result (outcome) as desired? Was the result good or bad?
* Did you and the nurse have timely and effective communication?
* What went well? What were the problems?
* Does the care plan need to change (Chapter 7)?
* Did the nurse give feedback? *Feedback* means *to respond.* The nurse tells you what you did correctly and about any errors. Feedback helps you learn and improve the care you give.

See *Focus on Communication: Follow-Up and Feedback.*

FOCUS ON **COMMUNICATION**

Follow-Up and Feedback

Feedback helps you learn and improve in your role as a nursing assistant. Receive feedback in a respectful manner.

* Listen carefully.
* Have good eye contact.
* Consider ways you can improve.
* Avoid arguing or being defensive.
* Thank the nurse for the feedback.

Your Role in Delegation

You must protect the person from harm. You have 2 choices when delegated a task. You either *accept* or *refuse* a task. Use the *Five Rights of Delegation* in Box 3-5.

BOX 3-5 The *Five Rights of Delegation* for Nursing Assistants

The Right Task
* Does your state allow you to perform the task?
* Is the task in your job description?
* Were you trained to do the task?

The Right Circumstance
* Do you have experience with the task given the person's condition and needs?
* Do you understand the purposes of the task for the person?
* Can you perform the task safely under the current circumstances?
* Do you have needed equipment and supplies?
* Do you know how to use the equipment and supplies?

The Right Person
* Are you comfortable performing the task?
* Do you have concerns about performing the task?

The Right Directions and Communication
* Did the nurse give clear directions and instructions?
* Did you review the task with the nurse?
* Did you ask the nurse about questions you have?
* Do you understand what the nurse expects?

The Right Supervision and Evaluation
* Is a nurse available to answer questions?
* Is a nurse available if the person's condition changes or if problems occur?
* Did the nurse evaluate the result?

Modified from National Council of State Boards of Nursing, Inc.: *The five rights of delegation,* as referenced in *National guidelines for nursing delegation,* Chicago, April 29, 2019, National Council of State Boards of Nursing and American Nurses Association.

Accepting a Task. When you agree to perform a task, you are responsible for your actions. What you do or fail to do can harm the person. *You must complete the task safely.* Ask for help if you are unsure or have questions. Report to the nurse what you did and your observations.

Refusing a Task. You have the right to refuse and not accept a delegated task. You should refuse when:

- The task is beyond the range of functions for nursing assistants allowed by your state.
- The task is not in your job description.
- You were not trained to do the task.
- The task could harm the person.
- The person's condition has changed.
- You do not know how to use the supplies or equipment.
- Directions are not ethical or legal.
- Directions are against agency policies.
- Directions are not clear or complete.
- A nurse is not available to guide and assist you as needed.

Use common sense. This protects you and the person. Ask yourself if what you are doing is safe for the person.

Never ignore an order or a request to do something. Share your concerns with the nurse. For tasks within the legal limits of your role and in your job description, the nurse can help increase your comfort.

The nurse can:

- Answer your questions.
- Demonstrate the task.
- Show you how to use supplies and equipment.
- Observe you doing the task and help as needed.
- Check on you often.
- Arrange for needed training.

Do not refuse a task because you do not like it or do not want to do it. You must have sound reasons. Otherwise, you place the person at risk for harm. You could lose your job. See *Focus on Communication: Refusing a Task.*

FOCUS ON **COMMUNICATION**

Refusing a Task

A nurse may delegate a task that was not part of your training. The task is in your job description. You can say:

> I know this task is in my job description, but I did not learn it in school. Can you show me what to do and then observe me doing it? That would really help me.

A nurse may ask you to do something that is not in your job description. With respect, firmly refuse the nurse's request. For example, the nurse sets a cup of pills in the room and asks you to give them to the person when you finish brushing the person's teeth. You can say:

> I'm sorry, but I cannot give a person drugs. I was not trained to give drugs, and the task is not in my job description. Can I help you with something else?

FOCUS ON P R I D E

The Person, Family, and Yourself

P ersonal and Professional Responsibility

Personal and professional qualities allow you to do your job well. Communication skills, patience, compassion, and teamwork are examples. You will learn about other qualities when you study work ethics in Chapter 5.

R ights and Respect

Most NATCEPs involve practice in a clinical setting. Sometimes a patient or resident refuses to have a student. Or the person refuses to allow a student to watch a procedure. The person's right to refuse must be respected.

I ndependence and Social Interaction

You will practice many skills in the classroom or laboratory before going to the clinical setting. Practice as if you are with a real patient or resident. Practice what to say and how to act. Practice the skill many times. This will help you feel more comfortable and confident in the clinical setting.

D elegation and Teamwork

Good teamwork improves the delegation process. Staff interactions matter. The person and nursing team benefit when staff:

- Communicate openly.
- Trust, help, and encourage each other.
- Work toward a common goal.

E thics and Laws

Some nursing assistants work in more than 1 setting. Some are also emergency medical technicians (EMTs). EMTs give emergency care outside of health care settings. State laws and rules for EMTs and nursing assistants differ. For example, you work as an EMT and a nursing assistant. Your state laws allow EMTs to start intravenous (IV) lines. Nursing assistants do not start IVs.

The ability to do something does not give the right to do so in all settings. There are legal limits to your role. Be proud of the advanced skills and training you may have. But when working as a nursing assistant, follow your state's laws and rules for nursing assistants.

FOCUS ON PRIDE: *Application*

How do staff interactions affect the delegation process? Explain how good teamwork benefits the nursing team and the person.

Circle the BEST answer.

1 What state law affects what nursing assistants can do?
   a Standards for nursing assistants
   b Medicaid
   c OBRA
   d Nurse practice act

2 You do not pass your state's competency evaluation on the first attempt. You
   a Are not allowed to re-test
   b Must repeat your training program to re-test
   c May re-take the test
   d Are not allowed to repeat a training program

3 OBRA requires a nursing assistant registry. You are placed on the registry after
   a Completing the classroom part of your training program
   b Working as a nursing assistant for 1 year
   c Paying a registration fee
   d Successfully completing a state-approved NATCEP

4 Your nursing assistant certification (license, registration) can be revoked for
   a Refusing a nursing task for moral reasons
   b Asking the nurse questions
   c Performing acts beyond your role
   d Keeping the person's information confidential

5 You have not worked as a nursing assistant for 3 years (36 months). You can work as a nursing assistant again if
   a You meet your state's requirements for competency evaluation
   b You worked as a nursing assistant for at least 5 years
   c The agency waives your need for re-training
   d You repeat a background check

6 As a nursing assistant, you
   a Can take verbal or phone orders from doctors
   b Report observations to the nurse
   c Can remove tubes from the person's body
   d Can ignore a nursing task if it is not in your job description

7 Giving drugs is outside of the nursing assistant range of functions. Which is *true*?
   a Giving drugs can be included in your job description.
   b The nurse can ask you to give a person's drugs.
   c You cannot give drugs.
   d The nurse is not responsible for knowing your range of functions.

8 Who assigns and supervises your work?
   a A nurse
   b The health team
   c Another nursing assistant
   d You

9 You are responsible for
   a Supervising other nursing assistants
   b Telling the person his or her diagnosis
   c Knowing what you can safely do
   d Deciding what treatments are needed

10 You perform a task not allowed by your state. Which is *true*?
    a If a nurse asked you to do the task, there is no legal problem.
    b You could be practicing nursing without a license.
    c You can perform the task if it is in your job description.
    d If you complete the task safely, there is no legal problem.

11 A patient begins having trouble swallowing. The nurse decides not to delegate feeding to you. Why?
    a The task is beyond the legal limits of your role.
    b You are not trained to do the task.
    c The nurse does not trust you to do the task safely.
    d The person's condition has changed.

12 In the delegation process, communication involves
    a Observing care
    b Determining who should perform a task
    c Deciding if the task was successful
    d Asking questions about a task

13 Which statement about guidance and assistance is *true*?
    a The nurse must make sure you complete tasks correctly.
    b The nurse must be with you when you give care.
    c Simple tasks require more assistance than complex ones.
    d More guidance is needed when the person's condition is stable.

14 You can refuse to perform a task if
    a The task is within the legal limits of your role
    b The task is in your job description
    c You do not like the task
    d A nurse is not available to guide or assist you as needed

15 You decide to refuse a task. What should you do?
    a Communicate your concerns to the nurse.
    b Delegate the task to a nursing assistant.
    c Ignore the request.
    d Talk to the director of nursing.

Answers to Chapter 3 questions are on p. 587.

Answers to Chapter 3 questions are on p. 587.

FOCUS ON **PRACTICE**

Problem Solving

A nurse asks you to do a task that you have not done before. The task is in your job description. What will you do? How can the nurse help increase your comfort level?

Ethics and Laws

OBJECTIVES

- Define the key terms and key abbreviations in this chapter.
- Describe ethical conduct.
- Describe a code of conduct for nursing assistants.
- Explain how to maintain professional boundaries.
- Explain how standards of care relate to negligence.
- Give examples of unintentional and intentional torts.

- Describe how to protect the right to privacy.
- Explain the correct use of electronic communications.
- Explain the purpose of informed consent.
- Describe elder abuse, child abuse and neglect, and intimate partner violence.
- Explain how to promote PRIDE in the person, the family, and yourself.

KEY TERMS

abuse
- The willful infliction of injury, unreasonable confinement, intimidation, or punishment that results in physical harm, pain, or mental anguish
- Depriving the person (or the person's caregiver) of the goods or services needed to attain or maintain well-being

assault Intentionally attempting or threatening to touch a person's body without the person's consent

battery Touching a person's body without consent

boundary crossing
- A brief act or behavior of being over-involved with the person
- The intent of the act or behavior is to meet the person's needs

boundary sign An act, behavior, or thought that warns of a boundary crossing or boundary violation

boundary violation An act or behavior that meets your needs, not the person's

child abuse and neglect The intentional harm or mistreatment of a child under 18 years old that:
- Involves any recent act or failure to act on the part of a parent or caregiver
- Results in death, serious physical or emotional harm, sexual abuse, or exploitation
- Presents a likely or immediate risk for harm

civil law Laws concerned with relationships between people

crime An act that violates a criminal law

criminal law Laws concerned with offenses against the public and society in general

defamation Injuring a person's name and reputation by making false statements to a third person

elder abuse Any knowing, intentional, or negligent act by a caregiver or any other person to an older adult that causes harm or serious risk of harm

ethics Knowledge of what is right conduct and wrong conduct

false imprisonment Unlawful restraint or restriction of a person's freedom of movement

fraud Saying or doing something to trick, fool, or deceive a person

informed consent The process by which a person receives and understands information about a treatment or procedure and is able to decide to receive or refuse the treatment or procedure

intimate partner violence (IPV) Physical violence, sexual violence, stalking, or psychological aggression by a current or former partner

invasion of privacy Violating a person's right not to have his or her name, photo, or private affairs exposed or made public without giving consent

law A rule of conduct made by a government body

libel Making false statements in print, in writing (including e-mail and text messages), through pictures or drawings, through broadcast (radio, TV, or video), posted on-line on websites, or through video sites and social media sites

KEY TERMS—cont'd

malpractice Negligence by a professional person

neglect When a caregiver or responsible person fails to:
- Protect a vulnerable person from harm
- Provide food, water, clothing, shelter, health care, or basic activities of daily living to a vulnerable person

negligence An unintentional wrong in which a person did not act in a reasonable and careful manner and a person or the person's property was harmed

professional boundary That which separates helpful actions and behaviors from those that are not helpful

professional sexual misconduct A violation of professional interactions with an act, behavior, or comment that is sexual in nature

protected health information Identifying information and information about the person's health care that is maintained or sent in any form (paper, electronic, oral)

self-neglect A person's behaviors and way of living that threaten the person's own health, safety, and well-being

slander Making false statements through the spoken word, sounds, sign language, or gestures

standard of care The skills, care, and judgments required by a health team member under similar conditions

vulnerable adult A person 18 years old or older who has a disability or condition that causes the person to be at risk for harm

KEY ABBREVIATIONS

CDC	Centers for Disease Control and Prevention	**IPV**	Intimate partner violence
HIPAA	Health Insurance Portability and Accountability Act of 1996	**OBRA**	Omnibus Budget Reconciliation Act of 1987

Nurse practice acts, your training and job description, and safe delegation serve to protect patients and residents from harm (Chapter 3). Protecting them from harm also involves laws, rules, and standards of conduct. They form the ethical and legal aspects of care.

ETHICAL ASPECTS

Ethics is knowledge of what is right conduct and wrong conduct. Ethics involves choices or judgments about what should or should not be done. An ethical person behaves and acts in the right way. The person does not harm others.

Ethical behavior also involves not being prejudiced or biased. To be *prejudiced* or *biased* means *making judgments and having views before knowing the facts.* Judgments and views often are based on one's values and standards. They are based on culture, religion, education, and experiences. The person's situation and yours may be very different. For example:
- Children think their mother needs nursing home care. In your culture, children care for older parents at home.
- An older man does not want life-saving measures. You believe that everything must be done to save a life.

Do not judge the person by your values and standards. Do not avoid persons whose standards and values differ from your own.

Ethical problems involve making choices. You must decide what is the right thing to do.

Codes of Ethics

Professional groups have codes of ethics. A *code of ethics* has rules, or standards of conduct, for group members to follow. Also called *codes of conduct*, professional nursing organizations have codes of ethics for nurses. The rules of conduct in Box 4-1 can guide your thinking, actions, and behavior. See Chapter 5 for student and work ethics.

BOX 4-1 Code of Conduct for Nursing Assistants

- Respect each person as an individual.
- Know the limits of your role and knowledge.
- Perform only the tasks within the legal limits of your role.
- Perform only the tasks that you have been trained to do.
- Perform no act that will harm the person.
- Take drugs only if prescribed and supervised by a health care provider (doctor, advanced practice registered nurse).
- Follow the nurse's directions to your best possible ability.
- Follow agency policies and procedures.
- Complete each task safely.
- Be loyal to your employer and co-workers.
- Act as a responsible citizen at all times.
- Keep the person's information confidential.
- Protect the person's privacy.
- Protect the person's property.
- Consider the person's needs to be more important than your own.
- Report errors and incidents honestly and at once.
- Be responsible for your actions.

Professional Boundaries

As a nursing assistant, you enter into a helping relationship with patients or residents and families. In this relationship, you are trusted with the person's care and with private information. The proper focus is on meeting the needs of the person and family.

A *boundary* limits or separates something. *Professional boundaries separate helpful actions and behaviors from those that are not helpful* (Fig. 4-1, p. 32). Professional interactions involve helpful behaviors that meet the person's needs. Some behaviors are not helpful. They result in being *under-involved* or *over-involved* with the person.

Professional Boundaries

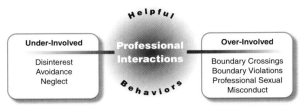

FIGURE 4-1 Professional boundaries guide your actions and behavior. Your focus is on helping the person. Being under-involved or over-involved is not helpful. (Modified from National Council of State Boards of Nursing, Inc.: *A nurse's guide to professional boundaries,* Chicago, 2018, Author.)

If you are under-involved, the following can occur.

- Disinterest—you lack interest in the person.
- Avoidance—you avoid the person.
- Neglect—you do not properly care for the person (p. 36).

If you are over-involved, the following can occur.

- *Boundary crossing*—*a brief act or behavior of being over-involved with the person. The intent of the act or behavior is to meet the person's needs.* The act or behavior may be thoughtless or something you did not mean to do. Or it could have purpose if it meets the person's needs. For example, you give a crying patient a hug. The hug meets the person's needs at the time. If the hug meets your needs, the act is wrong. Also, it is wrong to hug the person every time you see him or her.
- *Boundary violation*—*an act or behavior that meets your needs, not the person's.* The act or behavior is not ethical. It violates the code of conduct in Box 4-1. The person can be harmed. Boundary violations include:
  - Abuse (p. 35).
  - Giving a lot of information about yourself. You tell the person about your personal relationships or problems.
  - Keeping secrets with the person.
- *Professional sexual misconduct*—*a violation of professional interactions with an act, behavior, or comment that is sexual in nature.* It is sexual misconduct even if the person consents or makes the first move. (To *consent* means *to give permission.*)

Some boundary violations and some types of professional sexual misconduct also are crimes. To maintain professional boundaries, follow the rules in Box 4-2. Be alert to boundary signs. *Boundary signs* are *acts, behaviors, or thoughts that warn of a boundary crossing or boundary violation* (see Box 4-2).

See *Focus on Communication: Professional Boundaries.*

FOCUS ON **COMMUNICATION**

Professional Boundaries

Some patients, residents, and families send thank-you cards and letters. Some offer thank-you gifts—candy, cookies, money, gift cards, flowers, and so on. Accepting gifts is a boundary violation. When offered a gift, you can say:

- "Thank you for thinking of me. It's very kind of you. However, it is against center policy to accept gifts. I do appreciate your offer."
- "Thank you for wanting me to have the flowers from your friend. They are lovely. However, it is against hospital policy to receive gifts. May I help you find a way to take them home?"

BOX 4-2 **Professional Boundaries**

Maintaining Professional Boundaries

- Follow the code of conduct in Box 4-1. Maintain a professional relationship at all times.
- Talk to the nurse if you sense a boundary sign, crossing, or violation.
- Avoid caring for family, friends, and people you know. This may be hard to do in a small community. Tell the nurse if you know the person. The nurse may change your assignment.
- Do not make sexual comments or jokes.
- Do not use offensive language.
- Use touch correctly (Chapter 6). Touch or handle sexual and genital areas only for needed care. The areas include the breasts, nipples, perineum, buttocks, thighs, and anus.
- Do not visit or spend extra time with someone who is not part of your assignment.
- The following apply to patients, residents, and families.
  - Do not date, flirt with, kiss, or have a sexual relationship with them.
  - Do not discuss your sexual relationships with them.
  - Do not say or write things that could suggest a romantic or sexual relationship with them.
  - Do not accept gifts, loans, money, credit cards, or other valuables from them.
  - Do not give gifts, loans, money, credit cards, or other valuables to them.
  - Do not borrow from them. This includes money, personal items, and transportation.
  - Do not develop a personal relationship or friendship with them.
  - Do not share personal or financial information with them.
  - Do not help with their finances.
  - Do not take a person home with you. This includes for holidays or other events.
- Ask yourself these questions before you date or marry a person whom you cared for. Be aware of the risk for professional sexual misconduct.
  - When were you involved with the person's care?
  - Was the person's care short-term or long-term?
  - What kind and how much information do you have about the person? How will that information affect your relationship with the person?
  - Will the person need more care in the future?
  - Does dating or marrying the person place the person at risk for harm?

Boundary Signs

- You think about the person when not at work.
- You visit with the person during breaks, meal times, when off duty, and so on.
- You give more attention to the person at the expense of others.
- You think no one else understands the person's needs.
- The person gives you gifts or money.
- You give the person gifts or money.
- You share information about yourself or your work situation with the person.
- You flirt with the person.
- You make comments with a sexual message.
- You notice more touch between you and the person.
- You use vulgar or offensive language when with the person.
- You do not like questions about your care or your relationship with the person.
- You change your appearance when you will see the person.
- You have contact with the person after discharge from the agency.

LEGAL ASPECTS

Ethics is about what you *should or should not do*. Laws tell you what you *can and cannot do*. A *law is a rule of conduct made by a government body*. The U.S. Congress and state legislatures make laws. Enforced by the government, laws protect the public welfare.

Criminal laws are concerned with offenses against the public and society in general. An act that violates a criminal law is called a crime. If found guilty of a crime, the person is fined or sent to prison. Murder, robbery, stealing, rape, kidnapping, and abuse (p. 35) are crimes.

Civil laws are concerned with relationships between people. Contracts and nurse practice acts are examples. A person found guilty of breaking a civil law usually has to pay a sum of money to the injured person.

Tort comes from the French word meaning *wrong*. Torts are part of civil law. A *tort is a wrong committed against a person or the person's property.* Some torts are *unintentional*. Harm was not intended. *Intentional* torts are done on purpose. Harm was intended.

What you do or do not do can lead to legal action if you harm a person or a person's property. You are legally responsible *(liable)* for your own actions. Sometimes refusing to follow the nurse's directions is your right and duty (Chapter 3).

Unintentional Torts

Health team members are expected to give care at a certain level. A *standard of care refers to the skills, care, and judgments required by a health team member under similar conditions.*

Standards of care come from laws, job descriptions (Chapter 3), agency policies and procedures (Chapter 1), and manufacturer's instructions for use of equipment and supplies. Approval (regulatory) agencies such as the Centers for Medicare & Medicaid Services (CMS) and accrediting agencies set standards (Chapter 1). Standards and guidelines also come from other government agencies like the Centers for Disease Control and Prevention (CDC).

Negligence is a risk when standards of care are not met. *Negligence is an unintentional wrong. The negligent person did not act in a reasonable and careful manner. A person or the person's property was harmed.* The person causing the harm did not intend or mean to cause harm. The person failed to do what a reasonable and careful person *would have done.* Or the person did what a reasonable and careful person *would not have done.*

Malpractice is negligence by a professional person. A person has professional status because of education and services provided. Nurses, doctors, dentists, and pharmacists are examples.

Intentional Torts

Intentional torts are meant to be harmful and may be crimes.

- *Defamation is injuring a person's name and reputation by making false statements to a third person.*
  - *Libel is making false statements in print, in writing (including e-mail and text messages), through pictures or drawings, through broadcast (radio, TV, or video), posted on-line on websites, or through video sites and social media sites.* See "Wrongful Use of Electronic Communications" on p. 34.
  - *Slander is making false statements through the spoken word, sounds, sign language, or gestures.*
- Invasion of privacy. See "Invasion of Privacy" on p. 34.
- *Fraud is saying or doing something to trick, fool, or deceive a person.* The act is fraud if it does or could harm a person or the person's property. Telling someone that you are a nurse is fraud. So is giving wrong or incomplete information on a job application.
- *False imprisonment is the unlawful restraint or restriction of a person's freedom of movement.* It involves:
  - Threatening to restrain a person
  - Restraining a person
  - Preventing a person from leaving the agency
- *Assault is intentionally attempting or threatening to touch a person's body without the person's consent.* The person fears bodily harm. Threatening to "tie down" a person is an example of assault.
- *Battery is touching a person's body without consent.* The person must consent to any procedure, treatment, or other act that involves touching the body. The person has the right to withdraw consent at any time. See "Informed Consent" on p. 35.

See *Promoting Safety and Comfort: Intentional Torts.*

PROMOTING SAFETY AND COMFORT

Intentional Torts

Safety

To protect yourself from defamation, never make false statements about a patient, resident, family member, visitor, co-worker, or any other person. This includes:

- Through e-mails or text messages
- On websites, video sites, or social media sites
- In newspapers, magazines, or other print sources
- Through broadcasts (TV, radio, or film)
- With words, sounds, signs, gestures, or any form of communication

Also protect yourself from being accused of assault and battery. Explain to the person what you are going to do and get the person's consent. Consent may be verbal—"yes" or "okay." Or it can be a gesture—a nod, turning over for a back massage, or holding out an arm for you to take a pulse.

Invasion of Privacy. Patients and residents have the right to personal privacy (Chapter 2). This involves privacy of the person's body, private affairs, and information about care, treatment, and condition. *Invasion of privacy is violating a person's right not to have his or her name, photo, or private affairs exposed or made public without giving consent.*

You must treat the person with respect and ensure privacy. See Box 4-3 for measures to protect privacy.

See *Focus on Communication: Invasion of Privacy.*

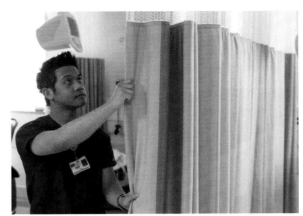

FIGURE 4-2 Pulling the privacy curtain around the bed helps protect the person's privacy.

BOX 4-3 Protecting the Right to Privacy

- Keep all information about the person confidential.
- Cover the person when in hallways and elevators.
- Ask visitors to leave the room when care is given.
- Screen the person. Close the privacy curtain as in Figure 4-2. Close the room door and window coverings to give care.
- Close the bathroom door for elimination or hygiene.
- Expose only the body part involved in a task.
- Do not discuss the person or the person's treatment with anyone except the nurse supervising your work.
- Do not open the person's mail.
- Allow the person to visit with others in private.
- Allow the person to use the phone in private.
- Follow agency policies and procedures to protect privacy.

FOCUS ON COMMUNICATION

Invasion of Privacy

The *Health Insurance Portability and Accountability Act of 1996 (HIPAA)* protects the privacy and security of a person's health information. **Protected health information** *refers to identifying information and information about the person's health care that is maintained or sent in any form (paper, electronic, oral).* Failure to follow HIPAA rules can result in fines, penalties, and criminal actions including jail time.

To avoid HIPAA violations:
- Always follow agency policies and procedures.
- *Never take photos or videos of patients or residents or any person in the health care setting.* Sharing photos or videos or posting them on video sites or social media sites is a very serious violation of HIPAA.
- *Never send an e-mail or text message or post anything on a website, video site, or social media site about a patient, resident, family member, or visitor.* Sharing information is a very serious violation of HIPAA.
- *Never write anything for a newspaper, magazine, or print source about a patient, resident, family member, or visitor.*
- *Never broadcast (through TV, radio, or video) anything about a patient, resident, family member, or visitor.*
- *Only discuss the person's health information with staff directly involved in the person's care.*
- See "Wrongful Use of Electronic Communications."

You may be asked questions about the person or the person's care. Direct such questions to the nurse. Also follow the rules for using computers and other electronic devices (Chapter 7).

Wrongful Use of Electronic Communications

Electronic communications include e-mail, text messages, faxes, websites, video sites, and social media sites. Video and social media sites include Facebook, Twitter, LinkedIn, YouTube, Instagram, and so on. Other forms of electronic communications are expected in the future.

Correct use of electronic communications is essential in your personal life and as a nursing assistant. Follow the rules in Box 4-4. Do so whether using a computer, phone, camera, or other electronic device at home, at school, at work, or in any other setting. Wrongful use of electronic communications can result in job loss and loss of your certification (license, registration).

Wrongful use also can result in:
- Civil action resulting in a fine
- Criminal action resulting in a fine or jail time

See *Focus on Communication: Wrongful Use of Electronic Communications.*

FOCUS ON COMMUNICATION

Wrongful Use of Electronic Communications

The following are examples of wrongful use of electronic communications.
- Laura is a nursing assistant student. On the last day of clinical, she asks 2 residents if she can take a photo with them. Laura posts the photo on a social media site with this comment: "Done with clinical! I'll miss my residents."
- Justin works on a cancer unit. A patient posts on a blog about a tiring day of treatments. Justin posts: "Chemo can wear you down. Maybe the new medicine will help you rest. Hope you feel better tomorrow. See you then."

What did Laura do wrong? What did Justin do wrong?

Often wrongful use of electronic communications is not intentional. You must be very careful. Your communication must protect privacy and confidentiality at all times.

BOX 4-4 Electronic Communications

- Follow agency policies for using electronic communications.
- Remember that:
  - Anything you send or post electronically can be sent to or shared with someone other than the intended person.
  - Electronic communications last forever. They can be retrieved for legal purposes.
  - Private information shared with the intended person still violates the rights to privacy and confidentiality.
  - Referring to a person by nickname, room number, diagnosis, or other means but not by name still violates the rights to privacy and confidentiality.
- Protect privacy and maintain confidentiality at all times.
- Never take photos or videos of the person or any part of the person's body.
- Never send in any way information about the person or images (photos, videos, art) of the person.

- Never identify patients or residents by name.
- Never share information that can lead to the person being identified.
- Maintain professional boundaries. Avoid electronic contact with patients and residents, former patients and residents, and their family members.
- Do not use electronic communications to share or discuss workplace issues or co-workers.
- Tell the nurse at once if you may have violated the person's right to privacy or confidentiality. If you suspect that a co-worker has done so, also tell the nurse.
- See "Gossip" in Chapter 5.
- See "Unethical Student Behavior" in Chapter 5.
- See "Electronic Devices" in Chapter 7.

Modified from National Council of State Boards of Nursing: *A nurse's guide to the use of social media*, Chicago, 2018, Author.

Informed Consent

A person has the right to decide what will be done to his or her body and who can touch his or her body. The doctor is responsible for informing the person about all aspects of treatment. *Informed consent is the process by which a person receives and understands information about a treatment or procedure and is able to decide to receive or refuse the treatment or procedure. (Refuse means to decline or not accept.)* Consent is informed when the person clearly understands all aspects of treatment.

Persons under legal age (usually 18 years) cannot give consent. Nor can persons who are mentally unable. This includes persons who are unconscious, sedated, or confused. Or they have certain mental health disorders. Informed consent is given by a responsible party—a spouse, parent, adult child, guardian, or legal representative.

You are never responsible for obtaining written consent. In some agencies, you can witness the signing of a consent. When a witness, you are present when the person signs the consent.

See *Focus on Communication: Informed Consent.*

REPORTING ABUSE

Some persons are mistreated or harmed on purpose. This is abuse. Abuse is a crime. *Abuse is:*

- *The willful infliction of injury, unreasonable confinement, intimidation, or punishment that results in physical harm, pain, or mental anguish.* **Intimidation** means *to make afraid with threats of force or violence.* Abuse includes involuntary seclusion (Chapter 2).
- *Depriving the person (or the person's caregiver) of the goods or services needed to attain or maintain well-being.*

Abuse can occur at home or in a health care agency. All persons must be protected from abuse. This includes persons in a coma (Chapter 6).

The abuser is often a family member or caregiver—spouse, partner, adult child, and others. The abuser can be a friend, neighbor, landlord, or other person. Both men and women are abusers. Both men and women are abused.

See *Focus on Communication: Reporting Abuse.*
See *Focus on Surveys: Reporting Abuse,* p. 36.

FOCUS ON COMMUNICATION

Informed Consent

There are different ways to give consent.
- *Written consent.* The person signs a form agreeing to a treatment or procedure. You are not responsible for obtaining written consent.
- *Verbal consent.* The person states aloud that consent is given. "Yes" and "okay" are examples.
- *Implied consent.* For example, you ask if you can check a person's blood pressure. The person extends an arm. The movement implies consent.

Before any procedure or task, explain the steps to the person. This is how you obtain verbal or implied consent. Also explain each step during a procedure. This allows the person to refuse at any time.

FOCUS ON COMMUNICATION

Reporting Abuse

Abused persons may confide in you. They may ask you to keep it a secret. For example, a person says: "If I tell you something, will you promise not to tell anyone?" Never promise to keep abuse a secret from the nurse. Be honest. Do not say you will keep a secret and then report it to the nurse. You can say: "For your safety, some things I must tell the nurse. What did you want to tell me?" If the person refuses to tell you, notify the nurse.

If you suspect abuse, tell the nurse. Give as much detail as you can. For example: "I am concerned about Ms. Sloan. She is very quiet today. When I asked about her visit with her family, she didn't answer. She refused her bath. And when I helped her to the bathroom, I saw bruises on her back."

Vulnerable Adults

Vulnerable comes from the Latin word *vulnerare*, which means *to wound*. A *vulnerable adult is a person 18 years old or older who has a disability or condition that causes the person to be at risk for harm.* Such persons have problems caring for or protecting themselves due to:
- A mental, emotional, physical, intellectual, or developmental disability
- Brain damage
- Changes from aging

All patients and residents, regardless of age or care setting, are vulnerable. Older persons are at risk for abuse. See *Focus on Older Persons: Vulnerable Adults.*

Elder Abuse

An *elder*, as defined by the CDC, is an older adult 60 years of age or older. *Elder abuse is any knowing, intentional, or negligent act by a caregiver or any other person to an older adult. The act causes harm or serious risk of harm.* Elder abuse can take these forms. Often more than 1 form of abuse is present.
- *Physical abuse.* This is the intentional use of physical force that results in illness, injury, pain, impaired function, distress, or death. See Figure 4-3 and Box 4-5 for signs of and examples of physical abuse.
- *Neglect. Neglect is when a caregiver or responsible person fails to protect a vulnerable person from harm. Or the person fails to provide food, water, clothing, shelter, health care, or basic activities of daily living to a vulnerable person.* Leaving a person lying in urine or feces and failing to answer call lights are examples.
- *Financial abuse.* The older person's resources (money, property, assets) are mis-used or stolen. Terms that may be used include:
  - *Exploitation*—mis-use of a person's money, property, or assets.
  - *Misappropriation*—the illegal, dishonest, unfair, or wrongful use of a person's money, property, or assets for one's own use.
- *Emotional or psychological abuse.* This is any verbal (oral or written) or nonverbal behavior that causes mental pain, anguish, fear, or distress. Humiliation, harassment, insults, and threats of punishment are examples. Isolation (seclusion) and control (withholding needed resources) are other examples.
- *Sexual abuse.* This is forced or unwanted sexual interaction of any kind with an older adult or incapacitated person. (*Incapacitated* means *being unconscious or lacking awareness.*) The interaction may be completed or attempted. It may involve touching or non-touching. Unwanted touching, forced nudity, and taking photos or videos are forms of sexual abuse. So is harassing the person about sex or sexuality.
- *Abandonment. Abandon* means *to leave or desert someone.* The person is deserted by someone who is supposed to provide care. Abandonment involves the following 4 points.
  - You accept an assignment to care for a person or group of persons.
  - You accept the assignment for a certain time period.
  - You remove yourself from the care setting—hospital, nursing center, or other agency.
  - You do not report off to a staff member who will assume responsibility for care.

There are many signs of elder abuse. The abused person may show only some of the signs in Box 4-6.

Reporting Elder Abuse. Federal and state laws require the reporting of elder abuse. If you suspect abuse, share your concerns and observations with the nurse. Be as detailed as possible. The nurse contacts health team members and community agencies as needed. Sometimes the police or courts are involved.

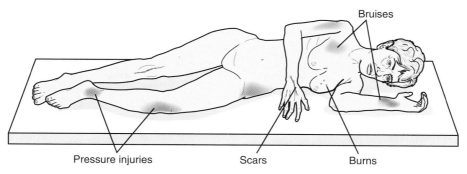

FIGURE 4-3 Some signs of physical elder abuse.

BOX 4-5 Examples of Physical Abuse

- Biting
- Burning
- Choking, suffocation
- Corporal punishment—punishment inflicted directly on the body (beatings, lashings, whippings, and so on)
- Depriving of a basic need—food, water, shelter, and so on (Chapter 6)
- Force-feeding
- Grabbing, pinching, scratching
- Hair-pulling
- Hitting, kicking, punching, slapping
- Pushing, shaking, shoving
- Restraint—physical or chemical (Chapter 13)
- Striking with or without an object

BOX 4-6 Signs of Elder Abuse

- The person reports mistreatment.
- Living conditions are not safe, clean, or adequate.
- Personal and oral hygiene are lacking (Chapters 21 and 22). The person is not clean. Clothes are dirty.
- Weight loss—signs of poor nutrition and poor fluid intake.
- Adaptive (assistive) devices are missing or broken—eyeglasses, hearing aids, dentures, cane, walker, and so on.
- Medical needs are not met.
- The person cannot reach toilet facilities, food, water, and other needed items.
- Drugs are not taken properly. Drugs are not bought. Or too much or too little of the drug is taken.
- Frequent injuries—injuries are strange or seem impossible.
- Old and new injuries—bruises, pressure marks, welts, scars, fractures, punctures, and so on.
- Problems walking or sitting.
- Bleeding, bruising, irritation, itching, or pain around the breasts, inner thighs, or genital or anal area.
- Torn, stained, or bloody under-garments.
- Burns on the feet, hands, buttocks, or other parts of the body. Cigarettes and cigars cause small circle-like burns.
- Pressure injuries (Chapter 36) or contractures (Chapter 32).
- Emotional problems (Chapter 41):
  - Panic attacks
  - Post-traumatic stress disorder
  - Quiet, withdrawn from others and normal activities
  - Does not want to talk or answer questions
  - Depression
  - Suicide thoughts or attempts
  - Fear, anxiety, or agitation
  - Inappropriate, unusual, or aggressive sexual behavior
- Sudden changes in alertness.
- Sudden changes in finances.
- The person is restrained. Or the person is locked in a certain area for long periods.
- Private conversations are not allowed. The caregiver is present during all conversations.
- Strained or tense relationships with a caregiver.
- Frequent arguments with a caregiver.
- The person seems anxious to please the caregiver.
- Emergency room visits may be frequent.
- The person may change doctors often. Some people do not have a doctor.

OBRA Requirements. The *Omnibus Budget Reconciliation Act of 1987 (OBRA)* requires these actions if abuse is suspected within the center.

- The matter is reported at once to the administrator. It also is reported at once to other officials as required by federal and state laws.
- All claims of abuse are thoroughly investigated.
- The center must prevent further potential for abuse while the investigation is in progress.
- Investigation results are reported to the center administrator and required agencies within 5 days of the incident.
- Corrective actions are taken if the claim is found to be true.

Child Abuse and Neglect

Child abuse and neglect is the intentional harm or mistreatment of a child under 18 years old. It:

- *Involves any recent act or failure to act on the part of a parent or caregiver.*
- *Results in death, serious physical or emotional harm, sexual abuse, or exploitation.*
- *Presents a likely or immediate risk for harm.*

Child abuse is complex. It can occur in many forms. Often more than 1 type is present. See Table 4-1, p. 38. You must be alert for signs of child abuse.

All states require the reporting of suspected child abuse. If you suspect child abuse, share your concerns with the nurse. Give as much detail as you can. The nurse contacts health team members and child protection agencies as needed.

TABLE 4-1 Child Abuse and Neglect—Types and Signs

Type and Description	Signs of Abuse—Child	Signs of Abuse—Parent or Parent and Child
General behaviors—may be present with any type of mistreatment	**The Child** • Reports bad treatment or abuse by a parent or caregiver. • Has sudden changes in behavior. • Has sudden changes in school performance. • Has learning problems or problems concentrating. The problem is not caused by a physical or mental health disorder. • Has untreated health problems. • Seems watchful; seems to wait for something bad to happen. • Lacks adult supervision. • Is overly agreeable or obedient. • Is quiet, withdrawn, or uninvolved. • Arrives early at school or stays late. • Does not want to go home from school, activities, or someone's house. • Fears a parent or certain person; does not want to be around a parent or certain person.	**The Parent** • Denies that the child has problems at school or home. • Blames the child for problems at school or home. • Asks teachers or caregivers to use harsh discipline. • Describes the child as bad, worthless, or a burden. • Demands physical or academic performance above the child's abilities. • Shows little concern for the child. • Relies on the child for care, attention, or emotional satisfaction. **The Parent and Child** • Rarely touch or look at each other. • View their relationship as poor or bad. • State that they do not like each other.
Physical abuse—injuring the child on purpose	**The Child** • Has injuries that are not explained—burns, bites, bruises, broken bones, black eyes. • Has fading bruises or other marks after being gone from school. • Is scared, anxious, depressed, withdrawn, or aggressive. • Fears parents and does not want to go home. • Shrinks (cowers) when an adult approaches. • Has changes in eating and sleeping habits. • Reports injury by a parent or caregiver. • Abuses animals or pets.	**The Parent** • Gives different or confusing stories about an injury. Or does not give an explanation. • Uses harsh discipline. • Has a history of abusing animals or pets.
Neglect—failing to provide for the child's basic needs (food, clothing, shelter, supervision, health care, education, affection and attention)	**The Child** • Begs or steals food or money. • Is dirty or has a severe body odor. • Lacks the correct clothing for the weather. • Abuses alcohol or drugs. • States that no one is at home to provide care. • Is often absent from school. • Lacks medical or dental care. Does not have needed eyeglasses.	**The Parent** • Seems to have little interest in the child. • Shows little or no emotion or is depressed. • Has behaviors that are bizarre or not logical. • Abuses alcohol or drugs.
Sexual abuse—using, persuading, or forcing the child to engage in any sexual contact, activity, or behavior or exposing a child to sexual acts	**The Child** • Has trouble walking or sitting. • Has bleeding, bruising, or swelling in sexual areas. • Refuses to go to school. • Has nightmares or wets the bed. • Has a sudden change in appetite. • Has sexual knowledge or behavior that is unusual or does not fit with the child's age. • Is pregnant or has a sexually transmitted disease (Chapter 40), especially under the age of 14. • Runs away. • Reports sexual abuse. • Attaches to strangers or new adults quickly.	**The Parent** • Tries to be the child's friend instead of a parent. • Makes up excuses to be alone with the child. • Tells the child about personal problems or relationships.
Emotional abuse—injuring the child mentally or damaging the child's sense of self-worth	**The Child** • Has extremes in behavior—overly agreeable or demanding, quiet and withdrawn, or aggressive. • Acts much younger or older than the child's actual age. For example, the child shows infant-like behaviors (rocking, head-banging). Or the child acts like a parent to other children. • Has physical or emotional developmental delays. • Is depressed. • Has suicidal thoughts. • Has trouble bonding with others.	**The Parent** • Blames, criticizes, or scolds the child often. • Describes the child negatively. • Rejects the child.

Modified from Child Welfare Information Gateway: *What is child abuse and neglect: recognizing the signs and symptoms*, Washington, DC, April 2019, Children's Bureau.

Intimate Partner Violence

The CDC describes *intimate partner violence (IPV)* *as physical violence, sexual violence, stalking, or psychological aggression by a current or former partner.* Also called domestic abuse, domestic violence, intimate partner abuse, partner abuse, and spousal abuse—IPV occurs in relationships. IPV includes dating violence and teen dating violence. In IPV, 1 partner has power and control over the other through abuse. The abuse may range from 1 event to chronic, severe violence over several years. Rarely is IPV a 1-time event.

IPV causes fear and harm. Usually more than 1 type of IPV is present.

- *Physical violence*—a person hurts or tries to hurt a partner using physical force (hitting, kicking, and so on).
- *Sexual violence*—a person forces or attempts to force a partner to take part in a sex act, sexual touching, or a non-physical sexual event. The partner does not or cannot give consent.
- *Stalking*—there is a pattern of repeated, unwanted attention and contact that causes fear or concern for one's safety or the safety of another (family, friend).
- *Psychological aggression*—a person uses verbal and nonverbal communication to harm a partner mentally or emotionally. The intent may be to control the person.

Both men and women can be victims. Patients and residents can suffer from IPV. For example, a partner is insulted and slapped during a visit. You, yourself, may be a victim of IPV. Warning signs include:

- Unwanted physical or sexual contact
- Threats to you, your children, family members, or pets
- Threats of suicide to get you to do something
- Using or threatening to use a weapon against you
- Keeping or taking your paycheck
- Saying things to put you down or make you feel bad
- Keeping you from seeing family or friends
- Keeping you from going to work

Intimate partner violence is a complex safety issue. The victim often hides the abuse. State laws vary about reporting IPV. However, the health team has an ethical duty to give information about safety and community resources. If you suspect IPV, tell the nurse. The nurse gathers information to help the person.

See *Promoting Safety and Comfort: Intimate Partner Violence.*

PROMOTING SAFETY AND COMFORT

Intimate Partner Violence

Safety

Intimate partner violence occurs in relationships. Partners may be:

- Married
- Not married but living together
- Dating
- Divorced or separated
- Female and male; male and male; female and female

If you are a victim of abuse, call 911 or the police. Tell the police everything that happened—the abuser, what happened, marks on your body, and so on. Answer their questions honestly and completely. The police can help you and your children to a safe place. They can give you information about IPV, IPV programs and shelters, and how to develop a personal safety plan.

OTHER LAWS

See "Ethics and Laws" in the *Focus on PRIDE: The Person, Family, and Yourself* boxes at the end of each chapter. They describe other laws affecting your work as a nursing assistant.

FOCUS ON P R I D E

The Person, Family, and Yourself

P ersonal and Professional Responsibility

States have laws about who must report abuse and neglect. Such persons are called *mandatory reporters*. *Mandatory* means *required*. For example, most states require that health care providers report suspected abuse or neglect of children, vulnerable adults, and elders. Tell the nurse if you suspect abuse or neglect.

R ights and Respect

The person has the right to be free from abuse, mistreatment, and neglect. Abuse can take many forms. For example:
- A person constantly crying out for help is left alone with the door closed.
- A person is told to be nice or care will not be given.
- A person is turned in a rough and hurried manner.
- A person lies in a wet and soiled bed all night.
- A person uses the call light a lot. It is removed from the room.
- A person is told that family does not visit because the person is mean.

I ndependence and Social Interaction

You will interact closely with patients, residents, and families. You may begin to know them well. Social and professional relationships differ. Use good judgment when interacting with patients, residents, and families. Maintain professional boundaries.

D elegation and Teamwork

Working within the limits of your role protects persons from harm. You must understand your roles and responsibilities to know when a task is outside these limits. Accepting a task beyond the legal limits of your role can lead to negligence.

E thics and Laws

Negligence is a risk when standards of care are not met. For example:
- You fail to test the water temperature for a shower. The water is too hot. The person is burned.
- You do not answer a call light promptly. The person gets up without help. The person falls and breaks an arm.
- You do not follow the manufacturer's instructions for a mechanical lift. The person slips out of the lift and falls. The person fractures a hip.
- You do not identify the person before a procedure. You perform the procedure on the wrong person. Both residents are harmed. One had a procedure that was not ordered. The other did not have a needed procedure.

Your training helps you develop the skills and judgment needed to give safe care. Take pride in protecting persons from harm.

FOCUS ON PRIDE: *Application*

A code of conduct guides your thinking and behavior. Write a personal code of conduct stating what you expect of yourself as a nursing assistant.

REVIEW QUESTIONS

Circle the BEST answer.

1 Which is ethical behavior?
   a Sharing information about a person with a friend
   b Accepting gifts from a resident's family
   c Reporting errors
   d Calling your family before answering a call light

2 On your days off, you call the agency to check on a patient. This is a
   a Professional boundary
   b Tort
   c Boundary violation
   d Boundary sign

3 To maintain professional boundaries, focus on
   a Helping the person
   b Meeting your needs
   c Being biased
   d Showing that you care

4 You help with a friend's hospital care. This is a
   a Professional boundary
   b Boundary crossing
   c Tort
   d Crime

5 If a harmful act was intentional, it was
   a Attempted but not completed
   b Done by a professional person
   c Accidental
   d Done on purpose

6 These statements are about negligence. Which is *true*?
   a It is an intentional tort.
   b The negligent person acted in a reasonable manner.
   c The person or the person's property was harmed.
   d A prison term is likely.

7 You do not tell the nurse about a patient's chest pain. The patient dies from a heart attack. You
   a Did nothing wrong
   b Could face negligence charges
   c Are not legally responsible
   d Are guilty of fraud

8 You tell others that you are a nurse. This is
   a Negligence
   b Fraud
   c Libel
   d Slander

9 Restraining a person's freedom of movement is
   a Neglect
   b Invasion of privacy
   c Defamation
   d False imprisonment

10 Threatening to touch the person's body without the person's consent is
   a Assault
   b Battery
   c Defamation
   d False imprisonment

11 Sharing a resident's photo on a social media site is
   a Fraud
   b Allowed with the family's consent
   c A violation of HIPAA
   d Allowed if you obtain informed consent

12 Informed consent is when the person
   a Fully understands all aspects of treatment
   b Signs a consent form
   c Is admitted to the agency
   d Agrees to a procedure

13 Self-neglect is when
   a A caregiver harms a person
   b The person's behaviors put him or her at risk for harm
   c A person is deprived of food, clothing, hygiene, and shelter
   d The person does not receive attention or affection

14 You scold an older person for not eating lunch. This is
   a Physical abuse
   b Neglect
   c Battery
   d Emotional or psychological abuse

15 Which is a sign of elder abuse?
   a Stiff joints and joint pain
   b Weight gain
   c Poor personal hygiene
   d Forgetfulness

16 An older adult has a black eye and bruises on the face. These are signs of
   a Physical abuse
   b Sexual abuse
   c Neglect
   d Substance abuse

17 Depriving a child of food, clothing, and shelter is
   a Physical abuse
   b Emotional abuse
   c Negligence
   d Neglect

18 Bruising around a child's genitalia is a sign of
   a Physical abuse
   b Sexual abuse
   c Neglect
   d Substance abuse

19 Which statement about intimate partner violence is *true*?
   a It always involves physical harm.
   b It is usually a 1-time event.
   c One partner has control over the other partner.
   d Only 1 type of abuse is usually present.

20 You suspect a resident was abused. You should
   a Tell the nurse
   b Call the police
   c Tell the family
   d Ask the person about the abuse

Answers to Chapter 4 questions are on p. 587.

FOCUS ON **PRACTICE**

Problem Solving

A resident in your nursing center asks you to bring your children to visit. How will you respond? How do professional boundaries protect the person?

CHAPTER 5

Student and Work Ethics

OBJECTIVES

- Define the key terms and key abbreviations in this chapter.
- Describe the qualities and traits of a successful nursing assistant.
- Describe good health and hygiene practices.
- Explain how to look professional.
- Explain how to prepare for school and work.
- Explain how to function as a safe and effective member of a team.
- Explain how to manage stress.

- Explain how to problem solve and deal with conflict.
- Explain the aspects of harassment.
- Explain how to resign from a job.
- Identify the common reasons for losing a job.
- Explain the reasons for drug testing.
- Describe unethical student behavior and possible consequences.
- Explain how to promote PRIDE in the person, the family, and yourself.

KEY TERMS

bullying Repeated attacks or threats of fear, distress, or harm by a bully toward a target
burnout A job stress resulting in being physically or mentally exhausted, having doubts about your abilities, and having doubts about the value of your work
confidentiality Trusting others with personal and private information
gossip To spread rumors or talk about the private matters of others
harassment To trouble, torment, offend, or worry a person by one's behavior or comments

priority The most important thing at the time
professionalism Following laws, being ethical, having good work ethics, and having the skills to do your work
stress The response or change in the body caused by any emotional, psychological, physical, social, or economic factor
teamwork Staff members work together as a group; everyone does their part to give safe and effective care
work ethics Behavior in the workplace

KEY ABBREVIATIONS

ID Identification

NATCEP Nursing assistant training and competency evaluation program

As a student and a nursing assistant, you must act and function in a professional manner. *Professionalism involves following laws, being ethical, having good work ethics, and having the skills to do your work.* Certain behaviors (conduct), choices, and judgments are expected. *Work ethics deals with behavior in the workplace.* Your conduct reflects your choices and judgments.

Work ethics involves:
- How you look
- What you say
- How you behave
- How you treat and work with others
- The qualities and traits shown and described in Figure 5-1

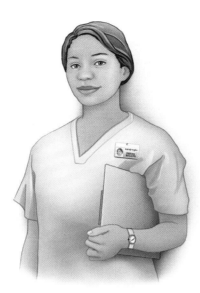

Caring—having concern for the person; making the person's life happier, easier, or less painful

Cheerful—greeting and talking to others in a pleasant manner

Conscientious—being careful, alert, and exact in following instructions; giving thorough care; protecting the person's property

Considerate—respecting the person's physical and emotional feelings; being kind to patients, residents, families, and the health team

Cooperative—helping and working with others willingly; willing to do more during busy and stressful times

Courteous—being polite to patients, residents, families, and the health team

Dependable—reporting to work on time and as scheduled; completing assignments; keeping obligations and promises

Empathy—seeing things from the person's point of view; putting yourself in the person's place

Enthusiastic—being eager, interested, and excited about your work

Honest—reporting the care given, your observations, and any errors accurately

Patient—coping with problems and delays; staying calm rather than getting upset, annoyed, or angry; not rushing the person or a co-worker

Respectful—treating the person with respect and dignity at all times; respecting the person's rights, values, beliefs, and feelings; showing respect for the health team

Self-aware—knowing your feelings, strengths, and weaknesses; understanding yourself so you can understand patients and residents

Trustworthy—keeping information confidential; not gossiping about patients, residents, families, or the health team

FIGURE 5-1 Good work ethics involves these qualities and traits.

In this chapter, *work ethics* also applies to you as a student. For student success, practice good work ethics in the classroom and clinical setting and with instructors and fellow students.

HEALTH, HYGIENE, AND APPEARANCE

Patients, residents, families, and visitors expect you to look, act, and be healthy. For example, a person must stop smoking. Yet because you smoke, you and your clothes smell of smoke. If you do not look or smell clean, people wonder if you give good care. Your health, hygiene, and appearance need careful attention.

Your Health

To learn and give safe and effective care, you must be physically and mentally healthy. The following affect your health.

- *Diet.* You need a balanced diet for good nutrition (Chapter 28).
- *Sleep and rest.* Most adults need 7 to 8 hours of sleep daily.
- *Exercise.* Exercise promotes muscle tone, circulation, and weight control.
- *Your eyes.* You must read instructions and measurements correctly. Wrong readings and measurements can harm the person. Have your eyes checked. Wear needed eyeglasses or contact lenses. Have good lighting for reading and fine work.

- *Smoking.* Smoke odors stay on your breath, hands, clothing, and hair. Hand-washing and good hygiene are needed.
- *Drugs.* Some drugs affect thinking, feeling, behavior, and function. Working under the influence of drugs affects the person's safety and yours. Take only prescribed drugs in the prescribed way.
- *Alcohol.* Alcohol is a drug that affects thinking, balance, coordination, and alertness. Never go to work under the influence of alcohol. Do not drink alcohol while working.
- *Body mechanics.* You will bend, carry heavy objects, and move and turn persons. Use your muscles correctly (Chapter 16).

Your Hygiene

Your hygiene needs careful attention. Bathe daily. Use a deodorant or antiperspirant to prevent body odors. Brush your teeth often—upon awakening, before and after meals, and at bedtime. Use mouthwash to prevent breath odors. Shampoo often. Keep fingernails clean, short, and smoothly and neatly shaped.

Menstrual hygiene is important. Change tampons or sanitary pads often, especially for heavy flow. Wash your genital area with soap and water at least once a day. Also practice good hand-washing.

Foot care prevents odors and infection. Wash your feet daily. Dry thoroughly between the toes. Cut toenails straight across after bathing or soaking them.

Your Appearance

How you look affects what people think about you and the agency. If staff or students are clean and neat, people think the agency is clean and neat. If staff or students are messy and unkempt, people may question the agency's cleanliness and quality of care.

You need to look clean, neat, and professional. See Box 5-1 and Figure 5-2.

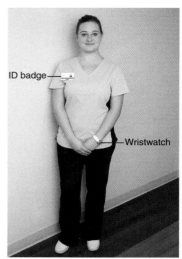

FIGURE 5-2 The nursing assistant is well groomed. The uniform and shoes are clean. Hair has a simple style—away from the face and off of the collar. Jewelry is not worn.

BOX 5-1 Professional Appearance

- Practice good hygiene.
- Follow the dress code of your agency or training program for:
  - Uniforms
  - Jewelry
  - Shoes
  - Hair
  - Nails, make-up, and fragrances

Uniforms

- Wear required uniforms. Do not wear home or social attire at work or as a student in the clinical setting. This includes tight, revealing, or sexual clothing. Halter tops, tank tops, low-cut tops, tops with arm slits, jeans, shorts, short skirts, low-rise pants, leggings, yoga pants, or high-cut pants are not worn.
- Uniforms fit well and are modest in length and style. Do not wear tight, revealing, or sexual-looking uniforms.
  - Women—do not show cleavage, tops of breasts, or upper thighs.
  - Men—do not wear tight pants. Do not expose your chest. Open just the top button of your shirt.
- Keep uniforms clean, pressed, and mended. Sew on buttons. Repair zippers, tears, and hems.
- Wear a clean uniform and clean under-garments daily.
- Wear appropriate under-garments for your body shape and uniform.
  - Under-garments are clean and fit properly.
  - Under-garments are the correct color for your skin tone.
  - Colored (red, pink, blue, and so on) and patterned under-garments are not worn. They can be seen through white and light-colored uniforms.
- Wear clean socks or stockings that fit well. Change them daily.
- Wear your name badge or photo ID (identification) according to the dress code. The badge or ID is usually worn above the waist where it can be seen by others (see Fig. 5-2). Agencies may use first and last names or only first names. Your student ID will have your school's name.
- Cover tattoos (body art) with your uniform. Tattoos (body art) may offend others.

Jewelry

- Wear only allowed jewelry.
  - Wedding and engagement rings may be allowed. Do not wear rings that can scratch a person.
  - Bracelets are not allowed. They can scratch a person.
  - Necklaces and dangling earrings are not allowed. Confused or combative persons might pull on them.
  - One set of small, simple earrings is usually allowed.
- Do not wear jewelry in visible piercings—eyebrows, nose, lips, cheek, tongue, or other sites.
- Wear a wristwatch with a second (sweep) hand (Fig. 5-3).

Shoes

- Wear shoes that fit, are comfortable, give needed support, and have slip-resistant soles.
  - Do not wear sandals or open-toed shoes.
- Wear clean shoes. Wash or replace shoes and laces as needed.

Hair

- Have a simple, attractive hair-style.
  - Hair is off your collar and away from your face. This includes men with long hair.
- Use simple pins, barrettes, hair ties, clips, bands, or other devices to keep long hair up and in place. This includes men with long hair.
- Keep beards and mustaches clean and trimmed.

Nails, Make-Up, and Fragrances

- Keep fingernails clean, short, and smoothly and neatly shaped. Long or jagged nails can scratch a person.
- Do not wear nail polish. Chipped nail polish may provide a place for microbes to grow.
  - If nail polish is allowed, wear only a light-colored polish.
- Do not wear non-natural nails. Fake and artificial nails and nail extenders are examples. Nails must be natural.
- Use make-up that is modest in amount and moderate in color. Avoid a painted and severe look.
- Do not wear perfume, cologne, or after-shave lotion. The scents (fragrances) may offend, nauseate, or cause breathing problems in patients and residents.

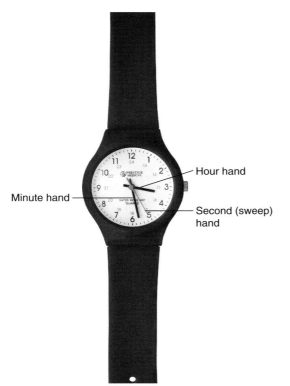

FIGURE 5-3 A watch with a second (sweep) hand. (Courtesy Prestige Medical, Northridge, Calif.)

PREPARING FOR SCHOOL OR WORK

Being dependable is important as a student and as an employee. As a student, you are preparing yourself for work. The classroom and clinical settings help you develop dependable behaviors.

To be dependable as a student:
* Arrive on time for class and clinical experiences. Arrive early to store your things, use the restroom, and gather needed items for class or clinical. Be ready for class or clinical to start.
* Complete and turn in assignments on time.
* Pay attention and follow directions.
* Stay for the entire class or clinical experience.

To be dependable in the work setting, you must:
* Work when scheduled.
* Get to work on time. See "Attendance."
* Stay the entire shift.

Absences and tardiness (being late) can affect your success in school. Your state's nursing assistant training and competency evaluation program (NATCEP) requires a certain number of hours. You must complete the required number of hours.

Absences and tardiness are also common reasons for losing a job. Childcare and transportation issues often interfere with getting to school and work. You need to plan carefully.

Childcare

Someone needs to care for your children when you leave for school or work, while you are at school or work, and before you get home. Also plan for emergencies.
* Your childcare provider is ill or cannot care for your children that day.
* A child becomes ill or injured while you are at school or work.
* You will be late getting home from school or work.

Transportation

Plan for getting to and from school or work. If you drive, keep your car in good working order. Keep enough gas in the car. Or leave early to get gas.

Carpooling is an option. Carpoolers depend on each other. If the driver is late, everyone is late for school or work. If 1 person is not ready, everyone is late for school or work. Carpool with people you trust to be ready on time. Be on time as a driver and as a passenger.

Know bus or train schedules. Know what bus or train to take if delays occur. Always carry enough money for fares to and from school or work.

Have a back-up transportation plan. Your car may not start, the carpool driver may not be going that day, or public transportation may not run.

TEAMWORK

Teamwork means that staff members work together as a group. Everyone does their part to give safe and effective care. Teamwork involves:
* Working when scheduled
* Being cheerful and friendly
* Completing assignments
* Helping others willingly
* Being kind to others

You are an important member of the health and nursing teams. Quality of care is affected by how you work with others and how you feel about your job.

Attendance

Report to work when scheduled and on time. The entire unit is affected when just 1 person is late. Call the agency if you will be late or cannot go to work. Follow the attendance policy in your employee handbook. Poor attendance can cause you to lose your job.

You must be dependable. Be *ready to work* when your shift starts.
* Store your things before your shift starts.
* Use the restroom when you arrive at the agency.
* Arrive on your nursing unit a few minutes early. Greet others and settle yourself.

You must stay the entire shift. Watching the clock for your shift to end gives a bad image. You may need to work over-time. Prepare to stay longer if necessary. When it is time to leave, report off duty to the nurse.

See *Focus on Communication: Attendance*, p. 46.

Your Attitude

You need a good attitude. Show that you enjoy your work. Listen to others. Be willing to learn. Stay busy and use your time well.

Always think before you speak. These statements signal a bad attitude.

- "That's not my resident (patient)."
- "I can't. I'm too busy."
- "I didn't do it."
- "I don't feel like it."
- "It's not my fault."
- "Don't blame me."
- "It's not my turn. I did it yesterday."
- "Nobody told me."
- "That's not my job."
- "You didn't say that you needed it right away."
- "I did more than they did."
- "I work harder than anyone else."
- "No one appreciates what I do."
- "I'm tired of this place."
- "Is it time to leave yet?"
- "Good luck. I had a horrible day."

Gossip

To *gossip means to spread rumors or talk about the private matters of others.* Gossiping is unprofessional and hurtful. To avoid gossip:

- Remove yourself from where people are gossiping.
- Do not make or repeat any comment that can hurt a person—patient or resident, family member, visitor, co-worker, fellow student, instructor, the school or agency, and so on.
- Do not make or write false statements about another person. See Chapter 4.

- Do not talk about patients, residents, family members, visitors, co-workers, fellow students, instructors, the school or agency, or others at home or in social settings.
- Do not send or post comments about others or the school or agency by e-mail, instant messaging, text messaging, video sites, social media, or other electronic means. This is especially true of hurtful, false, or private comments. See "Wrongful Use of Electronic Communications" in Chapter 4.

Confidentiality

The person's information is private and personal. *Confidentiality means trusting others with personal and private information.* The person's information is shared only among staff involved in the person's care. The person has the right to privacy and confidentiality. Agency, family, co-worker, and student information also is confidential.

Share information only with the nurse or your instructor. Do not talk about patients, residents, families, the agency, or co-workers when others are present. Do not talk about them in hallways, elevators, dining areas, or outside the agency. Others may over-hear you and eavesdrop. To *eavesdrop* means *to listen in or over-hear what others are saying.* It invades a person's privacy.

Many agencies have intercom systems. They allow for communication between the bedside and the nurses' station (Chapter 19). Be careful what you say. The intercom is like a loud speaker. Others nearby can hear what you are saying.

See *Focus on Communication: Confidentiality.*

Speech and Language

Your speech and language must be professional. Some words used in home and social settings are not proper in class, the clinical setting, and at work. Such words may offend patients, residents, families, visitors, and co-workers. Remember:

- Do not swear or use foul, vulgar, slang, sexual, or abusive language.
- Speak softly and gently.
- Speak clearly. Hearing problems are common.
- Do not shout or yell.
- Do not fight or argue with a patient or resident, family member, visitor, co-worker, your instructor, or a fellow student.

Courtesies

A *courtesy* is a polite, considerate, or helpful comment or act. Courtesies take little time or energy. Even the smallest kind act can brighten someone's day.

- Address others by Miss, Mrs., Ms., Mr., or Doctor. Or use the name the person prefers. Do not call your instructor by his or her first name.
- Say "please." Begin or end each request with "please."
- Say "thank you" when someone does something for you or helps you.
- Apologize. Say "I'm sorry" when you make a mistake or hurt someone. Even little things—like bumping someone in the hallway—need an apology.
- Be thoughtful. Compliment others. Wish others a happy birthday, day or weekend off, or holiday.
- Wish the person and family well when they leave the agency. "Stay well" and "stay healthy" are examples.
- Hold doors and elevator doors open for others. If you are at the door first, open the door and let others pass through.
- Let patients, residents, families, and visitors enter elevators first.
- Stand to greet families and visitors.
- Help others willingly when asked.
- Give praise. When a co-worker or student does something that impresses you, tell that person. Also tell your co-workers or other students.
- Do not take credit for another person's deeds. Give the person credit for the action.

Attention

Your attention (focus) matters. At work, distractions can affect quality of care and safety. You must focus on your work. See "Personal Matters."

As a student, being distracted affects your ability to learn. Distracting (disruptive) behaviors also interfere with other students' learning. Such behaviors do not show respect for your instructor or other students. The following are examples of distracting (disruptive) behaviors.

- Talking while the instructor or another student is talking.
- Talking while other students are finishing an assignment or examination.
- Making unnecessary noises (tapping or clicking an object, sighing, and so on).
- Fidgeting or moving a lot.
- Not participating in learning activities. Or doing something other than what is expected.
- Bringing children to class.
- Sleeping in class.
- Arriving late or leaving early.
- Using electronic devices during class.

Listen well, participate (be involved), and take notes in class. When you take notes, you write about what is read or presented. Ask questions about what you do not understand. These actions help you focus and learn.

Personal Matters

Personal matters must not interfere with your training or job. To keep personal matters out of school and the workplace:

- Make phone calls during meals and breaks.
- Do not let family and friends visit you at school or on the unit. If they must see you, meet them during a meal or break.
- Make appointments (doctor, dentist, lawyer, and others) for your days off.
- Do not use school or agency computers, printers, fax machines, copiers, or other equipment for your personal use.
- Do not take the school's or agency's supplies (pens, paper, and others) for your personal use.
- Do not discuss personal problems.
- Control your emotions. If you need to cry or express anger, do so in private. Get yourself together quickly and return to your work.
- Do not borrow money from or lend it to co-workers or fellow students.
- Do not sell things or engage in fund-raising.
- Turn off personal phones and other electronic devices.
- Do not send or check e-mails, text messages, or other electronic messages.

Job Safety

You must protect patients, residents, families, visitors, co-workers, and yourself from harm. Negligent acts affect the safety of others (Chapter 4). Safety practices are presented throughout this book. These guidelines apply to everything you do.

- Understand the roles, functions, and responsibilities in your job description.
- Follow agency rules, policies, and procedures.
- Know what is right and wrong conduct.
- Know what you can and cannot do.
- Develop the desired qualities and traits in Figure 5-1.
- Follow the nurse's directions and instructions.
- Question unclear directions and things you do not understand.
- Help others willingly when asked.
- Ask for any training you might need.
- Report accurately—measurements, observations, the care given, the person's complaints, and any errors (Chapters 7 and 11).
- Be responsible for your actions. Admit when you are wrong or make mistakes. Do not blame others. Do not make excuses. Learn what you did wrong and why. Try to learn from your mistakes.
- Handle the person's property carefully and prevent damage.
- Follow the safety measures in Chapter 11 and throughout this book. Also see the *Promoting Safety and Comfort* boxes throughout this book.

Meals and Breaks

Meal breaks are usually 30 minutes. Other breaks are usually 15 minutes. Meals and breaks are scheduled so that some staff are always on the unit. Staff on the unit cover for the staff on break.

Staff members depend on each other. Leave for and return from breaks on time. Other staff need their turn. Do not take longer than allowed. Tell the nurse when you leave and return to the unit.

Planning Your Work

Some care measures and nursing unit tasks are done at certain times. Others are done at the end of the shift. Deciding what to do and when is called *priority setting*. A *priority* is the most important thing at the time. To set your priorities, decide:

- Who has the greatest or most life-threatening needs.
- What task the nurse or person needs done first.
- What tasks need to be done at a certain time.
- What tasks need to be done when your shift starts and at the end of your shift.
- How long it takes to complete a task.
- How much help you need to complete a task.
- Who can help you and when.

Priorities change as the person's needs change. A person's condition can improve or worsen. New patients and residents are admitted. Others are transferred to other nursing units or discharged. These and many other factors can change priorities.

Setting priorities becomes easier with experience. Plan your work to give safe, thorough care and to use your time well (Box 5-2).

See *Focus on Communication: Planning Your Work.*

BOX 5-2 Planning Your Work

- Discuss priorities with the nurse.
- Know the routine of your shift and nursing unit.
- Follow unit policies for shift reports. In an *end-of-shift report*, the nurse gives a report to the on-coming shift (Chapter 7).
- List tasks that are on a schedule. For example, some persons are turned or offered the bedpan every 2 hours.
- Judge how much time you need for each person and task.
- Identify tasks to do while patients and residents are eating, visiting, or involved with activities or therapies.
- Plan care around meal times, visiting hours, and therapies. Also consider recreation and social activities.
- Identify when you will need help from a co-worker. Ask a co-worker to help you. Give the time when you will need help and for how long.
- Schedule equipment or rooms for the person's use. The shower room is an example.
- Review your assignment sheet (Chapter 7). Gather needed supplies ahead of time.
- Do not waste time. Stay focused on your work.
- Leave a clean work area. Make sure rooms and utility areas are neat and orderly.
- Be a self-starter. Have initiative. Ask others if they need help. Follow unit routines, stock supply areas, and clean utility rooms. Stay busy.

FOCUS ON COMMUNICATION

Planning Your Work

You can ask your instructor or the nurse to help you set priorities. Communicate what you know—what you need to do and which tasks are time sensitive (must be done at a certain time). Ask your instructor or the nurse to help you plan. For example, you say to the nurse:

I have 2 showers to give after breakfast—Mr. Lim's and Ms. Parker's. I also need to measure Ms. Parker's vital signs. Mr. Lim needs to be ready for his appointment at 9:30 AM. Do you need Ms. Parker's vital signs by a certain time? Would you like me to check them before giving Mr. Lim's shower?

STRESS

Stress is the response or change in the body caused by any emotional, psychological, physical, social, or economic factor. Stress is normal. It occurs every minute of every day in everything you do. No matter the cause—pleasant or unpleasant—stress affects the whole person.

- Physically—sweating, rapid heart rate, faster and deeper breathing, increased blood pressure, dry mouth, and so on
- Mentally—anxiety, fear, anger, dread, apprehension, and defense mechanisms (Chapter 41)
- Socially—changes in relationships, avoiding others, needing others, blaming others, and so on
- Spiritually—changes in beliefs and values and strengthening or questioning one's beliefs in God or a higher power

Prolonged or frequent stress threatens physical and mental health. Some problems are often minor—headaches, stomach upset, sleep problems, muscle tension, and so on. Others are life-threatening—high blood pressure, heart attack, stroke, ulcers, and so on.

School, job, and personal stresses can affect your family, friends, studies, and work. Stress affects you, the care you give, the person's quality of life, and how you relate to co-workers.

Burnout

Burnout is a job stress resulting in:
- *Being physically or mentally exhausted*
- *Having doubts about your abilities*
- *Having doubts about the value of your work*

Burnout occurs over time. Causes, signs, and symptoms are listed in Box 5-3. Burnout can cause physical and mental health problems. They include fatigue, sleep problems, depression, anxiety, alcohol or substance use disorders, heart disease, diabetes, stroke, and weight gain. Problems can develop at home and with personal relationships.

BOX 5-3 Burnout—Causes, Signs, and Symptoms

Causes of Burnout
- Schedules, assignments, or workloads that you find difficult
- Not being comfortable with your supervisor or co-workers
- Being harassed, bullied, or heavily criticized by your supervisor or a co-worker
- Conflicts with how problems and grievances are handled
- Not liking your job or the agency
- Having skills that are greater than or lesser than what the job requires
- Lacking emotional support at work, at home, or socially
- Lacking balance between work and home, family, and social life

Signs and Symptoms of Burnout
- Lack of energy
- Sense of dread about going to work; not wanting to go to work
- Sleep problems
- Forgetfulness
- Problems concentrating
- Frequent illness—infection, cold, influenza
- Physical symptoms:
  - Chest pain
  - Rapid or irregular heartbeat
  - Shortness of breath
  - Gastro-intestinal pain
  - Dizziness
  - Fainting
  - Headaches
  - Loss of appetite
- Anxiety
- Anger
- Depression
- Irritability
- Wanting to be alone
- Calling in sick; going to work late

Managing Stress

To reduce or cope with stress:
- Exercise regularly.
- Get enough rest and sleep.
- Eat healthy.
- Plan personal and quiet time for you.
- Use common sense about what you can and cannot do. Do not try to do everything that others ask you to do.
- Do 1 thing at a time. Set priorities.
- Do not judge yourself harshly. Do not try to be perfect or expect too much from yourself.
- Give yourself praise. You do good and wonderful things every day.
- Have a sense of humor. Laugh at yourself. Laugh with others. Spend time with those who make you laugh.
- Have a social life that does not include co-workers.
- Talk to the nurse if your work or a person is causing too much stress. The nurse can help you deal with the matter.

Dealing With Conflict

People bring their values, attitudes, opinions, experiences, and expectations to school and work settings. Differences often lead to conflict. *Conflict* is a clash between opposing interests or ideas. People disagree and argue. There are misunderstandings and unrest.

Conflicts arise over issues or events. Work schedules, absences, and the amount and quality of work are examples. The problems must be resolved (settled, worked out, solved). Otherwise, unkind words or actions may occur. The learning or work setting becomes unpleasant. Care is affected.

Resolving Conflict. *Problem solving* steps are used to resolve conflict.
- Step 1: Define the problem. *A nurse ignores me.*
- Step 2: Collect information about the problem. Do not include unrelated information. *The nurse does not look at me. The nurse does not talk to me. The nurse does not respond when I ask for help. The nurse does not ask me to help with tasks that require 2 people. The nurse talks to other staff members.*
- Step 3: Identify possible solutions. *Ignore the nurse. Talk to my supervisor. Talk to co-workers about the problem. Change jobs.*
- Step 4: Select the best solution. *Talk to my supervisor.*
- Step 5: Carry out the solution. *See below.*
- Step 6: Evaluate the results. *See below.*

Communication and good work ethics help prevent and resolve conflicts. Identify and solve problems before they become major issues. To deal with conflict:
- Ask your instructor or supervisor for time to talk privately. Explain the problem. Give facts and specific examples. Ask for advice to solve the problem.
- Approach the person with whom you have the conflict. Ask to talk privately. Be polite and professional.
- Agree on a time and place to talk.
- Talk in a private setting. No one should hear you or the other person.
- Explain the problem and what is bothering you. Give facts and specific behaviors. Focus on the problem. Do not focus on the person.
- Listen to the person. Do not interrupt.
- Identify ways to solve the problem. Offer your thoughts. Ask for the other person's ideas.
- Set a date and time to review the matter.
- Thank the person for meeting with you.
- Carry out the solution.
- Review the matter as scheduled.
  See *Focus on Communication: Resolving Conflict,* p. 50.

FOCUS ON COMMUNICATION

Resolving Conflict

Dealing with conflict is hard for many people. However, letting the problem continue will make the matter worse. The following may help you start talking to the person. Always ask the person involved if you can talk privately.

- "You say 'no' when I ask you to help me. I help you when asked. Can we talk about this privately for a few minutes?"
- "I heard you tell Sam that I was sitting in a resident's room. You seemed angry when you said it. Can we talk privately? I want to explain why I was sitting. If it bothers you, you can tell me why."
- "The new schedule shows me working every weekend this month. Please tell me why. The employee handbook says that we work every other weekend."
- "We were late for class 2 times this week when you drove. How can I help so that we are not late?"

HARASSMENT

Harassment means to trouble, torment, offend, or worry a person by one's behavior or comments. Harassment can involve age, race, ethnic background, gender identity (Chapter 6), sexuality, religion, or disability. Respect others. Do not offend others with gestures, remarks, use of touch, or through electronic communications. Do not offend others with jokes, photos, or other images (pictures, drawings, cartoons, and so on). Harassment is not legal.

You have the right not to be harassed. No student (in your NATCEP or otherwise) should be allowed to harass or bully you. The same applies to instructors and other school staff, clinical staff, and co-workers. If you believe that you are being harassed or bullied, talk to your instructor, school counselor, or work supervisor. Follow the steps in "Resolving Conflict."

See *Focus on Communication: Harassment.*

FOCUS ON COMMUNICATION

Harassment

You have the right to feel safe and not threatened. If comments make you uncomfortable, you can say: "Please don't say things like that. It's unprofessional." If someone's actions make you uneasy, you can say: "Please don't do that. It's unprofessional." Leave the area. Report the person's statements or actions to the nurse or your instructor.

Sexual Harassment

Sexual harassment involves unwanted sexual behaviors by another. The behavior may be a sexual advance or a request for a sexual favor. Some remarks, comments, and touch are sexual. The behavior affects work and comfort. In extreme cases, a job (or grade) is threatened if sexual favors are not granted.

Sexual harassment can take the form of sexting. *Sexting* combines the words *sex* and *texting*. Sexting involves creating, sending, and posting sexual text messages, photos, or videos of oneself or others. Phones and other electronic devices are used.

Victims of sexual harassment may be men or women. Men harass women or men. Women harass men or women. If you feel sexually harassed, report the matter to the nurse and the human resources officer. As a student, tell your instructor and school counselor.

Be careful about what you say or do. Even innocent remarks and behaviors can be viewed as sexual harassment. You might not be sure about your own or another person's remarks or behaviors. If so, talk to your instructor or the nurse. You cannot be too careful.

Bullying

Bullying is repeated attacks or threats of fear, distress, or harm by a bully toward a target. A bully tries to gain power and control over a target. Bullying may be:

- Physical—hitting, tripping, and so on
- Verbal—name calling, insults, teasing
- Emotional—spreading rumors, shunning, excluding
- Cyber-bullying—sending or sharing hurtful things through electronic means
- Sexual—targeting a person with repeated and harmful actions of a sexual nature
- Prejudicial—targeting a person because of race, ethnicity, religion, gender identity, or sexual orientation

Bullying can occur in work, classroom, clinical, or social settings. Cyber-bullying occurs through electronic means (including phones)—phone calls and voice messages, e-mail, chat rooms, instant messaging, text messaging, videos, photos, and social media sites.

Bullying can result in injury, emotional distress, and even death. Victims of bullying are at risk for depression, anxiety, sleep problems, and poor school or work performance. Those who bully are at risk for substance use disorders, school or work problems, and violence. If you need help with a bullying situation, talk to your instructor or supervisor.

RESIGNING FROM A JOB

A job closer to home, better pay, or new opportunities may prompt you to leave your job. School, children, and illness are other reasons. Whatever your reason for resigning, tell your employer. Agency policy may require:

- A written notice.
- A resignation letter.
- Completing a form in the human resources office.

A 2-week notice is a good practice. Do not leave without notice. Include the following in your notice.

- Reason for leaving
- The last date you will work
- Comments thanking the employer for the opportunity to work in the agency

LOSING A JOB

You must perform your job well and protect patients and residents from harm. No pay raise or losing your job results from poor performance. Failing to follow agency policy is often grounds for termination. So is failing to get along with others. Box 5-4 lists many reasons why you can lose your job. To protect your job, function at your best. Always practice good work ethics.

DRUG TESTING

Drug and alcohol use affect patient, resident, and staff safety. Quality of care suffers. Being late to or absent from work is more common. Many agencies have drug testing policies. Review your agency's policy for when and how you might be tested.

UNETHICAL STUDENT BEHAVIOR

Your NATCEP and school will likely have a code of conduct (Chapter 4). Violating the code of conduct is unethical behavior. Many of the reasons listed in Box 5-4 are violations of your school's and NATCEP's code of conduct. As a result, your school and NATCEP may take 1 or more of the following actions.

- Dismiss you from the school or NATCEP
- Issue a failing grade
- Not recommend that you take the competency evaluation (written and skills tests)

Act in an ethical manner at all times. Always try to do the right thing. If you do, you will be a successful nursing assistant.

BOX 5-4 Common Reasons for Losing a Job

- Poor attendance—not going to work or excessive tardiness (being late).
- Abandonment—leaving the job during your shift.
- Falsifying a record—job application or a person's record.
- Violent behavior in the workplace.
- Weapons in the workplace—guns, knives, explosives, or other dangerous items.
- Having, using, or distributing alcohol or drugs in the work setting. This excludes having or using drugs ordered by your doctor.
- Taking a person's drugs for your own use or giving them to others.
- Harassment.
- Offensive speech and language.
- Stealing or destroying the agency's or a person's property.
- Disrespect to patients, residents, families, visitors, co-workers, or supervisors.
- Abusing or neglecting a person.
- Invading a person's privacy.
- Failing to maintain patient, resident, family, agency, or co-worker confidentiality.
- Wrongful use of electronic communications (Chapter 4).
- Using the agency's supplies and equipment for your own use.
- Defamation—see Chapter 4 and "Gossip" (p. 46).
- Abusing meal breaks and break time.
- Sleeping on the job.
- Violating the agency's dress code.
- Violating any agency policy or care procedure.
- Tending to personal matters while on duty.

FOCUS ON P R I D E

The Person, Family, and Yourself

P ersonal and Professional Responsibility

Your job as a nursing assistant is important. You can help persons feel safe, secure, and cared for. Through good work ethics, you can make others' lives happier, easier, and less painful. Take pride in your work ethics. Your work affects quality of life.

R ights and Respect

Conflict with other students and co-workers will arise. Do not gossip, put others down, or talk about people behind their backs. These behaviors are disrespectful and not professional. Deal with conflict in a respectful and mature way.

I ndependence and Social Interaction

Smile and greet patients and residents by name. Politely introduce yourself. Display a caring and friendly manner all the time. Remain calm and helpful in stressful situations. These actions promote good relationships and reflect well on you and the agency.

D elegation and Teamwork

Your work ethics affect the team. Greet co-workers pleasantly. Help others willingly. After completing tasks, ask if you can help with anything else. Be someone others enjoy working with.

E thics and Laws

As a student and as a nursing assistant, you are responsible for following the ethical guidelines in this chapter. Patients, residents, families, visitors, and co-workers depend on you for safe and effective care.

FOCUS ON PRIDE: Application

Think of a person you enjoy working with. What qualities do you value in a co-worker? How will you apply these qualities in your work?

REVIEW QUESTIONS

Circle the BEST answer.

1 You show honesty when you
   a Help others complete tasks
   b Report mistakes
   c Remain calm
   d Are polite

2 Which will help you do your job well?
   a Sleeping 3 to 4 hours daily
   b Not wearing needed eyeglasses
   c Using drugs and alcohol
   d Exercising regularly

3 Which is a good hygiene practice?
   a Bathing weekly
   b Wearing strongly scented perfume or cologne
   c Brushing teeth after meals
   d Having long and polished fingernails

4 You are getting ready for clinical. Which is a good practice?
   a Styling hair up and off your collar
   b Wearing jewelry
   c Wearing your name badge at waist level
   d Having tattoos exposed

5 You show you are dependable as a student when you
   a Arrive 5 minutes late for class
   b Turn in incomplete assignments
   c Leave class early for a personal matter
   d Follow directions

6 Which statement reflects a good attitude?
   a "It's not my fault."
   b "I can help you."
   c "That's not my job."
   d "I did it yesterday. It's your turn."

7 A co-worker tells you that a doctor and nurse are dating. You should
   a Not repeat the comment to others
   b Ask your co-worker for more details
   c Ask other staff if they know about it
   d Text the comment to a friend you trust

8 You can share information about a patient
   a In a private conversation on social media
   b During a meal with your family
   c With the nurse
   d With staff not involved in the person's care

9 Which is professional speech and language?
   a Using vulgar words
   b Shouting
   c Arguing
   d Speaking clearly

10 Which is a courteous act?
    a Telling co-workers they did a good job
    b Calling a resident "honey"
    c Taking credit for a co-worker's work
    d Closing an elevator door as a person approaches

11 Talking to another student while your instructor is teaching
    a Shows interest   c Is distracting
    b Shows respect   d Improves learning

12 Sending text messages while working
    a Shows good time management
    b Can lead to neglect and job loss
    c Helps prevent burnout
    d Is allowed at the nurses' station

13 You are on a meal break. Which is *true*?
    a You cannot make personal phone calls.
    b Family members cannot meet you.
    c The nurse needs to know that you are off the unit.
    d You can take a few extra minutes if needed.

14 When planning your work
    a Discuss priorities with the nurse
    b Delegate tasks you will not have time to do
    c Do not ask co-workers for help
    d Plan care so that you can watch the person's TV

15 These statements are about stress. Which is *true*?
    a Personal stress does not affect work.
    b Stress affects the whole person.
    c All stress is unpleasant.
    d Stress is abnormal.

16 Thinking about work makes you doubt your abilities and feel anxious. Which action is *best*?
    a Ignore the feelings.
    b Resign from your job.
    c Call in absent.
    d Try healthy methods to reduce stress.

17 You have extra work because a co-worker is often late. To resolve the conflict
    a Explain the problem to your supervisor
    b Refuse to work with the person
    c Ignore the problem
    d Complain about the person to co-workers

18 Which statement about harassment is *true*?
    a Giving a resident a compliment is harassment.
    b Joking about a person's religion is not harassment.
    c Harassment can occur through text messages.
    d Only women are victims of harassment.

19 You are often late for work. Which is *true*?
    a Tardiness is excused if you give the reason.
    b You may be fined.
    c You can make up the time by skipping your break.
    d You can lose your job.

20 You show good ethics as a student when you
    a Ask your instructor not to record your tardiness
    b Follow your training program's dress code
    c Use class time for personal matters
    d Tell your family about residents at your clinical site

Answers to Chapter 5 questions are on p. 587.

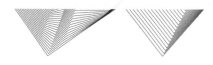

FOCUS ON **PRACTICE**

Problem Solving

A co-worker did not show up for work. You and the other staff members have extra work. How do you respond? How will you plan, prioritize, and manage the extra work?

CHAPTER 6

Communicating With the Person

OBJECTIVES

- Define the key terms in this chapter.
- Identify the parts that make up the whole person.
- Explain how to properly address the person.
- Explain Abraham Maslow's theory of basic needs.
- Explain the importance of understanding the person's culture and religion.
- Identify factors that influence health care beliefs and practices.
- Identify the elements needed for good communication.
- Describe how to use verbal and nonverbal communication.

- Explain the methods and barriers to good communication.
- Describe how behavior is a form of communication.
- List ways to manage difficult behaviors.
- Explain how to communicate with persons who have special needs.
- Explain why family and visitors are important to the person.
- Explain how to promote PRIDE in the person, the family, and yourself.

KEY TERMS

body language Messages sent through facial expressions, gestures, posture, hand and body movements, gait, eye contact, and appearance

comatose Being unable to respond to stimuli; unconscious

communication The exchange of information—a message sent is received and correctly interpreted by the intended person

culture The characteristics of a group of people—language, values, beliefs, habits, likes, dislikes, customs—passed from 1 generation to the next

disability Any lost, absent, or impaired physical or mental function

esteem The worth, value, or opinion one has of a person

gender identity A person's sense or feelings of being male, female, a combination of male and female, or neither male nor female

holism A concept that considers the whole person; the whole person has physical, psychological, social, and spiritual parts that are woven together and cannot be separated

need Something necessary or desired for maintaining life and mental well-being

nonverbal communication Communication that does not use words

paraphrasing Re-stating the person's message in your own words

religion Spiritual beliefs, needs, and practices

risk factor Something that increases the chance of illness or injury

self-esteem Thinking well of oneself and seeing oneself as useful and having value

verbal communication Communication that uses written or spoken words

Each person is unique and has value. Your care becomes more personal (individualized) as you better understand the person. Understanding the whole person helps you communicate with the person better.

THE WHOLE PERSON

Holism means *whole.* **Holism** *is a concept that considers the whole person. The whole person has physical, psychological, social, and spiritual parts. These parts are woven together and cannot be separated* (Fig. 6-1, p. 54).

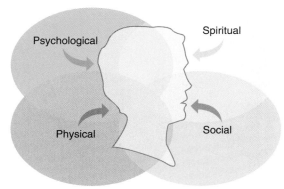

FIGURE 6-1 A person is a physical, psychological, social, and spiritual being. The parts over-lap and cannot be separated.

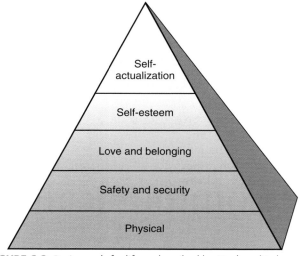

FIGURE 6-2 Basic needs for life as described by Maslow. (Redrawn from Maslow AH, Frager RD (Editor), Fadiman J (Editor): *Motivation and personality*, ed 3. © 1987. Reprinted with permission of Ann Kaplan.)

Each part relates to and depends on the others. As a social being, a person speaks and communicates with others. Physically, the brain, mouth, tongue, lips, and throat structures must function for speech. Communication is also psychological. It involves thinking and reasoning.

To consider only the physical part is to ignore the person's ability to think, make decisions, and interact with others. It also ignores experiences, life-style, culture, religion, joys, sorrows, and needs.

Addressing the Person

You must know and respect the whole person for effective, quality care. Too often a person is referred to as a room number. For example: "12A needs the bedpan" rather than "Mrs. Olson in 12A needs the bedpan." This strips the person of his or her identity.

To address patients and residents with dignity and respect:

- Greet the person by title—Mrs. Jones, Mr. Wills, Miss Parker, Ms. Norris, or Dr. Gonzalez. Then ask what name the person prefers.
- Do not use their first names or any other name unless they ask you to.
- Do not call them grandma, papa, sweetheart, honey, or other names.

Gender Identity. *Gender identity refers to a person's sense or feelings of being male, female, a combination of male and female, or neither male nor female.* Sometimes a person's biological sex (male or female) does not fit with the person's gender identity. There may be name and pronoun changes. For example, Jamie and "she" and "her" are used instead of James and "he" and "him." Or Allison is changed to Allen with pronoun changes.

Use the person's preferred name and pronouns. These are included in the person's care plan (Chapter 7).

BASIC NEEDS

A *need is something necessary or desired for maintaining life and mental well-being.* According to psychologist Abraham Maslow, basic needs must be met for a person to survive and function. The needs are arranged in order of importance (Fig. 6-2). Lower-level needs must be met before higher-level needs.

Basic needs, from the lowest level to the highest level, are:

- *Physical needs.* Oxygen, food, water, elimination, rest, and shelter are needed to live and survive. A person dies within minutes without oxygen. Without food or water, weakness and illness occur within hours. The kidneys and intestines must function. If not, poisonous wastes build up in the blood and can cause death. Without enough rest and sleep, a person becomes very tired. Without shelter, the person is exposed to extremes of heat and cold.
- *Safety and security needs.* The person needs to feel safe from harm, danger, and fear. Health care often involves strange equipment, pain, and discomfort. People feel more secure if they know what will happen. For each task, even a simple bath, the person should know:
  - Why it is needed
  - Who will do it
  - How it will be done
  - What sensations or feelings to expect
- *Love and belonging needs.* These needs relate to love, closeness, affection, and meaningful relationships with others. Family and friends meet love and belonging needs. The health team can also provide meaningful interaction.
- *Self-esteem needs.* **Esteem** *is the worth, value, or opinion one has of a person.* **Self-esteem** *means to think well of oneself and to see oneself as useful and having value.* People often lack self-esteem when ill, injured, older, or disabled.
- *The need for self-actualization.* *Self-actualization* means *experiencing one's potential.* It involves learning, understanding, and creating to the limit of a person's ability. This is the highest need. Rarely, if ever, is it totally met. Most people constantly try to learn and understand more. This need can be postponed and life will continue.

CULTURE AND RELIGION

Culture is the characteristics of a group of people—language, values, beliefs, habits, likes, dislikes, and customs. They are passed from 1 generation to the next. Culture affects thinking and behavior when health care is needed.

People come from many cultures, races, and nationalities. Their family practices and food choices may differ from yours. So might their hygiene habits and clothing styles. Some speak a foreign language. Some cultures have beliefs about what causes and cures illness. They may perform rituals to rid the body of disease. Many cultures have health beliefs and rituals about dying and death (Chapter 44). Culture also is a factor in communication.

Religion relates to spiritual beliefs, needs, and practices. Religions may have beliefs about daily living, behaviors, relationships with others, diet, healing, days of worship, birth and birth control, drugs, and death.

Many people find comfort and strength from religion during illness. They may want to pray and observe religious practices. Hospitals and nursing centers offer religious services and have areas for prayer. Assist the person to attend services as needed.

A person may not follow all the beliefs and practices of his or her culture or religion. Some people do not practice a religion. Each person is unique. Do not judge the person by your standards. And do not force your ideas on the person.

See *Caring About Culture: Culture and Religion.*
See *Focus on Communication: Culture and Religion.*

HEALTH CARE BELIEFS AND PRACTICES

Many factors affect a person's health care beliefs and practices. Age, gender, culture, and religion are some. Family and work roles, education, income, family and social support, and community resources are others. Past health problems and family history of illness also shape a person's thoughts and behaviors.

These and other factors influence the person's:
- Life-style choices
- Thoughts about risk
- Practices to promote health and prevent illness and injury
- Decisions about treatment
- Access to care
- Ability to follow through with a treatment plan

The nurse asks questions to better understand the person's beliefs and practices. The nurse teaches the person about risk factors. A *risk factor is something that increases the chance of illness or injury.* Some risk factors can be controlled. Others cannot. For example, a person has a family history of heart disease. The nurse teaches the person about diet, exercise, and not smoking. The goal is to promote health and decrease the risk of illness and injury.

See *Caring About Culture: Health Care Beliefs and Practices,* p. 56.

 CARING ABOUT CULTURE

Culture and Religion

The following guidelines will help you communicate with persons from different cultures.
- Determine your own beliefs. Do not let your own ideas, attitudes, beliefs, or values negatively affect care.
- Learn about the person's culture. You can ask the nurse and the person. The person's family may be another valuable source.
- Remember that each person is unique. A person may not follow all of the beliefs and practices of his or her culture.
- Consider how culture affects communication. Modify your approach to meet the person's needs. For example, it is important to learn how listening (p. 59) is communicated in the person's culture.
- Be alert to signs of fear, anxiety, or confusion.
- Be kind and attentive to needs.
- Have an attitude of interest, respect, and flexibility.
- Be patient and develop trust. Listen well and allow time for the person to respond. If the person gives "extra" information, listen with interest. Give the person your full attention.
- See "Verbal Communication" on p. 56 for communicating with persons who speak a foreign language.

Modified from Giger JN: *Transcultural nursing: assessment and intervention,* ed 7, St Louis, 2017, Mosby.

FOCUS ON **COMMUNICATION**

Culture and Religion

The person's care plan (Chapter 7) communicates practices to include in his or her care. Check the care plan for the person's preferences.

Show interest in the person's culture and religion. You can ask about beliefs or practices important to the person. Be respectful. For example:
- "Do you have any cultural or religious practices that should be part of your care?"
- "Your cross is pretty. Does it have special meaning for you?"
- "I see that you like your food prepared a certain way. I am interested in why it is important to you."
- "I understand that you speak Spanish and English. Can you teach me some Spanish words?"

CARING ABOUT CULTURE

Health Care Beliefs and Practices

Culture can influence beliefs about the cause of illness and how to treat illness. The following are examples.

Some *Chinese* cultures believe in a balance of 2 forces—*yin* and *yang*. Body organs are in either a yin or a yang group. Foods have either yin (cold) or yang (hot) qualities. Foods can cause or treat illness. The opposite force is used for treatment. For example, a person believes an infection (caused by yang forces) can be treated with green vegetables and fruits (foods with yin qualities). Spacial arrangements (the practice of *feng shui*), colors, and numbers may also be believed to affect health and life.

The hot-cold balance is also a belief of some *Vietnamese* groups. Illnesses, food, drugs, and herbs have hot or cold qualities. Hot is given to balance cold illnesses. Cold is given for hot illnesses. Folk practices include *cao gio* ("rub wind")—rubbing the skin with a coin to treat the common cold. Skin pinching,

known as *bat gio* ("catch wind"), may be done for headaches and sore throats. Herbs, oils, and soups are used for many signs and symptoms.

In *Mexican* culture, some believe that outside forces (luck or God) control health. Some believe that health and illness are related to a balance of certain forces (hot, cold, wet, dry). The opposite force is used to cure an illness. Older adults may believe that health problems are a result of age and not seek treatment. Seeking care from a family member with knowledge of folk medicine or a folk healer is common in *Mexican* culture. An herbalist (*yerbero, yerbera*) uses herbs and spices to prevent or cure disease. A healer (*curandero, curandera*) may give care for serious illness.

NOTE: *Each person is unique. A person may not follow all of the beliefs and practices of his or her culture. Follow the care plan.*

Modified from Giger JN: *Transcultural nursing: assessment and intervention,* ed 7, St Louis, 2017, Mosby.

EFFECTIVE COMMUNICATION

Good communication is needed to give effective care. **Communication** *is the exchange of information—a message sent is received and correctly interpreted by the intended person.*

You communicate with the person every time you give care. You give information to the person. The person gives information to you. For effective communication between you and the person, follow the rules in Box 6-1.

See *Focus on Older Persons: Effective Communication.*

BOX 6-1 Communicating With the Person

- Use words that have the same meaning for you and the person.
- Avoid medical terms and words not familiar to the person.
- Communicate in a logical and orderly manner. Do not wander in thought.
- Give facts and be specific.
- Be brief and concise.
- Understand and respect the patient or resident as a person.
- View the person as a physical, psychological, social, and spiritual human being.
- Appreciate the person's problems and frustrations.
- Respect the person's rights, religion, and culture.
- Give the person time to understand the information that you give.
- Repeat information as often as needed. Repeat what you said. Use the exact same words. Do not give the person a new message to process. If the person does not seem to understand after repeating, re-phrase the message. This is very important for persons with hearing problems.
- Ask questions to see if the person understood you.
- Be patient. People with memory problems may ask the same question many times. Do not say that you are repeating information.
- Include the person in conversations when others are present. This includes when a co-worker is assisting with care.

FOCUS ON OLDER PERSONS

Effective Communication

Communicating with persons who have dementia can be hard. The Alzheimer's and Related Dementias Education and Referral Center (ADEAR) recommends the following.
- Gain the person's attention before speaking. Say the person's name. Make eye contact.
- Be aware of your voice tone and body language (p. 58).
- Choose simple words and short sentences. Give simple, step-by-step instructions.
- Use a gentle, calm voice. Show a caring manner.
- Do not talk to the person as you would a baby.
- Do not talk about the person as if he or she is not there.
- Keep distractions and noise to a minimum.
- Repeat instructions as needed. Be patient.
- Give the person time to respond. Do not interrupt.
- Try to provide the word the person is struggling to find.
- State questions and instructions in a positive way. For example, "please do this" instead of "don't do that."

You will learn more about how to communicate with persons with Alzheimer's disease and other types of dementia in Chapter 42.

Verbal Communication

Verbal communication uses written or spoken words. Most verbal communication involves the spoken word. Follow these rules.
- Face the person. Look directly at the person.
- Position yourself at the person's eye level. Sit or squat by the person as needed.
- Control the loudness and tone of your voice.
- Speak clearly, slowly, and distinctly.
- Do not use slang or vulgar words.
- Repeat information as needed.
- Ask 1 question at a time. Wait for an answer.
- Do not shout, whisper, or mumble.
- Be kind, courteous, and friendly.

You use the written word when the person cannot speak or hear but can read. The nurse and care plan tell you how to communicate with the person (Fig. 6-3). The person may have poor vision. When writing messages:
- Keep them simple and brief.
- Use a black felt pen on white paper.
- Print in large letters.
- Use black and a large font (print size) if using a computer or other electronic device.

Some persons cannot speak or read. Ask questions that have "yes" or "no" answers. The person can nod, blink, or use other gestures for "yes" and "no." Follow the care plan. Persons who are deaf may use sign language. See Chapter 39.

See *Caring About Culture: Verbal Communication.*

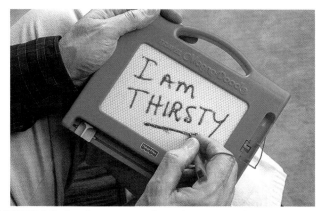

FIGURE 6-3 A written message is used to communicate.

CARING ABOUT CULTURE

Verbal Communication

Persons from different cultures may speak a language you do not understand. The following are helpful when communicating with a person who speaks a different language.
- Convey comfort by your voice tone and body language (p. 58).
- Speak slowly and clearly. Do not speak loudly or shout.
- Keep messages short and simple.
- Use words that you know the person understands. Avoid using medical terms and abbreviations.
- Use a language dictionary or a list of common words and phrases. See *Evolve Student Learning Resources* for a "Spanish Vocabulary and Phrases Audio Glossary."

- Use gestures or pictures to communicate (Fig. 6-4).
- Be alert for signs that the person does not understand. A confused or concerned look is an example. Or the person may pretend to understand. Nodding and answering "yes" to all questions may signal that the person does not understand.
- Repeat the message as often as needed. Say the message in another way if needed.

When health care staff cannot speak the person's language, a translator (interpreter) is used. If used, speak as if speaking to the person, not the translator. Digital translators (electronic language translators) offer another means of communication.

Modified from Giger JN: *Transcultural nursing: assessment and intervention*, ed 7, St Louis, 2017, Mosby.

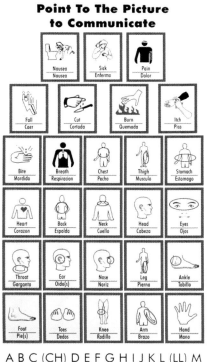
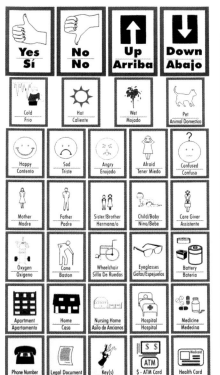
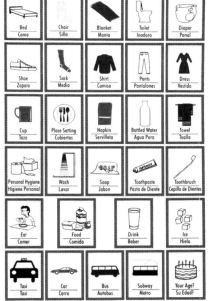

FIGURE 6-4 A picture board in English and Spanish.

Nonverbal Communication

Nonverbal communication does not use words. Gestures, facial expressions, posture, body movements, touch, and smell are used. Nonverbal messages more accurately reflect a person's feelings than words do. They are usually involuntary and hard to control. A person may say one thing but act another way. Watch the person's eyes, hand movements, gestures, posture, and other actions. They may tell you more than words.

Touch. Touch is an important form of nonverbal communication. It conveys comfort, caring, love, affection, interest, trust, concern, and reassurance. Touch means different things to different people. The meaning depends on age, gender, experiences, and culture.

Some people do not like being touched. However, touching an arm or shoulder or holding a hand can comfort a person. Touch should be gentle—not hurried, rough, or sexual. To use touch, follow the person's care plan. Remember to maintain professional boundaries.

See *Caring About Culture: Touch.*

CARING ABOUT CULTURE

Touch

Touch practices vary among cultural groups. The following are examples.

- For *Americans*, hugs are common among family and friends. A pat on the shoulder is often a gesture of friendship. A firm hand-shake can show good character and be a sign of strength.
- In some *American Indian* groups, a firm, lengthy hand-shake may be seen as aggressive and offend the person. Instead, there is a light touch, grasp, or just the passing of hands.
- In the *East Indian Hindu* culture, showing public affection is usually considered disrespectful. A common greeting is to bow with clasped hands and say the word *namaste* ("I bow to thee").
- In *Japanese* culture, touch is often minimal, especially among adults. Likewise, in *Chinese* culture, people do not usually touch each other while speaking. Touching a person's head is very rude.
- Touch is often used in *Mexican* cultures. A hug or hand-holding while walking is common among close friends.

  Note: *Each person is unique. A person may not follow all of the beliefs and practices of his or her culture. Follow the care plan.*

Modified from Giger JN: *Transcultural nursing: assessment and intervention,* ed 7, St Louis, 2017, Mosby.

Body Language. With *body language, messages are sent through facial expressions, gestures, posture, hand and body movements, gait, eye contact, and appearance.* Appearance includes clothing, hygiene, jewelry, perfume, cosmetics, body art and piercings, and so on.

Many messages are sent through body language. Slumped posture may mean the person is not happy or not feeling well. A person may deny pain but stand, sit, or lie in a certain way to protect a body part.

Your actions, movements, and facial expressions send messages. Your body language should show interest, caring, respect, and enthusiasm.

Often you will need to control your body language. Control reactions to odors from body fluids or the person's body. The person cannot control some odors. Embarrassment increases if you react to odors.

See *Caring About Culture: Body Language.*

CARING ABOUT CULTURE

Body Language

Facial Expressions

Through facial expressions, *Americans* may communicate:

- *Coldness*—there is a constant stare. Face muscles do not move.
- *Fear*—eyes are wide open. Eyebrows are raised. The mouth is tense with the lips drawn back.
- *Anger*—eyes are fixed in a hard stare. Upper lids are lowered. Eyebrows are drawn down. Lips are slightly compressed.
- *Tiredness*—eyes are rolled upward.
- *Disapproval*—eyes are rolled upward.
- *Disgust*—eyes are narrowed. The upper lip is curled. There are nose movements.
- *Embarrassment*—eyes are turned away or down. The face is flushed. Pretending to smile; rubbing the eyes, nose, or face; and twitching the hair, beard, or mustache are common.
- *Surprise*—the person has a direct gaze with raised eyebrows.

  Italian, Jewish, African American, and *Hispanic* persons are known to smile readily. They may use many facial expressions and gestures for happiness, pain, or displeasure. *Irish, English,* and *Northern European* persons tend to have less facial expression.

  In some cultures, facial expressions mean the opposite of what the person feels. For example, *Asians* may conceal negative emotions with a smile.

Eye Contact

In the *American* culture, eye contact usually signals a good self-concept. It also shows openness, interest in others, attention, honesty, and warmth. Lack of eye contact can mean:

- Shyness
- Lack of interest
- Humility
- Guilt
- Embarrassment
- Low self-esteem
- Rudeness
- Dishonesty

  For some *Asian* and *American Indian* cultures, eye contact is impolite. It is an invasion of privacy. In certain *Indian* cultures, eye contact is avoided with persons of higher or lower socio-economic class. Long, direct eye contact may be avoided in *African American* cultures.

  Note: *Each person is unique. A person may not follow all of the beliefs and practices of his or her culture. Follow the care plan.*

Modified from Giger JN: *Transcultural nursing: assessment and intervention,* ed 7, St Louis, 2017, Mosby.

Communication Methods

Certain methods help you communicate with others. They result in better relationships. More information is gained about the person.

Listening. Listening means to focus on verbal and nonverbal communication. You use sight, hearing, touch, and smell. You focus on what the person is saying. You observe nonverbal clues. They can support or not support what the person says. For example, a person says: "I want to stay here so my family won't have to care for me." You see tears. The person looks away from you. The person's verbal says *happy;* nonverbal shows *sadness.*

Listening requires that you care and have interest. Follow these guidelines.
* Face the person.
* Make eye contact.
* Lean toward the person (Fig. 6-5). Do not sit back with your arms crossed.
* Respond to the person. Nod your head. Say: "uh huh," "mmm," and "I see." Ask questions. Repeat what you heard. See "Paraphrasing."
* Avoid the communication barriers (p. 60). See *Caring About Culture: Listening.*

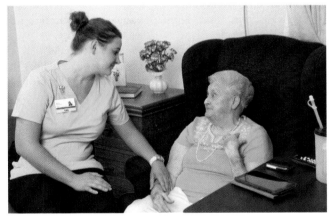

FIGURE 6-5 Listen by facing the person. Have good eye contact. Lean toward the person.

CARING ABOUT CULTURE

Listening

Communicating respect is important in all cultural groups. This can be shown in how you listen. Giving the person your attention and showing kindness and interest communicate respect. In some cultures, eye contact communicates listening. In others, the listener turns an ear to listen.

Modified from Giger JN: *Transcultural nursing: assessment and intervention,* ed 7, St Louis, 2017, Mosby.

Paraphrasing. *Paraphrasing is re-stating the person's message in your own words.* You use fewer words than the person did. Paraphrasing:
* Shows you are listening.
* Lets the person see if you understand the message.
* Promotes more communication.

The person usually responds to your statement. For example:

> *Mrs. Hayes:* I grew up on a farm. I never liked having to get up so early in the morning. The days were long and tiring.
> *You:* You like to sleep in?
> *Mrs. Hayes:* Yes, I would much rather stay up later and sleep until the sun rises.

Direct Questions. Direct questions focus on certain information. You ask what you need to know. Some direct questions have "yes" or "no" answers. Others require more information. For example:

> *You:* Mr. Walker, do you want to shower this morning?
> *Mr. Walker:* Yes.
> *You:* Mr. Walker, when would you like to do that?
> *Mr. Walker:* Could we start in 15 minutes? I want to call my son first.
> *You:* Yes, we can start in 15 minutes. You said you didn't eat much breakfast. What did you eat?
> *Mr. Walker:* I had toast and coffee. I didn't feel like eating.

Open-Ended Questions and Statements. Open-ended questions and statements lead or invite the person to share thoughts, feelings, or ideas. The topic is broad. The person controls the information given. Answers require more than a "yes" or "no." For example:
* "What do you like about living with your son?"
* "Tell me about your grandchildren."
* "What do you like about being retired?"

Clarifying. Clarifying helps you understand the message. You can ask the person to repeat the message, say you do not understand, or re-state the message. For example:
* "Could you say that again?"
* "I'm sorry. I don't understand what you mean."
* "Are you saying that you want to go home?"

Focusing. Focusing deals with a certain topic. It is useful when a person rambles or wanders in thought. For example, a person talks at length about places to eat. You need to know why the person did not eat much breakfast. To focus on breakfast you say: "Let's talk about breakfast. You said you didn't feel like eating."

Silence. Silence is a powerful way to communicate. Sometimes you do not need to say anything. This is true during sad times. Just being there shows you care.

At other times, silence gives time to think, organize thoughts, or choose words. It also helps when the person is upset and needs to gain control. Silence on your part shows caring and respect for the person's situation and feelings.

Pauses or long silences may seem uncomfortable. You do not need to talk when the person is silent. The person may need silence.

Communication Barriers

Communication barriers prevent the sending and receiving of messages. Communication fails.

- *Unfamiliar language.* You and the person may speak different languages. Or you use words the person does not understand. Slang, medical terms, and abbreviations are examples.
- *Cultural differences.* The person may attach different meanings to verbal and nonverbal communication.
- *Changing the subject.* Someone changes the subject when the topic is uncomfortable.
- *Giving your opinion.* Opinions involve judging values, behaviors, or feelings. Let others express feelings and concerns without adding your opinion. Do not make judgments or jump to conclusions.
- *Talking a lot when others are silent.* Talking too much is usually from nervousness and discomfort with silence.
- *Failure to listen.* Do not pretend to listen. It shows lack of interest and caring. This causes poor responses. You miss important information or symptoms to report to the nurse.
- *Pat answers.* "Don't worry." "Everything will be okay." "Your doctor knows best." These show a lack of caring about the person's concerns, feelings, and fears.
- *Illness and disability.* Speech, hearing, vision, cognitive function, and body movements are often affected. Verbal and nonverbal communication is affected.
- *Age.* Values and communication styles vary among age-groups.

See *Focus on Communication: Communication Barriers.*

FOCUS ON **COMMUNICATION**

Communication Barriers

Some persons who need a translator may normally have a family member translate. However, in health care settings, the nurse may prefer to use a translator from the agency. Trained translators know medical terms. Family or friends may state something other than what was meant. Receiving wrong information is a risk.

Having family or friends translate also violates the right to privacy. The *Health Insurance Portability and Accountability Act of 1996 (HIPAA)* protects the right to privacy and security of a person's health information (Chapter 4). Privacy is protected when using the agency's translator.

The *Patient Protection and Affordable Care Act of 2010* requires health care agencies to provide access to language assistance services. Qualified interpreters and written information in other languages are examples.

BEHAVIOR

Behaviors communicate needs. Understanding some of the causes of the following behaviors can help you give better care.

- *Anger.* Causes include fear, pain, and dying and death. Loss of function and loss of control over health and life are causes. Anger is a symptom of some diseases that affect thinking and behavior. Verbal outbursts, shouting, raised voices, and rapid speech are common. Some people are silent. Others are not cooperative. Nonverbal signs include rapid movements, pacing, clenched fists, and a red face. Glaring and getting close to you when speaking are other signs. Violent behaviors can occur.
- *Demanding and self-centered behavior.* Nothing seems to please the person. The person is impatient, critical, and wants care at a certain time and in a certain way. The person thinks others' needs are less important. The person expects time and attention from others. Loss of independence, loss of health, and loss of control of life are causes. So are unmet needs.
- *Aggressive behavior.* The person may swear, bite, hit, pinch, scratch, or kick. Fear, anger, pain, and dementia are causes. Protect the person, others, and yourself from harm (Chapter 11).
- *Withdrawal.* There is little or no contact with others. The person spends time alone and does not take part in social or group events. This may signal physical illness or depression. Some people are not social. They prefer to be alone.
- *Inappropriate sexual behavior.* Some people make inappropriate sexual remarks. Or they touch others in the wrong way. Some disrobe or masturbate in public. These behaviors may be on purpose. Or they are caused by disease, confusion, dementia, or drug side effects.

Such behaviors can be difficult to manage. You cannot avoid the person or lose control. Good communication is needed. Behaviors are addressed in the care plan. The care plan may include some of the guidelines in Box 6-2.

See *Focus on Communication: Behavior.*
See *Focus on Older Persons: Behavior.*

BOX 6-2 Managing Difficult Behavior

- Recognize frustrating and frightening situations. Put yourself in the person's situation. How would you feel? How would you want to be treated?
- Treat the person with dignity and respect.
- Answer questions clearly and thoroughly. Ask the nurse to answer questions you cannot answer.
- Keep the person informed. Tell the person what you are going to do and when.
- Anticipate (expect) the person's needs.
- Do not keep the person waiting. Answer call lights promptly. If you tell the person that you will do something, do it promptly.
- Explain the reason for long waits. Ask if you can get or do something to increase the person's comfort.
- Stay calm and professional, especially if the person is angry or hostile. Often the person is angry at another person or situation, not at you.
- Do not argue with the person.
- Listen and use silence. The person may feel better if able to express feelings.
- Protect yourself from violent behaviors (Chapter 11).
- Report the person's behavior to the nurse. Discuss how to help the person.

FOCUS ON COMMUNICATION

Behavior

Anger is a common response to illness and disability. The person may be angry with the situation. You might have problems dealing with anger directed at you. Act professionally. Stay calm. Listen to the person's concerns. Give needed care. Try not to take angry statements personally. If a person says hurtful things, you can kindly say: "Please don't say those things. I'm trying to help you." Tell the nurse about the person's behavior.

Caring for demanding or angry persons can be hard. Ask the nurse or co-workers to help if needed.

FOCUS ON OLDER PERSONS

Behavior

Changes in the brain with Alzheimer's disease and other forms of dementia can affect communication and judgment. Unable to communicate needs as usual, the brain uses other methods. Caregivers and staff must remember that behaviors communicate needs. For example, a person is hot. Instead of saying "I am hot," the person begins taking off clothes in the dining room. You will learn about behavior changes and how to provide for the person's needs in Chapter 42.

PERSONS WITH SPECIAL NEEDS

Each person is unique. Special knowledge and skills may be required to meet the person's needs.

The Person Who Is Comatose

Comatose (unconscious) means being unable to respond to stimuli. (A *stimulus* is something that causes a person to change, react, or respond.) The person is not alert (awake). The person cannot respond to others. Often the person can hear and can feel touch and pain. Pain may be shown by grimacing or groaning. Assume that the person hears and understands you. Use touch and give care gently. Practice these measures.

- Knock before entering the person's room.
- Tell the person your name, the time, and the place every time you enter the room.
- Follow the same schedule every day.
- Explain what you are going to do. Explain care measures step-by-step as you do them.
- Use touch to communicate care, concern, and comfort.
- Tell the person when you are completing care.
- Tell the person what time you will return.
- Tell the person when you are leaving the room.

Persons With Disabilities

A *disability is any lost, absent, or impaired physical or mental function.* Temporary or permanent, a disability can develop at any age. Disease and injury are common causes. Common courtesies and manners *(etiquette)* apply to any person with a disability. See Box 6-3 for disability etiquette.

BOX 6-3 Disability Etiquette

- Show the same courtesies to the person as you do to anyone else.
- Provide for privacy.
- Touch or handle the person's wheelchair only with consent.
- Do not hang on or lean on a person's wheelchair.
- Treat adults as adults. Use the person's first name only when asked to do so. Do the same for others present.
- Do not pat a person who is in a wheelchair on the head.
- Speak directly to the person. Do not direct questions for the person to a companion.
- Do not be embarrassed for using words that relate to the disability. For example, you say: "See you later." to a person with a vision problem.
- Sit or squat to talk to a person in a wheelchair or in a chair. You and the person are at eye level.
- Ask if help is needed before acting. If the answer is "no," respect the person's wishes. If the person wants help, ask what to do and how to do it.
- Think before giving directions to a person in a wheelchair. Think about distances, weather conditions, stairs, curbs, steep hills, and other obstacles.
- Let the person set the pace in walking, talking, or other activities.
- See Chapter 39 for persons with hearing or vision problems.

Modified from Easter Seals, *Disability etiquette*, 2022.

Persons With Bariatric Needs

Bariatrics focuses on *the treatment and control of obesity.* *Obesity* means *having an excess amount of total body fat.* Bariatric persons are at risk for many serious health problems. Heart disease, high blood pressure, stroke, cancer, and diabetes are examples. Physical and emotional needs are common. Special equipment and furniture are needed to meet the person's needs.

FAMILY AND FRIENDS

Family and friends help meet basic needs. They offer support and comfort. The presence or absence of family or friends affects the person's quality of life.

The person has the right to visit with others in private and without unneeded interruptions. You may need to give care when visitors are there. Protect the right to privacy. Do not expose the person's body in front of others. Politely ask them to leave the room. Show them where to wait. Promptly tell them when they can return. A partner or family member may want to help you. If the patient or resident consents, you can let the person stay.

Treat family and friends with courtesy and respect. They have concerns about the person's condition and care. They need support and understanding. However, do not discuss the person's condition with them. Refer their questions to the nurse.

Visiting rules depend on agency policy and the person's condition. Know your agency's visiting policies and what is allowed for the person.

Visitors may have questions about the chapel, gift shop, lounge, dining room, or business office. Know the location, special rules, and hours of these areas.

A visitor may upset or tire a person. Report your observations to the nurse. The nurse will speak with the visitor about the person's needs.

FOCUS ON P R I D E

The Person, Family, and Yourself

P ersonal and Professional Responsibility

Improving communication is on-going. You may be uncomfortable with patient or resident interactions at first. To develop communication skills:

- Use methods such as listening and clarifying.
- Pay attention to the nonverbal messages you send.
- Avoid the communication barriers.
- Learn from your mistakes.
  With practice, you will communicate more effectively. This is a valuable skill.

R ights and Respect

Some persons seem demanding and self-centered when needs are not met properly. When needs are met, they can be grateful and kind. Ask about the person's preferences. Say that you want to do the task the way the person wants it done. Listen and follow the person's preferences as much as is safely possible.

Showing respect can develop rapport. *Rapport* means you have a trusting relationship. You communicate well and have positive interactions. This can lessen or stop demanding and self-centered behaviors.

I ndependence and Social Interaction

Normal, daily activities bring pleasure, worth, and contact with others. With illness and disability, such activities may be hard or impossible. The person may feel angry and useless when help is needed with routine functions. The need for hospital or long-term care can bring feelings of isolation and loneliness. Self-esteem is affected.

To provide a sense of identity, worth, and belonging:

- Greet each person by name. Smile and show that you are happy to see the person.
- Talk to the person while giving care.
- Take an extra minute to talk or just listen.
- Encourage as much independence as possible. This often takes more time. Plan and be patient. Encouragement and independence improve self-esteem.
- Focus on the person's abilities, not the disabilities.
- Allow private time with visitors.

D elegation and Teamwork

Your co-workers are valuable resources. If you have questions or need advice, ask. For example, a resident shows anger when told it is time to shower. You ask the nurse if the task is difficult for other nursing assistants. The nurse shares advice about timing of the shower, words to say and avoid, and distraction techniques. You try, and the person is calmer.

Value your co-workers. Thank them for helpful advice.

E thics and Laws

You will care for persons with different ideas, values, and life-styles. These shape the person's character and identity. Each person is unique and has value. Do not insult the person or force your views and beliefs on the person. Respect the person as a whole.

FOCUS ON PRIDE: Application

Imagine yourself as a patient or resident. What would you want the staff to know about you? Ask 1 or 2 others what would be important to them. How does understanding the person help you give better care?

Circle the BEST answer.

1 You apply holism when you focus on
   a What the family thinks the person needs
   b What you think the person needs
   c The person's physical, psychological, social, and spiritual needs
   d The person's health care problems

2 Which basic need is the *most* essential?
   a The need to feel safe
   b The need to feel valued
   c The need for affection
   d The need for food

3 A person says: "I'm falling!" Which needs are *most* important at the time?
   a Self-actualization needs
   b Safety and security needs
   c Love and belonging needs
   d Self-esteem needs

4 Which statement about culture and religion is *true*?
   a Cultural and religious practices are not allowed in nursing centers.
   b A person must follow all beliefs and practices of his or her culture or religion.
   c Culture and religion influence health care practices.
   d Culture and religion do not influence food choices.

5 A patient is talking about her culture. You should
   a Listen with interest
   b Change the subject
   c Give your opinion
   d Pretend to listen

6 A person has risk factors for illness. The nurse teaches about risk factors to
   a Help the person form healthy practices
   b Control the person's decisions
   c Show that the person has been making bad choices
   d Earn the person's trust

7 Which is *true*?
   a Nonverbal communication uses the written or spoken word.
   b Verbal communication is the truest reflection of a person's feelings.
   c Body language cannot be controlled.
   d Touch means different things to different people.

8 You touch a person on the forearm and smile. Which response shows the touch was received well?
   a The person pulls the arm away.
   b The person moves your hand off of the arm.
   c The person pats your hand and smiles back.
   d The person says "ouch" and grabs the arm.

9 Which shows that you are listening?
   a You sit with your arms crossed.
   b You have eye contact with the person.
   c You avoid asking questions.
   d You use communication barriers.

10 Which is an open-ended question?
   a "What hobbies do you enjoy?"
   b "Do you want to wear your red sweater?"
   c "Would you like eggs and toast for breakfast?"
   d "Do you want to sit in your chair?"

11 You ask: "What name do you prefer?" This is
   a A communication barrier
   b A direct question
   c Paraphrasing
   d An open-ended question

12 Which promotes communication?
   a "Don't worry."
   b "Everything will be fine."
   c "This is a good nursing center."
   d "Go ahead. I'm listening."

13 Which is a barrier to communication?
   a Focusing
   b Asking questions
   c Talking a lot when others are silent
   d Using familiar language

14 A person wants care given at a certain time and in a certain way. Nothing seems to please the person. Which response is *best*?
   a "Please stop being so picky."
   b "I'm sorry. I don't have time for this."
   c "Please tell me what you would like done."
   d "You are never happy with what I do."

15 A person is angry. You should
   a Put yourself in the person's situation
   b Ignore the behavior
   c Ask the person to be nicer
   d Avoid the person

16 A person is comatose. Which action is *correct*?
   a You assume that the person cannot hear.
   b You explain what you are going to do.
   c You use listening and silence to communicate.
   d You enter the room without knocking.

17 A person uses a wheelchair. For effective communication, you should
   a Lean on the wheelchair
   b Pat the person on the head
   c Direct questions to the companion
   d Sit or squat next to the person

18 A visitor seems to tire a person. What should you do?
   a Ask the person to leave.
   b Tell the nurse.
   c Stay in the room to observe the person and visitor.
   d Find out the visitor's relationship to the person.

Answers to Chapter 6 questions are on p. 587.

FOCUS ON **PRACTICE**

Problem Solving

A resident was admitted to the center last month. The resident is withdrawn, impatient, and angry toward the staff. Explain possible reasons for the behaviors. How will you manage the behaviors and provide quality care?

CHAPTER 7

Health Team Communications

OBJECTIVES

- Define the key terms and key abbreviations in this chapter.
- Explain why health team members need to communicate.
- Describe the rules for good communication.
- Explain the purpose, parts, and information found in the medical record.
- Describe the legal and ethical aspects of medical records.
- Describe the 5 steps in the nursing process.
- Explain your role in the nursing process.
- Explain the difference between objective and subjective data (signs and symptoms).

- List the observations and information you need to report to the nurse.
- List the rules for recording.
- Explain how electronic devices are used in health care.
- Explain how to protect the right to privacy when using electronic devices.
- Describe how to answer phones.
- Use the 24-hour clock.
- Explain how to promote PRIDE in the person, the family, and yourself.

KEY TERMS

assessment Collecting information about the person; see "nursing process"

chart See "medical record"

electronic health record (EHR) An electronic version of a person's medical record; electronic medical record

electronic medical record (EMR) See "electronic health record"

end-of-shift report A report that the nurse gives at the end of the shift to the on-coming shift; change-of-shift report

evaluation To measure if goals in the planning step were met; see "nursing process"

implementation To perform or carry out nursing interventions (nursing measures, nursing actions, nursing tasks) in the care plan; see "nursing process"

medical record The legal account of a person's condition and response to treatment and care; chart

nursing care plan A written guide about the person's nursing care; care plan

nursing diagnosis A health problem that can be treated by nursing measures; see "nursing process"

nursing intervention An action or measure taken by the nursing team to help the person reach a goal; nursing action, nursing measure, nursing task

nursing process The method nurses use to plan and deliver nursing care; its 5 steps are assessment, nursing diagnosis, planning, implementation, and evaluation

objective data Information that is seen, heard, felt, or smelled by an observer; signs

observation Using the senses of sight, hearing, touch, and smell to collect information

planning Setting priorities and goals; see "nursing process"

recording The written account of care and observations; charting, documentation

reporting The oral account of care and observations

signs See "objective data"

subjective data Things a person tells you about that you cannot observe through your senses; symptoms

symptoms See "subjective data"

KEY ABBREVIATIONS

ADL	Activities of daily living	EMR	Electronic medical record
BM	Bowel movement	EPHI; ePHI	Electronic protected health information
CMS	Centers for Medicare & Medicaid Services	MDS	Minimum Data Set
EHR	Electronic health record	PHI	Protected health information

Communication is needed for coordinated and effective care. Health team members share information about:
- What was done for the person
- What needs to be done for the person
- The person's response to treatment

For example, a patient needs comfort measures. The nurse plans to give a pain-relief drug and asks you to position the person. The nurse explains the plan to you and the patient. The nurse tells you when the drug is given and evaluates the person's response. You position the person. The nurse records about pain. You report and record the care you gave. The nurse reports observations and care to the next nurse on duty.

Communication and care were coordinated. The person knew what to expect. Care was reported and recorded so team members know what was done.

You need to practice the aspects and rules of communication. Then you can communicate effectively with the nursing and health teams. For good communication, see Box 7-1.

THE MEDICAL RECORD

The *medical record (chart) is the legal account of a person's condition and response to treatment and care.* Medical records are written on paper forms or electronically with computers or other electronic devices. An *electronic health record (EHR) or electronic medical record (EMR) is an electronic version of a person's medical record.* Most agencies use EHRs (EMRs) (Fig. 7-1).

The health team uses the medical record to communicate information about the person. The record is a permanent legal document. Often it is used months or years later if the person's health history is needed. It can be used in court as legal evidence of the person's problems, treatment, and care.

Government and accrediting agencies review medical records to see if license, certification, or accrediting standards have been met. The record is also used to determine the amount paid for services (Chapter 1).

The record has different parts (Table 7-1, p. 66). Each part has the person's name, identification (ID) number, room and bed number, and other identifying information. The record tells about care provided and the person's response.

BOX 7-1 Communication Rules

- Use words that have the same meaning for you and the message receiver. Avoid words with more than 1 meaning. Does "far" mean 50 feet or 100 feet?
- Ask about messages you do not understand. You will learn medical terms (Chapter 8). If you do not know a term, ask what it means. Or use a dictionary. You must understand the message for communication to occur.
- Be brief and concise. Do not add unrelated or unnecessary information. Stay on the subject. Do not wander in thought or get wordy.
- Give information in a logical and orderly way. Organize your thoughts. Present them step-by-step.
- Give facts and be specific. Reporting a pulse rate of 110 is more specific than "the pulse is fast."

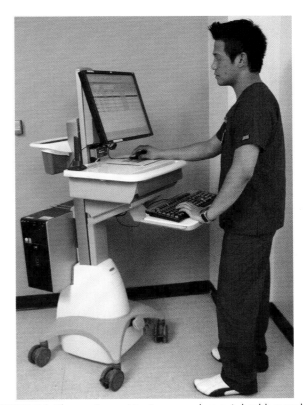

FIGURE 7-1 The nursing assistant uses an electronic health record (electronic medical record).

TABLE 7-1 Parts of a Medical Record

Part	Description
Admission record	Completed on admission (entry) into the agency. Contains personal and identifying information—legal name, birth date, age, biological sex (male or female), address, insurance information, marital status, nearest relative and legal representative, religion, place of worship, employer, diagnoses, date and time of admission, doctor's name. A signed general consent for treatment is included.
Advance directives	A document stating a person's wishes about end-of-life care (Chapter 44).
Health history	A record of the person's medical history. • Chief complaint—reason for seeking health care • History of current illness—onset (time, sudden or gradual) and signs and symptoms • Past health problems, surgeries, and injuries • Childhood illnesses • Allergies and type of reaction • Current drugs • Vaccinations • Family health history • Life-style—habits, diet, sleep, hobbies • Adaptive (assistive) devices used—dentures, eyeglasses, contact lenses, hearing aids, cane, walker, wheelchair, and so on • Ability to perform *activities of daily living (ADL)*—the activities usually done during a normal day in a person's life • Education and occupation
Nursing assessment	Data collected during the nurse's physical assessment (p. 68).
Nursing care plan; care plan	A guide about the person's nursing care (p. 70).
Nursing progress notes	*Progress notes* describe the care given and the person's response and progress (Fig. 7-2). For example, the nurse records: • Signs and symptoms • Information about treatments and drugs • Information about teaching and counseling • Procedures performed • Visits by health team members
Flow sheets and graphic sheets	Used for frequent care measures, measurements, and observations (Fig. 7-3). • Hygiene and grooming measures • Activity and positioning • Vital signs—temperature, pulse, respirations, blood pressure, and pulse oximetry (Chapters 31 and 37) • Weight • Intake and output (Chapter 30) • Urinary and bowel elimination
Medication administration record (MAR); electronic medication administration record (eMAR)	A record of drugs ordered, given, and not taken.
Physical examination	Information collected during the physical examination. The examination is done by a doctor or advanced practice registered nurse (APRN).
Orders	Directions from the doctor or APRN about tests and care measures to be performed.
Progress notes (health team)	Reports from the health team—medical (doctor, APRN); physical, occupational, speech-language, and recreational therapies; dietary; social services; and others.
Laboratory results	Results of tests done on blood, urine, and other body fluids and tissues.
X-ray reports	Results of x-ray tests.
Therapy records	Records for intravenous (IV), respiratory, wound care, and other therapies.
Consultation reports	Reports from other health care providers consulted by the person's doctor.
Special consents	Signed permissions for surgeries and procedures needing informed consent (Chapter 4).
Discharge summary	Information and instructions for the person when leaving the agency—wound care; drug prescriptions and changes; rest, activity, and exercise; diet; signs and symptoms to report; follow-up appointments.

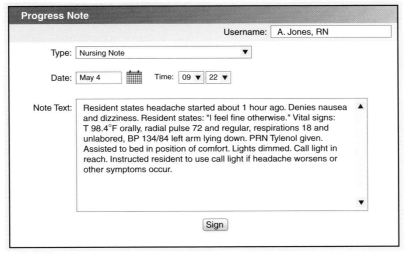

Progress Note

Username: A. Jones, RN

Type: Nursing Note ▼

Date: May 4 📅   Time: 09 ▼ 22 ▼

Note Text: Resident states headache started about 1 hour ago. Denies nausea and dizziness. Resident states: "I feel fine otherwise." Vital signs: T 98.4°F orally, radial pulse 72 and regular, respirations 18 and unlabored, BP 134/84 left arm lying down. PRN Tylenol given. Assisted to bed in position of comfort. Lights dimmed. Call light in reach. Instructed resident to use call light if headache worsens or other symptoms occur.

Sign

FIGURE 7-2 A sample progress note.

		06/16 12:00	06/16 13:00	06/16 13:10	06/16 13:20	06/16 15:00	06/16 15:10	06/16 15:15			
Vital Signs	Temperature	98.4									
	Pulse	72									
	Respiration	18									
	Blood Pressure	118/76									
	O2SAT	99									
	O2 L/M										
Intake/Output	P.O. ORAL	240									
	New Intake										
	VOIDED URINE			250			200				
	New Output										
	NUTRITION:	SELF									
	ELIMINATION:			TOILET			TOILET				
Activity	ACTIVITY:	CHAIR	CHAIR	BATH	BED	AMBUL	BATH	BED			
	POSITIONING:	SELF			BACK		RIGHT				
	HYGIENE:		ORAL	PERI			PERI				
Safety	SAFETY:	CALL	CALL	BELT	CALL	BELT	BELT	CALL			

Ready   Interface   CHART MENU   Reflex   Completed   Room: 274-1   Exit

FIGURE 7-3 A sample flow sheet. (Courtesy Abraham Lincoln Memorial Hospital, Lincoln, Ill.)

Legal and Ethical Aspects

Agencies have policies about medical records and who can see them. Policies address:

- Who records
- When to record
- Ink color (paper charting)
- Abbreviations
- How to make and sign entries
- How to correct errors

Some agencies allow nursing assistants to record observations and care. Others do not. Follow your agency's policies.

Professional staff involved in a person's care can review charts. Cooks and laundry, housekeeping, and office staff do not need to read charts. Some agencies let nursing assistants read charts. If not, the nurse shares needed information.

You have an ethical and legal duty to keep information confidential. If not involved in the person's care, you have no right to read the person's chart. Doing so is an invasion of privacy.

Patients and residents have the right to the information in their medical records. The person or the person's legal representative may ask to see the chart. Tell the nurse. The nurse handles the request.

THE NURSING PROCESS

The *nursing process* is the method nurses use to plan and deliver nursing care. It has 5 steps.

- *Assessment*
- *Nursing diagnosis*
- *Planning*
- *Implementation*
- *Evaluation*

The person and nursing team need good communication. With good communication, nursing care is organized and has purpose. All nursing team members do the same things for the person. They focus on the same goals for the person.

The nursing process is on-going. New information is gathered and the person's needs may change. However, the steps are the same. You will see how the nursing process is continuous as each step is explained (Fig. 7-4, p. 68).

The nurse is responsible for the nursing process. You assist through the observations you make and the care you give.

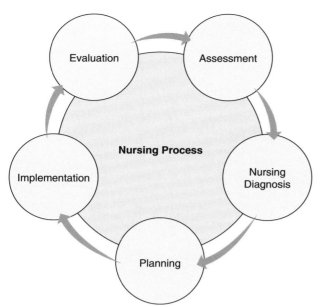

FIGURE 7-4 The nursing process is continuous.

Assessment

Assessment involves collecting information about the person. The nurse takes a health history about current and past health problems. The family's health history is important. Information from the doctor is reviewed. So are test results and past medical records.

The nurse assesses the person's body systems and mental status. You assist with assessment. You make observations as you give care and talk to the person.

Observation is using the senses of sight, hearing, touch, and smell to collect information.

- You *see* how the person lies, sits, or walks. You see flushed or pale skin. You see red and swollen body areas.
- You *listen* to the person breathe, talk, and cough. You use a stethoscope to measure blood pressure.
- Through *touch*, you feel if the skin is hot or cold, or moist or dry. You use touch to take a pulse.
- *Smell* is used to detect body, wound, and breath odors. You also smell odors from urine and bowel movements (BMs).

The word *data* relates to information that is collected and used for decision making. *Objective data (signs) are seen, heard, felt, or smelled by an observer.* You can feel a pulse. You can see urine color. *Subjective data (symptoms) are things a person tells you about that you cannot observe through your senses.* You cannot feel or see the person's pain, fear, or nausea.

Box 7-2 lists observations to report at once (right away). You will also learn about signs and symptoms of conditions that require emergency care in Chapter 43. Box 7-3 lists the basic observations to make and report to the nurse. Note your observations as you make them. Use your notes when reporting to the nurse (p. 72).

You do not assess. The nurse performs the assessment step of the nursing process. However, what you observe helps the nurse with assessment.

See *Focus on Communication: Assessment.*

The Minimum Data Set. The Centers for Medicare & Medicaid Services (CMS) requires the *Minimum Data Set (MDS)* for nursing center residents (Appendix C, p. 592). The MDS is an assessment tool. It provides information about the person. Examples include memory, communication, hearing and vision, physical function, and activities.

The nurse uses your observations for the MDS. The MDS is started when the person is admitted to the center. The MDS is updated before each care conference (p. 70). A new MDS is done once a year and for a significant change (decline or improvement) in the person's health status.

Nursing Diagnosis

The nurse uses assessment information (data) to make a nursing diagnosis. A *nursing diagnosis describes a health problem that can be treated by nursing measures.* Nursing diagnoses deal with the person's physical, emotional, social, and spiritual needs.

Nursing diagnoses and medical diagnoses are not the same. A *medical diagnosis* is the identification of a disease or condition by a doctor. Cancer, stroke, heart attack, and diabetes are examples. Doctors use drugs, therapies, and surgery to cure or heal.

BOX 7-3 Basic Observations

Ability to Respond
- Is the person easy or hard to wake up?
- Can the person give his or her name, the time, and location when asked?
- Does the person identify others correctly?
- Does the person answer questions correctly?
- Does the person speak clearly?
- Are instructions followed correctly?
- Is the person calm, restless, or excited?
- Is the person conversing, quiet, or talking a lot?

Movement
- Can the person squeeze your fingers with each hand?
- Can the person move arms and legs?
- Are movements shaky or jerky?
- Does the person complain of stiff or painful joints?
- Are there areas of weakness?
- Does the person complain of fatigue (feeling tired)?

Pain or Discomfort
- Where is the pain located? (Have the person point to the pain.)
- Does the pain go anywhere else?
- How does the person rate the severity of the pain—mild, moderate, severe?
- How does the person rate the pain on a scale of 0 to 10 (Chapter 33)?
- When did the pain begin?
- What was the person doing when the pain began?
- How long does the pain last?
- How does the person describe the pain?
  - Sharp
  - Severe
  - Stabbing
  - Dull
  - Burning
  - Aching
  - Comes and goes
  - Depends on position
- Was a pain-relief drug given?
- Did the pain-relief drug relieve pain? Is pain still present?
- Can the person sleep and rest?
- What is the position of comfort?

Skin
- Is the skin pale or flushed?
- Is the skin cool, warm, or hot?
- Is the skin moist or dry?
- Does the skin appear mottled (blotchy, spotted with color)?
- What color are the lips and nail beds?
- Is the skin intact? Are there broken areas? If so, where?
- Are sores or reddened areas present? If yes, where?
- Are bruises present? If yes, where?
- Does the person complain of itching? If yes, where?

Eyes, Ears, Nose, and Mouth
- Is there drainage from the eyes? Drainage color?
- Are the eyelids closed? Do they stay open?
- Are the eyes reddened?
- Does the person complain of spots, flashes, or blurring?
- Is the person sensitive to bright lights?
- Is there drainage from the ears? Drainage color?
- Can the person hear? Is repeating necessary? Are questions answered correctly?
- Is there drainage from the nose? Drainage color?

Eyes, Ears, Nose, and Mouth—cont'd
- Can the person breathe through the nose?
- Is there breath odor?
- Does the person complain of a bad taste in the mouth?
- Does the person complain of painful gums or teeth?
- Do the person's gums bleed with oral hygiene (Chapter 21)?
- Does the person with dentures say that the dentures are loose or do not fit well?

Respirations
- Do both sides of the chest rise and fall with respirations?
- Is breathing noisy?
- Does the person complain of pain or difficulty breathing?
- What is the amount and color of sputum?
- How often does the person cough? Is the cough dry or productive?

Bowels and Bladder
- Is the abdomen firm or soft?
- Does the person complain of gas?
- Which does the person use: toilet, commode, bedpan, or urinal?
- What are the amount, color, and consistency of bowel movements (BMs)?
- What is the frequency of BMs?
- Can the person control BMs?
- Does the person have pain or difficulty urinating?
- What is the amount of urine?
- What is the color of urine?
- Is the urine clear? Are there particles in the urine?
- Does urine have a foul smell?
- Can the person control the passage of urine?
- What is the frequency of urination?

Appetite
- Does the person like the food served?
- How much of the meal is eaten?
- What foods does the person like?
- Can the person chew food?
- What is the amount of fluid taken?
- What fluids does the person like?
- How often does the person drink fluids?
- Can the person swallow food and fluids?
- Does the person cough when swallowing?
- Does the person complain of nausea?
- What is the amount and color of vomitus?
- Does the person have hiccups?
- Is the person belching?

Activities of Daily Living
- Can the person perform personal care without help?
  - Bathing?
  - Brushing teeth?
  - Combing and brushing hair?
  - Shaving?
- Does the person need help with feeding?
- Can the person walk?
- What amount and kind of help is needed?
- Does the person have problems using adaptive (assistive) devices? Examples include devices for mobility (walker, cane, wheelchair), devices for hygiene and grooming (Chapters 22 and 23), and devices for eating (Chapter 29).

Bleeding
- Is the person bleeding? If yes, from where and how much?

A person can have many nursing diagnoses. For example, a person is unable to bathe, move in bed, and walk without help. Nursing diagnoses address each of these issues. Nursing diagnoses may change as assessment information changes. Or new ones are added.

Planning

Planning involves setting priorities and goals.
- *Priorities*—what is most important for the person.
- *Goals*—what is desired for or by a person as a result of nursing care. Also called *objectives*, goals are aimed at the person's highest level of well-being and function.

Nursing interventions are chosen after goals are set. An *intervention* is an *action or measure*. A **nursing intervention** *(nursing action, nursing measure, nursing task) is an action or measure taken by the nursing team to help the person reach a goal.* A nursing intervention does not need a doctor's order. Actions to prevent falls, provide hygiene, and promote comfort are examples.

The **nursing care plan** *(care plan) is a written guide about the person's nursing care.* It has the person's nursing diagnoses and goals. It also has the nursing measures or actions for each goal. A communication tool, the care plan:
- Communicates what care to give
- Helps ensure that nursing team members give the same care

The care plan is found in the written or electronic medical record. The plan is carried out. It may change as nursing diagnoses change.

See *Focus on Surveys: Planning.*

Care Conferences. Care conferences are held to share information and ideas about the person's care. The purpose is to develop or revise the nursing care plan. Effective care is the goal. Nursing assistants may take part in the conference.

See *Focus on Communication: Care Conferences.*

The Comprehensive Care Plan. The CMS requires a *comprehensive care plan.* It is a guide about the person's care. The plan has the person's problems, nursing diagnoses, goals, and actions to take.

For example, the MDS shows that a resident cannot do activities of daily living (ADL). A care plan is developed to solve the problem. The goal is for the resident to perform ADL. Actions to reach the goal are:
- Occupational therapy for ADL daily
- Physical therapy for exercises daily
- Nursing staff to walk the resident 20 yards twice daily

The care plan also has the person's strengths. For example, the resident can eat without help. This strength increases independence. The health team helps the resident to continue to eat without help.

Implementation

To *implement* means *to perform or carry out.* In the **implementation** *step, nursing interventions (nursing measures, nursing actions, nursing tasks) in the care plan are performed or carried out.* Care is given.

Nursing care ranges from simple to complex. The nurse delegates tasks within your legal limits and job description. The nurse may delegate or ask you to assist with complex measures.

Assignment Sheets. The nurse communicates delegated tasks to you. An assignment sheet is used for this purpose (Fig. 7-5). The assignment sheet tells you about:
- Each person's care.
- What nursing interventions and tasks to do.
- Which nursing unit tasks to do. Cleaning utility rooms and stocking shower rooms are examples.

Talk to the nurse about an unclear assignment. Also check the care plan for more information.

See *Focus on Communication: Assignment Sheets.*

Evaluation

Evaluate means *to measure.* The **evaluation** *step involves measuring if the goals in the planning step were met.* Progress is evaluated. Goals may be met totally, in part, or not at all. Assessment information is used for this step. Changes in nursing diagnoses, goals, and the care plan may result.

Assignment Sheet

Date: _9–10_
Shift: _Day_
Nursing assistant: _J. Reed_
Supervisor: _M. Garcia, RN_

Breaks: _1000_   _1400_
Lunch: _1230_
Unit Tasks: _Pass drinking water at 0900_
Clean utility room at 1430

*Check the care plan for other care measures and information

Room # _501A_ Name: _Mrs. Ann Lopez_ ID Number: _S1514491530_ Date of birth: _11/04/1934_ VS: _Daily at 0700_ T _____ P _____ R _____ BP _____ Wt: _Weekly (Monday at 0700)_ _____ Intake _____ Output _____ BM _____ Bath: _Complete bed bath_ Shampoo Bed rails	**Functional status/ care measures and procedures** Total assist with ADL Full-sling mechanical lift transfer Uses wheelchair with footplates Incontinent of bowel and bladder – uses briefs Passive ROM exercises to extremities twice daily Turn and re-position q2h when in bed Wears eyeglasses and dentures Diet: High fiber (total assist)
Room # _510B_ Name: _Mr. Mark Lee_ ID Number: _D4468947762_ Date of birth: _12/29/1940_ VS: _2 times daily, at 0700 and 1500_ 0700: T _____ P _____ R _____ BP _____ 1500: T _____ P _____ R _____ BP _____ Wt: _Daily at 0700_ _____ Intake _____ Output _____ BM _____ Bath: _Shower_	**Functional status/ care measures and procedures** Independent with ADL Independent with ambulation Attends exercise group every morning Continent of bowel and bladder – q4h bathroom schedule to maintain continence Wears eyeglasses Coughing and deep-breathing exercises q4h Diet: Sodium-controlled (independent)

FIGURE 7-5 A sample assignment sheet. NOTE: This assignment sheet is a computer printout.

Your Role

You have key roles in the nursing process. Your observations are used for nursing diagnoses and planning. You may help develop care plans. In the implementation step, you perform tasks in the care plan. Your assignment sheet tells you what to do. Your observations are used for the evaluation step.

REPORTING AND RECORDING

The health team communicates by reporting and recording. **Reporting** *is the oral account of care and observations.* **Recording** *(charting, documentation) is the written account of care and observations.*

Reporting and Recording Time

The 24-hour clock (military time or international time) has 4 digits (Fig. 7-6, *A*). The first 2 digits are for the hours. The last 2 digits are for the minutes. A colon and AM and PM are not used.

The 24-hour clock is shown in Figure 7-6, *B*. The clock begins at midnight. After the noon hour (1200), the hours keep counting up (13, 14, and so on) instead of starting over at 1 (as done with conventional time). When midnight is reached (2400 or 0000), a new day begins. Follow agency policy for whether to use 2400 or 0000 for midnight. Box 7-4 (p. 72) shows how conventional time is written in 24-hour time.

See *Focus on Math: Reporting and Recording Time*, p. 72.
See *Focus on Communication: Reporting and Recording Time*, p. 72.

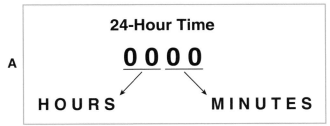

A

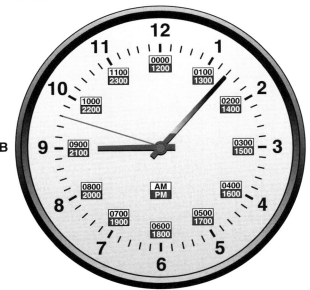

B

FIGURE 7-6 24-hour time. **A,** In 24-hour time, there are 4 digits. The first 2 are for the hours. The last 2 are for the minutes. A colon and AM and PM are not used. **B,** The 24-hour clock. NOTE: 12:00 AM (midnight) is 0000 (or 2400 in some agencies); 12:00 PM (noon) is 1200.

BOX 7-4 24-Hour Time

AM		PM	
Conventional Time	24-Hour Time	Conventional Time	24-Hour Time
12:00 MIDNIGHT	0000 or 2400	12:00 NOON	1200
1:00 AM	0100	1:00 PM	1300
2:00 AM	0200	2:00 PM	1400
3:00 AM	0300	3:00 PM	1500
4:00 AM	0400	4:00 PM	1600
5:00 AM	0500	5:00 PM	1700
6:00 AM	0600	6:00 PM	1800
7:00 AM	0700	7:00 PM	1900
8:00 AM	0800	8:00 PM	2000
9:00 AM	0900	9:00 PM	2100
10:00 AM	1000	10:00 PM	2200
11:00 AM	1100	11:00 PM	2300

FOCUS ON COMMUNICATION

Reporting and Recording Time

Reading and saying 24-hour time is different than conventional time.

- When a 24-hour time begins with zero (0), read or say the "0" as "zero" or "oh."
- When the last 2 digits (minutes) end in "00," read or say the numbers as "hundred" or "hundred hours."
- When the last 2 digits are numbers other than 2 zeros (00), read or say the first 2 numbers (hours) and the last 2 numbers (minutes).

  The following are examples of how to say 24-hour times.
- 0200: "zero two hundred (hours)" or "oh two hundred (hours)"
- 1700: "seventeen hundred (hours)"
- 0620: "zero six twenty" or "oh six twenty"
- 1215: "twelve fifteen"

FOCUS ON MATH
Reporting and Recording Time

A *digit* is any number from 0 to 9. With conventional time, 3 or 4 digits are used with a colon and AM or PM (7:30 AM, 7:45 PM, 10:15 PM). With 24-hour time, 4 digits are used without a colon and without AM or PM (0730, 1945, 2215).

When changing from conventional time to 24-hour time, the hours from 1:00 PM to 11:00 PM require math. Twelve (12) is added to the hours digit(s). The minutes digits do not change. See Figure 7-7.

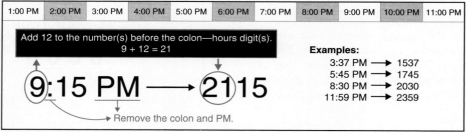

FIGURE 7-7 From 1:00 PM to 11:00 PM, add 12 to the hours digit(s) to change from conventional time to 24-hour time. Remove the colon and PM.

Reporting

Report care and observations to the nurse.

- When there is a change from normal or a change in the person's condition. Report these changes at once.
- When the nurse asks you to do so.
- Before leaving the unit for meals, breaks, or other reasons.
- Before the end-of-shift report. See "End-of-Shift Report."
- After the end-of-shift report and before reporting off duty.

  When reporting, follow the rules in Box 7-5.

BOX 7-5 Rules for Reporting

- Be prompt, thorough, and accurate.
- Give the person's name and room and bed number.
- Give the time you made the observations or gave care. Use 24-hour time or conventional time (AM or PM) according to agency policy.
- Report only what you observed and did yourself.
- Report care measures that the person might need. For example, the person may need the bedpan during your meal break.
- Report expected changes in the person's condition. For example, the person may be tired after lunch.
- Give reports as often as the person's condition requires. Also give them when the nurse asks you to.
- Report at once any changes from normal or changes in the person's condition.
- Use your written notes for a specific, concise, and clear report.

End-of-Shift Report. *The nurse gives a report at the end of the shift to the on-coming shift. This is called the* **end-of-shift report** *or change-of-shift report.* The nurse reports about:

- The care given
- The care to give during other shifts
- The person's current condition
- Likely changes in the person's condition
- New or changed orders

Some agencies have the entire nursing team hear the end-of-shift report as they come on duty. In other agencies, only nurses hear the report. After the report, nursing assistants receive needed information.

See *Promoting Safety and Comfort: End-of-Shift Report.*

PROMOTING SAFETY AND COMFORT

End-of-Shift Report

Safety

You may not hear the end-of-shift report as you come on duty. You answer call lights and give care before the nurse shares information with you. For safe care:

- Check the care plan before granting a request. The person's condition or care plan may have changed. There may be new orders.
- Ask a nurse about the care needs of new patients or residents. If the need is urgent, politely interrupt the end-of-shift report to ask your questions.
- Do not take directions or orders from another nursing assistant. Remember, nursing assistants cannot supervise or delegate to other nursing assistants.

You may answer call lights during the end-of-shift report as you go off duty. Be sure to report observations, care measures, requests, and so on before you leave. For example, you assist a resident onto the bedpan before going home. The nursing team of the on-coming shift needs to know so they can check on the person. Otherwise the person could be left on the bedpan for a long time, causing the person harm.

Recording

When recording (documenting, charting), you must communicate clearly and thoroughly. Follow the rules in Box 7-6. Anyone reading your charting should know:

- What you observed
- What you did
- The person's response

See *Focus on Communication: Recording.*

FOCUS ON COMMUNICATION

Recording

"Small," "moderate," "large," "long," and "short" mean different things to different people. Measurements and descriptions like "dime-sized" or "quarter-sized" are clearer. If not sure how to describe something, ask the nurse for help.

BOX 7-6 Rules for Recording

General Rules

- Follow agency policies and procedures for recording. Ask for needed training.
- Check the name and identifying information on the chart. You must record on the correct chart.
- Include the date and time for each recording. Use 24-hour time or conventional time (AM or PM) according to agency policy.
- Use only agency-approved abbreviations (see "Abbreviations" in Chapter 8).
- Use correct spelling, grammar, and punctuation.
- Do not use ditto (") marks.
- Record only what you observed and did yourself. Do not record for another person.
- Never chart a procedure, treatment, or care measure until after it is completed.
- Be accurate, concise, and factual. Do not record judgments or interpretations. For example, "The person felt sad" is a judgment. "The person was crying" is factual.
- Record in a logical manner and in sequence.
- Be descriptive. Avoid terms with more than 1 meaning.
- Use the person's exact words when possible. Use quotation marks ("…") for a direct quote.
- Chart changes from normal or changes in the person's condition. Also chart that you told the nurse (include the nurse's name), what you said, and the time you made the report.
- Do not omit (leave out) information.
- Record safety measures. Examples include placing the call light within reach, assisting the person when up, or reminding a person not to get out of bed.
- Sign or save all entries as required by agency policy.

On Computer

- Log in (sign in) using your username and password (Fig. 7-8, p. 74). Do not use another person's username.
- Check the time your entry is made. Make sure it is the right time.
- Check for accuracy. Review your entry before saving.
- Save your entries. Un-saved data will be lost. You click an icon or button to save the entry. If you forget, most systems have a reminder. You can choose to log off without saving (delete the entry) or save the entry.
- Follow the manufacturer's instructions to change or un-chart a mistaken entry. Most electronic systems keep a record of original entries and changes.
- Log off after charting. This prevents others from charting under your username.
- See "Electronic Devices" on p. 75.

On Paper

- Make sure each form and page has the person's name and other identifying information.
- Always use ink. Use the ink color required by the agency.
- Make sure writing is readable and neat.
- Follow agency policy for correcting errors. Never erase or use correction fluid (white out). Draw a line through the incorrect part. Date and initial the line. Write "mistaken entry" over it if this is agency policy. Then re-write the part. See Figure 7-9, p. 74.
- Sign your entry. Include your name and title at the end (see Fig. 7-9).
- Do not skip lines. Draw a line through the blank space of a partially completed line or to the end of the page (see Fig. 7-9). This prevents others from recording in a space with your signature.

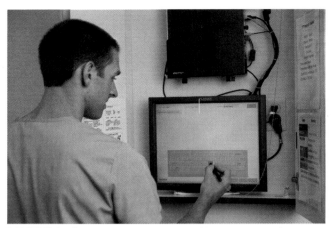

FIGURE 7-8 The nursing assistant enters his username and password to log in to a medical record.

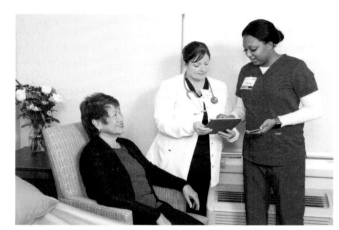

Date	Time	Nursing Margin / Other Depts Margin
7/26	1045	Requested assistance to lie down. States, "I don't feel well. I have a little upset stomach."
		Denies pain. VS taken. T-99(0). P-76 regular rate and rhythm. R-18 unlabored.
		BP 134/84 L arm lying down. Call light within reach. Paula Jones, RN notified at 1040.
		Mary Jensen, CNA
7-26	1100	Asleep in bed. Appears to be resting comfortably. Color good. No signs of
		discomfort or distress noted at this time. Paula Jones, RN
7-26	1145	Refused to go to the dining room for lunch. Reports nausea.
		Denies abdominal pain. Has not had an emesis. Abdomen soft to
		palpation. Good bowel sounds. VS taken. T~98.2~ 99.2. P-76 regular (Mistaken entry 7-26, PJ)
		rate and rhythm. R-18 unlabored. BP-134/84. States she will try to
		eat something. Full liquid room tray ordered. Paula Jones, RN

FIGURE 7-9 Progress note on paper. A mistaken entry is corrected by drawing a single line through the incorrect part.

Electronic Recording. Electronic health (medical) records improve access to medical records. Recording may be done in patients' or residents' rooms, in hallways, at the nurses' station, or on portable or hand-held devices (Fig. 7-10).

Users log in (sign in) to access or record on the person's medical record. You will be trained to use your agency's system. An electronic charting sample is shown in Figure 7-11.

FIGURE 7-10 Hand-held electronic devices are used to access and record on the person's medical record.

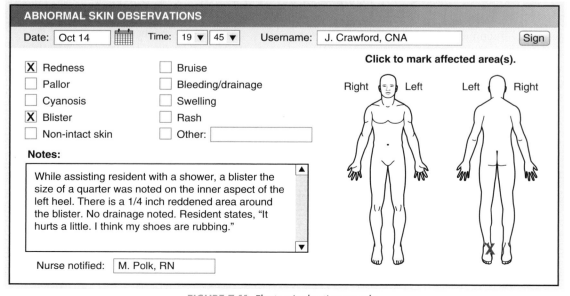

FIGURE 7-11 Electronic charting sample.

ELECTRONIC DEVICES

Electronic devices are used to store and send information to the health team. Computers and portable and hand-held devices are common. Fax machines are used to send and receive paper documents.

Follow agency policies when using electronic devices. Use only your username and password. You must keep protected health information (PHI) and electronic protected health information (EPHI; ePHI) confidential. Follow the rules in Box 7-7 and the ethical and legal rules about privacy, confidentiality, and defamation (Chapters 4 and 5) when using electronic devices.

PHONE COMMUNICATIONS

You will answer phones at the nurses' station or in the person's room. Use good communication skills. Your tone of voice, speech clarity, and attitude are important. Be professional and courteous. Also practice good work ethics. Follow the agency's policy and the guidelines in Box 7-8 (p. 76).

BOX 7-7 Electronic Devices

Computers and Portable and Hand-Held Devices
- See "Wrongful Use of Electronic Communications" in Chapter 4.
- Do not tell anyone your username or password. With your information, others can access, record, send, receive, or store PHI (EPHI; ePHI) under your name. It will be hard to prove you did not do so.
- Do not write down, post, or expose your username or password. This is for your security. For example, do not write them on a note pad or post them at your work station.
- Change your password often. Follow agency policy.
- Do not use another person's username or password.
- Follow the rules for recording (see Box 7-6).
- Enter data carefully. Double-check your entries.
- Prevent others from seeing the screen.
  - Place the screen so it cannot be seen by others.
  - Be aware of anyone standing behind you.
  - Stand or sit with your back to the wall if using a mobile computer.
  - Do not leave a device unattended.
- Log off after making an entry.
- Do not leave printouts where others can read or pick them up.
- Shred or destroy printouts, assignment sheets, or worksheets. Place such documents in a wastebasket marked *CONFIDENTIAL INFORMATION* for shredding. Follow agency policy.
- Send e-mail and messages only to those needing the information.
- Do not e-mail information or messages that require immediate reporting. Give the report in person. The person may not read the e-mail in a timely manner.
- Do not use e-mail or messages to report confidential information. This includes addresses, phone numbers, and Social Security numbers. The computer system may not be secure.
- Remember that any communication can be read or heard by someone other than the intended person.
- Remember that deleted communications can be retrieved by authorized staff.

Computers and Portable and Hand-Held Devices—cont'd
- Do not use agency devices for personal use. Do not:
  - Send personal e-mail messages.
  - Send or receive e-mail or messages that are offensive, not legal, or sexual.
  - Send or receive e-mail for illegal activities, jokes, politics, gambling (including football and other pools), chain letters, or other non-work activities.
  - Post information, opinions, or comments on websites or video or social media sites.
  - Upload, download, or send materials containing a copyright, trademark, or patent.
- Remember that the agency has the right to monitor your use of electronic devices. This includes Internet use.
- Do not open another person's e-mail or messages.
- Follow agency policy for mis-directed e-mails.

Faxes
- See "Wrongful Use of Electronic Communications" in Chapter 4.
- Use the agency's "cover sheet." The sheet has instructions about:
  - The confidentiality of PHI (EPHI; ePHI)
  - The receiver's responsibilities about PHI (EPHI; ePHI)
  - The receiver's responsibilities for a fax received in error (mis-directed fax)
- Complete the "cover sheet" according to agency policy. The following are common.
  - Name of the person to receive the fax
  - Receiver's fax number
  - Date
  - Number of pages being faxed
  - Department name
  - Name and phone number of the person sending the fax
- Follow agency policy for a mis-directed fax.
- Do not leave sent or received faxes unattended in the fax machine or lying around.

BOX 7-8 Answering Phones

- Answer the call after the first ring if possible. Be sure to answer by the fourth ring.
- Do not answer in a rushed or hasty manner.
- Give a courteous greeting. Identify the agency or nursing unit and give your name and title. For example: "Good morning, 3 center. Pat Wills, nursing assistant."
- Follow agency policy for answering phones in patient or resident rooms.
- Note this information to take a message.
  - The caller's name and phone number (include the area code and extension number)
  - The date and time
  - Who the message is for
- Repeat the message and phone number back to the caller.
- Ask the caller to "Please hold" if necessary. First find out who is calling and the caller's number. Then ask if the caller can hold. Do not put callers with an emergency on hold.
- Do not lay the phone down or cover the receiver with your hand when not speaking to the caller. The caller may over-hear confidential conversations.
- Return to a caller on hold within 30 seconds. Ask if the caller can wait longer or if the call can be returned.
- Do not give confidential information to any caller. Patient, resident, and employee information is confidential. Refer such calls to the nurse.
- Transfer the call if appropriate.
  - Tell the caller that you are going to transfer the call.
  - Give the name of the department or the name of the person who should answer the phone if appropriate.
  - Get the caller's name and number in case the call gets disconnected.
  - Give the caller the phone number to call in case the call gets disconnected or the line is busy. Include the extension number if needed.
- End the conversation politely. Thank the person for calling and say good-bye.
- Give the message to the appropriate person.

FOCUS ON PRIDE

The Person, Family, and Yourself

Personal and Professional Responsibility

You are responsible for what you report and record. It must be accurate and timely. Remember:
- Document what you did. If you do not, it is assumed that the task was not done.
- Never document that something *was* done when it really *was not* done.
- Record a task *after* completing it, not before.

Rights and Respect

The person has the right to take part in care planning. The person also has the right to refuse actions suggested by the nursing and health teams. The goal is a plan of care that meets the person's needs and preferences.

Independence and Social Interaction

Health team communications are not limited to reporting and recording. You interact in the nurses' station, patient and resident rooms, hallways, break room, cafeteria, parking lot, and so on. Treat co-workers with kindness and respect. Have a good attitude. Be someone others enjoy working with!

Delegation and Teamwork

The end of shift requires good teamwork. Your attitude is important. Greet your co-workers politely. If going off duty, avoid saying or thinking:
- "I'm ready to go home. Let them do it."
- "It's their turn. I've been here all day (evening or night)."
- "No one helped us when we came on duty."

Some agencies have clear duties for the 2 shifts. For example, those going off duty know about the patients or residents. They continue to answer call lights. Waiting to receive report, the on-coming shift performs routine tasks and collects needed supplies and equipment.

Teamwork goes beyond those you work with at a certain time of the day. Treat co-workers on different shifts as part of the team.

Ethics and Laws

Assignment sheets have confidential information. Keep your sheets with you. Do not leave them lying around for others to find. This violates the *Health Insurance Portability and Accountability Act of 1996* (Chapter 4). Before leaving work, place your assignment sheets in a wastebasket marked *CONFIDENTIAL INFORMATION* for shredding. Take pride in protecting the privacy and security of protected health information.

FOCUS ON PRIDE: Application

Explain why accurate and timely reporting and recording are important. What problems may occur from incorrect or delayed reporting or recording?

Circle the BEST answer.

1 To communicate well, you should
   a Use terms with many meanings
   b Give long descriptions
   c Use unfamiliar terms
   d Give facts and be specific

2 A person is discharged from the agency. The medical record is
   a Destroyed
   b Sent home with the family
   c Permanent
   d No longer private

3 You help with Mr. Hild's care. If you record on his medical record, you have
   a Violated his right to privacy
   b Provided a record of what care was given
   c The right to access his wife's medical records too
   d To give him your username so he can read what you wrote

4 You measured a person's vital signs and re-positioned the person. You should
   a Record your care on the flow sheet in the person's medical record
   b Only record if there is something abnormal
   c Not record because these are routine care measures
   d Ask the nurse to record it in the health history part of the chart

5 Which statement about the nursing process is *correct*?
   a Assessment involves gathering information.
   b Medical diagnoses and nursing diagnoses are the same thing.
   c Implementation involves planning goals and priorities.
   d The person is discharged when the evaluation step is reached.

6 You measure a person's temperature and pulse. You have
   a Performed an assessment
   b Completed the nursing process
   c Collected subjective data
   d Collected objective data

7 Which is a symptom?
   a Skin redness
   b Vomiting
   c Pain
   d Yellow urine

8 Which should you report at once?
   a The person can no longer move a body part.
   b The person answers questions correctly.
   c The person has a breath odor.
   d The person walked to the dining room.

9 The care plan
   a Is written by the doctor
   b Communicates what care to give
   c Is the same for all persons
   d Does not change after it is developed

10 To communicate delegated tasks to you, the nurse uses
   a The care plan
   b The Minimum Data Set
   c An assignment sheet
   d Care conferences

11 Your role in the nursing process involves
   a Reporting observations
   b Making nursing diagnoses
   c Writing the care plan
   d Evaluating if goals are met

12 In the evening, the clock shows 9:26. In 24-hour clock time this is
   a 9:26 PM
   b 1926
   c 0926
   d 2126

13 In the morning, the clock shows 7:45. In 24-hour clock time this is
   a 0745
   b 1945
   c 745
   d 7:45 AM

14 Which is a safe recording practice?
   a Recording a task at 1330 that you plan to do at 1400
   b Checking the identifying information on the chart before recording
   c Asking another nursing assistant to chart something for you
   d Using a co-worker's username and password to log in

15 Which entry is descriptive and concise?
   a "Mrs. Jones ate some of her breakfast."
   b "Mrs. Jones ate half of her oatmeal and half of her fruit."
   c "Mrs. Jones ate fairly well."
   d "Mrs. Jones ate as much as she usually eats."

16 You type a correct entry into an electronic medical record. You click the button to log off. A message pops up asking "Do you want to save your entry?" You should
   a Try to log off again
   b Turn off the computer
   c Click "No"
   d Click "Yes"

17 You have access to the agency's computer. Which is *true*?
   a The agency can monitor your computer use.
   b E-mail is used for reports the nurse needs at once.
   c You can post your username and password in your work area.
   d You can use the computer for your personal needs.

18 A phone rings at the nurses' station. Which greeting is *best*?
   a "Good morning. This is Joey."
   b "North hall."
   c "Good morning, North hall. Joey Wilson, nursing assistant, speaking."
   d "Hello."

Answers to Chapter 7 questions are on p. 587.

FOCUS ON **PRACTICE**

Problem Solving

You measure a patient's vital signs. You continue with other tasks before reporting or recording them. An hour later, the nurse asks for the measurements. You say: "They were fine." What problems do you notice? Can harm result? How can communication be improved?

CHAPTER 8

Medical Terminology

OBJECTIVES

- Define the key terms in this chapter.
- Identify the word parts that make up medical terms.
- Explain how to define medical terms.
- Locate the 4 abdominal quadrants.
- Identify the directional terms used to describe the locations of body parts.
- Identify the terms used to describe the position of the body when lying down.
- Define common abbreviations and health care terms.
- Explain how to promote PRIDE in the person, the family, and yourself.

KEY TERMS

abbreviation A shortened form of a word or phrase
prefix A word element at the beginning of a word; it changes the meaning of the word
root A word element that contains the basic meaning of the word

suffix A word element at the end of a word; it changes the meaning of the word
word element A part of a word

Medical terms and abbreviations are used in health care. Understanding the basics of medical terminology is important for your training and work.

If you do not understand a word, phrase, or abbreviation, ask a nurse for its meaning. Otherwise, communication does not occur. A medical dictionary is useful to learn new words.

MEDICAL TERMS

Like all words, medical terms are made up of *parts of words or word elements*—prefixes, roots, and suffixes. Most are from Greek or Latin. Word elements are combined to form medical terms (Fig. 8-1).

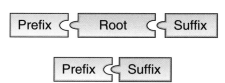

FIGURE 8-1 Prefixes, roots, and suffixes are combined to form medical terms. (Modified from Leonard PC: *Building a medical vocabulary with Spanish translations,* ed 10, St Louis, 2018, Elsevier.)

Prefixes, Roots, and Suffixes

A *prefix is a word element at the beginning of a word. It changes the meaning of the word.* For example, the prefix *hemi-* (half) is placed before *-plegia* (paralysis) to make *hemiplegia.* It means paralysis on half of the body. Prefixes are used with other word elements. Prefixes are not used alone.

The *root is the word element that contains the basic meaning of the word.* It is combined with another root, a prefix, or a suffix. A vowel (an *o* or an *i*) may be added when 2 roots are combined or when a suffix that begins with a consonant is added to a root. (A consonant is any letter other than a vowel.) The vowel *(combining vowel)* makes the word easier to pronounce.

A *suffix is a word element at the end of a word. It changes the meaning of the word.* Suffixes are not used alone. For example, *colonoscopy* means examination of the large intestine using a scope. It is formed by combining the root *colon (o)* (colon, large intestine) and the suffix *-scopy* (examination using a scope).

Learning Word Elements. Studying word elements will help you understand the meanings of medical terms.

See Table 8-1 for a list of common prefixes. The prefixes in the table are followed by a hyphen (hyper-).

See Table 8-2 (p. 81) for a list of common roots. Each root is followed by its combining vowel in parentheses [hem (o)].

See Table 8-3 (p. 82) for a list of common suffixes. The suffixes in the table are written with a hyphen at the beginning (-itis).

TABLE 8-1 Word Elements—Prefixes

Prefix	Meaning	Prefix	Meaning
a-, an-	without, no, not, lack of	intra-	within
ab-	away from	intro-	into, within
ad-	to, toward, near	leuko-	white
ante-	before, forward, in front of	macro-	large
anti-	against	mal-	bad, illness, disease
auto-	self	meg-	large
bi-	double, two (2), twice	micro-	small
brady-	slow	mono-	one (1), single
circum-	around	neo-	new
contra-	against, opposite	non-	not
cyan-	blue	olig-	small, scant
de-	down, from, off, opposite	para-	beside, beyond, after
dia-	across, through, apart	per-	by, through
dis-	apart, free from	peri-	around
dys-	bad, difficult, abnormal, painful	poly-	many, much
ecto-	outer, outside	post-	after, behind
en-	in, into, within	pre-	before, in front of, prior to
endo-	inner, inside	pro-	before, in front of
epi-	on, upon, over (Fig. 8-2, p. 80)	re-	again, backward
erythro-	red	retro-	backward, behind
eu-	normal, good, well, healthy	semi-	half
ex-	out, out of, from, away from	sub-	beneath, under (see Fig. 8-2)
hemi-	half	super-	above, over, excess
hyper-	excessive, too much, high	supra-	above, over
hypo-	under, decreased, less than normal	tachy-	fast, rapid
in-	in, into, within, not	trans-	across
inter-	between	uni-	one (1)

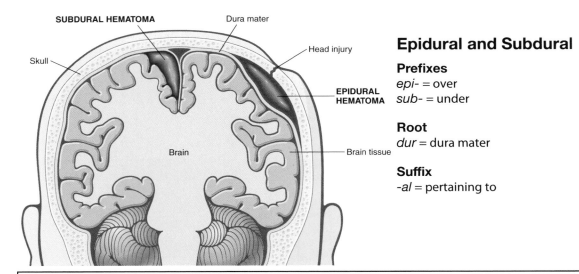

Epidural and Subdural

Prefixes
epi- = over
sub- = under

Root
dur = dura mater

Suffix
-al = pertaining to

A *prefix* is at the beginning of the word.
Changing the prefix changes the meaning of the word.

epi- + *dur* + *-al* = pertaining to <u>over</u> the dura mater (outer lining of the brain and spinal cord)

sub- + *dur* + *-al* = pertaining to <u>under</u> the dura mater (outer lining of the brain and spinal cord)

FIGURE 8-2 A prefix is at the beginning of the word. This figure shows hematomas in 2 areas of the brain. *Hematoma* means a mass of blood (*hemat* + *-oma*). *Epidural* and *subdural* describe the locations. Changing the prefix changes the meaning of the word. (Modified from Chabner D-E: *Medical terminology: a short course,* ed 8, St Louis, 2018, Elsevier.)

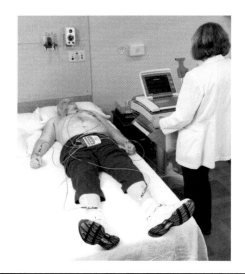

Electrocardiogram

Roots
electr (o) = electricity
cardi (o) = heart

Suffix
-gram = record

A *root* contains the basic meaning of the word.
A word can have more than 1 root.

electr (o) + ***cardi (o)*** + *-gram* = A record of the electricity in the heart

---

FIGURE 8-3 A root contains the basic meaning of the word. A word can have more than 1 root. *Electrocardiogram* has the roots *electr (o)* (meaning electricity) and *cardi (o)* (meaning heart). An electrocardiogram is a test that records the heart's electrical activity.

TABLE 8-2 Word Elements—Roots

Root (Combining Vowel)	Meaning	Root (Combining Vowel)	Meaning
abdomin (o)	abdomen	men (o)	menstruation
aden (o)	gland	my (o)	muscle
adren (o)	adrenal gland	myel (o)	spinal cord, bone marrow
angi (o)	vessel	necr (o)	death
arteri (o)	artery	nephr (o)	kidney
arthr (o)	joint	neur (o)	nerve
bronch (o)	bronchus, bronchi	ocul (o)	eye
carcin (o)	cancerous, cancer	onc (o)	tumor
card, cardi (o)	heart (Fig. 8-3)	oophor (o)	ovary
cephal (o)	head	ophthalm (o)	eye
cerebr (o)	cerebrum (largest part of the brain)	orth (o)	straight, normal, correct
chole, chol (o)	bile	oste (o)	bone
chondr (o)	cartilage	ot (o)	ear
col, colon (o)	colon, large intestine	path (o)	disease
cost (o)	rib	ped (o)	child, foot
crani (o)	skull	pharyng (o)	pharynx (throat)
cyst (o)	bladder, cyst	phleb (o)	vein
cyt (o)	cell	pneum (o)	lung, air, gas
dent (i)	tooth	proct (o)	rectum
derm, dermat (o)	skin	psych (o)	mind
duoden (o)	duodenum (part of the small intestine)	pulmon (o)	lung
dur (o)	dura mater (outer lining of the brain and spinal cord) (see Fig. 8-2)	py (o)	pus
electr (o)	electricity (see Fig. 8-3)	rect (o)	rectum
encephal (o)	brain	ren (o)	kidney
enter (o)	intestines	rhin (o)	nose
fibr (o)	fiber, fibrous	salping (o)	eustachian tube, fallopian tube
gastr (o)	stomach	splen (o)	spleen
gloss (o)	tongue	stern (o)	sternum
gluc (o)	sweetness, glucose (Fig. 8-4, p. 82)	stomat (o)	mouth
glyc (o)	sugar	therm (o)	heat
gyn, gyne, gynec (o)	woman	thorac (o)	chest
hem, hema, hem (o), hemat (o)	blood	thromb (o)	clot, thrombus
hepat (o)	liver	thyr (o)	thyroid
hydr (o)	water	toxic (o)	poison, poisonous
hyster (o)	uterus	trache (o)	trachea (windpipe)
ile (o)	ileum (part of the small intestine)	urethr (o)	urethra
ili (o)	ilium (part of the hip bone)	urin (o)	urine
jejun (o)	jejunum (part of the small intestine)	ur (o)	urine, urinary tract, urination
lapar (o)	abdomen, loin, flank	uter (o)	uterus
laryng (o)	larynx (voice box)	vas (o)	blood vessel, vas deferens
lith (o)	stone	vascul (o)	blood vessel
mamm, mast (o)	breast, mammary gland	ven (o)	vein
		vertebr (o)	spine, vertebrae

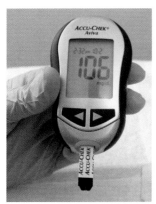

Glucometer

Root
gluc (o) = glucose

Suffix
-meter = measuring instrument

> **A *suffix* is at the end of the word.**
>
> *gluc (o)* + ***-meter*** = a measuring instrument for glucose

FIGURE 8-4 A suffix is at the end of the word. The suffix *-meter* means measuring instrument. A *glucometer* is a device used to measure blood glucose.

TABLE 8-3 Word Elements—Suffixes

Suffix	Meaning	Suffix	Meaning
-ac, -al	pertaining to (see Fig. 8-2)	-oma	tumor, mass
-algia	pain	-opsy	to view
-asis	condition, usually abnormal	-osis	condition
-cardia	heart action or location	-pathy	disease
-cele	hernia, herniation, pouching	-penia	lack, deficiency
-centesis	surgical puncture to remove fluid	-phagia	to eat or consume, swallowing
-cyte	cell	-phasia	speaking, speech
-ectasis	dilation, stretching	-phobia	an exaggerated fear
-ectomy	excision, removal of	-plasty	surgical repair or re-shaping
-emesis	vomiting	-plegia	paralysis
-emia, -emic	blood condition	-pnea	breathing, respiration
-genesis	development, production, creation	-ptosis	falling, sagging, dropping down
-genic	producing, causing	-rrhage, rrhagia	excessive flow
-gram	record (see Fig. 8-3)	-rrhaphy	stitching, suturing
-graph	a diagram, a recording instrument	-rrhea	flow, discharge
-graphy	making a recording	-sclerosis	hardening
-iasis	condition of	-scope	examination instrument
-ic	pertaining to	-scopy	examination using a scope
-ism	a condition	-stasis	maintenance, maintaining a constant level, controlling, stopping
-itis	inflammation		
-logy	the study of	-stenosis	narrowing
-lysis	breakdown, destruction of, decomposition	-stomy, -ostomy	creation of an opening
-megaly	enlargement	-tomy, -otomy	incision, cutting into
-mentia	condition of the mind	-trophy	growth, development, nourishment
-meter	measuring instrument (see Fig. 8-4)	-uria	urine

Defining Medical Terms

Medical terms are formed by combining word elements. Remember, prefixes are at the beginning. Suffixes are at the end. A root can be combined with prefixes, roots, and suffixes. Some words have only a prefix and suffix.

The combining vowel of a root is usually used between roots and when the suffix begins with a consonant. When the suffix begins with a vowel (a, e, i, o, u), the combining vowel is not used.

To define a term, separate the word into its elements (Table 8-4). To read the meaning:

1 Begin with the suffix. Read the meaning of the suffix.
2 Go to the beginning of the word. Read the meaning of each word part up to the suffix.

For some terms with only a prefix and suffix, it is easier to read the meaning of the prefix first. Then read the meaning of the suffix.

TABLE 8-4 Defining Medical Terms

Medical Term	Word Elements	Definition
Aphasia	*a-* (without, lack of) + *-phasia* (speaking) [prefix] [suffix]	Lack of speaking ability
Cyanosis	*cyan-* (blue) + *-osis* (condition) [prefix] [suffix]	Condition of having a bluish color
Dysphagia	*dys-* (difficult) + *-phagia* (swallowing) [prefix] [suffix]	Difficulty swallowing
Dyspnea	*dys-* (difficult, painful) + *-pnea* (breathing) [prefix] [suffix]	Difficult or painful breathing
Endocarditis	*endo-* (inner) + *card* (heart) + *-itis* (inflammation) [prefix] [root] [suffix]	Inflammation of the inner part of the heart
Gastroenterology	*gastr (o)* (stomach) + *enter (o)* (intestines) + *-logy* (the study of) [root] [root] [suffix]	The study of the stomach and intestines
Gastrostomy	*gastr* (stomach) + *-ostomy* (creation of an opening) [root] [suffix]	A surgically created opening in the stomach
Mastectomy	*mast* (breast) + *-ectomy* (excision or removal) [root] [suffix]	Removal of a breast
Nephritis	*nephr* (kidney) + *-itis* (inflammation) [root] [suffix]	Inflammation of the kidney
Oliguria	*olig-* (scant, small amount) + *-uria* (urine) [prefix] [suffix]	A small amount of urine

ABDOMINAL QUADRANTS

The abdomen can be divided into 4 quadrants. *Quad* means *four*. The quadrants are used to describe the location of body structures, pain, or discomfort. The quadrants are shown in Figure 8-5. They are:

- Right upper quadrant (RUQ)—contains much of the liver, the gallbladder, part of the pancreas, and parts of the small and large intestines
- Left upper quadrant (LUQ)—contains the rest of the liver, the stomach, the spleen, the rest of the pancreas, and parts of the small and large intestines
- Right lower quadrant (RLQ)—contains parts of the small and large intestines, the appendix, and part of the bladder
- Left lower quadrant (LLQ)—contains parts of the small and large intestines and part of the bladder

You will learn about the body structures found in these areas in Chapter 9.

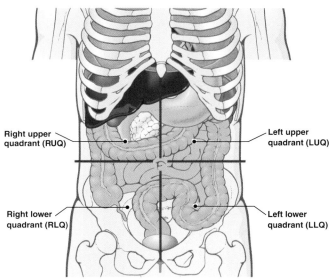

FIGURE 8-5 The 4 abdominal quadrants. (From Chabner D-E: *The language of medicine*, ed 12, St Louis, 2021, Elsevier.)

DIRECTIONAL TERMS

Certain terms describe the location of 1 body part in relation to another. These terms give the direction of the body part when a person is standing and facing forward. The arms are stretched out with the thumbs pointing outward. See Figure 8-6.

- *Anterior (ventral)*—at or toward the front of the body or body part
- *Posterior (dorsal)*—at or toward the back of the body or body part
- *Proximal*—the part nearest to the center or to the point of attachment
- *Distal*—the part farthest from the center or from the point of attachment
- *Lateral*—away from the mid-line; at the side of the body or body part
- *Medial*—at or near the middle or mid-line of the body or body part
- *Superior*—above another structure
- *Inferior*—below another structure
- *Superficial*—on the surface
- *Deep*—below the surface

Directional terms are also used to describe the location of observations (Chapter 7). For example, you report that a person has a reddened area the size of a quarter on the medial aspect (part) of the right knee. This is descriptive and concise.

POSITIONAL TERMS

These terms describe the position of the body when lying down (Chapter 16).

- *Supine*—lying flat and facing up
- *Prone*—lying flat and facing down
- *Lateral*—lying on the side
- *Fowler's*—lying on the back with the head of the bed raised

In Fowler's position, the head of the bed is raised between 45 and 60 degrees. Variations of Fowler's include *semi-Fowler's* (the head of the bed is only raised 30 degrees) and *high-Fowler's* (the head of the bed is raised 60 to 90 degrees). See Chapter 16.

ABBREVIATIONS

Abbreviations are shortened forms of words or phrases. They save time and space when recording. Each agency has a list of allowed abbreviations. Obtain the list when you are hired. Use only those on the list. If not sure about an abbreviation, write the term out in full. This promotes clear communication.

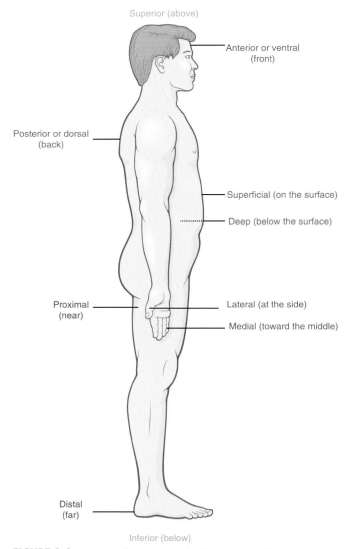

FIGURE 8-6 Directional terms describe the location of 1 body part in relation to another. (Modified from Chabner D-E: *The language of medicine*, ed 12, St Louis, 2021, Elsevier.)

See Table 8-5 for a list of common abbreviations that you may see. Most chapters in this book contain a "Key Abbreviations" list. See p. 602 for a full list of all of the Key Abbreviations used in the book.

TABLE 8-5 Common Abbreviations

Abbreviation	Meaning	Abbreviation	Meaning
abd	abdomen	lt; L	left
AC; a.c.	before meals	meds	medications
ADL	activities of daily living	mid noc	midnight
ad lib	as desired	min	minute
AIDS	acquired immunodeficiency syndrome	mL	milliliter
AM	morning	neg	negative
AMB; amb	ambulate (to walk); ambulatory (able to walk)	noc	night
amt	amount	NPO; npo	nothing by mouth (nil per os)
ap; AP	apical	O_2	oxygen
BM; bm	bowel movement	OOB	out of bed
BP	blood pressure	OR	operating room
BRP	bathroom privileges	os	mouth
$\overline{c}$	with	OT	occupational therapy
C	centigrade; Celsius	oz; OZ	ounce
cal	calories	PC; p.c.	after meals
cath	catheter	per	by, through
CBR	complete bed rest	PM	afternoon
C/O; c/o	complains of	PO; po	by mouth; orally
CPR	cardiopulmonary resuscitation	prep	preparation
CS	central service; central supply	prn	when necessary
drsg	dressing	Pt; pt	patient
Dx	diagnosis	PT	physical therapy
ECG; EKG	electrocardiogram	q	every
ER; ED	emergency room; emergency department	qh	every hour
F	Fahrenheit	q2h, q3h, etc.	every 2 hours, every 3 hours, and so on
fl; fld	fluid	R	rectal temperature, respiration
Fx	fracture	R/O	rule out
GI	gastro-intestinal	ROM	range of motion; range-of-motion
h; hr	hour	rt; R	right
H_2O	water	$\overline{s}$	without
HIV	human immunodeficiency virus	Spec; spec	specimen
ht	height	stat	at once, immediately
hx	history	tbsp	tablespoon
ICU	intensive care unit	TPR	temperature, pulse, and respirations
I&O	intake and output	tsp	teaspoon
IV	intravenous	U/a; U/A; u/a	urinalysis
L	liter	UTI	urinary tract infection
Lab	laboratory	VS; vs	vital signs
lb	pound	w/c	wheelchair
LOC	level of consciousness	Wt; wt	weight

COMMON TERMS AND PHRASES

Some terms and phrases apply to basic care, safety, or the person's condition. Because they are used throughout this book, they are defined in Table 8-6. Some are presented as key terms in other chapters.

TABLE 8-6 Common Health Care Terms and Phrases

Term	Definition
abnormal	Different from what is normal or usual
activities of daily living (ADL)	The activities usually done during a normal day in a person's life
adaptive (assistive) device	Any item used by the person or staff to promote the person's function or safety (hand rails, grab bars, mechanical lifts, canes, walkers, wheelchairs, devices for eating or dressing, and so on)
aphasia	The total or partial loss (a) of the ability to use or understand language (phasia)
atrophy	The decrease (a) in size or the wasting away of tissue (trophy)
biological sex	Male or female
call light	Part of the call system allowing the person to signal the nurses' station for help
care plan	A written guide about the person's care
chronic	An on-going illness that is slow or gradual in onset; it has no known cure; it can be controlled and complications prevented with proper treatment
cognitive function	Involves memory, thinking, reasoning, ability to understand, judgment, and behavior
contracture	The lack of joint mobility caused by abnormal shortening of a muscle
dementia	The loss (de) of cognitive and social function (mentia) caused by changes in the brain
drug	A substance taken by mouth, injected, or applied to treat or prevent a disease or condition; medication, medicine
dysphagia	Difficulty (dys) swallowing (phagia)
dyspnea	Difficult, labored, or painful (dys) breathing (pnea)
feces	The semi-solid mass of waste products in the colon that is expelled through the anus; stool or stools
fever	Elevated body temperature
incontinence	Not being able to control urination (urinary incontinence) or bowel movements (fecal incontinence)
mobility	The ability to move
orientation; oriented	Awareness of one's self and others, one's location, and the time; or awareness of one's surroundings
perineal	The genital and anal areas
pressure injury	Localized damage to the skin and underlying soft tissue; the injury is usually over a bony prominence or related to a medical or other device and results from pressure or pressure in combination with shear
range of motion (ROM)	The movement of a joint to the extent possible without causing pain
stool	Excreted feces
unconscious	Being unaware of one's setting and being unable to react or respond to people, places, or things
vital signs	Temperature, pulse, respirations, and blood pressure (and pulse oximetry [Chapter 37] and pain in some agencies)
voiding	Emptying urine from the bladder; urinating, urination

FOCUS ON P R I D E

The Person, Family, and Yourself

P ersonal and Professional Responsibility

To communicate in health care you must learn medical terms. You may feel overwhelmed at first. Begin by learning the word elements. Study a little at a time. Use a medical dictionary for words you do not understand and to learn new words. You will understand more as you study body structure, care measures, and disorders.

R ights and Respect

The person must be given information in understandable language. The person may not know medical terms. Use familiar words when talking to the patient or resident.

I ndependence and Social Interaction

Only use abbreviations allowed by your agency. Social media and texting abbreviations are not used in your work.

D elegation and Teamwork

Assignment sheets often include medical terms and abbreviations. (See "Assignment Sheets" in Chapter 7.) Review the assignment sheet example on p. 71. Do you understand the sheet better? Take pride in learning.

E thics and Laws

Never be afraid to ask for a term or abbreviation to be explained. You must know the meaning to provide safe care. A careful person asks for needed help. Negligence results when reasonable care is not taken and the person is harmed.

FOCUS ON PRIDE: *Application*

Identify ways to study word elements and medical terms. How do you plan to study? Do you study better alone or with someone? Ask other students how they plan to learn.

REVIEW QUESTIONS

Circle the BEST answer.

1 To define a medical term, what do you do *first*?
   a Read the meaning of the root.
   b Read the meaning of the suffix.
   c Separate the word into its parts.
   d Read the meaning of the prefix.

2 A suffix is
   a Placed at the beginning of a word
   b Placed at the end of a word
   c A shortened form of a word or phrase
   d The main meaning of the word

3 The prefix *hypo-* means
   a Less than normal
   b Difficult
   c Large
   d Half

4 The root *vascul (o)* means
   a Vertebrae
   b Air
   c Blood vessel
   d Heat

5 The suffix *-algia* means
   a Paralysis
   b Pain
   c Disease
   d Removal of

6 Which word means a blood condition involving too much sugar?
   a Hepatitis (hepat-itis)
   b Tachycardia (tachy-cardia)
   c Hyperglycemia (hyper-glyc-emia)
   d Hemolysis (hemo-lysis)

7 Which word means an excessive flow of blood?
   a Hemiplegia (hemi-plegia)
   b Cyanosis (cyan-osis)
   c Laparoscopy (laparo-scopy)
   d Hemorrhage (hemo-rrhage)

8 Which word means examination of the bladder using a scope?
   a Ileostomy (ileo-stomy)
   b Colonoscopy (colono-scopy)
   c Tracheostomy (tracheo-stomy)
   d Cystoscopy (cysto-scopy)

Continued

9 The stomach is located in the abdomen's
  a RUQ (right upper quadrant)
  b LUQ (left upper quadrant)
  c RLQ (right lower quadrant)
  d LLQ (left lower quadrant)

10 Which description is *correct*?
  a Proximal means far away.
  b Inferior means inside.
  c Anterior means toward the back.
  d Lateral means at the side.

11 You are studying the heart. A structure is described as "superior." This means it is
  a Below another structure
  b Above another structure
  c More important than other structures
  d Inside another structure

12 Which is *true*?
  a The shoulder is proximal and the wrist is distal.
  b The toes are posterior.
  c The brain is superficial.
  d The thumb is on the medial side of the hand.

13 You are told to place a person in the lateral position. You
  a Help the person lie flat
  b Raise the head of the bed
  c Turn the person onto the side
  d Move the person to the side of the bed

14 You must complete a task *stat*. "Stat" means
  a At once, immediately
  b As desired
  c Without moving the person
  d When necessary, as needed

15 What are ADL?
  a The activities a person does daily
  b Devices used to assist with care
  c Foods allowed on the person's diet
  d Drugs a person takes daily

16 You see I&O on your assignment sheet. I&O means
  a Inside and outside
  b Intervention and outcome
  c Intake and output
  d Inspect and observe

17 Your assignment sheet says VS q4h. You will
  a Refuse the task because it involves giving drugs
  b Have the person void 4 times during your shift
  c Do a visual safety check 4 times an hour
  d Measure vital signs every 4 hours

18 Exercising a person's joints to the extent possible without causing pain is called
  a Physical therapy (PT)
  b Range of motion (ROM)
  c Cardiopulmonary resuscitation (CPR)
  d Occupational therapy (OT)

19 A person with dementia has
  a Difficulty swallowing
  b Painful or difficult breathing
  c Damage to the skin and tissues
  d Loss of cognitive and social function

20 Which definition is *correct*?
  a *Contracture* is the decrease in size or wasting away of tissue.
  b *Perineal* is the genital and anal areas.
  c *Feces* is an elevated body temperature.
  d *Pressure injury* is a lack of joint mobility caused by shortening of a muscle.

21 Incontinence is a term meaning
  a Inability to control urination or bowel movements
  b Lack of awareness of surroundings
  c Damage to the skin and tissues
  d Inability to use or understand language

22 A care plan lists care measures for aphasia and dysphagia. You know that
  a These mean the same thing
  b *a-* means 1 and *dys-* means without
  c *-phasia* means speaking and *-phagia* means swallowing
  d *-phasia* means breathing and *-phagia* means speaking

Answers to Chapter 8 questions are on p. 587.

FOCUS ON **PRACTICE**

Problem Solving

You are training in the clinical setting. A person has an *NPO* sign above the bed. You do not remember what "NPO" means. What will you do? Why is it important for you to know?

CHAPTER 9

Body Structure and Function

OBJECTIVES

- Define the key terms and key abbreviations in this chapter.
- Identify the basic structures of the cell.
- Explain how cells divide.

- Identify the structures and functions of each body system.
- Explain how to promote PRIDE in the person, the family, and yourself.

KEY TERMS

artery A blood vessel that carries blood away from the heart

capillary A very tiny blood vessel; nutrients, oxygen, and other substances pass from capillaries into the cells

cell The basic unit of body structure

digestion The process that breaks down food physically and chemically so it can be absorbed for use by the cells

hemoglobin The substance in red blood cells that carries oxygen and gives blood its red color

hormone A chemical substance secreted by the endocrine glands into the bloodstream

immunity Protection against a disease or condition; the person will not get or be affected by the disease

joint The point at which 2 or more bones meet to allow movement

menstruation The process in which the lining of the uterus (endometrium) breaks up and is discharged from the body through the vagina

metabolism How the body uses nutrients to provide energy and maintain body functions

organ Groups of tissue that function together

peristalsis Involuntary muscle contractions in the digestive system that move food down the esophagus through the alimentary canal

reflex The body's response (function or movement) to a stimulus

respiration The process of supplying cells with oxygen and removing carbon dioxide from them

stimulus Anything that excites or causes a body part to function, become active, or respond

system Organs that work together to perform special functions

tissue A group of cells with similar functions

vein A blood vessel that returns blood to the heart

KEY ABBREVIATIONS

CNS	Central nervous system	**O₂**	Oxygen
CO₂	Carbon dioxide	**PNS**	Peripheral nervous system
GI	Gastro-intestinal	**RBC**	Red blood cell
mL	Milliliter	**WBC**	White blood cell

Ideally, the human body is in *homeostasis*—a steady state. *(Homeo* means *sameness. Stasis* means *maintenance.)* Various body functions and processes work to promote health and survival. Homeostasis is affected by illness, disease, and injury.

Knowing the body's normal structure *(anatomy)* and function *(physiology)* will help you understand signs, symptoms, and the reasons for care and procedures. You will give safe and more effective care.

See Chapter 10 for the changes in body structure and function that occur with aging.

ORGANIZATION OF THE BODY

Cells are the most basic structure in the body. Groups of cells form *tissues.* Groups of tissue form *organs.* Organs that work together form *body systems.* See Figure 9-1.

Cells

*The basic unit of body structure is the **cell**.* Cells have the same basic structure. Function, size, and shape may differ. Cells are very small. You need a microscope to see them. Cells need water, oxygen (O_2), and nutrients to live and function. Nutrients include proteins, fats, carbohydrates, vitamins, and minerals (Chapter 28).

Figure 9-2 shows the cell and its structures. The *cell membrane* is the outer covering. It encloses the cell and helps hold the cell's shape. The *nucleus* is the control center of the cell. It directs the cell's activities. The nucleus is in the center of the cell. The *cytoplasm* is a gelatin-like substance much like an egg white that surrounds the nucleus. Cytoplasm contains small structures that perform cell functions.

Chromosomes are thread-like structures in the nucleus. Each cell has 46 chromosomes. Chromosomes contain *genes.* Genes control the traits children inherit from their parents. Height, eye color, and skin color are examples.

The nucleus controls cell reproduction. Cells reproduce by dividing in half. The process of cell division is called *mitosis* (Fig. 9-3). It is needed for tissue growth and repair. During mitosis, the 46 chromosomes arrange themselves in 23 pairs. As the cell divides, the 23 pairs are pulled in half. The 2 new cells are identical. Each has 46 chromosomes.

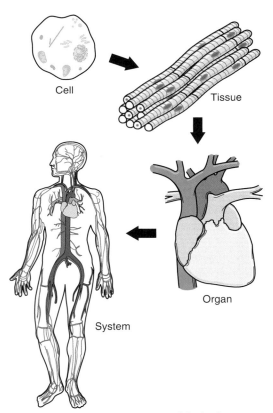

FIGURE 9-1 Organization of the body.

Cell

Tissue

Organ

System

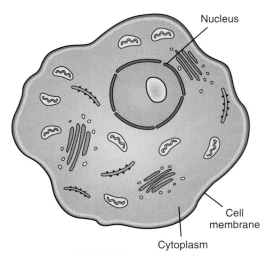

FIGURE 9-2 Parts of a cell.

Nucleus

Cell membrane

Cytoplasm

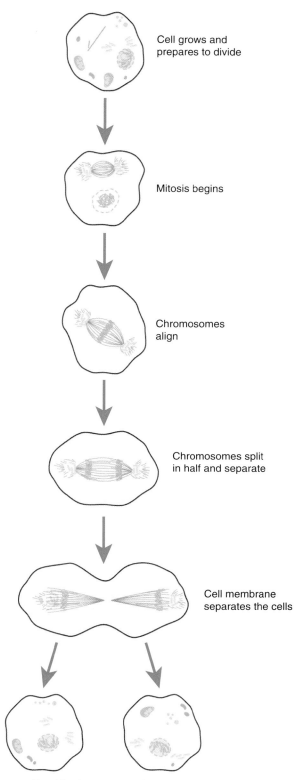

Cell grows and prepares to divide

Mitosis begins

Chromosomes align

Chromosomes split in half and separate

Cell membrane separates the cells

Two identical cells are formed

FIGURE 9-3 The process of cell division.

Tissues

Cells are the body's building blocks. *Groups of cells with similar functions combine to form* **tissues.**

- *Epithelial tissue* covers internal and external body surfaces. Tissue lining the nose, mouth, respiratory tract, stomach, and intestines is epithelial tissue. So are the skin, hair, nails, and glands. *Glands* secrete (release) substances that perform specific functions in the body.
- *Connective tissue* anchors, connects, and supports other tissues. It is in every part of the body. Bones, tendons, ligaments, and cartilage are connective tissue. Blood is a form of connective tissue.
- *Muscle tissue* stretches and contracts to let the body move.
- *Nerve tissue* receives and carries impulses to the brain and back to body parts.

A *membrane* is a thin sheet of epithelial or connective tissue. Membranes cover body surfaces and organs and line body cavities (areas that contain organs). *Mucous membranes* are 1 type of membrane. These membranes line areas of the body that open to the outside. The linings of the ears, nose, and mouth are examples. Mucous membranes secrete *mucus*—a watery substance that coats and protects cells. In some areas, mucus helps trap contaminants.

Organs and Body Systems

Groups of tissue that function together form **organs.** An organ has 1 or more functions. Examples of organs are the heart, brain, liver, lungs, and kidneys. **Systems** *are formed by organs that work together to perform special functions* (see Fig. 9-1).

This chapter explains the basic structure and function of the:

- Integumentary system (p. 92)
- Musculo-skeletal system (p. 92)
- Nervous system (p. 95)
- Circulatory system (p. 98)
- Lymphatic system (p. 100)
- Respiratory system (p. 100)
- Digestive system (p. 101)
- Urinary system (p. 102)
- Reproductive system (p. 102)
- Immune system (p. 104)
- Endocrine system (p. 105)

THE INTEGUMENTARY SYSTEM

The *integumentary system*, or *skin*, is the largest system. *Integument* means *covering*. The skin covers the body. It has epithelial, connective, and nerve tissue. It also has oil glands and sweat glands. There are 2 skin layers (Fig. 9-4).

- The *epidermis* is the outer layer. It has living cells and dead cells. The dead cells were once deeper in the epidermis. They were pushed upward as the cells divided. Dead cells constantly flake off. They are replaced by living cells. Living cells die and flake off. Living cells of the epidermis contain *pigment*. Pigment gives skin its color. The epidermis has no blood vessels and few nerve endings.
- The *dermis* is the inner layer. It is made up of connective tissue. Blood vessels, nerves, sweat glands, and oil glands are found in the dermis. So are hair roots.

The epidermis and dermis are supported by *subcutaneous tissue*. The subcutaneous tissue is a thick layer of fat and connective tissue.

Oil glands and *sweat glands*, *hair*, and *nails* are skin appendages.

- Hair—covers the entire body, except the palms of the hands and the soles of the feet. Hair in the nose and ears and around the eyes protects these organs from dust, insects, and other foreign objects.
- Nails—protect the tips of the fingers and toes. Nails help fingers pick up and handle small objects.
- Sweat glands *(sudoriferous glands)*—help the body regulate temperature. Sweat consists of water, salt, and a small amount of wastes. Sweat is secreted through pores in the skin. The body is cooled as sweat evaporates.
- Oil glands *(sebaceous glands)*—lie near the hair shafts. They secrete an oily substance into the space near the hair shaft. Oil travels to the skin surface. This helps keep the hair and skin soft and shiny.

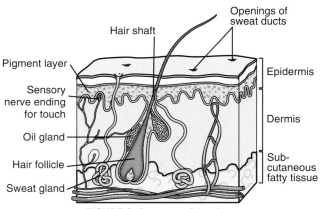

FIGURE 9-4 Layers of the skin.

Functions of the Skin

The skin has many functions.
- It is the body's protective covering.
- It prevents microorganisms and other substances from entering the body.
- It prevents excess amounts of water from leaving the body.
- It protects organs from injury.
- Nerve endings in the skin sense both pleasant and unpleasant stimulation. Nerve endings are over the entire body. They sense cold, pain, touch, and pressure to protect the body from injury.
- It helps regulate body temperature. Blood vessels *dilate* (widen) when temperature outside the body is high. More blood is brought to the body surface for cooling during evaporation. When blood vessels *constrict* (narrow), the body retains heat. This is because less blood reaches the skin.
- It stores fat and water.

THE MUSCULO-SKELETAL SYSTEM

The *musculo-skeletal system* provides the framework for the body. It lets the body move. This system also protects internal organs and gives the body shape.

Bones

The human body has 206 *bones* (Fig. 9-5). There are 4 types of bones.
- *Long bones* bear the body's weight. Leg bones are long bones.
- *Short bones* allow skill and ease in movement. Bones in the wrists, fingers, ankles, and toes are short bones.
- *Flat bones* protect the organs. They include the ribs, skull, pelvic bones, and shoulder blades.
- *Irregular bones* are the vertebrae in the spinal column. They allow various degrees of movement and flexibility.

Bones are hard, rigid structures. They are made up of living cells. Calcium and phosphorus are needed for bone formation and strength. Bones store these minerals for use by the body.

Bones are covered by a membrane called *periosteum*. Periosteum contains blood vessels that supply bone cells with O_2 and nutrients. Inside the hollow centers of the bones is a substance called *bone marrow*. Blood cells are formed in the bone marrow.

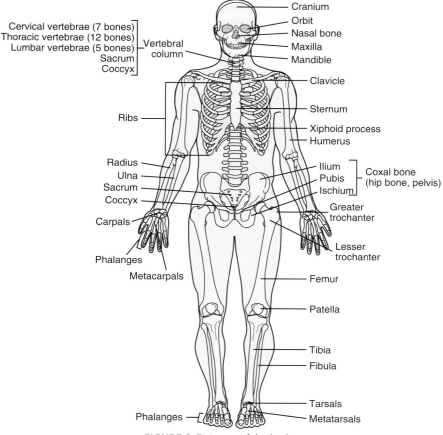

FIGURE 9-5 Bones of the body.

Joints

A *joint* is the point at which 2 or more bones meet. Joints allow movement (Chapter 32). *Cartilage* is connective tissue at the end of the long bones. It cushions the joint so that the bone ends do not rub together. The *synovial membrane* lines the joints. It secretes *synovial fluid.* Synovial fluid acts as a lubricant so the joint can move smoothly. Bones are held together at the joint by strong bands of connective tissue called *ligaments.*

There are 3 major types of joints (Fig. 9-6).

- A *ball-and-socket joint* allows movement in all directions. It is made of the rounded end of 1 bone and the hollow end of another bone. The rounded end of 1 fits into the hollow end of the other. The joints of the hips and shoulders are ball-and-socket joints.
- A *hinge joint* allows movement in 1 direction. The elbow is a hinge joint.
- A *pivot joint* allows turning from side to side. A pivot joint connects the skull to the spine.

Some joints cannot move. They connect the bones of the skull.

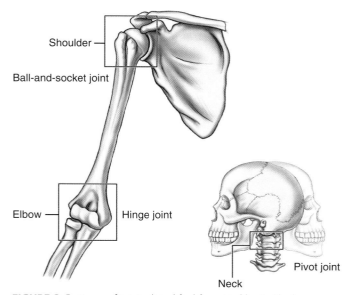

FIGURE 9-6 Types of joints. (Modified from Herlihy B: *The human body in health and illness,* ed 6, St Louis, 2018, Elsevier.)

Muscles

The body has over 500 *muscles* (Figs. 9-7 and 9-8). Some are voluntary. Others are involuntary.

- *Voluntary muscles* can be consciously controlled. Muscles attached to bones *(skeletal muscles)* are voluntary. Arm muscles do not work unless you move your arm; likewise for leg muscles. Skeletal muscles are *striated*. That is, they look striped or streaked.
- *Involuntary muscles* work automatically. You cannot control them. They control the action of the stomach, intestines, blood vessels, and other body organs. Involuntary muscles also are called *smooth muscles*. They look smooth, not streaked or striped.
- *Cardiac muscle* is in the heart. It is an involuntary muscle. However, it appears striated like skeletal muscle.

Muscles have 3 functions.

- Movement of body parts
- Maintenance of posture or muscle tone
- Production of body heat

Strong, tough connective tissues called *tendons* connect muscles to bones. When muscles *contract* (shorten), tendons at each end of the muscle cause the bone to move. The body has many tendons. See the Achilles tendon in Figure 9-8. Some muscles constantly contract to maintain posture. When muscles contract, they use energy. Heat is produced. The more muscle activity, the greater the amount of heat produced. Shivering is how the body produces heat when exposed to cold. Shivering is from rapid, general muscle contractions.

Sphincters are circular bands of muscle fibers. They *constrict* (narrow) a passage. Or they close a natural body opening. For example:

- The *lower esophageal sphincter* (Fig. 9-9) is between the esophagus and the stomach. It prevents food from moving back up into the esophagus.
- The *pyloric sphincter* (see Fig. 9-9) is an opening from the stomach into the small intestine. Closed, it holds food in the stomach for partial digestion. It opens to allow partially digested food to enter the small intestine.
- The *anal sphincter* keeps the anus closed. It opens for a bowel movement.
- *Urethral sphincters* seal off the bladder. This allows urine to collect in the bladder. The sphincters open for urination.

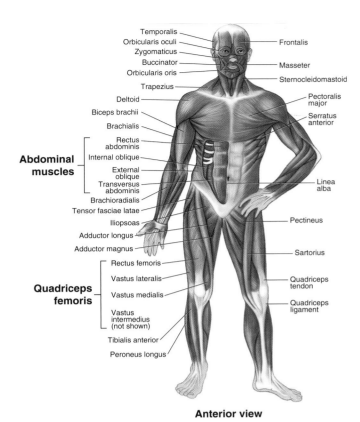

Anterior view

FIGURE 9-7 Anterior view of the muscles of the body. (Modified from Herlihy B: *The human body in health and illness,* ed 6, St Louis, 2018, Elsevier.)

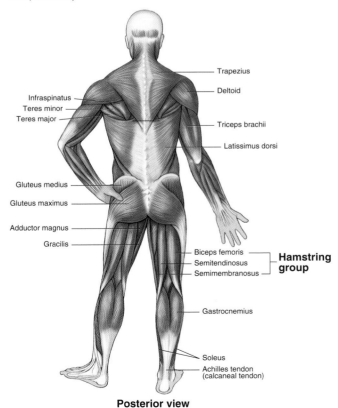

Posterior view

FIGURE 9-8 Posterior view of the muscles of the body. (From Herlihy B: *The human body in health and illness,* ed 6, St Louis, 2018, Elsevier.)

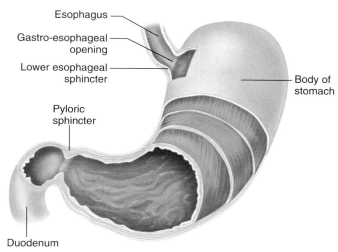

FIGURE 9-9 Pyloric sphincter. (Redrawn from Patton KT, Thibodeau GA: *The human body in health and disease*, ed 7, St Louis, 2018, Elsevier.)

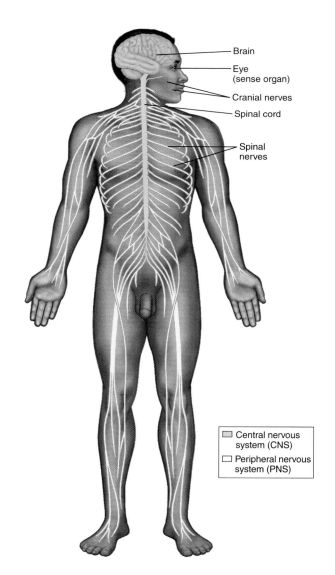

FIGURE 9-10 The nervous system is divided into the central nervous system and the peripheral nervous system. (Modified from Patton KT: *Anatomy and physiology*, ed 10, St Louis, 2019, Elsevier.)

THE NERVOUS SYSTEM

The *nervous system* controls, directs, and coordinates body functions. Its 2 main divisions are shown in Figure 9-10.

- The *central nervous system (CNS)* consists of the brain and spinal cord.
- The *peripheral nervous system (PNS)* involves the nerves throughout the body.

Nerves connect to the spinal cord. Nerves carry messages or impulses to and from the brain. A ***stimulus*** *is anything that excites or causes a body part to function, become active, or respond.* A ***reflex*** *is the body's response (function or movement) to a stimulus.* A stimulus causes a nerve impulse. A reflex results. For example, eye irritation (stimulus) causes the eyelid to blink (reflex). Reflexes are involuntary, unconscious, and immediate. The person cannot control reflexes.

Nerves are easily damaged and take a long time to heal. Some nerve fibers have a protective covering called a *myelin sheath.* The myelin sheath also insulates the nerve fiber. Nerve fibers covered with myelin conduct impulses faster than those fibers without it.

The Central Nervous System

The *brain* and *spinal cord* make up the central nervous system (Fig. 9-11). The brain is covered by the skull. The 3 main parts of the brain are the *cerebrum,* the *cerebellum,* and the *brainstem* (Fig. 9-12, p. 96).

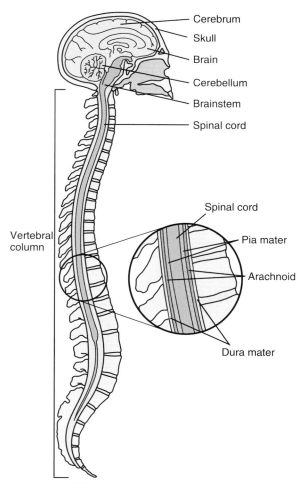

FIGURE 9-11 Central nervous system.

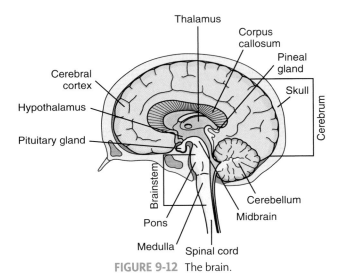

FIGURE 9-12 The brain.

The Peripheral Nervous System

Peripheral relates to the outer part or surrounding area of something. The nerves that spread throughout the body make up the peripheral nervous system.

- *Cranial nerves* conduct impulses between the brain and the head, neck, chest, and abdomen. They conduct impulses for smell, vision, hearing, taste, pain, touch, temperature, and pressure. They also conduct impulses for voluntary and involuntary muscles. There are 12 pairs of cranial nerves.
- *Spinal nerves* carry impulses from the skin, extremities, and internal structures not supplied by the cranial nerves. There are 31 pairs of spinal nerves named for where they come out of the vertebral column. See Figure 9-13.

The cerebrum is the largest part of the brain. It is the center of thought and intelligence. The cerebrum is divided into 2 halves called *right* and *left hemispheres.* The right hemisphere controls movement and activities on the body's left side. The left hemisphere controls the right side.

The outside of the cerebrum is called the *cerebral cortex.* It controls the highest functions of the brain. These include reasoning, memory, consciousness, speech, voluntary muscle movement, vision, hearing, sensation, and other activities.

The cerebellum regulates and coordinates body movements. It controls balance and the smooth movements of voluntary muscles. Injury to the cerebellum results in jerky movements, loss of coordination, and muscle weakness.

The brainstem connects the cerebrum to the spinal cord. The brainstem contains the *midbrain, pons,* and *medulla.* The midbrain and pons relay messages between the medulla and the cerebrum. The medulla controls heart rate, breathing, blood vessel size, swallowing, coughing, and vomiting. The brain connects to the spinal cord at the lower end of the medulla.

The spinal cord lies within the spinal column. The cord is 17 to 18 inches long. It contains pathways that conduct messages to and from the brain.

The brain and spinal cord are covered and protected by 3 layers of connective tissue called *meninges* (see Fig. 9-11).
- The outer layer is a tough covering called the *dura mater.*
- The middle layer is the *arachnoid.*
- The inner layer is the *pia mater.*

The space between the middle layer (arachnoid) and inner layer (pia mater) is the *arachnoid space.* The space is filled with *cerebrospinal fluid.* It circulates around the brain and spinal cord. Cerebrospinal fluid protects the central nervous system. It cushions shocks that could easily injure brain and spinal cord structures.

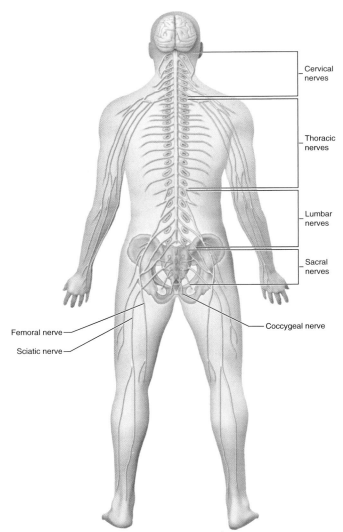

FIGURE 9-13 Spinal nerves and major nerve branches of the peripheral nervous system. (Modified from Solomon EP: *Introduction to human anatomy and physiology,* ed 4, St Louis, 2016, Saunders.)

The Autonomic Nervous System. The *autonomic nervous system* is part of the peripheral nervous system. This system controls involuntary muscles and certain body functions. The functions include the heartbeat, blood pressure, intestinal contractions, and glandular secretions. These functions occur automatically.

The autonomic nervous system is divided into the *sympathetic nervous system* and the *parasympathetic nervous system*. They balance each other. The sympathetic nervous system speeds up functions. The parasympathetic nervous system slows functions. When you are angry, scared, excited, or exercising, the sympathetic nervous system is stimulated. The parasympathetic system is activated when you relax or when the sympathetic system is stimulated for too long.

The Sense Organs

The 5 senses are *sight*, *hearing*, *taste*, *smell*, and *touch*. Receptors for taste are in the tongue. They are called *taste buds*. Receptors for smell are in the nose. Touch receptors are in the dermis, especially in the toes and fingertips.

The Eye. Receptors for vision are in the eyes (Fig. 9-14). The eye is easily injured. Bones of the skull, eyelids and eyelashes, and tears protect the eyes from injury.

The eye has 3 layers.
* The *sclera*, the white of the eye, is the outer layer. It is made of tough connective tissue.
* The *choroid* is the second layer. Blood vessels, the *ciliary muscle*, and the *iris* make up the choroid. The iris gives the eye its color. The opening in the middle of the iris is the *pupil*. Pupil size varies with the amount of light entering the eye. The pupil constricts (narrows) in bright light. It dilates (widens) in the dark.
* The *retina* is the inner layer. It has receptors for vision and the nerve fibers of the *optic nerve*. The *macula* is a portion of the retina responsible for central vision.

Light enters the eye through the *cornea*. It is the transparent part of the outer layer that lies over the eye. Light rays pass to the *lens*, which lies behind the pupil. The light is then reflected to the retina. Light is carried to the brain by the optic nerve.

The *aqueous chamber* separates the cornea from the lens. The chamber is filled with a fluid called *aqueous humor*. The fluid helps the cornea keep its shape and position. The *vitreous humor* is behind the lens. It is a gelatin-like substance that supports the retina and maintains the eye's shape.

The Ear. The *ear* is a sense organ (Fig. 9-15). It functions in hearing and balance. The ear has 3 parts—the *external ear*, *middle ear*, and *inner ear*.

The external ear (outer part) is called the *pinna* or *auricle*. Sound waves are guided through the external ear into the *auditory canal*. Glands in the auditory canal secrete a waxy substance called *cerumen*. The auditory canal extends about 1 inch into the *eardrum*. The eardrum (*tympanic membrane*) separates the external and middle ear.

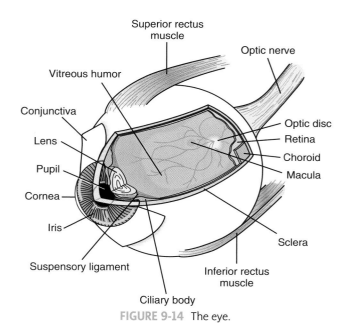
FIGURE 9-14 The eye.

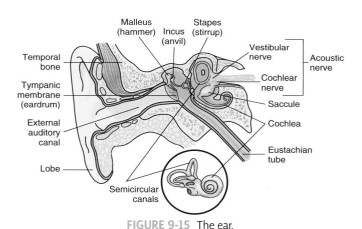
FIGURE 9-15 The ear.

The middle ear contains the *eustachian tube* and 3 small bones called *ossicles*. The eustachian tube connects the middle ear and the throat. Air enters the eustachian tube so there is equal pressure on both sides of the eardrum. The ossicles amplify sound received from the eardrum and transmit the sound to the inner ear. The 3 ossicles are:
* The *malleus*—looks like a hammer.
* The *incus*—looks like an anvil.
* The *stapes*—shaped like a stirrup.

The inner ear consists of *semicircular canals* and the *cochlea*. The cochlea contains fluid. The fluid carries sound waves from the middle ear to the *acoustic nerve*. The acoustic nerve then carries messages to the brain.

The 3 semicircular canals are involved with balance. They sense the head's position and changes in position. They send messages to the brain.

THE CIRCULATORY SYSTEM

The *circulatory system (cardiovascular system)* is made up of the *blood*, *heart*, and *blood vessels*. The heart pumps blood through the blood vessels. The circulatory system has many functions.

- Blood carries nutrients, hormones, and other substances to the cells.
- Blood transports (carries) the gases of respiration (p. 100). It brings O_2 to the cells.
- Blood removes waste products from cells.
- Blood plays a role in maintaining the body's fluid balance.
- Blood and blood vessels help regulate body temperature. The blood carries heat from muscle activity to other body parts. Blood vessels in the skin dilate to cool the body. They constrict to retain heat.
- The system produces and carries cells that defend the body from microbes that cause disease.

The Blood

The *blood* consists of blood cells and *plasma*. Plasma is mostly water. It carries blood to other body cells. Plasma also carries substances that cells need to function. This includes nutrients, hormones (p. 105), and chemicals.

Red blood cells (RBCs) are called *erythrocytes*. *Hemoglobin is a substance in RBCs that carries oxygen and gives blood its red color.* As RBCs circulate through the lungs, hemoglobin picks up O_2. Hemoglobin carries O_2 to the cells. When blood is bright red, hemoglobin in the RBCs is filled with O_2. As blood circulates through the body, O_2 is given to the cells. Cells release carbon dioxide (CO_2, a waste product). It is picked up by the hemoglobin. RBCs filled with CO_2 make the blood look dark red.

The body has about 25 trillion (25,000,000,000,000) RBCs. About $4\frac{1}{2}$ to 5 million cells are in a cubic millimeter of blood (the size of a tiny drop). RBCs live for 3 to 4 months. They are destroyed by the liver and spleen as they wear out. New RBCs are formed in the bone marrow. About 1 million RBCs are produced every second.

White blood cells (WBCs) are called *leukocytes*. They have no color. They protect the body against infection. There are about 5,000 to 10,000 WBCs in a cubic millimeter of blood. At the first sign of infection, WBCs rush to the infection site and multiply rapidly. The number of WBCs increases when there is an infection. Formed by the bone marrow, WBCs live for about 9 days.

Platelets (thrombocytes) are needed for blood clotting. They are formed by the bone marrow. There are about 200,000 to 400,000 platelets in a cubic millimeter of blood. A platelet lives for about 4 days.

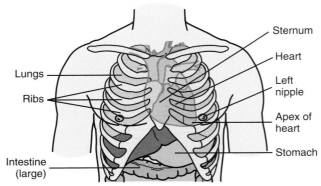

FIGURE 9-16 Location of the heart in the chest cavity.

The Heart

The *heart* is a muscle. It pumps blood through the blood vessels to the tissues and cells. The heart lies in the middle to lower part of the chest cavity toward the left side (Fig. 9-16) and is hollow with 3 layers (Fig. 9-17).

- The *pericardium* is the outer layer. It is a thin sac covering the heart.
- The *myocardium* is the second layer. It is the thick, muscular part of the heart.
- The *endocardium* is the inner layer. A membrane, it lines the inner surface of the heart.

The heart has 4 chambers (see Fig. 9-17). Upper chambers receive blood and are called *atria*. The *right atrium* receives blood from body tissues. The *left atrium* receives blood from the lungs. Lower chambers are called *ventricles*. Ventricles pump blood. The *right ventricle* pumps blood to the lungs for O_2. The *left ventricle* pumps blood to all parts of the body.

Valves are between the atria and ventricles. The valves allow blood flow in 1 direction. They prevent blood from flowing back into the atria from the ventricles. The *tricuspid valve* is between the right atrium and the right ventricle. The *mitral valve (bicuspid valve)* is between the left atrium and left ventricle.

Heart action has 2 phases.

- *Diastole.* It is the resting phase. Heart chambers fill with blood.
- *Systole.* It is the working phase. The heart contracts. Blood is pumped through the blood vessels when the heart contracts.

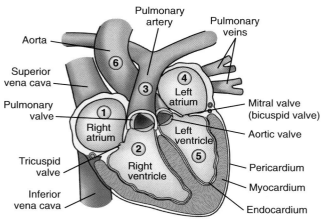

1. Venous blood, poor in O_2, enters the right atrium.

2. Blood flows through the tricuspid valve into the right ventricle.

3. The right ventricle pumps blood through the pulmonary artery to the lungs to pick up O_2.

4. Oxygen-rich blood from the lungs enters the left atrium.

5. Blood flows through the mitral valve into the left ventricle.

6. The left ventricle pumps blood through the aorta to other arteries.

FIGURE 9-17   Structures of the heart and blood flow through the heart.

The Blood Vessels

Blood flows to body tissues and cells through the blood vessels. There are 3 groups of blood vessels: *arteries,* *capillaries,* and *veins.*

Arteries are blood vessels that carry blood away from the heart. Arterial blood is rich in O_2. The *aorta* is the largest artery. It receives blood directly from the left ventricle. The aorta branches into other arteries that carry blood to all parts of the body (Fig. 9-18). These arteries branch into smaller parts within the tissues. The smallest branch of an artery is an *arteriole.*

Arterioles connect to capillaries. *Capillaries are very tiny blood vessels. Nutrients, oxygen, and other substances pass from capillaries into the cells.* The capillaries pick up waste products (including CO_2) from the cells. Veins carry waste products back to the heart.

Veins are blood vessels that return blood to the heart. They connect to the capillaries by *venules.* Venules are small veins. Venules branch together to form veins. The many veins also branch together as they near the heart to form 2 main veins—the *inferior vena cava* and the *superior vena cava* (see Fig. 9-18). Both empty into the right atrium. The inferior vena cava carries blood from the legs and the trunk (torso—chest and abdomen). The superior vena cava carries blood from the head and the arms. Venous blood is dark red. It has little O_2 and a lot of CO_2.

Blood flow through the heart is shown in Figure 9-17. From there:

1. Arterial blood is carried to the tissues by arterioles and to the cells by capillaries.

2. Cells and capillaries exchange O_2 and nutrients for CO_2 and waste products.

3. Capillaries connect with venules. Venules carry blood that has CO_2 and waste products.

4. Venules form veins.

5. Veins return blood to the heart.

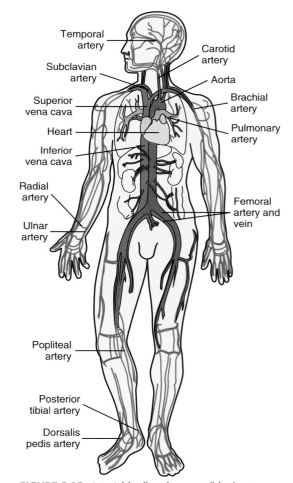

FIGURE 9-18   Arterial (red) and venous (blue) systems.

THE LYMPHATIC SYSTEM

The lymphatic (lymph) system is a complex network that transports lymph throughout the body (Fig. 9-19). *Lymph* is a clear, thin, watery fluid. Lymph contains proteins and fats from the intestines. Lymph also contains WBCs.

The lymphatic system:

- Collects extra lymph from the tissues and returns it to the blood. This helps maintain fluid balance. Water, proteins, and other substances normally leak out of the capillaries. The lymphatic system drains the extra fluid from the tissues. Otherwise, the tissues swell.
- Defends the body against infection by producing lymphocytes. *Lymphocytes* are a type of WBC that defends the body against microorganisms that cause infection (Chapter 14).
- Absorbs fats from the intestines and transports them to the blood.

Lymph is formed in the tissues. Lymph is transported by *lymphatic vessels*—lymphatic capillaries to lymphatic venules to the right lymphatic duct and the thoracic duct. Lymph then enters the blood in veins near the neck.

- The *right lymphatic duct* collects lymph from the right arm and from the right side of the head, neck, and chest. It empties into a vein on the right side of the neck.
- The *thoracic duct (left lymphatic duct)* collects lymph from the pelvis, abdomen, lower chest, and the rest of the body. It empties into a vein on the left side of the neck.

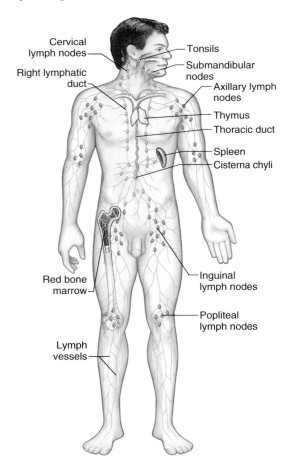

FIGURE 9-19 Lymphatic system. (From Patton KT, Thibodeau GA: *The human body in health and disease,* ed 7, St Louis, 2018, Elsevier.)

Lymph nodes are shaped like beans. They range from the size of a pinhead to as large as a lima bean. They are found in the neck, underarm, groin area, chest, abdomen, and pelvis. Usually, you cannot see or feel lymph nodes. They swell when producing more lymphocytes to fight infection.

Lymph enters lymph nodes through the lymphatic vessels. The lymph nodes filter bacteria, cancer cells, and damaged cells from the lymph. This prevents such substances from circulating throughout the body.

See Figure 9-19 for the location of the *thymus (thymus gland)*. Certain lymphocytes—T lymphocytes (T cells)—develop in the thymus. Such lymphocytes are important for immune system function (p. 104). The thymus reaches full growth at puberty. Then thymus tissue is slowly replaced by fat and connective tissue. By age 80, it is usually gone.

The *tonsils* are in the back of the throat. *Adenoids* are behind the nose. These structures trap microorganisms in the mouth and nose to help prevent infection.

The *spleen* is the largest structure in the lymphatic system. It is about the size of a fist. The spleen has a rich blood supply—about 500 milliliters (mL) (1 pint) of blood. The spleen:

- Filters and removes bacteria and other substances.
- Destroys old RBCs.
- Saves the iron found in hemoglobin when RBCs are destroyed.
- Stores blood. When needed, the blood is returned to the circulatory system.

THE RESPIRATORY SYSTEM

Oxygen (O_2) is needed to live. Every cell needs O_2. Air contains about 21% O_2. This meets the body's needs under normal conditions. The respiratory system (Fig. 9-20) brings O_2 into the lungs and removes carbon dioxide (CO_2). *Respiration is the process of supplying cells with oxygen and removing carbon dioxide from them.* Respiration involves *inhalation* (breathing in) and *exhalation* (breathing out). The terms *inspiration* (breathing in) and *expiration* (breathing out) also are used.

Air enters the body through the *nose*. The air then passes into the *pharynx* (throat). It is a tube-shaped passage-way for air and food. Air passes from the pharynx into the *larynx* (voice box). A piece of cartilage, the *epiglottis*, acts like a lid over the larynx. The epiglottis prevents food from entering the airway during swallowing. During inhalation the epiglottis lifts up to let air pass over the larynx. Air passes from the larynx into the *trachea* (windpipe).

The trachea divides into the *right bronchus* and the *left bronchus*. Each bronchus enters a lung. Upon entering the lungs, the bronchi divide many times into smaller branches called *bronchioles*. The bronchioles subdivide. They end up in tiny 1-celled air sacs called *alveoli*.

Alveoli look like small clusters of grapes. They are supplied by capillaries. The alveoli and capillaries exchange O_2 and CO_2. Blood in the capillaries picks up O_2 from the alveoli. Then the blood is returned to the left side of the heart and pumped to the rest of the body. Alveoli pick up CO_2 from the capillaries for exhalation.

The lungs are filled with alveoli, blood vessels, and nerves. Each lung is divided into lobes. The right lung has 3 lobes; the left lung has 2. The lungs are separated from the abdominal cavity by a muscle called the *diaphragm*.

Each lung is covered by a 2-layered sac called the *pleura*. One layer is attached to the lung and the other to the chest wall. The pleura secretes a very thin fluid that fills the space between the layers. The fluid prevents the layers from rubbing together during inhalation and exhalation. A bony framework made up of the ribs, sternum, and vertebrae protects the lungs.

THE DIGESTIVE SYSTEM

Digestion is the process that breaks down food physically and chemically so it can be absorbed for use by the cells. The digestive system is also called the gastro-intestinal (GI) system. The system also removes solid wastes from the body.

The digestive system involves the *alimentary canal (GI tract)* and the accessory organs of digestion (Fig. 9-21). The alimentary canal is a long tube. It extends from the mouth to the anus. Its major parts are the mouth, pharynx, esophagus, stomach, small intestine, and large intestine. Accessory organs are the teeth, tongue, salivary glands, liver, gallbladder, and pancreas.

Digestion begins in the *mouth (oral cavity)*. It receives food and prepares it for digestion. Using chewing motions, the *teeth* cut, chop, and grind food into small particles for digestion and swallowing. The *tongue* aids in chewing and swallowing. *Taste buds* on the tongue's surface contain nerve endings. Taste buds allow sweet, sour, bitter, and salty tastes to be sensed. *Salivary glands* in the mouth secrete *saliva*. Saliva moistens food particles to ease swallowing and begin digestion. During swallowing, the tongue pushes food into the *pharynx*.

The pharynx (throat) is a muscular tube. Swallowing continues as the pharynx contracts. Contraction of the pharynx pushes food into the *esophagus*. The esophagus is a muscular tube about 10 inches long. It extends from the pharynx to the *stomach*. *Involuntary muscle contractions in the digestive system move food down the esophagus through the alimentary canal* (**peristalsis**).

The stomach is a muscular, pouch-like sac. It is in the upper left part of the abdominal cavity. Strong stomach muscles stir and churn food to break it up into even smaller particles. A mucous membrane lines the stomach. It contains glands that secrete *gastric juices*. Food is mixed and churned with the gastric juices to form a semi-liquid substance called *chyme*. Through peristalsis, the chyme is pushed from the stomach into the small intestine.

The *small intestine* is about 20 feet long. It has 3 parts. The first part is the *duodenum*. There, more digestive juices are added to the chyme. One is called *bile*. Bile is a greenish liquid made in the *liver*. Bile is stored in the *gallbladder*. Juices from the *pancreas* and small intestine are added to the chyme. Digestive juices chemically break down food into nutrients to be absorbed.

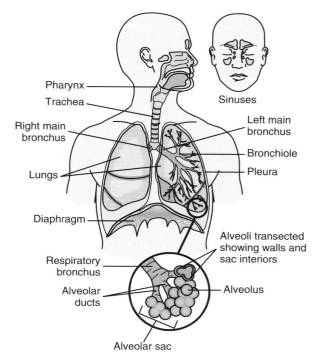

FIGURE 9-20 Respiratory system.

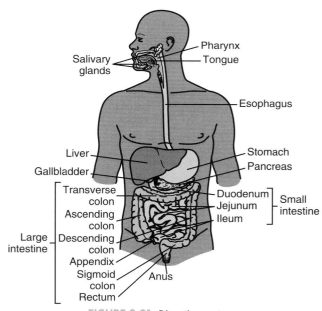

FIGURE 9-21 Digestive system.

Peristalsis moves the chyme through the 2 other parts of the small intestine: the *jejunum* and the *ileum*. Tiny projections called *villi* line the small intestine. Villi absorb nutrients into the capillaries. Most nutrient absorption takes place in the small intestine.

Undigested chyme passes from the small intestine into the *large intestine (large bowel* or *colon)*. The colon absorbs most of the water from the chyme. The remaining semi-solid material is called *feces*. Feces contain a small amount of water, solid wastes, and some mucus and germs. These are the waste products of digestion. Feces pass through the colon into the *rectum* by peristalsis. Feces pass out of the body through the *anus*.

THE URINARY SYSTEM

The digestive system rids the body of solid wastes. The lungs rid the body of CO_2. Water and other substances leave the body through sweat. There are other waste products in the blood.

The urinary system (Fig. 9-22):
- Removes waste products from the blood.
- Maintains water balance within the body.
- Maintains electrolyte balance. *Electrolytes* are substances that dissolve in water—sodium, potassium, calcium, and magnesium.
  - Sodium is needed for fluid balance. The body retains water if sodium levels are high. Loss of sodium (through vomiting, diarrhea, some drugs, and so on) can result in dehydration.
  - Potassium is needed for the proper function of skeletal and cardiac muscles.
  - Calcium and magnesium are needed for normal nerve and muscle function and for bone and teeth formation.
- Maintains acid-base balance. A pH scale measures if a substance is acidic, neutral, or basic. A pH of 7 is neutral. Anything below 7 is acidic. Anything above 7 is basic. The blood must remain within a certain pH range (7.35–7.45) for normal body function.

The *kidneys* are 2 bean-shaped organs in the upper abdomen. Protected by the lower edge of the ribs, the kidneys lie against the back muscles on each side of the spine.

Each kidney has over a million tiny *nephrons* (Fig. 9-23). Each nephron is the basic working unit of the kidney. Each nephron has a *convoluted tubule*, which is a tiny coiled tubule. Each convoluted tubule has a *Bowman's capsule* at 1 end. The capsule partly surrounds a cluster of capillaries called a *glomerulus*. Blood passes through the glomerulus and is filtered by the capillaries.

The fluid part of the blood is squeezed into the Bowman's capsule. The fluid then passes into the tubule. Most of the water and other needed substances are re-absorbed by the blood. The rest of the fluid and the waste products form *urine* in the tubule. Urine flows through the tubule to a *collecting tubule*. All collecting tubules drain into the *renal pelvis* in the kidney.

A tube called the *ureter* is attached to the renal pelvis of the kidney. Each ureter is about 10 to 12 inches long. The ureters carry urine from the kidneys to the *bladder*. The bladder is a hollow, muscular sac. It lies toward the front in the lower part of the abdominal cavity.

Urine is stored in the bladder until the need to urinate is felt. This usually occurs when there is about a half pint (250 mL) of urine in the bladder. Urine passes from the bladder through the *urethra*. The opening at the end of the urethra is called the *meatus*. Urine passes from the body through the meatus. Urine is a clear, yellowish fluid.

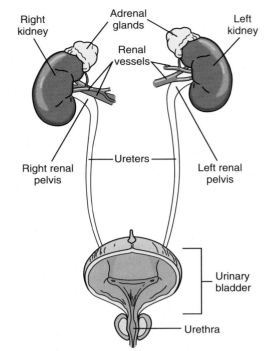

FIGURE 9-22 Urinary system.

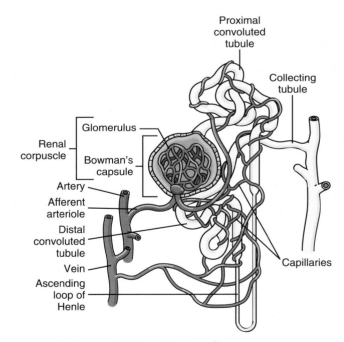

FIGURE 9-23 A nephron.

THE REPRODUCTIVE SYSTEM

Human reproduction results from the union of a male sex cell and a female sex cell. The male and female reproductive systems are different. This allows for the process of reproduction.

The Male Reproductive System

The male reproductive system is shown in Figure 9-24. The *testes (testicles)* are the male sex glands. Sex glands also are called *gonads*. The 2 testes are oval or almond-shaped glands. Male sex cells *(sperm)* are produced in the testes.

Testosterone, the male hormone, is produced in the testes. This hormone is needed for reproductive organ function. It also is needed for the development of male secondary sex characteristics. There is facial hair; pubic and axillary (underarm) hair; and hair on the arms, chest, and legs. Neck and shoulder sizes increase.

The testes are suspended between the thighs in a sac called the *scrotum*. The scrotum is made of skin and muscle.

The *epididymis* is a coiled tube on top and to the side of each testis. Sperm travel from the testis to the epididymis. From the epididymis, sperm travel through a tube called the *vas deferens*. Each vas deferens joins a *seminal vesicle*. The 2 seminal vesicles store sperm and produce *semen*. Semen is a fluid that carries sperm from the male reproductive tract. The ducts of the seminal vesicles unite to form the *ejaculatory duct*. It passes through the *prostate gland*.

The prostate gland lies just below the bladder. It is shaped like a donut. The gland secretes fluid into the semen. As the ejaculatory ducts leave the prostate, they join the *urethra*. The urethra runs through the prostate gland. The urethra is the outlet for urine and semen. The urethra is contained within the *penis*.

The penis is outside of the body. The *glans* is at the end of the penis. The urethra opens at the end of the glans. A fold of skin (*prepuce* or *foreskin*) is at the end of the penis (Chapter 22).

The penis has *erectile* tissue. When a man is sexually excited, blood fills the erectile tissue. The penis enlarges and becomes hard and erect. The erect penis can enter a female's vagina. *Cowper's glands* are 2 pea-sized glands under the prostate. They produce a clear, colorless fluid before ejaculation (release of semen). The fluid cleanses the urethra, protects sperm from damage, and provides some lubrication for intercourse. With ejaculation, semen—containing sperm—is released into the vagina.

The Female Reproductive System

Figure 9-25 shows the female reproductive system. The female gonads are 2 almond-shaped glands called *ovaries*. An ovary is on each side of the uterus in the abdominal cavity.

The ovaries contain eggs called *ova*. Ova are the female sex cells. One ovum (egg) is released monthly during the woman's reproductive years. Release of an ovum is called *ovulation*.

The ovaries secrete the female hormones *estrogen* and *progesterone*. These hormones are needed for reproductive system function. They also are needed for the development of female secondary sex characteristics. These include increased breast size, pubic and axillary (underarm) hair, slight deepening of the voice, and widening and rounding of the hips.

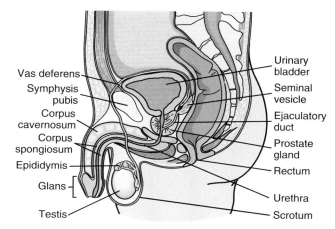

FIGURE 9-24 Male reproductive system.

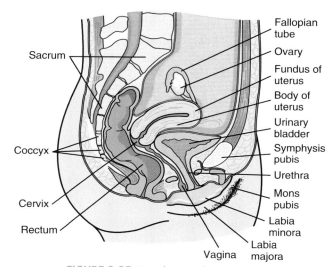

FIGURE 9-25 Female reproductive system.

When an ovum is released from an ovary, it travels through a *fallopian tube*. There are 2 fallopian tubes, 1 on each side. The tubes are attached at 1 end to the *uterus*. The ovum travels through the fallopian tube to the uterus.

The uterus is a hollow, muscular organ shaped like a pear. It is in the center of the pelvic cavity behind the bladder and in front of the rectum. The main part of the uterus is the *fundus*. The neck or narrow section of the uterus is the *cervix*. Tissue lining the uterus is the *endometrium*. The endometrium has many blood vessels. If sex cells from the male and female unite into 1 cell, that cell implants into the endometrium. There, the cell grows into a *fetus* (unborn baby) and receives nourishment.

The cervix of the uterus projects into a muscular canal called the *vagina*. The vagina opens to the outside of the body. It is just behind the urethra. The vagina receives the penis during intercourse. It also is part of the birth canal. Glands in the vaginal wall keep it moistened with secretions. The external vaginal opening is partially closed by a membrane called the *hymen*. The hymen can stretch or tear (rupture) from intercourse, injury, or surgery.

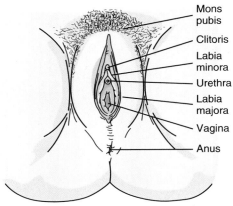

FIGURE 9-26 External female genitalia.

The external female genitalia are called the *vulva* (Fig. 9-26).

- The *mons pubis* is a rounded, fatty pad over a bone called the *symphysis pubis*. The mons pubis is covered with hair in the adult female.
- The *labia majora* and *labia minora* are 2 folds of tissue on each side of the vaginal opening.
- The *clitoris* is a small organ composed of erectile tissue. It becomes hard when sexually stimulated.

Menstruation. The endometrium is rich in blood to nourish the cell that grows into a fetus. If pregnancy does not occur, menstruation begins. *Menstruation is the process in which the lining of the uterus (endometrium) breaks up and is discharged from the body through the vagina.* It occurs about every 28 days. Therefore it is called the *menstrual cycle.*

The first day of the menstrual cycle begins with menstruation. Blood flows from the uterus through the vaginal opening. Menstrual flow usually lasts 3 to 7 days. Ovulation occurs during the next phase. An ovum matures in an ovary and is released. Ovulation usually occurs on or about day 14 of the cycle.

Meanwhile, estrogen and progesterone (the female hormones) are secreted by the ovaries. These hormones cause the endometrium to thicken for pregnancy. If pregnancy does not occur, the hormones decrease in amount. This causes the blood supply to the endometrium to decrease. The endometrium breaks up. It is discharged through the vagina. Another menstrual cycle begins.

Mammary Glands. The *mammary glands (breasts)* secrete milk after childbirth. Breasts are made up of glandular tissue and fat. The milk *(breast-milk)* drains into ducts that open onto the *nipple.*

Fertilization

To reproduce, a male sex cell (sperm) must unite with a female sex cell (ovum). The uniting of the sperm and ovum into 1 cell is called *fertilization.* A sperm has 23 chromosomes. An ovum has 23 chromosomes. When the 2 cells unite, the fertilized cell has 46 chromosomes.

During intercourse, millions of sperm are deposited into the vagina. Sperm travel up the cervix, through the uterus, and into the fallopian tubes. If a sperm and an ovum unite in a fallopian tube, fertilization results. Pregnancy occurs. The fertilized cell travels down the fallopian tube to the uterus. After a short time, the fertilized cell implants into the thick endometrium and grows during pregnancy.

THE IMMUNE SYSTEM

The immune system protects the body from disease and infection. Abnormal body cells can grow into tumors. Sometimes the body produces substances that cause the body to attack itself. Microorganisms (bacteria, viruses, and other germs) can cause an infection. The immune system defends against threats inside and outside the body.

The immune system gives the body immunity. *Immunity means that a person has protection against a disease or condition. The person will not get or be affected by the disease.*

- *Specific immunity* is the body's reaction to a certain threat.
- *Non-specific immunity* is the body's reaction to anything it does not recognize as a normal body substance. Special cells and substances function to produce immunity.
- *Antibodies*—normal body substances that recognize other substances. They are involved in destroying abnormal or unwanted substances.
- *Antigens*—substances that cause an immune response. Antibodies recognize and bind with unwanted antigens. This leads to the destruction of unwanted substances and the production of more antibodies.
- *Phagocytes*—white blood cells (WBCs) that digest and destroy microorganisms and other unwanted substances (Fig. 9-27).
- *Lymphocytes*—WBCs that produce antibodies. Lymphocyte production increases as the body responds to an infection.
  - *B lymphocytes (B cells)*—cause the production of antibodies that circulate in the plasma. The antibodies react to specific antigens.
  - *T lymphocytes (T cells)*—destroy invading cells. *Killer T cells* produce poisons near the invading cells. Some T cells attract other cells. The other cells destroy the invaders.

When the body senses an antigen from an unwanted substance, the immune system acts. Phagocyte and lymphocyte production increases. Phagocytes destroy the invaders through digestion. The lymphocytes produce antibodies that identify and destroy the unwanted substances.

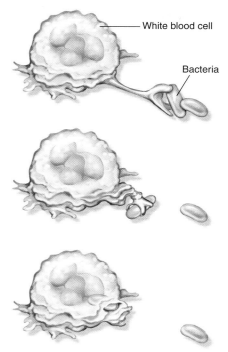

FIGURE 9-27 A phagocyte digests and destroys a microorganism. (From Patton KT, Thibodeau GA: *Structure & function of the body*, ed 16, St Louis, 2020, Elsevier.)

THE ENDOCRINE SYSTEM

The endocrine system is made up of glands called the *endocrine glands* (Fig. 9-28). *The endocrine glands secrete chemical substances called* **hormones** *into the bloodstream.* Hormones regulate the activities of other organs and glands in the body. See Table 9-1.

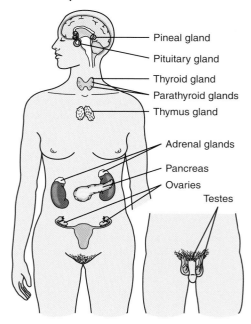

FIGURE 9-28 Endocrine system.

TABLE 9-1 Endocrine System	
Gland	**Hormones and Actions**

Pituitary gland (master gland)
• Small, cherry-sized gland at the base of the brain behind the eyes
• 2 parts:
  ◦ *Anterior pituitary lobe*
  ◦ *Posterior pituitary lobe*
	Anterior pituitary lobe secretes:
	• *Growth hormone (GH)*—stimulates the growth of muscles, bones, and organs.
	• *Thyroid stimulating hormone (TSH)*—stimulates thyroid gland function.
	• *Adrenocorticotropic hormone (ACTH)*—stimulates adrenal gland function.
	• Hormones regulating growth, development, and function of the male and female reproductive systems.
	Posterior pituitary lobe secretes:
	• *Antidiuretic hormone (ADH)*—prevents the kidneys from excreting too much water.
	• *Oxytocin*—causes uterine contractions during childbirth.

Thyroid gland • Butterfly-shaped gland in the neck below the larynx (voice box)	*Thyroid hormone (TH, thyroxine)* regulates **metabolism**—*how the body uses nutrients to provide energy and maintain body functions.* • Too little TH causes slow body processes, slow movements, and weight gain. • Too much TH causes increased metabolism, excess energy, and weight loss.
Parathyroid glands • 4 total—2 lie on each side of the thyroid gland	*Parathormone* regulates calcium use. Calcium is needed: • For nerve and muscle function • To prevent *tetany*—a state of severe muscle contraction and spasm that can lead to death
Thymus • Gland in the upper chest behind the sternum	*Thymosin*—needed for development and function of the immune system.
Pancreas • Gland in the abdomen behind the stomach	*Insulin*—regulates the amount of sugar in the blood available for use by the cells. Without insulin, sugar cannot enter the cells. Excess sugar builds up in the blood causing *diabetes*.

Adrenal glands
• 2 glands—1 on top of each kidney
• Each gland has 2 parts:
  ◦ *Adrenal medulla* (inner part)
  ◦ *Adrenal cortex* (outer part)
	Adrenal medulla secretes:
	• *Epinephrine and norepinephrine*—stimulate the body to quickly produce energy during emergencies. Heart rate, blood pressure, muscle power, and energy increase.
	Adrenal cortex secretes:
	• *Glucocorticoids*—regulate metabolism of carbohydrates and control the body's response to stress and inflammation.
	• *Mineralocorticoids*—regulate the amount of salt and water absorbed and lost by the kidneys.
	• Small amounts of male and female sex hormones.

Gonads • *Testes*—male sex glands • *Ovaries*—female sex glands	• Male glands (testes) secrete *testosterone*. • Female glands (ovaries) secrete *estrogen* and *progesterone*.

FOCUS ON P R I D E

The Person, Family, and Yourself

P ersonal and Professional Responsibility

Taking care of yourself is a personal and professional responsibility. A healthy diet, exercise, and rest are needed. To care for others, you need a strong and healthy body.

R ights and Respect

Patients and residents have the right to make decisions about their bodies. You may not agree with those decisions. But you must respect the person's choices. If the decision will cause no harm, comply with the request. For example, a person does not want to wear a sweater today.

If the person's decision may cause harm, tell the nurse at once. For example, a person refuses to eat. You tell the nurse. The person cannot be forced to eat. But the nurse can talk with the person about the decision, the consequences, and possible solutions.

I ndependence and Social Interaction

The body does not always work right. People become ill or injured. Sometimes the health team cannot prevent loss of function. Take pride in helping each person regain or maintain the highest level of function possible.

D elegation and Teamwork

The body works like a team. Each system has independent functions. But all systems interact and depend on each other. When a person has a problem with 1 body system, other systems are affected. Understanding each system and how the systems interact helps you provide better care.

E thics and Laws

Sometimes a person is not able to make health care decisions. Spouses, parents, family members, or legal representatives may make decisions. Some persons have an advance directive (Chapter 44). Sometimes the court appoints a guardian for a short time. Finally, the agency's ethics committee may address complex issues. The person's safety and best interests must guide care decisions.

FOCUS ON PRIDE: *Application*

Body systems interact for normal function. Explain how the circulatory and respiratory systems interact. How might a problem in 1 system affect the other?

REVIEW QUESTIONS

Circle the BEST answer.

1 The basic unit of body structure is the
   a Cell
   b Neuron
   c Nephron
   d Ovum

2 The process of cell division is called
   a Physiology
   b Mitosis
   c Homeostasis
   d Metabolism

3 Which is a function of the skin?
   a Provides the protective covering for the body
   b Transports lymph
   c Forms blood cells
   d Provides the shape and framework for the body

4 Which allows movement?
   a Bone marrow
   b Mucous membranes
   c Joints
   d Ligaments

5 Skeletal muscles
   a Are under involuntary control
   b Appear smooth
   c Are under voluntary control
   d Appear striped and smooth

6 The central nervous system is made up of
   a The brain and spinal cord
   b Cranial nerves and spinal nerves
   c Cervical, thoracic, and lumbar nerves
   d The midbrain, pons, and medulla

7 Which statement about the autonomic nervous system is *correct*?
   a The sympathetic nervous system slows down functions.
   b The parasympathetic nervous system speeds up functions.
   c It controls voluntary actions.
   d It is part of the peripheral nervous system.

8 The ear is involved with
   a Regulating body movements
   b Balance
   c Smoothness of body movements
   d Controlling involuntary muscles

9 Which statement about the phases of heart action is *correct?*
   a Diastole is the working phase.
   b Systole is the resting phase.
   c The heart contracts (pumps) during systole.
   d Diastole and systole occur at the same time.

10 Which part of the heart pumps blood to the body?
   a Right atrium
   b Left atrium
   c Right ventricle
   d Left ventricle

11 Which carry blood away from the heart?
   a Capillaries
   b Veins
   c Venules
   d Arteries

12 Which statement about the lymphatic system is *correct?*
   a The tonsils are the largest structures in the lymphatic system.
   b Lymph transports oxygen and nutrients to cells.
   c The spleen filters and removes bacteria.
   d Extra lymph from the blood is moved to the tissues.

13 Oxygen and carbon dioxide are exchanged
   a In the bronchi
   b Between the alveoli and capillaries
   c Between the lungs and pleura
   d In the trachea

14 Digestion begins in the
   a Mouth
   b Stomach
   c Small intestine
   d Colon

15 Most nutrient absorption takes place in the
   a Stomach
   b Small intestine
   c Colon
   d Large intestine

16 Urine is formed by the
   a Jejunum
   b Kidneys
   c Bladder
   d Liver

17 Urine passes from the body through the
   a Ureters
   b Urethra
   c Anus
   d Nephrons

18 Which statement about the reproductive system is *correct?*
   a The male sex gland is the prostate.
   b The female sex gland is the uterus.
   c Male sex cells are called sperm.
   d Female sex cells are called ovaries.

19 The discharge of the lining of the uterus is called
   a The endometrium
   b Ovulation
   c Fertilization
   d Menstruation

20 The immune system protects the body from
   a Low blood sugar
   b Disease and infection
   c Loss of fluid
   d Stunted growth

21 The endocrine glands secrete
   a Hormones
   b Mucus
   c Semen
   d Antibodies

22 The pancreas
   a Has digestive and endocrine functions
   b Secretes thyroid hormone
   c Is a gland in the brain
   d Regulates calcium use

Answers to Chapter 9 questions are on p. 587.

FOCUS ON **PRACTICE**

Problem Solving

A patient has a disorder that affects the immune system. How does this affect body function? How will you provide care in a way that protects the person?

The Older Person

- Define the key terms and key abbreviation in this chapter.
- Identify developmental tasks throughout life.
- Identify the psychological and social changes common in late adulthood.
- Describe the physical changes from aging and the care required.
- Describe the gains and losses related to long-term care.
- Explain why sexuality is important throughout life.
- Explain how to deal with inappropriate sexual behavior.
- Explain how to promote PRIDE in the person, the family, and yourself.

development Changes in mental, emotional, and social function
developmental task A skill that must be completed during a stage of development for development to continue
geriatrics The care of aging people
gerontology The study of the aging process
growth The physical changes that are measured and that occur in a steady, orderly manner

menopause The time when menstruation stops and menstrual cycles end; there has been at least 1 year without a menstrual period
sexuality The physical, emotional, social, cultural, and spiritual factors that affect a person's feelings, attitudes, and behaviors about one's gender identity and sexual behavior

UTI Urinary tract infection

Late adulthood ranges from 65 years of age and older. The oldest-old are 85 years of age and older. Aging is normal. *Gerontology is the study of the aging process.* Normal changes occur in body structure and function. Psychological and social changes also occur. Often changes are slow.

The risk for illness, injury, and disability increases with aging. *Geriatrics is the care of aging people.* Many older persons have 1 or more chronic diseases and disabilities. Disabilities can become more severe with aging and as the disease progresses. Quality of life is affected when disabilities interfere with every-day activities.

GROWTH AND DEVELOPMENT

Growth is the physical changes that are measured and that occur in a steady, orderly manner. Growth is measured in weight, height, and changes in appearance and body functions.

Development relates to changes in mental, emotional, and social function. A person behaves and thinks in certain ways in each stage of development. For example, babies depend on adults for basic needs. Adults can meet most of their basic needs without help.

Growth and development occur in a sequence, order, and pattern. Certain skills are completed during each stage. A *developmental task is a skill that must be completed during a stage of development for development to continue.* A stage cannot be skipped. Each stage is the basis for the next stage. See Box 10-1.

BOX 10-1 Developmental Tasks

Infancy (Birth to 1 Year)
- Learning to walk
- Learning to eat solid foods
- Beginning to talk and communicate with others
- Learning to trust
- Beginning to have emotional relationships with parents, brothers, and sisters
- Developing stable sleep and feeding patterns

Toddlerhood (1 to 3 Years)
- Tolerating separation from the primary caregiver
- Gaining control of bowel and bladder function
- Using words to communicate
- Becoming less dependent on the primary caregiver

Preschool (3 to 6 Years)
- Increasing the ability to communicate and understand others
- Performing self-care
- Learning gender differences and developing sexual modesty
- Learning right from wrong and good from bad
- Learning to play with others
- Developing family relationships

School Age (6 to 9 or 10 Years)
- Developing the social and physical skills needed for playing games
- Learning to get along with persons of the same age-group and background *(peers)*
- Learning behaviors and attitudes common for one's gender
- Learning basic reading, writing, and math skills
- Developing a conscience and morals
- Developing a good feeling and attitude about oneself

Late Childhood (9 or 10 to 12 Years)
- Becoming independent of adults and learning to depend on oneself
- Developing and keeping friendships with peers
- Understanding physical, psychological, and social changes
- Developing moral and ethical behavior
- Developing greater muscular strength, coordination, and balance
- Learning how to study

Adolescence (12 to 18 Years)
- Accepting changes in the body and appearance
- Developing appropriate relationships with others and beginning to attract partners
- Becoming independent from parents and adults
- Preparing for marriage and family life
- Preparing for a career
- Developing morals, attitudes, and values needed to function in society

Young Adulthood (18 to 40 Years)
- Choosing education and a career
- Selecting a partner
- Learning to live with a partner
- Becoming a parent and raising children
- Developing a satisfactory sex life

Middle Adulthood (40 to 65 Years)
- Adjusting to physical changes
- Adjusting to having grown children
- Developing leisure-time activities
- Adjusting to aging parents

Late Adulthood (65 Years and Older)
- Adjusting to decreased strength and loss of health
- Adjusting to retirement and reduced income (Fig. 10-1)
- Coping with a partner's death
- Developing new friends and relationships
- Preparing for one's own death

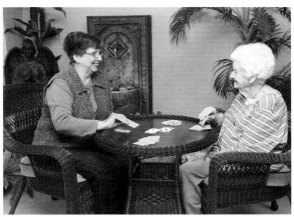

FIGURE 10-1 This retired woman is a nursing center volunteer.

PSYCHOLOGICAL AND SOCIAL CHANGES

Graying hair, wrinkles, and slow movements are physical reminders of aging. They threaten self-esteem, self-image, self-worth, and independence.

Social roles change. For example, a parent may rely on an adult child for care. Social changes include:

- *Retirement.* Retirement is when a person stops working. Retirement allows time to relax and enjoy life. Some people retire because of poor health or disability. Some persons continue part-time jobs or do volunteer work (see Fig. 10-1). Work helps meet love, belonging, and self-esteem needs. The person feels useful and forms friendships.
- *Reduced income.* Retirement often means reduced income. Social Security may provide the only income. House or rent payments continue. Food, clothing, utility bills, and taxes are other expenses. Car expenses, home repairs, drugs, and health care are other costs. Money problems can result. Some people have income from savings, investments, retirement plans, and insurance.
- *Social relationships.* Social relationships change throughout life. Children grow up, leave home, and have families. Some live far away. Family members and friends die, move away, or are disabled. Yet many older people have regular contact with children, grandchildren, family, and friends. Companionship with people their own age is important (Fig. 10-2). Hobbies, religious and community events, and new friends provide enjoyment.
- *Children as caregivers.* Sometimes parents and children change roles. The child cares for the parent. The older person may feel more secure or unwanted, in the way, and useless. Some lose dignity and self-esteem. Tensions may occur among the child, parent, and other household members. Lack of privacy and loss of independence are causes. So are disagreements and criticisms about housekeeping, raising children, meals, and friends.
- *Death and grieving.* A person may try to prepare for a loss, but death and grief are still devastating. Feelings of loneliness and emptiness are common after the death of a partner. As people live longer, some out-live their adult children. Parents of any age experience grief when a child dies. Emotional needs are great. Life changes and physical and mental health problems are common.

See *Focus on Communication: Psychological and Social Changes.*

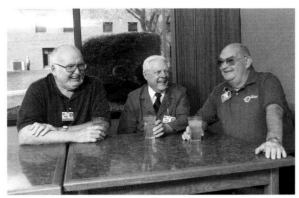

FIGURE 10-2 Older people enjoy being with others of their own age.

FOCUS ON COMMUNICATION

Psychological and Social Changes

The social changes of aging can cause loneliness. With nursing center care, the loneliness can seem greater. You can help the person feel less lonely.

- Suggest calling a family member or friend. Offer to help with phone numbers and dialing.
- Keep the phone within reach. Calls or text messages can be placed or answered with greater ease.
- Suggest reading cards and letters. Offer to assist.
- Visit with the person a few times during your shift.
- Introduce new residents to other residents and staff.
- Encourage e-mailing or video calls with family and friends. Some residents have electronic devices with center-provided Internet access.

PHYSICAL CHANGES

Physical changes of aging happen to everyone (Table 10-1). Body processes slow. Energy level and body efficiency decline. The rate and degree of changes vary with each person. They depend on diet, health, exercise, stress, environment, heredity, and other factors. Changes are slow over many years. Often they are not seen for a long time.

TABLE 10-1   The Aging Process—Physical Changes and Care Measures

Physical Changes	Care Measures

Nervous System
 • Brain and spinal cord lose nerve cells
 • Nerve cells send messages at a slower rate
 • Reflexes slow
 • Reduced blood flow to the brain
 • Abnormal structures can form in the brain
 • Brain tissue may shrink *(atrophy)*
 • Changes in brain cells affect personality and mental function
 • Shorter memory; forgetfulness; confusion may occur
 • Trouble recalling recent events; long-ago events are easier to recall
 • Slower ability to respond
 • Dizziness
 • Sleep patterns change
  ◦ Difficulty falling asleep
  ◦ Waking during the night
  ◦ Less sleep is needed
  ◦ Going to sleep early and waking early are common
 • Reduced sensitivity to pain, pressure, and touch
 • Smell and taste decrease
 • Eyes and vision change
  ◦ Eyelids thin and wrinkle
  ◦ Less tear secretion
  ◦ Pupils less responsive to light
  ◦ Decreased vision at night or in dark rooms
  ◦ Problems seeing green and blue colors
  ◦ Poor vision; problems focusing on close objects
 • Hearing loss
  ◦ Changes in acoustic nerve
  ◦ Eardrums atrophy
  ◦ High-pitched sounds are hard to hear
  ◦ Earwax hardens and thickens; impacted earwax (earwax wedged in the ear) can cause hearing loss
	• Practice safety measures to prevent injuries and falls.
	 • Remind the person to get up slowly from bed or chair.
	 • Follow the care plan to assist with memory, personality, or mental changes.
	 • Follow safety measures for heat and cold.
	 • Check for signs of skin breakdown and pressure injuries.
	 • Give good skin care.
	 • Prevent skin tears and pressure injuries.
	 • Follow the care plan to promote sleep. Day-time naps and rest may be needed.
	 • Have the person wear eyeglasses, contact lenses, and hearing aids as needed.
	 • Provide good room lighting and night-lights.
	 • See the following chapters for care measures.
	  ◦ Chapters 11 and 12—safety and preventing falls
	  ◦ Chapter 17—turning and moving
	  ◦ Chapter 18—getting in and out of bed or chair
	  ◦ Chapter 33—sleep
	  ◦ Chapter 35—heat and cold
	  ◦ Chapter 39—eyeglasses, contact lenses, and hearing aids
	  ◦ Chapters 41 and 42—confusion and mental changes

Integumentary System
 • Skin becomes less elastic
 • Skin loses strength
 • Brown spots *(age spots* or *liver spots)* on the wrists and hands
 • Fewer nerve endings affect temperature, pressure, and pain sensation
 • Fewer blood vessels
 • Fatty tissue layer is lost
 • Skin thins and sags
 • Skin is fragile and easily injured or burned
 • Folds, lines, and wrinkles appear
 • Blood vessels become more fragile
 • Decreased secretion of oil and sweat glands
 • Dry, itchy skin
 • More sensitive to cold
 • Nails become thick and tough
 • Whitening or graying hair
 • Facial hair in some women
 • Loss or thinning of hair
 • Drier hair
	• Protect from drafts and cold.
	 • Provide sweaters, lap blankets, socks, and extra blankets.
	 • Check thermostat settings. Higher settings are helpful.
	 • Provide for hygiene—shower or bath 2 times a week; partial baths on other days.
	 • Use mild soaps or soap substitutes to clean the underarms, genitals, and under the breasts. Soap may be avoided on the face, arms, legs, back, chest, and abdomen.
	 • Apply lotions and creams to prevent drying and itching.
	 • Provide nail and foot care.
	 • Prevent burns. Do not use hot water bottles or heating pads on the feet.
	 • Brush and shampoo hair as needed for hygiene and comfort. Shampoo frequency often decreases with age.
	 • Protect from prolonged sun exposure.
	 • See the following chapters for care measures.
	  ◦ Chapter 11—preventing burns
	  ◦ Chapters 22 and 23—hygiene, skin care, and grooming
	  ◦ Chapter 35—skin tears
	  ◦ Chapter 36—pressure injuries

Continued

TABLE 10-1   The Aging Process—Physical Changes and Care Measures—cont'd

Physical Changes	Care Measures
Musculo-Skeletal System • Muscles shrink *(atrophy)* • Muscle strength, tone, and contractility decrease • Bone mass decreases • Bones become weaker • Bones become brittle; can break easily • Vertebrae shorten • Joints become stiff and painful • Hip and knee joints become flexed (bent) • Gradual loss of height; trunk (torso) becomes shorter • Decreased mobility	• Promote exercise and activity as ordered to prevent atrophy and loss of strength. • Assist with range-of-motion exercises as ordered (Chapter 32). • Encourage a diet high in protein, calcium, and vitamins as ordered. • Practice safety measures to prevent injuries and falls (Chapters 11 and 12). • Turn and move the person gently and carefully. • Assist the person in getting out of bed or chair as needed. • Provide support when walking as needed (Chapter 32).

Circulatory System
 • Heart pumps with less force
 • Heart valves thicken and become stiff
 • Heart rate may slow
 • Abnormal heart rhythms may occur
 • Heart may enlarge slightly
 • Heart walls thicken
 • Arteries narrow and become stiffer
 • Less blood flows through narrowed arteries
 • Weakened heart works harder to pump blood through narrowed vessels
 • Number of red blood cells decreases
 • Fatigue
	• Follow the person's activity limits.
	  ○ Promote exercise as ordered. Encourage the person to be as active as possible. Moderate daily exercise helps maintain health and well-being.
	  ○ Assist with range-of-motion exercises as ordered.
	  ○ Avoid over-exertion. The person should not walk far, climb many stairs, or carry heavy things. Encourage rest periods.
	  ○ Follow orders for bed rest if it is needed (Chapter 32). *Bed rest* means *being confined to bed.*
	 • Keep personal care items, TV controls, phone, and other needed items within reach.

Respiratory System • Respiratory muscles weaken • Some lung tissue is lost • Lung tissue becomes less elastic • Chest is less able to stretch to breathe • Difficulty breathing *(dyspnea)* • Decreased strength for coughing and clearing the airway	• Promote normal breathing. • Position the person for easier breathing. Semi-Fowler's or Fowler's position (Chapter 16) may be preferred. • Assist with coughing and deep-breathing exercises as ordered (Chapter 37). • Avoid heavy bed linens over the chest. • Turn and position the person according to the care plan. Persons on bed rest are re-positioned often. • Encourage activity as ordered.
Digestive System • Decreased saliva production • Difficulty swallowing *(dysphagia)* • Decreased appetite • Decreased secretion of digestive juices • Difficulty digesting fried and fatty foods • Indigestion • Loss of teeth • Decreased peristalsis causing *flatulence* (gas) and constipation	• Provide oral hygiene and denture care to improve taste (Chapter 21). • Encourage diet as ordered (Chapters 28 and 29). Dry, fried, fatty, and hard-to-chew foods are avoided. The person may need food ground, chopped, or pureed. • Promote fluid intake as ordered (Chapter 30). Thickened liquids may be needed for persons with swallowing problems. • Follow the care plan to prevent *flatulence* (gas) and constipation (Chapter 27). High-fiber foods help prevent constipation. Some are hard to chew and irritate the intestines. Apricots, celery, and fruits and vegetables with skins and seeds are avoided.
Urinary System • Kidney function decreases • Reduced blood supply to kidneys • Kidneys atrophy • Bladder tissues less able to stretch • Bladder muscles weaken • Bladder may not empty completely • Urinary tract infections (UTIs) may occur • Urinary frequency, urgency, incontinence (loss of bladder control), or night-time urination may occur • Prostate gland enlarges (men)	• Answer call lights promptly (Chapter 19). • Promote normal urination (Chapter 25). Provide the bedpan, urinal, or commode as needed. • Follow the care plan to manage incontinence (Chapter 25). • Provide catheter care according to the care plan (Chapter 26). • Encourage fluids as ordered to prevent UTIs. Most fluids should be taken before 5:00 PM (1700) to reduce the need to urinate at night. • Follow the person's bladder training program (Chapter 25).

TABLE 10-1 The Aging Process—Physical Changes and Care Measures—cont'd	
Physical Changes	Care Measures

Immune System
• Fewer immune cells
• Immune response slows
  ◦ Increased risk for infection
  ◦ Different signs of infection than usual
• Healing slows
• Ability to detect and correct cell defects (problems) declines
  ◦ Increased cancer risk
	• Practice measures to prevent infection (Chapters 14 and 15).
	• Monitor closely for signs of infection.
	  ◦ Usual signs are lessened or absent. The person may have only a slight *fever* (elevated body temperature) or no fever.
	  ◦ Confusion, mood changes, a change in level of consciousness, or a recent fall may signal infection.
	• Prevent injuries and falls (Chapters 11 and 12).
	• Promote exercise as ordered (Chapter 32) and a healthy diet (Chapter 28). Exercise and good nutrition strengthen the immune system.
	• Follow the care plan for wound care measures and pressure injury prevention (Chapters 35 and 36).
	• The nurse teaches about healthy life-style choices and illness prevention.
	  ◦ Smoking slows healing and weakens the immune system.
	  ◦ Vaccines may prevent certain infections. Influenza and pneumonia are examples (Chapter 40).

Reproductive System
• Men
  ◦ Testosterone decreases slightly
  ◦ Erections take longer
  ◦ Longer phase between erection and orgasm
  ◦ Less forceful orgasms
  ◦ Erections lost quickly
  ◦ Longer time between erections
• Women
  ◦ **Menopause**—*the time when menstruation stops and menstrual cycles end; there has been at least 1 year without a menstrual period*
  ◦ Estrogen and progesterone decrease
  ◦ Uterus, vagina, and genitalia atrophy
  ◦ Thinning of vaginal walls
  ◦ Vaginal dryness
  ◦ Arousal takes longer
  ◦ Less intense orgasms
  ◦ Quicker return to pre-excitement state
	• Follow the care plan for the person with reproductive changes.

NURSING CENTER CARE

Nursing centers are options for persons who cannot care for themselves (Chapter 1). Aging changes and safety needs are considered in the center's design. Programs and services meet basic needs. The setting is as home-like as possible (Fig. 10-3). Some people stay in nursing centers until death. Others return home.

The person needing nursing center care may suffer some or all of these losses.

• Loss of identity as a productive member of a family and community
• Loss of possessions—home, household items, car, and so on
• Loss of independence
• Loss of real-world experiences—shopping, traveling, cooking, driving, hobbies, and so on
• Loss of health and mobility

Feeling useless, powerless, and hopeless are common emotions. The health team helps the person cope with loss and improve quality of life. Treat the person with dignity and respect. Also practice good communication skills. Follow the care plan.

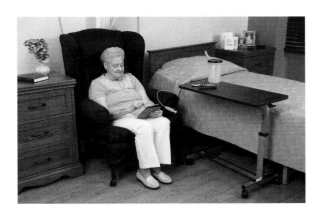

FIGURE 10-3 A nursing center is as home-like as possible. Some centers allow residents to bring their own bed and furniture from home.

SEXUALITY

Sexuality is the physical, emotional, social, cultural, and spiritual factors that affect a person's feelings, attitudes, and behaviors about one's gender identity and sexual behavior. Gender identity refers to a person's sense of being male, female, a blend of both, or neither. Sexuality is more than *sex*—the physical interactions between people involving the body and reproductive organs. It involves the personality and the body—how a person behaves, thinks, dresses, and responds to others.

Older persons love, fall in love, and have intimate relationships and activities. Reproductive organs change with aging (see Table 10-1). Frequency of sex may decrease. Besides life events, reasons relate to weakness, fatigue, and pain. Reduced mobility, aging, and chronic illness are other factors. Some men experience *erectile dysfunction (ED)*—the inability to have or maintain an erection. ED can be treated with drugs.

Some older people do not have intercourse. This does not mean loss of sexual needs or desires. Needs are often expressed in other ways. They hold hands, touch, caress, and embrace. These bring closeness and intimacy.

Sexuality Needs

Love, affection, and intimacy are important throughout life (Fig. 10-4). The measures in Box 10-2 show respect for the person's sexuality needs.

Married couples in nursing centers can share the same room. This is a requirement of the *Omnibus Budget Reconciliation Act of 1987 (OBRA)*. Non-married persons may have roommate preferences.

Sometimes relationships develop between residents. They are allowed time together, not kept apart. To protect against sexual abuse, relationships must be consensual (Chapter 4). *Consensual* involves *giving consent*.

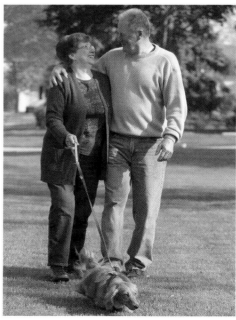

FIGURE 10-4 Love and affection are important to persons of all ages.

BOX 10-2 Respecting Sexuality Needs

- Let the person practice grooming routines. Assist as needed. See Chapter 23.
- Let the person choose clothing. Patient gowns can embarrass the person. Street clothes are worn if the person's condition permits.
- Protect the right to privacy. Do not expose the person. Drape and screen the person.
- Treat the person with dignity and respect. The person may not share your sexual attitudes, values, or practices. Do not gossip about or insult the person.
- Allow privacy. If the person has a private room, close the door for privacy. Some agencies have *DO NOT DISTURB* signs for doors. Let the person and partner know how much time they have alone. For example, remind them about meal times and care measures. Tell other staff that the person wants time alone.
- Knock before you enter any room. This simple courtesy shows respect for privacy.
- Consider the person's roommate. Privacy curtains do not block sound. Arrange for privacy when the roommate is out of the room. A roommate may offer to leave for a while. Or the nurse finds a private area.
- Allow privacy for masturbation. It is a normal form of sexual expression. Close the privacy curtain and the door. Knock before you enter the room. This saves you and the person embarrassment. Sometimes confused persons masturbate in public areas. Lead the person to a private area. Or distract the person with an activity.

Inappropriate Sexual Behavior

Patients and residents may have inappropriate sexual behaviors. Such behaviors may be innocent and non-aggressive. Others are aggressive.

Some persons flirt or make sexual advances or comments. Some expose themselves or touch staff. Often there are reasons for the person's behavior. Understanding this helps you deal with the matter.

Inappropriate sexual behaviors have many causes. They include:
- Nervous system disorders
- Confusion, disorientation, and dementia
- Drug side effects
- Fever
- Poor vision

Some behaviors are innocent. The person may mistake another person as a partner. Or the person cannot control the behavior. The healthy person controls sexual urges. Changes in the brain and mental function make control difficult.

Sometimes touch is used to gain attention. For example, a person cannot speak or move the right side. Your buttocks are within reach. To get your attention, the person touches your buttocks. The behavior is not sexual.

Touching the genitals may signal a health problem or a need. Urinary or reproductive system disorders can cause genital soreness and itching. So can poor hygiene and being wet or soiled from urine or feces. Some persons touch or grab at their clothing to communicate an elimination need. Such behaviors are not sexual. They communicate needs.

Sexually aggressive behaviors—touching, grabbing, offensive comments—may be about power, control, or fears about sexual function. For example, a person wants to prove attractiveness and the ability to perform sexually. You must be professional about the matter.

- Ask the person not to touch you. State the places where you were touched.
- Tell the person what you will not do.
- Tell the person what behaviors make you uncomfortable. Politely ask the person not to act that way.
- Allow privacy if the person is becoming aroused. Provide for safety. Complete a safety check of the room (see the inside of the back cover). Tell the person when you will return.
- Discuss the matter with the nurse. The nurse can help you understand the behavior.
- Follow the care plan. It has measures to deal with sexually aggressive behaviors. They are based on the cause of the behavior.

See *Focus on Communication: Inappropriate Sexual Behavior.*

FOCUS ON **COMMUNICATION**

Inappropriate Sexual Behavior

Dealing with sexually inappropriate behavior is hard for new and experienced staff. Consider:

- Does the person have a health problem that affects impulse control? If yes, the behavior may not have a sexual purpose.
- Is the person's behavior on purpose? Is the intent sexual? If yes, you must confront the behavior. Be direct and matter-of-fact. For example, you can say:
  - "You brushed your hand across my breast (or other body part) twice this morning. Please don't do that again."
  - "No, I cannot kiss you. It would be unprofessional."
  - "You exposed yourself to me again today. Please do not do that again."

The sexually aggressive person needs the nurse's attention. Report what happened and when. Also report what you said and did. The nurse must deal with the problem. If other staff report such behaviors, the problem is viewed in a broader way.

Protecting the Person

The person must be protected from unwanted sexual comments and advances. This is sexual abuse (Chapter 4). Tell the nurse right away. No one is allowed to sexually abuse another person. This includes staff members, patients, residents, family members or other visitors, and volunteers.

FOCUS ON P R I D E

The Person, Family, and Yourself

P ersonal and Professional Responsibility

All older persons are not the same. Each person is unique. Treat each person as an individual.

R ights and Respect

Simple actions promote dignity and respect for the older person. For example:

- Greet the person by name. Make eye contact and smile. Be pleasant.
- Treat the person as an adult, not a child.
- Speak to the person, not just to a caregiver or family member.
- Listen to the person (Chapter 6).
- Promote independence and a sense of control. Offer choices. Follow the person's preferences.

I ndependence and Social Interaction

Older persons may feel lonely and isolated. Loss of friends and loved ones, a new home setting, reduced income, and physical changes are causes. To promote social interaction:

- Encourage the person to talk about friends and family.
- Ask about hobbies and interests.
- Use touch to show caring. For example, gently place your hand on the person's shoulder or arm. Remember to maintain professional boundaries (Chapter 4).
- Take time to listen. Avoid seeming rushed.

Some persons prefer quiet and privacy. They may avoid social contacts. Respect their wishes for privacy. Take pride in considering social needs.

D elegation and Teamwork

The health team must try to determine the cause of inappropriate sexual behaviors. If the cause can be corrected, the behavior may stop. If not, the care plan includes measures to manage the behavior. A professional response is always needed.

Tell the nurse about aggressive behaviors. The problem cannot be ignored. Rely on the nursing team for advice, guidance, and support.

E thics and Laws

The changes of aging can affect the person's ability to do normal daily tasks. The older person may need help from family or caregivers. Watch for signs of abuse.

- The person is treated like an infant or child.
- The person is not spoken to.
- The person is insulted, scolded, or criticized.
- Threats to with-hold care are made.
- Mis-use or theft of money or possessions is suspected.
- The person lacks needed care or has poor hygiene.
- The person has signs of physical abuse—bruises, scars, burns, and so on.

See "Elder Abuse" in Chapter 4. If you suspect abuse, tell the nurse. The person must be protected from mistreatment.

FOCUS ON PRIDE: *Application*

List 5 changes that can occur with aging. Describe how each affects the person. How would you modify care to meet the person's needs?

Circle the BEST answer.

1 Development in late adulthood involves
   a Developing coordination and balance
   b Adjusting to decreased strength
   c Developing a satisfactory sex life
   d Performing self-care

2 Retirement usually results in
   a Lowered income
   b Nursing center care
   c Less free time
   d Financial security

3 Which causes loneliness in older persons?
   a Having hobbies
   b Children moving away
   c Attending community events
   d Contact with other older persons

4 Which statement about a partner's death is *true?*
   a The surviving partner's life will not likely change.
   b Preparing for the event lessens grief.
   c Grief cannot cause physical problems.
   d Feelings of loss and emptiness occur.

5 Aging causes changes in the nervous system. Which is *true?*
   a Sleep patterns change.
   b Recent memories are easier to recall than past memories.
   c Sensitivity to pressure increases.
   d Confusion occurs in all older persons.

6 Changes occur in the eyes with aging. Which is *true?*
   a Tear secretion increases.
   b There is no change in seeing colors.
   c There is more trouble focusing on far objects.
   d Vision is poor at night and in dark rooms.

7 Which is *true* of hearing loss in older persons?
   a Low-pitched sounds are hard to hear.
   b Acoustic nerve changes affect hearing.
   c Earwax cannot affect hearing.
   d Ear infections often cause hearing loss.

8 Skin changes occur with aging. Care should include
   a Keeping the room cool
   b A daily bath with soap
   c Applying lotion
   d Bathing in hot water

9 Musculo-skeletal changes occur with aging. Which is *true?*
   a Bones become firm.
   b Exercise promotes muscle atrophy.
   c Joints become stiff and painful.
   d Bed rest prevents loss of strength.

10 An older person has circulatory changes. Which care measure would you question?
   a Keep needed items nearby
   b Get a moderate amount of daily exercise
   c Avoid over-exertion
   d Take long walks

11 Respiratory changes occur with aging. Which is *true?*
   a Heavy bed linens are used.
   b The person is turned often if on bed rest.
   c The side-lying position is best for breathing.
   d Deep breathing is avoided.

12 Older persons should avoid dry foods because of
   a Decreases in saliva and difficulty swallowing
   b Appetite changes
   c Increased amounts of digestive juices
   d Increased peristalsis

13 An older person is at risk for a urinary tract infection (UTI). The doctor ordered increased fluid intake. You should
   a Give most of the fluid before 1700 (5:00 PM)
   b Question the order
   c Start a bladder training program
   d Insert a catheter

14 Immune system changes from aging
   a Do not affect signs of illness
   b Lower the risk of infection
   c Cause high fevers in mild illness
   d Cause slower healing

15 A person is masturbating in the dining room. You should
   a Do nothing
   b Scold the person
   c Quietly take the person to his or her room
   d Restrain the person

16 A person touches you sexually. You should
   a Ignore the behavior
   b Push the person away from you
   c Tell your co-workers
   d Ask the person not to touch you

Answers to Chapter 10 questions are on p. 587.

FOCUS ON **PRACTICE**

Problem Solving

A person has urinary incontinence and swallowing problems due to changes from aging. A co-worker uses the term "diaper" to describe incontinence products and "bib" for clothing protectors. The co-worker threatens to with-hold privileges if the person does not finish meals.

Why should you treat the person as an adult and not a child? Describe ways to provide age-appropriate care. How will you respond to your co-worker's statements and actions?

CHAPTER 11

Safety Needs

OBJECTIVES

- Define the key terms and key abbreviations in this chapter.
- Describe accident risk factors.
- Explain why you identify a person before giving care.
- Explain how to correctly identify a person.
- Describe the safety measures to prevent burns, poisoning, and suffocation.
- Identify the signs and causes of choking.
- Explain how to prevent equipment accidents.

- Explain how to handle hazardous chemicals.
- Describe how agencies prepare for disasters.
- Describe fire prevention measures and oxygen safety.
- Explain what to do during a fire.
- Explain how to protect yourself from workplace violence.
- Describe your role in risk management.
- Perform the procedures described in this chapter.
- Explain how to promote PRIDE in the person, the family, and yourself.

KEY TERMS

coma A prolonged state of unconsciousness

dementia The loss of cognitive and social function caused by changes in the brain

disaster A harmful event that can affect the agency, patient or resident population, community, or larger geographic area

elopement When a patient or resident leaves the agency without staff knowledge

hazard Anything in the person's setting that could cause injury or illness

hazardous chemical Any chemical that is a physical hazard or a health hazard

incident Any event that has harmed or could harm a patient, resident, visitor, or staff member

paralysis Loss of muscle function

poison Any substance harmful to the body when ingested, inhaled, injected, or absorbed through the skin

suffocation When breathing stops from the lack of oxygen; asphyxia

unconscious Being unaware of one's setting and being unable to react or respond to people, places, or things

workplace violence Violent acts (including assault or threat of assault) directed toward persons at work or while on duty

KEY ABBREVIATIONS

AED	Automated external defibrillator
CDC	Centers for Disease Control and Prevention
CMS	Centers for Medicare & Medicaid Services
CPR	Cardiopulmonary resuscitation
EMS	Emergency Medical Services
FBAO	Foreign-body airway obstruction
ID	Identification

OSHA	Occupational Safety and Health Administration
PASS	*Pull* the safety pin, *aim* low, *squeeze* the lever, *sweep* back and forth
PPE	Personal protective equipment
RACE	Rescue, alarm, confine, extinguish
RRS	Rapid Response System
SDS	Safety data sheet

Safety is a basic need. Patients and residents are at great risk for accidents and falls. (See Chapter 12 for falls.) Some accidents and injuries cause death. You must protect patients, residents, visitors, co-workers, and yourself from harm.

The goal is to prevent accidents and injuries without limiting the person's mobility and independence. Safety measures must not interfere with the person's rights (Chapter 2).

This chapter covers general safety. The care plan lists specific safety measures for the person.

See *Focus on Surveys: Safety Needs.*

See *Promoting Safety and Comfort: Safety Needs.*

FOCUS ON SURVEYS

Safety Needs

A survey team will observe the agency setting and patient or resident rooms. Surveyors look for:

- Potential or actual hazards. A **hazard** *is anything in the person's setting that could cause injury or illness.* Examples include spills, loose hand rails, unanswered call lights, burnt-out bulbs, unsafe equipment, and other safety issues described in this chapter and other chapters.
- How staff respond to potential or actual hazards.
- If the care plan was followed on each shift for persons at risk.
- How staff supervise persons at risk.
- If a hazard was changed or removed.

During staff interviews, a surveyor may ask:

- About measures in the person's care plan to reduce the risk for an accident.
- When and how you report risks and hazards.
- When and how you correct an immediate hazard. A spill is an example.
- The agency's procedures for removing or reducing a hazard.

Always provide for safety. Know what to do if you find a hazard. Remember to give surveyors complete and honest answers. Surveys protect patients and residents.

PROMOTING SAFETY AND COMFORT

Safety Needs

Safety

The safety measures in this chapter apply to all health care settings and every-day life. You may see something unsafe. Correct the matter right away if it is something you can do. For example:

- Wipe up spills. Do so even if you did not cause the spill.
- A person is sliding out of a wheelchair. Position the person correctly. Do so even if a co-worker is responsible for the person's care.
- A person has problems holding a coffee cup. Offer to help the person.

Follow agency policy to report problems that you cannot correct. They include:

- Electrical outlets or switches that do not work or are coming out of the wall
- Water leaks from windows, doors, ceilings, pipes, faucets, tubs, showers, toilets, water heaters, and other sources
- Toilets that do not work properly
- Water from faucets that does not warm up or is very hot
- Broken or damaged windows or furniture
- Windows, doors, knobs, or handles that are broken or do not work properly
- Hand rails and grab bars that are loose or need repair
- Odd smells, odors, and sounds
- Signs of rodents, flies, ants, or other pests
- Lights and lamps that do not work or have burnt-out bulbs
- Flooring (carpeting, tiles, hardwood flooring) needing repair

---

ACCIDENT RISK FACTORS

Some people cannot protect themselves. They present dangers to themselves and others. Certain factors increase the risk of accidents and injuries.

- *Awareness of surroundings and ability to respond.* Confused and disoriented persons may not understand what is happening to and around them. A *disoriented* person lacks awareness of 1 or more of the following—the self or others, time, location or surroundings. Changes in level of consciousness can occur from illness or injury.
  - **Unconscious**—*being unaware of one's setting and being unable to react or respond to people, places, or things*
  - **Coma**—*a prolonged state of unconsciousness*
- *Agitated and aggressive behaviors.* Pain can cause these behaviors. So can confusion, decreased awareness of surroundings, and fear of what may happen.
- *Vision loss.* Persons with poor vision can fall or trip over toys, rugs, equipment, furniture, and cords. Some cannot read container labels. Poisoning can result.
- *Hearing loss.* Persons with hearing loss may not hear warning signals or fire alarms. Some cannot hear approaching meal carts, drug carts, stretchers, or wheelchairs. They do not know to move to safety.
- *Impaired smell and touch.* Illness and aging affect smell and touch. The person may not detect smoke or gas odors. Burns are a risk from impaired touch. The person has problems sensing heat and cold. Some people have a decreased sense of pain. They may be unaware of injury.
- *Impaired mobility. Mobility* is the ability to move (Chapter 32). Some diseases and injuries affect mobility. The person may not be able to move to safety. Some persons cannot walk or propel wheelchairs. Some persons are paralyzed. **Paralysis** *means loss of muscle function.* Loss of sensation can also occur. Paralysis may involve just the lower body (*paraplegia*), the upper and lower body (*quadriplegia* or *tetraplegia*), or 1 side of the body (*hemiplegia*). See Chapter 40.
- *Drugs.* Drug side effects may include loss of balance, drowsiness, and poor coordination. Reduced awareness, confusion, and disorientation may occur.
- *Age.* Children and older persons are at risk for injuries. See *Focus on Older Persons: Accident Risk Factors.*

FOCUS ON OLDER PERSONS

Accident Risk Factors

Changes from aging increase the risk for falls and other injuries. See Chapter 10.

Some persons have dementia. **Dementia** *is the loss of cognitive and social function caused by changes in the brain* (Chapter 42). (*Cognitive* relates to *knowledge.*) Memory and the ability to think and reason are affected.

Persons with dementia may be confused and disoriented. Awareness of surroundings is often reduced. They may not understand what is happening to and around them. Judgment may be poor. Some no longer know safety from danger. They may access closets, cupboards, or other unsafe and unlocked areas. They may eat or drink cleaning products, drugs, or poisons. Accidents and injuries are great risks.

IDENTIFYING THE PERSON

Each person has different treatments, therapies, and activity limits. The wrong care can threaten life and health.

The person may receive an identification (ID) bracelet when admitted to the agency (Fig. 11-1). The bracelet has the person's name, ID number, room and bed number, date of birth (DOB), age, and doctor. Other identifying information and numbers are included. A medical record number (MRN)—used to identify the person's medical record—is an example.

You use the ID bracelet to identify the person before giving care. Your assignment sheet states what care to give. To identify the person:

- Compare identifying information on the assignment sheet with that on the ID bracelet (Fig. 11-2). Carefully check the information. Some people have the same first and last names. For example, John Smith is a very common name.
- Use at least 2 identifiers. Some agencies require the person to state and spell his or her name and give his or her birth date. Others require checking the person's ID number. You cannot use the person's room or bed number. Always follow agency policy.
- Call the person by name when checking the ID bracelet. This is a courtesy as you touch the person and before giving care. Just calling the person by name is not enough for identification. Confused, disoriented, drowsy, hard of hearing, or distracted persons may answer to any name.

See *Focus on Communication: Identifying the Person.*
See *Promoting Safety and Comfort: Identifying the Person.*

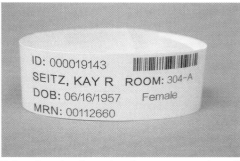

FIGURE 11-1 ID bracelet. (ID—identification; DOB—date of birth; MRN—medical record number.)

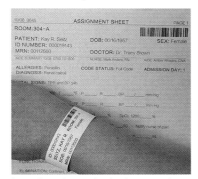

FIGURE 11-2 The ID bracelet is checked against the assignment sheet to accurately identify the person.

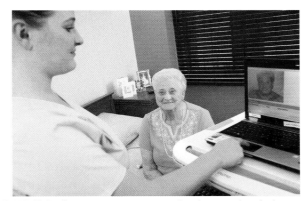

FIGURE 11-3 The nursing assistant uses the photo to identify the person.

Identifying Nursing Center Residents

Alert and oriented residents may not wear ID bracelets. This is noted on the person's care plan. Follow center policy and the care plan to identify the person.

Some nursing centers use photo ID systems (Fig. 11-3). The person's photo is taken on admission for the medical record. If your center uses such a system, learn to use it safely.

FOCUS ON **COMMUNICATION**

Identifying the Person

To identify the person, call the person by name. Ask to see the ID bracelet. For example: "Hello, Mr. Hall. May I see your ID bracelet?" Then ask for 2 identifiers. You can say: "Please tell me your full name and birth date." Compare the identifiers with the information on the ID bracelet and your assignment sheet.

Identifying oneself over and over again can be annoying. The person may say: "Do I have to say it again? You know who I am." Be polite. Explain why you check identity. You can say: "It is important to check so I give care to the right person. It is for your safety." Thank the person. Use the person's title and name. For example: "Thank you, Mr. Hall."

PROMOTING SAFETY AND COMFORT

Identifying the Person

Safety

Always identify the person before giving care. Do not identify the person and then leave the room for supplies and equipment. You could go to the wrong room and give care to the wrong person. The person needing care would not receive it. Harm could result.

Water, spilled food and fluids, and every-day wear and tear can damage ID bracelets. If you cannot read the information on the ID bracelet, tell the nurse. The nurse can have a new bracelet made.

Comfort

Make sure ID bracelets are not too loose or too tight. You should be able to slide 1 or 2 fingers under a bracelet. If it is too loose or too tight, tell the nurse.

PREVENTING BURNS

Smoking, spilled hot liquids, electrical items, and very hot water (sinks, tubs, showers) are common causes of burns. The safety measures in Box 11-1 can prevent burns.

See *Focus on Older Persons: Preventing Burns.*

BOX 11-1 Preventing Burns

Eating and Drinking
- Assist with eating and drinking as needed. Spilled hot food or liquids can cause burns.
- Be careful when carrying hot food and liquids.
- Keep hot food and liquids away from counter and table edges. Use the center of the counter or table.
- Do not pour hot liquids near a person.

Water
- Turn on cold water first, then hot water (for a 2-handled faucet). Turn off hot water first, then cold water.
- Measure bath or shower water temperature (Chapter 22). Check it before the person gets into the tub or shower.
- Check for "hot spots" in bath water. Move your hand back and forth in the water.

Electrical Equipment
- See "Preventing Equipment Accidents" (p. 124).
- Do not let the person sleep with a heating pad or an electric blanket.

Smoking
- Be sure patients and residents smoke only in smoking areas.
- Do not leave smoking materials at the bedside.
- Supervise the smoking of persons who cannot protect themselves.
- Do not allow smoking in bed.
- Do not allow smoking where oxygen is used or stored (Chapter 37).
- Be alert to ashes that may fall onto a person.

Other
- See "Fire Safety" (p. 126).
- Follow safety guidelines when applying heat and cold (Chapter 35).

FOCUS ON OLDER PERSONS

Preventing Burns

Older persons are at risk for burns. Risk factors include decreased skin thickness, decreased sensitivity to heat, slowed reaction time, decreased mobility, communication problems, confusion, and dementia. The measures in Box 11-1 help to prevent burns.

PREVENTING POISONING

A *poison is any substance harmful to the body when ingested, inhaled, injected, or absorbed through the skin.* Drugs and household products are common poisons. Poisoning in adults may be from carelessness, confusion, or poor vision when reading labels. As a result, a person may take too much of a drug or ingest a harmful substance. To prevent poisoning:
- Make sure patients and residents cannot reach harmful products.
- Keep harmful products in their original containers.
- Leave the original label on harmful products.
- Store personal care items according to agency policy. Soap, mouthwash, lotion, deodorant, and shampoo are examples. These products are harmful when swallowed.
- Read all labels carefully before using the product.
- Do not leave harmful products unattended when in use.
- Store harmful products according to agency policy.

Poisoning is an emergency. The Poison Control Center provides free 24-hour guidance for poison emergencies. The number is 1-800-222-1222. See Chapter 43 for the emergency care for poisoning.

See *Promoting Safety and Comfort: Preventing Poisoning.*

PROMOTING SAFETY AND COMFORT

Preventing Poisoning

Safety

Keep emergency numbers by the phone and stored in your phone. If you call 911 or the Poison Control Center (1-800-222-1222), give the following information.
- Your location, name, phone number, and distance to the nearest hospital
- The person's signs and symptoms, condition (breathing; not breathing), and health problems
- The person's age and weight
- The substance, containers, or bottles involved
- How you think the substance entered the body—swallowed, inhaled or smelled, injected, skin contact, splashed into the eyes
- When you think the substance entered the body
- If the person has vomited
- Emergency care given (Chapter 43)

Follow the rules for basic emergency care in Chapter 43. Follow the directions given by the Poison Control Center.

PREVENTING SUFFOCATION

Suffocation (asphyxia) is when breathing stops from the lack of oxygen. Death occurs if the person does not start breathing. Common causes include choking, drowning, inhaling gas or smoke, strangulation, and electrical shock (p. 124). (See "Altered Respiratory Function" in Chapter 37.)

Measures to prevent suffocation are listed in Box 11-2. Clear the airway if the person is choking.

BOX 11-2 Preventing Suffocation

- Make sure dentures fit properly and are in place.
- Report loose teeth or dentures.
- Check the care plan for swallowing problems before serving food (including snacks) or fluids. The person may have special food (fluid) orders (Chapter 29). Make sure the person is able to chew and swallow what is served.
- Cut foods into small, bite-sized pieces for persons who cannot do so themselves.
- Tell the nurse at once if the person has swallowing problems.
- Do not give oral foods or fluids to persons with feeding tubes (Chapter 29).
- Follow aspiration precautions (Chapter 29).
- Do not leave a person unattended in a bathtub or shower.
- Move all persons from the area if you smell smoke.
- Position the person in bed properly.
- Prevent entrapment in the bed system (Chapter 19).
- Use bed rails correctly (Chapter 12).
- Practice safe use of restraints if they must be used for protection. Restraints can cause strangulation. See Chapter 13.
- Do not use power strips for care equipment.
- See "Preventing Equipment Accidents" (p. 124).

Choking

A foreign body (food or object) can obstruct (block) the airway. This is called *choking* or *foreign-body airway obstruction (FBAO)*. Air cannot pass through the airways into the lungs. The body does not get enough oxygen. Death can result.

Choking often occurs during eating. A large, poorly chewed piece of meat is a common cause. Laughing and talking while eating also are common causes. So is excessive alcohol intake.

Unconscious persons can choke. Common causes are aspiration of vomitus and the tongue falling back into the airway.

See *Focus on Older Persons: Choking.*

FOCUS ON OLDER PERSONS

Choking

Older persons are at risk for choking. Weakness, dentures that fit poorly, *dysphagia* (difficulty swallowing), and chronic illness are common causes.

Mild and Severe Airway Obstruction. Foreign bodies can cause mild (partial) or severe (complete) airway obstruction. With *mild airway obstruction*, some air moves in and out of the lungs. The person is conscious and usually can speak. Often forceful coughing can remove the object. Breathing may sound like wheezing between coughs. For mild airway obstruction:

- Stay with the person.
- Encourage the person to keep coughing to expel the object.
- Do not interrupt the person's efforts to clear the airway. If the person is breathing and coughing, abdominal thrusts are not needed.
- If the obstruction persists, call for help.

A person with *severe airway obstruction* has difficulty breathing. Air does not move in and out of the lungs. The person may not be able to breathe, speak, or cough. If able to cough, the cough is of poor quality. When the person tries to inhale (breathe in), there is no noise or a high-pitched noise. The person may appear pale and *cyanotic* (bluish color). Severe airway obstruction is an emergency.

Relieving Choking. When choking, the conscious person usually clutches at the throat (Fig. 11-4). Clutching at the throat is often called the *universal sign of choking.* The conscious person is very frightened. If the obstruction is not removed, the person will die.

Abdominal thrusts are used to relieve severe airway obstruction. Abdominal thrusts are quick, upward thrusts to the abdomen. Also known as the *Heimlich maneuver*, the thrusts force air out of the lungs and create an artificial cough. They are done to try to expel the foreign body from the airway.

You may observe a person choking. And you may perform emergency measures to relieve choking. Relief of choking occurs when the foreign body is removed. Or it occurs when you feel air move and see the chest rise and fall when giving rescue breaths (Chapter 43).

If you assist a choking person, report and record what happened. Include what you did and the person's response.

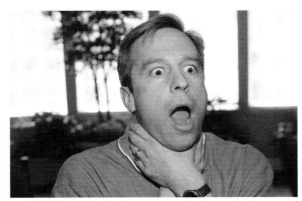

FIGURE 11-4 A choking person clutches at the throat.

Chest thrusts are used for obese or pregnant persons (Fig. 11-5). If you are alone and choking, perform self-administered abdominal thrusts. See Box 11-3.

See procedure: *Relieving Choking—Adult or Child (Over 1 Year of Age).*

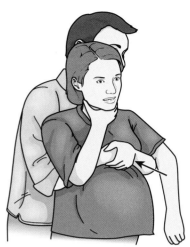

FIGURE 11-5 Chest thrusts to relieve choking in a pregnant woman.

BOX 11-3 Relieving Choking

Chest Thrusts for Obese or Pregnant Persons
1 Stand behind the person.
2 Place your arms under the person's underarms. Wrap your arms around the person's chest.
3 Make a fist. Place the thumb side of the fist on the middle of the sternum (breastbone).
4 Grasp the fist with your other hand.
5 Give chest thrusts until the object is expelled or the person becomes unresponsive.
6 If the person becomes unresponsive, have someone activate the Emergency Medical Services (EMS) system or the agency's Rapid Response System (RRS) if not already done. An RRS is a team that quickly responds to give care in life-threatening situations. Start cardiopulmonary resuscitation (CPR). See Chapter 43.

Self-Administered Abdominal Thrusts
1 Make a fist with 1 hand.
2 Place the thumb side of the fist above your navel and below the lower end of the sternum.
3 Grasp your fist with your other hand.
4 Press inward and upward quickly.
5 Press the upper abdomen against a hard surface if the thrust did not relieve the obstruction. Use the back of a chair, a table, or a railing.
6 Use as many thrusts as needed.

Guidelines for emergency care are updated as new information becomes available. You are responsible for following current guidelines. Updates can be found on-line at the American Heart Association's website.

Relieving Choking—Adult or Child (Over 1 Year of Age)

Procedure

1 Ask the person: "Are you choking?"
   a *If the person can cough or talk,* see p. 121 for mild airway obstruction.
   b *If the person is unresponsive,* you may not know the cause. Call for help and begin CPR. See Chapter 43.
   c *If the person nods "yes" and cannot talk,* continue to step 2.
2 Have someone call for help if another person is available. If not, continue to step 3.
   a *In a public area,* have someone call 911 to activate the EMS system. Send someone to get an automated external defibrillator (AED) (Chapter 43).
   b *In an agency,* have someone call the agency's RRS and get a defibrillator (AED).
3 Give abdominal thrusts.
   a Stand or kneel behind the person.
   b Wrap your arms around the person's waist.
   c Make a fist with 1 hand.
   d Place the thumb side of the fist against the abdomen. The fist is slightly above the navel in the middle of the abdomen and well below the end of the sternum (breastbone). See Figure 11-6, A.
   e Grasp your fist with your other hand (Fig. 11-6, B).
   f Press your fist into the abdomen with a quick, upward thrust (Fig. 11-7).
   g Repeat thrusts until the object is expelled or the person becomes unresponsive.
4 *If the object is dislodged,* encourage hospital care. Injuries can occur from abdominal thrusts.

5 *If the person becomes unresponsive:*
   a Lower the person to the floor or ground. Position the person supine (lying flat on the back).
   b Make sure the EMS or RRS was called.
      1) *If alone with a phone,* call while giving care.
      2) *If alone without a phone,* give about 2 minutes of CPR first. Then call the EMS or RRS and get an AED.
   c Start CPR. See Chapter 43. Do not check for a pulse.
      1) Give 30 chest compressions.
      2) Open the airway with the head tilt–chin lift method (Fig. 11-8). Open wide the person's mouth. Look for an object. Remove the object if you can see it and can remove it easily.
      3) Give 2 breaths.
      4) Continue cycles of 30 chest compressions followed by 2 breaths. Look for an object every time you open the airway.
   d *If choking is relieved,* check for a response, breathing, and a pulse. (NOTE: Choking is relieved when you feel air move and see the chest rise and fall when giving breaths.)
      1) *If no response, no normal breathing, and no pulse*—continue CPR. Use the AED as soon as possible (Chapter 43).
      2) *If no response and no normal breathing but there is a pulse*—give rescue breaths. For an adult, give 1 breath every 6 seconds. For a child, give 1 breath every 2 to 3 seconds. Check for a pulse about every 2 minutes. If no pulse, begin CPR.
      3) *If the person has normal breathing and a pulse*—place the person in the recovery position if there is no response (Chapter 43). Continue to check the person until help arrives. Encourage hospital care.

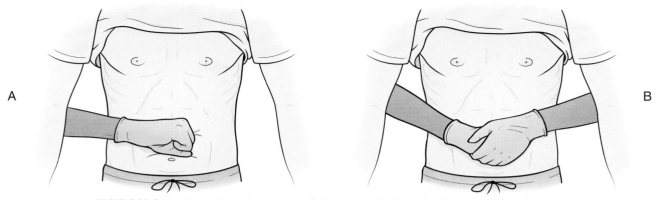

FIGURE 11-6 Hand positioning for abdominal thrusts. **A,** The fist is slightly above the navel in the mid-line of the abdomen. **B,** The other hand clasps the fist.

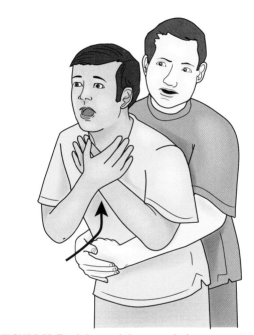

FIGURE 11-7 Abdominal thrusts with the person standing.

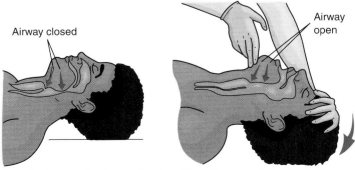

FIGURE 11-8 The head tilt–chin lift method opens the airway. One hand is on the person's forehead. Pressure is applied to tilt the head back. The chin is lifted with the fingers of the other hand.

PREVENTING EQUIPMENT ACCIDENTS

All equipment is unsafe if broken, not used correctly, not working properly, or in need of repair. This includes hospital beds. Inspect all equipment before use. Check all items for cracks, chips, and sharp or rough edges. They can cause cuts, stabs, or scratches. Follow the safety measures in Box 11-4.

See *Promoting Safety and Comfort: Preventing Equipment Accidents.*

PROMOTING SAFETY AND COMFORT

Preventing Equipment Accidents

Safety

Beds, chairs, wheelchairs, stretchers, toilets, commodes, and other equipment usually have a weight capacity of 250 to 350 pounds. Bariatric patients and residents can weigh from 250 pounds to over 1000 pounds. Bariatric equipment is labeled:

- "Bariatric"
- "EC" for "expanded capacity"
- With the weight limit suggested by the manufacturer

Do not use the item if the person's weight is greater than the weight capacity. Follow the nurse's directions and the care plan.

Electrical Equipment

Frayed cords (Fig. 11-10, *A*) and over-loaded electrical outlets (Fig. 11-10, *B*) can cause fires, burns, and electrical shocks. *Electrical shock* is when electrical current passes through the body. It can burn the skin, muscles, nerves, and other tissues. It can affect the heart and cause death.

Warning signs of a faulty electrical item include:

- Shocks
- Loss of power or a power surge
- Dimming or flickering lights
- Sparks
- Sizzling or buzzing sounds
- Burning odor
- Loose plugs

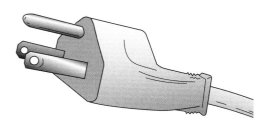

FIGURE 11-9 A three-pronged plug.

BOX 11-4 Preventing Equipment Accidents

General Safety

- Follow agency policies and procedures.
- Follow the manufacturer's instructions. Use equipment correctly.
- Read all caution and warning labels.
- Do not use an unfamiliar item. Ask for training. Also ask a nurse to supervise you the first time you use the item.
- Use an item only for its intended purpose.
- Make sure the item works before you begin.
- Have all needed equipment before you begin.
- Do not use broken or damaged items.
- Do not give broken or damaged items to patients or residents.
- Do not try to repair broken or damaged items.
- Show a broken or damaged item to the nurse. Follow the nurse's instructions and agency policies for discarding items or sending them for repair.

Electrical Safety

- Check cords and equipment for damage. Make sure they are in good repair.
- Use 3-pronged plugs on all electrical devices (Fig. 11-9). Make sure all prongs are intact.
- Avoid using extension cords. If you must use an extension cord, use it for only 1 device. This prevents over-loading a circuit.
- Do not use power strips for care equipment.
- Do not cover or run any cord under rugs, carpets, linens, or other materials.
- Connect a bed power cord directly to a wall outlet. Do not connect a bed power cord to an extension cord or power strip.
- Do not use the person's electrical items until they have been approved for safety by the maintenance staff.
- Keep electrical items away from water.
- Keep work areas clean and dry. Wipe up spills right away.
- Do not touch electrical items if you are wet, if your hands are wet, if you are in water, or if you are standing in water. This includes using a phone when it is plugged into a charger.
- Do not put a finger or any item into an outlet.
- Turn off equipment before unplugging it. Sparks occur when electrical items are unplugged while turned on.
- Hold on to the plug (not the cord) when removing it from an outlet.
- Do not give showers or tub baths during storms. Lightning can travel through pipes.
- Do not use electrical items or phones during storms.
- Do not use water to put out an electrical fire. If possible, turn off or unplug the item. Call 911 at once.
- Do not touch a person who is having an electrical shock. If possible, turn off or unplug the item. Call 911 or the RRS.
- Keep electrical cords away from heating vents and other heat sources.
- Turn off the device when done using the item.
- Unplug all devices when not in use.

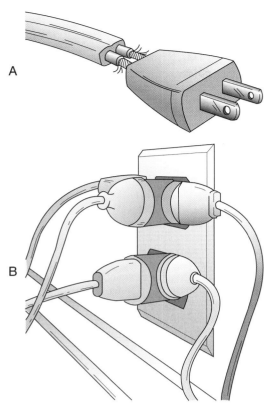

FIGURE 11-10 **A,** A frayed electrical cord. **B,** An over-loaded electrical outlet.

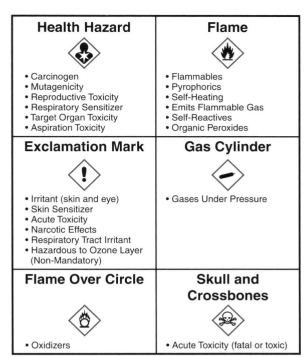

Health Hazard	Flame
• Carcinogen • Mutagenicity • Reproductive Toxicity • Respiratory Sensitizer • Target Organ Toxicity • Aspiration Toxicity	• Flammables • Pyrophorics • Self-Heating • Emits Flammable Gas • Self-Reactives • Organic Peroxides
Exclamation Mark	**Gas Cylinder**
• Irritant (skin and eye) • Skin Sensitizer • Acute Toxicity • Narcotic Effects • Respiratory Tract Irritant • Hazardous to Ozone Layer (Non-Mandatory)	• Gases Under Pressure
Flame Over Circle	**Skull and Crossbones**
• Oxidizers	• Acute Toxicity (fatal or toxic)

FIGURE 11-11 Some pictograms from the Occupational Safety and Health Administration. Depending on the chemical, the warning label contains the necessary pictograms and associated hazards. (Redrawn from OSHA Quick Card™, OSHA® Occupational Safety and Health Administration, U.S. Department of Labor, Washington, DC.)

Wheelchair and Stretcher Safety

Wheelchairs are useful for people who cannot walk or who have severe problems walking. Stretchers are used to transport persons who cannot sit up or must lie down. Stretchers are used in hospitals and by emergency medical personnel.

The person can fall from the wheelchair or stretcher. Or the person can fall during transfers to and from the wheelchair or stretcher. See Chapter 18 for wheelchair and stretcher safety.

HAZARDOUS CHEMICALS

A *hazardous chemical* is any chemical that is a physical hazard or a health hazard. *Physical hazards* can cause fires or explosions. *Health hazards* can cause health problems. Health hazards can:

* Cause cancer.
* Affect blood cell formation and function.
* Damage the kidneys, nervous system, lungs, skin, eyes, or mucous membranes.
* Cause birth defects, miscarriages, and fertility problems.

Exposure to hazardous chemicals can occur from equipment failures, container ruptures, or the release of a hazard into the workplace. Workplace hazards include:

* Equipment containing latex (Chapter 15)
* Thermometers and blood pressure equipment containing mercury (Chapter 31)
* Cleaners and disinfectants (Chapter 14)

Your agency provides hazardous chemical training. It also provides eyewash and total body wash stations where hazardous chemicals are used.

Labeling

Hazardous chemical containers have warning labels. The warning labels contain *pictograms*—symbols used to communicate specific information about a chemical hazard. See Figure 11-11 for examples.

If a warning label is removed or damaged, do not use the substance. Show the container to the nurse and explain the problem. Do not leave the container unattended.

Safety Data Sheets

Every hazardous chemical has a *safety data sheet (SDS)*. Some agencies use the term *material safety data sheet (MSDS)*. Information provided includes:

* Name and common names
* Hazards about the chemical
* Chemical ingredients
* Emergency measures
* Fire-fighting measures
* Accidental release measures
* Safe handling and storage measures
* Personal protection measures

Check the SDS before using a hazardous chemical, cleaning up a leak or spill, or disposing of the substance. Call for the nurse about a leak or spill right away. Do not leave a leak or spill unattended.

DISASTERS

A *disaster* is a harmful event that can affect the agency, patient or resident population, community, or larger geographic area. The following are examples.

- Natural disasters—tornados, hurricanes, blizzards, earthquakes, volcano eruptions, floods, some fires
- Human-made disasters—auto, bus, train, and airplane accidents; fires; bombings; power plant accidents; gas or chemical leaks; explosions; wars
- Power failures
- Communication failures and cyber-attacks (criminal activity involving information systems)
- Infectious disease threats (see "Pandemics" on p. 128)
- Missing residents (see "Elopement" on p. 128)

Communities and fire and police departments have disaster plans. The Centers for Medicare & Medicaid Services (CMS) requires that health care agencies have an *emergency preparedness program* in place. The program describes the agency's approach to meeting health, safety, and security needs of patients or residents, staff, and the community before, during, and after a disaster.

Planning for disasters includes development of an *emergency plan*.

- Potential hazards are identified.
- Policies and procedures are formed and implemented (carried out).
- A communication plan is developed.
- Staff are trained and the plan is tested.

Your agency provides training on policies and procedures and your role in responding in an emergency.

See *Focus on Surveys: Disasters.*

FOCUS ON SURVEYS

Disasters

Drills are used to prepare for real emergencies. Staff learn and practice how to respond. Their actions are evaluated. Surveyors observe for a quick and appropriate response to drills. During a disaster drill, you need to respond as if it is a real emergency.

You may also be asked about being prepared for a disaster. For example, a surveyor may ask you:

- About fire safety. See "Fire Safety." This includes:
  - What to do if a fire alarm goes off.
  - What to do if you find a fire in a person's room.
  - Where to find fire alarms and fire extinguishers.
  - How to use a fire extinguisher.
- What to do if a patient or resident is missing. See "Elopement" on p. 128.

Bomb Threats

Follow agency procedures for a bomb threat or if you find an item that looks or sounds strange. Bomb threats can be sent by phone, mail, e-mail, text message, messenger, or other means. Or the person can leave a bomb in the agency. If you see a stranger or strange item or package in the agency, tell the nurse at once. You cannot be too safe.

Fire Safety

Faulty electrical equipment and wiring, over-loaded electrical circuits, and smoking are major causes of fires. The health team must prevent fires and act quickly during a fire. See Box 11-5.

BOX 11-5 Fire Prevention Measures

- Follow the safety measures:
  - For oxygen use (see "Fire and Oxygen")
  - To prevent equipment accidents (p. 124)
  - To prevent burns (p. 120)
- Practice smoking and ashtray safety.
  - Smoke only where allowed to do so.
  - Supervise persons who smoke. This is very important for persons who are confused, disoriented, or sedated.
  - Do not smoke or light matches or lighters around flammable liquids or materials or oxygen equipment (Chapter 37). Alcohol-based hand sanitizer (Chapter 14) is flammable (it can catch on fire).
  - Provide ashtrays.
  - Empty ashtrays only when sure that all ashes, cigars, cigarettes, and other smoking materials are out (extinguished).
  - Empty ashtrays into a metal container partially filled with sand or water. Do not empty ashtrays into plastic containers or wastebaskets lined with paper or plastic bags.
- Keep matches, lighters, and flammable liquids and materials away from children and confused or disoriented persons.
- Light matches carefully.
  - Be alert for sparks when lighting a match. The sparks can ignite materials that can burn.
  - Keep your hair, clothing, and anything that will burn away from the match and flame.
- Do not leave cooking unattended on stoves, in ovens, or in microwave ovens.

Fire and Oxygen. Three things are needed for a fire—a spark or flame, a material that will burn, and oxygen. Air has some oxygen. However, some people need extra oxygen (Chapter 37). Safety measures are needed where oxygen is used and stored.

- *NO SMOKING* signs are on the door and near the bed.
- No one can smoke in the room.
- Smoking materials (cigarettes, electronic cigarettes, cigars, and pipes), matches, and lighters are removed from the room.
- Safety measures to prevent equipment accidents are followed (see Box 11-4).
- Wool blankets and synthetic fabrics that cause static electricity are removed from the room.
- The person wears a cotton gown or pajamas.
- Lit candles and other open flames are not allowed.
- Materials that ignite easily are removed from the room—oil, grease, nail polish remover, and so on.

See *Focus on Communication: Fire and Oxygen.*

What to Do During a Fire. Know your agency's fire emergency and evacuation procedures. Know where to find fire alarms, fire extinguishers, and emergency exits. Fire drills are held to practice emergency fire procedures. Remember the word *RACE* (Fig. 11-12).

- *R*—for *rescue*. Rescue persons in immediate danger. Move them to a safe place.
- *A*—for *alarm*. Sound the nearest fire alarm. Call 911 or activate the agency's fire response system.
- *C*—for *confine*. Close doors and windows to confine the fire. Turn off oxygen or electrical items used in the general area of the fire.
- *E*—for *extinguish*. Use a fire extinguisher on a small fire that has not spread to a larger area.

Clear equipment from all normal and emergency exits. *Do not use elevators if there is a fire.*

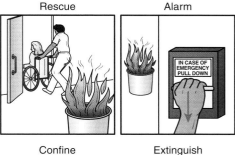
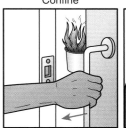
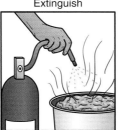

FIGURE 11-12 During a fire, remember *RACE*: Rescue, Alarm, Confine, Extinguish.

Using a Fire Extinguisher. Different extinguishers are used for different kinds of fires.

- Oil and grease fires
- Electrical fires
- Paper and wood fires

A general procedure for using a fire extinguisher follows.

See procedure: *Using a Fire Extinguisher.*

Using a Fire Extinguisher

Procedure

1 Pull the fire alarm.
2 Get the nearest fire extinguisher.
3 Carry it upright.
4 Take it to the fire.
5 Follow the word *PASS*.
  a *P*—for *pull the safety pin* (Fig. 11-13, *A*). This unlocks the handle.
  b *A*—for *aim low* (Fig. 11-13, *B*). Direct the hose (nozzle) at the base of the fire. Do not try to spray the tops of the flames.
  c *S*—for *squeeze the lever* (Fig. 11-13, *C*). Squeeze or push down on the lever, handle, or button to start the stream. Release the lever, handle, or button to stop the stream.
  d *S*—for *sweep back and forth* (Fig. 11-13, *D*). Sweep the stream back and forth (side to side) at the base of the fire.

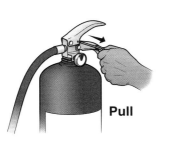
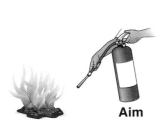
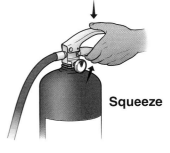
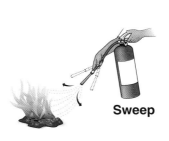

A **B** **C** **D**

FIGURE 11-13 Using a fire extinguisher. *A, Pull* the safety pin. *B, Aim* the hose at the base of the fire. *C, Squeeze* the top handle down. *D, Sweep* back and forth.

Pandemics

An *epidemic* occurs when a disease spreads within a large number of people in a community or region at the same time. A *pandemic* occurs when the disease spreads over several countries or continents. The CMS includes infectious disease threats among the hazards to be considered when preparing for disasters and emergencies.

The CMS, Centers for Disease Control and Prevention (CDC), and Occupational Safety and Health Administration (OSHA) have plans and guidance for managing pandemics. Proper hand hygiene and infection control practices (Chapters 14 and 15) and social distancing help reduce the spread of infection. *Social distancing (physical distancing)* measures limit person-to-person contact and maintain a distance of at least 6 feet from others. Screening measures for persons within and entering the agency and personal protective equipment (PPE) requirements are other safety practices. (See "Personal Protective Equipment" in Chapter 15.)

Practice the measures to prevent the spread of infection in Chapters 14 and 15. Follow local, state, and federal guidance in response to a pandemic. Also follow agency policies and procedures.

Elopement

Elopement is when a patient or resident leaves the agency without staff knowledge. The person who leaves a safe setting is at risk for many dangers. Heat or cold exposure, dehydration, drowning, and being struck by a vehicle are examples.

The agency must:
- Identify persons at risk for elopement.
- Monitor and supervise persons at risk.
- Address elopement in the person's care plan.
- Have a plan to find a missing patient or resident.

WORKPLACE VIOLENCE

Workplace violence is violent acts (including assault or threat of assault) directed toward persons at work or while on duty. It includes:
- Murders
- Beatings, stabbings, and shootings
- Rapes and sexual assaults
- Use of weapons—firearms, bombs, knives, and so on
- Kidnapping
- Robbery
- Threats—obscene phone calls; threatening oral, written, or body language
- Harassment of any kind (Chapter 5)—including being followed, sworn at, or shouted at

Staff in health care settings are at risk for workplace violence. The nursing staff has regular contact with patients, residents, and visitors. See Box 11-6 for risk factors in the health care setting.

OSHA has guidelines for preventing workplace violence. Work-site hazards are identified. Prevention measures are followed. Also, staff receive safety and health training. Box 11-6 has some safety measures to prevent or control workplace violence. You need to:
- Follow your agency's workplace violence prevention program.
- Follow safety and security measures.
- Voice safety and security concerns.
- Report suspicious persons right away.
- Report violent incidents promptly and accurately.
- Serve on committees that review workplace violence.
- Attend training programs to recognize and manage agitation, assaultive behavior, and criminal intent.

BOX 11-6 Workplace Violence—Risk Factors and Safety Measures

Risk Factors
- Working with persons (or family members) who have a history of violence, have substance use disorders (Chapter 41), or are gang members
- Transporting patients and residents
- Working alone
- Working in a setting where a staff member cannot see or escape from danger or a violent situation
- Poorly lit hallways, rooms, parking lots, and other areas
- Lacking a way to communicate an emergency situation
- People having access to firearms, knives, and other weapons
- Working in areas with high crime rates
- Lacking policies and training to recognize and manage hostile and assaultive behaviors from patients, residents, visitors, and staff
- Low staff levels during meal times and visiting hours
- High staff turn-over rates
- Not enough security and mental health staff
- Long waits for patients or residents
- Over-crowded and uncomfortable waiting rooms
- Visitors being able to go anywhere in the agency
- A sense that violence is tolerated and that victims cannot contact the police or press charges

Safety Measures
Agitated or Aggressive Persons
- Stand away from the person. Judge the length of the person's arms and legs. Stand far enough away that the person cannot hit or kick you.
- Be able to exit the room. Do not become trapped in the room.
- Identify items in the room that can be used as weapons. Move away from such objects. Vases, phones, radios, letter openers, paper weights, and belts are examples.
- Know where to find and how to use panic buttons, call lights, alarms, closed-circuit monitors, and other security devices.
- Keep your hands free.
- Stay calm. Talk to the person in a calm manner. Do not raise your voice or argue, scold, or interrupt the person.
- Be aware of your body language. Do not point a finger or glare at the person. Do not put your hands on your hips.
- Do not touch the person.
- Say that you will get the nurse to speak to the person.
- Leave the room as soon as you can. Make sure the person is safe.
- Tell the nurse and security officer about the matter at once. Report items in the room that can be used as weapons.

BOX 11-6 Workplace Violence—Risk Factors and Safety Measures—cont'd

Safety Measures—cont'd

Weapons

- Jewelry and scarves are not worn. They can be used as weapons. For example, a person can grab earrings and bracelets. Or a person can strangle someone with a necklace or scarf.
- Long hair is worn up and off the collar (Chapter 5). A person can pull long hair and cause head injuries.
- Keys, scissors, pens, or other items that could be used as weapons are not within the person's reach.
- Pictures, vases, and other items that could be used as weapons are limited (few in number).
- Tools or items left by maintenance staff or visitors are removed if they could be used as weapons.

Safety Measures—cont'd

Staff Safety Measures

- Staff work together when caring for persons with agitated or aggressive behaviors. Staff do not work alone.
- Staff wear ID badges that prove employment. IDs do not have last names or addresses.
- Staff use a "buddy system" when using elevators, stairways, restrooms, and low-traffic areas.
- Uniforms fit well. Tight uniforms limit running. An attacker can grab loose uniforms.
- Shoes are slip-resistant and fit well. Shoes that cause slipping limit running.
- Vehicles are locked and in good repair.
- Security escort services are used for walking to vehicles, bus stops, or train stations.

Risk factors modified from Occupational Safety and Health Administration: *Guidelines for preventing workplace violence for healthcare and social service workers*, U.S. Department of Labor, OSHA publication 3148.

RISK MANAGEMENT

Risk management involves identifying and controlling risks and safety hazards affecting the agency. The intent is to:

- Protect all in the agency—patients, residents, visitors, and staff.
- Protect agency property from harm or danger.
- Protect the person's valuables.
- Prevent accidents and injuries.
  Risk management deals with these and other safety issues.
- Accident and fire prevention
- Negligence, malpractice, and abuse (Chapter 4)
- Workplace violence
- Federal and state requirements

Risk managers look for patterns and trends in incidents, complaints (patients, residents, staff, visitors), and accident and injury investigations. Unsafe situations are corrected. Procedure and training changes are made as needed.

Color-Coded Wristbands

Color-coded wristbands promote the person's safety and prevent harm. They quickly communicate an alert or warning (Fig. 11-14). The type of alert is printed on the band. The printing is useful in dim lighting and for persons who are color blind.

These colors are common.

- Red—for an "allergy alert." Red is a warning to "stop." A red wristband warns of allergies to food, drugs, treatment supplies such as tape or latex gloves, and so on. Allergies are not listed on the wristband.
- Yellow—for a "fall risk." Yellow implies "caution." Yellow wristbands are used for persons with a history of falls. Or they are used for persons at risk for falls because of dizziness, balance problems, confusion, and so on.
- Purple—for a "Do Not Resuscitate" (DNR) order. See Chapter 44.

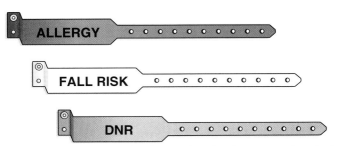

FIGURE 11-14 Color-coded wristband examples. The alert is printed on the band.

Some agencies have colors for other alerts. For example, pink is for a "limb alert." This means that an arm or leg is not used for blood pressure measurements, blood draws, or intravenous infusions.

To safely use color-coded wristbands:

- Know the colors used in your agency. Colors may vary among agencies.
- Check the care plan and your assignment sheet when you see a color-coded wristband. You need to know the reason for the wristband and the care measures needed. Ask the nurse if you have questions.
- Do not confuse "social cause" bands with your agency's color-coded wristbands. "Live Strong" is an example.
- Check for wristbands on persons transferred from another agency. That agency may use different colors. Or the meanings may differ from those in your agency. The nurse needs to remove wristbands from another agency.
- Tell the nurse if you think a person needs a color-coded wristband.

Personal Belongings

The person's belongings must be kept safe. Often valuables are sent home with the family. A personal belongings list is completed. Each item is listed and described. The staff member and the person sign the completed list.

A valuables envelope is used for jewelry and money. Each jewelry item is listed and described on the envelope. Describe what you see. For example, describe a ring as having a white stone with 4 prongs in a yellow setting. Do not assume the stone is a diamond in a gold setting. For valuables:

- Count money with the person.
- Put money and each jewelry item in the envelope. Have the person watch. Seal and sign the envelope like a personal belongings list.
- Give the envelope to the nurse. Have a witness. The nurse takes it to the safe or sends it home with the family.

Dentures, eyeglasses, hearing aids, watches, some jewelry, radios and music players, phones, and other electronic devices are kept at the bedside. Items kept at the bedside are listed in the person's record. Some people keep money for newspapers and personal items. The amount kept is noted in the person's record.

In nursing centers, clothing and shoes are labeled with the person's name. So are other items brought from home. Follow center procedures to label items.

Reporting Incidents

An *incident* is any event that has harmed or could harm a patient, resident, visitor, or staff member. This includes:

- Accidents involving patients, residents, visitors, or staff.
- Errors in care—giving the wrong care, giving care to the wrong person, not giving care.
- Broken or lost items owned by the person. Dentures, hearing aids, and eyeglasses are examples.
- Lost money or clothing.
- Hazardous chemical incidents.
- Workplace violence incidents.

Report accidents and errors at once. Complete an *incident report* as soon as possible. Incident reports are reviewed by a risk management committee. The committee looks for patterns and trends in accidents or errors. For example, are falls occurring on the same shift and on the same unit? Are lost or missing items being reported on the same shift or same unit? Are residents injured on the same shift or same unit? There may be new policies and procedures to prevent future incidents.

FOCUS ON P R I D E

The Person, Family, and Yourself

P ersonal and Professional Responsibility

Some persons are at risk for choking. Persons with developmental disabilities, young children, and older persons are examples. Safety measures must be taken to avoid harm.

You can help prevent choking. Know who is at risk. Ask the nurse or check the care plan. Monitor those persons closely. Check that they have the right diet. See Chapter 29 for more precautions.

R ights and Respect

If you value safety, you will perform safety measures. For example, you will:
- Identify the person before giving care.
- Check water temperature before bathing.
- Use and store harmful products safely.
- Cut food into small pieces.
- Observe for swallowing problems and signs of choking.
- Use equipment correctly.
- Know what to do during a fire or disaster.
- Report concerns and incidents.

Show respect for others' well-being. Take pride in providing safe care.

I ndependence and Social Interaction

Older persons often cannot do things they used to do. They still may want to try. Respect the desire to maintain independence. Listen and let the person do as much as is safely possible. Kindly communicate safety limits. Discuss letting the person do the task with help. Tell the nurse about safety concerns.

D elegation and Teamwork

Personal safety practices protect you and co-workers. Work as a team for the safety of all staff arriving at and leaving the agency.
- Wait for a person finishing work a few minutes late.
- Walk with others to and from the parking area.
- Walk in well-lit areas at night.
- Do not leave the parking area until your co-workers are safely in their vehicles. Have them do the same for you.
- Offer to call security escort services for a co-worker going to a different location. For example, a person is walking to a bus stop.

E thics and Laws

Accidents happen. Errors occur. No matter how much you try, mistakes are made. Do not lie or try to hide the incident. You must:
- Be honest.
- Tell the nurse.
- Fill out an incident report.

Incident reports are used to improve systems and promote safety. Information gained signals areas for improvement. Processes may be changed to make mistakes more difficult. Or they are changed to make it easier to do the right thing.

Always do your best to give safe care. When errors or accidents happen, take responsibility. Take pride in doing the right thing by honest reporting.

FOCUS ON PRIDE: Application

As a student or new nursing assistant, it is normal to have fears of causing harm. What concerns do you have? How will you overcome your fears?

REVIEW QUESTIONS

Circle the BEST answer.

1. Safety measures are meant to prevent accidents and injuries while
   a. Protecting rights
   b. Limiting mobility
   c. Limiting independence
   d. Saving staff time

2. Which is *safe?*
   a. Not wearing needed eyeglasses
   b. Having hearing problems
   c. Being disoriented
   d. Being able to sense pain

3. An unconscious person
   a. Has suffered an electrical shock
   b. Has dementia
   c. Is unaware of surroundings
   d. Has stopped breathing

4. Dementia increases the risk for accidents and injuries because it affects
   a. Vision and hearing
   b. Thinking and reasoning
   c. Pain sensation
   d. Muscle function

Continued

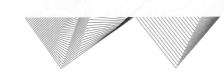

5 To identify a person, you
  a Call the person by his or her first name
  b Ask the person for his or her ID number
  c Compare information on the ID bracelet against your assignment sheet
  d Check that you entered the correct room number

6 To prevent burns
  a Keep smoking materials at the person's bedside
  b Pour hot liquids near a person
  c Turn on hot water first
  d Check water temperature before the person enters the shower

7 Which helps to prevent poisoning?
  a Keeping harmful products in low storage areas
  b Keeping harmful products in their original containers
  c Removing product labels
  d Storing harmful products near food

8 Which can cause suffocation?
  a Checking for loose teeth or dentures
  b Using electrical items that are in good repair
  c Cutting food into small, bite-sized pieces
  d Restraints

9 If severe airway obstruction occurs, the person usually
  a Clutches at the throat
  b Can speak, cough, and breathe
  c Is calm
  d Has a seizure

10 These statements are about FBAO. Which is *correct*?
  a A person is coughing forcefully. Give abdominal thrusts.
  b A person is pregnant. Give abdominal thrusts.
  c Injuries can occur from abdominal or chest thrusts.
  d Unconscious persons cannot choke.

11 How do you know that a new resident's electric shaver is safe to use?
  a You turn the device on.
  b The maintenance staff checks and approves the device.
  c You check the SDS.
  d You ask the resident if it is working properly.

12 You are using an electrical device. Which measure is *unsafe*?
  a Unplugging the item while it is turned on
  b Keeping the item away from water and spills
  c Holding on to the plug (not the cord) when unplugging it
  d Following the manufacturer's instructions

13 Which is *unsafe*?
  a A chair's weight capacity exceeds the person's weight.
  b A person's weight exceeds a wheelchair's weight capacity.
  c A person who cannot walk uses a wheelchair.
  d A person who cannot sit up is transported by stretcher.

14 You spilled a hazardous substance. Which action is *correct*?
  a Follow the instructions on the safety data sheet.
  b Cover the spill and go tell the nurse.
  c Wipe up the spill with paper towels.
  d Leave the spill for housekeeping.

15 You work in a nursing center. In a severe weather alert, you should
  a Take cover
  b Follow the center's emergency plan
  c Make sure your family is safe
  d Pull the fire alarm

16 The fire alarm sounds. Which action is *correct*?
  a Leave oxygen on.
  b Use elevators.
  c Open doors and windows.
  d Move residents to a safe place.

17 Social distancing is a safety measure used during
  a A pandemic
  b Workplace violence
  c Elopement
  d A fire

18 A person is agitated and aggressive. Which is *unsafe*?
  a Standing away from the person
  b Standing so the person does not block your exit
  c Using touch to show you care
  d Talking to the person without raising your voice

19 Risk managers
  a Look for patterns or trends in accidents and errors
  b Prevent legal problems when injuries occur
  c Are only responsible for staff safety
  d Are the same as surveyors

20 You see a resident with a color-coded wristband. You should
  a Remove it
  b Ask the person what it means
  c Check the person's care plan
  d Apply wristbands to the other residents

21 A resident brought a phone from home. To prevent property loss
  a Send the item home with the family
  b Label the item with the person's name
  c Put the item in a safe
  d Store it at the nurses' station

22 You gave a person the wrong treatment. Which is *correct*?
  a Report the error at the end of the shift.
  b Take action only if the person was injured.
  c You are guilty of negligence.
  d You must complete an incident report.

Answers to Chapter 11 questions are on p. 587.

FOCUS ON PRACTICE

Problem Solving

A person begins to cough loudly during a meal. The person can speak a few words. You hear wheezing between breaths. What do you do? The person is suddenly unable to cough, speak, or breathe. What do you do?

CHAPTER 12

Preventing Falls

OBJECTIVES

- Define the key terms and key abbreviations in this chapter.
- Identify the causes and risk factors for falls.
- Describe the safety measures that prevent falls.
- Explain how to use position change alarms safely.
- Explain how to use bed rails safely.
- Explain the purpose of hand rails and grab bars.
- Explain how to use wheel locks (brakes) safely.
- Describe how to use transfer/gait belts.
- Explain how to help the person who is falling.
- Perform the procedures described in this chapter.
- Explain how to promote PRIDE in the person, the family, and yourself.

KEY TERMS

bed rail A device that serves as a guard or barrier along the side of the bed; side rail
gait belt See "transfer belt"

position change alarm Any physical or electronic device that monitors a person's movement and alerts staff of movement
transfer belt A device applied around the waist and used to support a person who is unsteady or disabled; gait belt

KEY ABBREVIATIONS

CDC   Centers for Disease Control and Prevention
CMS   Centers for Medicare & Medicaid Services

ID   Identification

The risk of falling increases with age. Persons older than 65 years are at risk. A history of falls increases the risk of falling again. Falls are the most common accidents in nursing centers.

According to the Centers for Disease Control and Prevention (CDC):

- Each year, over a quarter (¼) of adults age 65 and older fall.
- Falls are the main cause of injuries and injury-related deaths in older adults.
- Falls can cause serious injuries.
  - Broken bones. Wrist, arm, ankle, and hip fractures are common. Hip fractures are very serious. Recovery can be hard. Many people are not able to live on their own afterward.
  - Head injuries. Head injuries are very serious, especially if the person takes anticoagulant drugs (drugs that slow blood clotting).
- A fall often causes a fear of falling again, even if the person was not injured. The person may limit daily activities to prevent falling. Less active, the person becomes weaker. This increases the risk of falling. See *Focus on Surveys: Preventing Falls.*

FOCUS ON SURVEYS
Preventing Falls

The Centers for Medicare & Medicaid Services (CMS) defines a *fall* as:

- Unintentionally coming to rest on the ground, floor, or other lower level. Force, such as being pushed, was not involved.
- When a person loses balance and would have fallen if staff did not act to prevent the fall.
- When a person is found on the floor unless matters suggest otherwise.
- When a person falls but is not injured. A fall without injury is still a fall.

The survey team will observe and interview staff about:

- Fall risk factors described in this chapter.
- The hazards described in this chapter and in Chapter 11.
- Safety measures to prevent falls.
- The safe use of bed rails, hand rails and grab bars, and wheel locks (brakes).
- The safe use of adaptive (assistive) devices. Canes, walkers, and transfer/gait belts (p. 139) are examples.
- Safe transfer and ambulation (walking) procedures. See Chapters 18 and 32.
- Answering call lights promptly.
- Following the person's care plan and meeting care needs.

CAUSES AND RISK FACTORS FOR FALLS

Most falls are caused by many risk factors. The more risk factors present, the greater the risk of falling. The accident risk factors described in Chapter 11 can lead to falls. The problems listed in Box 12-1 increase a person's risk of falling.

See *Focus on Older Persons: Causes and Risk Factors for Falls.*

BOX 12-1 Fall Risk Factors

Care Setting
- Bed height: too low or too high
- Care equipment: IV (intravenous) poles, drainage tubes and bags, and others
- Floors: cluttered, wet, slippery, or uneven
- Furniture out of place
- Lighting: poor or glares
- No hand rails or grab bars
- Restraint use
- Setting: new, strange, and unfamiliar
- Throw rugs or other tripping hazards
- Wet and slippery bathtubs and showers
- Wheelchairs, walkers, canes, and crutches: improper use or fit

The Person
- Age: over 65 years
- Alcohol: over-use
- Balance problems
- Blood pressure: low or high
- Confusion; disorientation
- Depression
- Dizziness or light-headedness; dizziness on standing
- Drug side effects
  - Confusion and disorientation
  - Coordination: poor
  - Diarrhea
  - Dizziness
  - Drowsiness
  - Fainting
  - Low blood pressure when standing or sitting
  - Unsteadiness
  - Urination: frequent
- Elimination: incontinence (urinary or fecal), frequency, urgency, urinating at night (*nocturia*)
- Falls: history of; fear of falling
- Foot problems; foot pain
- Gait: unsteady
- Joint pain and stiffness
- Judgment: poor
- Memory problems
- Mobility: impaired
- Reaction time: slow
- Shoes that fit poorly; no shoes or shoes without slip-resistant surfaces
- Sleep problems
- Vision problems
- Weakness; leg weakness

FOCUS ON OLDER PERSONS

Causes and Risk Factors for Falls

Nursing center residents are at increased risk for falls. Weakness and walking problems are common causes. Care setting hazards are other causes—poor lighting, wet floors, incorrect bed height. Other risk factors are transfer problems (Chapter 18), shoes that fit poorly, and improper use or fit of wheelchairs, walkers, canes, and other devices. See Box 12-1.

FALL PREVENTION PROGRAMS

Agencies have fall prevention programs. Meeting the person's basic needs is an essential part of fall prevention. Make sure that:
- Food and fluid needs are met.
- Needed items are within reach.
- Help is given with elimination needs. Assist the person to the bathroom or with the bedpan, urinal, or commode.
- The bedpan, urinal, or commode is kept within reach if the person can use the device without help.
- A warm drink, soft lights, or a back massage is used to calm the person who is agitated.
- The person is properly positioned in bed or in a chair or wheelchair. Use pillows or other positioning devices as the nurse and care plan direct (Chapters 16 and 32).
- Correct procedures and equipment are used for transfers and ambulation (walking). See Chapters 18 and 32. Follow the care plan. Explain tasks before and while performing them.
- The person is involved in meaningful activities.
- Exercise programs are followed. They help improve balance, strength, walking, and physical function.
- The person's setting is safe. Complete a safety check before leaving the room. (See the inside of the back cover.)

The measures listed in Box 12-2 may be part of the agency's program and the person's care plan. The care plan also lists measures for the person's specific risk factors. The goal is to prevent falls without decreasing quality of life.

See *Focus on Communication: Fall Prevention Programs.*

See *Promoting Safety and Comfort: Fall Prevention Programs*, p. 136.

FOCUS ON COMMUNICATION

Fall Prevention Programs

A person can fall when reaching for needed items. The person reaches too far and falls. Or the person tries to get up without help. To prevent falls, ask the person:
- "What things would you like near you?"
- "Can I move this closer to you?"
- "Can you reach the call light?"
- "Can you reach your cane?" (Walker and wheelchair are other examples.)
- "Do you need to use the bathroom?"
- "Do you need anything else before I leave the room?"

BOX 12-2 Measures to Help Prevent Falls

Bathrooms and Shower/Tub Rooms
- Showers and tubs have slip-resistant surfaces or slip-resistant bath mats.
- The person uses grab bars (safety bars) in bathrooms and showers (p. 138).
- Shower chairs are used (Chapter 22).
- Safety measures for tub baths and showers are followed (Chapter 22).

Floors, Stairs, and Hallways
- Carpeting (if used) is wall-to-wall or tacked down.
- Scatter, area, and throw rugs are not used.
- Flooring is 1 color. Bold designs can cause dizziness in older persons.
- Floors have non-glare, slip-resistant surfaces.
- Non-skid wax is used on hardwood, tiled, or linoleum floors.
- Slip-resistant strips are on the floor next to the bed and in the bathroom. They are intact.
- Loose floor boards and tiles are reported. So are frayed rugs and carpets.
- Floors and stairs are free of clutter, cords, and other items that can cause tripping.
- Floors are free of spills. Wipe up spills at once. Put a *WET FLOOR* sign by the wet area.
- Floors are free of excess furniture and equipment.
- Electrical and extension cords are out of the way. This includes power strips.
- Equipment and supplies are kept on 1 side of the hallway.
- Barriers are used to prevent wandering (Fig. 12-1, p. 136).
- Hand rails (p. 138) are on both sides of stairs and hallways.
- The person uses hand rails when walking or using stairs.

Furniture
- Furniture is placed for easy movement.
- Furniture is kept in place. It is not re-arranged.
- Chairs have armrests. Armrests give support when standing or sitting.
- A phone, lamp, and personal belongings are within reach.

Beds and Other Equipment
- The bed is at the correct height for the person. Follow the care plan. The bed is raised for bedside care. Then it is lowered to a safe and comfortable level for the person. The distance from the bed to the floor is reduced if the person falls or gets out of bed.
- Bed rails (p. 137) are used according to the care plan.
- A mattress, special mat, or floor cushion is on the floor by the bed (Fig. 12-2, p. 136). This reduces the chance of injury if the person falls or gets out of bed.
- Wheelchairs, walkers, canes, and crutches fit properly. They are in good repair. Another person's equipment is not used.
- Crutches, canes, and walkers have slip-resistant tips.
- Wheelchair and stretcher safety is followed (Chapter 18).
- Wheel locks (brakes) on beds (p. 138), wheelchairs, stretchers, commodes, and shower chairs are in working order. Wheels are locked (braked) for transfers.
- Linens are checked for sharp objects and for the person's property (dentures, eyeglasses, hearing aids, and so on).

Lighting
- Rooms, hallways, and stairways have good lighting. So do bathrooms and shower/tub rooms.
- Light switches are within reach and easy to find.
- Night-lights are in bedrooms, hallways, and bathrooms.

Shoes and Clothing
- Slip-resistant footwear is worn. Socks (without other footwear), bedroom slippers, and long shoelaces are avoided.
- Shoes fit well. They do not slip up and down on the feet. All shoelaces and straps are fastened.
- Clothing fits properly. Clothing is not loose or dragging on the floor.
- Belts are tied or secured in place.

Call Lights and Alarms
- The person is taught how to use the call light (Chapter 19).
- The call light is always within the person's reach. This includes when sitting in the chair or on the commode and when in the bathroom and shower/tub room.
- The person is asked to use the call light when help is needed.
  - To get out of bed or a chair or return to bed
  - To walk
  - To get to or from the bathroom
  - To get on or off the toilet, bedpan, or commode
  - To stand to use the urinal
- Call lights are answered promptly. The person may not wait for help.
- Bed, chair, door, floor mat, and belt alarms are used as directed in the care plan. Such devices do not stop the person from falling. They sense when the person tries to get up, get out of bed, or open a door. See "Position Change Alarms" on p. 136.
- Alarms are responded to at once.

Observation
- The person is checked often. This may be every 15 minutes or as required by the care plan. Careful and frequent observation is important.
- Frequent checks are made on persons with poor judgment or memory. This may be every 15 minutes or as required by the care plan.
- Persons at risk for falls are close to the nurses' station.
- Family and friends are asked to visit during busy times. Meal times and shift changes are examples. They are also asked to visit during the evening and night shifts.
- Sitters, companions, or volunteers are provided to stay with the person.

Other
- Color-coded alerts warn of a fall risk. Yellow is common for a fall alert. Besides wristbands (Chapter 11), some agencies also use color-coded blankets, slip-resistant footwear, socks, and magnets or stickers on room doors.
- Caution is used when turning corners, entering corridor intersections, and going through doors. You could injure a person coming from the other direction.
- Pull (do not push) wheelchairs, stretchers, carts, and other wheeled equipment through doorways. You lead the way and can see where you are going.
- A safety check is made of the room after visitors leave. (See the inside of the back cover.) They may have lowered a bed rail, moved a call light, or moved a walker out of reach. Or they may have brought an item that could harm the person.

PROMOTING SAFETY AND COMFORT

Fall Prevention Programs

Safety

Some people have vision and hearing problems. Be sure eyeglasses and hearing aids are worn as needed. Reading glasses are not worn when up and about. Besides the measures in Box 12-2, other safety measures may be needed to prevent falls. See Chapter 39.

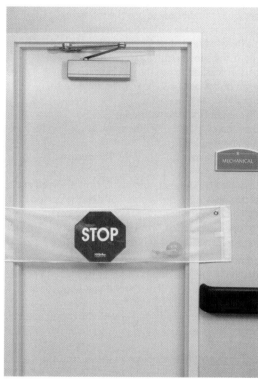

FIGURE 12-1 Barriers are used to prevent wandering.

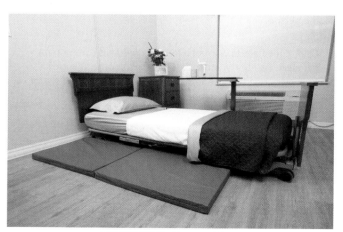

FIGURE 12-2 Floor cushion.

Position Change Alarms

The CMS describes a *position change alarm as any physical or electronic device that monitors a person's movement and alerts staff of movement.* Position change alarms do not include door and elevator alarms that monitor wandering. Types include:

- Chair and bed sensor pads (Fig. 12-3)
- Bedside alarm mats
- Alarms clipped to clothing
- Seat-belt alarms
- Wireless motion sensors

To alert staff, the device makes a sound—alarm, beep, chime, music, and so on. Some play a recorded message. For example: "Please do not get up. Sit down and use your call light for help."

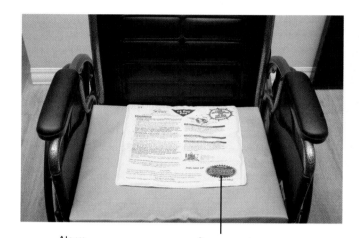

Alarm   Sensor pad

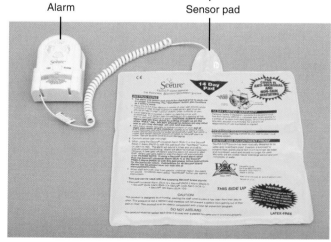

FIGURE 12-3 A position change alarm. This device has a sensor pad connected to an alarm. The alarm sounds when the person moves off of the pad. (NOTE: Position change alarms do not replace close observation. Careful and frequent observation is needed.)

Using Position Change Alarms. To use position change alarms safely:

- Follow the manufacturer's instructions.
- Mount the alarm securely out of the person's reach.
- Place the alarm at least 2 feet away from the person's ear. Alarms are loud.
- Test the alarm before leaving the person. If the device does not work, stay with the person. Call for the nurse.
- Respond to alarms at once.
  For an alarm with a cord that attaches (clips) to clothing:
- Attach the clip securely out of the person's reach. The clip is at the back near the shoulder. Check that clothing is not frayed or torn.
- Check the cord. The cord should allow movement for comfort but be short enough to sound if the person moves from the safe area. The cord must not be tangled in bed rails, linens, chair parts, and so on.

Alarms do not replace close observation. Persons at risk for falls are checked often. Careful and frequent observation is important.

See *Promoting Safety and Comfort: Using Position Change Alarms.*

PROMOTING SAFETY AND COMFORT

Using Position Change Alarms

Safety
If position change alarms are used:
- Patterns and routines are monitored. For example, do alarms sound at certain times? Before or after meals, at bedtime, or when needing to use the bathroom are examples.
- Enough supervision is provided for the person's needs.
- Staff must respond to an alarm at once. False alarms are common. As a result, staff do not always respond or do not respond promptly. This increases the risk for falls.

Comfort
Alarms that limit freedom of movement may be considered a restraint (Chapter 13). For example, a person avoids moving because the alarm disrupts staff and other patients or residents. Alarms can cause:
- Embarrassment
- Loss of dignity
- Decreased mobility
- Incontinence
- Sleep problems from the sound of the alarm or fear of moving in bed
- Confusion, fear, agitation, anxiety, or irritation when the alarm sounds

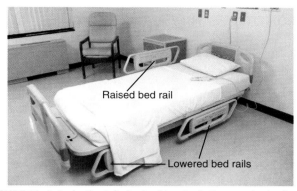

FIGURE 12-4 Bed rails. A far bed rail is raised. The near bed rails are lowered.

Bed Rails

A *bed rail (side rail) is a device that serves as a guard or barrier along the side of the bed.* Bed rails are on both sides of the bed. They are raised and lowered (Fig. 12-4). They lock in place with levers, latches, or buttons. Bed rails are quarter (¼), half (½), three quarters (¾), or the full length of the bed. When half-length rails are used, each side has 1 or 2 rails (see Fig. 12-4).

The nurse and the care plan tell you when to raise bed rails. They are needed by persons who are unconscious or sedated with drugs. Some confused or disoriented people need them. When bed rails are needed, keep them up at all times except when giving bedside care.

Bed rails present hazards. When raised, the person cannot get out of bed. The person can fall if trying to climb over them. *Entrapment* is also a risk (Chapter 19). That is, the person can get caught, trapped, entangled, or strangled.

Bed rails are considered to be restraints (Chapter 13) if:
- The person cannot get out of bed.
- They cannot or will not be lowered to allow the person to leave the bed.

Bed rails cannot be used unless needed to treat a medical symptom. They must be in the person's best interest. Some people feel safer with bed rails up. Others use them for position changes in bed. The person or legal representative must give written consent for raised bed rails. The need for bed rails is carefully noted in the person's medical record and care plan.

The procedures in this book include bed rails. This helps you learn to use them correctly. The nurse, the care plan, and your assignment sheet tell you who uses bed rails. If a person does not use them, omit the "raise bed rails" and "lower bed rails" steps.

Check the person often. Tell the nurse that you checked the person. If allowed to chart, record when you checked the person and your observations.

See *Promoting Safety and Comfort: Bed Rails*, p. 138.

PROMOTING SAFETY AND COMFORT
Bed Rails

Safety

You raise the bed to give care. Follow these safety measures to prevent falling.

- *For a person who uses bed rails:* Always raise the far bed rail(s) if you are working alone. Raise bed rails on both sides and lower the bed if you need to leave the bedside.
- *For a person who does not use bed rails:* Ask a co-worker to help you. The co-worker stands on the far side of the bed to protect the person from falling.
- Never leave the person alone when the bed is raised.
- Lower the bed to a comfortable and safe level for the person after giving care. Follow the care plan.

Comfort

The person has to reach over raised bed rails for items on the bedside stand and over-bed table (Chapter 19). That is unsafe. Adjust the over-bed table so needed items (water mug, tissues, phone, TV and light controls) are within reach. Ask what other items to place nearby. Always make sure needed items, including the call light, are within reach.

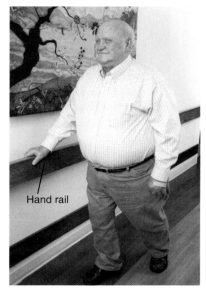

FIGURE 12-5 Hand rails provide support when walking.

Hand Rails and Grab Bars

Hand rails are in hallways and stairways (Fig. 12-5). They give support to persons who are weak or unsteady when walking.

Grab bars (safety bars) are in bathrooms and in shower/tub rooms (Fig. 12-6). They provide support to sit down or get up from a toilet. They also are used when standing in the shower and to get in and out of the shower or tub.

Wheel Locks

Bed wheels let the bed move easily. Wheels have locks (brakes) to prevent the bed from moving (Fig. 12-7). Wheels are locked (braked) at all times except when moving the bed. Make sure bed wheels are locked (braked):
- When giving bedside care
- When you transfer a person to and from bed

Wheelchair and stretcher wheels also are locked (braked) during transfers (Chapter 18). You or the person can be injured if the bed, wheelchair, or stretcher moves.

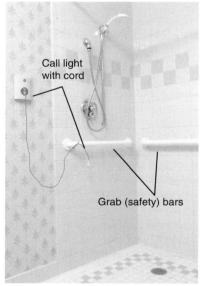

FIGURE 12-6 Grab bars (safety bars) in a shower.

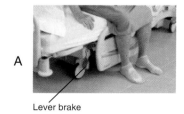 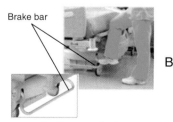

FIGURE 12-7 Examples of bed wheel locks (brakes). **A,** Lever brake. **B,** Brake bar. (Courtesy © Hill-Rom Services, Inc. Reprinted with permission. All rights reserved.)

◢ TRANSFER/GAIT BELTS

A *transfer belt (gait belt)* is a device applied around the waist and used to support a person who is unsteady or disabled (Fig. 12-8). It helps prevent falls and injuries.

• When used to transfer a person (Chapter 18), it is called a *transfer belt.*
• When used to help a person walk, it is called a *gait belt.*

The belt goes around the waist. Grasp the belt from underneath for support. Use an *upward* grasp (see Fig. 12-8). A downward grasp at the top of the belt is not secure. If the belt has handles, grasp the belt by the handles (Fig. 12-9).

See *Promoting Safety and Comfort: Transfer/Gait Belts.*
See procedure: *Using a Transfer/Gait Belt,* p. 140.

PROMOTING SAFETY AND COMFORT

Transfer/Gait Belts

Safety

Transfer/gait belts are routinely used in nursing centers. If the person needs help, a belt is required. For safe use, always follow the manufacturer's instructions.

Do not use a broken or soiled belt. Before use, check the belt for damage.

• Broken stitches or parts
• Torn, cut, or frayed material
• Broken or cracked buckles
• A buckle that does not hold securely

Some transfer/gait belts have a quick release buckle (Fig. 12-10). Position the buckle at the back where the person cannot reach or release it. Injury could result if the buckle is released.

Do not leave excess strap dangling. Tuck the excess strap into the belt (see Fig. 12-8).

Remove the belt after the procedure. Do not leave the person alone while wearing a transfer/gait belt.

The standard-sized transfer/gait belt fits waist sizes up to 51 inches. Bariatric-sized belts fit waist sizes up to 71 inches. The nurse and care plan tell you what size to use. If the person's waist size is greater than 71 inches, follow the nurse's directions and the care plan.

Using a transfer/gait belt is unsafe for some persons. The belt could cause pressure or rub against care equipment. Check with the nurse and the care plan before using a transfer/gait belt if the person has:

• An ostomy—colostomy or ileostomy (Chapter 27)
• A gastrostomy tube (Chapter 29)
• Chronic obstructive pulmonary disease (Chapter 40)
• An abdominal or chest wound, incision, or drainage tube
• Monitoring equipment
• A hernia (Part of an organ protrudes or projects through an opening in a muscle wall. Hernias often involve a loop of bowel or the stomach.)
• Other conditions or equipment involving the chest or abdomen

Comfort

A transfer/gait belt is always applied over clothing—never over bare skin. Also, it is applied around the waist and under the breasts. Breasts must not be caught under the belt. The belt buckle is never positioned over the person's spine.

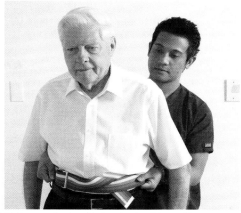

FIGURE 12-8   Transfer/gait belt. The buckle is off-center. Excess strap is tucked into the belt. The nursing assistant grasps the belt from underneath with an upward grasp.

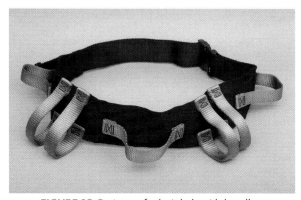

FIGURE 12-9   A transfer/gait belt with handles.

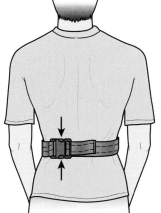

To release the buckle:
1) Press the buttons on both sides of the buckle together.
2) Pull the buckle apart.

FIGURE 12-10   A transfer/gait belt with a quick release buckle. The buckle is positioned off-center at the back.

Using a Transfer/Gait Belt

Quality of Life

- Knock before entering the person's room.
- Address the person by name.
- Introduce yourself by name and title.

- Explain the procedure before starting and during the procedure.
- Protect the person's rights during the procedure.
- Handle the person gently during the procedure.

Pre-Procedure

1 See *Promoting Safety and Comfort: Transfer/Gait Belts,* p. 139.
2 Practice hand hygiene.
3 Obtain a transfer/gait belt of the correct type and size.

4 Identify the person. Check the identification (ID) bracelet against the assignment sheet. Use 2 identifiers (Chapter 11). Also call the person by name.
5 Provide for privacy.

Procedure

6 Assist the person to a sitting position. Apply slip-resistant footwear if not already on.
7 Apply the belt. Hold the belt by the buckle. Wrap the belt around the person's waist over clothing. Do not apply it over bare skin.
  a For a belt with a metal buckle:
    1) Insert the belt's metal tip into the buckle. Pass the belt through the side with the teeth first (Fig. 12-11, A).
    2) Bring the belt tip across the front of the buckle. Insert the tip through the buckle's smooth side (Fig. 12-11, B).
  b For a belt with a quick release buckle, push the belt ends together to secure the buckle.

8 Tighten the belt so it is snug. It should not cause discomfort or impair breathing. You should be able to slide your open, flat hand under the belt. Ask about the person's comfort. If the belt is too loose or too tight, adjust the belt as needed.
9 Make sure that the person's breasts are not caught under the belt.
10 Place the buckle off-center in the front (Fig. 12-11, C) or off-center in the back (see Fig. 12-10) for the person's comfort. A quick release buckle is in the back, out of the person's reach. The buckle is not over the spine.
11 Tuck any excess strap into the belt (see Fig. 12-11, C).
12 Complete the transfer (Chapter 18) or ambulation procedure (Chapter 32). Grasp the belt from underneath with 2 hands (see Fig. 12-8). Use an upward grasp. Or grasp the belt by the handles.

Post-Procedure

13 Remove the belt after the procedure in step 12. The person is not left alone wearing the belt.
  a For a belt with a metal buckle:
    1) Bring the belt strap back through the buckle's smooth side.
    2) Pull the belt through the side with the teeth.
  b For a belt with a quick release buckle, push inward on the quick release buttons (see Fig. 12-10).
  c Remove the belt from the person's waist. Do not drag the belt across the back or waist.
14 Provide for comfort. (See the inside of the back cover.)

15 Place the call light and other needed items within reach.
16 Follow the care plan and the person's preferences for privacy measures to maintain. Leaving the privacy curtain, window coverings, and door open or closed are examples.
17 Complete a safety check of the room. (See the inside of the back cover.)
18 Return the transfer/gait belt to its proper place.
19 Practice hand hygiene.
20 Report and record your care and observations.

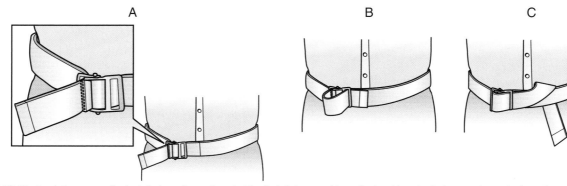

FIGURE 12-11 Applying a transfer/gait belt at the waist. **A,** The belt is inserted into the buckle. The belt goes through the side with the teeth first. **B,** The belt is inserted into the buckle's smooth side. **C,** The buckle is off-center in the front. Excess strap is tucked into the belt.

THE FALLING PERSON

A person may start to fall when standing or walking. The person may be weak, light-headed, or dizzy. Fainting may occur (Chapter 43).

Do not try to prevent the fall. You could injure yourself and the person while twisting and straining to prevent the fall. You could lose your balance. You both could fall. Head, wrist, arm, hip, knee, and back injuries could occur.

If a person starts to fall, bring the person close to your body. Ease the person to the floor. This lets you control the direction of the fall. You can also protect the person's head. Do not let the person move or get up before the nurse checks for injuries. Reassure the person and explain that the nurse will check for injuries before the person is helped up.

If you find a person on the floor, do not move the person. Stay with the person. Call for the nurse.

An incident report is completed after all falls (Chapter 11). The nurse may have you help with the report.

See *Focus on Older Persons: The Falling Person.*
See *Promoting Safety and Comfort: The Falling Person.*
See procedure: *Helping the Falling Person.*

FOCUS ON OLDER PERSONS

The Falling Person

Some older persons are confused. Confused persons may not understand why you do not want them to move or get up after a fall. Forcing a person not to move may injure the person and you. You may need to let the person move. Never use force to hold a person down. Stay calm and protect the person from injury. Talk to the person in a quiet, soothing voice. Call for help.

PROMOTING SAFETY AND COMFORT

The Falling Person

Safety

If a bariatric person starts to fall, there is little that you can do. For the person's safety and yours:

- Do *not* use the procedure: *Helping the Falling Person.*
- Move items that could cause injury out of the way. Do so as fast as possible.
- Try to protect the person's head from striking the floor, equipment, or other objects.
- Call for the nurse at once. Stay with the person.
- Assist the health team to move the person from the floor.

Helping the Falling Person

Procedure

1 Stand behind the person with your feet apart. Keep your back straight.
2 Bring the person close to your body as fast as possible (Fig. 12-12, A). Use the transfer/gait belt. Or wrap your arms around the person's waist. If necessary, hold the person under the arms.
3 Move your leg so the person's buttocks rest on it (Fig. 12-12, B).
4 Lower the person to the floor. The person slides down your leg to the floor (Fig. 12-12, C). Bend at your hips and knees as you lower the person.
5 Call a nurse to check the person. Stay with the person.
6 Help the nurse return the person to bed. Ask other staff to help if needed.

Post-Procedure

7 Provide for comfort. (See the inside of the back cover.)
8 Place the call light and other needed items within reach.
9 Raise or lower bed rails. Follow the care plan.
10 Complete a safety check of the room. (See the inside of the back cover.)
11 Practice hand hygiene.
12 Report and record the following.
  - How the fall occurred
  - If the person was standing or walking
  - How far the person walked
  - How activity was tolerated before the fall
  - Complaints before the fall
  - How much help the person needed while walking
13 Complete an incident report (Chapter 11).

A   B   C

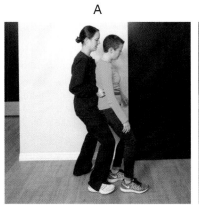 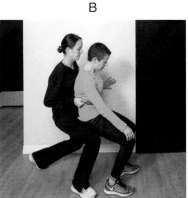 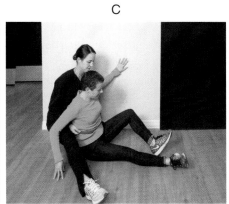

FIGURE 12-12 Helping the falling person. **A,** The falling person is supported with the gait belt. **B,** The person's buttocks rest on the nursing assistant's leg. **C,** The person is eased to the floor.

MOVING THE PERSON FROM THE FLOOR

After a fall, the nurse will assess the person for injuries. Special procedures are used to move a person with severe injuries. Assist as the nurse directs. If there are no injuries or minor injuries, follow the nurse's directions to move the person from the floor.

The Occupational Safety and Health Administration (OSHA) recommends minimal manual lifting or not lifting when possible. If the person can stand alone, the nurse has staff stand by as the person stands up. Or a transfer/gait belt is used to assist the person. A mechanical lift (Chapter 18) may be used (Fig. 12-13). The lift must reach the floor. If a manual lift is required, protect yourself from injury. See Chapter 16.

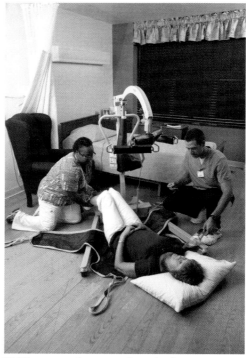

FIGURE 12-13 Moving the person from the floor using a mechanical lift.

FOCUS ON P R I D E

The Person, Family, and Yourself

P ersonal and Professional Responsibility

Safety measures can take time. Resist the urge to take short cuts. Take the time to:
- Find and use adaptive (assistive) devices.
- Put proper footwear on the person. Footwear is slip-resistant and fits well.
- Raise or lower the bed and bed rails as needed.
- Lock (brake) wheels on beds, stretchers, and wheelchairs.
- Ask for help.
  Take time for safety. Take pride in doing the right thing.

R ights and Respect

Fear of falling does not make a person feel safe. Before moving a person, explain what you will do and what the person needs to do. Also give step-by-step instructions. Good communication supports the person's right to safety and security.

I ndependence and Social Interaction

Some people feel that safety devices limit independence. Using a transfer/gait belt is an example. Listen to the person's concerns. Kindly explain the reason for the safety device. If the person still refuses, tell the nurse. Do not be talked out of a safety device. Safety is always a priority.

D elegation and Teamwork

Helping co-workers is part of teamwork. Communication is needed for safety. To help a co-worker's patient or resident, you must know:
- Is the person at risk for falls?
- Is the person weak? Can the person bear weight?
- Are there activity limits?
- How many staff are needed for the task?
- Are adaptive (assistive) devices needed? A cane, transfer belt, wheelchair, and walker are examples.
- Is other equipment needed? A mechanical lift (Chapter 18) is an example.

E thics and Laws

Falls are a serious matter. Failing to prevent injury can result in legal action. For example:
- A resident asked repeatedly for help and was told "I'm busy." The person tried to get up alone and fell.
- A person was using a shower chair (Chapter 22). The floor was wet. A nursing assistant transferred the person from the chair without shoes on the feet. The person slipped and fell.
- A nursing assistant did not lower the bed after working at the bedside. The patient fell out of bed and broke a hip.
  Follow the safety measures in this chapter. Take pride in protecting the person, yourself, and the agency.

FOCUS ON PRIDE: *Application*

A person is embarrassed about needing a transfer/gait belt and walker. How will you promote safety and dignity? What if the person refuses to use the devices?

Circle the BEST answer.

1 These statements are about falls. Which is *true*?
   a Most are caused by many risk factors.
   b Serious injuries are unlikely.
   c Falling indoors is not common.
   d Nursing center residents are at decreased risk.

2 Which person has the *lowest* risk of falls?
   a A 75-year-old with confusion
   b A 68-year-old with a history of falls
   c A 60-year-old with a hearing aid
   d An 80-year-old with urinary incontinence

3 A person's care plan includes fall prevention measures. Which should you question?
   a Assist with elimination needs.
   b Keep phone, lamp, and TV controls within reach.
   c Unlock bed wheels when giving bedside care.
   d Complete a safety check after visitors leave the room.

4 You observe the following in the person's room. Which is *unsafe*?
   a The lamp cord is by the chair.
   b The chair has armrests.
   c The night-light is on.
   d The bed is in a low position.

5 You note the following after a person is dressed. Which is *safe*?
   a Pant cuffs are dragging on the floor.
   b The person is wearing slip-resistant shoes.
   c The belt is not fastened.
   d The shirt is too big.

6 A resident's care plan includes use of a position change alarm. You hear the alarm sound. What should you do?
   a Find the resident's nursing assistant.
   b Tell the nurse.
   c Assist the person right away.
   d Wait for someone to respond to the alarm.

7 To help prevent falls, you need to report
   a Equipment and supplies being on 1 side of the hallway
   b A floor cushion beside the bed
   c A co-worker pulling a wheelchair through a doorway
   d A loose grab bar (safety bar) in a bathroom

8 Bed rails are used
   a For all persons
   b According to the care plan
   c When you want to use them
   d For persons at high risk for bed entrapment

9 Before transferring a person to bed, you must
   a Raise the bed rails
   b Get a grab bar
   c Lock (brake) the bed wheels
   d Remove the person's shoes

10 A transfer/gait belt is applied
   a To the skin
   b Over clothing at the waist
   c Over the breasts
   d Over a colostomy or ileostomy site

11 To safely use a transfer/gait belt, you must
   a Follow the manufacturer's instructions
   b Be able to slide a closed fist under the belt
   c Leave the belt on if the person is left alone
   d Position the buckle over the person's spine

12 You apply a transfer/gait belt. What should you do with the excess strap?
   a Cut it off.
   b Wrap it around the person's waist.
   c Tuck it into the belt.
   d Let it dangle.

13 A person starts to fall. Your *first* action is to
   a Try to prevent the fall
   b Call for help
   c Bring the person close to your body
   d Lower the person to the floor

14 When a bariatric person falls, you should
   a Try to stop the fall
   b Do nothing
   c Quickly pull the person close to you
   d Try to protect the person's head

15 You found a person lying on the floor. What should you do?
   a Lock the bed wheels.
   b Help the person back to bed.
   c Apply a transfer belt.
   d Call for the nurse.

Answers to Chapter 12 questions are on p. 587.

FOCUS ON **PRACTICE**

Problem Solving

You are assisting a resident in the bathroom. The resident is not to be left alone while in the bathroom. You hear a chair alarm sound in the hallway outside the door. What will you do?

CHAPTER 13

Restraint Alternatives and Restraints

OBJECTIVES

- Define the key terms and key abbreviations in this chapter.
- Describe the purpose of restraints.
- Identify restraint alternatives.
- Identify the risk factors related to restraint use.

- Explain the legal aspects of restraint use.
- Identify safety guidelines for restraint use.
- Perform the procedure described in this chapter.
- Explain how to promote PRIDE in the person, the family, and yourself.

KEY TERMS

chemical restraint Any drug used for discipline or convenience and not required to treat medical symptoms
enabler A device that limits freedom of movement but is used to promote independence, comfort, or safety

physical restraint Any manual method or physical or mechanical device, material, or equipment that:
- Is attached to or near the person's body
- Cannot be removed easily by the person
- Restricts freedom of movement or normal access to the body

KEY ABBREVIATIONS

CMS	Centers for Medicare & Medicaid Services	ROM	Range-of-motion
FDA	Food and Drug Administration	TJC	The Joint Commission
ID	Identification		

Chapters 11 and 12 have many safety measures. Some persons present dangers to themselves or others (including staff). Restraints are a last resort for protection. Safety is the priority.

The Centers for Medicare & Medicaid Services (CMS) has rules for restraint use. CMS rules protect the person's right to be free from restraint. Restraints may only be used for a brief time to treat a medical symptom that would require restraint use or for the immediate physical safety of the person or others.

Restraints may be used only when less restrictive measures fail to protect the person or others. They are not used without seeking to identify and address the condition causing the medical symptom. Restraints must be discontinued as soon as possible.

TERMS

The CMS uses the following terms and definitions regarding restraints (Box 13-1). A *physical restraint is any manual method or physical or mechanical device, material, or equipment that:*
- *Is attached to or near the person's body*
- *Cannot be removed easily by the person*
- *Restricts freedom of movement or normal access to the body*

A *chemical restraint is any drug used for discipline or convenience and not required to treat medical symptoms.* The drug or dose affects behavior or restricts movement and is not a standard treatment for the person's condition.

Physical restraints and drugs are used only when necessary to treat a medical symptom. *They are not used to discipline a person or for staff convenience.*

BOX 13-1 Restraint Terms and Definitions

- *Manual method*—to hold or limit voluntary movement by using body contact.
- *Remove easily*—the manual method, device, material, or equipment used to restrain the person can be removed intentionally by the person in the same manner it was applied by the staff. For example, a person can put bed rails down, untie a knot, or open a buckle. An item that the person *cannot* remove easily may be a restraint. See "Restraint Types" on p. 146.
- *Freedom of movement*—any change in place or position of the body or any part of the body that the person can control. An item that *restricts* freedom of movement or activity may be a restraint.
- *Discipline*—any action taken by the agency to punish or penalize a patient or resident. *Restraints are not used to discipline a person.*
- *Convenience*—any action taken to control or manage a person's behavior that requires less effort by the staff. The action is not in the person's best interests. *Restraints are not used for staff convenience.*
- *Medical symptom*—an indication or characteristic of a physical or psychological condition. A symptom may be physical, emotional, or behavioral.

Modified from Centers for Medicare & Medicaid Services: *State operations manual, appendix PP,* Baltimore, 2017, Author.

HISTORY OF RESTRAINT USE

Restraints were once used to *prevent* falls. However, there is no evidence that restraints prevent falls. Injuries are more serious from falls in restrained persons than in those not restrained.

Restraints were also used to prevent wandering or interfering with treatment. They were used for confusion, poor judgment, or behavior problems. Older persons were restrained more often than younger persons. Restraints were viewed as safety measures. However, they can cause serious harm, even death. See "Risks From Restraint Use" on p. 147.

Besides the CMS, the Food and Drug Administration (FDA), state agencies, and The Joint Commission (TJC—an accrediting agency) have restraint guidelines. They do not forbid restraint use. *All other appropriate alternatives must be considered or tried first.* See "Restraint Alternatives."

Every agency has policies and procedures for restraints. They include identifying persons at risk for harm, harmful behaviors, restraint alternatives, and proper restraint use. Staff training is required.

RESTRAINT ALTERNATIVES

Often there are causes and reasons for harmful behaviors. Knowing and treating the cause can prevent restraint use. The nurse tries to learn what the behavior means.

- Is the person in pain, ill, or injured?
- Is the person short of breath? Do cells have enough oxygen (Chapter 37)?
- Is the person afraid in a new setting?
- Does the person need to use the bathroom?
- Is the person uncomfortable, hot, cold, hungry, or thirsty?
- Are body fluids causing skin irritation?
- What are the person's life-long habits?
- Does the person have problems communicating?
- Is the person seeing, hearing, or feeling things that are not real (Chapters 41 and 42)?
- Is the person confused or disoriented (Chapter 42)?
- Are drugs causing the behaviors?

Restraint alternatives are identified in the care plan (Box 13-2). The care plan is changed as needed.

BOX 13-2 Restraint Alternatives

Physical Needs
- Life-long habits and routines are followed.
- Pillows and positioning devices are used.
- Food, fluid, hygiene, and elimination needs are met.
- Needed items are within reach.
- Comfort needs are met. Pain is controlled. See Chapter 33.
- A calm, quiet setting is provided.
- Exercise programs are provided.
- Outdoor time is planned for nice weather.
- Furniture meets the person's needs—lower bed, reclining chair, chair or wheelchair with lap-top tray (Fig. 13-1, p. 146).
- Observations and visits are made at least every 15 minutes or more often. Follow the care plan.
- The person's room is close to the nurses' station.
- Lighting meets the person's needs and preferences.
- Staff assignments are consistent.
- Sleep is not interrupted.

Safety and Security Needs
- The call light is within reach. The person is reminded to use the call light. Call lights are answered promptly.
- The person wanders in safe areas. Door alarms or knob guards are used to prevent access to unsafe areas.
- All staff are aware of persons who tend to wander.
- Falls and injuries are prevented (Chapter 12).
  - Padded hip protectors are worn (Fig. 13-2, p. 146).
  - The bed is lowered close to the floor. A soft mat or floor cushion is next to the bed.
  - Bolsters or roll guards are used. These padded devices are placed along the sides of the bed to prevent rolling out of bed.
- Walls and furniture corners are padded.
- Procedures and care measures are explained.
- Frequent explanations are given about equipment or devices.
- Confused persons are oriented to person, time, and place. (To *orient* means *to remind the person of his or her name and the date, time, and setting.*) Calendars and clocks are provided.

Love, Belonging, and Self-Esteem Needs
- Diversion is provided—music, games, relaxation, and so on.
- The person watches videos of family and friends.
- Time is spent in supervised areas (lounge, by the nurses' station).
- Family, friends, and volunteers visit.
- The person has companions or sitters.
- Time is spent with the person.
- Extra time is spent with a person who is restless.
- Reminiscing is done with the person.
- The person does jobs or tasks he or she enjoys and consents to.

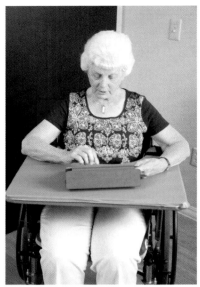

FIGURE 13-1 This lap-top tray is a restraint alternative. It is a restraint when used to prevent freedom of movement.

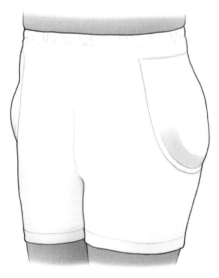

FIGURE 13-2 Hip protector. Worn under clothing, the garment helps prevent hip injuries from a fall.

RESTRAINT TYPES

A *physical restraint* confines the person to an area—bed or chair. Or it prevents movement of a body part. Holding a person down is a form of physical restraint. Some furniture or barriers prevent freedom of movement and meet the definition of a physical restraint. For example:

- A device (table, bar, lap-top tray, lap cushion, belt) is used to prevent a person from rising from a chair. The person cannot easily remove the device.
- A bed or chair is placed so close to the wall that the person cannot get out of it.
- Bed rails (Chapter 12) are raised to keep the person from getting out of bed. The person cannot lower the rails to get out of bed as desired.
- The design of a chair or mattress prevents a person from getting up.
- A sheet is tucked in so tightly that the person cannot get out of bed.
- Fabric or clothing is fastened in a way that restricts freedom of movement.
- A position change alarm (Chapter 12) is used to monitor movement. The person is afraid to move to avoid setting off the alarm.

Some devices are manufactured as physical restraints. They are applied to the chest (vest or jacket), waist (belt), wrists or ankles (limb holder), or hands (mitt). See "Laws, Rules, and Guidelines" on p. 148 and "Restraints" on p. 152.

Some drugs are restraints because they affect mood, behavior, or mental function. Drugs used to treat anxiety, depression, and psychotic disorders are examples (Chapter 41). Drugs or drug dosages are *chemical restraints* if they control behavior or restrict movement and are not standard treatment for the person's condition. For example, a drug that makes a person sleepy (sedated) and unable to function at his or her highest level is a chemical restraint.

Sometimes restraints are needed to protect the person or others. That is, a person may have violent or aggressive behaviors that are harmful to the self or others or that are threatening to others. Restraints are dangerous. The person has the right to freedom from restraint. Laws, rules, and guidelines for restraint use must be followed (p. 148).

See *Focus on Older Persons: Restraint Types.*

FOCUS ON OLDER PERSONS

Restraint Types

Dementia can affect behavior, mood, and personality. Symptoms such as aggression, agitation, delusions, and hallucinations can occur. In Chapter 42 you will learn about causes and care measures for persons with dementia. Care measures include:
- Identifying causes and triggers
- Understanding the person and following his or her routine
- Providing a calm setting
- Using distraction or an activity that is meaningful to the person

Drugs used for aggression, agitation, delusions, and hallucinations (antipsychotic drugs) can cause stroke and death in persons with dementia. Such drugs are not approved to treat dementia symptoms. They are very dangerous for persons with dementia.

Physical restraints can increase confusion and agitation. The person may try to get free from a restraint. Serious injury and death are risks.

Enablers

A device may be a restraint for 1 person but not for another. For example:

- A wheelchair with a lap-top tray is used for meals, writing, and so on (see Fig. 13-1). The person can lift the tray to exit the wheelchair.
- A person uses half (½) bed rails to move in bed and get out of bed. They do not prevent the person from leaving the bed.

In these examples, the device is an enabler, not a restraint. An ***enabler*** *is a device that limits freedom of movement but is used to promote independence, comfort, or safety.* Even though the device limits freedom of movement, the person chooses to use it to help with function. The person can remove the device easily. The person's care plan includes use of the device.

RISKS FROM RESTRAINT USE

Restraints can cause serious injury and death. Box 13-3 lists the risks from restraints. Injuries can occur as the person tries to get free of the restraint. Injuries also occur from using the wrong restraint, applying it wrong, or keeping it on too long. Cuts, bruises, and fractures are common. *The most serious risk is death from strangulation.* See Figures 13-3 and 13-4.

Restraints are medical devices. The *Safe Medical Devices Act* applies if a restraint causes illness, injury, or death. Also, the CMS requires the reporting of any death that occurs:

- While a person is in a restraint.
- Within 24 hours after a restraint was removed.
- Within 1 week after a restraint was removed. This applies if the restraint may have contributed directly or indirectly to the person's death.

See *Promoting Safety and Comfort: Risks From Restraint Use.*

BOX 13-3 Risks From Restraint Use

- Constipation
- Contractures
- Cuts and bruises
- Decline in physical function (ability to walk and muscle problems are examples)
- Dehydration
- Falls
- Fractures
- Head trauma
- Incontinence
- Infections: pneumonia and urinary tract
- Nerve injuries
- Pressure injuries
- Social and mental health problems: agitation, aggression, anger, anxiety, delirium, depression, loss of dignity, embarrassment and humiliation, mistrust, loss of self-respect, reduced social contact, withdrawal
- Strangulation

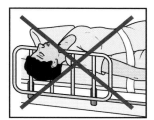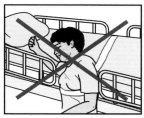

FIGURE 13-3 Restraints can cause injury and death. Incorrect application and trying to get free are causes. Here, the person is caught within and suspended between bed rails while a restraint is used.

PROMOTING SAFETY AND COMFORT

Risks From Restraint Use

Safety

If you find a person strangling from a restraint:

- Release the restraint. Or cut the strap if you have scissors in your pocket or within reach.
- Shout for help and a nurse as you are releasing the restraint.
- Stay with the person. Follow the guidelines for cardiopulmonary resuscitation (CPR) and rescue breathing (Chapter 43). Follow agency policy. Assist the nurse as directed.

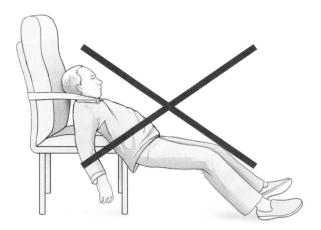

FIGURE 13-4 Death from strangulation is the most serious risk from restraint use.

LAWS, RULES, AND GUIDELINES

Federal and state laws and rules (CMS, FDA) for restraint use are followed. So are accrediting agency (TJC) guidelines. They are part of the agency's policies and procedures for restraint use.

- *Restraints must protect the person.* Restraints do not replace properly supervising the person. A restrained person requires more staff time for care and observation. When used, the restraint must be the best safety measure for the person. Restraints are not used to punish or penalize uncooperative persons.
- *A doctor's order is required.* The doctor gives the reason for the restraint, what body part to restrain, what to use, and how long to use it. This information is on the care plan and your assignment sheet. In an "immediate danger" emergency, the order must be obtained during or immediately after a restraint is applied.
- *The least restrictive method is used.* Some restraints restrict freedom of movement more than others. The method that allows the greatest amount of movement and body access is used.
- *Restraints are used only after other measures fail to protect the person* (see Box 13-2). The person's care plan lists specific measures to protect the person and others. Many fall prevention measures are restraint alternatives (Chapter 12).
- *Unnecessary restraint is false imprisonment* (Chapter 4). You must understand the reason for the restraint and its risks. If not, politely ask about its use. An unneeded restraint may lead to false imprisonment charges.
- *Informed consent is required.* The person must understand the reason for the restraint and possible risks. The person is told how the restraint will help medical treatment. If the person cannot give consent, his or her legal representative is given the information. Consent is needed before a restraint can be used. The doctor or nurse provides needed information and obtains consent. The person can refuse the restraint and withdraw consent at any time.

See *Focus on Surveys: Laws, Rules, and Guidelines.*

Safety Guidelines

The restrained person must be kept safe (Box 13-4). Also remember these key points.

- *Observe for increased confusion and agitation.* Whether confused or alert, people are aware of restricted movements. They may try to get out of the restraint or struggle to pull at it. Some restrained persons beg others to free or to help release them. These behaviors often are viewed as signs of confusion. Confusion can increase because of not understanding what is happening. Provide repeated explanations and reassurance. Spending time with them has a calming effect.
- *Protect the person's quality of life.* Restraints are used only for a brief time. The care plan must show how to reduce restraint use. You must meet the person's physical, emotional, and social needs.
- *Follow the manufacturer's instructions to safely apply and secure the restraint.* Tight restraints affect circulation and breathing. The person must be comfortable and able to move the restrained part to a limited and safe extent. Restraints must be applied and secured properly.
- *Apply restraints with enough help to protect the person and staff from injury.* In an emergency, restraints may need to be applied quickly. Combative and agitated people can hurt themselves and the staff when restraints are applied. Enough staff members are needed to complete the task safely and quickly.
- *Observe the person at least every 15 minutes or as often as directed by the nurse and the care plan.* Injuries and deaths can result from improper restraint use and poor observation. Prevent complications. Breathing and circulation problems are examples. Constant observation may be required for persons:
  - Who are aggressive, combative, or agitated.
  - At risk for aspiration—breathing food, fluid, vomitus, or an object into the lungs (Chapter 29). Persons who are supine (lying down) and unable to sit up are examples.
  - At risk for suicide (Chapter 41).
- *Remove or release the restraint, re-position the person, and meet basic needs at least every 2 hours. Or do so as often as noted in the care plan.* See Box 13-4.

FOCUS ON SURVEYS

Laws, Rules, and Guidelines

Agencies must have a policy about restraint use. Surveyors will try to learn how restraints were used. Surveyors may interview staff about:
- How staff members define "restraint."
- What restraint alternatives were used.
- The medical symptoms leading to restraint use. Could they be reversed or reduced?

- Were medical symptoms caused by failure to:
  - Meet the person's needs
  - Provide rehabilitation
  - Provide meaningful activities
  - Change the person's setting for safety
- If the least restrictive restraints were used.
- How long the restraints were used.

BOX 13-4 Safety Measures for Using Restraints

Before Applying Restraints

- Do not use sheets, towels, tape, rope, straps, bandages, Velcro, or other items to restrain a person.
- Apply a restraint only after learning about its proper use.
- Demonstrate correct application of the restraint before applying it.
- Use the correct restraint and size. Small restraints are tight. They cause discomfort and agitation and restrict breathing and circulation. Strangulation is a risk from big or loose restraints.
- Use only restraints that have the manufacturer's instructions and warning labels.
  - Read the warning labels. Note the front and back of the restraint.
  - Follow the instructions. Some restraints are safe for bed, chair, and wheelchair use. Others are used only with certain equipment.
- Use intact restraints.
  - Look for broken stitches, tears, cuts, or frayed fabric or straps.
  - Look for missing or loose buckles, locks, hooks, loops, or straps or other damage. The restraint must hold securely.
- Test zippers, buckles, locks, hooks, loops, and other closures. The device must fasten securely.
- Do not alter or repair a restraint.
- Do not use soiled or damaged restraints. Have the nurse inspect a damaged product.
- Do not use a restraint near a fire, a flame, smoking materials, or other heat sources.

Applying Restraints

- Follow agency policies and procedures and the manufacturer's instructions.
- Do not use a restraint to position a person:
  - On a toilet
  - On furniture that does not allow for correct application
- Position the person in good alignment before applying the restraint (Chapter 16). When in a chair, position the person so the hips are well to the back of the chair.
- Pad bony areas and the skin as directed by the nurse. This prevents pressure and injury from the restraint.
- Follow the manufacturer's application instructions. A restraint applied wrong or backward may cause serious injury or death. Death may occur from suffocation or strangulation.
  - *Vest restraint*—The "V" neck is in front.
  - *Jacket restraint*—The opening is in the back.
  - *Belt restraint when in a chair*—Apply the restraint at a 45-degree angle over the thighs (Fig. 13-5, p. 150).
- Do not criss-cross straps in the back unless required by the manufacturer's instructions (Fig. 13-6, p. 150). Straps may loosen when the person moves and cause serious injury.
- Secure restraints according to the manufacturer's instructions. Quick release buckles (Fig. 13-7, p. 150) or quick release knots (Fig. 13-8, p. 151) are used. Both are easy to release in an emergency.
- Leave 1 to 2 inches of slack in the straps if directed to do so by the nurse. This allows some movement of the part.
- Secure restraint straps to a safe and secure location out of the person's reach.
  - Bed—Secure the restraint to the movable part of the bed frame (Fig. 13-9, A, p. 151). This is the part of the bed frame that moves when raising or lowering the bed. *Never secure restraints to bed rails, head-boards, or foot-boards.*
  - Chair or wheelchair—Secure the straps under the seat (Fig. 13-9, B, p. 151).

Applying Restraints—cont'd

- Check for snugness after applying the restraint. The restraint should be snug but allow some movement of the restrained part. Follow the manufacturer's instructions. For example:
  - *If applied to the chest or waist*—Make sure the person can breathe easily. A flat hand should slide between the restraint and the person's body (Fig. 13-10, p. 152). Check with the nurse if you have very small or very large hands. Small or large hands could cause a tight or loose restraint.
  - *For limb holders and mitt restraints*—You should be able to slide 1 finger under the device. Check with the nurse if you have very small or very large fingers. Small or large fingers could cause a tight or loose restraint.
- Make sure that the straps cannot tighten, loosen, slip, slide, or cause too much slack. The straps can change if pulled on by the person. Changing the bed or seat (cushion) position can also change the straps. Injury or death can result from:
  - Tight straps that can impair breathing and cause suffocation.
  - Loose straps that allow the person to get free of the restraint.
  - Loose straps that allow the person to slip or slide off the bed or chair. The person can become suspended in the restraint (see Figs. 13-3 and 13-4). Chest compression and suffocation can result from strangulation.
- Use bed rail covers or gap protectors as instructed by the nurse (Fig. 13-11, p. 152). The person can become trapped or suspended (see Fig. 13-3) between:
  - The bars of a bed rail
  - The space between half-length (split) bed rails
  - The bed rail and mattress
  - The head-board or foot-board and mattress

After Applying Restraints

- Keep bed rails up when using a vest, jacket, or belt restraint. Also use bed rail covers or gap protectors. Otherwise the person could fall off the bed and strangle on the restraint. Or the person can get caught between half-length bed rails.
- Do not use back cushions when a person is restrained in a chair. If the cushion moves out of place, slack occurs in the straps. Strangulation is a risk if the person slides forward or down from the extra slack.
- Do not cover the person with a sheet, blanket, bedspread, or other covering. The restraint must be within plain view at all times.
- Check the person at least every 15 minutes for safety, comfort, and signs of injury. Or check the person more often as directed by the nurse and the care plan.
- Monitor persons in the supine (back-lying) position constantly. Aspiration is a great risk if vomiting occurs (Chapter 29). Call for the nurse at once.
- Keep scissors in your pocket. In an emergency such as strangulation, cutting the tie may be faster than releasing a knot or buckle. Never leave scissors where the person can reach them. Make sure the person cannot reach the scissors in your pocket.
- Keep the call light and other needed items within the person's reach. Record that this was done.
- Complete a safety check before leaving the room. (See the inside of the back cover.)

Continued

BOX 13-4 Safety Measures for Using Restraints—cont'd

After Applying Restraints—cont'd
- Check the person's circulation at least every 15 minutes or more often as directed by the nurse and the care plan.
  - *For limb holders or mitt restraints*—You should feel a pulse at a pulse site below the restraint. Fingers or toes should be warm and pink. Tell the nurse at once if:
    - You cannot feel a pulse.
    - Fingers or toes are cold, pale, or blue in color.
    - The person complains of pain, numbness, or tingling in the restrained part.
    - The skin is red or damaged.
  - *For a belt, jacket, or vest restraint*—The person should be able to breathe easily. Also check the position of the restraint, especially in the front and back.
- Remove or release the restraint and re-position the person every 2 hours or more often as noted in the care plan. The restraint is removed or released for at least 10 minutes.

After Applying Restraints—cont'd
- Meet the person's basic needs when the restraint is removed or released.
  - Measure vital signs.
  - Meet elimination needs.
  - Offer food and fluids.
  - Meet hygiene needs.
  - Give skin care.
  - Perform range-of-motion (ROM) exercises or help the person walk. Follow the care plan.
  - Provide for physical and emotional comfort. (See the inside of the back cover.)
- Report to the nurse every time you checked the person and removed or released the restraint. Report your observations and the care given. Follow agency policy for recording. See "Reporting and Recording" on p. 156.

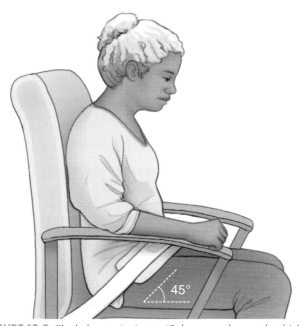

FIGURE 13-5 The belt restraint is at a 45-degree angle over the thighs.

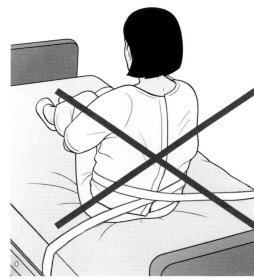

FIGURE 13-6 Never criss-cross vest or jacket straps in the back.

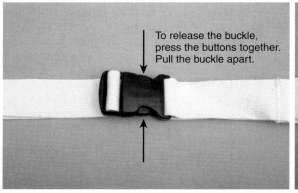
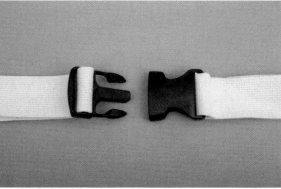

To release the buckle, press the buttons together. Pull the buckle apart.

FIGURE 13-7 Quick release buckle.

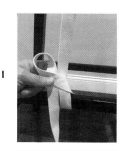

Bring the strap down across the front of the bar. Wrap the strap around to the back of the bar.

Cross the loose end over the front of the strap.

Make a loop.

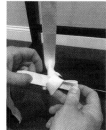

Pass the loop through the area where the strap crosses.

Pull to tighten.

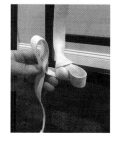

Make a second loop with the loose end.

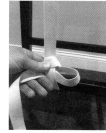

Pass the second loop through the first loop.

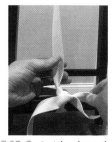

Pull to tighten.

Check that the strap is secure.

To untie, pull the loose end.

FIGURE 13-8 Quick release knot. (NOTE: This figure shows only the *method* for tying a quick release knot. The knot should be tied to a secure area out of the person's reach—a movable part of the bed frame or below the chair or wheelchair seat.)

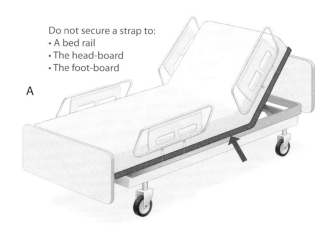

Do not secure a strap to:
• A bed rail
• The head-board
• The foot-board

A

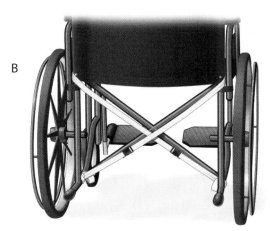

B

FIGURE 13-9 Locations for securing restraint straps. (NOTE: Straps are secured out of the person's reach.) **A,** On a bed, straps are secured to the movable part of the bed frame. This is the part that moves when raising or lowering the bed. *Do not secure a strap to a bed rail, head-board, or foot-board.* **B,** On a wheelchair, straps are secured to the frame below the seat.

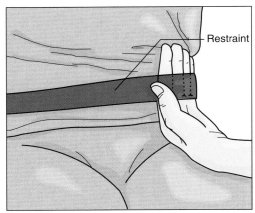

FIGURE 13-10 A flat hand slides between the restraint and the person.

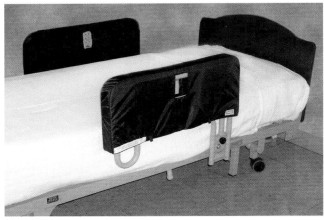

FIGURE 13-11 Bed rail protector. (From Perry AG, Potter PA, Ostendorf WR Laplante N: *Clinical nursing skills and techniques*, ed 10, St Louis, 2022, Elsevier.)

RESTRAINTS

Manufactured restraints are made of cloth or other durable materials. Cloth restraints (soft restraints) include limb holders, mitts, belts, vests, and jackets.

More restrictive, cuff-style restraints for limbs (arms and legs) are made of more durable materials. These are only used in situations of extreme danger.

Limb Holders

Limb holders applied to the wrists (wrist restraints) limit arm movement (Fig. 13-12). For a brief time, limiting such movement may be necessary if the person:

- Is at risk for pulling out tubes used for life-saving treatment (intravenous [IV] infusion, feeding tube).
- Is at risk for pulling at devices that monitor vital signs.
- Scratches at, pulls at, picks at, or peels the skin, a wound, or a dressing. This can damage the skin or the wound.

Mitt Restraints

Hands are placed in mitt restraints. They prevent finger use. They allow hand, wrist, and arm movements. They have the same purpose as wrist restraints. Most mitts are padded (Fig. 13-13).

Belt Restraints

Belt restraints prevent the person from getting out of bed or out of a chair. With some types, the person can turn from side to side and sit up in bed (Fig. 13-14).

The belt is applied around the waist and secured to the bed or chair (lap belt). It is applied over a garment. The person can release the quick release type. It is less restrictive than those that only staff can release. Such belts may be considered for persons at risk for falls.

Vest Restraints and Jacket Restraints

Vest and jacket restraints are applied to the chest. They prevent the person from getting out of bed or out of a chair. With some, the person cannot turn from side to side or sit up.

A jacket restraint is applied with the opening in the back. For a vest restraint, the "V" neck is in front (Fig. 13-15). If needed, the vest crosses in the front. The restraint is always applied over a garment. (*Note: The straps of vest and jacket restraints cross in the front. A vest or jacket restraint may have positioning slots in the back* [Fig. 13-16]. *If so, criss-cross straps following the manufacturer's instructions.*)

Vest and jacket restraints have life-threatening risks. Death can occur from strangulation. If caught in the restraint, it can become so tight that the person's chest cannot expand to inhale air. The person quickly suffocates and dies. Correct application is critical. *You are advised to only assist the nurse in applying vest and jacket restraints. The nurse should have full responsibility for applying these types of restraints.*

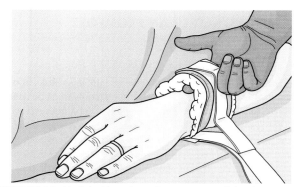

FIGURE 13-12 Limb holder. The soft part is toward the skin. One finger fits between the holder and the wrist.

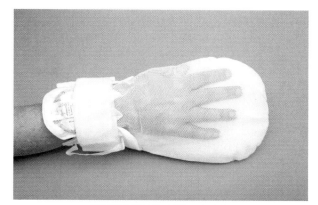

FIGURE 13-13 Mitt restraint.

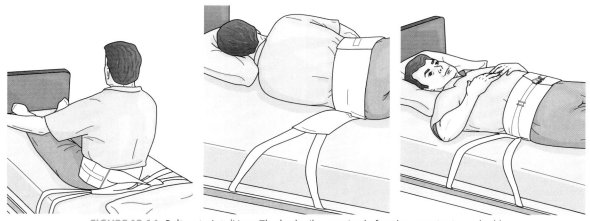

FIGURE 13-14 Belt restraint. (NOTE: The bed rails are raised after the restraint is applied.)

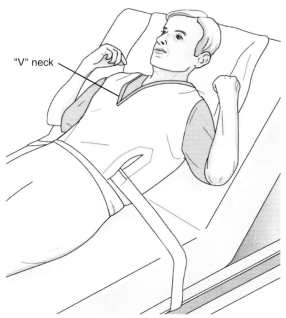

"V" neck

FIGURE 13-15 Vest restraint. The "V" neck is in front. (NOTE: The bed rails are raised after the restraint is applied.)

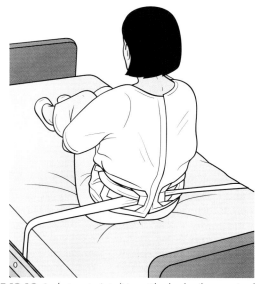

FIGURE 13-16 Jacket restraint. (NOTE: The bed rails are raised after the restraint is applied.)

APPLYING RESTRAINTS

Follow the restraint manufacturer's instructions for application and use. The procedure that follows may be used as a guide to practice applying and using:

- Wrist restraints (limb holders)
- Mitt restraints
- A belt restraint
- A vest restraint
- A jacket restraint

  See *Focus on Communication: Applying Restraints.*
  See *Delegation Guidelines: Applying Restraints.*
  See *Promoting Safety and Comfort: Applying Restraints.*
  See procedure: *Applying Restraints.*

FOCUS ON **COMMUNICATION**
Applying Restraints

If you do not know how to apply a certain restraint, do not do so. Ask the nurse to show you the correct way. You can say: "I've never applied this restraint before. Would you please show me how and then watch me apply it?" Thank the nurse for helping you.

Explain to the person what you will do. Then tell the person what you are doing step-by-step. Always check for safety and comfort.

Place the call light within reach. Make sure the person can use it with the restraint on. Remind the person to call for help if uncomfortable or if anything is needed. Do so as often as needed. For example:

- "How does the restraint feel? Is it too tight? Is it too loose?"
- "Please put your call light on. I want to make sure that you can reach and use it with the restraint on."
- "Please call for help right away if the restraint is too tight."
- "Please call for help right away if you feel pain in your fingers or hands. Also call for me if you feel numbness or tingling."
- "Please call for help right away if you are having problems breathing."
- "Please use your call light if you need anything."

PROMOTING SAFETY AND COMFORT
Applying Restraints

Safety

Restraints can cause serious harm, even death. (See "Risks from Restraint Use" on p. 147.) When needed, restraints must be used correctly and with caution. Application and safety measures vary with the restraint ordered and the manufacturer. *Always read and follow warning labels and follow the manufacturer's instructions for the restraint ordered.* Instructions for 1 restraint may not apply to another. The information, guidelines, and procedure in this chapter do not replace the manufacturer's instructions.

Never use force. Ask a co-worker to help if a person is confused or agitated. The manufacturer may have instructions for applying restraints on such persons. Report problems to the nurse at once.

Check the person at least every 15 minutes or more often as directed by the nurse and the care plan. Make sure the call light is within reach and the person can use it. Ask the person to use the call light at the first sign of problems or discomfort.

Never use a restraint as a seat belt in a car or other vehicle.

Mitt Restraints

Mitt restraints prevent finger use. Often they are not secured to the bed or chair. Therefore the person can raise the mitt to the mouth. Observe the person closely. Watch that the person does not:

- Use the teeth to remove or damage the device.
- Ingest (eat) any mitt material.

Persons with mitt restraints may be able to walk about. Falls are a risk. Practice safety measures to prevent falls (Chapter 12).

Belt, Vest, and Jacket Restraints

When a belt, vest, or jacket restraint is used, monitor the person's position. Risks include:

- Sliding forward or down in the chair or bed and becoming suspended or entrapped.
- Falling off the chair or mattress and becoming suspended or entrapped.

Comfort

Restraints limit movement. This affects position changes and reaching needed items. Position the person in good alignment before applying a restraint (Chapter 16). Make sure needed items are within reach—call light, water mug, tissues, phone, bed controls, and so on.

DELEGATION GUIDELINES
Applying Restraints

Before applying a restraint, you need this information from the nurse and the care plan.

- Why the doctor ordered the restraint.
- What type and size to use.
- Where to apply the restraint.
- How to safely apply the restraint. Have the nurse show you how to apply it. Then show correct application back to the nurse.
- How to correctly position the person.
- What bony areas to pad and how to pad them.
- If bed rail covers or gap protectors are needed.
- If bed rails are up or down.
- What special equipment is needed.
- If the person needs to be checked more often than every 15 minutes. If yes, how often?
- When to apply and release the restraint.
- What observations to report and record. See "Reporting and Recording" on p. 156.
- When to report observations.
- What patient or resident concerns to report at once (see Box 13-4).

Applying Restraints

Quality of Life

- Knock before entering the person's room.
- Address the person by name.
- Introduce yourself by name and title.
- Explain the procedure before starting and during the procedure.
- Protect the person's rights during the procedure.
- Handle the person gently during the procedure.

Pre-Procedure

1 Follow *Delegation Guidelines: Applying Restraints.* See *Promoting Safety and Comfort: Applying Restraints.*
2 Practice hand hygiene and get the following supplies as instructed by the nurse.
   - Correct type and size of restraint
   - Padding for skin and bony areas
   - Bed rail pads or gap protectors (if needed)
3 Arrange items in the person's room.
4 Practice hand hygiene.
5 Identify the person. Check the identification (ID) bracelet against the assignment sheet. Use 2 identifiers (Chapter 11). Also call the person by name.
6 Provide for privacy.

Procedure

7 Position the person for comfort and good alignment.
8 Put the bed rail pads or gap protectors (if needed) on the bed for the person in bed. Follow the manufacturer's instructions.
9 Pad bony areas. Follow the nurse's instructions and the care plan.
10 Read and follow the manufacturer's instructions. Note the front and back of the restraint.
11 *For limb holders to the wrists:*
   a Place the soft or foam part toward the skin.
   b Secure the holder so it is snug but not tight. Make sure you can slide 1 finger under the holder (see Fig. 13-12). Adjust the straps if the holder is too loose or too tight. Check for snugness again.
   c Secure the straps to the movable part of the bed frame out of the person's reach. Use the buckle or a quick release knot.
   d Repeat steps 11, a–c for the other wrist.
12 *For mitt restraints:*
   a Clean and dry the person's hands.
   b Insert the person's hand into the restraint with the palm down.
   c Wrap the wrist strap around the smallest part of the wrist. Secure the strap with the hook-and-loop or other closure.
   d Secure the restraint to the bed if directed to do so. Secure the straps to the movable part of the bed frame out of the person's reach. Use the buckle or a quick release knot.
   e Check for snugness. Slide 1 finger between the restraint and the wrist. Adjust the straps if the restraint is too loose or too tight. Check for snugness again.
   f Repeat steps 12, b–e for the other hand.
13 *For a belt restraint:*
   a Assist the person to a sitting position.
   b Apply the restraint.
   c Remove wrinkles or creases from the front and back.
   d Bring the ties through the slots in the belt if present.
   e Position the straps at a 45-degree angle between the wheelchair seat and sides (see Fig. 13-5). If in bed, help the person lie down.
   f Make sure the person is comfortable and in good alignment.
   g Secure the straps to the movable part of the bed frame. Use the buckle or a quick release knot. The buckle or knot is out of the person's reach. For a wheelchair, criss-cross and secure the straps as in Figure 13-9, *B.*

h Check for snugness. Slide an open hand between the restraint and the person. Adjust the restraint if it is too loose or too tight. Check for snugness again.
14 *For a vest restraint, assist the nurse as directed.*
   a Assist the person to a sitting position. If in a wheelchair:
      1) The person is as far back in the wheelchair as possible.
      2) The buttocks are against the chair back.
   b Apply the restraint. The "V" neck is in the front.
   c Bring the straps through the slots if the vest criss-crosses (see Fig. 13-17, p. 156).
   d Make sure the side seams are under the arms. Remove wrinkles in the front and back. Close the zipper if the device opens in the back. Or fasten with other closures.
   e Position the straps at a 45-degree angle between the wheelchair seat and sides. If in bed, help the person lie down.
   f Make sure the person is comfortable and in good alignment.
   g Secure the straps to the movable part of the bed frame at waist level. Use the buckle or a quick release knot. The buckle or knot is out of the person's reach. For a wheelchair, criss-cross and secure the straps as in Figure 13-9, *B.*
   h Check for snugness. Slide an open hand between the restraint and the person. Adjust the restraint if it is too loose or too tight. Check for snugness again.
15 *For a jacket restraint, assist the nurse as directed.*
   a Assist the person to a sitting position. If in a wheelchair:
      1) The person is as far back in the wheelchair as possible.
      2) The buttocks are against the chair back.
   b Apply the restraint. The jacket opening goes in the back.
   c Make sure the side seams are under the arms. Remove wrinkles in the front and back.
   d Close the back with the zipper or other closures.
   e Position the straps at a 45-degree angle between the wheelchair seat and sides. If in bed, help the person lie down.
   f Make sure the person is comfortable and in good alignment.
   g Secure the straps to the movable part of the bed frame at waist level. Use the buckle or a quick release knot. The buckle or knot is out of the person's reach. For a wheelchair, criss-cross and secure the straps as in Figure 13-9, *B.*
   h Check for snugness. Slide an open hand between the restraint and the person. Adjust the restraint if it is too loose or too tight. Check for snugness again.

Continued

Applying Restraints—cont'd

Post-Procedure

16 Position the person as the nurse directs.
17 Provide for comfort. (See the inside of the back cover.)
18 Place the call light and other needed items within the person's reach.
19 Raise or lower bed rails. Follow the care plan and the manufacturer's instructions for the restraint.
20 Follow the care plan and the nurse's instructions for privacy measures to maintain.
21 Complete a safety check of the room. (See the inside of the back cover.)
22 Practice hand hygiene.
23 Check the person and the restraint at least every 15 minutes or more often as directed by the nurse and the care plan. Report and record your observations.
  a *For limb holders or mitt restraints*: Check the pulse, color, and temperature of the restrained parts.
  b *For a belt, vest, or jacket restraint*: Check the person's breathing. Make sure the restraint is properly positioned in the front and back. *Release the restraint and call for the nurse at once if the person is not breathing or is having problems breathing.*

24 Do the following at least every 2 hours for at least 10 minutes.
  a Remove or release the restraint.
  b Measure vital signs.
  c Re-position the person.
  d Meet food, fluid, hygiene, and elimination needs.
  e Give skin care.
  f Perform ROM exercises or help the person walk. Follow the care plan.
  g Provide for physical and emotional comfort. (See the inside of the back cover.)
  h Re-apply the restraint.
25 Complete a safety check of the room. (See the inside of the back cover.)
26 Practice hand hygiene.
27 Report and record your care and observations.

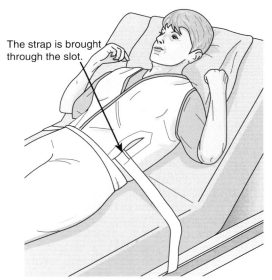

The strap is brought through the slot.

FIGURE 13-17 This vest criss-crosses in front. The straps are brought through the slots. (Note: The bed rails are raised after the restraint is applied.)

REPORTING AND RECORDING

Restraint information is recorded in the person's medical record (Fig. 13-18). If you apply restraints or care for a restrained person, report and record:

- The restraint type and body part or parts restrained
- Safety measures taken (for example, bed rails padded and up, call light within reach)
- The time you applied the restraint
- The time you removed or released the restraint and for how long
- The person's vital signs
- The care given when the restraint was removed and for how long
- Skin color and condition
- Condition of the extremities
- The pulse felt in the restrained part
- Changes in the person's behavior
  Report the following at once.
- Difficulty breathing
- Pain, numbness, or tingling in the restrained part
- Discomfort
- A tight restraint

Restraint Type				
☐ Limb holders (wrists)	☒ Mitt restraints (hands)	☐ Belt restraint	☐ Vest restraint	☐ Jacket restraint

Safety and Care Measures

☒ Restraints released/removed	☒ Food/fluid needs met	☒ Comfort measures
Duration: 20 minutes	☒ ROM/exercise/activity	☒ Skin care and hygiene
☒ Restraints re-applied	☒ Urinary/bowel elimination	☒ Bed rails up and padded
☐ Measures refused	☒ Positioning	☐ Other: _____
Notified nurse: E. Scott, RN	☒ Call light and needed items in reach	

Vital Signs

Temp 98.4 °F	Pulse 70	R 14	BP 116 / 72 mm Hg	Pain 0 /10

Circulation Observations (Normal in blue)

Color: ☒ Pink ☐ Pale ☐ Cyanotic (bluish)
Temperature: ☐ Hot ☒ Warm ☐ Cool ☐ Cold
Sensation: ☒ Good sensation ☐ Numbness/tingling ☐ No sensation
Movement: ☒ Able to move extremities ☐ Unable to move extremities
Pulses: ☒ Pulses present in all extremities ☐ Pulse faint/absent in any extremity

Tell the nurse at once if any observations are abnormal.
Notified Nurse: _____

FIGURE 13-18 Charting sample.

FOCUS ON PRIDE
The Person, Family, and Yourself

P ersonal and Professional Responsibility

Restraints have many risks. See Box 13-3. Therefore restraint use brings many responsibilities. You must:
- Promote safety and comfort.
- Apply the restraint properly.
- Observe the person closely.
- Meet basic needs.
- Report any concerns to the nurse.

R ights and Respect

You may be asked to assist with restraint alternatives (see Box 13-2). Make a true effort. Be honest. Do not tell the nurse you tried if you did not. Do your best to allow the person the right to freedom from restraint.

I ndependence and Social Interaction

All restraints limit movement. Independence is restricted. To promote independence:
- Keep the call light within reach at all times. Make sure the person can use it. Tell the person to signal for you if anything is needed. Answer the call light and meet the person's needs promptly.
- Keep needed items within reach. This is most important with restraints that allow hand and arm use. Belt, vest, and jacket restraints are examples.
- Allow choice. For example, let the person choose what to eat and drink when you release the restraint and meet needs.
- Let the person do as much as is safely possible.
Personal choice and freedom of movement promote independence, dignity, and self-esteem. Provide care that gives restrained persons the independence they deserve.

D elegation and Teamwork

Care conferences are held to meet the person's safety and care needs. Your input has value. Share your observations and ideas. For example, a person does not try to get out of a chair when looking at photos or reading a book. You share this with the team for the person's care plan.

E thics and Laws

Imagine the following.
- You need to use the bathroom. Your arms are restrained. You cannot get up or use your call light. You soil yourself with urine.
- You are uncomfortable. You have a vest restraint. You cannot move or turn in bed.
- You are thirsty. Your wrists are restrained. You cannot reach the water mug.
- You hear the fire alarm. You have on a restraint. You cannot get up to move to a safe place. You must wait to be rescued.
What would you do? Would you calmly lie or sit there? Would you try to get free from the restraint? Would you yell for help? Would the staff think that you are uncomfortable? Or would they think that you are agitated and uncooperative? Would you feel angry, embarrassed, or humiliated?

Restraints lessen dignity and freedom. Put yourself in the person's situation. Then you can better understand how the person feels. Treat the person like you would want to be treated—with kindness, caring, respect, and dignity.

FOCUS ON PRIDE: Application

Describe 3 scenarios involving behavior that is dangerous or that interferes with treatment. List ideas for managing the behavior without using restraints.

Circle the BEST answer.

1 Restraints
   a Promote dignity
   b Limit freedom of movement
   c Are a safe fall prevention measure
   d Are calming

2 Restraints may be used
   a For staff convenience
   b For discipline
   c For a person's specific medical symptom
   d When you think they are needed

3 Which is a restraint alternative?
   a Positioning the person's chair close to the wall
   b Using a chair that prevents the person from rising
   c Giving a drug that restricts movement
   d Padding walls and corners of furniture

4 Which is a restraint?
   a A padded hip protector that is worn under clothing
   b Bed rails that prevent the person from leaving the bed
   c A supervised lounge area near the nurses' station
   d A floor cushion on the floor next to the bed

5 Physical restraints
   a Can be removed easily by the person
   b Are not allowed by the CMS
   c Require a doctor's order
   d Are safer than chemical restraints

6 Which statement about restraints is *true*?
   a Some drugs are restraints.
   b A device must be attached to the body to be a restraint.
   c Restrained persons require less supervision than others.
   d You can apply a restraint if a restraint alternative fails.

7 An unneeded restraint is applied. Which is *true*?
   a This can lead to charges of false imprisonment.
   b Recording in the medical record is not required.
   c Releasing the restraint every 2 hours is not needed.
   d There is no harm if the restraint was applied properly.

8 The following can occur from restraints. Which is the *most* serious?
   a Fractures
   b Strangulation
   c Pressure injuries
   d Urinary tract infections

9 Which of the following is *safe*?
   a A vest restraint is applied with the "V" neck in the back.
   b Bed rails are left down when a vest restraint is used.
   c A jacket restraint is used to position a person on a toilet.
   d Limb holder straps are secured with a quick release knot.

10 A restraint is applied to a person in bed. Where are the straps secured?
   a To the bed rails
   b To the head-board
   c To the movable part of the bed frame
   d To the foot-board

11 A person has a restraint. You check the person and the position of the restraint at least every
   a 15 minutes
   b 30 minutes
   c Hour
   d 3 hours

12 A person has mitt restraints. Which will you report to the nurse at once?
   a The hands are clean, warm, and dry.
   b The person has numbness in the hands.
   c You removed the restraints for 10 minutes.
   d You felt a pulse in both arms.

13 When applying restraints, you should
   a Know when to apply and release them
   b Use force if the person is agitated
   c Allow plenty of slack in the straps
   d Apply a restraint you have not used before

14 A person has a vest restraint. To check for snugness, slide
   a A fist between the vest and the person
   b 1 finger between the vest and the person
   c An open hand between the vest and the person
   d 3 fingers between the vest and the person

15 The correct way to apply any restraint is to follow the
   a Nurse's directions
   b Doctor's orders
   c Care plan
   d Manufacturer's instructions

Answers to Chapter 13 questions are on p. 587.

FOCUS ON **PRACTICE**

Problem Solving

A person uses a wheelchair and often tries to get up without help. The person is at risk for falls. What are some alternatives to restraints that may be tried? If a restraint is needed, how will you provide for the person's basic needs?

CHAPTER 14

Preventing Infection

OBJECTIVES

- Define the key terms and key abbreviations in this chapter.
- Identify what microbes need to live and grow.
- List the signs and symptoms of infection.
- Explain the chain of infection.
- Describe healthcare-associated infections and the persons at risk.
- Describe the principles of asepsis.

- Explain the rules of hand hygiene.
- Identify 5 moments for hand hygiene during routine care.
- Explain how to care for equipment and supplies.
- Describe disinfection and sterilization methods.
- Explain the Bloodborne Pathogen Standard.
- Perform the procedures described in this chapter.
- Explain how to promote PRIDE in the person, the family, and yourself.

KEY TERMS

antibiotic A drug that kills bacteria

asepsis The absence *(a)* of disease-producing microbes; *sepsis* means *infection*

biohazardous waste Items contaminated with blood or other potentially infectious materials (OPIM); regulated medical waste, infectious waste

bloodborne pathogens Microbes that are present in blood and can cause infection

carrier A human or animal that is a reservoir for microbes but does not develop the infection

clean technique See "medical asepsis"

communicable disease A disease caused by a pathogen that can spread to others; contagious disease

contagious disease See "communicable disease"

contamination The process of becoming unclean

cross-contamination Passing microbes from 1 person to another by contaminated hands, equipment, or supplies

disinfection The process of killing pathogens

healthcare-associated infection (HAI) An infection that develops in a person cared for in any setting where health care is given; the infection is related to receiving health care

infection A disease state resulting from the invasion and growth of microbes in the body

infection control Practices and procedures that prevent the spread of infection

medical asepsis Practices used to reduce the number of microbes and prevent their spread from 1 person or place to another person or place; clean technique

microbe See "microorganism"

microorganism A small *(micro)* living thing *(organism)* seen only with a microscope; microbe

non-pathogen A microbe that does not usually cause an infection

normal flora Microbes that live and grow in a certain area

pathogen A microbe that is harmful and can cause an infection

sterile The absence of *all* microbes

sterile technique See "surgical asepsis"

sterilization The process of destroying *all* microbes

surgical asepsis Practices used to remove *all* microbes; sterile technique

KEY ABBREVIATIONS

CDC	Centers for Disease Control and Prevention	MRSA	Methicillin-resistant *Staphylococcus aureus*
E. coli	*Escherichia coli*	OPIM	Other potentially infectious materials
GI	Gastro-intestinal	OSHA	Occupational Safety and Health Administration
HAI	Healthcare-associated infection	PPE	Personal protective equipment
HBV	Hepatitis B virus	VRE	Vancomycin-resistant *Enterococci*
HIV	Human immunodeficiency virus	WHO	World Health Organization
MDRO	Multidrug-resistant organism		

An *infection is a disease state resulting from the invasion and growth of microbes in the body.* Infection is a major safety and health hazard. Minor infections are short-term. Some infections are serious and can cause death. Older and disabled persons are at risk. Certain *practices and procedures prevent the spread of infection (infection control).* The goal is to protect patients, residents, visitors, and staff from infection.

MICROORGANISMS

A *microorganism (microbe) is a small* (micro) *living thing* (organism) *seen only with a microscope.* Commonly called *germs,* microbes are everywhere—mouth, nose, respiratory tract, stomach, and intestines. They are on the skin and in the air, soil, water, and food. They are on animals, clothing, and furniture. Bacteria, fungi, and viruses are 3 types of microbes.

Microbes that are harmful and can cause infections are called **pathogens.** *Non-pathogens are microbes that do not usually cause an infection.*

Microbes that live and grow in a certain area are called **normal flora.** They are non-pathogens where they normally live and grow. When transmitted to another site or host, they become pathogens. For example, bacteria normally present in the colon enter the urinary system and cause an infection.

Requirements of Microbes

Microbes need a *reservoir* (host). The reservoir is the place where the microbe lives and grows. People, plants, animals, the soil, food, and water are common reservoirs. Microbes need *water* and *nourishment* from the reservoir. Most need *oxygen* to live. A *warm* and *dark* environment is needed. Most grow best at body temperature. They are destroyed by heat and light.

Multidrug-Resistant Organisms

Multidrug-resistant organisms (MDROs) are microbes that can resist the effects of antibiotics. *Antibiotics are drugs that kill bacteria.* Sometimes bacteria can change their structures, making them harder to kill. They can live in the presence of antibiotics. Therefore the infections they cause are hard to treat.

MDROs are caused by prescribing antibiotics when not needed (over-prescribing). Not taking antibiotics for the length of time prescribed is another cause.

Common MDROs are:

- *Methicillin-resistant Staphylococcus aureus (MRSA).* *Staphylococcus aureus* ("staph") is found in the nose and on the skin. MRSA is resistant to antibiotics often used for "staph" infections. MRSA can cause serious wound and bloodstream infections and pneumonia.
- *Vancomycin-resistant Enterococci (VRE). Enterococcus* is found in the intestines and in feces. It can be transmitted to other sites by contaminated hands, toilet seats, care equipment, and other items that the hands touch. Enterococci can cause urinary tract, wound, pelvic, and other infections. Enterococci resistant to vancomycin (an antibiotic) are called *vancomycin-resistant Enterococci (VRE).*

INFECTION

People can be sick with signs and symptoms of an infection. Or they can have a pathogen present but not have signs or symptoms. This is called *colonization.* A colonized person can still pass the microbe on to others.

For an infection to occur, microbes must enter the body, invade tissues, multiply, and cause the body to respond. A *local infection* is in a body part. A *systemic infection* involves the whole body. (*Systemic* means *entire.*) The person has some or all of the signs and symptoms listed in Box 14-1.

See *Focus on Older Persons: Infection.*

BOX 14-1 Infection—Signs and Symptoms

- *Fever* (elevated body temperature)
- Pulse and respirations: increased
- Chills
- Pain, tenderness, or limited use of a body part
- Fatigue and loss of energy
- Appetite: loss of (*anorexia*)
- Nausea and vomiting
- Diarrhea
- Rash
- Sores on mucous membranes
- Redness and swelling of a body part
- Discharge or drainage from the infected area
- Heat or warmth in a body part
- Headache
- Muscle aches
- Joint pain
- Confusion

The Chain of Infection

Communicable diseases (contagious diseases) are diseases caused by pathogens that can spread to others. Understanding how infections occur can help prevent the spread of the pathogens that cause them.

The *chain of infection* explains how infections occur. See Figure 14-1. The chain of infection involves a:

- Source—A pathogen.
- Reservoir—The pathogen needs a place to grow and multiply. A *carrier is a human or animal that is a reservoir for microbes but does not develop the infection.* The person is colonized with the microbe. Carriers can pass pathogens to others.
- Portal of exit—The pathogen needs a way to leave the reservoir. Exits are the respiratory, gastro-intestinal (GI), urinary, and reproductive tracts; breaks in the skin; and blood.
- Method of transmission—The pathogen is *transmitted* to another host (Fig. 14-2). In health care settings, the major transmission methods are:
  - Contact (touch). For example, staff touch a contaminated item or surface and then give care without cleaning the hands.
  - Droplets (splashes or sprays). This occurs through coughing and sneezing. Droplets carry microbes short distances. Microbes can transfer to another person's eyes, nose, or mouth.
  - Airborne (inhalation). Some microbes can spread over longer distances through the air.
  - Sharps injuries. The skin barrier is broken by a used needle or other used sharp instrument. Pathogens present in blood can transmit infections (p. 170).
- Portal of entry—The pathogen enters the body. Portals of entry and exit are the same—the respiratory, GI, urinary, and reproductive tracts; breaks in the skin; and blood.
- Susceptible host—The transmitted microbe needs a host where it can grow and multiply. Susceptible hosts are at risk for infection (p. 162).

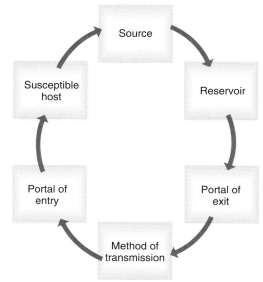

FIGURE 14-1 The chain of infection. (Redrawn and modified from Potter PA, Perry AG, Stockert PA, Hall AM: *Fundamentals of nursing,* ed 10, St Louis, 2021, Elsevier.)

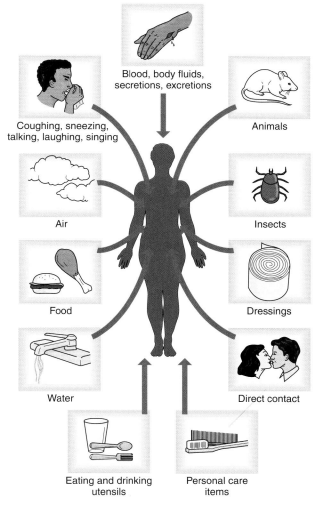

FIGURE 14-2 Methods of transmitting microbes.

Susceptible Hosts. Susceptible hosts include persons who:
- Are very young or who are older.
- Are ill.
- Were exposed to the pathogen.
- Have weakened immune systems.
- Are not immune (by vaccination or naturally). An *immune* person has protection against a certain disease. The person will not get the disease.
- Have extra ways for microbes to enter the body. Medical devices inserted in the body and surgical openings are examples.
- Do not follow practices to prevent infection.

The ability to resist infection relates to age, nutrition, stress, fatigue, and health. Drugs, disease, and injury also are factors. Infection can be deadly for:
- *Burn patients.* Burns destroy the skin, providing a portal of entry for microbes.
- *Transplant patients.* A *transplant* involves transferring an organ or tissue from 1 person to another person or from 1 body part to another body part. The body's normal immune response is to attack (reject) the new organ or tissue. Drugs are given to prevent rejection. They suppress (prevent) the immune system from producing antibodies. Antibodies are needed to fight infection.
- *Chemotherapy patients.* Some chemotherapy drugs given to treat cancer (Chapter 40) affect the production of white blood cells (WBCs). WBCs are needed to fight infection.

Healthcare-Associated Infections

A *healthcare-associated infection (HAI) is an infection that develops in a person cared for in any setting where health care is given. The infection is related to receiving health care.* HAIs also are called nosocomial infections. *(Nosocomial* comes from the Greek word for *hospital.)*

HAIs are caused by normal flora. Or they are caused by microbes from other sources. For example, *Escherichia coli (E. coli)* is normally in the colon and feces. Poor wiping after bowel movements can cause *E. coli* to enter the urinary system. With poor hand-washing, *E. coli* spreads to any body part, thing, or person the hands touch.

Microbes can enter the body from care equipment and supplies. Such items must be free of microbes. Staff can transfer microbes from 1 person to another and from themselves to others. Common sites for HAIs are:
- The urinary system
- The respiratory system
- Wounds and surgical sites
- The bloodstream

The health team uses the practices that follow and those in Chapter 15 to prevent infection and stop the spread of infection once it occurs.

ASEPSIS

Microbes are everywhere. Measures are needed to prevent microbes from causing infection. *Asepsis is the absence* (a) *of disease-producing microbes.* (Sepsis *means* infection.) The health team practices measures to achieve asepsis.

Medical asepsis (clean technique) is the practices used to:
- *Reduce the number of microbes.*
- *Prevent microbes from spreading from 1 person or place to another person or place.*

Extra precaution must be taken any time the skin or tissues are entered. During surgery is an example. *All* microbes must be removed, not just pathogens. *Surgical asepsis (sterile technique) is the practices used to remove* all *microbes. Sterile means the absence of* all *microbes.* Pathogens and non-pathogens are removed.

Contamination is the process of becoming unclean.
- In medical asepsis, an item or area is *clean* when it is free of pathogens. The item or area is *contaminated* when pathogens are present.
- A sterile item or area is *contaminated* when pathogens or non-pathogens are present.

Cross-contamination is passing microbes from 1 person to another by contaminated hands, equipment, or supplies (Fig. 14-3). Medical asepsis and surgical asepsis prevent cross-contamination.

Common Aseptic Practices

Aseptic practices break the chain of infection. You practice them in your daily life. You will learn how aseptic practices apply to your work. For example, to prevent the spread of microbes, you wash your hands:
- After elimination.
- After changing tampons or sanitary pads.
- After contact with your own or another person's blood or body fluids—saliva, vomit, urine, feces (stools), vaginal discharge, mucus, semen, wound drainage, pus, or respiratory secretions.
- After coughing, sneezing, or blowing your nose.
- Before and after handling, preparing, or eating food.
- After smoking.
  These measures also protect yourself and others.
- Provide all persons with their own linens and personal care items.
- Cover your nose and mouth when coughing, sneezing, or blowing your nose. If without tissues, cough or sneeze into your upper arm (Fig. 14-4). Do not cough or sneeze into your hands.
- Bathe, wash hair, and brush your teeth regularly.
- Wash fruit and raw vegetables before eating or serving them.
- Wash cooking and eating utensils with soap and water after use.

See *Focus on Older Persons: Common Aseptic Practices.*

…

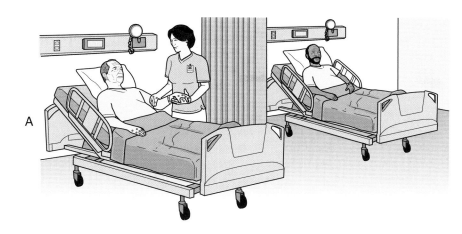

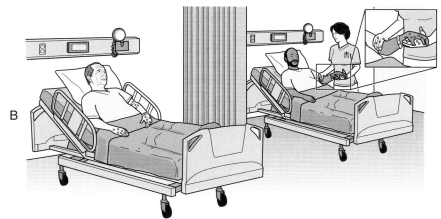

FIGURE 14-3 Cross-contamination. **A,** Microbes on the person's skin are transmitted to the nursing assistant's hands. **B,** The nursing assistant's contaminated hands transmit microbes from 1 person to another.

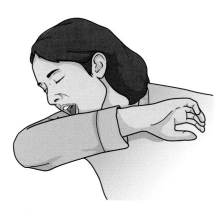

FIGURE 14-4 Sneezing into the upper arm.

FOCUS ON OLDER PERSONS

Common Aseptic Practices

Dementia can affect a person's judgment. Persons with dementia may no longer practice their own aseptic measures well. They need reminders and help. Assist them with hand-washing:

- After elimination
- After coughing, sneezing, or blowing the nose
- Before and after they eat or handle food
- Any time their hands are soiled

Check and clean their hands and fingernails often. They may not tell you when soiling occurs. Some are unable to tell you.

Hand Hygiene

Hand hygiene is the easiest and most important way to prevent the spread of microbes and infection. You use your hands for almost everything. They are easily contaminated. They can spread microbes to other persons or items (see Fig. 14-3).

There are 2 common methods for practicing hand hygiene.

- Using soap and water. This method removes microbes.
- Using an alcohol-based hand sanitizer. This method kills microbes.

At home and in community settings, using soap and water is best. You should scrub the hands with soap and water for at least 20 seconds. Alcohol-based hand sanitizer is useful when soap and water are not available. Use a product that contains at least 60% (percent) alcohol. This is listed on the product's label.

The Centers for Disease Control and Prevention (CDC) has guidelines for hand hygiene in health care settings. The CDC recommends the use of alcohol-based hand sanitizer for most health care situations (unless hands are visibly soiled). According to the CDC, hand sanitizer is effective at reducing the number of microbes that may be on the hands of staff. Also, staff are often more compliant with using hand sanitizer compared to soap and water.

There are times when soap and water should be used instead of hand sanitizer in health care settings. See Box 14-2 for the rules of hand hygiene.

See *Focus on Surveys: Hand Hygiene*, p. 166.
See *Promoting Safety and Comfort: Hand Hygiene*, p. 166
See procedure: *Hand-Washing*, p. 166.
See procedure: *Using an Alcohol-Based Hand Sanitizer*, p. 167.

BOX 14-2 Rules for Hand Hygiene in Health Care Settings

When to Use Soap and Water
Wash your hands (with soap and water):
- When they are visibly dirty or soiled. Soiling may be from blood or a body fluid. Body fluids include secretions such as saliva or nasal secretions and excretions such as urine, feces (stools), or vomit.
- Before eating.
- After using the restroom.
- After caring for a person with known or suspected infectious diarrhea. *Clostridioides difficile (C. diff)* is discussed in Chapter 27.
- After known or suspected exposure to spores. (Spores are bacteria protected by a hard shell.) *C. diff* and anthrax spores are examples.
- If an alcohol-based hand sanitizer is not available.

When to Use Alcohol-Based Hand Sanitizer
Use alcohol-based hand sanitizer for hand hygiene if your hands are not visibly soiled:
- Before touching a patient or resident.
- Before performing a clean or aseptic task. Such tasks involve contact with mucous membranes, non-intact skin, or an invasive medical device. (*Invasive* means *entering the body*.)
- Before moving from a soiled body site to a clean body site on the same person.
- After contact with blood, body fluids, or contaminated items or surfaces.
- After touching a patient or resident.
- After touching items close to a patient or resident. This includes equipment.
- After removing gloves.

How to Use Soap and Water
Follow these rules for washing your hands with soap and water. See procedure: *Hand-Washing*, p. 166.
- Wash your hands under warm running water. Do not use hot water. Hot water can dry the skin.
- Stand away from the sink. Do not let your hands, body, or uniform touch the sink. The sink is contaminated. See Figure 14-5.
- Do not touch the inside of the sink at any time.

How to Use Soap and Water—cont'd
- Keep your hands and forearms lower than your elbows. If you hold your hands and forearms up, dirty water runs from your hands to your forearms and elbows. Those areas become contaminated.
- Wet your hands with water first. Then apply the amount of soap recommended by the manufacturer.
- Rub your palms together (Fig. 14-6) and interlace your fingers (Fig. 14-7) to work up a good lather. The rubbing action helps remove microbes and dirt.
- Pay attention to areas often missed during hand-washing—thumbs, knuckles, sides of the hands, little fingers, and under the nails.
- Clean fingernails by rubbing the fingertips against your palms (Fig. 14-8).
- Use a nail file or orangewood stick to clean under fingernails (Fig. 14-9). Microbes grow easily under the fingernails.
- Wash your hands for at least 20 seconds. Wash longer if they are dirty or soiled. Use your judgment and follow agency policy.
- Use clean, dry paper towels to dry your hands.
- Dry your hands starting at the fingertips. Work up to your forearms (Fig. 14-10). You will dry the cleanest area first.
- Use a clean, dry paper towel for each faucet to turn the water off (Fig. 14-11, p. 166). Faucets are contaminated. The paper towels prevent you from contaminating your clean hands.

How to Use Alcohol-Based Hand Sanitizer
Follow these rules when decontaminating your hands with an alcohol-based hand sanitizer. See procedure: *Using an Alcohol-Based Hand Sanitizer*, p. 167.
- Apply the product to the palm of 1 hand. Follow the manufacturer's instructions for the amount to use.
- Rub your hands together.
- Cover all surfaces of your hands and fingers.
- Continue rubbing your hands together until your hands are dry. It should take about 20 seconds.

Lotions and Creams
- Use hand lotion or cream to prevent the skin from chapping and drying. Skin breaks can occur in chapped and dry skin. Skin breaks are portals of entry for microbes.
- Use an agency-approved lotion. Other lotions can interfere with hand sanitizing products.

Modified from Centers for Disease Control and Prevention: Guidelines for hand hygiene in health-care settings, *Morbidity and Mortality Weekly Report* 51 (RR-16), October 2002. (Note: Updated from Centers for Disease Control and Prevention: *Frequent questions about hand hygiene*, last reviewed August 10, 2021, and *Hand hygiene in healthcare settings: healthcare providers*, last reviewed January 8, 2021.)

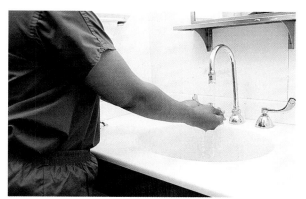

FIGURE 14-5 The uniform does not touch the sink. Hands are lower than the elbows. Hands do not touch the inside of the sink.

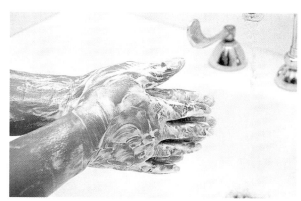

FIGURE 14-6 The palms are rubbed together to work up a good lather.

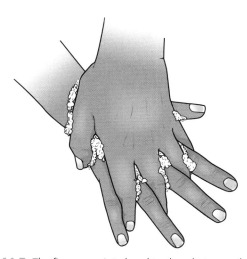

FIGURE 14-7 The fingers are interlaced to clean between the fingers.

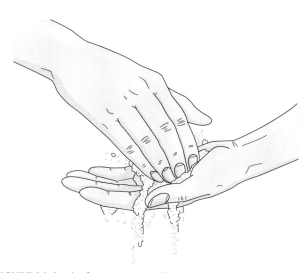

FIGURE 14-8 The fingertips are rubbed against the palms to clean under the fingernails.

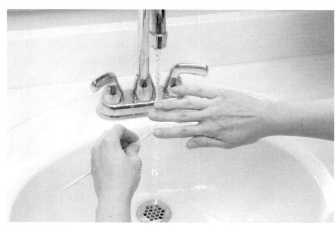

FIGURE 14-9 An orangewood stick is used to clean under the fingernails.

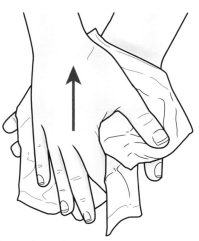

FIGURE 14-10 Hands are dried starting at the fingertips and working up to the forearms.

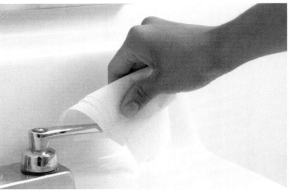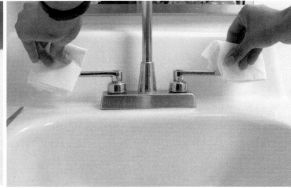

FIGURE 14-11 A paper towel is used to turn off each faucet.

NATCEP VIDEO

Hand-Washing

Procedure

1 See *Promoting Safety and Comfort: Hand Hygiene.*
2 Make sure you have soap, paper towels, an orangewood stick or nail file, and a wastebasket. Get any missing items.
3 Push your watch up your arm 4 to 5 inches. Push long uniform sleeves up too.
4 Stand away from the sink so your clothes do not touch the sink (see Fig. 14-5). Stand so the soap and faucet are easy to reach. Do not touch the inside of the sink at any time.
5 Turn on and adjust the water until it feels warm.
6 Wet your wrists and hands. Keep your hands lower than your elbows. Be sure to wet the area 3 to 4 inches above your wrists.
7 Apply about 1 teaspoon of soap to your hands. Follow the manufacturer's instructions for the amount to use.
8 Rub your palms together and interlace your fingers to work up a good lather (see Fig. 14-6). Lather your wrists, hands, and fingers. Keep your hands lower than your elbows. Steps 8 through 10 should last at least 20 seconds.

9 Wash each hand and wrist thoroughly. Clean the back of your fingers and between your fingers (see Fig. 14-7).
10 Clean under the fingernails. Rub your fingertips against your palms (see Fig. 14-8).
11 Clean under the fingernails with a nail file or orangewood stick (see Fig. 14-9). Do this for the first hand-washing of the day and when your hands are visibly soiled.
12 Rinse your wrists, hands, and fingers well. Water flows from above the wrists to your fingertips.
13 Repeat steps 7 through 12, if needed.
14 Dry your fingers, hands, and wrists with clean, dry paper towels. Pat dry starting at your fingertips (see Fig. 14-10).
15 Discard the paper towels into the wastebasket.
16 Turn off faucets with clean, dry paper towels. This prevents you from contaminating your hands (see Fig. 14-11). Use a clean paper towel for each faucet. Or use knee or foot controls to turn off the faucet.
17 Discard the paper towels into the wastebasket.

Using an Alcohol-Based Hand Sanitizer

Procedure

1 See *Promoting Safety and Comfort: Hand Hygiene.*
2 Apply a palmful of an alcohol-based hand sanitizer into a cupped hand (Fig. 14-12). Follow the manufacturer's instructions for the amount to use.
3 Rub your hands together. Cover all surfaces of the hands and fingers (see Fig. 14-12).
  a Rub your palms together.
  b Rub the palm of 1 hand over the back of the other. Do the same for the other hand.

c Rub your palms together with your fingers interlaced.
d Interlock your fingers. Rub your fingers back and forth.
e Rub the thumb of 1 hand in the palm of the other. Do the same for the other thumb.
f Rub the fingers of 1 hand into the palm of the other hand. Use a circular motion. Do the same for the fingers of the other hand.
4 Continue rubbing your hands until they are dry.

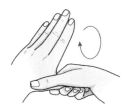

Apply a palmful of an alcohol-based hand sanitizer into a cupped hand.

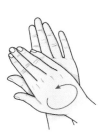

Rub the palms together.

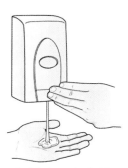

Rub the palm of 1 hand over the back of the other hand. Repeat for the other hand.

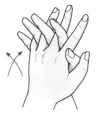

Rub the palms together with the fingers interlaced.

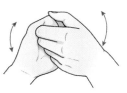

Interlock the fingers and rub back and forth.

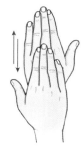

Rub the thumb of 1 hand in the palm of the other hand. Repeat for the other thumb.

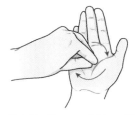

Rub the fingers of 1 hand into the palm of the other hand with circular motions. Repeat for the fingers on the other hand.

FIGURE 14-12 Using an alcohol-based hand sanitizer.

Your 5 Moments
for Hand Hygiene

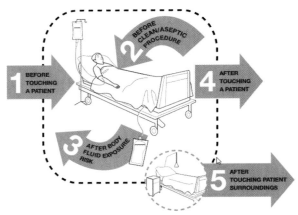

FIGURE 14-13 WHO's 5 Moments for Hand Hygiene. (Note: Dashed lines mark the separation of the zones. The "patient zone" is within the dashed lines. The "health-care area" is outside the dashed lines.) (From World Health Organization: *SAVE LIVES: Clean your hands*, 2022.)

Moments for Hand Hygiene. The World Health Organization (WHO) has promoted "5 Moments for Hand Hygiene" in an effort to improve health care worker hand hygiene (Fig. 14-13). The WHO's model describes 2 "zones"—the "patient zone" and the "health-care area."

The "patient zone" includes the patient or resident and his or her close surroundings. This zone typically involves a bed. However, it also applies to other situations. A patient or resident seated in a chair is an example. The "patient zone" involves:

- *The person and his or her intact skin*
- *Items the person touches or has direct contact with*—bed rails, the bedside table, bed linens, medical equipment near the person
- *Objects frequently touched by health care workers while caring for the person*—bed controls; other buttons, monitors, or controls; other frequently touched objects

In the "patient zone," it is assumed that the patient's normal flora quickly contaminate the area. Also, that area is cleaned before another patient or resident uses it.

The "health-care area" includes all objects outside of the "patient zone." The health care facility and other patients or residents within their "patient zones" are part of the "health-care area." The "health-care area" is considered to be contaminated with microbes that may be harmful if brought into a "patient zone."

The WHO has identified 5 moments when hand hygiene is essential. See Box 14-3 and Figure 14-13. During routine care, always practice hand hygiene at these times. If 2 moments occur together, a single act of hand hygiene covers both moments.

See *Promoting Safety and Comfort: Moments for Hand Hygiene.*

BOX 14-3 WHO's 5 Moments for Hand Hygiene

Moment 1: Before touching a patient or resident
- This moment occurs between the last contact with an object in the health care area and the first contact with the person.
- This protects the person. It prevents the transfer of microbes from the health care setting to the person.
- For example, you touch the door handle to enter the room. You practice hand hygiene before touching the arm to check the person's identification (ID) bracelet.

Moment 2: Before a clean/aseptic procedure
- This moment occurs between the last contact with any object (even within the patient zone) and before a task involving contact with mucous membranes, non-intact skin, or invasive medical devices.
- This protects the person. It prevents the transfer of microbes to a site that can cause an infection.
- For example, you had contact with items near the person. You practice hand hygiene immediately before performing oral care.

Moment 3: After body fluid exposure risk
- This moment occurs after a task that exposes the hands to body fluids. Hand hygiene must occur before contact with any other object (even within the patient zone).
- This protects others. It prevents the transfer of microbes to the health care worker and then to others. It also prevents transmission of microbes between a soiled and a clean body site on the same person.
- For example, you had contact with urine during bathing. You practice hand hygiene before touching clean clothes to dress the person.

Moment 4: After touching a patient or resident
- This moment occurs after contact with the person and before touching an object in the health care area.
- This protects others. It prevents the transfer of microbes to the health care area and then to others.
- For example, you turn and re-position a patient. You practice hand hygiene after touching the person. You leave the room.

Moment 5: After touching patient or resident surroundings
- This moment occurs after touching any object in the patient zone and before touching any object in the health care area. Hand hygiene is needed even if the person is not touched.
- This protects others. It prevents the transfer of microbes to the health care area and then to others.
- For example, you bring a resident fresh water and move the over-bed table closer to the bed. You practice hand hygiene after touching the over-bed table. You leave the room.

Modified from World Health Organization: *WHO guidelines on hand hygiene in health care*, 2009.

PROMOTING SAFETY AND COMFORT

Moments for Hand Hygiene

Safety

Depending on the procedure and care setting, some supplies and equipment are gathered outside of the "patient zone." For the procedures in this book, hand hygiene is indicated at the following times when supplies are likely to be gathered outside of the "patient zone":

- Before gathering supplies and equipment
- Before touching the person

Supplies and Equipment

Disposable supplies and equipment help prevent the spread of infection. Discard single-use items after use. A person uses multi-use items many times. They include plastic bedpans, urinals, wash basins, and water mugs. Label multi-use items with the person's name and room and bed number. Do not "borrow" them for another person.

Non-disposable items are cleaned and then disinfected. Then they are sterilized, usually by the supply department.

Cleaning. Cleaning reduces the number of microbes present. It also removes organic matter such as food, blood, and body fluids. *Organic matter* comes from living plants and animals and will decay.

To clean equipment:
- Wear personal protective equipment (PPE) to clean items contaminated with blood or body fluids. PPE includes gloves, a mask, a gown, and goggles or a face shield. See Chapter 15.
- Work from *clean* to *dirty* areas. If you work from a *dirty* to *clean* area, the *clean* area becomes contaminated (*dirty*).
- Rinse the item in cold water to remove organic matter. Heat makes organic matter thick, sticky, and hard to remove.
- Wash the item with soap and hot water.
- Scrub thoroughly. Use a brush if necessary.
- Rinse the item in warm water. Dry the item.
- Disinfect the item. Or have it sterilized.
- Disinfect equipment and the sink used for cleaning.
- Discard PPE.
- Practice hand hygiene.

Disinfection. *Disinfection is the process of killing pathogens.* Disinfectants are used to clean objects and surfaces. A *disinfectant* is a liquid chemical that can kill many or all pathogens. Disinfectants are used to clean counters, tubs, showers, and re-usable items. Such items include:
- Blood pressure cuffs
- Commodes and bedpans
- Shower chairs
- Wheelchairs and stretchers
- Furniture
  See *Promoting Safety and Comfort: Disinfection.*

PROMOTING SAFETY AND COMFORT

Disinfection

Safety

Disinfectants can burn and irritate the skin. Wear utility gloves or rubber household gloves to prevent skin irritation. These gloves are waterproof. Do not wear disposable gloves.

Some disinfectants have special measures for use and storage. Check the safety data sheet (SDS) before handling a disinfectant. See Chapter 11.

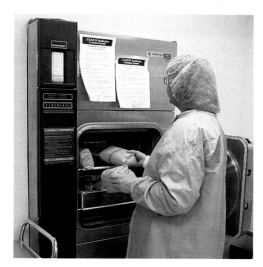

FIGURE 14-14 An autoclave.

Sterilization. *Sterilization is the process of destroying* all *microbes* (pathogens and non-pathogens). Very high temperatures are used. Heat destroys microbes.

Boiling water, radiation, liquid or gas chemicals, dry heat, and *steam under pressure* are sterilization methods. An autoclave (Fig. 14-14) is a pressure steam sterilizer. Glass, surgical items, and metal items are autoclaved. High temperatures destroy plastic and rubber items. They are not autoclaved.

Antiseptics

Antiseptics kill, slow the growth of, or reduce the amount of microbes on the skin or mucous membranes. (*Anti* means *against. Sepsis* means *infection*.) Antiseptic products have a variety of uses. For example:
- Alcohol-based hand sanitizer is used during routine care.
- An antiseptic is applied to a patient's skin before surgery.
- A nurse applies an antiseptic to the area around a patient's urethra before inserting a urinary catheter (Chapter 26).
- You use antiseptic wipes to clean the parts of your stethoscope that are placed in your ears and on the person (Chapter 31).

Other Aseptic Measures

Hand hygiene, cleaning, disinfection, and sterilization are important aseptic measures used in health care settings. So are the measures listed in Box 14-4, p. 170. They are also useful at home and in every-day life.

BOX 14-4 Aseptic Measures

Controlling Reservoirs (Hosts—You or the Person)
- Provide for hygiene needs (Chapter 22).
- Wash contaminated areas with soap and water. Feces (stools), urine, blood, and other body fluids (including secretions and excretions) can contain microbes.
- Use leak-proof plastic bags for soiled tissues, linens, and other items.
- Keep tables, counters, wheelchair trays, and other surfaces clean and dry.
- Label bottles with the person's name and the date the bottle was opened.
- Keep bottles and fluid containers tightly capped or covered.
- Keep drainage containers below the drainage site (Chapter 26).
- Empty drainage containers and dispose of drainage following agency policy. Usually drainage containers are emptied every shift. The nurse may have you empty them more often.

Controlling Portals of Exit
- Cover your nose and mouth to cough or sneeze.
- Provide the person with tissues to use when coughing or sneezing.
- Wear PPE as needed (Chapter 15).

Controlling Transmission
- Provide all persons with their own personal care equipment. This includes wash basins, bedpans, urinals, commodes, and eating and drinking utensils.
- Do not take equipment from 1 person's room to use for another person. Even if un-used, do not take the item from 1 room to another.
- Hold equipment and linens away from your uniform (Fig. 14-15).
- Practice hand hygiene. See Box 14-2.
- Assist the person with hand-washing.
  - Before and after eating
  - After elimination
  - After changing tampons, sanitary napkins, or other personal hygiene products
  - After contact with blood or body fluids (including secretions or excretions)

Controlling Transmission—cont'd
- Prevent dust movement. Do not shake linens or equipment. Use a damp cloth for dusting.
- Clean from *clean* to *dirty* areas. This prevents soiling a clean area.
- Clean away from your body. Do not dust, brush, or wipe toward yourself. Otherwise you transmit microbes to your skin, hair, and clothing.
- Flush urine and feces (stools) down the toilet. Avoid splatters and splashes.
- Pour contaminated liquids directly into sinks or toilets. Avoid splashing onto other areas.
- Do not sit on the person's bed or chair. You will pick up microbes and transfer them to other surfaces that you sit on.
- Do not use items on the floor. The floor is contaminated.
- Follow agency disinfection procedures to clean:
  - Tubs, showers, and shower chairs after each use
  - Bedpans, urinals, and commodes after each use
- Report pests—ants, spiders, mice, and so on.

Controlling Portals of Entry
- Provide good skin care and oral hygiene (Chapters 21 and 22). This promotes intact skin and mucous membranes.
- Protect the skin from injury.
  - Do not let the person lie on tubes or other items.
  - Make sure linens are dry and wrinkle-free (Chapter 20).
  - Turn and re-position the person as directed by the nurse and care plan (Chapters 17 and 18).
- Assist with or clean the genital area after elimination. (See "Perineal Care" in Chapter 22.) Wipe and clean from the urethra (cleanest area) to the rectum (dirtiest area). This helps prevent urinary tract infections.
- Make sure drainage tubes are properly connected. This prevents microbes from entering the drainage system.

Protecting the Susceptible Host
- Follow the care plan to meet nutrition and fluid needs (Chapters 28, 29, and 30). This helps prevent infection.
- Assist with deep-breathing and coughing exercises as directed (Chapter 37). This helps prevent respiratory infections.

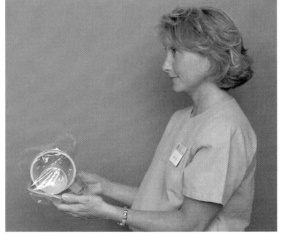

FIGURE 14-15 Hold equipment away from your uniform.

BLOODBORNE PATHOGEN STANDARD

Bloodborne pathogens are microbes that are present in blood and can cause infection. The human immunodeficiency virus (HIV) and the hepatitis B virus (HBV) are examples (Chapter 40). Persons who come into contact with bloodborne pathogens are at risk for infection and illness.

The goal of the Occupational Safety and Health Administration (OSHA) is to ensure safe working conditions. The *Bloodborne Pathogen Standard* is a regulation of OSHA. It protects the health team from exposure to bloodborne pathogens.

The standard has requirements for employers to follow in order to protect workers who may be exposed to blood or other potentially infectious materials (OPIM) in their work. OPIM may contain blood. Body fluids such as semen, vaginal secretions, saliva in dental procedures, and any body fluid visibly contaminated with blood are some OPIM.

The following body fluids are generally *not* considered OPIM—urine, feces (stools), nasal secretions, sputum, vomit, breast-milk, and saliva (other than in dental procedures). Standard Precautions (Chapter 15) are used for contact with such body fluids. Standard Precautions assume that every person is infected or colonized with a pathogen that can be transmitted in the health care setting. Precautions are used when handling such body fluids. However, they are generally not considered a source of bloodborne pathogens unless blood is visible. See "Standard Precautions" in Chapter 15.

Staff at risk for exposure to blood or OPIM receive free training. It occurs upon employment and yearly. Training is also done for new or changed tasks involving exposure to bloodborne pathogens.

Infection prevention and follow-up measures in the Bloodborne Pathogen Standard include:
- Vaccination against hepatitis B
- Engineering and work practice controls to reduce exposure
- The use of personal protective equipment (PPE)
- Regulations for equipment, work surfaces, biohazardous waste, and laundry
- Requirements for exposure incidents

Hepatitis B Vaccination

A *vaccination* involves giving a vaccine to produce immunity against an infectious disease. A *vaccine* is a preparation containing dead or weakened microbes. The hepatitis B vaccine produces immunity against hepatitis B. The hepatitis B vaccination involves 3 injections (shots). Injection 2 is given 1 month after the first. Injection 3 is given at least 4 months after the first one. The vaccination can be given before or after HBV exposure.

The agency must offer the hepatitis B vaccination after you are trained about the vaccine and within 10 days of your first working day. The agency pays for it. You can refuse the vaccination. If so, you must sign a statement refusing the vaccine. You can have the vaccination at a later date if you want.

Engineering and Work Practice Controls

Engineering controls isolate or remove bloodborne pathogen hazards from the workplace. For example, broken glass is safely cleaned up and discarded using a brush and dust pan. Pieces are placed in a puncture-resistant container. The hands (even gloved hands) are not used to pick up broken glass.

Work practice controls reduce the likelihood of exposure. All tasks involving blood or OPIM are done in ways to limit splatters, splashes, and sprays. Producing droplets also is avoided.

Health care workers:
- Do not eat, drink, smoke, apply cosmetics or lip balm, or handle contact lenses in areas of exposure.
- Do not store food or drinks where blood or OPIM are kept.
- Practice hand hygiene after removing gloves.
- Wash hands as soon as possible after skin contact with blood or OPIM.
- Never re-cap, bend, or remove needles by hand. A mechanical means (forceps) or a 1-handed method is used.
- Never shear or break needles.
- Discard needles and sharp instruments (such as razors) in containers that are closable, puncture-resistant, and leakproof. Containers have the *BIOHAZARD* symbol. See Figure 14-16. The color red is used to designate a hazard. Containers must be upright and not allowed to over-fill.

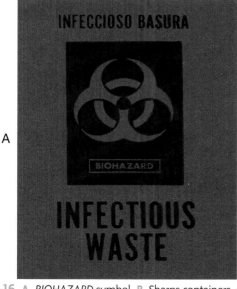
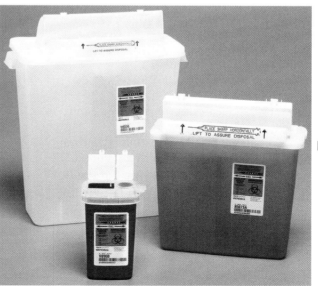

FIGURE 14-16 **A,** *BIOHAZARD* symbol. **B,** Sharps containers. Containers are leak-proof and puncture-resistant. (B from Warekois RS, Robinson R: *Phlebotomy worktext and procedures manual,* ed 4, St Louis, 2016, Elsevier.)

Personal Protective Equipment (PPE)

Personal protective equipment (PPE) is the clothing or equipment worn by staff for protection against a hazard (Chapter 15). This includes gloves, goggles, face shields, masks, laboratory coats, gowns, shoe covers, and surgical caps. Blood or OPIM must not pass through them. They protect your clothes, under-garments, skin, eyes, mouth, and hair.

PPE is free to staff. OSHA requires these measures.
- Remove PPE before leaving the work area.
- Remove PPE when it becomes contaminated.
- Place used PPE in marked areas or containers when being stored, washed, decontaminated, or discarded.
- Wear gloves for contact with blood or OPIM.
- Wear gloves to handle or touch contaminated items or surfaces.
- Replace worn, punctured, or contaminated gloves.
- Never wash or decontaminate disposable gloves for re-use.
- Discard utility gloves that show signs of cracking, peeling, tearing, or puncturing. Utility gloves are decontaminated for re-use if the process will not ruin them.

Equipment and Work Surfaces

Contaminated equipment and work surfaces are cleaned and decontaminated with a proper disinfectant.
- Upon completing tasks
- At once for obvious contamination
- At the end of your work shift when surfaces became contaminated since the last cleaning

Biohazardous Waste

Some waste is hazardous. Also known as *regulated medical waste or infectious waste*, **biohazardous waste** *involves items contaminated with blood or other potentially infectious materials (OPIM). (Bio means life. Hazardous means dangerous or harmful.)* Such waste requires special handling.

Closable, puncture-resistant, leak-proof containers that are color-coded in red with the *BIOHAZARD* symbol (see Fig. 14-16, *A*) are used to collect:
- Liquid or semi-liquid blood or OPIM
- Items contaminated with blood or OPIM
- Items caked with blood or OPIM
- Contaminated sharps (needles, syringes, razors, and other sharp items)

State and local guidelines and regulations determine what is considered biohazardous waste. The amount of soiling is a factor. Follow agency policies and procedures for handling contaminated trash, equipment, and supplies.

Laundry

OSHA requires these measures for laundry soiled with blood or OPIM.
- Handle it as little as possible.
- Wear gloves or other needed PPE.
- Bag contaminated laundry where it is used.
- Mark laundry bags or containers with the *BIOHAZARD* symbol for laundry sent off-site.
- Place wet, contaminated laundry in leak-proof containers before transport. The containers are color-coded in red or have the *BIOHAZARD* symbol. See *Focus on Surveys: Laundry.*

FOCUS ON SURVEYS
Laundry

Surveyors will observe how staff handle, store, process, and transport linens. For example, do staff:
- Handle linens according to agency policies and procedures?
- Store and transport linens properly?

Exposure Incidents

An *exposure incident* is any eye, mouth, other mucous membrane, non-intact skin, or parenteral contact with blood or OPIM. *Parenteral* means *piercing the mucous membranes or the skin.* Causes include needle-sticks, human bites, cuts, and abrasions.

Report an exposure incident at once. Medical evaluation, follow-up, and testing are free. Your blood is tested for HIV and HBV. If you refuse testing, the blood sample is kept for at least 90 days. Testing is done later if you desire.

You are told about medical conditions related to the exposure that may need treatment. You receive a written opinion within 15 days after the evaluation is complete.

The *source individual* is the person whose blood or body fluids are the source of an exposure incident. The source's blood is tested for HIV and HBV. The agency informs you about laws affecting the source's identity and test results.

FOCUS ON P R I D E

The Person, Family, and Yourself

P ersonal and Professional Responsibility

Your actions affect the person's risk for infection. You are responsible for following the guidelines in this chapter. Practice good hand hygiene at the correct times. This is the most important way to prevent the spread of microbes.

R ights and Respect

The person and visitors have the right to ask health care workers about hand hygiene. Many agencies encourage them to ask. The CDC has posters and brochures with messages such as:

- "It's OK to ask for protection from infection."
- "Ask for safe care. Ask for clean hands."
- "Speak up for clean hands."
- "Clean hands count."

Think about what you will say and do if a patient, resident, or visitor asks you about hand hygiene. Will you be angry, embarrassed, or annoyed? Or will you kindly thank the person for the reminder? Your attitude matters. Show a good attitude in your interactions with the person and visitors.

I ndependence and Social Interaction

Patients and residents often cannot perform their usual hygiene measures. Hand hygiene is an example. Ask patients and residents if they would like to clean their hands. Ask often and assist as needed.

The CDC lists these important times for the person to perform hand hygiene.

- Before eating
- Before touching the eyes, nose, or mouth
- Before and after changing bandages on wounds
- After elimination

- After coughing, sneezing, or blowing the nose
- After touching doorknobs
- After touching bed rails, bedside tables, remote controls, or the phone

Hand hygiene is important for patients and residents. Encourage it and make it a routine part of the person's care.

D elegation and Teamwork

Precautions must be taken to contain (isolate) pathogens and prevent their spread. Chapter 15 discusses the precautions used for all persons and those used for persons with certain types of infections. You will also learn about the use of PPE.

Consistency is key. All team members must follow the rules. Even one careless act can spread microbes. The health team must work together to prevent the spread of microbes and infection.

E thics and Laws

When assisting with or performing a procedure, do not use items that become contaminated. If necessary, stop and get new supplies. Do not use a contaminated item. For example, a washcloth falls on the floor. Do not use the washcloth.

You may be alone. Be honest with yourself. Be responsible. Do the right thing, even if other staff are not present.

FOCUS ON PRIDE: *Application*

Consider your every-day actions. How do they prevent infection? Give some examples. Identify areas to improve. How might your attitude affect how you prevent infection at work?

REVIEW QUESTIONS

Circle the BEST answer.

1 Which area is *best* for a pathogen to live and grow?
   a A cold and wet area
   b A warm and dark area
   c A hot and bright area
   d A dry area without oxygen

2 Which statement about microbes is *true*?
   a A pathogen can cause an infection.
   b Normal flora are pathogens in their natural sites.
   c Microbes cannot invade other body parts.
   d Antibiotics are used to kill viruses.

3 A microbe is resistant to drugs used to treat it. This means
   a Infection with the microbe will have no signs or symptoms
   b Hand hygiene will not prevent its spread
   c Infection caused by the microbe is harder to treat
   d Infection caused by the microbe does not need to be treated

4 Which is a sign of infection?
   a A bruise
   b Redness in a body part
   c Warm, dry, and intact skin
   d A bleeding wound

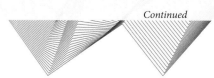

Continued

5 Medical asepsis involves practices to
   a Sterilize items before surgery
   b Diagnose and treat infections
   c Prevent staff from getting a healthcare-associated infection
   d Reduce the number of microbes and prevent microbe spread

6 Hand hygiene and disinfection are measures used to prevent cross-contamination.
   a True
   b False

7 If an item is "sterile," this means that
   a There are only non-pathogens on the item
   b The item has been cleaned with soap and hot water
   c There are no microbes on the item
   d The item has been cleaned with a disinfectant

8 Unless hands are visibly soiled, which is used for hand hygiene in *most* health care situations?
   a Soap and water
   b Alcohol-based hand sanitizer
   c Disinfectant spray
   d Hot water

9 You have blood on your hand. What should you do?
   a Wash your hands with soap and water.
   b Use an alcohol-based hand sanitizer.
   c Rinse your hands.
   d Wash your hands with a disinfectant.

10 You move from a soiled body site to a clean body site. Your hands are not visibly soiled. What should you do?
   a Wash your hands after the next task.
   b Use an alcohol-based hand sanitizer.
   c Rinse your hands with water.
   d Continue care without hand hygiene.

11 When washing your hands with soap and water, you should
   a Stand with your body against the sink
   b Hold your hands and forearms up
   c Scrub the hands for 10 seconds
   d Dry from the fingertips toward the forearms

12 Hand hygiene is performed before touching a person. This prevents the transfer of microbes from the health care setting to the person.
   a True
   b False

13 Why do you practice hand hygiene immediately before a procedure that involves mucous membranes?
   a To protect yourself
   b To protect the person
   c To protect other staff
   d To protect other patients or residents

14 You touch items in the person's room but do not touch the person. You are going to leave the room. Hand hygiene
   a Is optional
   b Is not needed if the person was not touched
   c Is not needed if there was no contact with body fluids
   d Is needed after touching items in the person's room

15 To use an alcohol-based hand sanitizer correctly
   a Wash your hands before applying the hand sanitizer
   b Rinse your hands after applying the hand sanitizer
   c Rub the product only on the palms of your hands
   d Rub your hands together until they are dry

16 When cleaning equipment
   a Rinse the item in hot water before cleaning
   b Wash the item with soap and cold water
   c Use a brush if necessary
   d Work from dirty to clean areas

17 To control a portal of exit
   a Cover the mouth and nose when coughing
   b Position drainage containers above the drainage site
   c Clean the genital area from the rectum to the urethra
   d Leave an open wound uncovered

18 Which measure prevents the transmission of microbes?
   a Sharing personal care equipment
   b Holding linens against your uniform
   c Disinfecting a shower chair after use
   d Sitting on the person's bed

19 The Bloodborne Pathogen Standard is a regulation of OSHA to protect workers from exposure to pathogens present in blood.
   a True
   b False

20 Bloodborne pathogens are spread through
   a Only blood
   b Blood and other potentially infectious materials
   c Close contact
   d Coughing and sneezing

21 According to the Bloodborne Pathogen Standard, you should
   a Wear PPE home so you can clean it
   b Discard a used razor in a wastebasket
   c Wear a torn glove
   d Get a hepatitis B vaccine

22 Blood splashed in your eye at work. Which is *true*?
   a You do not have to report the exposure.
   b You pay for required tests after the exposure.
   c You can refuse HIV and HBV testing.
   d The source individual is not tested for HIV or HBV.

Answers to Chapter 14 questions are on p. 587.

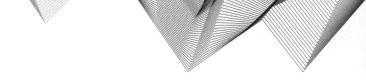

FOCUS ON PRACTICE

Problem Solving

Two residents share a room. You make both beds without practicing hand hygiene between beds. Why is this a problem? When should you practice hand hygiene? Can you use an alcohol-based hand sanitizer?

CHAPTER 15

Isolation Precautions

OBJECTIVES

- Define the key terms and key abbreviations in this chapter.
- Identify when Standard Precautions and Transmission-Based Precautions are used.
- Explain the purpose of Standard Precautions.
- Describe how to follow Standard Precautions.
- Explain the purpose of Transmission-Based Precautions.
- Identify 3 types of Transmission-Based Precautions.
- Describe the rules for Transmission-Based Precautions.

- Explain how to use personal protective equipment.
- Describe infection control measures for handling used laundry, supplies, and equipment.
- Describe infection control measures when collecting specimens and transporting persons.
- Perform the procedure described in this chapter.
- Explain how to promote PRIDE in the person, the family, and yourself.

KEY TERMS

infection control Practices and procedures that prevent the spread of infection

personal protective equipment (PPE) The clothing or equipment worn by staff for protection against a hazard

KEY ABBREVIATIONS

CDC   Centers for Disease Control and Prevention
PPE   Personal protective equipment

TB   Tuberculosis

Infection control is the practices and procedures that prevent the spread of infection. A goal is to isolate (contain) and prevent the spread of pathogens. In health care settings, the *Guideline for Isolation Precautions: Preventing Transmission of Infectious Agents in Healthcare Settings 2007* is followed. It is a guideline of the Centers for Disease Control and Prevention (CDC).

The CDC guideline has 2 tiers of precautions.

- *Standard Precautions*—used in all situations for all persons.
- *Transmission-Based Precautions*—used when persons have or may have certain infections. More precautions are needed.

STANDARD PRECAUTIONS

Standard Precautions are basic precautions used in health care settings (Box 15-1, p. 176). They:

- Reduce the risk of spreading pathogens.
- Reduce the risk of spreading known and unknown infections.

  Standard Precautions are used for all persons whenever care is given. Standard Precautions prevent the spread of infection from:

- Blood.
- All body fluids (except sweat). This includes secretions and excretions even if blood is not visible. Nasal secretions, saliva, sputum, urine, feces (stools), vomit, and breast-milk are examples. Sweat is not known to spread infection.
- Non-intact skin (skin with open breaks).
- Mucous membranes.

BOX 15-1 Standard Precautions

Hand Hygiene
- Follow the rules of hand hygiene. See Chapter 14.
- Touch surfaces close to the person only when necessary. This prevents contaminating clean hands from room or care setting surfaces. It also prevents transmitting pathogens from contaminated hands to other surfaces.
- Do not wear fake nails or nail extenders for contact with persons at risk for infection or other adverse outcomes. Microbes can live under fake nails even after hand hygiene. (NOTE: Non-natural nails are not allowed in some agencies.)
- Keep natural nail tips less than ¼ (one-quarter) inch long.

Personal Protective Equipment (PPE) (p. 180)
- Wear personal protective equipment (PPE) when contact with blood or body fluids is likely.
- Do not contaminate your clothing or skin when removing PPE.
- Remove and discard PPE before leaving the person's room or care setting.

Gloves
- Wear gloves when contact with the following is likely.
  - Blood or other potentially infectious materials (Chapter 14)
  - Body fluids (including secretions and excretions)
  - Mucous membranes
  - Non-intact skin
  - Skin or equipment that may be contaminated (for example, from urine or feces [stools])
- Wear gloves that fit and are needed for the task.
  - Wear disposable gloves for direct care.
  - Wear disposable gloves or utility gloves to clean equipment or care settings.
- Remove gloves after contact with:
  - The person
  - The person's care setting
  - Equipment used in the person's care or other care equipment
- Remove gloves after contact with a person and before going to another person. Do not wear the same pair of gloves for the care of more than 1 person.
- Do not wash gloves for re-use.
- Change gloves during care if your hands will move from a soiled body site to a clean body site.

Gowns
- Wear a gown to protect your skin and clothing when contact with blood or body fluids is likely.
- Wear a gown for direct contact with a person who has uncontained secretions or excretions.
- Remove the gown and perform hand hygiene before leaving the person's room or care setting.
- Do not re-use gowns, even for repeat contact with the same person.

Mouth, Nose, and Eye Protection
- Wear PPE—masks, goggles, face shields, or a combination of each—for procedures and tasks that are likely to cause splashes and sprays of blood or body fluids.
- Wear the correct PPE for the procedure or task.
- Wear gloves, a gown, and 1 of the following for procedures or tasks likely to cause sprays of respiratory secretions.
  - A face shield that fully covers the front and sides of the face
  - A mask with attached shield
  - A mask and goggles

Respiratory Hygiene/Cough Etiquette
- Instruct persons with respiratory symptoms to:
  - Cover the nose and mouth to cough or sneeze.
  - Use tissues to contain respiratory secretions.
  - Dispose of tissues in the nearest no-touch waste container.
  - Perform hand hygiene after contact with respiratory secretions.
- Provide visitors with masks according to agency policy.

Care Equipment
- Wear the correct PPE to handle:
  - Care equipment that is visibly soiled with blood or body fluids
  - Care equipment that may have been in contact with blood or body fluids
- Remove organic material before disinfection and sterilization procedures. Follow agency policy for using cleaning agents.

Care of the Environment
- Follow agency procedures to clean and maintain surfaces. Care setting surfaces and care equipment are examples. Surfaces near the person may need frequent cleaning and maintenance—door knobs, bed rails, over-bed tables, walker and cane handles, toilet surfaces and areas, and so on.
- Follow agency procedures to clean and disinfect multi-use electronic equipment. This includes:
  - Items used by patients and residents
  - Items used to give care
  - Mobile devices that are moved in and out of patient or resident rooms
- Follow these rules for children's toys. This includes toys in waiting areas.
  - Select toys that are easy to clean and disinfect.
  - Do not allow stuffed, furry toys if they will be shared.
  - Clean and disinfect large stationary toys (for example, climbing equipment) at least weekly and when visibly soiled.
  - Rinse toys with water after disinfection if they are likely to be mouthed by children. Or wash them in a dishwasher.
  - Clean and disinfect a toy at once when it needs cleaning. Or store the toy in a labeled container away from toys that are clean and ready for use.

Textiles and Laundry
- Handle used textiles and fabrics (linens) with minimal (the least amount of) agitation. This prevents contamination of air, surfaces, and other persons.

Worker Safety
- Protect yourself and others from exposure to bloodborne pathogens. This includes handling needles and other sharps. See "Bloodborne Pathogen Standard" in Chapter 14.
- Use a mouthpiece, resuscitation bag, or other ventilation device for resuscitation to prevent contact with the person's mouth and oral secretions. See Chapter 43.

Patient or Resident Placement
- A private room is preferred if the person is at risk for transmitting infection to others.
- Follow the nurse's directions if a private room is not available.

Modified from Siegel JD, Rhinehart E, Jackson M, Chiarello L, and the Healthcare Infection Control Practices Advisory Committee: *Guideline for isolation precautions: preventing transmission of infectious agents in healthcare settings 2007*, Atlanta, last update July 2019, Centers for Disease Control and Prevention.

TRANSMISSION-BASED PRECAUTIONS

With some infections, transmission is not prevented with Standard Precautions alone. When a person is known or suspected to have such an infection, Transmission-Based Precautions are needed along with Standard Precautions. Transmission-Based Precautions are commonly called "isolation precautions."

There are 3 types of Transmission-Based Precautions. Some infections require more than 1 type of precaution.

* *Contact*—involves touch. The pathogen spreads through touching the person or items and surfaces near the person.
* *Droplet*—involves respiratory droplets. The pathogen spreads through close contact with respiratory secretions.
* *Airborne*—involves air. The pathogen is able to suspend in the air. It can be transmitted over long distances.

Personal protective equipment (PPE) is required. Needed PPE depends on how the pathogen is spread. Gloves, a gown, a mask or respirator, and goggles or a face shield may be needed. The CDC provides guidelines on what PPE to wear and how to safely apply and remove it. See "Personal Protective Equipment" on p. 180.

Disposable (single-use) equipment is used when possible. Or dedicated equipment is kept in the room. *Dedicated equipment* is only used for 1 person. For example, a thermometer and blood pressure equipment are kept in the room. The equipment is not removed for use on another person. Equipment that must be shared is disinfected after use. A mechanical lift (Chapter 18) is an example.

In this chapter, "isolation room" refers to the room of a person who needs Transmission-Based Precautions. The nurse may have you help set up an isolation room. Follow agency procedures. The following are common.

* PPE is in a cart or cabinet outside the room (Fig. 15-1). Re-stock supplies as needed.
* A sign is posted outside the room to alert staff and visitors of needed precautions (Fig. 15-2).
* A wastebasket and linen cart are inside the room. Color-coded or red bags with the *BIOHAZARD* label are used (Chapter 14).
* Dedicated equipment, leak-proof plastic bags, and a disinfectant are supplied.

See Box 15-2 (p. 178) for the CDC's guidelines for the 3 types of Transmission-Based Precautions. Agency policies may differ from those in this text. The rules in Box 15-3 (p. 179) are a guide for giving safe care when using Transmission-Based Precautions.

See *Focus on Communication: Transmission-Based Precautions,* p. 179.

See *Focus on Surveys: Transmission-Based Precautions,* p. 179.

See *Delegation Guidelines: Transmission-Based Precautions,* p. 179.

See *Promoting Safety and Comfort: Transmission-Based Precautions,* p. 179.

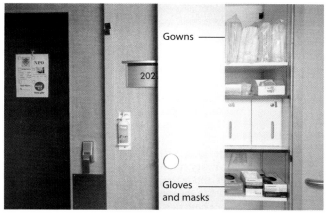

FIGURE 15-1 Personal protective equipment is in a cabinet outside the person's room.

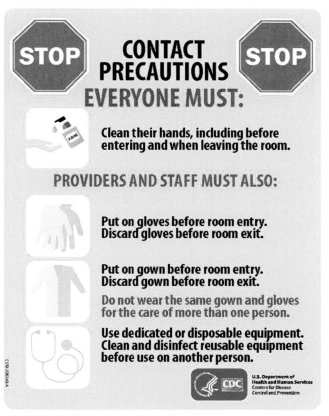

FIGURE 15-2 Sample sign for Contact Precautions. The sign is posted outside the room to alert staff and visitors of needed precautions. (From Centers for Disease Control and Prevention, Department of Health and Human Services.)

BOX 15-2 Transmission-Based Precautions

Contact Precautions
- Used for persons with known or suspected infections or conditions that increase the risk of contact (touch) transmission.
- Patient or resident placement:
  - A single room is preferred.
  - If a room is shared with another person not infected with the same agent:
    - Keep the persons separated—more than 3 feet apart.
    - Keep the privacy curtain between the beds closed.
    - Change PPE and practice hand hygiene between contact with persons in the same room. Do so regardless of whether 1 or both persons are on Contact Precautions.
- Gloves:
  - Don (put on) gloves upon entering the person's room or care setting.
  - Wear gloves to touch the person's intact skin.
  - Wear gloves to touch surfaces or items near the person.
- Gown:
  - Wear a gown when clothing may have direct contact with the person.
  - Wear a gown when contact is likely with surfaces or equipment near the person.
  - Don the gown upon entering the person's room.
  - Remove the gown and practice hand hygiene before leaving the person's room.
  - Make sure your clothing and skin do not touch potentially contaminated surfaces after removing the gown.
- Patient or resident transport:
  - Limit transport and movement of the person outside of the room to medically-necessary purposes.
  - Cover the infected area of the person's body.
  - Remove and discard contaminated PPE and practice hand hygiene before transporting the person.
  - Don clean PPE to handle the person at the transport destination.
- Care equipment:
  - Follow Standard Precautions.
  - Use disposable equipment when possible. If possible, leave non-disposable equipment in the person's room.
  - Clean and disinfect non-disposable and multiple-use equipment before use on another person.

Droplet Precautions
- Used for persons known or suspected to be infected with pathogens transmitted by respiratory droplets. Such droplets come from coughing, sneezing, or talking.
- Patient or resident placement:
  - A single room is preferred.
  - If a room is shared with another person who is not infected with the same agent:
    - Keep the persons separated—more than 3 feet apart. Some infections require at least 6 feet of separation.
    - Keep the privacy curtain between the beds closed.
    - Change PPE and practice hand hygiene between contact with persons in the same room. Do so regardless of whether 1 or both persons are on Droplet Precautions.
- PPE:
  - Don a mask upon entering the person's room.
  - Wear other PPE as required for the pathogen or as required by agency policy.
- Patient or resident transport:
  - Limit transport and movement of the person outside of the room to medically-necessary purposes.
  - Have the person wear a mask.
  - Instruct the person to follow Respiratory Hygiene/Cough Etiquette (see Box 15-1).
  - No mask is required for staff transporting the person.

Airborne Precautions
- Used for persons known or suspected to be infected with pathogens transmitted person-to-person by the airborne route. Tuberculosis (TB), measles, chicken pox, and smallpox are examples.
- The person is placed in an airborne infection isolation room (AIIR). If not available, the person is transferred to an agency with an AIIR. The room door is kept closed except when someone enters or leaves the room.
- Staff susceptible to the infection do not enter the room (if immune staff members are available to give care).
- PPE:
  - An agency-approved respirator is worn on entering the room when TB or smallpox is suspected or confirmed.
  - Agency policy is followed for respiratory protection for other airborne infections.
  - Other PPE is worn as required for the pathogen or as required by agency policy.
- Patient or resident transport:
  - Limit transport and movement of the person outside of the room to medically-necessary purposes.
  - Have the person wear a surgical mask.
  - Instruct the person to follow Respiratory Hygiene/Cough Etiquette (see Box 15-1).
  - Cover skin lesions infected with the microbe.
  - No mask or respirator is required for staff transporting the person if the person is wearing a mask and skin lesions are covered.

Modified from Siegel JD, Rhinehart E, Jackson M, Chiarello L, and the Healthcare Infection Control Practices Advisory Committee: *Guideline for isolation precautions: preventing transmission of infectious agents in healthcare settings 2007*, Atlanta, last update July 2019, Centers for Disease Control and Prevention.

BOX 15-3 Rules for Transmission-Based Precautions

- Tell the nurse if you have any cuts, open skin areas, a sore throat, vomiting, or diarrhea.
- Collect all needed items before entering the room.
- Do not touch your hair, nose, mouth, eyes, or other body parts.
- Do not touch any clean area or object if your hands are contaminated.
- Wash your hands with soap and water if they are visibly dirty or contaminated with blood or body fluids (including secretions and excretions).
- Place clean items on paper towels.
- Do not shake linens.
- Use paper towels to handle contaminated items.
- Use paper towels to turn faucets on and off.
- Use a paper towel to open the door to the person's room. Discard it after use.
- Do not contaminate equipment and supplies. Floors are contaminated. So is any object on the floor or that falls to the floor.
- Clean floors with mops wetted with a disinfectant solution. Floor dust is contaminated.
- Prevent drafts. Drafts can carry some microbes in the air.
- Remove items from the room in leak-proof plastic bags.
- Follow agency procedures to remove and transport re-usable and disposable items. For meal trays:
  - Place re-usable dishes, drinking vessels, eating utensils, and trays in a leak-proof plastic bag (p. 186).
  - Discard disposable dishes, drinking vessels, eating utensils, and trays in the waste container in the person's room.

FOCUS ON COMMUNICATION
Transmission-Based Precautions

The health team and visitors must know what PPE to use. Signs are a common way to communicate the type of precaution and the needed PPE (see Fig. 15-2). Signs are posted at the person's doorway. In long-term care settings, signs may instruct visitors to see the nurse before entering the person's room.

Visitors may ask why PPE is needed. Some visitors ignore signs or requests to wear PPE. Politely communicate with the person and visitors about PPE. For example, you can say: "Please wear this mask. It is our policy to protect you, your family member, and others." Tell the nurse if the person or visitors have more questions. Also tell the nurse if someone refuses to wear PPE.

If you see a staff member not wearing needed PPE, remind the person. You can also offer to get the person PPE. For example, you can say:
- "I'll get you the mask that you need."
- "Here are gloves and a gown that you need."
Be polite. Tell the nurse if the person refuses.

FOCUS ON SURVEYS
Transmission-Based Precautions

When a person requires Transmission-Based Precautions, surveyors will observe if staff:
- Wash their hands correctly and at the correct times.
- Change gloves after providing personal care.
- Don, wear, and dispose of PPE correctly.

DELEGATION GUIDELINES
Transmission-Based Precautions

If a person needs Transmission-Based Precautions, review the type with the nurse. Also check with the nurse and care plan about:
- What PPE to use
- What special measures are needed
- What equipment to use—disposable or dedicated

PROMOTING SAFETY AND COMFORT
Transmission-Based Precautions

Safety

Preventing the spread of infection is important. Transmission-Based Precautions protect everyone—patients, residents, visitors, staff, and you. If you are careless, everyone's safety is at risk.

Meeting Basic Needs

With Transmission-Based Precautions, the person is more isolated and knows the disease can spread to others. Visitors might avoid the person. Staff may not enter as often because of needed PPE. Without intending to, visitors and staff can make the person feel ashamed, guilty, or dirty. Sadness and loneliness are common.

Do not avoid the person. When giving care, talk to the person. Show kindness and respect. See *Focus on PRIDE: The Person, Family, and Yourself* (p. 187) for other ways to meet love, belonging, and self-esteem needs.

See *Focus on Communication: Meeting Basic Needs.*
See *Focus on Older Persons: Meeting Basic Needs.*

FOCUS ON COMMUNICATION
Meeting Basic Needs

Some questions or statements can make the person feel dirty or ashamed. Be careful what you say. For example, do not say:
- "How did you get that?"
- "I'm afraid to touch you."
- "Don't breathe on me."

FOCUS ON OLDER PERSONS
Meeting Basic Needs

Some older persons have dementia. PPE may increase confusion and cause fear and agitation. These measures can help.
- Tell the person who you are and what you need to do.
- Use a calm, soothing voice.
- Do not rush the person.
- Use touch to reassure the person.
- Follow the care plan and the nurse's instructions for other measures to help the person.
- Report signs of increased confusion or behavior changes.

PERSONAL PROTECTIVE EQUIPMENT

Personal protective equipment (PPE) is the clothing or equipment worn by staff for protection against a hazard. PPE protects you and prevents the spread of microbes.

- For Standard Precautions, PPE is worn when contact with blood or body fluids is likely. The task determines what is needed.
- For Transmission-Based Precautions, PPE is worn regularly when giving care. The infection determines what is needed.

PPE includes gowns, masks and respirators, goggles and face shields, and gloves. If you are unsure of what PPE to wear, ask the nurse.

Gowns

Gowns protect your clothes and body from contact with blood and body fluids. They also protect against splashes and sprays. Gowns are worn with gloves and with other PPE as needed.

A gown must completely cover your body front from the neck to the knees. The long sleeves have tight cuffs. The gown opens at the back and wraps around your back to cover your uniform. It is tied in the back at the neck and waist. *The gown front and sleeves are considered contaminated.*

Gowns are used once. A wet gown is contaminated. Hold water basins and wet items out away from the gown. Avoid contact with wet surfaces. Remove a wet gown and put on a dry one. Discard disposable gowns after use.

Masks and Respirators

You wear disposable masks:

- To prevent contact with infectious materials from the person. Respiratory secretions and sprays of blood or body fluids are examples.
- To protect the person from infectious agents carried in your mouth or nose during sterile procedures.

A wet or moist mask is contaminated. Breathing can cause masks to become wet or moist. Apply a new mask when contamination occurs.

A mask fits snugly over your nose and mouth. Practice hand hygiene before putting on a mask. To remove a mask, touch only the ties or the elastic bands. *The front of the mask is contaminated.*

Agency-approved respirators (Fig. 15-3) are worn when caring for persons with infections spread by the airborne route. TB is an example (Chapter 40). A respirator must fit securely. Employers provide fit testing and training on how to check for a proper seal.

Goggles and Face Shields

Splashes and sprays can occur when you give care, clean items, or dispose of fluids. Goggles protect your eyes from splashing or spraying of blood and body fluids. Face shields protect your eyes and other areas of your face.

The front (outside) of goggles or a face shield is contaminated. The headband, ties, or ear-pieces used to secure the device are *clean.* Use them to remove the device after hand hygiene

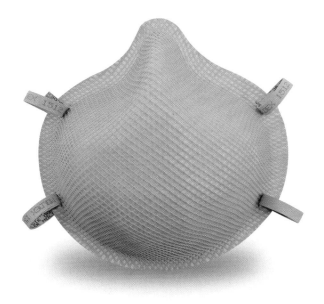

FIGURE 15-3   A respirator. (© Moldex.)

when they are safe to touch with bare hands. Lift the ties or ear-pieces from the back when removing the device.

Discard disposable goggles or face shields after use. Re-usable eyewear is cleaned before re-use. It is washed with soap and water. Then a disinfectant is used.

See *Promoting Safety and Comfort: Goggles and Face Shields.*

PROMOTING SAFETY AND COMFORT

Goggles and Face Shields

Safety

Eyeglasses and contact lenses do not provide eye protection. The face shield must fit over eyeglasses with minimal gaps.

Goggles do not provide splash or spray protection to other parts of your face.

Gloves

A natural barrier, the skin prevents microbes from entering the body. Small skin breaks on the hands and fingers are common and may be hard to see. Disposable gloves provide a barrier. They protect:

- You from the person's pathogens
- The person from microbes on your hands

Wear gloves when contact with blood, body fluids (including secretions and excretions), mucous membranes, or non-intact skin is likely. Contact may be directly with blood or body fluids. Or contact may be with contaminated items or surfaces.

Wearing gloves is the most common measure for Standard Precautions and Transmission-Based Precautions. See Box 15-4 for guidelines to follow when using gloves.

See *Promoting Safety and Comfort: Gloves.*

BOX 15-4 Rules for Glove Use

When to Wear Gloves
- Wear gloves when contact with blood, body fluids (including secretions and excretions), mucous membranes, or non-intact skin is likely. This includes items that are or may be soiled with blood or body fluids.
- Wear gloves as required by Transmission-Based Precautions.

Applying Gloves
- Apply to dry hands. Gloves are easier to put on dry hands.
- Do not tear gloves when putting them on (Fig. 15-4). Carelessness, long fingernails, and rings can tear gloves. Blood and body fluids can enter the glove through a tear. This contaminates your hand.
- Put on gloves last when worn with other PPE.
- Make sure gloves cover your wrists. If you wear a gown, gloves cover the cuffs (Fig. 15-5).

When to Remove or Change Gloves
- Remove damaged gloves at once. Torn, cut, or punctured gloves need to be removed. Practice hand hygiene. Apply a new pair.
- Remove gloves when hand hygiene is needed during care (Chapter 14). Practice hand hygiene. Apply clean gloves if they are needed for the next task. During care, hand hygiene is needed:
  - Before clean or aseptic tasks
  - Before moving from a soiled body site to a clean body site on the same person
  - After tasks involving contact with blood or body fluids
- Remove gloves and practice hand hygiene before touching portable computer keyboards or other equipment that is moved from room to room.
- Remove gloves and practice hand hygiene before contact with another person. Never wear the same pair of gloves for the care of more than 1 person.

Removing Gloves
- *Consider the outside of gloves to be contaminated.* Remove gloves so the inside part is on the outside. The inside is *clean.*
- Discard gloves after use. Gloves are only worn once.
- Practice hand hygiene after removing gloves.

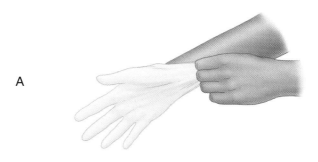

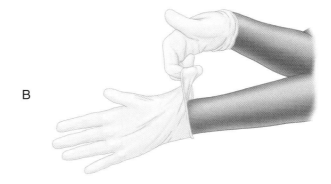

FIGURE 15-4 Applying (donning) gloves. **A,** Grasp the first glove at the wrist area. Carefully pull on the glove. **B,** Grasp the second glove at the wrist area. Carefully pull on the glove. Avoid touching your wrist and forearm with the gloved hand. Do not tear the gloves.

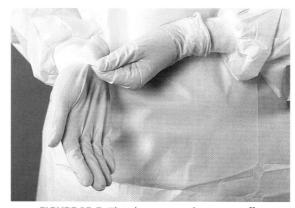

FIGURE 15-5 The gloves cover the gown cuffs.

PROMOTING SAFETY AND COMFORT

Gloves

Safety

Some gloves are made of latex (a rubber product). Latex allergies can cause skin rashes. Difficulty breathing and shock are more serious problems. Report skin rashes, breathing problems, or symptoms of shock (Chapter 43) to the nurse at once.

You may have a latex allergy. Some patients and residents are allergic to latex. This is noted on the care plan and your assignment sheet. Latex-free gloves are worn for latex allergies.

Comfort

Gloves are needed when contact with blood, body fluids, mucous membranes, or non-intact skin is likely. Gloves are not needed when such contact is not likely. Back massages and brushing and combing hair are examples if the skin is intact. To reduce exposure to latex, wear gloves only when needed.

Donning and Removing PPE

The PPE worn depends on the task to be done or the type of Transmission-Based Precautions needed. Non-sterile gloves are the most common PPE used. See Figure 15-4 for how to apply gloves. Any time a gown is worn, gloves are also needed. Gloves cover the gown cuffs (see Fig. 15-5).

According to the CDC, PPE may safely be donned (put on) using more than 1 method. You need training and practice using your agency's equipment and procedures.

Practice hand hygiene before donning PPE. The CDC lists the following order for donning as an example. See Figure 15-6.

1 Gown
2 Mask or respirator
3 Eyewear (goggles or face shield)
4 Gloves

PPE should not be adjusted while giving care. For example, do not retie a gown or adjust a mask or respirator. Be sure PPE is applied correctly before giving care.

PPE is removed at the doorway before leaving the person's room. If a respirator is worn, it is removed after leaving the person's room and closing the door. Sometimes goggles or a face shield is also removed at this time after hand hygiene. Follow your agency's procedures.

PPE is removed slowly and carefully to avoid contaminating your body and uniform. More than 1 method may be used to safely remove PPE. The CDC gives 2 examples.

See Figure 15-7, *A* for Method 1:

1 Gloves
2 Eyewear (goggles or face shield)
3 Gown
4 Mask or respirator

See Figure 15-7, *B* (p. 184) for Method 2:

1 Gown and gloves
2 Eyewear (goggles or face shield)
3 Mask or respirator

Practice hand hygiene after removing PPE. Practice hand hygiene between steps if your hands become contaminated. Then practice hand hygiene again after removing all PPE.

See *Promoting Safety and Comfort: Donning and Removing PPE.*

See procedure: *Donning and Removing Personal Protective Equipment*, p. 185.

PROMOTING SAFETY AND COMFORT

Donning and Removing PPE

Safety

Some severe and deadly infections require additional PPE—full face shield, helmet, or headpiece; coveralls with socks or special gowns; double gloving; boot or shoe covers; and aprons. Special training is needed to care for such patients and for donning and removing the PPE.

Some states and agencies have different procedures for donning or removing PPE. Follow your state's procedures for your state competency exam. Follow your agency's procedures when working.

SEQUENCE FOR PUTTING ON PERSONAL PROTECTIVE EQUIPMENT (PPE)

The type of PPE used will vary based on the level of precautions required, such as standard and contact, droplet or airborne infection isolation precautions. The procedure for putting on and removing PPE should be tailored to the specific type of PPE.

1. GOWN

- Fully cover torso from neck to knees, arms to end of wrists, and wrap around the back
- Fasten in back of neck and waist

2. MASK OR RESPIRATOR

- Secure ties or elastic bands at middle of head and neck
- Fit flexible band to nose bridge
- Fit snug to face and below chin
- Fit-check respirator

3. GOGGLES OR FACE SHIELD

- Place over face and eyes and adjust to fit

4. GLOVES

- Extend to cover wrist of isolation gown

USE SAFE WORK PRACTICES TO PROTECT YOURSELF AND LIMIT THE SPREAD OF CONTAMINATION

- Keep hands away from face
- Limit surfaces touched
- Change gloves when torn or heavily contaminated
- Perform hand hygiene

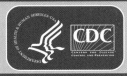

FIGURE 15-6 Donning PPE. (From Centers for Disease Control and Prevention, Department of Health and Human Services.)

HOW TO SAFELY REMOVE PERSONAL PROTECTIVE EQUIPMENT (PPE) EXAMPLE 1

There are a variety of ways to safely remove PPE without contaminating your clothing, skin, or mucous membranes with potentially infectious materials. Here is one example. **Remove all PPE before exiting the patient room** except a respirator, if worn. Remove the respirator **after** leaving the patient room and closing the door. Remove PPE in the following sequence:

A

1. GLOVES
- Outside of gloves are contaminated!
- If your hands get contaminated during glove removal, immediately wash your hands or use an alcohol-based hand sanitizer
- Using a gloved hand, grasp the palm area of the other gloved hand and peel off first glove
- Hold removed glove in gloved hand
- Slide fingers of ungloved hand under remaining glove at wrist and peel off second glove over first glove
- Discard gloves in a waste container

2. GOGGLES OR FACE SHIELD
- Outside of goggles or face shield are contaminated!
- If your hands get contaminated during goggle or face shield removal, immediately wash your hands or use an alcohol-based hand sanitizer
- Remove goggles or face shield from the back by lifting head band or ear pieces
- If the item is reusable, place in designated receptacle for reprocessing. Otherwise, discard in a waste container

3. GOWN
- Gown front and sleeves are contaminated!
- If your hands get contaminated during gown removal, immediately wash your hands or use an alcohol-based hand sanitizer
- Unfasten gown ties, taking care that sleeves don't contact your body when reaching for ties
- Pull gown away from neck and shoulders, touching inside of gown only
- Turn gown inside out
- Fold or roll into a bundle and discard in a waste container

4. MASK OR RESPIRATOR
- Front of mask/respirator is contaminated — DO NOT TOUCH!
- If your hands get contaminated during mask/respirator removal, immediately wash your hands or use an alcohol-based hand sanitizer
- Grasp bottom ties or elastics of the mask/respirator, then the ones at the top, and remove without touching the front
- Discard in a waste container

5. WASH HANDS OR USE AN ALCOHOL-BASED HAND SANITIZER IMMEDIATELY AFTER REMOVING ALL PPE

OR

PERFORM HAND HYGIENE BETWEEN STEPS IF HANDS BECOME CONTAMINATED AND IMMEDIATELY AFTER REMOVING ALL PPE

CDC

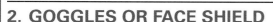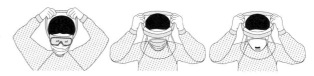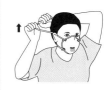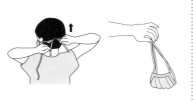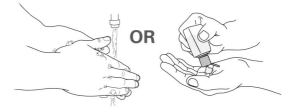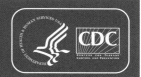

FIGURE 15-7 A, Removing PPE: Method 1.

Continued

HOW TO SAFELY REMOVE PERSONAL PROTECTIVE EQUIPMENT (PPE) EXAMPLE 2

Here is another way to safely remove PPE without contaminating your clothing, skin, or mucous membranes with potentially infectious materials. **Remove all PPE before exiting the patient room** except a respirator, if worn. Remove the respirator **after** leaving the patient room and closing the door. Remove PPE in the following sequence:

1. GOWN AND GLOVES

- Gown front and sleeves and the outside of gloves are contaminated!
- If your hands get contaminated during gown or glove removal, immediately wash your hands or use an alcohol-based hand sanitizer
- Grasp the gown in the front and pull away from your body so that the ties break, touching outside of gown only with gloved hands
- While removing the gown, fold or roll the gown inside-out into a bundle
- As you are removing the gown, peel off your gloves at the same time, only touching the inside of the gloves and gown with your bare hands. Place the gown and gloves into a waste container

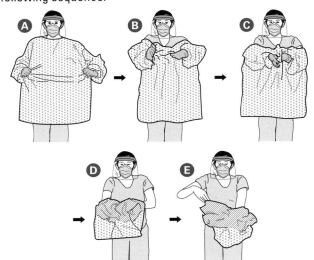

2. GOGGLES OR FACE SHIELD

- Outside of goggles or face shield are contaminated!
- If your hands get contaminated during goggle or face shield removal, immediately wash your hands or use an alcohol-based hand sanitizer
- Remove goggles or face shield from the back by lifting head band and without touching the front of the goggles or face shield
- If the item is reusable, place in designated receptacle for reprocessing. Otherwise, discard in a waste container

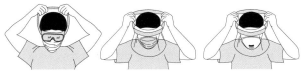

3. MASK OR RESPIRATOR

- Front of mask/respirator is contaminated — DO NOT TOUCH!
- If your hands get contaminated during mask/respirator removal, immediately wash your hands or use an alcohol-based hand sanitizer
- Grasp bottom ties or elastics of the mask/respirator, then the ones at the top, and remove without touching the front
- Discard in a waste container

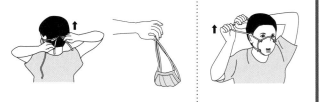

4. WASH HANDS OR USE AN ALCOHOL-BASED HAND SANITIZER IMMEDIATELY AFTER REMOVING ALL PPE

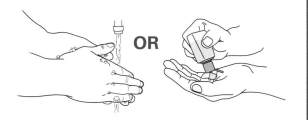

PERFORM HAND HYGIENE BETWEEN STEPS IF HANDS BECOME CONTAMINATED AND IMMEDIATELY AFTER REMOVING ALL PPE

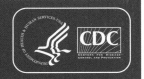

CS250672-E

FIGURE 15-7, cont'd B, Removing PPE: Method 2. (From Centers for Disease Control and Prevention, Department of Health and Human Services.)

Donning and Removing Personal Protective Equipment

Procedure

1 Follow *Delegation Guidelines: Transmission-Based Precautions,* p. 179. See *Promoting Safety and Comfort:*
   a *Transmission-Based Precautions,* p. 179
   b *Goggles and Face Shields,* p. 180
   c *Gloves,* p. 181
   d *Donning and Removing PPE,* p. 182
2 Remove your watch and all jewelry.
3 Roll up uniform sleeves.
4 Practice hand hygiene.
5 Put on a gown (see Fig. 15-6).
   a Hold a clean gown out in front of you.
   b Unfold the gown. Face the back (opening) of the gown. Do not shake it.
   c Put your hands and arms through the sleeves.
   d Make sure the gown covers you from your neck to your knees. It must cover your arms to the end of your wrists.
   e Tie the strings at the back of the neck.
   f Over-lap the back of the gown. Make sure it covers your uniform. The gown should be snug, not loose.
   g Tie the waist strings. Tie them at the back or the side. Do not tie them in front.
6 Put on a mask or respirator (see Fig. 15-6 and Fig. 15-8, p. 186).
   a Pick up a mask by its upper ties. Do not touch the part that will cover your face.
   b Place the mask over your nose and mouth (Fig. 15-8, A).
   c Place the upper strings above your ears. Tie them at the back in the middle of your head (Fig. 15-8, B).
   d Tie the lower strings at the back of your neck (Fig. 15-8, C). The lower part of the mask is under your chin.
   e Pinch the metal band around your nose. The top of the mask must be snug over your nose. If you wear eyeglasses, the mask must be snug under the bottom of the eyeglasses.
   f Make sure the mask is snug over your face and under your chin.
7 Put on goggles or a face shield (if needed and if not part of the mask) (see Fig. 15-6).
   a Place the device over your face and eyes.
   b Adjust the device to fit.
8 Put on gloves (see Fig. 15-4). Make sure the gloves cover the wrists of the gown (see Fig. 15-5).
9 Provide care.
10 Remove and discard the PPE. Practice hand hygiene between each step if your hands become contaminated.
   a *Method 1: Remove gloves, goggles or face shield, gown, mask or respirator* (see Fig. 15-7, A).
      1) Remove and discard the gloves (Fig. 15-9, p. 186).
         i Make sure that glove touches only glove.
         ii Grasp a glove at the palm (Fig. 15-9, A). Grasp it on the outside.
         iii Pull the glove down over your hand so it is inside-out (Fig. 15-9, B).
         iv Hold the removed glove with your other gloved hand.
         v Reach inside the other glove. Use the first 2 fingers of the ungloved hand (Fig. 15-9, C).
         vi Pull the glove down (inside-out) over your hand and the other glove (Fig. 15-9, D).
         vii Discard the gloves.

      2) Remove and discard the goggles or face shield if worn.
         i Lift the headband or ear-pieces from the back. Do not touch the front of the device.
         ii Discard the device. If re-usable, follow agency procedures.
      3) Remove and discard the gown. Do not touch the outside of the gown.
         i Untie the neck and the waist strings.
         ii Pull the gown down and away from your neck and shoulders. Only touch the inside of the gown.
         iii Turn the gown inside-out as it is removed. Hold it at the inside shoulder seams and bring your hands together.
         iv Fold or roll up the gown away from you. Keep it inside-out. Do not let the gown touch the floor.
         v Discard the gown.
      4) Remove and discard the mask if worn. (NOTE: Remove a respirator after leaving the room and closing the door.)
         i Untie the lower strings of the mask.
         ii Untie the top strings.
         iii Hold the top strings. Remove the mask without touching the front of the mask.
         iv Discard the mask.
   b *Method 2: Remove gown and gloves, goggles or face shield, mask or respirator* (see Fig. 15-7, B).
      1) Remove and discard the gown and gloves.
         i Grasp the gown in front with your gloved hands. Pull away from your body so the ties break. Only touch the outside of the gown.
         ii Fold or roll the gown inside-out into a bundle while removing the gown. Keep it inside-out. Do not let the gown touch the floor.
         iii Peel off your gloves as you remove the gown. Only touch the inside of the gloves and gown with your bare hands.
         iv Discard the gown and gloves.
      2) Remove and discard the goggles or face shield.
         i Lift the headband or ear-pieces from the back. Do not touch the front of the device.
         ii Discard the device. If re-usable, follow agency procedures.
      3) Remove and discard the mask if worn. (NOTE: Remove a respirator after leaving the room and closing the door.)
         i Untie the lower strings of the mask.
         ii Untie the top strings.
         iii Hold the top strings. Remove the mask without touching the front of the mask.
         iv Discard the mask.
11 Practice hand hygiene after removing all PPE.

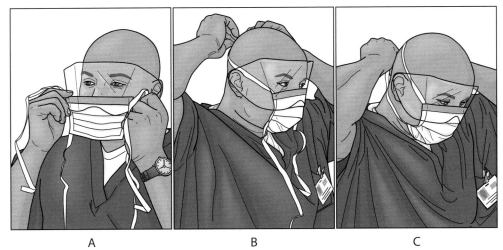

FIGURE 15-8 Donning a mask. (NOTE: The mask has a face shield.) **A,** The mask covers the nose and mouth. **B,** Upper strings are tied at the back of the head. **C,** Lower strings are tied at the back of the neck.

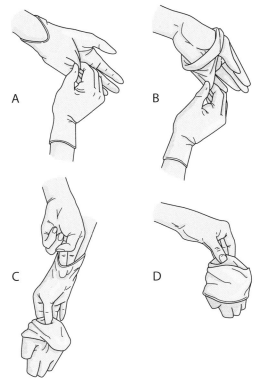

FIGURE 15-9 Removing gloves. **A,** Grasp the glove at the palm. **B,** Pull the glove down over the hand. The glove is inside-out. **C,** Insert the fingers of the ungloved hand inside the other glove. **D,** Pull the glove down and over the other hand and glove. The glove is inside-out.

USED LAUNDRY

Laundry commonly includes bed linens, towels and wash-cloths, and personal clothing or patient gowns. Standard Precautions are used to prevent the transmission of microbes when handling used laundry. Wear gloves if contact with blood or body fluids is likely. Hold laundry away from your body and uniform. Do not shake items, place them on the floor, or place them on a clean item or surface. Place used laundry in leak-proof containers or bags where it was used.

Follow agency policies and procedures for collecting and disposing of used laundry in an isolation room. A second bag (double-bagging) is used only if the outside of the first bag is visibly soiled or if the contents have leaked through and the bag is wet.

USED SUPPLIES AND EQUIPMENT

See Chapter 14 for the measures used to clean and disinfect or sterilize re-usable supplies and equipment. Follow agency policies and procedures to:
- Handle, contain, and transport supplies and equipment contaminated with blood or body fluids.
- Remove re-usable items from an isolation room. To bag items:
  - Have a co-worker stand outside the door with an open, leak-proof, clean plastic bag.
  - Place the item inside the bag without contaminating the outside of the bag.
  - Have your co-worker seal the bag and take the item to the appropriate area for cleaning and disinfection.

COLLECTING SPECIMENS

Blood and body fluids often require laboratory testing (Chapter 34). Wear PPE as required for the task to collect the specimen. Place the specimen container in a plastic specimen bag labeled with the *BIOHAZARD* symbol (Chapter 14) for transport to the laboratory. Do not let the specimen container touch the outside of the bag.

Follow agency policies and procedures to collect and transport specimens for persons needing Transmission-Based Precautions. The following method is common.
- Leave the biohazard bag outside the room.
- Place the specimen container on a paper towel inside the room.
- Collect the specimen (Chapter 34). Do not contaminate the outside of the container. Secure the lid.
- Remove and discard PPE. Practice hand hygiene.
- Use a paper towel to pick up the container. Place the specimen in the biohazard bag. Do not contaminate the outside of the bag.
- Discard the paper towel.
- Practice hand hygiene.

TRANSPORTING PERSONS

To *transport* means *to move from 1 place to another*. Patients and residents often need to go to other areas for treatments or tests that cannot be done in the person's room. Wheelchairs and stretchers (Chapter 18) are commonly used to move the person. Follow agency policies and procedures for disinfecting equipment used for transport.

Persons needing Transmission-Based Precautions usually do not leave their rooms unless it is necessary. If transport is needed, follow agency procedures. A safe transport protects others from the infection.
- Staff in the receiving area need to know that the person requires isolation precautions. They need to know the type of precaution and the PPE needed.
- The person wears a clean gown or pajamas.
- Barriers are used as needed (see Box 15-2). For example:
  - Tissues and a leak-proof bag are provided for respiratory secretions. Used tissues are placed in the bag.
  - Skin lesions or infected or draining areas are covered.
  - The person wears a mask as required.
- Staff do not wear contaminated PPE during the transport.
- Only the person and transport staff enter an elevator when 1 is needed. This prevents others from exposure to infection.
- Staff don clean PPE to handle the person at the transport destination.
- Transport equipment is disinfected after use.

FOCUS ON P R I D E

The Person, Family, and Yourself

P ersonal and Professional Responsibility

Standard Precautions and Transmission-Based Precautions are important for the safety of the person, others, and you. Other chapters will remind you to follow these precautions. Be sure you understand this information and the rules of hand hygiene in Chapter 14 well. Ask your instructor if you have questions. At work, ask the nurse if you have questions about needed PPE.

R ights and Respect

Caring for persons who need Transmission-Based Precautions can be a challenge. Extra time and effort are needed to apply and remove PPE and clean equipment used in the room. The person must not feel like a burden. You must:
- Watch your verbal and nonverbal communication (Chapter 6).
- Avoid complaining.
- Practice good teamwork and time management.
- Tell the nurse if you are feeling overwhelmed.

I ndependence and Social Interaction

The person on Transmission-Based Precautions may feel isolated and lonely. To help the person:
- Provide newspapers, magazines, books, or other reading matter.
- Provide hobby materials if possible.
- Suggest that the person call family and friends.
- Visit and interact pleasantly with the person.

Remember, items brought into the person's room become contaminated. Disinfect or discard the items according to agency policy.

D elegation and Teamwork

Good teamwork is helpful when patients or residents need Transmission-Based Precautions. You can tie a gown for a co-worker. You can answer call lights while co-workers provide care in an isolation room. And you can bring any needed supplies to the doorway of the room.

Communicate with co-workers when you will be in a room for a long period of time. Politely ask if they can answer call lights for you. Thank them for their help.

E thics and Laws

When a person has an infectious disease, remember that the pathogen is undesirable, not the person. Show kindness and respect. Treat the person with dignity.

FOCUS ON PRIDE: Application

Explain the emotional and social effects of Transmission-Based Precautions. How can you help meet these needs?

REVIEW QUESTIONS

Circle the BEST answer.

1 Which statement about Standard Precautions is *true*?
   a They are used for all persons.
   b The 3 types are contact, droplet, and airborne.
   c They are used only in hospitals.
   d They require a doctor's order.

2 Transmission-Based Precautions are used for
   a All persons
   b Persons who have or may have certain infections
   c Persons recovering from surgery
   d Staff who are at risk for infection

3 What PPE is needed to move and position a patient requiring Contact Precautions?
   a A gown and gloves
   b A gown, mask, and gloves
   c A gown, mask, goggles, and gloves
   d None

4 A patient requires Droplet Precautions. There is 1 mask left outside the room. You should
   a Not use the mask
   b Use the mask and return it for re-use
   c Use the mask and re-stock the masks
   d Wait until a co-worker re-stocks the masks to give care

5 A resident requires Transmission-Based Precautions. You can
   a Use linens that fall on the floor
   b Touch your hair and face in the person's room
   c Use a leak-proof plastic bag to remove a meal tray from the room
   d Keep PPE on when leaving the room to get supplies

6 To remove a gown safely
   a Roll the gown so the outside of the gown is on the outside of the roll
   b Touch the inside with gloved hands
   c Touch the ties with gloved hands
   d Do not touch the front and sleeves with ungloved hands

7 A mask
   a Is removed before other PPE is removed
   b Is contaminated when moist
   c Is the same as a respirator
   d Should fit loosely for breathing

8 To use PPE correctly
   a Never change gloves in the person's room
   b Tie a gown's waist strings in front
   c Don gloves first when applying PPE
   d Apply new PPE for each person

9 Which task requires gloves?
   a Measuring blood pressure
   b Giving a back massage
   c Providing denture care
   d Moving the person up in bed

10 A glove tears while giving care. You should
   a Continue giving care with the glove
   b Apply a second glove over the torn glove
   c Remove gloves and finish the task without gloves
   d Remove gloves, practice hand hygiene, and apply new gloves

11 You assist a person with wiping after having a bowel movement. Then you provide oral care. Which is *correct*?
   a Hand hygiene and clean gloves are needed for oral care.
   b Gloves are not needed for either task.
   c You can wear the same pair of gloves for both tasks.
   d You can change gloves without practicing hand hygiene.

12 Which can contaminate your skin when removing gloves?
   a You touch the inner part of a glove with an ungloved finger.
   b You touch the outer part of a glove with an ungloved hand.
   c You touch the outer part of a glove with a gloved hand.
   d You roll a glove inside-out as it is removed.

13 Goggles or a face shield is worn
   a For Contact Precautions
   b When splashing of body fluids may occur
   c If you have an eye infection
   d When assisting with sterile procedures

14 Which shows you understand how to handle laundry safely?
   a You shake a blanket to remove crumbs from it.
   b You hold linens against your uniform.
   c You place used linens on the floor.
   d You wear gloves to handle a sheet soiled with urine.

15 A person on Droplet Precautions needs a specimen collected. You need to
   a Avoid contaminating the outside of the biohazard bag
   b Wear PPE to deliver the specimen to the laboratory for testing
   c Transport the person to the laboratory to collect the specimen
   d Have the person wear a mask while collecting the specimen

Answers to Chapter 15 questions are on p. 587.

FOCUS ON **PRACTICE**

Problem Solving

You plan to do the following for 1 patient. Identify when to practice hand hygiene and apply gloves. Do you need to change gloves before any tasks?

- Help the person move from the bed to a chair.
- Empty urine from the person's urinal (a container that holds urine).
- Brush and floss the person's teeth.

CHAPTER 16

Body Mechanics

OBJECTIVES

- Define the key terms and key abbreviations in this chapter.
- Explain the purpose and rules of body mechanics.
- Identify the risk factors for work-related injuries.
- Identify the activities at high risk for work-related injuries, including back injuries.

- Identify the causes, signs, and symptoms of back injuries.
- Explain how to prevent work-related injuries.
- Position persons in the basic bed positions and in a chair.
- Explain how to promote PRIDE in the person, the family, and yourself.

KEY TERMS

base of support The area on which an object rests
body alignment The way the head, trunk, arms, and legs align with one another; posture
body mechanics Using the body in an efficient and careful way
dorsal recumbent position The back-lying or supine position
ergonomics The science of designing a job to fit the worker; *ergo* means *work, nomos* means *law*
Fowler's position A semi-sitting position; the head of the bed is raised between 45 and 60 degrees
high-Fowler's position A variation of Fowler's position; the head of the bed is raised 60 to 90 degrees
lateral position The person lies on 1 side or the other; side-lying position

left semi-prone position The person lies on the left side of the abdomen; the upper leg (right leg) is sharply flexed (bent) so it is not on the lower leg (left leg); the lower arm (left arm) is behind the person
musculo-skeletal disorders (MSDs) Injuries and disorders of the muscles, tendons, ligaments, joints, and cartilage
posture See "body alignment"
prone position The person lies on the abdomen with the head turned to 1 side
semi-Fowler's position A variation of Fowler's position; the head of the bed is raised 30 degrees
side-lying position See "lateral position"
supine position The back-lying or dorsal recumbent position

KEY ABBREVIATIONS

MSD Musculo-skeletal disorder

OSHA Occupational Safety and Health Administration

Body mechanics *means using the body in an efficient and careful way.* It involves good posture, balance, and using your strongest and largest muscles for work. Fatigue and injury can result from the incorrect use and positioning of the body during activity or rest.

The principles of body mechanics, safe handling, and proper positioning help protect you and the person from injury.

PRINCIPLES OF BODY MECHANICS

Body alignment (posture) is the way the head, trunk, arms, and legs align with one another. (The *trunk [torso]* is the chest and abdomen.) Good alignment lets the body move and function with strength and efficiency. Standing, sitting, and lying down require good alignment.

Base of support is the area on which an object rests. A good base of support is needed for balance (Fig. 16-1, p. 190).

When standing, your feet are your base of support. Stand with your feet apart for a wider base of support and more balance.

Your strongest and largest muscles are in the shoulders, upper arms, hips, and thighs. Use these muscles to handle and move persons and heavy objects. Otherwise, you place strain and exertion on the smaller and weaker muscles. This causes fatigue and injury. *Back injuries are a major risk.* For good body mechanics:

- Bend your knees and squat to lift a heavy object (Fig. 16-2). Do not bend from your waist. Bending from the waist places strain on small back muscles.
- Hold items close to your body and base of support (see Fig. 16-2). This involves upper arm and shoulder muscles. Holding objects away from the body places strain on small muscles in the lower arms.

All activities require good body mechanics. Follow the rules in Box 16-1.

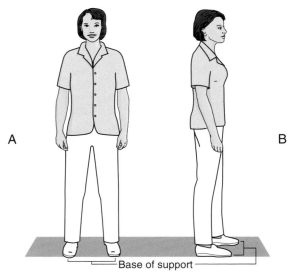

FIGURE 16-1 **A,** Anterior (front) view of an adult in good body alignment. The feet are apart for a wide base of support. **B,** Lateral (side) view of an adult with good posture and alignment.

BOX 16-1 Rules of Body Mechanics

- Keep your body in good alignment with a wide base of support. Your feet are at least 12 inches apart or shoulder-width apart.
- Use an upright working posture. Bend your legs. Do not bend your back.
- Use the stronger and larger muscles in your shoulders, upper arms, thighs, and hips.
- Keep objects close to your body to lift, move, or carry them (see Fig. 16-2).
- Avoid bending and reaching. Raise the bed and over-bed table to waist level or to a comfortable working height.
- Face your work area. This prevents twisting.
- Push, slide, or pull heavy objects when you can rather than lifting them. Pushing is easier than pulling.
- Widen your base of support to push or pull. Move your front leg forward when pushing. Move your rear leg back when pulling (Fig. 16-3).
- Use both hands and arms to lift, move, or carry objects.
- Turn your whole body to change direction. Do not twist.
- Work with smooth and even movements. Avoid sudden or jerky motions.
- Do not lean over a person to give care.
- *Get help from a co-worker to move persons or heavy objects. Do not lift or move them by yourself.*
- Bend your hips and knees to lift heavy objects from the floor (see Fig. 16-2). Straighten your back as the object reaches thigh level. Your leg and thigh muscles work to raise the item off the floor and to waist level.
- Do not lift objects higher than chest level. Do not lift above your shoulders. Use a step stool or ladder to reach an object higher than chest level.

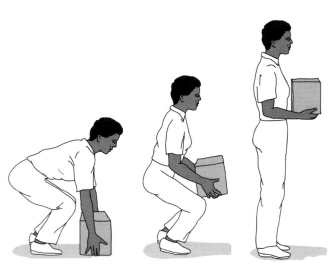

FIGURE 16-2 Picking up a box using good body mechanics.

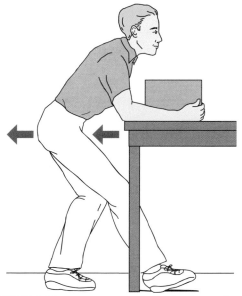

FIGURE 16-3 Move your rear leg back when pulling.

WORK-RELATED INJURIES

Musculo-skeletal disorders (MSDs) are injuries and disorders of the muscles, tendons, ligaments, joints, and cartilage. They can be caused or made worse by the work setting. The lower back and shoulders are often affected. Injuries can involve the nervous system.

Sprains and strains are common.

- *Sprain*—ligaments are stretched or torn. (*Ligaments* are strong bands of connective tissue that connect bones.) Symptoms include pain, bruising, swelling, and not being able to use the joint.
- *Strain*—muscles or tendons are stretched or torn. (*Tendons* are strong bands of connective tissue that connect muscles to bones.) Symptoms include pain, muscle spasms, swelling, cramping, and problems moving.

MSDs can develop slowly over weeks, months, and years. Or they can occur from 1 event. Early signs and symptoms include pain, difficulty moving, or swelling. Numbness, tingling, stiff joints, and muscle weakness can occur. Disabilities can result. Time off work is often needed.

MSD Risk Factors

The Occupational Safety and Health Administration (OSHA) has identified MSD risk factors. An MSD is more likely if risk factors are combined. For example, a task involves both force and repeating actions.

- *Force*—the amount of physical effort needed for a task. Lifting or transferring heavy persons, preventing falls, and sudden motions are examples.
- *Repeating action*—doing the same motion or series of motions often or continually. Re-positioning persons and transfers to and from beds, chairs, and commodes without adequate rest breaks are examples.
- *Awkward postures*—assuming positions that place stress on the body. Examples are reaching above shoulder height, kneeling, squatting, leaning over a bed, bending, or twisting the torso while lifting.
- *Heavy lifting*—manually lifting people who cannot move themselves.

According to the U.S. Department of Labor, nursing assistants are at great risk. The tasks listed in Box 16-2 are high risk for MSDs.

Back Injuries. Back injuries are major threats. Back injuries can occur from repeated activities or from 1 event. Signs and symptoms include:

- Pain when trying to assume a normal posture
- Decreased mobility
- Pain when standing or rising from a seated position

Follow the rules and safety measures in this chapter to prevent back injuries. Be very careful during tasks associated with back injuries.

See *Promoting Safety and Comfort: Back Injuries.*

BOX 16-2 Musculo-Skeletal Disorders—Risk Factors for Nursing Assistants

- Transfers—to and from beds, chairs, wheelchairs, toilets, stretchers, and bathtubs
- Trying to stop a person from falling
- Picking up a person from the floor to the bed
- Lifting alone
- Lifting persons who are confused or uncooperative
- Lifting persons who cannot support their own weight
- Lifting heavy persons
- Weighing a person
- Moving a person up in bed
- Re-positioning a person in a bed or in a chair
- Changing an incontinence product
- Making beds
- Dressing and undressing a person
- Feeding a person in bed
- Giving a bed bath
- Applying anti-embolism stockings
- Prolonged holding of a body part for care measures—arm, leg, abdomen, skin fold

---

PROMOTING SAFETY AND COMFORT

Back Injuries

Safety

The activities listed in Box 16-2 are related to back injuries. Use good body mechanics. Get help and avoid lifting and bending the back when possible. Protect yourself from injury.

Preventing MSDs

A safe work setting is free of hazards that cause or may cause death or serious physical harm to staff. The employer must make reasonable attempts to prevent or reduce hazards.

Ergonomics is the science of designing a job to fit the worker. (Ergo *means* work. Nomos *means* law.) It involves changing the task, work station, equipment, and tools to help reduce stress on the worker's body. The goal is to eliminate a serious work-related MSD.

Your employer has a role in preventing MSDs. So do you. Moving and transfer procedures are major risk factors for injury. Use the guidelines in Box 16-3 (p. 192) to prevent work-related injuries during moving and transfer procedures.

Always report a work-related injury as soon as possible. Early attention can prevent the problem from becoming worse. Also, injuries are often less serious and less costly to treat with early attention.

BOX 16-3 Preventing Work-Related Injuries

General Guidelines

- Wear shoes with good traction. Avoid shoes with worn-down soles or sides. Good traction helps prevent slips or falls.
- Use assist equipment and devices (Chapters 17 and 18) when possible instead of lifting and moving the person manually. Follow the care plan.
- Get help from other staff. The nurse and care plan tell you the number of staff needed for a task.
- Plan and prepare for the task. For example, know what equipment is needed, where to place chairs or wheelchairs, and what side of the bed to work on.
- Schedule harder tasks early in your shift.
- Balance lighter and harder tasks. Plan to complete a lighter task after a harder one.
- Lock (brake) bed wheels and wheelchair or stretcher wheels.
- Tell the person how to help. Give clear, simple instructions. Give the person time to respond.
- Do not hold or grab the person under the underarms.
- Do not let the person hold or grasp you around your neck.

Manual Lifting

- *Minimize or eliminate manual lifting when possible.*
- Stand with good posture. Keep your back straight.
- Bend your legs, not your back.
- Use the large muscles in your legs to do the work.
- Face the person.
- Do not twist or turn. Pick up your feet. Pivot your whole body in the direction of the move.
- Keep what you are moving close to you.
- Move the person toward you, not away from you.
- Use a wide, balanced base of support. Stand with 1 foot slightly ahead of the other.
- Use smooth, even movements. Avoid jerking movements.
- Lift on the "count of 3" when lifting with others. Everyone lifts at the same time.

Moving the Person in Bed (Chapter 17)

- Adjust the bed to a safe and comfortable working height.
- Lower the bed rail.
- Work on the side where the person will be closest to you.
- Place equipment or other items close to you at waist level or at a comfortable working height.
- Use friction-reducing devices (Chapters 17 and 18).

Transfer/Gait Belts (Chapter 12)

- Keep the person as close to you as possible.
- Avoid bending your back, reaching, or twisting for these and other nursing tasks:
  - Applying or removing a transfer/gait belt
  - Lowering the person to the chair, bed, toilet, or floor
  - Helping the person walk
- Use a gentle rocking motion to help the person stand. The rocking motion gives strength and force as you help the person stand.

Stand and Pivot Transfers (Chapter 18)

- Use assist devices as directed. Follow the care plan.
- Use a transfer belt as directed. The nurse may have you use a transfer belt with handles. See Chapter 12.
- Plan the transfer so the person's strong side moves first.
- Lower the bed so the person can place the feet on the floor.

Stand and Pivot Transfers (Chapter 18)—cont'd

- Get the person close to the edge of the bed or the chair.
- Block the person's weak leg with your legs or knees. If the position is awkward:
  - Use a transfer belt with handles.
  - Straddle your legs around the person's weak leg.
- Keep your feet at least shoulder-width apart.
- Bend your legs. Do not bend your back.
- Have the person lean forward slightly. Use a gentle rocking motion to help the person stand. The rocking motion gives strength and force as you help the person stand.
- Pivot (turn) with your feet. Do not twist.

Lateral Transfers (Chapter 18)

- Position surfaces close to each other. (A lateral transfer involves 2 horizontal surfaces. For example, a person is moved from a bed to a stretcher.)
- Adjust surfaces to about waist height or to a comfortable working height. Do 1 of the following as directed by the nurse and care plan.
  - Adjust the surfaces to the same level.
  - Adjust the receiving surface so it is slightly lower (about $\frac{1}{2}$ inch) than the surface the person is on. This allows the use of gravity. For example, the stretcher surface (receiving surface) is slightly lower than the bed for a bed to stretcher transfer.
- Have staff on both sides—staff on the receiving side and staff at the side of the surface the person is on.
- Lower bed rails and stretcher side rails.
- Use friction-reducing devices. Get a good hand-hold. Roll up the sides of the device. Or use a device with handles.
- Kneel on the bed or stretcher if needed to prevent extended reaches and bending your back.
- Move the person on the "count of 3." Use a smooth, push-pull motion. Do not reach across the person.

Transporting the Person and Equipment

- Push, do not pull.
- Keep the load close to your body.
- Use an upright posture.
- Push with your whole body, not just your arms.
- Move down the center of the hallway. This helps avoid collisions.
- Watch out for door handles and high thresholds on floors. These can cause abrupt stops.

Transferring the Person From the Floor

- Avoid manual lifting when possible. Assist as the nurse directs. See Chapter 12.
- See "Manual Lifting" if a manual lift is required and there are no injuries or minor injuries.
  - Roll the person onto the side.
  - Position an assist device. A blanket or drawsheet are examples. Avoid reaching across the person.
  - Have at least 2 staff members on each side. The larger the person, the more staff are needed.
  - Bend your knees, not your back. Do not twist.
  - For the lift:
    - Kneel on 1 knee.
    - Grasp the drawsheet, blanket, or other device.
    - Lift smoothly with your legs as you stand. Stand together on the "count of 3." Do not bend your back.

Modified from Cal/OSHA: *A back injury prevention guide for health care providers*, Sacramento, Calif., 1997, Author; and Occupational Safety and Health Administration: *Guidelines for nursing homes: ergonomics for the prevention of musculoskeletal disorders*, Washington, DC, revised March 2009, Author.

Safe Handling Programs. *Proper body mechanics alone do not prevent injury.* Health care agencies must plan other ways to protect workers. *Safe handling programs* help reduce the risk of injury to staff and patients or residents from transferring, lifting, re-positioning, and other moving activities.

A safe handling program begins at the management level. OSHA identifies the following elements of an effective program.

- Management is committed to implementing a safe handling program. Policies are in place. Management and departments support the program.
- Staff are involved in the process of planning and implementing the program.
- Hazards are identified and addressed with safety measures.
- Transfer and lifting devices are part of the plan. Staff are involved in the selection of patient or resident handling devices.
- Staff have the needed equipment to avoid manual lifting. Assist devices and mechanical lifts are examples (Chapters 17 and 18).
- Care planning includes safe moving and transfer procedures.
- Staff are trained. Training includes hazard awareness, safe use of transfer and lift equipment and other devices, and safe practices for patient or resident handling.
- The program is reviewed and evaluated.
  See *Promoting Safety and Comfort: Safe Handling Programs.*

PROMOTING SAFETY AND COMFORT
Safe Handling Programs

Safety
Transfer and lifting devices do not only benefit staff. Such devices can help protect patients and residents from falls, bruising, and skin tears (Chapter 35).

Comfort
Patients, residents, and their families are more at ease when taught about how transfer and lifting devices can prevent injury. The nurse provides this teaching. You must explain a move or transfer before you perform the procedure. See Chapters 17 and 18.

POSITIONING THE PERSON

The person must be positioned correctly at all times. Regular position changes and good alignment promote comfort and well-being. Breathing is easier. Circulation is promoted. Pressure injuries and contractures are prevented. A *contracture* is the lack of joint mobility caused by the abnormal shortening of a muscle (Chapter 32).

Many patients and residents are able to move and turn when in a bed or a chair. Some need reminding or help to adjust their positions. Others depend entirely on the nursing team for position changes.

Whether in a bed or a chair, the person is re-positioned at least every 2 hours or more often. Follow the nurse's instructions and the care plan. To safely position a person:

- Use good body mechanics.
- Follow the care plan for use of assist devices (Chapters 17 and 18).
- Ask a co-worker to help you if needed.
- Explain the procedure to the person.
- Provide for privacy.
- Be gentle when moving the person.
- Use pillows as directed by the nurse for support and alignment.
- Provide for comfort after positioning. (See the inside of the back cover.)
- Place the call light and other needed items within reach after positioning.
- Complete a safety check before leaving the room. (See the inside of the back cover.)
  See *Focus on Communication: Positioning the Person.*
  See *Delegation Guidelines: Positioning the Person.*
  See *Promoting Safety and Comfort: Positioning the Person,* p. 194.

FOCUS ON **COMMUNICATION**
Positioning the Person

Moving can be painful. Some older persons have painful joints. Pain is common after surgery or an injury. Avoid causing pain when positioning the person. Explain what you will do before and during the procedure. Move the person slowly and gently. Give the person time to tell you if a movement is painful. Make sure the person is comfortable. You can say:

- "Am I hurting you?"
- "Please tell me if I'm moving you too fast."
- "Please tell me if you feel pain or discomfort."
- "Do you need a pillow adjusted?"
- "Are you comfortable?"
- "How can I help make you more comfortable?"

DELEGATION GUIDELINES
Positioning the Person

Many tasks involve positioning and re-positioning. You need this information from the nurse and the care plan.

- Position or positioning limits ordered by the doctor
- How often to turn and re-position the person
- How many staff members need to help you
- What assist devices to use (Chapters 17 and 18)
- What skin care measures to perform (Chapter 22)
- What range-of-motion exercises to perform (Chapter 32)
- Where to place pillows
- What positioning and protective devices are needed and how to use them (Chapters 32 and 36)
- What observations to report and record
- When to report observations
- What patient and resident concerns to report at once

PROMOTING SAFETY AND COMFORT

Positioning the Person

Safety

Pressure injuries are serious threats from lying or sitting too long in 1 place. Wet, soiled, and wrinkled linens are other causes. When you re-position a person, make sure linens are clean, dry, and wrinkle-free. Change or straighten linens as needed. Follow the care plan for prevention measures and protective devices to use. See Chapter 36.

Contractures can develop from staying in 1 position too long (Chapter 32). Re-positioning, exercise, and activity help prevent contractures.

Comfort

Pillows and positioning devices (Chapter 32) support body parts and provide good alignment. This promotes comfort. Place pillows and positioning devices as directed by the nurse and the care plan.

Older persons may have limited range of motion in their necks and other joints. (*Range of motion* is the movement of a joint to the extent possible without causing pain. See Chapter 32.) Some positions may not be comfortable for them. Ask about comfort. Do not leave the person in an uncomfortable position.

Fowler's Positions

Fowler's position is a semi-sitting position. The head of the bed is raised between 45 and 60 degrees (Fig. 16-4). The knees may be slightly elevated. *Variations of Fowler's position include:*
- *Semi-Fowler's position—the head of the bed is raised 30 degrees.* In some agencies, semi-Fowler's position includes raising the knee portion of the bed 15 degrees.
- *High-Fowler's position—the head of the bed is raised 60 to 90 degrees.*
  For good alignment:
- The spine is straight.
- The head is supported with a small pillow.
- The arms are supported with pillows.

The nurse may have you place small pillows under the lower back, thighs, and ankles. Persons with heart and respiratory disorders usually breathe easier in Fowler's position.

See *Focus on Math: Fowler's Positions.*

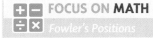

FOCUS ON MATH
Fowler's Positions

When 2 lines meet, an angle is formed. Angles are measured in degrees (°). Degrees range from 0 to 360. With bed positions, you need a basic understanding of angle measurements between 0° and 90°.

To estimate the angle:
1. Use the bed frame and the head of the bed as the 2 lines.
2. Estimate the angle from the bed frame to the head of the bed. See Figure 16-5.

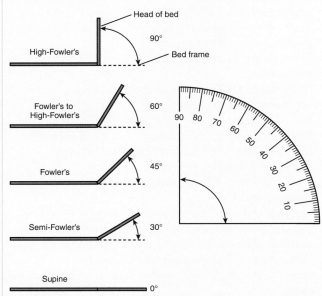

FIGURE 16-5 Measuring bed angles. The angle is measured from the bed frame to the back of the head of the bed. As the head of the bed rises, the angle increases.

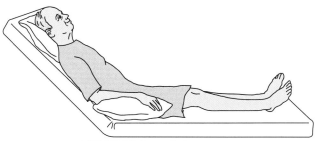

FIGURE 16-4 Fowler's position.

Supine Position

The ***supine position (dorsal recumbent position)*** *is the back-lying position* (Fig. 16-6).

- The bed is flat.
- The head and shoulders are supported on a pillow.
- Arms and hands are at the sides. You can support the arms with regular pillows. Or you can support the hands on small pillows with the palms down.

The nurse may have you place a small pillow under the lower back and thighs. A pillow under the lower legs lifts the heels off of the bed. This prevents the heels from rubbing on the sheets.

Prone Position

In the ***prone position,*** *the person lies on the abdomen with the head turned to 1 side.*

- The bed is flat.
- Small pillows are under the head, abdomen, and lower legs (Fig. 16-7).
- Arms are flexed at the elbows with the hands near the head.

You also can position a person with the feet hanging over the end of the mattress (Fig. 16-8). A pillow is not needed under the feet.

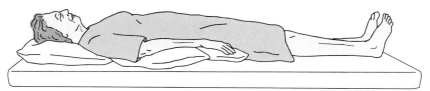

FIGURE 16-6   Supine position.

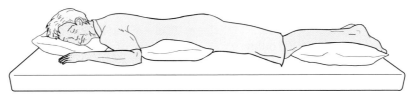

FIGURE 16-7   Prone position.

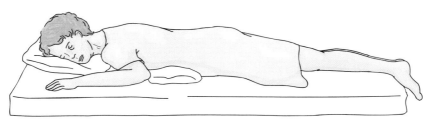

FIGURE 16-8   Prone position with the feet hanging over the edge of the mattress.

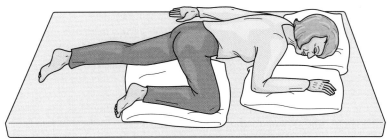

FIGURE 16-9 Left semi-prone position.

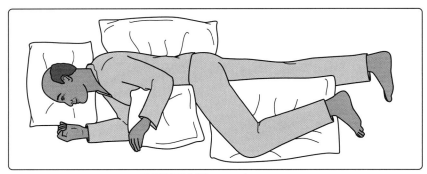

FIGURE 16-10 Lateral position.

Left Semi-Prone Position

In the *left semi-prone position, the person lies on the left side of the abdomen. The upper leg (right leg) is sharply flexed (bent) so it is not on the lower leg (left leg). The lower arm (left arm) is behind the person* (Fig. 16-9). This position may be used for certain procedures involving the bowel (Chapter 27). In this position:

- The bed is flat.
- A pillow is under the person's head and shoulder.
- The upper leg (right leg) is supported with a pillow.
- A pillow is under the upper arm (right arm) and hand (right hand).

Lateral Position

In the *lateral position (side-lying position), the person lies on 1 side or the other* (Fig. 16-10).

- The bed is flat.
- A pillow is under the head and neck.
- The upper (top) leg is flexed (bent) in front of the lower (bottom) leg. The upper (top) leg does not rest on the lower (bottom) leg.
- The upper (top) leg is supported with a pillow. The ankle is supported.
- A pillow is against the person's back. The person rolls back against the pillow so that the back is at a 45-degree angle with the mattress.
- A small pillow is under the upper (top) arm. The hand is supported.

Chair Position

A person in a chair must hold the upper body and head upright. If not, poor alignment results. For good alignment:

- The person's back and buttocks are against the back of the chair.
- Feet are flat on the floor or wheelchair footplates. Never leave feet unsupported.
- Backs of the knees and calves are slightly away from the edge of the seat (Fig. 16-11).

The nurse may have you put a small pillow between the person's lower back and the chair. This supports the lower back. *Remember, a pillow is not used behind the back if restraints are used* (Chapter 13).

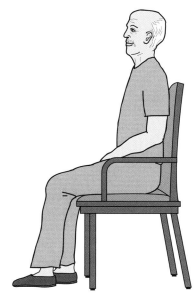

FIGURE 16-11 Chair position.

Support Devices. Sliding down in the seat, leaning forward, and leaning to the side cause poor alignment. Some persons need postural support devices. Special cushions, back supports, side (lateral) supports, and padded footrests are examples.

Weak or paralyzed arms are supported. Pillows or elevated armrests are used. Some persons have positioners (Fig. 16-12). The nurse may have you position the wrists at a slight upward angle.

The health team selects the best products for the person's needs. Safety, dignity, and function are considered. The nurse or therapist teaches how to use devices properly.

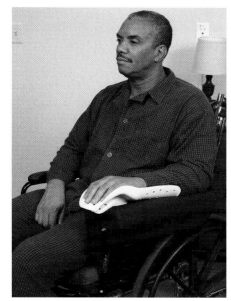

FIGURE 16-12 Elevated armrest and positioner.

FOCUS ON PRIDE
The Person, Family, and Yourself

Personal and Professional Responsibility

You make decisions daily about protecting yourself.
- Do you bend at the waist or the hips and knees to lift objects?
- Do you reach or use a step stool to get high objects?
- Do you exercise for strength and endurance?
- Do you raise the bed when giving bedside care?
- Do you move a person alone or get help?

Your decisions affect the safety of yourself and others. Use good judgment at home and in the workplace. Protect yourself from harm.

Rights and Respect

OSHA requires a safe work setting. You have the right to ask employers about safety plans to reduce your risk of injury. Ask about the agency's safe handling program, staff training, and safety practices.

Independence and Social Interaction

Talk with the person before and during positioning. Explain what you will do. Ask what the person prefers. Doing so promotes comfort, independence, and social interaction.

Delegation and Teamwork

Know which tasks increase your risk for injury. Use caution when doing them. Get help when needed.

Thinking that injuries happen only to others is dangerous. Anyone can be injured. Your safety is important. Take pride in working carefully.

Ethics and Laws

Failure to move and position the person correctly places the person at risk. For example, a person develops a pressure injury after being slumped in a chair for 3 hours. Or a person is injured from being moved without enough help. You must give care in a way that maintains or improves quality of life, health, and safety.

FOCUS ON PRIDE: *Application*

What changes will you make in your daily life to protect yourself from injury? How do you plan to protect yourself in the workplace?

REVIEW QUESTIONS

Circle the BEST answer.

1 Good body mechanics involve
   a Having an upright posture
   b Having a narrow base of support
   c Using the muscles in the back and lower arms
   d Lifting a heavy object alone

2 Which is an example of good alignment?
   a Being slumped in a bed
   b Sitting upright in a chair
   c Leaning to the side in a wheelchair
   d Walking with the head down and the back bent forward

3 Which action shows poor body mechanics?
   a Holding an object close to your body
   b Facing the direction you are working to prevent twisting
   c Leaning over a raised bed rail to give care
   d Using both hands and arms to lift an object

4 You need to move a large chair in a resident's room. You should
   a Push or slide the chair
   b Lift and carry the chair
   c Ask the nurse to move the chair for you
   d Pull the chair using quick, jerking motions

5 The purpose of ergonomics is to
   a Reduce stress on the worker's body
   b Safely position the person
   c Promote quality of life
   d Use good body mechanics

6 Risk of MSDs decreases with
   a Repeating actions
   b Awkward postures
   c Avoiding manual lifting when possible
   d Greater force

7 Which statement about back injuries is *true*?
   a Back injuries cannot be prevented.
   b Pain when assuming a normal posture is a symptom.
   c Nursing center staff are at low risk.
   d Bending when making beds does not cause back injuries.

8 Regular work tasks include moving persons in bed, transfers to and from bed, dressing, and giving bed baths. These activities
   a Place you at risk for injury
   b Are safe if you usually use good body mechanics
   c Cannot be included in safe handling program planning
   d Cannot be done safely

9 You ask about safe handling practices during a job interview. Which reply communicates a commitment to safe handling?
   a "You will not get hurt if you use good body mechanics."
   b "Why do you ask? Do you have back problems?"
   c "You look healthy. I am sure you will be fine."
   d "Staff are trained on hazards and how to safely use equipment to prevent injury."

10 Which statement about positioning is *true*?
    a Re-positioning helps prevent pressure injuries and contractures.
    b Circulation is not affected by positioning.
    c Position changes are avoided if moving causes pain.
    d Persons in chairs do not need to be re-positioned.

11 A resident is to be re-positioned at least every 2 hours. You last re-positioned the person at 0800. At 0900 the person is slumped in bed. You should
    a Wait until 1000 to re-position the person
    b Re-position the person when it is convenient
    c Re-position the person at 0900
    d Wait until the person asks to be re-positioned

12 You position a resident in the lateral position. Where do you place the call light?
    a At the foot of the bed
    b At the head of the bed
    c Behind the person
    d Within the person's reach

13 For Fowler's position
    a The bed is flat
    b The head of the bed is raised 45 to 60 degrees
    c The person's head is turned to 1 side
    d The feet hang over the edge of the mattress

14 The back-lying position is called
    a The prone position
    b The supine position
    c The lateral position
    d High-Fowler's position

15 A pillow is placed against the person's back in
    a A chair while restraints are used
    b The prone position
    c The lateral position
    d The left semi-prone position

16 For proper alignment in a chair, the person's feet
    a Are flat on the floor
    b Are able to touch the floor with the toes
    c Are dangling (do not touch the floor)
    d Are positioned on pillows

Answers to Chapter 16 questions are on p. 587.

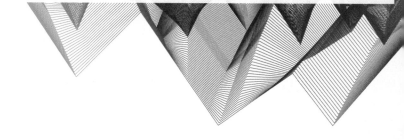

FOCUS ON **PRACTICE**

Problem Solving

To complete tasks quickly, you do not raise the bed to a comfortable working height. You move persons alone instead of getting help. You lean over the bed instead of moving to the other side. Why do these actions put you at increased risk for injury?

You now have back pain. Your walking is affected. How does this affect your work and daily life? How could you have avoided this problem?

CHAPTER 17

Moving the Person

OBJECTIVES

- Define the key terms and key abbreviation in this chapter.
- Explain how to prevent work-related injuries during moving procedures.
- Identify the delegation information needed before moving the person.

- Identify comfort and safety measures for moving the person.
- Explain how to plan and prepare for a safe move.
- Explain the purpose of friction-reducing devices.
- Perform the procedures described in this chapter.
- Explain how to promote PRIDE in the person, the family, and yourself.

KEY TERMS

bed mobility How a person moves to and from a lying position, turns from side to side, and re-positions in a bed or other sleeping furniture
friction The rubbing of 1 surface against another

logrolling Turning the person as a unit, in alignment, with 1 motion
shearing When the skin sticks to a surface while muscles slide in the direction the body is moving

KEY ABBREVIATION

ID   Identification

You will move persons often. You will assist with bed mobility. *Bed mobility is how a person moves to and from a lying position, turns from side to side, and re-positions in a bed or other sleeping furniture.* You also position the person in chairs and wheelchairs.

Moving procedures involve lifting, awkward postures, and repeated motions. These increase your risk for injury. You must prevent work-related injuries during moving procedures. See Chapter 16.

Good body mechanics alone will not prevent injury. The Occupational Safety and Health Administration (OSHA) recommends:
- Minimizing manual lifting in all cases
- Eliminating manual lifting when possible

You must work carefully to protect yourself and the person from injury.

See *Focus on Communication: Moving the Person.*
See *Delegation Guidelines: Moving the Person*, p. 200.
See *Promoting Safety and Comfort: Moving the Person*, p. 200.

FOCUS ON **COMMUNICATION**

Moving the Person

Moving can be painful after an injury or surgery. Many older persons have painful joints. Provide for comfort and avoid causing pain. You can say:
- "Please tell me when you feel pain or discomfort."
- "Do you need a pillow adjusted?"
- "Are you comfortable?"
- "How can I make you more comfortable?"

DELEGATION GUIDELINES

Moving the Person

Many tasks involve moving persons. Before moving a person, you need this information from the nurse and the care plan.
- The person's height and weight.
- How much help the person needs. These terms may be used.
  - *Independent*—moves without help.
  - *Supervision*—moves without help but needs supervision or cues. To *cue* means *to remind the person what to do.*
  - *Limited assistance*—staff guide (but do not lift) the arms or legs. The person moves on his or her own.
  - *Extensive assistance*—staff provide weight-bearing support to help the person move.
  - *Total dependence*—staff move the person.
- The person's physical abilities. Does the person have strength in the arms and legs?
- If the person has a weak side. If yes, which side?
- If the person has problems that increase the risk of injury. Weakness, dizziness, confusion, hearing or vision problems, recent surgery, and fragile skin are examples.
- The person's ability to follow directions.
- Possible behavior problems. Combative, agitated, uncooperative, and unpredictable behaviors are examples.
- The number of staff needed to complete the task safely.
- Any doctor's orders for moving the person.
- What procedure to use.
- What equipment or devices to use.
- What observations to report and record:
  - Who helped you with the move
  - How much help the person needed
  - How the person tolerated the move
  - How you positioned the person
  - Complaints of pain or discomfort
  - Signs of skin breakdown or pressure injury (Chapter 36)
- When to report observations.
- What patient or resident concerns to report at once.

PROMOTING SAFETY AND COMFORT

Moving the Person

Safety

For all moving procedures, you need to move the person carefully. Keep the person in good alignment during and after the move. Make sure the face, nose, and mouth are not obstructed (blocked) by a pillow or other device.

Comfort

Explain what you will do and how the person can help. Be courteous. Treat the person with dignity. Screen and cover the person for privacy. These measures promote mental comfort.

Use pillows and other positioning and protective devices as directed by the nurse and the care plan (Chapters 32 and 36). If a pillow is allowed under the person's head, position it so it supports the head and neck.

PLANNING A SAFE MOVE

Each person is different. Careful planning is needed to move the person safely. You must know about the person's physical abilities and the number of staff needed. The number of staff depends on the person's height, weight, cognitive function, and physical abilities.

The nurse and care plan tell you what procedure to use and the equipment or devices needed. Always follow the manufacturer's instructions. You should be trained to use your agency's equipment and devices safely. Ask for any needed training. Use equipment and devices correctly.

See *Focus on Communication: Planning a Safe Move.*
See *Promoting Safety and Comfort: Planning a Safe Move.*

FOCUS ON **COMMUNICATION**

Planning a Safe Move

Before beginning a procedure, tell the person what you and your co-workers will do. Also explain what the person needs to do. Just before the move, remind the person what will happen.

The procedures in this chapter have you move the person on the "count of 3." Staff smoothly move the person at the same time. One co-worker leads by counting. Decide who will count before the move. Be sure the person and staff know who is leading and what to do. You can say:

We will help you move up in bed. I will count "1, 2, 3." When I say "3," push against the bed with your feet. We will help you move when I say "3."

PROMOTING SAFETY AND COMFORT

Planning a Safe Move

Safety

Decide how to move the person before the procedure. Ask needed staff to help before you begin. To prevent injury:
- Follow the rules of body mechanics (Chapter 16). Stand with a wide base of support and good posture. Bend your hips and knees, not your back.
- Have help to move persons who cannot move alone. Use friction-reducing devices as instructed by the nurse and the care plan.

Beds are raised to move persons in bed. This reduces bending and reaching. You must:
- Use the bed correctly.
- Protect the person from falling when the bed is raised (Chapter 12). Follow the care plan for bed rail use. Ask a co-worker to help you if needed. Never leave the person alone when the bed is raised.
- Lower the bed to a comfortable and safe level for the person after giving care. Follow the care plan.

You need to plan how to protect tubes and devices connected to the person. Intravenous (IV) tubing (Chapter 30) and a urine drainage system (Chapter 26) are examples.

PROTECTING THE SKIN

Friction and shearing injure the skin. Both cause infection and pressure injuries (Chapter 36).

- *Friction* is the rubbing of 1 surface against another. When moved in bed, the person's skin rubs against the sheet.
- *Shearing* is when the skin sticks to a surface while muscles slide in the direction the body is moving (Fig. 17-1). It occurs when the person slides down in bed or is moved in bed.

Older persons are at great risk for shearing. Their fragile skin is easily torn. Protect the skin during moving procedures. Ask a co-worker to help you. Move the person carefully and gently. Use a friction-reducing device.

See *Focus on Surveys: Protecting the Skin.*

Friction-Reducing Devices

Friction-reducing devices (assist devices) protect the person's skin from injury. They also help prevent work-related injuries. Examples include:

- Turning pads or turning sheets (Fig. 17-2)
- Slide sheets (Fig. 17-3)
- Drawsheets (Chapter 20) or flat sheets folded in half
- Large re-usable waterproof under-pads (Chapter 20)

With these devices, the person is moved evenly. Shearing and friction are reduced. At least 2 staff members are needed to move a person with a friction-reducing device. See "Moving Persons in Bed" on p. 202.

When able, the person moves alone or helps with the move. The person may use a trapeze (Fig. 17-4) to move in bed alone or with the help of staff and a friction-reducing device.

See *Promoting Safety and Comfort: Friction-Reducing Devices.*

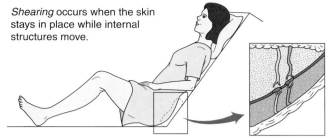

FIGURE 17-1 Shearing can damage the skin, tissues, and blood vessels.

Shearing occurs when the skin stays in place while internal structures move.

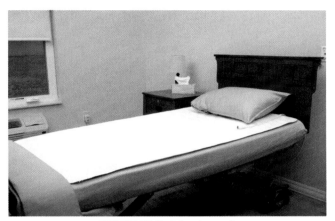

FIGURE 17-2 A turning pad.

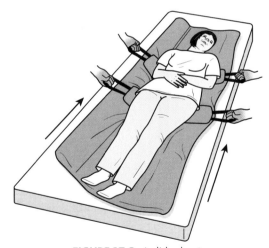

FIGURE 17-3 A slide sheet.

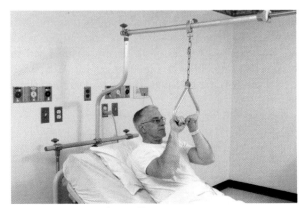

FIGURE 17-4 A trapeze.

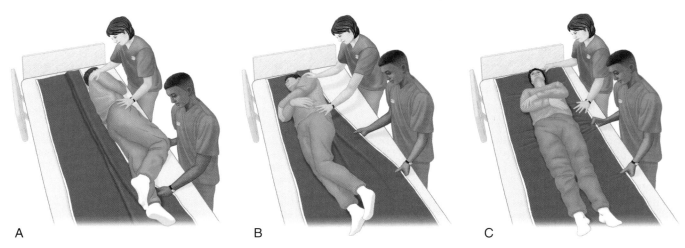

A   B   C

FIGURE 17-5 Turning the person to position a friction-reducing device. **A,** The person is turned to the side. The device is placed on the bed and fan-folded toward the person. **B,** The person is rolled to the other side. The device is pulled tightly. **C,** The person is rolled onto the back. The person is lying on the device.

Positioning Friction-Reducing Devices. For a device manufactured as a friction-reducing device, use it following the manufacturer's instructions.

Some slide sheets can be positioned with the person lying flat. The device is folded, placed under the person beginning at the head or foot, and unfolded beneath the person. Follow the manufacturer's instructions to position the device.

Turning (rolling) to position a device is common (Fig. 17-5). You and at least 1 co-worker:

1   Turn the person to 1 side. See "Turning Persons" on p. 206.
2   Place the device on the bed. Open and fan-fold it toward the person. The device is positioned from the head to above the knees or lower.
3   Tell the person that he or she will roll over a "bump." Assure the person that he or she will not fall.
4   Turn the person to the other side. The person rolls over the device.
5   Pull the device tightly. Smooth any wrinkles.
6   Roll the person onto the back. The person is lying on the device.

MOVING PERSONS IN BED

Some persons can move and turn in bed without help. Others need help from at least 1 person. Those who are weak, unconscious, paralyzed, or in casts need help. Sometimes 2 or 3 people or a mechanical lift (Chapter 18) is needed. Follow the guidelines in Box 17-1 to move persons in bed.

See *Focus on Older Persons: Moving Persons in Bed.*
See *Delegation Guidelines: Moving Persons in Bed.*

BOX 17-1 Guidelines for Moving Persons in Bed

- Follow the rules to prevent work-related injuries (Chapter 16).
- Know how much help and what equipment or friction-reducing devices you need. Follow the nurse's directions and the care plan. The nurse uses the person's weight to plan a safe move.
  - *Persons fully able to assist*—staff assistance is not needed. Staff stand by for safety and provide cues as needed.
  - *Persons partially able to assist:*
    - *The person weighs less than 200 pounds*—2 to 3 staff members and a friction-reducing device are used.
    - *The person weighs more than 200 pounds*—at least 3 staff members and a friction-reducing device are used.
  - *Persons unable to assist*—a mechanical lift and at least 2 staff members are needed. See "Using a Mechanical Lift" in Chapter 18.

Modified from Occupational Safety and Health Administration: *Guidelines for nursing homes: ergonomics for the prevention of musculoskeletal disorders,* Washington, DC, revised March 2009, Author.

FOCUS ON **OLDER PERSONS**

Moving Persons in Bed

Persons with dementia may not understand what you are doing. They may resist your efforts. The person may shout, grab you, or try to hit you. Always have a co-worker help you. Do not force the person. The person's care plan has measures for safe care. For example:

- Proceed slowly. Do not rush.
- Use a calm, pleasant voice.
- Distract the person. For example, let the person hold a washcloth or other soft object. This helps distract the person and keeps the hands busy.

Tell the nurse at once if you have problems moving the person.

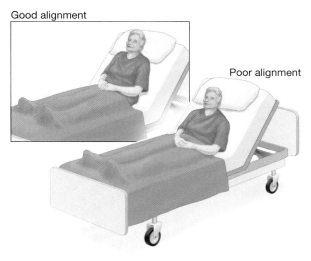

Good alignment

Poor alignment

FIGURE 17-6 A person in poor alignment after sliding down in bed.

Moving the Person Up in Bed

When the head of the bed is raised, it is easy to slide down toward the middle and foot of the bed (Fig. 17-6). Moving the person up in bed promotes good alignment and comfort.

Persons who are fully able to assist can move up in bed alone. Some need cues (direction) from staff. For example, a person uses a trapeze and pushes off of the bed with the feet. You lower the head of the bed and direct the person in the move. Then you position pillows and raise the head of the bed for comfort.

For persons needing help, 2 or more staff members are needed. Having enough staff is especially important when the person has pain with movement or is heavy, weak, or older. Using a friction-reducing device promotes safety and comfort. Always protect the person and yourself from injury.

See *Promoting Safety and Comfort: Moving the Person Up in Bed.*

See procedure: *Moving the Person Up in Bed With a Friction-Reducing Device*, p. 204.

Moving the Person Up in Bed With a Friction-Reducing Device

Quality of Life

- Knock before entering the person's room.
- Address the person by name.
- Introduce yourself by name and title.

- Explain the procedure before starting and during the procedure.
- Protect the person's rights during the procedure.
- Handle the person gently during the procedure.

Pre-Procedure

1 Follow *Delegation Guidelines:*
  a *Moving the Person,* p. 200
  b *Moving Persons in Bed,* p. 203
  See *Promoting Safety and Comfort:*
  a *Moving the Person,* p. 200
  b *Planning a Safe Move,* p. 200
  c *Friction-Reducing Devices,* p. 201
  d *Moving the Person Up in Bed,* p. 203
2 Ask at least 1 co-worker to help you.

3 Practice hand hygiene and get the needed friction-reducing device if not already positioned under the person.
4 Identify the person. Check the identification (ID) bracelet against the assignment sheet. Use 2 identifiers (Chapter 11). Also call the person by name.
5 Provide for privacy.
6 Lock (brake) the bed wheels.
7 Raise the bed for body mechanics. Bed rails are up if used.

Procedure

8 Lower the head of the bed to a level appropriate for the person. It is as flat as possible.
9 Stand on 1 side of the bed. Your co-worker stands on the other side.
10 Lower the bed rails if up.
11 Remove pillows as directed by the nurse. Place a pillow upright against the head-board if the person can be without it.
12 Position the friction-reducing device. (See "Positioning Friction-Reducing Devices" on p. 202.)
13 Roll the sides of the device up close to the person. (NOTE: Omit this step if the device has handles.)

14 Grasp the device firmly near the person's shoulders and hips (Fig. 17-7). Or grasp it by the handles. Be sure the person's head is supported.
15 Stand with a wide base of support and good posture. Bend your hips and knees, not your back. Position the leg near the head of the bed slightly forward in the direction of the move.
16 Move the person up in bed on the "count of 3." Shift your weight from your rear leg to your front leg. Use the strong muscles in your legs.
17 Repeat steps 15 and 16 if necessary.
18 Unroll the sides of the device. (NOTE: Omit this step if the device has handles.) Remove the slide sheet if used.

Post-Procedure

19 Put the pillow under the person's head and neck. Straighten linens.
20 Position the person in good alignment. Raise the head of the bed to a level appropriate for the person.
21 Provide for comfort. (See the inside of the back cover.)
22 Place the call light and other needed items within reach.
23 Lower the bed to a safe and comfortable level. Follow the care plan.

24 Raise or lower bed rails. Follow the care plan.
25 Follow the care plan and the person's preferences for privacy measures to maintain. Leaving the privacy curtain, window coverings, and door open or closed are examples.
26 Complete a safety check of the room. (See the inside of the back cover.)
27 Practice hand hygiene.
28 Report and record your care and observations.

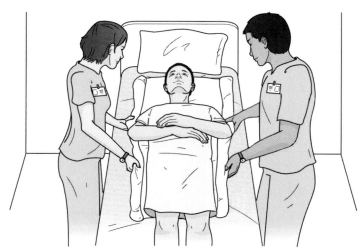

FIGURE 17-7 A drawsheet is used to move the person up in bed. It extends from the person's head to above the knees. Rolled close to the person, the drawsheet is held near the shoulders and hips.

Moving the Person to the Side of the Bed

Re-positioning and care procedures require moving the person to the side of the bed. For example, bathing in a bed may require reaching over the person. You reach less if the person is near you.

Before turning the person into the lateral (side-lying) position, you move the person to the side of the bed. Otherwise, after turning, the person lies on the side of the bed—not in the middle.

In 1 method, the person is moved in segments (Fig. 17-8). Sometimes you can do this alone if the person is small in size. Using a friction-reducing device helps prevent pain, skin damage, and injury to the bones, joints, and spinal cord. Follow the guidelines for moving persons in bed (Box 17-1). A mechanical lift (Chapter 18) may be needed.

See *Promoting Safety and Comfort: Moving the Person to the Side of the Bed.*

See procedure: *Moving the Person to the Side of the Bed.*

PROMOTING SAFETY AND COMFORT

Moving the Person to the Side of the Bed

Safety

Use the method and equipment that are best for the person. The nurse and the care plan tell you which method to use. The wrong method could cause injury. This is very important for persons who are older, have painful joints, or have spinal cord involvement.

Only move the person alone in segments if the person is small in size and you are comfortable doing so. To move the person in segments, move the person toward you, not away from you. Stand with a wide base of support and good posture. Bend your hips and knees, not your back. Position 1 leg in front of the other. When moving, shift your weight to your rear leg.

To use a friction-reducing device, you need at least 1 co-worker to help you. More staff members may be needed. Remove a slide sheet after use.

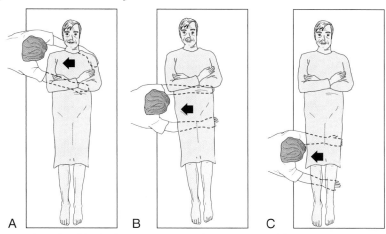

FIGURE 17-8 Moving the person to the side of the bed in segments. A, The upper part of the body is moved. B, The lower part of the body is moved. C, The legs and feet are moved.

Moving the Person to the Side of the Bed

Quality of Life

- Knock before entering the person's room.
- Address the person by name.
- Introduce yourself by name and title.

- Explain the procedure before starting and during the procedure.
- Protect the person's rights during the procedure.
- Handle the person gently during the procedure.

Pre-Procedure

1 Follow *Delegation Guidelines:*
  a *Moving the Person,* p. 200
  b *Moving Persons in Bed,* p. 203
  See *Promoting Safety and Comfort:*
  a *Moving the Person,* p. 200
  b *Planning a Safe Move,* p. 200
  c *Friction-Reducing Devices,* p. 201
  d *Moving the Person to the Side of the Bed*
2 Ask at least 1 co-worker to help you if using a friction-reducing device.

3 Practice hand hygiene and get the needed friction-reducing device if not already positioned under the person. (This procedure uses a drawsheet.)
4 Identify the person. Check the ID bracelet against the assignment sheet. Use 2 identifiers (Chapter 11). Also call the person by name.
5 Provide for privacy.
6 Lock (brake) the bed wheels.
7 Raise the bed for body mechanics. Bed rails are up if used.

Procedure

8 Lower the head of the bed to a level appropriate for the person. It is as flat as possible.
9 Stand on the side of the bed to which you will move the person.

10 Lower the bed rail near you if bed rails are used. (Both bed rails are lowered for Method 2.)
11 Remove pillows as directed by the nurse.

Continued

Moving the Person to the Side of the Bed—cont'd

Procedure—cont'd

12 Cross the person's arms over the chest.
13 Stand with a wide base of support and good posture. Bend your hips and knees, not your back. One foot is in front of the other.
14 *Method 1—moving the person in segments:*
   a Place your arm under the person's neck and shoulders. Grasp the far shoulder.
   b Place your other arm under the mid-back.
   c Move the upper part of the person's body toward you. Rock backward. Shift your weight to your rear leg (see Fig. 17-8, *A*).
   d Place 1 arm under the person's waist and 1 under the thighs.
   e Rock backward to move the lower part of the person toward you (see Fig. 17-8, *B*).

   f Repeat the procedure for the legs and feet (see Fig. 17-8, *C*). Your arms should be under the person's thighs and calves.
15 *Method 2—moving the person with a drawsheet:*
   a Position the drawsheet if it is not already under the person.
   b Roll up the drawsheet close to the person (see Fig. 17-7).
   c Grasp the rolled-up drawsheet near the person's shoulders and hips. Your co-worker does the same. Be sure the person's head is supported.
   d Rock backward on the "count of 3," moving the person toward you. Your co-worker rocks backward slightly and then forward toward you while keeping the arms straight.
   e Unroll the drawsheet. Remove any wrinkles.

Post-Procedure

16 Put the pillow under the person's head and neck. Straighten linens.
17 Turn and position the person on the side. See "Turning Persons." Or return the person to the center of the bed after completing care at the side of the bed.
18 Position the person in good alignment.
19 Provide for comfort. (See the inside of the back cover.)
20 Place the call light and other needed items within reach.
21 Lower the bed to a safe and comfortable level. Follow the care plan.

22 Raise or lower bed rails. Follow the care plan.
23 Follow the care plan and the person's preferences for privacy measures to maintain. Leaving the privacy curtain, window coverings, and door open or closed are examples.
24 Complete a safety check of the room. (See the inside of the back cover.)
25 Practice hand hygiene.
26 Report and record your care and observations.

 ## TURNING PERSONS

Turning persons onto their sides helps prevent complications from immobility and bed rest (Chapter 32). Procedures and care measures often require the side-lying position. You also may turn the person to position and remove friction-reducing devices.

You turn the person toward you or away from you (Fig. 17-9). The direction depends on the person's condition and the situation.

Many older persons have painful joints and arthritis in their spines, hips, and knees. Less painful, logrolling (p. 208) is preferred for turning these persons.

See *Delegation Guidelines: Turning Persons.*
See *Promoting Safety and Comfort: Turning Persons.*
See procedure: *Turning and Positioning the Person on the Side.*

DELEGATION GUIDELINES

Turning Persons

Before turning and positioning a person, you need this information from the nurse and the care plan.
• How much help the person needs
• The number of staff needed for safety
• The person's comfort level and painful body parts
• If logrolling is needed (p. 208)
• What friction-reducing device to use (if needed)
• What positioning and protective devices to use (Chapters 32 and 36)
• Where to place pillows
• What observations to report and record (see *Delegation Guidelines: Moving the Person*, p. 200)
• When to report observations
• What patient or resident concerns to report at once

PROMOTING SAFETY AND COMFORT

Turning Persons

Safety
Do not turn a person away from you with the far bed rail down. You can do 1 of the following instead.
• Turn the person toward a co-worker positioned on the other side of the bed.
• Raise the bed rail on the side near you. Go to the other side of the bed. Turn the person toward you.

When positioned on the side, the person does not lie on the lower (bottom) arm. The upper (top) leg is flexed (bent) in front of the lower leg and supported. This prevents contact between the knees and ankles that can cause pressure injuries (Chapter 36). Make sure the person's face, nose, and mouth are not obstructed (blocked) by a pillow or other device.

Comfort
Move the person to the side of the bed (p. 205) before turning and positioning the person on the side. Move the person to the side of the bed opposite to where you will turn. The person is in the center of the bed after the turn.

After turning, position the person in good alignment. Use pillows as directed to support the person in the lateral (side-lying) position. Placing a pillow in the following places is common for comfort and alignment.
• Under the head and neck
• Against the back
• Supporting the upper (top) arm and hand
• Supporting the upper (top) leg and ankle

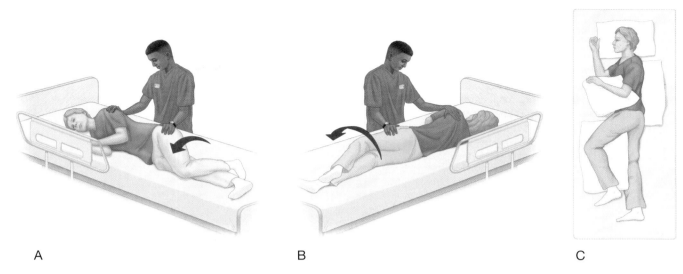

A   B   C

FIGURE 17-9 Turning and positioning the person on the side (lateral position). **A,** Turning the person away from you. **B,** Turning the person toward you. **C,** Positioning on the side with pillows for support.

Turning and Positioning the Person on the Side

Quality of Life

- Knock before entering the person's room.
- Address the person by name.
- Introduce yourself by name and title.

- Explain the procedure before starting and during the procedure.
- Protect the person's rights during the procedure.
- Handle the person gently during the procedure.

Pre-Procedure

1 Follow *Delegation Guidelines:*
  a *Moving the Person,* p. 200
  b *Moving Persons in Bed,* p. 203
  c *Turning Persons*
  See *Promoting Safety and Comfort:*
  a *Moving the Person,* p. 200
  b *Planning a Safe Move,* p. 200
  c *Moving the Person to the Side of the Bed,* p. 205
  d *Turning Persons*

2 Practice hand hygiene.
3 Identify the person. Check the ID bracelet against the assignment sheet. Use 2 identifiers (Chapter 11). Also call the person by name.
4 Provide for privacy.
5 Lock (brake) the bed wheels.
6 Raise the bed for body mechanics. Bed rails are up if used.

Procedure

7 Lower the head of the bed to a level appropriate for the person. It is as flat as possible.
8 Stand on the side of the bed opposite to where you will turn the person.
9 Lower the bed rail.
10 Move the person to the side near you. (See procedure: *Moving the Person to the Side of the Bed,* p. 205.)
11 Cross the person's arms over the chest. Cross the leg near you over the far leg.
12 *Turning the person away from you:*
  a Stand with a wide base of support and good posture. Bend your hips and knees, not your back. One foot is in front of the other.
  b Place 1 hand on the person's shoulder. Place the other on the hip near you.
  c Roll the person gently away from you toward the raised bed rail (see Fig. 17-9, *A*). Shift your weight from your rear leg to your front leg. If the person can assist with the turn, have the person grasp the far bed rail when able.

13 *Turning the person toward you:*
  a Raise the bed rail.
  b Go to the other side of the bed. Lower the bed rail.
  c Stand with a wide base of support and good posture. Bend your hips and knees, not your back. One foot is in front of the other.
  d Place 1 hand on the person's shoulder. Place the other on the far hip.
  e Roll the person gently toward you (see Fig. 17-9, *B*). Shift your weight from your front leg to your rear leg.
14 Position the person (see Fig. 17-9, *C*). Follow the nurse's directions and the care plan. For a lateral (side-lying) position:
  a Place a pillow under the head and neck.
  b Adjust the shoulder. The person should not be on an arm.
  c Position a pillow against the back.
  d Place a small pillow under the upper (top) arm and hand.
  e Flex (bend) the upper (top) hip and knee. Position the upper (top) leg in front of the lower (bottom) leg. Support the upper (top) leg and ankle on a pillow.

Continued

Turning and Positioning the Person on the Side—cont'd

Post-Procedure

15 Provide for comfort. (See the inside of the back cover.)
16 Place the call light and other needed items within reach.
17 Lower the bed to a safe and comfortable level. Follow the care plan.
18 Raise or lower bed rails. Follow the care plan.
19 Follow the care plan and the person's preferences for privacy measures to maintain. Leaving the privacy curtain, window coverings, and door open or closed are examples.

20 Complete a safety check of the room. (See the inside of the back cover.)
21 Practice hand hygiene.
22 Report and record your care and observations.

 ## Logrolling

Logrolling is turning the person as a unit, in alignment, with 1 motion. The head, neck, and spine are kept straight. The procedure is used to turn:

- Older persons with painful joints or arthritis of the spine, hip, or knee.
- Persons recovering from hip fractures.
- Persons with spinal cord injuries or after spinal cord surgery. The head, neck, and spine are kept straight at all times after a spinal cord injury or surgery.
  See *Promoting Safety and Comfort: Logrolling.*
  See procedure: *Logrolling the Person.*

PROMOTING SAFETY AND COMFORT

Logrolling

Safety

For logrolling, 2 or 3 staff members are needed. If the person is tall or heavy, at least 3 are needed. You may use a friction-reducing device (p. 201).

After spinal cord injury or surgery, the head, neck, and spine are kept straight. A device on the neck (cervical collar) helps maintain alignment. The doctor or nurse stands at the head of the bed and holds the head, neck, and spine straight during the move. The nurse directs the move and tells you what to do step-by-step. Assist the nurse as directed.

Comfort

After spinal cord injury or surgery, the doctor orders positioning limits. Follow the nurse's directions and the care plan to position the person and use pillows.

Logrolling the Person

Quality of Life

- Knock before entering the person's room.
- Address the person by name.
- Introduce yourself by name and title.

- Explain the procedure before starting and during the procedure.
- Protect the person's rights during the procedure.
- Handle the person gently during the procedure.

Pre-Procedure

1 Follow *Delegation Guidelines:*
   a *Moving the Person,* p. 200
   b *Moving Persons in Bed,* p. 203
   c *Turning Persons,* p. 206
   See *Promoting Safety and Comfort:*
   a *Moving the Person,* p. 200
   b *Planning a Safe Move,* p. 200
   c *Friction-Reducing Devices,* p. 201
   d *Turning Persons,* p. 206
   e *Logrolling*

2 Ask a co-worker to help you.
3 Practice hand hygiene and get the needed friction-reducing device if not already positioned under the person. (This procedure uses a turning pad.)
4 Identify the person. Check the ID bracelet against the assignment sheet. Use 2 identifiers (Chapter 11). Also call the person by name.
5 Provide for privacy.
6 Lock (brake) the bed wheels.
7 Raise the bed for body mechanics. Bed rails are up if used.

Logrolling the Person—cont'd

Procedure

8 Make sure the bed is flat.
9 Stand on the side opposite to which you will turn the person. Your co-worker stands on the other side.
10 Lower the bed rails if used.
11 Position the turning pad or other friction-reducing device if needed.
12 Move the person as a unit to the side of the bed near you. Use the turning pad. (If the person has a spinal cord injury or had spinal cord surgery, assist the nurse as directed.)
13 Place the person's arms across the chest. Place a pillow between the knees.
14 Raise the bed rail if used.
15 Go to the other side.
16 Stand near the shoulders and chest. Your co-worker stands near the hips and thighs.
17 Stand with a wide base of support and good posture. Bend your hips and knees, not your back. One foot is in front of the other.
18 Ask the person to hold the body rigid.
19 Grasp the turning pad as shown in Figure 17-10, *A.* Or position your hands as shown in Figure 17-10, *B* if a friction-reducing device is not used.
20 Roll the person toward you. Turn the person as a unit.
21 Position the person in good alignment. Use pillows as directed by the nurse and care plan.

Post-Procedure

22 Provide for comfort. (See the inside of the back cover.)
23 Place the call light and other needed items within reach.
24 Lower the bed to a safe and comfortable level. Follow the care plan.
25 Raise or lower bed rails. Follow the care plan.
26 Follow the care plan and the person's preferences for privacy measures to maintain. Leaving the privacy curtain, window coverings, and door open or closed are examples.
27 Complete a safety check of the room. (See the inside of the back cover.)
28 Practice hand hygiene.
29 Report and record your care and observations.

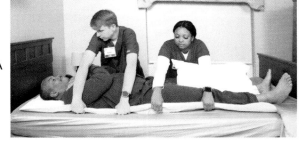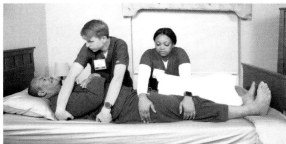

FIGURE 17-10 Logrolling. A pillow is between the person's legs. The arms are crossed on the chest. The person is on the far side of the bed. The person is turned as a unit. **A,** With a turning pad. **B,** Without a turning pad.

SITTING ON THE SIDE OF THE BED (DANGLING)

You will assist patients and residents to sit on the side of the bed *(dangle).* The procedure is part of some tasks—assisting the person to stand, transferring from bed to chair, partial bath, and others. While dangling the legs, the person coughs and deep breathes. Moving the legs back and forth in circles stimulates circulation.

Patients and residents may become dizzy or faint when getting out of bed too fast. Activity may increase in stages—lying flat, to lying with the head of the bed raised, to dangling, to sitting in a chair, and then to walking. This is common after surgery. The person may need to sit on the side of the bed for 1 to 5 minutes before transferring or walking.

Persons with weakness or balance problems need support. If dizziness or fainting occurs while in bed, lay the person down. If standing, have the person sit or lie down. Tell the nurse at once. See "The Falling Person" in Chapter 12 for safety measures for falling. See Chapter 43 for fainting.

See *Focus on Older Persons: Dangling.*
See *Delegation Guidelines: Dangling,* p. 210.
See *Promoting Safety and Comfort: Dangling,* p. 210.
See procedure: *Sitting on the Side of the Bed (Dangling),* p. 210.

FOCUS ON **OLDER PERSONS**

Dangling

Older persons may have circulatory changes. They may become dizzy or faint when getting up too fast. Let them sit on the side of the bed for a few minutes before standing.

DELEGATION GUIDELINES
Dangling

The nurse may ask you to help a person sit on the side of the bed. Before the dangling procedure, you need this information from the nurse and the care plan.

- Areas of weakness. For example, if the arms are weak, the person cannot hold on to the mattress for support. If the left side is weak, turn the person onto the stronger right side. The person uses the right arm to help move from the lying to sitting position.
- The amount of help the person needs.
- If you need a co-worker to help you.
- If the bed is raised or in a low position. If the person will walk or transfer to a chair, the bed is in a low position safe for a transfer (Chapter 18).
- How long the person needs to sit on the side of the bed.
- What exercises are to be done while dangling.
  - Range-of-motion exercises (Chapter 32)
  - Deep-breathing and coughing exercises (Chapter 37)
- What observations to report and record:
  - Pulse and respiratory rates (Chapter 31)
  - Pale or bluish skin color (cyanosis)
  - Complaints of dizziness, light-headedness, or difficulty breathing
  - How long the person dangled
  - The observations listed in Delegation Guidelines: Moving the Person, p. 200
- When to report observations.
- What patient or resident concerns to report at once.

PROMOTING SAFETY AND COMFORT
Dangling

Safety
Weakness and balance problems can occur after illness, injury, surgery, and bed rest. Some disabilities affect sitting and balance. Support the person who is sitting on the side of the bed. Have a co-worker help you. This protects the person from falling and other injuries.

As the person sits on the side of the bed, you observe the person. Lay the person down and tell the nurse at once if the person:

- Is dizzy or light-headed.
- Has an abnormal pulse or respirations.
- Has difficulty breathing.
- Has pale or bluish skin.

Do not leave the person alone. Provide support at all times.

Comfort
Provide for warmth during the procedure. Help the person put on a robe. Or cover the shoulders and back with a bath blanket (Chapter 20).

The person may want to perform hygiene measures while sitting on the side of the bed. Oral hygiene and washing the face and hands are examples. These measures are refreshing and stimulate circulation. Follow the nurse's directions and the care plan.

Sitting on the Side of the Bed (Dangling)

Quality of Life

- Knock before entering the person's room.
- Address the person by name.
- Introduce yourself by name and title.
- Explain the procedure before starting and during the procedure.
- Protect the person's rights during the procedure.
- Handle the person gently during the procedure.

Pre-Procedure

1 Follow Delegation Guidelines:
  a Moving the Person, p. 200
  b Dangling
  See Promoting Safety and Comfort:
  a Moving the Person, p. 200
  b Planning a Safe Move, p. 200
  c Dangling
2 Ask a co-worker to help you if needed.

3 Practice hand hygiene.
4 Identify the person. Check the ID bracelet against the assignment sheet. Use 2 identifiers (Chapter 11). Also call the person by name.
5 Provide for privacy.
6 Decide which side of the bed to use.
7 Move furniture to provide moving space.
8 Lock (brake) the bed wheels.
9 Raise the bed for body mechanics. Bed rails are up if used.

Procedure

10 Lower the bed rail if up.
11 Position the person in a side-lying position facing you (Fig. 17-11, A). The person lies on the strong side. The lower (bottom) arm is flat on the bed. The upper (top) arm is crossed over the chest. The hips and knees are flexed (bent).
12 Raise the head of the bed. If possible, raise it to a sitting position.
13 Stand by the person's hips.
14 Slide 1 arm under the person's shoulder. Place your other hand over the thighs near the knees (see Fig. 17-11, A).
15 Stand with a wide base of support. Bend your hips and knees, not your back.

16 Move the person's legs over the side of the bed. Assist the person to an upright position (Fig. 17-11, B).
  a If the person can assist, have the person push off of the mattress to help move from the lying to the sitting position.
  b If the person cannot assist, the procedure is best done with a co-worker. You move the upper body. Your co-worker moves the lower body.
17 Have the person hold on to the edge of the mattress. This supports the person in the sitting position. If possible, raise a half-length bed rail (on the person's strong side) for the person to grasp. Have your co-worker support the person at all times.

Use the following method if the person is alert and cooperative. The person must be able to follow directions. And the person must have the strength to help.

1 Lock (brake) the wheelchair wheels. Remove or swing front rigging out of the way. See Chapter 18 for wheelchair safety.
2 Position the person's feet flat on the floor.
3 Apply a transfer belt (Chapter 12).
4 Position the person's arms on the armrests.
5 Stand in front of the person. Block the person's knees and feet with your knees and feet.
6 Grasp the transfer belt on each side while the person leans slightly forward.
7 Ask the person to push with the feet and arms on the "count of 3."
8 Move the person back into the chair on the "count of 3" as the person pushes with the feet and arms (Fig. 17-13).
9 Remove the transfer belt.

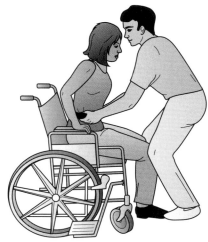

FIGURE 17-13 Re-positioning the person in a wheelchair. A transfer belt is used to move the person to the back of the chair.

FOCUS ON P R I D E

The Person, Family, and Yourself

P ersonal and Professional Responsibility

You will practice moving and positioning procedures in your training program. Practice with other students. Be willing to act as the patient or resident to help other students practice. Use your practice time wisely.

R ights and Respect

How would you feel if these statements were made to you?
• "You're too heavy. I need to get help to move you."
• "I'll get hurt if I try to move you."
    What you say affects the person's self-esteem. Choose your words carefully. Show respect in what you say.

I ndependence and Social Interaction

Persons who need help moving may feel embarrassed or helpless. To promote independence and self-esteem:
• Focus on the person's abilities.
• Encourage the person.
• Let the person help as much as safely possible.
• Tell the person when you notice even small improvements.

D elegation and Teamwork

Moving is safer when done by 2 or more workers. This is very important when caring for bariatric persons. Moving a person without enough help can harm you, your co-workers, and the person. Work as a team to protect yourself and others from injury.

E thics and Laws

Before a move, explain what you will do and what the person needs to do. Ask if the person has any questions or preferences. The person may suggest an easier or more comfortable method. Always listen. Ignoring the person is wrong. If the method is not safe, explain why. Ask the nurse if you do not know how to answer or if you are unsure how to safely move the person.

FOCUS ON PRIDE: Application

Most moving procedures require a team effort. How well do you work with others? What can you improve?

Circle the BEST answer.

1. You move the person on the "count of 3" to
   a. Save time
   b. Distract the person from the move
   c. Move the person smoothly
   d. Move the person slowly

2. Which term describes needing the *most* assistance with a move?
   a. Independent
   b. Supervision
   c. Limited assistance
   d. Total dependence

3. Good body mechanics alone will prevent injury when moving persons.
   a. True
   b. False

4. A resident with dementia needs to be moved up in bed. You should
   a. Avoid rushing
   b. Wait until the person is asleep
   c. Move the person alone
   d. Continue if the person resists the move

5. Drawsheets and slide sheets are used to
   a. Promote privacy
   b. Reduce friction
   c. Promote independence
   d. Improve posture

6. When used to move a person in bed, a waterproof under-pad is placed so that it
   a. Covers the person's body
   b. Extends from the mid-back to mid-thigh level
   c. Is under the head to above the knees
   d. Covers the entire mattress

7. You need to turn a person to position a friction-reducing device. The person has painful joints and cannot assist. You should
   a. Move the person without the device
   b. Position the device by yourself
   c. Get help and logroll the person to position the device
   d. Refuse to move the person

8. A person is fully able to assist with moving up in bed. You should
   a. Stand by and provide cues as needed
   b. Move the person up in bed by yourself
   c. Ask 1 co-worker to help move the person
   d. Ask 2 co-workers to help move the person

9. A person is partially able to assist with moving up in bed. You should
   a. Stand by for safety but not assist
   b. Move the person up in bed by yourself
   c. Tell the person not to assist to avoid injury
   d. Ask for help and get a friction-reducing device

10. Before turning a person onto the side, you
    a. Move the person to the middle of the bed
    b. Move the person to the side of the bed
    c. Raise the head of the bed 30 degrees
    d. Position a pillow against the back

11. A patient with a spinal cord injury is turned with
    a. The logrolling procedure
    b. A transfer belt
    c. A mechanical lift
    d. A pillow under the head and neck

12. You turn and position a person on the side. Which is *safe*?
    a. The pillow under the upper (top) arm is covering the face.
    b. The person is lying on the lower (bottom) arm.
    c. The upper (top) leg is flexed and supported so the knees and ankles do not touch.
    d. The person's face is up against the bed rail.

13. You are helping an older person sit on the side of the bed before standing. Which is *true*?
    a. The person should sit only for a few seconds before standing.
    b. Circulatory changes can cause dizziness.
    c. Difficulty breathing during the procedure is normal.
    d. Moving the person quickly promotes comfort.

14. To protect the person's rights during dangling
    a. Leave the room as the person dangles
    b. Perform the procedure alone
    c. Do not ask how the person feels
    d. Close the privacy curtain

15. A person is able to help move. To re-position the person in a wheelchair
    a. Pull the person from behind
    b. Unlock the wheelchair wheels
    c. Position the person's feet flat on the floor
    d. Position the person's arms across the chest

Answers to Chapter 17 questions are on p. 587.

FOCUS ON **PRACTICE**

Problem Solving

A person with right-sided weakness needs to sit on the side of the bed (dangle). Which side of the bed is best—right, left, or either? Why? The person becomes pale and dizzy while dangling. What will you do?

CHAPTER 18

Transferring the Person

OBJECTIVES

- Define the key terms and key abbreviation in this chapter.
- Explain how to prevent work-related injuries during transfers.
- Identify the delegation information needed to transfer a person.
- Identify comfort and safety measures for transferring the person.
- Explain wheelchair and stretcher safety.
- Perform the procedures described in this chapter.
- Explain how to promote PRIDE in the person, the family, and yourself.

KEY TERMS

lateral transfer When a person moves between 2 horizontal surfaces

pivot To turn one's body from a set standing position
transfer How a person moves to and from a surface

KEY ABBREVIATION

ID   Identification

Patients and residents are moved to and from surfaces such as beds, chairs, wheelchairs, shower chairs, commodes, toilets, and stretchers. A *transfer is how a person moves to and from a surface.* The amount of help needed and the method used vary with the person's abilities. You will assist with transfers often.

Rules for body mechanics and the safety measures for preventing work-related injuries apply to transfers (Chapter 16). So do the rules for moving persons (Chapter 17). Protect yourself and the person from injury. Use your body and transfer devices and equipment correctly.

See *Focus on Communication: Transferring the Person.*

See *Delegation Guidelines: Transferring the Person.*

See *Promoting Safety and Comfort: Transferring the Person.*

> ### FOCUS ON **COMMUNICATION**
> *Transferring the Person*
>
> Transfers can be painful for older persons and after an injury or surgery. Ask about comfort. Remind the person to tell you about discomfort.
> - "Please tell me if you feel pain or discomfort."
> - "Tell me to stop if you feel pain."
>
> Before any transfer, tell the person what you and your co-workers will do. Also explain what the person needs to do. Give step-by-step instructions during the procedure.
>
> The procedures in this chapter explain how to transfer on the "count of 3." You and the person or you and your co-workers move at the same time. For example:
>
> *I will help you transfer to the chair. I will count "1, 2, 3." When I say "3," push on the mattress with your hands and stand. I will steady you with the transfer belt as you stand. You will turn so your legs touch the seat's edge. Grab the chair's armrests. I will help you sit.*

DELEGATION GUIDELINES

Transferring the Person

Transfer procedures include stand and pivot transfers (p. 217), lateral transfers (p. 223), and transfers using a mechanical lift (p. 224). Before transferring a person, you need information from the nurse and care plan.

- What procedure to use.
- The person's weight and height.
- How much help the person needs. These terms may be used.
  - *Independent*—the person transfers without help.
  - *Supervision*—the person transfers without help but needs supervision or cues.
  - *Limited assistance*—staff guide (but do not lift) the arms or legs. The person transfers on his or her own.
  - *Extensive assistance*—staff or a mechanical lift provides weight-bearing support to help the person transfer.
  - *Total dependence*—staff transfer the person with a mechanical lift.
- The person's physical abilities.
  - Can the person sit up, stand up, or walk without help?
  - Does the person have strength in the arms and legs?
  - Does the person have a weak side? If yes, which side?
- If the person has problems that increase the risk of injury. Dizziness, confusion, hearing or vision problems, recent surgery, and fragile skin are examples.
- The person's ability to follow directions.
- If behavior problems are likely. Combative, agitated, uncooperative, and unpredictable behaviors are examples.
- The number of staff needed for a safe transfer.
- What equipment or devices to use.
  - *Stand and pivot transfer*—transfer belt, wheelchair, stand-assist device (p. 217), positioning devices, wheelchair cushion, position change alarm, and so on
  - *Lateral transfer*—friction-reducing device (Chapter 17) or other lateral transfer device (p. 223)
  - *Mechanical lift transfer*—stand-assist mechanical lift or full-sling mechanical lift (p. 224)
- What observations to report and record:
  - The amount of help needed to transfer the person
  - How the person helped with the procedure
  - How the person tolerated the transfer
  - How you positioned the person
  - The person's pulse, respirations, and blood pressure if asked to measure them before, during, or after the procedure
  - Complaints of dizziness, pain, discomfort, difficulty breathing, weakness, or fatigue
  - Who helped you with the transfer
- When to report observations.
- What patient or resident concerns to report at once.

PROMOTING SAFETY AND COMFORT

Transferring the Person

Safety

To prevent injury to fragile bones and joints:

- Follow the rules of body mechanics and the safety measures for preventing work-related injuries (Chapter 16).
- Have help to transfer the person.
- Use assist devices as directed by the nurse and the care plan. Wheelchair, walker or cane (Chapter 32), and transfer belt (Chapter 12) are examples.
- Transfer the person carefully and in good alignment.
  Decide how to transfer the person before beginning. Ask needed staff to help. Arrange the room to allow enough space for a safe transfer. Correctly place the chair, wheelchair, or other device. Also plan to protect tubes or devices connected to the person.
  Raise or lower the bed to a safe and comfortable level for the transfer. If the person will stand, the feet must be flat on the floor. For a lateral transfer, the bed is at a safe working height for staff.

Comfort

To promote mental comfort:

- Explain what you will do and how the person can help.
- Screen and cover the person for privacy.
- Reassure the person that mechanical lifts (p. 224) are safe.
  To promote physical comfort:
- Keep the person in good alignment.
- Do not pull on any part of the person's body.
- Raise the head of the bed as soon as possible. Lying flat for too long can cause discomfort and trouble breathing.
- Use pillows and other positioning devices as directed by the nurse and the care plan.

WHEELCHAIR AND STRETCHER SAFETY

Wheelchairs are useful for people who cannot walk or who have severe problems walking (Fig. 18-1, p. 216). You use the hand grips/push handles to move the wheelchair. Or the person moves it using the hand rims or with the feet. Stretchers are used to transport persons who cannot sit up or who are very ill.

Follow the safety measures in Box 18-1 (p. 216) to use wheelchairs and stretchers. The person can fall from the wheelchair or stretcher. Or the person can fall during transfers to and from the wheelchair or stretcher.

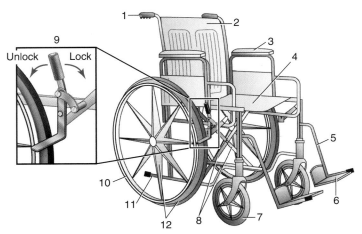

1 Hand grip/push handle
2 Back upholstery
3 Armrest
4 Seat upholstery
5 Front rigging
6 Footplate
7 Caster
8 Crossbrace
9 Wheel lock/brake
10 Wheel and hand rim
11 Tipping lever
12 Tire and wheel spokes

FIGURE 18-1 Parts of a wheelchair.

BOX 18-1 Wheelchair and Stretcher Safety

Wheelchair Safety

Maintenance
- Check that you can lock and unlock the wheel locks (brakes).
- Check for flat or loose tires. A wheel lock (brake) will not work on a flat or loose tire.
- Make sure wheel spokes are intact. Damaged, broken, or loose spokes can interfere with moving the wheelchair or locking (braking) the wheels.
- Make sure the casters point forward. This keeps the wheelchair balanced and stable.
- Clean the wheelchair according to agency policy.
- Follow the safety measures to prevent equipment accidents (Chapter 11).

Transfers
- Lock (brake) both wheels before you transfer a person to or from the wheelchair (see Fig. 18-1). Make sure bed wheels are locked.
- Remove the near armrest (if removable) for lateral transfers to and from the bed, toilet, commode, tub, or car (p. 223). Leave the armrests in place if the person will push off of them to stand.
- Remove or swing front rigging out of the way for transfers to and from the wheelchair (Fig. 18-2). Raise the footplates.
- Do not let the person stand on the footplates.
- Do not let the footplates fall back onto the person's legs.
- Position the person's feet on the footplates after the transfer. The feet must not touch or drag on the floor when the chair is moving.
- Provide needed wheelchair accessories—safety belt, pouch, tray, lap-board, cushion.

Transport
- Follow the care plan for the number of staff needed for a safe transport. This depends on:
  - The person's weight
  - If the person is cooperative
  - If the wheelchair is motorized

Wheelchair Safety—cont'd

Transport—cont'd
- Push the chair forward to transport the person. Do not pull the chair backward unless going through a doorway or down a steep ramp or incline.
- Follow the nurse's or physical therapist's instructions on how to move a wheelchair up and down a ramp and over a curb.
  - *Going up*—The wheelchair is pushed forward.
  - *Going down*—The wheelchair is pulled backward.
- Follow the care plan for keeping the wheels locked (braked) when not moving the wheelchair. Locking (braking) the wheels prevents the chair from moving when the person moves to or from the chair. (Locking the wheelchair may be viewed as a restraint. See Chapter 13.)

Stretcher Safety
- Have 2 or more co-workers help you transfer the person to or from the stretcher.
- Lock (brake) the stretcher wheels before the transfer.
- Follow the care plan for the number of staff needed for a safe transport. As many as 4 staff members may be needed. This depends on:
  - The person's weight
  - If the person is cooperative
- Use safety straps if the stretcher has them. Fasten the safety straps when the person is properly positioned on the stretcher.
- Raise the side rails. Keep them up during the transport.
- Make sure the person's arms, hands, legs, and feet do not dangle through the side rail bars.
- Stand at the head of the stretcher. Another staff member may be positioned near the foot to help guide the stretcher.
- Move the stretcher feet first (Fig. 18-3). The staff member at the head of the stretcher watches the person's breathing and color during the transport.
- Do not leave the person alone.
- Follow the safety measures to prevent equipment accidents (Chapter 11).

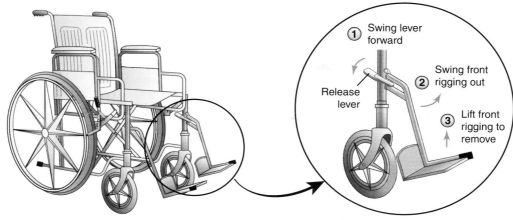

FIGURE 18-2 Removing wheelchair front rigging.

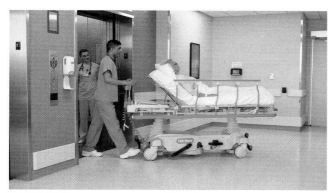

FIGURE 18-3 A stretcher is moved feet first. (Courtesy © Hill-Rom Services, Inc. Reprinted with permission. All rights reserved.)

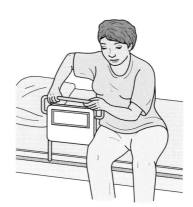

FIGURE 18-4 Stand-assist bed attachment.

STAND AND PIVOT TRANSFERS

Some persons can stand and pivot. *Pivot means to turn one's body from a set standing position.* A stand and pivot transfer is used if:

- The legs are strong enough to bear (support) some or all of the person's weight.
- The person can cooperate and follow directions.
- The person can assist with the transfer.

  See *Promoting Safety and Comfort: Stand and Pivot Transfers.*

Transfer Belts

Transfer belts (gait belts) are discussed in Chapter 12. They are used to:

- Support patients and residents during transfers.
- Re-position persons in chairs and wheelchairs (Chapter 17).
- Assist with ambulation (Chapter 32).

  Wider belts have padded handles. They are easier to grip and allow better control should the person fall.

PROMOTING SAFETY AND COMFORT

Stand and Pivot Transfers

Safety

You need to know about any areas of weakness. For example, if the arms are weak, the person cannot hold on to the mattress for support. If the left side is weak, the person should get out of bed on the stronger right side. The person uses the right arm to help move.

The person wears slip-resistant footwear for stand and pivot transfers. Such footwear helps prevent slipping, sliding, and falls. Tie shoelaces securely. Otherwise the person can trip and fall.

Long gowns and robes can cause the person to trip and fall. Also avoid robes with long ties.

Lock (brake) bed and wheelchair wheels and wheels on other devices. This prevents the bed and the device from moving during the transfer. Otherwise the person can fall. You also are at risk for injury.

The person must not put his or her arms around your neck. Otherwise the person can pull you forward or cause you to lose balance. Neck, back, and other injuries are possible. To stand, the person pushes off the mattress or the chair or wheelchair armrests. Or the person uses a bed rail or stand-assist device (Fig. 18-4). Follow the care plan and the nurse's directions.

Comfort

After the transfer, position the person in good alignment. Place the call light and other needed items within reach.

Bed to Chair or Wheelchair Transfers

Safety is important for chair and wheelchair transfers. Help the person out of bed on the person's strong side. If the left side is weak and the right side is strong, get the person out of bed on the right side. The strong side moves first. It pulls the weaker side along. Transfers from the weak side are awkward and unsafe.

See *Focus on Surveys: Bed to Chair or Wheelchair Transfers.*

See *Promoting Safety and Comfort: Bed to Chair or Wheelchair Transfers.*

See procedure: *Transferring the Person to a Chair or Wheelchair.*

FOCUS ON SURVEYS

Bed to Chair or Wheelchair Transfers

Agencies must ensure that nursing assistants can safely perform the skills needed for safe care. Surveyors will observe how nursing assistants function. One skill of focus is transferring a person from the bed to a wheelchair.

PROMOTING SAFETY AND COMFORT

Bed to Chair or Wheelchair Transfers

Safety

The chair or wheelchair must support the person's weight. The number of staff needed depends on the person's abilities, condition, and size (weight and height). Sometimes you need a mechanical lift (p. 224).

If not using a mechanical lift, use a transfer belt. It is safer for the person and you. Putting your arms around the person and grasping the shoulder blades is another method. This can cause the person discomfort and be stressful for you. Use this method only if the nurse and the care plan direct and you are comfortable doing so.

Bed and wheelchair wheels are locked (braked) for a safe transfer. After the transfer, unlock the wheelchair wheels (release the brakes) to position the wheelchair as the person prefers.

Then lock (brake) the wheels or keep them unlocked according to the care plan. Locked wheels may be viewed as restraints if the person cannot unlock them to move the wheelchair (Chapter 13). However, falls and other injuries are risks if the person tries to stand when the wheels are unlocked.

Comfort

Most wheelchairs and bedside chairs have vinyl seats and backs. Vinyl holds body heat. The person becomes warm and perspires (sweats) more. If the nurse allows, cover the back and seat with a folded bath blanket. This increases comfort.

Some people have wheelchair cushions or positioning devices. Follow the manufacturer's instructions for how to use and place a device. Ask the nurse if you need help.

Transferring the Person to a Chair or Wheelchair

Quality of Life

- Knock before entering the person's room.
- Address the person by name.
- Introduce yourself by name and title.

- Explain the procedure before starting and during the procedure.
- Protect the person's rights during the procedure.
- Handle the person gently during the procedure.

Pre-Procedure

1. Follow *Delegation Guidelines: Transferring the Person, p. 215.*
   See *Promoting Safety and Comfort:*
   a *Transfer/Gait Belts* (Chapter 12)
   b *Transferring the Person, p. 215*
   c *Stand and Pivot Transfers, p. 217*
   d *Bed to Chair or Wheelchair Transfers*
2. Practice hand hygiene and get the following supplies.
   - Wheelchair or arm chair
   - Bath blanket or cushion (if needed)
   - Lap blanket (if used)
   - Robe (if needed) and slip-resistant footwear
   - Paper towel or towel (if needed)
   - Transfer belt (if needed)

3. Arrange items in the person's room.
4. Practice hand hygiene.
5. Identify the person. Check the identification (ID) bracelet against the assignment sheet. Use 2 identifiers (Chapter 11). Also call the person by name.
6. Provide for privacy.
7. Decide which side of the bed to use. Move furniture for a safe transfer.

Transferring the Person to a Chair or Wheelchair—cont'd

Procedure

8   Raise the wheelchair footplates. Remove or swing front rigging out of the way if possible. Position the chair or wheelchair beside the bed on the person's strong side.
  a   If at the head of the bed, it faces the foot of the bed.
  b   If at the foot of the bed, it faces the head of the bed.
  c   The armrest almost touches the bed.
9   Place a folded bath blanket or cushion on the seat (if needed and allowed).
10   Lock (brake) the wheelchair wheels. Make sure bed wheels are locked.
11   Fan-fold top linens to the foot of the bed.
12   Place the paper towel or towel under the person's feet. (This protects linens from footwear.) Put footwear on the person. Or apply footwear when the person is seated on the side of the bed (step 14).
13   Lower the bed to a safe and comfortable level for the person. Follow the care plan.
14   Help the person sit on the side of the bed (Chapter 17). Feet must be flat on the floor.
15   Be sure the person's clothing will properly cover the person during the transfer. Help the person put on a robe if needed.
16   Apply the transfer belt if needed (Chapter 12). It is applied at the waist over clothing.
17   *Method 1—using a transfer belt:*
  a   Stand in front of the person.
  b   Have the person hold on to the mattress.
  c   Make sure the feet are flat on the floor.
  d   Have the person lean slightly forward.
  e   Grasp the transfer belt at each side. Grasp the handles or grasp the belt from underneath. Hands are in an upward position (upward grasp). See Chapter 12.
  f   Prevent the person from sliding or falling. Do 1 of the following.
    1)   Brace your knees against the person's knees. Block the feet with your feet (Fig. 18-5, p. 220).
    2)   Use the knee and foot of 1 leg to block the person's weak leg or foot. Place your other foot slightly behind you for balance.
    3)   Straddle your legs around the weak leg.
  g   Explain the following.
    1)   You will count "1, 2, 3."
    2)   The move will be on "3."
    3)   On "3," the person pushes down on the mattress and stands.
  h   Ask the person to push down on the mattress and stand on the "count of 3." Assist the person to a standing position as you straighten your knees (Fig. 18-6, A, p. 220).

18   *Method 2—no transfer belt:* (Note: Use this method only if directed by the nurse and the care plan and you are comfortable doing so.)
  a   Follow steps 17, a–c.
  b   Place your hands under the person's arms. Your hands are around the person's shoulder blades (Fig. 18-6, B, p. 220).
  c   Have the person lean slightly forward.
  d   Prevent the person from sliding or falling using 1 of the methods in step 17, f.
  e   Explain the "count of 3." See step 17, g.
  f   Ask the person to push down on the mattress and to stand on the "count of 3." Assist the person to a standing position as you straighten your knees.
19   Support the person in the standing position. Hold the transfer belt or keep your hands around the shoulder blades. Steady the person to prevent sliding or falling.
20   Help the person pivot (turn). Have the person grasp the far arm of the chair or wheelchair (Fig. 18-7, p. 220). The legs will touch the edge of the seat.
21   Continue to help the person pivot (turn) until the other armrest is grasped.
22   Lower the person into the chair or wheelchair as you bend your hips and knees (Fig. 18-8, p. 220). The person leans slightly forward and bends the elbows and knees.
23   Make sure the hips are to the back of the seat. Position the person in good alignment.
24   Attach wheelchair front rigging. Position the person's feet on the footplates.
25   Cover the person's lap and legs with a lap blanket (if used). Keep the blanket off the floor and the wheels.
26   Remove the transfer belt if used.
27   Position the chair as the person prefers. Lock (brake) the wheelchair wheels according to the care plan.

Post-Procedure

28   Provide for comfort. (See the inside of the back cover.)
29   Place the call light and other needed items within reach.
30   Follow the care plan and the person's preferences for privacy measures to maintain. Leaving the privacy curtain, window coverings, and door open or closed are examples.
31   Complete a safety check of the room. (See the inside of the back cover.)
32   Practice hand hygiene.
33   Report and record your care and observations.
34   See procedure: *Transferring the Person From a Chair or Wheelchair to Bed* (p. 221) to return the person to bed.

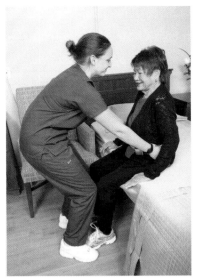

FIGURE 18-5 The person's knees and feet are blocked by the nursing assistant's knees and feet.

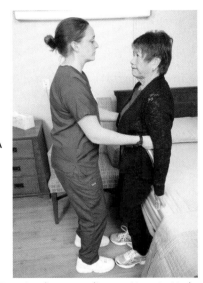

A

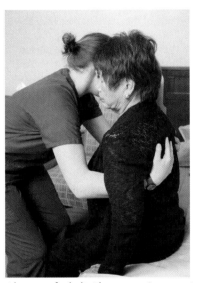

B

FIGURE 18-6 The person is assisted to a standing position. **A,** Method 1—with a transfer belt. The person is supported with the transfer belt. **B,** Method 2—without a transfer belt. The hands are under the person's arms and around the shoulder blades.

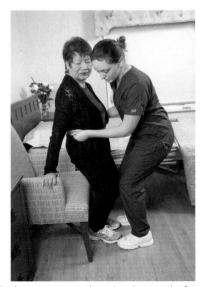

FIGURE 18-7 The person pivots (turns) and grasps the far arm of the chair.

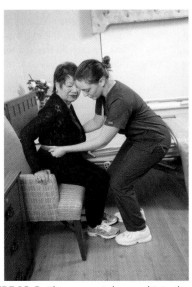

FIGURE 18-8 The person is lowered into the chair.

Chair or Wheelchair to Bed Transfers

Chair or wheelchair to bed transfers have the same rules as bed to chair transfers. If the person is weak on 1 side, transfer the person so that the strong side moves first. Position the person so the strong side is near the bed. See Figure 18-9. The strong side moves first.

You may have to move the chair or wheelchair. If you cannot safely move a chair alone, have help to move the chair or to transfer the person.

For example, a resident's right side is weak. The left side is strong. To transfer out of bed, the wheelchair was on the left side of the bed. The resident's left side (strong side) moved first. Now you will transfer the resident back to bed. With the wheelchair on the left side of the bed, the resident's weak right side is near the bed. Move the wheelchair to the other side of the bed or turn it around. The resident's stronger left side will be near the bed for a safer transfer.

See procedure: *Transferring the Person From a Chair or Wheelchair to Bed.*

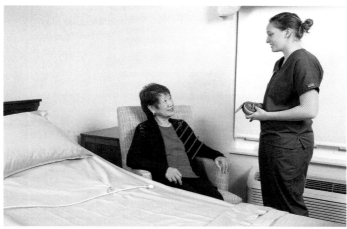

FIGURE 18-9 The chair is positioned so the person's strong side is near the bed. (*Note: The "weak" side is indicated by slash marks.*)

Transferring the Person From a Chair or Wheelchair to Bed

Quality of Life

- Knock before entering the person's room.
- Address the person by name.
- Introduce yourself by name and title.
- Explain the procedure before starting and during the procedure.
- Protect the person's rights during the procedure.
- Handle the person gently during the procedure.

Pre-Procedure

1 Follow *Delegation Guidelines: Transferring the Person,* p. 215.
  See *Promoting Safety and Comfort:*
  a *Transfer/Gait Belts* (Chapter 12)
  b *Transferring the Person,* p. 215
  c *Stand and Pivot Transfers,* p. 217
  d *Bed to Chair or Wheelchair Transfers,* p. 218

2 Practice hand hygiene and get a transfer belt if needed.
3 Identify the person. Check the ID bracelet against the assignment sheet. Use 2 identifiers (Chapter 11). Also call the person by name.
4 Provide for privacy.

Procedure

5 Move furniture for moving space.
6 Raise the head of the bed to a sitting position. Be sure the bed is at a safe and comfortable level for the person. Follow the care plan. When the person transfers to the bed, the feet must be flat on the floor when sitting on the side of the bed.
7 Move the call light so it is on the strong side when the person is in bed.
8 Position the chair or wheelchair so the person's strong side is next to the bed (see Fig. 18-9). Have a co-worker help you if necessary.
9 Lock (brake) the wheelchair and bed wheels.
10 Remove and fold the lap blanket.

11 Lift the person's feet from the footplates. Raise the footplates. Remove or swing front rigging out of the way. Put slip-resistant footwear on the person if not already done.
12 Apply the transfer belt if needed.
13 Make sure the person's feet are flat on the floor.
14 Stand in front of the person.
15 Have the person hold on to the armrests. (If the nurse directs you to do so, place your arms under the person's arms. Your hands are around the shoulder blades.)
16 Have the person lean slightly forward.

Continued

Transferring the Person From a Chair or Wheelchair to Bed—cont'd

Procedure—cont'd

17 Grasp the transfer belt on each side if using it. Grasp underneath the belt. Hands are in an upward position (upward grasp).
18 Prevent the person from sliding or falling. Do 1 of the following.
  a Brace your knees against the person's knees. Block the feet with your feet.
  b Use the knee and foot of 1 leg to block the person's weak leg or foot. Place your other foot slightly behind you for balance.
  c Straddle your legs around the person's weak leg.
19 Explain the "count of 3." See procedure: *Transferring the Person to a Chair or Wheelchair,* p. 218.
20 Ask the person to push down on the armrests on the "count of 3." Assist the person into a standing position as you straighten your knees.

21 Support the person in the standing position. Hold the transfer belt or keep your hands around the shoulder blades. Steady the person to prevent sliding or falling.
22 Help the person pivot (turn) to reach the edge of the mattress. The legs will touch the mattress. The person can reach the mattress with both hands.
23 Lower the person onto the bed as you bend your hips and knees. The person leans slightly forward and bends the elbows and knees.
24 Remove the transfer belt.
25 Remove the robe (if worn) and footwear.
26 Help the person lie down.

Post-Procedure

27 Provide for comfort. (See the inside of the back cover.)
28 Place the call light and other needed items within reach.
29 Raise or lower bed rails. Follow the care plan.
30 Arrange furniture to meet the person's needs.
31 Follow the care plan and the person's preferences for privacy measures to maintain. Leaving the privacy curtain, window coverings, and door open or closed are examples.

32 Complete a safety check of the room. (See the inside of the back cover.)
33 Practice hand hygiene.
34 Report and record your care and observations.

Transferring the Person To and From the Toilet

Using the bathroom for elimination promotes privacy, dignity, self-esteem, and independence. However, bathrooms are often small with little room for you or a wheelchair. Therefore transfers with wheelchairs and toilets are often hard. Falls and work-related injuries are risks.

Sometimes mechanical lifts (p. 224) are used for toilet transfers. The following procedure can be used if the person can stand and pivot from the wheelchair to the toilet.

See *Promoting Safety and Comfort: Transferring the Person To and From the Toilet.*

See procedure: *Transferring the Person To and From the Toilet.*

PROMOTING SAFETY AND COMFORT

Transferring the Person To and From the Toilet

Safety

Make sure the person has an elevated (raised) toilet seat. The toilet seat and wheelchair are at the same level.

Have the person use grab bars (Chapter 12). They are used to get on and off the toilet. Check that they are secure. If loose, tell the nurse. Do not transfer the person to the toilet if the grab bars are not secure.

Follow Standard Precautions. Wear gloves and practice hand hygiene as needed.

Transferring the Person To and From the Toilet

Quality of Life

- Knock before entering the person's room.
- Address the person by name.
- Introduce yourself by name and title.

- Explain the procedure before starting and during the procedure.
- Protect the person's rights during the procedure.
- Handle the person gently during the procedure.

Pre-Procedure

1 Follow *Delegation Guidelines: Transferring the Person,* p. 215.
  See *Promoting Safety and Comfort:*
  a *Transfer/Gait Belts* (Chapter 12)
  b *Transferring the Person,* p. 215
  c *Stand and Pivot Transfers,* p. 217
  d *Bed to Chair or Wheelchair Transfers,* p. 218
  e *Transferring the Person To and From the Toilet*

2 Practice hand hygiene and get the following supplies.
  • Transfer belt
  • Slip-resistant footwear (if not already on)
3 Provide for privacy.

Transferring the Person To and From the Toilet—cont'd

Procedure

4 Put slip-resistant footwear on the person.

5 Position the wheelchair next to the toilet if there is enough room. Or position the chair at a right angle (90-degree angle) to the toilet (Fig. 18-10). (See *Focus on Math: Fowler's Positions* in Chapter 16 to learn about angles.) It is best to have the person's strong side near the toilet.

6 Lock (brake) the wheelchair wheels.

7 Raise the footplates. Remove or swing front rigging out of the way.

8 Apply the transfer belt.

9 Help the person unfasten clothing.

10 Use the transfer belt to help the person stand and pivot (turn) to the toilet. (See procedure: *Transferring the Person From a Chair or Wheelchair to Bed*, p. 221.) The person uses the grab bars to pivot (turn) to the toilet.

11 Support the person with the transfer belt while he or she lowers clothing. Or have the person hold on to the grab bars for support. Lower the person's clothing.

12 Use the transfer belt to lower the person onto the toilet seat. Check for proper positioning on the toilet.

13 Remove the transfer belt.

14 Tell the person you will stay nearby. Remind the person to use the call light or call for you when help is needed. Stay with the person if required by the care plan.

15 Close the bathroom door for privacy.

16 Stay near the bathroom. Complete other tasks in the person's room. Check on the person every 5 minutes.

17 Knock on the bathroom door when the person calls for you.

18 Help with wiping, perineal care (Chapter 22), flushing, and hand-washing as needed. Wear gloves and practice hand hygiene after removing the gloves.

19 Apply the transfer belt.

20 Use the transfer belt to help the person stand.

21 Help the person raise and secure clothing as needed.

22 Use the transfer belt to transfer the person to the wheelchair. See procedure: *Transferring the Person to a Chair or Wheelchair*, p. 218.

23 Make sure the person's buttocks are to the back of the seat. Position the person in good alignment.

24 Position the feet on the footplates.

25 Remove the transfer belt.

26 Cover the lap and legs with a lap blanket. Keep the blanket off the floor and wheels.

27 Position the chair as the person prefers. Lock (brake) the wheelchair wheels according to the care plan.

Post-Procedure

28 Provide for comfort. (See the inside of the back cover.)

29 Place the call light and other needed items within reach.

30 Follow the care plan and the person's preferences for privacy measures to maintain. Leaving the privacy curtain, window coverings, and door open or closed are examples.

31 Complete a safety check of the room. (See the inside of the back cover.)

32 Practice hand hygiene.

33 Report and record your care and observations.

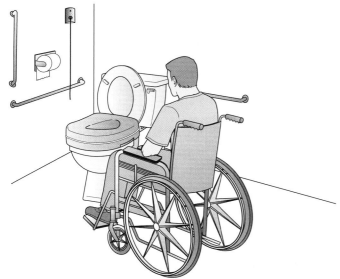

FIGURE 18-10 The wheelchair is at a right angle (90-degree angle) to the toilet.

LATERAL TRANSFERS

A *lateral transfer moves a person between 2 horizontal surfaces.* The person slides from 1 surface to the other. A transfer from a bed to a stretcher is an example.

Friction and shearing injure the skin (Chapter 17). Infection and pressure injuries can result (Chapter 36). Friction-reducing devices protect the skin during lateral transfers. They also protect staff from injury.

Lateral transfer devices to reduce friction include:

- Turning pads or turning sheets (Chapter 17)
- Slide sheets or other lateral sliding aids (lateral transfer devices) (Fig. 18-11, p. 224)
- Drawsheets (Chapter 20)
- Large re-usable waterproof under-pads (Chapter 20)

A transfer board (sliding board) (Fig. 18-12, p. 224) may be used for seated lateral transfers if:

- The person has upper body strength.
- The person has good sitting balance.
- There is enough room to position the 2 surfaces close together.

See *Promoting Safety and Comfort: Lateral Transfers*, p. 224.

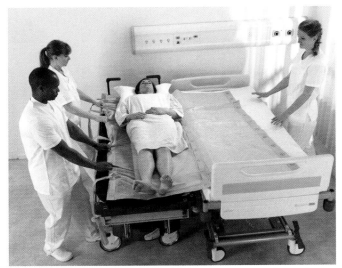

FIGURE 18-11 A slide sheet is used to transfer a person from a bed to a stretcher. (Image used with permission of Arjo Inc.)

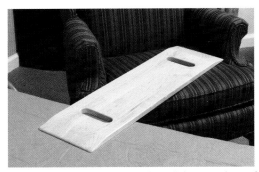

FIGURE 18-12 Transfer board (sliding board) for seated transfers to and from surfaces.

PROMOTING SAFETY AND COMFORT

Lateral Transfers

Safety

Protect yourself and the person from injury. Make sure you have enough help. At least 2 or 3 staff are needed to transfer to or from a stretcher (see Fig. 18-11). Practice good body mechanics and follow the guidelines for preventing work-related injuries (Chapter 16). Avoid extended reaches and bending your back.

Position the 2 surfaces as close as possible to each other. For a stretcher transfer, follow the rules for stretcher safety. See Box 18-1. Make sure the bed and stretcher wheels are locked (braked).

Follow the manufacturer's instructions for placing and using a lateral transfer device.

MECHANICAL LIFTS

Mechanical lifts are used for transfers to and from beds, chairs, wheelchairs, stretchers, tubs, shower chairs, toilets, commodes, whirlpools (tubs), or vehicles. They are used for persons who:
- Need weight-bearing support to transfer
- Cannot assist with transfers
- Are too heavy for staff to move

There are manual, battery-operated, and electric lifts. Two types are common.
- Stand-assist mechanical lifts (Fig. 18-13, *A* and Fig. 18-14, *A*)—for persons who require some help with transfers and can:
  - Bear (support) some weight.
  - Follow directions.
  - Sit on the side of the bed with or without help.
  - Bend the hips, knees, and ankles.
- Full-sling mechanical lifts (Fig. 18-13, *B* and Fig. 18-14, *B*)—for persons who:
  - Cannot assist with transfers.
  - Are partially able or unable to bear (support) weight.
  - Are heavy.
  - Have physical limits preventing other types of transfers.

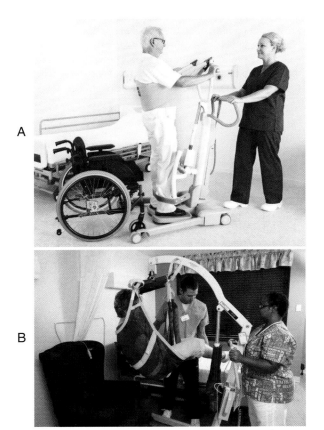

FIGURE 18-13 **A,** A stand-assist mechanical lift supports the upper body. **B,** A full-sling mechanical lift supports the entire body. (A, Used with permission of Arjo Inc.)

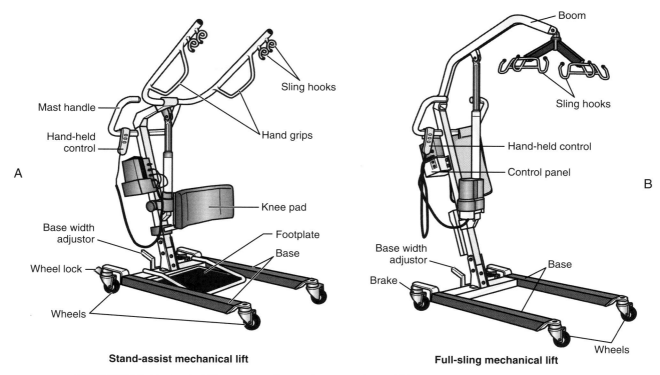

A

Sling hooks

Mast handle

Hand grips

Hand-held control

Knee pad

Base width adjustor

Footplate

Base

Wheel lock

Wheels

Stand-assist mechanical lift

Boom

Sling hooks

Hand-held control

Control panel

B

Base width adjustor

Base

Brake

Wheels

Full-sling mechanical lift

FIGURE 18-14 Mechanical lifts. **A,** Parts of a stand-assist mechanical lift. **B,** Parts of a full-sling mechanical lift.

Slings

The sling used depends on the lift type and the person's size, condition, and care needs. Slings are padded, unpadded, or made of mesh. Stand-assist slings support the upper body (see Fig. 18-13, *A*). Full-slings support the entire body (see Fig. 18-13, *B*). There are many types of full-slings.

- *Standard full-sling*—for normal transfers (Fig. 18-15).
- *Bathing sling*—for transfers from the bed or chair into a bathtub. Depending on the manufacturer's instructions, the sling may be left in place and attached to the lift during the bath.
- *Toileting sling*—the sling bottom is open.
- *Amputee sling*—for the person who has had both legs amputated.
- *Bariatric sling*—for use with a bariatric lift.

The nurse and care plan tell you what type and size sling to use. You must use a sling designed for use with the mechanical lift. Follow agency policy and the manufacturer's instructions for using slings and washing contaminated slings. A sling is contaminated if it:

- Has any visible sign of blood or body fluids.
- Is used on a person's bare skin.
- Is used to bathe a person.

▲ Using a Mechanical Lift

Before using a lift:

- You must be trained in its use.
- It must work.
- The sling, straps, hooks, or chains must be in good repair.
- The person's weight must not exceed the lift's capacity.
- You need enough help. At least 2 staff members are needed for most lifts. Follow agency policy and the person's care plan.

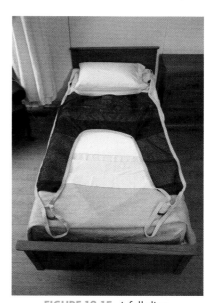

FIGURE 18-15 A full-sling.

There are different types of mechanical lifts. Always follow the manufacturer's instructions. The procedures that follow are used as a guide.

See *Delegation Guidelines: Using a Mechanical Lift*, p. 226.

See *Promoting Safety and Comfort: Using a Mechanical Lift*, p. 226.

See procedure: *Transferring the Person Using a Stand-Assist Mechanical Lift*, p. 226.

See procedure: *Transferring the Person Using a Full-Sling Mechanical Lift*, p. 228.

DELEGATION GUIDELINES

Using a Mechanical Lift

Before using a mechanical lift, you need the information in *Delegation Guidelines: Transferring the Person*, p. 215. You also need the following information from the nurse and the care plan.

- What lift to use—stand-assist mechanical lift or full-sling mechanical lift
- The lift's weight limit. Do not exceed the lift's weight limit.

- What type of sling to use.
- What size sling to use.
- If you need to apply an abdominal binder (Chapter 35). For the person with bariatric needs, an abdominal binder may be needed.

PROMOTING SAFETY AND COMFORT

Using a Mechanical Lift

Safety

Always follow the manufacturer's instructions. Knowing how to use 1 lift does not mean that you know how to use others. If you have not used a certain lift before, ask for training. Ask the nurse to help you until you are comfortable using the lift.

The lift's base widens (opens). The base closes (narrows) to fit under the bed and move through narrow areas. The lift is most stable with the base in the wide (open) position. Position the base in the wide (open) position when lifting, lowering, and moving when possible. If you must close (narrow) the base, do so briefly. Return the base to the wide (open) position as soon as possible.

For many lifts, the wheels are unlocked during lifting and lowering. This allows the lift to stabilize (become steady). For some stand-assist lifts, the wheels are locked (braked) when lifting and lowering. Follow the manufacturer's instructions for when to lock (brake) the lift's wheels. Bed and wheelchair wheels must be locked (braked).

Mechanical lifts must work correctly. Battery-powered lifts must have well-charged batteries. Tell the nurse when a lift needs repair or does not work properly.

One or 2 staff members are needed for a stand-assist mechanical lift. Follow the manufacturer's instructions and agency policy. Two staff members are needed to safely use a full-sling mechanical lift. Federal guidelines require that at least 1 staff member be 18 years of age or older.

Always stay with the person when using a mechanical lift. Never leave the person unattended (alone) in the lift.

Floor thresholds, uneven floor surfaces, and thick carpets can cause:

- Difficulty rolling the lift
- Imbalance of the lift
- More exertion (work) for staff

Use the handles to move the lift. Do not push on other parts of the lift. This may cause the lift to tilt.

Comfort

The person is lifted up and off the bed or chair. Falling is a common fear. For mental comfort, always explain the procedure before you begin. Also show the person how the lift works.

Transferring the Person Using a Stand-Assist Mechanical Lift

Quality of Life

- Knock before entering the person's room.
- Address the person by name.
- Introduce yourself by name and title.

- Explain the procedure before starting and during the procedure.
- Protect the person's rights during the procedure.
- Handle the person gently during the procedure.

Pre-Procedure

1 Follow *Delegation Guidelines:*
   a *Transferring the Person*, p. 215
   b *Using a Mechanical Lift*
   See *Promoting Safety and Comfort:*
   a *Transferring the Person*, p. 215
   b *Using a Mechanical Lift*
2 Ask a co-worker to help you (if needed).
3 Practice hand hygiene and get the following supplies.
   - Stand-assist mechanical lift and sling
   - Arm chair or wheelchair

- Slip-resistant footwear
- Bath blanket or cushion (if needed)
- Lap blanket (if used)
4 Arrange items in the person's room.
5 Practice hand hygiene.
6 Identify the person. Check the ID bracelet against the assignment sheet. Use 2 identifiers (Chapter 11). Also call the person by name.
7 Provide for privacy.

Procedure

8 Place the chair (wheelchair) at the head of the bed. It is even with the head-board and about 1 foot away from the bed. Lock (brake) the wheelchair wheels. Place a folded bath blanket or cushion in the seat if needed.

9 Assist the person to a seated position on the side of the bed. See procedure: *Sitting on the Side of the Bed (Dangling)* in Chapter 17. The person's feet are flat on the floor. Bed wheels are locked.
10 Put footwear on the person.

Transferring the Person Using a Stand-Assist Mechanical Lift—cont'd

Procedure—cont'd

11 Apply the sling.
  a Position the sling at the lower back.
  b Bring the straps around to the front of the chest. The straps are positioned under the arms.
  c Secure the waist belt around the person's waist. Adjust the belt so it is snug but not tight.
12 Position the lift in front of the person.
13 Widen the lift's base.
14 Lock (brake) the lift's wheels.
15 Have the person place the feet on the footplate and the knees against the knee pad. Assist as needed. If the lift has a knee strap, secure the strap around the legs. Adjust the strap so it is snug but not tight.
16 Attach the sling to the sling hooks.
17 Have the person grasp the lift's hand grips.
18 Unlock the lift's wheels (release the brakes) following the manufacturer's instructions.
19 Raise the person slightly off the bed. Check that the sling is secure, the feet are on the footplate, and the knees are against the knee pad (Fig. 18-16, A). If not, lower the person and correct the problem.

20 Raise the lift until the person is clear of the bed (Fig. 18-16, B). Or raise the person to a standing position (Fig. 18-16, C). Follow the care plan.
21 Adjust the base's width to move from the bed to the chair (wheelchair) if needed. Keep the base in the wide (open) position as much as possible.
22 Move the lift to the chair (wheelchair). The person's back is toward the seat.
23 Lower the person into the chair (wheelchair). Guide the person into the seat. See Figure 18-16, D and E.
24 Lock (brake) the lift's wheels following the manufacturer's instructions.
25 Unhook the sling from the sling hooks.
26 Unbuckle the waist belt. Remove the sling.
27 Unlock the lift's wheels (release the brakes).
28 Have the person lift the feet off of the footplate. Assist as needed. Move the lift. Position the feet flat on the floor or on the wheelchair footplates.
29 Cover the lap and legs with a lap blanket (if used). Keep it off the floor.

Post-Procedure

30 Provide for comfort. (See the inside of the back cover.)
31 Place the call light and other needed items within reach.
32 Follow the care plan and the person's preferences for privacy measures to maintain. Leaving the privacy curtain, window coverings, and door open or closed are examples.

33 Complete a safety check of the room. (See the inside of the back cover.)
34 Practice hand hygiene.
35 Report and record your care and observations.
36 Reverse the procedure to return the person to bed.

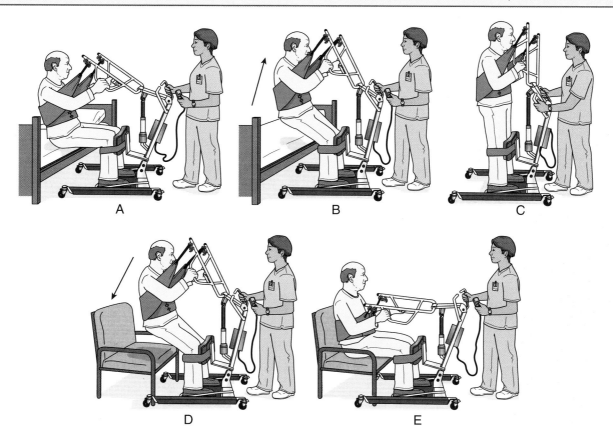

FIGURE 18-16 Using a stand-assist mechanical lift. A, The sling is around the person's lower back. The straps are under the arms. The waist belt is secure. Feet are on the footplate. The person holds the hand grips. B, The lift is raised. C, The person is in a standing position. D, The person is lowered into the chair. E, The person is seated. The back is against the back of the chair.

Transferring the Person Using a Full-Sling Mechanical Lift

Quality of Life

- Knock before entering the person's room.
- Address the person by name.
- Introduce yourself by name and title.

- Explain the procedure before starting and during the procedure.
- Protect the person's rights during the procedure.
- Handle the person gently during the procedure.

Pre-Procedure

1 Follow *Delegation Guidelines:*
  a *Transferring the Person*, p. 215
  b *Using a Mechanical Lift*, p. 226
  See *Promoting Safety and Comfort:*
  a *Transferring the Person*, p. 215
  b *Using a Mechanical Lift*, p. 226
2 Ask a co-worker to help you.
3 Practice hand hygiene and get the following supplies.
  - Full-sling mechanical lift and sling
  - Arm chair or wheelchair

  - Footwear
  - Bath blanket or cushion (if needed)
  - Lap blanket (if used)
4 Arrange items in the person's room.
5 Practice hand hygiene.
6 Identify the person. Check the ID bracelet against the assignment sheet. Use 2 identifiers (Chapter 11). Also call the person by name.
7 Provide for privacy.
8 Raise the bed for body mechanics. Bed rails are up if used.

Procedure

9 Lower the head of the bed to a level appropriate for the person. It is as flat as possible.
10 Stand on 1 side of the bed. Your co-worker stands on the other side.
11 Lower the bed rails if up. Lock (brake) the bed wheels.
12 Center the sling under the person (Fig. 18-17, *A*). To position the sling, turn the person from side to side (Chapter 17). Follow the manufacturer's instructions to position the sling.
13 Position the person in the semi-Fowler's position.
14 Place the chair (wheelchair) at the head of the bed. It is even with the head-board and about 1 foot away from the bed. Place a folded bath blanket or cushion in the seat if needed. Lock (brake) the wheelchair wheels.
15 Lower the bed so it is level with the chair.
16 Raise the lift to position it over the person.
17 Position the lift over the person (Fig. 18-17, *B*).
18 Widen the lift's base. Lock (brake) the lift wheels.
19 Attach the sling to the sling hooks (Fig. 18-17, *C*).
20 Raise the head of the bed to a comfortable level for the person.
21 Cross the person's arms over the chest.
22 Unlock the lift's wheels (release the brakes) following the manufacturer's instructions.
23 Raise the person slightly from the bed. Check that the sling is secure. If not, lower the person and correct the problem.

24 Raise the lift until the person and sling are free of the bed (Fig. 18-17, *D*).
25 Have your co-worker support the person's legs as you move the lift and the person away from the bed (Fig. 18-17, *E*).
26 Adjust the base's width to move from the bed to the chair (wheelchair) if needed. Keep the base in the wide (open) position as much as possible.
27 Position the lift so the person's back is toward the chair (wheelchair).
28 Adjust the position of the chair (wheelchair) as needed to lower the person into it. Lock (brake) the wheelchair wheels.
29 Lower the person into the chair (wheelchair). Guide the person into the seat (Fig. 18-17, *F*).
30 Lock (brake) the lift wheels following the manufacturer's instructions.
31 Unhook the sling. Unlock the lift's wheels (release the brakes). Move the lift away from the person. Remove the sling from under the person unless otherwise indicated.
32 Put footwear on the person. Position the feet flat on the floor or on the wheelchair footplates.
33 Cover the lap and legs with a lap blanket (if used). Keep it off the floor and wheels.
34 Position the chair (wheelchair) as the person prefers. Lock (brake) the wheelchair wheels according to the care plan.

Post-Procedure

35 Provide for comfort. (See the inside of the back cover.)
36 Place the call light and other needed items within reach.
37 Follow the care plan and the person's preferences for privacy measures to maintain. Leaving the privacy curtain, window coverings, and door open or closed are examples.
38 Complete a safety check of the room. (See the inside of the back cover.)
39 Practice hand hygiene.
40 Report and record your care and observations.

41 Reverse the procedure to return the person to bed. Follow the manufacturer's instructions to position a sling on a person seated in a chair or wheelchair. The following method is common.
  a Have the person lean forward. Have your co-worker help the person if needed.
  b Slide the sling behind the person's back. Tuck the sling down along the back to the seat of the chair or wheelchair.
  c Bring the leg straps around the sides of the person. The straps are at the sides of the legs.
  d Pass the leg straps under the legs.

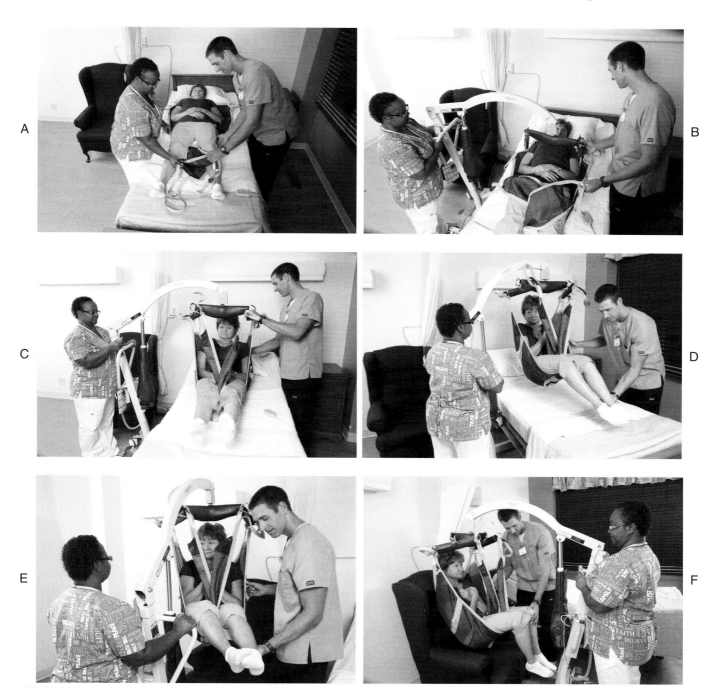

FIGURE 18-17 Using a full-sling mechanical lift. **A,** The sling is positioned under the person. **B,** The lift is over the person. **C,** The sling is attached to the lift. **D,** The lift is raised until the sling and person are off the bed. **E,** The legs are supported. The person and lift are moved away from the bed. **F,** The person is guided into a chair.

FOCUS ON P R I D E

The Person, Family, and Yourself

P ersonal and Professional Responsibility

Take time to plan and prepare for a transfer. Gather needed items. Organize the room and equipment. Remember to:

- Position the chair, wheelchair, stretcher, and so on for a safe transfer. Lock (brake) wheels.
- Remove wheelchair front rigging or swing it out of the way. Raise the footplates.
- Adjust the bed to a safe and comfortable height.
- Make sure a mechanical lift is charged.
- Move furniture or clutter out of the way.

R ights and Respect

Respect privacy during transfers. Close privacy curtains, doors, and window coverings. Properly cover the person. For example, a patient gown opens in the back. Apply a robe or another gown to cover the person's backside. Use a covering that is safe for transfers.

I ndependence and Social Interaction

How you speak to the person makes a difference. To give directions:

- Speak slowly and clearly.
- Talk loudly enough for the person to hear you.
- Speak calmly and kindly. Never yell at or insult the person.
- Face the person and use eye contact when possible.
- Give 1 direction at a time.
- Repeat directions as needed. Be patient.
- Ask if the person has questions before proceeding.
  Your speech and tone must convey dignity. Show you value the person through respectful interactions.

D elegation and Teamwork

You need help to transfer a person. Your co-workers are busy. Do you ask for help? Or do you try to move the person alone? Never be afraid to ask for help. Ask politely and say thank you. Work as a team for the person's safety and to protect yourself and others from injury.

E thics and Laws

The right way to transfer is not always the quickest way. Do not pull on the person's clothing or arm, underarm, or other body part. Choose to give care correctly. Take pride in giving care in a way that prevents harm and promotes comfort and safety.

FOCUS ON PRIDE: *Application*

Explaining procedures improves with practice. Practice explaining a transfer from the bed to a chair using:

- A stand and pivot transfer
- A stand-assist mechanical lift
- A full-sling mechanical lift

Circle the BEST answer.

1 To promote comfort during a transfer
   a Pull the person to a standing position
   b Explain the procedure
   c Let the person choose the procedure
   d Open the privacy curtain

2 For a safe transfer to a chair
   a Tell the person to grasp you around your neck
   b Hold the person under the underarms
   c Manually lift the person
   d Move furniture and equipment as needed

3 You are preparing to transfer a person. Which statement promotes comfort?
   a "I will move you quickly. The pain will be brief."
   b "I can leave the door open. This will not take long."
   c "Please tell me to stop if you feel pain."
   d "I'm nervous. I don't want to drop you."

4 A person uses a wheelchair. Which measure is *unsafe*?
   a The wheels are locked (braked) for transfers.
   b The chair is pulled backward for transport.
   c The feet are positioned on the footplates.
   d The casters point forward.

5 To use a stretcher safely
   a Lock (brake) the wheels for transfers to and from the stretcher
   b Transfer a person to a stretcher without help
   c Lower the side rails during a transport
   d Move the stretcher head first

6 A stand and pivot transfer is *unsafe* for a person who
   a Is hard of hearing but can follow directions
   b Can bear (support) some weight with the legs
   c Is confused and combative
   d Uses a transfer belt

7 A person has a weak side. For transfers,
   a The strong side moves first
   b The weak side moves first
   c Pillows are used for support
   d A transfer belt is not used

8 Which is *unsafe* for a stand and pivot transfer to a wheelchair?
   a The wheelchair's front rigging is removed.
   b The person's feet are flat on the floor.
   c The person is wearing slip-resistant footwear.
   d The wheelchair is behind you.

9 To transfer a person from a wheelchair to a toilet
   a Position the wheelchair facing the toilet
   b Remove the transfer belt when lowering clothing
   c Have the person hold on to the grab bar for support
   d Keep the bathroom door open

10 Which is used for a lateral transfer from a bed to a stretcher?
    a Slide sheet
    b Transfer belt
    c Stand-assist mechanical lift
    d Grab bar

11 When using a mechanical lift
    a Position the lift on the person's strong side
    b Collect a battery and transfer belt
    c Compare the person's weight to the lift's weight limit
    d Allow the person to control the lift

12 For a safe transfer with a full-sling mechanical lift, at least
    a 1 worker is needed
    b 2 workers are needed
    c 3 workers are needed
    d 4 workers are needed

13 You are using a stand-assist mechanical lift. Which is *unsafe*?
    a The person is holding the lift's hand grips.
    b The person's feet are on the footplate.
    c The lift's base is narrow when lifting.
    d The person's knees are against the knee pad.

14 After a transfer, which should you do *first*?
    a Report to the nurse.
    b Return the mechanical lift to the storage area.
    c Record the procedure.
    d Place the call light within reach.

Answers to Chapter 18 questions are on p. 588.

FOCUS ON **PRACTICE**

Problem Solving

You are preparing to transfer a resident using a stand and pivot transfer. Today the person is weaker than usual and unsteady. The person cannot bear (support) weight with the legs. What will you do?

19

The Person's Unit

- Define the key terms and key abbreviations in this chapter.
- Explain how to maintain the person's unit.
- Describe how to control the person's setting for comfort.
- Describe the basic bed positions.
- Identify the 7 hospital bed system entrapment zones.
- Identify the persons at risk for bed entrapment.

- Explain how to use the furniture and equipment in the person's unit.
- Explain how to safely use the call system.
- Describe how to promote safety, privacy, and comfort in the person's unit.
- Explain how to promote PRIDE in the person, the family, and yourself.

admission The official entry of a person into a health care setting
entrapment Getting caught, trapped, or entangled in spaces created by the bed rails, the mattress, the bed frame, the head-board, or the foot-board

full visual privacy Having the means to be completely free from public view while in bed
person's unit The space, furniture, and equipment used by the person in the agency

CMS	Centers for Medicare & Medicaid Services	**F**	Fahrenheit

The ***person's unit*** *is the space, furniture, and equipment used by the person in the agency* (Fig. 19-1). The person's unit is designed for comfort, safety, and privacy. In nursing centers, the person's unit is as personal and home-like as possible. Always treat the person's unit with respect.

A private room is for 1 person. Semi-private rooms have 2 units. Some rooms have 3 or 4 units.

The person's unit is kept clean, neat, safe, and comfortable. See Box 19-1.

See *Promoting Safety and Comfort: The Person's Unit.*

232

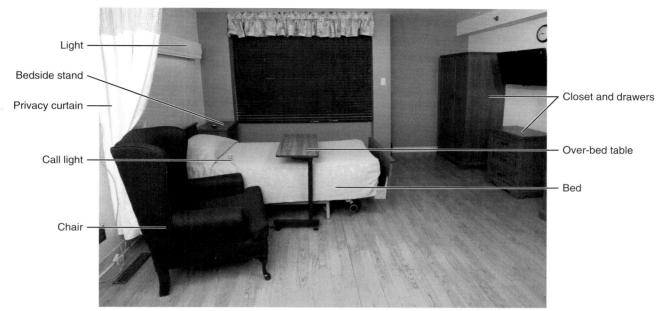

FIGURE 19-1   Furniture and equipment in a resident's unit.

BOX 19-1 Maintaining the Person's Unit

- Keep the following within the person's reach.
  - Call light (p. 240). *The call light is within reach at all times.*
  - Over-bed table and bedside stand (p. 239).
  - Phone, TV, bed, and light controls.
  - Tissues.
  - Other items as requested.
- Meet the needs of persons who cannot use the call system (p. 240).
- Adjust lighting, temperature, and ventilation for the person's comfort.
- Handle equipment carefully to prevent noise.
- Explain the causes of strange noises.
- Prevent odors. See p. 235.
- Use room deodorizers according to agency policy.
- Empty wastebaskets at least daily and when full. In some agencies, they are emptied every shift.
- Arrange personal items as the person prefers.
- Respect the person's belongings. An item may not be important to you. Yet even a scrap of paper can have great meaning to the person.
- Do not discard any items belonging to the person.
- Do not move furniture or the person's belongings. Persons with poor vision rely on memory or feel to find items.
- Straighten bed linens and towels as often as needed.
- Complete a safety check before leaving the room. (See the inside of the back cover.)

PROMOTING SAFETY AND COMFORT

The Person's Unit

Comfort

Admission *is the official entry of a person into a health care setting.* On admission to an agency, the nurse may have you orient the person and family to the area.

- Identify items in the person's unit. Explain the purpose of each.
- Explain how to use room furniture and equipment (p. 235).
  - Over-bed table
  - Call light
  - Bed, TV, and light controls
- Show the person the bathroom. Explain how to use the call light in the bathroom (p. 241).
- Explain how to use the agency's phone. Place the phone within reach.
- Explain how to connect to the Internet and show where to charge electronic devices.
- Explain where to find the nurses' station, lounge, chapel, dining room, and other areas.
- Identify staff—housekeeping, dietary, physical therapy, and others. Also identify students who are in the agency.
- Explain when meals and snacks are served.
- Explain visiting hours and policies.

Do not rush. Treat the person and family as guests. Be polite. Tell them good things about the agency. Introduce other nurses and nursing assistants. Help the person adjust to a new setting.

COMFORT

Comfort is a state of well-being (Chapter 33). Age, illness, and activity affect comfort. So do temperature, ventilation, noise, odors, and lighting. These factors are controlled to meet the person's needs.

See *Focus on Communication: Comfort.*

FOCUS ON COMMUNICATION

Comfort

What is comfortable for 1 person may not be for another. Ask about the person's comfort. You can say:
- "How is the temperature? Is it too hot or too cold?"
- "Is the noise level okay?"
- "Please let me know if you notice any bad odors."
- "How is the lighting? Is it too bright or too dark?"
- "Are you comfortable?"

Temperature and Ventilation

Most healthy people are comfortable with room temperatures between 68°F (Fahrenheit) and 74°F. This range may be too hot or too cold for others. Persons who are older or ill may need higher temperatures for comfort.

The Centers for Medicare & Medicaid Services (CMS) requires that nursing centers maintain a temperature of 71°F to 81°F. To protect patients and residents from cool areas and drafts:
- Have them wear enough of the correct clothing.
- Offer lap coverings (blankets, throws) to those in chairs and wheelchairs to cover the legs.
- Provide enough blankets for warmth.
- Cover them with bath blankets (Chapter 20) when giving care. A bath blanket provides warmth and privacy during care measures.
- Move them from drafty areas.
  See *Focus on Older Persons: Temperature and Ventilation.*

FOCUS ON OLDER PERSONS

Temperature and Ventilation

Poor circulation and loss of the skin's fatty tissue layer occur with aging. Therefore older persons are sensitive to cold (Chapter 10). They may wear extra clothing for warmth. Many wear sweaters or jackets in warm weather. Respect the person's wishes and choices.

Noise

According to the CMS, a "comfortable" sound level:
- Does not interfere with a person's hearing.
- Promotes privacy when privacy is desired.
- Allows the person to take part in social activities.

Common health care sounds can be disturbing. Examples include:
- Clanging and clattering equipment, dishes, and meal trays
- Loud voices, TVs, music, and so on
- Ringing phones
- Intercom systems and call lights
- Equipment or wheels needing repair or oil
- Cleaning and housekeeping equipment
  To decrease noise levels:
- Control your voice.
- Handle equipment carefully.
- Keep equipment in good working order.
- Answer phones, call lights, and intercoms promptly.
  See *Focus on Communication: Noise.*
  See *Focus on Older Persons: Noise.*
  See *Focus on Surveys: Noise.*

FOCUS ON COMMUNICATION

Noise

All staff must try to reduce noise. To reduce noise:
- Do not talk loudly in the hallways or nurses' station.
- Ask others to speak more softly if necessary. Ask politely.
- Avoid unnecessary conversation. Be professional. Do not discuss inappropriate topics at work. Others may over-hear and become offended.

FOCUS ON OLDER PERSONS

Noise

Persons with dementia may not understand what is happening around them. Common, every-day sounds can disturb them. For example, a person has an extreme reaction to a ring tone on a phone (Chapter 42). The reaction may be more severe at night. This is likely if the sound startles or suddenly awakens the person. A dark, strange room can make the problem worse.

FOCUS ON SURVEYS

Noise

Surveyors will observe for comfortable sound levels.
- Do background noises affect the person's ability to be heard or take part in activities?
- Do staff raise their voices to be heard?
- Are sound levels comfortable in the evening and during the night? Do your best to decrease noise and provide comfortable sound levels.

Odors

Odors occur in health care settings. To reduce odors:
- Empty, clean, and disinfect bedpans, urinals, commodes, and kidney basins promptly.
- Make sure toilets are flushed.
- Check incontinent persons often (Chapters 25 and 27).
- Clean persons who are wet or soiled from urine, feces (stools), vomitus, or wound drainage.
- Change wet or soiled linens and clothing promptly.
- Follow agency policy for where to place wet or soiled linens and clothing.
- Keep laundry containers closed.
- Dispose of incontinence and ostomy products promptly (Chapters 25 and 27).
- Provide good hygiene to prevent body and breath odors (Chapters 21 and 22).
- Use room deodorizers as needed and allowed by agency policy. Do not use sprays around persons with breathing problems. Ask the nurse if you are unsure.

Smoke odors present special problems. If you smoke, follow the agency's policy. Practice hand-washing after smoking, after handling smoking materials, and before giving care. Pay attention to your uniform, hair, and breath because of smoke odors.

Lighting

Safe and comfortable lighting:
- Lessens glares.
- Lets the person control the brightness, location, and direction of light.
- Lets visually impaired persons maintain or increase independent functioning.

Glares, shadows, and dull lighting can cause falls, headaches, and eyestrain. A bright room is cheerful. Dim light is better for relaxing and rest.

Adjust window coverings and lighting to meet the person's needs. The over-bed and ceiling lights provide soft, medium, or bright lighting. Always keep light controls within the person's reach. This protects the right to personal choice.

See *Focus on Older Persons: Lighting.*

FOCUS ON **OLDER PERSONS**

Lighting

Persons with dementia may become agitated or aggressive at times. There is often a reason for the reaction (Chapter 42). Lighting may be a factor. Adjust lighting for the person's needs. Soft, non-glare lights are relaxing. Brighter lighting lets the person see more clearly. This may improve orientation.

ROOM FURNITURE AND EQUIPMENT

Rooms are furnished and equipped for safety and to meet basic needs—comfort, sleep, elimination, nutrition, hygiene, and activity. There is equipment to communicate with staff. The right to privacy is considered.

The Bed

Beds have controls to:
- Raise and lower the whole bed (Fig. 19-2).
  - The bed is raised to give care and reduce bending and reaching.
  - The bed is lowered to let the person get out of bed with ease and to prevent injury from falls.
- Adjust the head and foot of the bed for comfort. The person is told of any position limits or restrictions. For example, lowering the head of the bed fully causes shortness of breath *(dyspnea)*. The care plan includes keeping the head of the bed raised at least 30 degrees.

Beds are manual or electric. Manual beds are controlled with cranks at the foot of the bed (Fig. 19-3, p. 236). The cranks are turned to raise and lower the whole bed or the head or foot of the bed. Electric beds are controlled with buttons. Electric beds are common.

Electric controls may be hand-held or on the bed rail (Fig. 19-4, p. 236). Sometimes controls are on the footboard. Some beds have pedals near the floor that can be controlled with the foot.

A
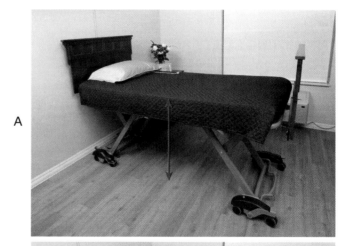

B
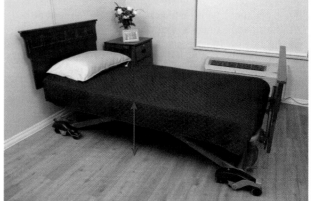

FIGURE 19-2 A, The bed is in a high position. **B,** The bed is in a low position.

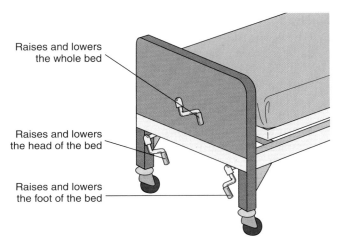

Raises and lowers the whole bed

Raises and lowers the head of the bed

Raises and lowers the foot of the bed

FIGURE 19-3 A manual bed has cranks at the foot of the bed.

Bed rail controls are often different on the inner and outer parts of the bed rail.

- Controls on the inner part are for patient or resident use (see Fig. 19-4, *B*). These controls are limited. This prevents the person from placing the bed in a dangerous position.
- Controls on the outer part are for staff use (see Fig. 19-4, *C*). These control all of the bed's functions. See *Promoting Safety and Comfort: The Bed.*

PROMOTING SAFETY AND COMFORT

The Bed

Safety

Most electric beds lock into any position. The person cannot adjust the bed to unsafe positions. Beds may be locked for persons:

- Restricted to certain positions
- With confusion or dementia

Bed wheels (Chapter 12) are locked (braked) at all times except when moving the bed. They must be locked to:

- Give bedside care.
- Transfer the person to and from the bed. The person can be injured if the bed moves. You could be injured too.

If using a manual bed, the cranks are pulled up for use. Cranks in the "up" position are safety hazards. Anyone walking past may bump into them. Return cranks to the "down" position after use.

Many people touch bed controls. Plan your care and use careful judgment to prevent the transmission of microbes to the person and others. Follow the guidelines for hand hygiene in Chapter 14. Remember to:

- Practice hand hygiene *before* tasks involving contact with mucous membranes, non-intact skin, or invasive medical devices. (Hand hygiene occurs just before the task, after contact with bed controls.)
- Practice hand hygiene *after* tasks that expose the hands to blood or body fluids. (Hand hygiene occurs before contact with bed controls.)

Comfort

Adjust the bed to meet the person's needs. Tell the nurse if the person complains about the bed or mattress.

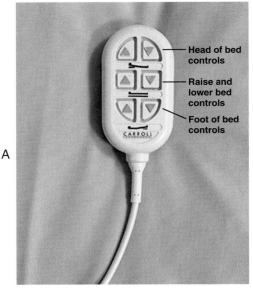

Head of bed controls

Raise and lower bed controls

Foot of bed controls

A

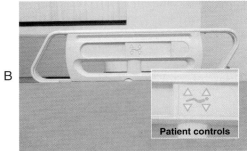

B

Patient controls

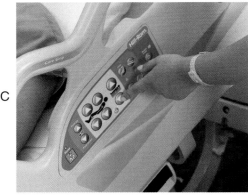

C

FIGURE 19-4 Electric bed controls. **A,** A hand-held bed control. **B,** Bed controls on the inner part of a bed rail. **C,** Bed controls on the outer part of a bed rail. (C, Courtesy © Hill-Rom Services, Inc. Reprinted with permission. All rights reserved.)

Bed Positions. The bed is often positioned flat for sleeping. The basic bed positions in Table 19-1 may be used for comfort or to treat a health problem. See Chapter 16 for proper alignment and positioning.

Some beds are able to convert into a chair position. See "Bariatric Beds" on p. 239.

TABLE 19-1 Bed Positions

Position	Description	Example
Semi-Fowler's position	The head of the bed is raised 30 degrees. In some agencies, the knee (foot) portion is also raised 15 degrees.	30°
Fowler's position	The head of the bed is raised 45 to 60 degrees.	45°
High-Fowler's position	The head of the bed is raised 60 to 90 degrees.	90°
Trendelenburg's position	The head of the bed is lowered. The foot of the bed is raised. The bed frame is tilted. A doctor orders this position.	
Reverse Trendelenburg's position	The head of the bed is raised. The foot of the bed is lowered. The bed frame is tilted. A doctor orders this position.	

Bed Safety. Bed safety involves the *hospital bed system*—the bed frame and its parts. The parts include the mattress, bed rails, head- and foot-boards, and bed attachments.

Hospital bed systems have 7 entrapment zones (Fig. 19-5). *Entrapment means getting caught, trapped, or entangled in spaces created by the bed rails, the mattress, the bed frame, the head-board, or the foot-board.* Head, neck, or chest entrapment can cause serious injuries and death. Arm and leg entrapment also can occur.

Persons at greatest risk for entrapment:
- Are older.
- Are frail.
- Are confused or disoriented.
- Are restless.
- Have uncontrolled body movements.
- Have poor muscle control.
- Are small in size.
- Are restrained (Chapter 13).

Always check the person for entrapment. If a person is caught, trapped, or entangled in the bed or any of its parts, try to release the person. Also call for the nurse at once.

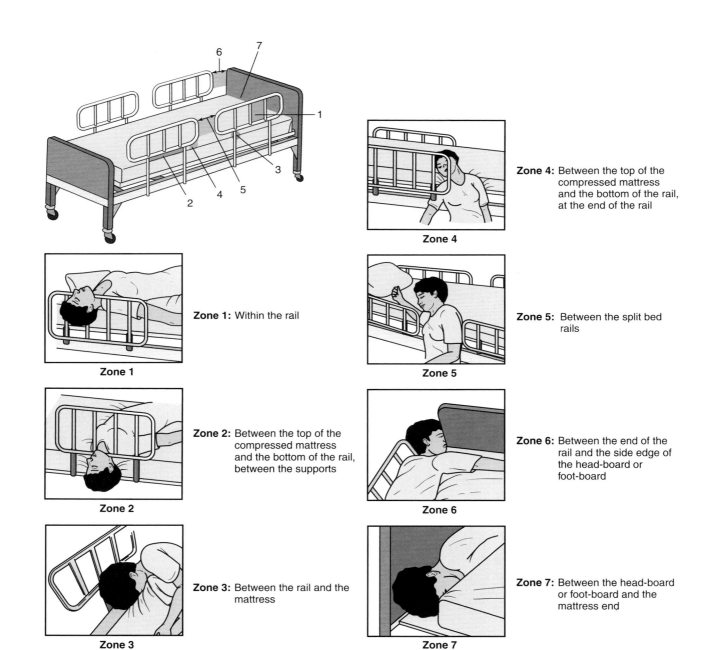

Zone 1: Within the rail

Zone 2: Between the top of the compressed mattress and the bottom of the rail, between the supports

Zone 3: Between the rail and the mattress

Zone 4: Between the top of the compressed mattress and the bottom of the rail, at the end of the rail

Zone 5: Between the split bed rails

Zone 6: Between the end of the rail and the side edge of the head-board or foot-board

Zone 7: Between the head-board or foot-board and the mattress end

FIGURE 19-5 Hospital bed system entrapment zones. (Redrawn from Food and Drug Administration: *Hospital bed system dimensional and assessment guidance to reduce entrapment,* March 10, 2006, content current as of August 23, 2018.)

Bed Rails. Bed rails are discussed in Chapter 12. Not all beds have bed rails. Not all persons use bed rails. Risk of entrapment and injury trying to exit the bed are hazards for some persons. If they prevent the person from exiting the bed, bed rails are considered restraints (Chapter 13). Use of bed rails must be in the person's best interest.

A lever, latch, or button releases the rail from the locked position to lower and raise the rail. Know how to use your agency's bed rails. Follow the safety measures in Chapter 12 for persons who use bed rails.

Bariatric Beds. Bariatric beds have a weight capacity from 500 to 1000 pounds (Fig. 19-6). Some bed frames adjust (shorten or lengthen) for the person's height. Bariatric beds vary depending on the model. Follow the manufacturer's instructions for safe use.

See *Focus on Communication: Bariatric Beds.*

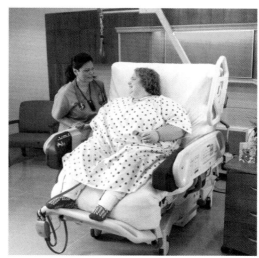

FIGURE 19-6 Bariatric bed converted to a chair. (Courtesy © Hill-Rom Services, Inc. Reprinted with permission. All rights reserved.)

FOCUS ON **COMMUNICATION**

Bariatric Beds

Comments about weight or size may offend some persons. Use other words. For example, do not say: "The nurse is getting a bed big enough for you." Instead, you can say: "The nurse is getting a bed that will be comfortable for you."

Be aware of your verbal and nonverbal communication. Your words and actions must show dignity and respect.

Over-Bed Tables and Bedside Stands

The over-bed table (Fig. 19-7) is moved over the bed by sliding the base under the bed. The table is raised or lowered for bed or chair use and to prevent bending when used as a work surface. Use the handle, crank, or lever to adjust the table's height.

The person uses the over-bed table for meals, writing, reading, and other activities. The nursing team uses the over-bed table as a work area.

The bedside stand is used for personal items and personal care equipment (Fig. 19-8).

- Stand top—used for tissues, clock, photos, phone, flowers, cards, and so on.
- Top drawer—used for eyeglass case, books, kidney basin (p. 240) with oral hygiene items.
- Middle drawer or shelf—stores the wash basin with personal care items (soap, lotion, washcloth and towels, and so on).
- Bottom drawer or lower shelf—stores the bedpan, urinal, and toilet paper.

Place only clean and sterile items on the over-bed table and bedside stand. Never place bedpans, urinals, or soiled linens on the top. Clean the over-bed table or bedside stand after use as a work surface. Clean the over-bed table before serving meal trays and after removing them.

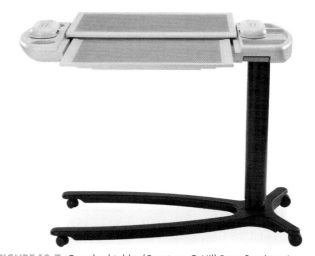

FIGURE 19-7 Over-bed table. (Courtesy © Hill-Rom Services, Inc. Reprinted with permission. All rights reserved.)

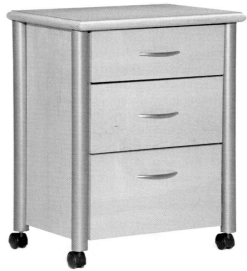

FIGURE 19-8 The bedside stand. (Courtesy © Hill-Rom Services, Inc. Reprinted with permission. All rights reserved.)

Chairs

The person's unit has at least 1 chair (see Fig. 19-1). It must be comfortable, sturdy, and not move or tip during transfers. The person should be able to get in and out of the chair with ease. It should not be too low or too soft. Nursing center residents may bring chairs from home.

Doors, Window Coverings, and Privacy Curtains

Each person has the right to *full visual privacy*—*having the means to be completely free from public view while in bed.*

The room door, bathroom door, and window coverings provide privacy. Close doors and window coverings before giving care. The privacy curtain (see Fig. 19-1) is pulled around the bed to provide privacy. *Always pull the curtain completely around the bed before giving care.* Privacy curtains do not block sounds or voices. Others in the room can hear sounds or talking behind the curtain.

Follow the care plan and the person's preferences for privacy measures to maintain after giving care.

Personal Care Items

Personal care items are used for hygiene and elimination (Fig. 19-9). A bedpan, urinal, or commode is provided as needed (Chapter 25). The agency also provides a wash basin, kidney basin, and water mug (see Fig. 19-9). Linens (Chapter 20) are provided.

Hygiene items are available. Some persons have their own oral and personal hygiene equipment and supplies. Respect the person's choices in personal care products.

The Call System

Whether in a room, bathroom, or bathing area, the person must be able to contact the staff. The call system lets the person signal for help.

The call light is at the end of a long cord (Fig. 19-10, A). It connects to a wall panel and attaches to the bed or chair with a clip. To get help, the person presses the button on the device. A light above the room door turns on (Fig. 19-10, B). A computer, light panel, or intercom system at the nurses' station notifies staff that the person needs help.

An intercom system lets the person communicate with staff from the nurses' station. The person says what is needed. Staff reply through the intercom. Persons who are hard of hearing may have problems using an intercom. Also, remember confidentiality. Persons nearby can hear what is said through an intercom.

Always keep the call light within the person's reach—in the room, bathroom, and shower or tub room. (See "The Bathroom" for call lights in bathrooms and shower and tub rooms.)

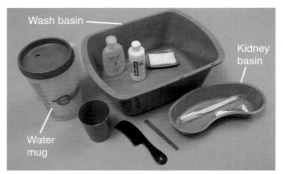

FIGURE 19-9 Personal care items.

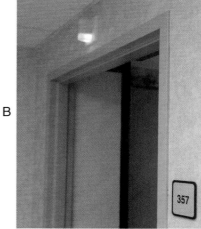

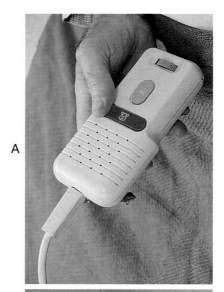

FIGURE 19-10 The call system. **A,** The call light button is pressed when help is needed. **B,** A light above the room door turns on. (NOTE: There are different types of call systems.)

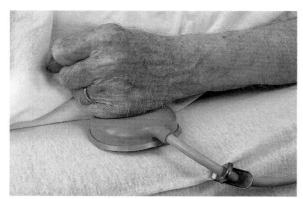

FIGURE 19-11 Call light for a person with limited hand movement.

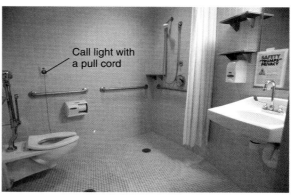

FIGURE 19-12 Bathroom in a person's room.

Some persons have limited hand movement and need a call light that is turned on with a tap of the hand or fist (Fig. 19-11). Some people cannot use call lights. Examples are persons who are confused or unconscious. The care plan lists special communication measures. Check these persons often. Make sure their needs are met.

See *Focus on Communication: The Call System.*

FOCUS ON **COMMUNICATION**

The Call System

You will answer call lights for patients and residents not assigned to you. To promote quality of life and safe care, you can say:

- "My name is Chris Hines. I'm a nursing assistant. How can I help you?"
- "I need to check your care plan before bringing you more salt. I'll be right back. Is there anything else I can do before I leave?"
- "I can take your meal tray. I'll tell your nursing assistant what you ate."
- "Do you use the bathroom or the bedpan?"

Sometimes patients and residents signal for help often. Do not delay in meeting their needs. Never take call lights away from them. This is not safe. Avoid statements that make a person feel like a burden. For example, do not say:

- "I just helped you to the bathroom. Can't you wait?"
- "I was just in your room. What do you want now?"

Do not discourage the person from asking for help. The person may try to do something alone. This could cause injury. Tell the nurse. Your co-workers can help you meet the person's needs.

Call System Safety. The phrase "call light" is used in this book when referring to the call system. You must:

- Keep the call light within the person's reach. Even if the person cannot use the call light, keep it within reach for use by visitors and staff. They may need to call for help.
- Place the call light on the person's strong side.
- Remind the person to signal when help is needed.
- Answer call lights promptly. For example, the person may have an urgent elimination need. Respond promptly to prevent embarrassing problems and complications from incontinence (Chapters 25 and 27). Infection, skin breakdown, pressure injuries, and falls are some examples.
- Answer bathroom and shower or tub room call lights at once.

The Bathroom

A toilet, sink, call light, and mirror are standard equipment in bathrooms (Fig. 19-12). Some bathrooms have showers.

Grab bars (safety bars) are by the toilet for getting on and off the toilet. Some bathrooms have higher toilets or elevated (raised) toilet seats. They make wheelchair transfers easier. They are helpful for persons with joint problems.

Towel racks, toilet paper, soap, paper towel dispenser, and a wastebasket are in the bathroom. They are within the person's reach.

The call light is a button or pull cord next to the toilet. The bathroom call light flashes red above the room door and at the nurses' station. To alert staff of bathroom use, the sound at the nurses' station is different from room call lights. Someone must respond at once when a person needs help in the bathroom.

Closet and Drawer Space

Closet and drawer space are provided (see Fig. 19-1). The CMS requires that nursing centers provide each person with closet space with shelves and a clothes rack. The person must be able to reach and have free access to the closet and its contents.

Sometimes people hoard items—drugs, napkins, straws, food, sugar, salt, pepper, and so on. Hoarding causes safety and health risks. The staff can inspect a person's closet or drawers if hoarding is suspected. The person is told of the inspection and is present when it takes place.

See *Promoting Safety and Comfort: Closet and Drawer Space.*

PROMOTING SAFETY AND COMFORT

Closet and Drawer Space

Safety

Closets and drawers contain the person's property. Ask the person's permission before opening them.

The nurse may ask you to inspect a person's closet, drawers, or personal items. If so, the person must be present. Also have a co-worker with you as a witness. This protects you if the person claims that something was stolen or damaged.

Other Equipment

Many agencies furnish rooms with a TV, radio, and clock. Many rooms have a phone and Internet access.

Other equipment in the room depends on the care setting. Blood pressure equipment, a wall outlet for delivering oxygen, and a pole for intravenous (IV) infusions are some of the equipment in hospital settings. A computer for accessing and recording on the medical record is included in some rooms.

Personal Belongings

Nursing center residents had furniture, appliances, and many belongings and treasures at home. Leaving one's home and living in a new place can be hard. The center is now the person's home. A home-like setting is important for quality of life.

Residents may bring personal items and some furniture from home. Photos, TVs, radios, books, religious items, and plants are examples. A chair, footstool, lamp, and small table are often allowed.

You can help the person choose the best place for personal items. Allow personal choice. Make sure the person's choices:

- Are safe.
- Will not cause falls or other accidents.
- Do not interfere with the rights of others.

FOCUS ON PRIDE

The Person, Family, and Yourself

Personal and Professional Responsibility

Reducing noise requires cooperation from all staff. It is not your responsibility alone. But you can help. Do your part to reduce noise. Politely remind others to speak softly if needed. Take pride in providing a quiet and comfortable setting.

Rights and Respect

You will need to move items in the person's setting when giving care. For example, you need to use the over-bed table as a work area. The person has items on the table. Ask permission to move personal items aside and use the table. Return items to their proper place before leaving the room. Ask if the placement meets the person's preferences. These actions show respect for the person.

Independence and Social Interaction

People want to be independent. Often accidents and injuries occur when the person tries to get needed items. The person has to reach too far and falls. Or the person tries to get up without help.

To promote independence and safety:
- Keep needed personal items within reach.
- Place adaptive (assistive) devices nearby. Walkers and canes are examples.
- Place the call light within the person's reach. Answer call lights and tend to the person's needs promptly.

Delegation and Teamwork

Some nursing units check on the person at regular times. For example, every hour staff ask about needs, positioning, comfort, and needed personal items. Needs are met. The person is reminded that staff will return in 1 hour. Nursing staff sign a form or record in the medical record each time. The person uses the call light for urgent needs.

If your unit uses this practice:
- Be prompt. Check on the person at the correct time.
- Be honest. Do not sign the form or record in the medical record if you did not check on the person. Also, do not sign or record before completing the check.
- Have a good attitude. Do not complain. Reasons for the practice may be to improve care, decrease call light use, or help nurses with time management.

Ethics and Laws

This chapter focuses on how objects and surroundings in the person's unit affect comfort and well-being. You are a part of that setting. Your words and actions are heard and seen by others. Your conduct affects quality of care. Always provide care in a way that promotes comfort, safety, and quality of life.

FOCUS ON PRIDE: *Application*

What makes your living space comfortable and personal? How would this change if you lived in a nursing center? What would change in a hospital setting? Why is it important to provide privacy, safety, and comfort?

REVIEW QUESTIONS

Circle the BEST answer.

1 To maintain the person's unit
   a Throw away items that do not look important
   b Remove cards from the bedside stand
   c Place personal items as you choose
   d Straighten bed linens as needed

2 To protect a person from drafts
   a Adjust the room temperature to 68°F
   b Use a bath blanket during a bed bath
   c Dress the person in light-weight clothing
   d Position the person near an open window

3 You get hot while giving a person a shower. You should
   a Open the bathroom door to cool off the room
   b Adjust the room temperature for your comfort
   c Bring a fan in the bathroom
   d Ask if the person is comfortable

4 To prevent odors
   a Place flowers in the room
   b Empty commodes at the end of your shift
   c Keep laundry containers open
   d Clean persons who are wet or soiled

5 To control noise
   a Answer phones after the third ring
   b Use the intercom system when possible
   c Handle equipment carefully
   d Talk with others in the hallway

6 Mr. Tanner is hard of hearing. He listens to the TV loudly. Residents playing cards nearby complain about the noise. You should
   a Ask Mr. Tanner to turn off his TV
   b Tell the residents playing cards to play somewhere else
   c Ask to close Mr. Tanner's door and ask if the noise level improved
   d Listen to the complaints but do nothing

7 The whole bed is raised to
   a Prevent bending and reaching when giving care
   b Promote the person's comfort
   c Prevent falls
   d Lock the bed in position

8 The head of the bed is raised 30 degrees. This is called
   a Semi-Fowler's position
   b Fowler's position
   c Trendelenburg's position
   d Reverse Trendelenburg's position

9 Which shows you understand how to safely use the person's bed?
   a You leave the room with the whole bed in the high position.
   b You follow the care plan for bed rail use.
   c You leave manual bed cranks in the up position.
   d You touch the bed controls with soiled gloves.

10 Which statement about hospital bed system entrapment is *true*?
   a Bed rails present the only risk for entrapment.
   b Serious injury and death can occur.
   c A person must be small in size for entrapment to occur.
   d Frail older persons have a lower risk of entrapment.

11 A person has right-sided weakness. You complete a safety check. Which do you need to correct before leaving the room?
   a The call light is on the right side of the bed.
   b The over-bed table is on the left side of the bed within reach.
   c The bed is in the low position.
   d Bed wheels are locked (braked).

12 You see the following on the person's over-bed table. Which should be moved?
   a A water mug
   b A TV remote control
   c A urinal
   d A cross-word puzzle

13 Which action is *correct* when using the over-bed table as a work surface?
   a You raise the table to a comfortable working height.
   b You place soiled linens on the table.
   c You replace personal items after use without cleaning it.
   d You place the bedpan on the table.

14 The privacy curtain is pulled around the bed
   a To prevent others from hearing conversations
   b To remind the person to stay in bed
   c To block sounds from the hallway
   d To prevent others from seeing the person

15 Call lights are answered
   a When you have time
   b At the end of your shift
   c Promptly
   d When you are near the person's room

Answers to Chapter 19 questions are on p. 588.

FOCUS ON **PRACTICE**

Problem Solving

Since your shift began an hour ago, a resident has called for help 6 times. You just left the room and are helping another resident. The call light is used again. What do you do?

   The resident uses the call light more often at night, after family visits, and when not checked on regularly. How might this information be helpful for the nurse in care planning?

243

CHAPTER 20

Bedmaking

OBJECTIVES

- Define the key terms and key abbreviation in this chapter.
- Describe closed, open, occupied, and surgical beds.
- Explain when to change bed linens.
- Identify the linens used for bedmaking.
- Explain the purposes of drawsheets and waterproof under-pads and how to use them.
- Handle linens following the rules of medical asepsis.
- Perform the procedures described in this chapter.
- Explain how to promote PRIDE in the person, the family, and yourself.

KEY TERMS

bath blanket A covering used for privacy and warmth during bathing, hygiene, and other care measures
drawsheet A small sheet placed over the middle of the bottom sheet to keep the mattress and bottom linens clean

occupied In use
waterproof under-pad An absorbent pad with a quilted top layer and a waterproof bottom layer

KEY ABBREVIATION

ID   Identification

Beds are made every day. Clean, dry, and wrinkle-free beds:
- Promote comfort.
- Prevent skin breakdown.
- Prevent pressure injuries (Chapter 36).

Beds are usually made in the morning after baths. Or they are made while the person is in the shower, up in the chair, or out of the room. To keep beds neat and clean:
- Change linens when they are wet, soiled, or damp.
- Straighten linens when loose or wrinkled and at bedtime.
- Check for and remove food and crumbs after meals and snacks.
- Check linens for dentures, eyeglasses, hearing aids, sharp objects, and other items.

TYPES OF BEDS
Beds are made in these ways.
- A *closed bed* is not in use (Fig. 20-1). The bed is ready for a new patient or resident. In nursing centers, closed beds are made for residents who are up during the day.
- An *open bed* is ready for use (Fig. 20-2). Top linens are fan-folded to the foot (end) of the bed so the person can get into bed.
- An *occupied bed* is made with the person in it (Fig. 20-3). *Occupied* means in use.
- A *surgical bed* is made to transfer a person from a stretcher to bed (Fig. 20-4). This includes an ambulance stretcher.

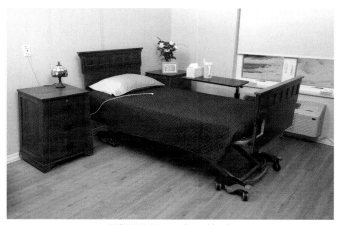

FIGURE 20-1 Closed bed.

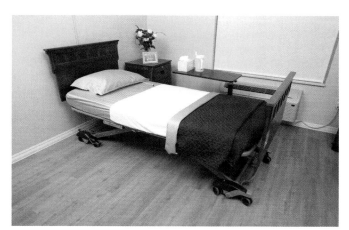

FIGURE 20-2 Open bed. Top linens are fan-folded to the foot of the bed.

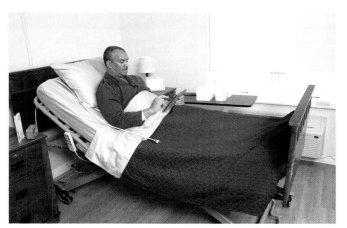

FIGURE 20-3 Occupied bed.

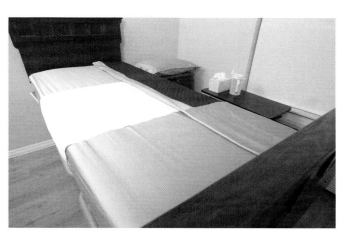

FIGURE 20-4 Surgical bed.

LINENS

Beds in health care settings are at least made with a bottom sheet, top sheet, bedspread, and a pillow with a pillowcase. Bottom sheets are flat (without elastic) or fitted. A fitted sheet has elastic in the sides of the sheet. The sheet is made to fit securely around the mattress. Fitted bottom sheets are common.

A mattress pad may be placed on top of the mattress for comfort and mattress protection. Drawsheets and waterproof under-pads are common. See "Drawsheets and Waterproof Under-Pads." An extra blanket may be applied for warmth. Personal items such as throw blankets, quilts, and decorative pillows are common in nursing centers.

Patient and resident rooms also need linens for personal hygiene. These include bath towels, hand towels, washcloths, gowns or pajamas, and bath blankets. A *bath blanket is a covering used for privacy and warmth during bathing, hygiene, and other care measures.* A bath blanket is used to cover the person when making an occupied bed (p. 254).

Drawsheets and Waterproof Under-Pads

A *drawsheet is a small sheet placed over the middle of the bottom sheet to keep the mattress and bottom linens clean* (Fig. 20-5, p. 246). The drawsheet absorbs moisture and reduces heat retention. A flat sheet folded in half can serve as a drawsheet. Drawsheets are often used as assist devices to move and transfer persons in bed (Chapters 17 and 18).

A *waterproof under-pad is an absorbent pad with a quilted top layer and a waterproof bottom layer* (Fig. 20-6, p. 246). "Soaker pad" and "chux pad" are other names. Waterproof under-pads come in different sizes. They are commonly used for incontinence (Chapter 25) to protect the bottom linens and mattress from being soiled. Disposable bed protectors may also be used (Fig. 20-7, p. 246).

A waterproof under-pad may be used for moving and transfers if the device is strong enough and large enough. Disposable bed protectors are not strong enough to be used for these purposes. See Chapter 17.

Drawsheets and waterproof under-pads are cleaned for re-use. They are placed in linen bags when wet, when soiled, or when it is time for a linen change. Disposable bed protectors are discarded in the trash.

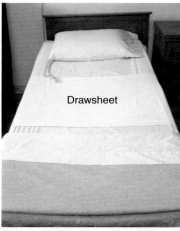

FIGURE 20-5 A drawsheet is placed across the middle of the bed on top of the bottom sheet.

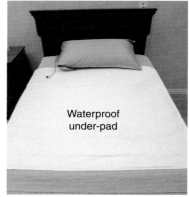

FIGURE 20-6 A waterproof under-pad is padded on top. It has an absorbent middle layer and a waterproof bottom layer.

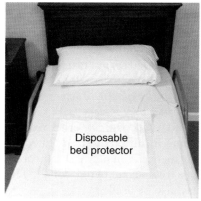

FIGURE 20-7 A disposable bed protector is discarded after use.

Collecting Linens

Do not collect unneeded linens. Once in the person's room, extra linens are considered contaminated. You cannot use them for another person.

Collect linens in the order of use. That way you avoid fumbling with linens for the piece you need. Linens stay neat and clean in your stack. Bed linens are used in the following order.

- Mattress pad (if needed)
- Bottom sheet (fitted or flat)
- Drawsheet (if needed)
- Waterproof under-pad (if needed)
- Top sheet
- Blanket (if needed)
- Bedspread
- Pillowcase(s)

When collecting linens for bedmaking, it is common to collect linens for personal hygiene. You may need to collect towels (bath and hand), washcloths, a gown or pajamas, and a bath blanket.

Use 1 hand to hold the linens. Use your other hand to pick them up. The first item to use is at the bottom of the stack. To get it on top, place your hand over the stack. Then turn the stack over onto the other hand (Fig. 20-8). The first item to use is now on top.

Handling Linens

When handling linens and making beds, practice medical asepsis. Your uniform is considered *dirty*. Always hold linens away from your body and uniform (see Fig. 20-8). Never shake linens. Shaking them spreads microbes. Place clean linens on a clean surface. Never put linens on the floor.

Used Linens. Used linens are handled carefully to prevent the spread of microbes. Remove used linens 1 piece at a time. Roll each piece away from you (Fig. 20-9). Roll soiled linens so the soiled side is inside the roll and away from you.

Leak-proof containers or bags (linen bags, laundry bags) are used to collect linens for transport to laundering areas. Some agencies have soiled linen hampers (containers, carts) in hallways or in a soiled utility room (Fig. 20-10). Others have hampers in each room. Some have laundry chutes.

The procedures in this chapter use a laundry bag. Follow agency policies and procedures for collecting and disposing of used linens. See Box 20-1 (p. 248) for guidelines for handling used linens.

See *Focus on Surveys: Used Linens*, p. 248.

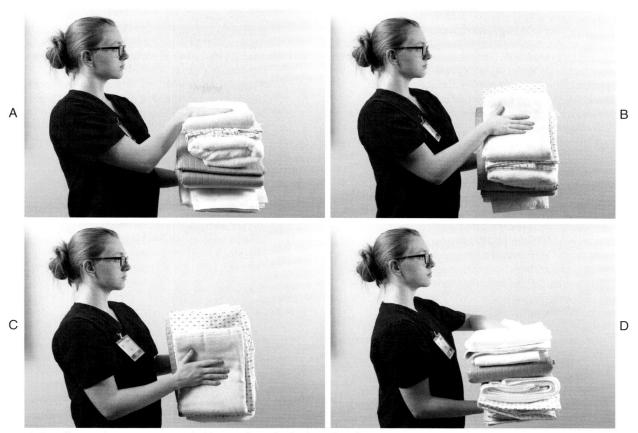

FIGURE 20-8 Collecting linens. Linens are held away from the body and uniform. A, One hand is placed over the top of the stack of linens. B, C, and D, The stack of linens is turned onto the other hand.

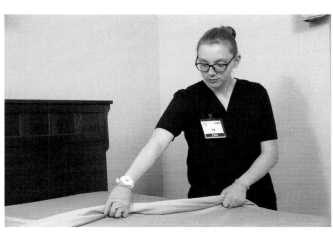

FIGURE 20-9 Used linens are rolled away from you.

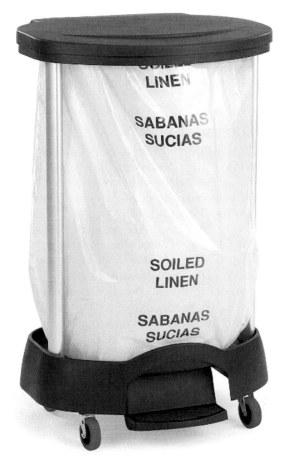

FIGURE 20-10 A hamper for used linens.

BOX 20-1 Guidelines for Handling Used Linens

- Follow Standard Precautions (Chapter 15) and the Bloodborne Pathogen Standard (Chapter 14). Wear gloves and any other needed personal protective equipment when handling soiled linens.
- Hold used linens away from your body and uniform.
- Handle linens carefully with minimal agitation. Never shake them. Shaking spreads microbes.
- Do not place used linens on the floor.
- Do not place used linens on clean linens or on a clean surface. The over-bed table is an example.
- Do not rinse or sort linens in the areas where they were used. For example, do not rinse a soiled waterproof under-pad in the person's bathroom.
- Bag used linens in the room where they were used.
  - Use a *BIOHAZARD* label (*BIOHAZARD* bag) for linens contaminated with blood or other potentially infectious materials (Chapter 14).
  - Follow agency policies and procedures for collecting and disposing of used linens when Transmission-Based Precautions are needed (Chapter 15).
  - Tie the bag securely.
  - Do not carry used linens un-bagged outside of the person's room.
- Place used linens in the correct container. Other containers in the same location may be for trash.
- Do not over-fill a hamper or laundry bag. The hamper's lid will not close. The person emptying the hamper or lifting the bag may be injured.
- Empty containers as needed. Some units assign a person to empty linen containers. Be helpful. Show good teamwork. If you see a full hamper, empty it. The person assigned the task may be busy.
- Clean up after yourself. If you fill a hamper, empty it. If you place an item inside that will cause an odor, empty the hamper.
- Do not place un-bagged linens in a laundry chute. Bag the items and tie the bag securely to prevent linens from falling out in the chute.

Used linens may contain microbes and blood or body fluids. You must help prevent the spread of infection. Surveyors will observe:
- How you transport linens.
- If you practice hand hygiene after handling used linens.
- If you use a second bag (double-bagging) when:
  - The outside of the laundry bag is visibly contaminated.
  - The contents have wet through to the outside of the bag.
- If you bag contaminated linens where they are used. The person's room and the shower room are examples.

MAKING BEDS

In hospitals, bottom and top sheets, the drawsheet, the waterproof under-pad (if used), and pillowcases are usually changed daily. If still clean, the bedspread can be re-used for the same person. If needed, mattress pads and blankets can also be re-used if still clean.

In nursing centers, linens are not changed every day. A complete linen change is usually done on the person's bath or shower day. This may be 1 or 2 times a week. On other days, the bed is made with the same linens.

Linens are not re-used if soiled, wet, or wrinkled. Change wet, damp, or soiled linens right away. Safety and medical asepsis are important for bedmaking. Follow the guidelines in Box 20-2.

Sometimes a special mattress is used to prevent or treat pressure injuries (Chapter 36). Air flows through the mattress for pressure relief. Follow the manufacturer's instructions and agency procedures for linens used with special mattresses.

See *Delegation Guidelines: Making Beds.*
See *Promoting Safety and Comfort: Making Beds.*

BOX 20-2 Bedmaking Guidelines

- Follow the guidelines for handling used linens in Box 20-1.
- Use good body mechanics at all times (Chapter 16).
- Follow the rules in Chapters 17 and 18 to safely move and transfer the person. You move the person when you make an occupied bed. You may transfer the person out of bed to make a closed or open bed.
- Practice hand hygiene before handling clean linens.
- Remove gloves and practice hand hygiene after removing soiled linens and before touching clean linens.
- Bring only needed linens to the person's room. Extra linens are considered contaminated. You cannot use extra linens for another person.
- Place clean linens on a clean surface. Use the bedside chair, over-bed table, or bedside stand. Place a barrier (towel, paper towel, disposable bed protector) between the clean surface and the linens if required by agency policy.
- Do not use torn or frayed linens.
- Never shake any linens—used or clean.
- Hold all linens away from your body and uniform. Do not let used or clean linens touch your uniform.
- Keep bottom linens tucked in and wrinkle-free.
- Straighten and tighten loose linens as needed.
- Move the bed and furniture as needed to allow room to move around the bed.
- Change wet, damp, or soiled linens right away.

DELEGATION GUIDELINES

Making Beds

Before making a bed, you need this information from the nurse and the care plan.
- What bed to make—closed, open, occupied, or surgical.
- If a drawsheet, waterproof under-pad, or disposable bed protector is needed.
- If the person uses bed rails.
- The person's treatment, therapy, and activity schedules. For example, change a resident's linens after a treatment. Or make a resident's bed while the person is in physical therapy.
- Position restrictions or the person's movement or activity limits.
- How to position the person and the positioning devices needed.
- If the bed needs to be locked into a certain position (Chapter 19).
- When to report observations.
- What patient or resident concerns to report at once.

PROMOTING SAFETY AND COMFORT

Making Beds

Safety

You need to raise the bed for body mechanics. The bed also is as flat as possible. Return the bed to the correct position when you are done. Lock the bed in position if ordered.

Bed wheels are locked (braked) during bedmaking. You may need to move the bed to avoid reaching. Unlock the wheels (release the brakes) to move the bed. Then lock (brake) the wheels.

Linens may contain blood or body fluids. Wear gloves to remove soiled linens from the bed. Follow Standard Precautions and the Bloodborne Pathogen Standard. The procedures in this chapter include glove use. (For skills tested in your state, wear gloves as required by your state's competency exam.) Practice hand hygiene after removing and discarding soiled gloves and before touching clean items or surfaces.

After making a bed, lower the bed to the correct level for the person. Follow the care plan. Raise or lower bed rails according to the care plan.

The Closed Bed

Closed beds are made for:
- Nursing center residents who are up for most or all of the day. Top linens are folded back at bedtime. Clean linens are used as needed.
- New patients and residents. The bed is made after the bed system (Chapter 19) is cleaned and disinfected. Clean linens are needed for the entire bed.

The procedure that follows shows how to make as much of 1 side of the bed as possible before moving to the other side. This saves time and energy. It also prepares you for what to do when the bed is occupied.

Another method is to place each item fully on the bed before moving to the next item. The bottom sheet is applied and fully tucked in on both sides, then the drawsheet is applied, and so on. This requires more trips from side to side. But for some it is easier to get linens tight and wrinkle-free.

See procedure: *Making a Closed Bed.*

Making a Closed Bed

Quality of Life

- Knock before entering the person's room.
- Address the person by name.
- Introduce yourself by name and title.
- Explain the procedure before starting and during the procedure.
- Protect the person's rights during the procedure.
- Handle the person gently during the procedure.

Pre-Procedure

1 Follow *Delegation Guidelines: Making Beds.* See *Promoting Safety and Comfort: Making Beds.*
2 Practice hand hygiene and get the following clean linens and supplies.
   - Mattress pad (if needed)
   - Bottom sheet (flat sheet or fitted sheet)
   - Drawsheet (if needed)
   - Waterproof under-pad (if needed)
   - Top sheet
   - Blanket (if needed)
   - Bedspread
   - A pillowcase for each pillow
   - Personal hygiene linens (as needed)—bath towel, hand towel, washcloth, gown or pajamas, bath blanket
   - Gloves
   - Laundry bag
   - Towel, paper towels, or disposable bed protector (as a barrier for clean linens)
3 Arrange items in the person's room. Place linens on a clean surface. First place the barrier between the clean surface and clean linens if required by agency policy.
4 Practice hand hygiene.
5 Raise the bed for body mechanics. Bed rails are down.

Continued

Making a Closed Bed—cont'd

Procedure

6 Put on gloves if contact with blood or body fluids may occur.
7 Remove linens. Roll each piece away from you. Place each piece in the laundry bag. (NOTE: If a disposable bed protector is used, discard it in the trash. Do not put it in the laundry bag.)
8 Clean the bed frame and mattress (if this is your job).
9 Remove and discard the gloves. Practice hand hygiene.
10 Move the mattress to the head of the bed.
11 Put the mattress pad on the mattress (if used). It is even with the head of the mattress.
12 Apply the bottom sheet to 1 side of the bed. Unfold the sheet length-wise. Place the center crease in the middle of the bed.
  a *For a flat sheet* (Figs. 20-11 and 20-12):
    1) Place the lower edge even with the foot of the mattress (see Fig. 20-11, A).
      i If there is a large and small hem, the large hem is at the head. The small hem is at the foot.
      ii Place the stitched side of the hem downward, away from the person. Hem-stitching can be rough. The smooth side is up, against the skin.
    2) Open and fan-fold the sheet to the other side of the bed (see Fig. 20-11, B).
    3) Tuck the top of the sheet under the mattress. Smooth the sheet from the head to the foot.
    4) Make a mitered corner at the top. Tuck in the sheet along the side of the mattress. See Figure 20-12.
  b *For a fitted sheet* (Fig. 20-13, p. 252):
    1) Open and fan-fold the sheet to the other side of the bed.
    2) Tuck the corners over the mattress at the head and the foot of the bed on 1 side.
13 Place the drawsheet (if used) on the bed. It is in the middle of the mattress. Open and fan-fold the drawsheet to the other side of the bed. Tuck it under the mattress.
14 Go to the other side of the bed.
15 Tuck in the bottom sheet on the other side of the bed. Make sure the sheet is smooth and tight without wrinkles.
  a *For a flat sheet*, miter the top corner. Tuck in the sheet along the side of the mattress.
  b *For a fitted sheet*, tuck the corners over the mattress at the head and the foot of the bed.
16 Pull the drawsheet tight so there are no wrinkles (Fig. 20-14, p. 252). Tuck in the drawsheet.
17 *If using a waterproof under-pad*, place the waterproof under-pad on the bed. It is in the middle of the mattress.

18 Put the top sheet on the bed.
  a Unfold it length-wise with the center crease in the middle.
  b Place the top edge even with the head of the mattress.
    1) If there is a large and small hem, the large hem is at the head. The small hem is at the foot.
    2) Place the stitched side of the hem outward, away from the person. The smooth side is down, against the skin.
  c Open and fan-fold the sheet to the other side of the bed. Do not tuck the sheet in yet. Never tuck top linens in on the sides.
19 Place the blanket on the bed (if used).
  a Unfold it with the center crease in the middle.
  b Put the top edge about 6 to 8 inches from the head of the mattress.
  c Open and fan-fold the blanket to the other side.
20 Place the bedspread on the bed (Fig. 20-15, p. 252).
  a Unfold it with the center crease in the middle.
  b Place the top edge even with the head of the mattress.
  c Open and fan-fold the bedspread to the other side.
  d Make sure the bedspread facing the door is even. It covers all top linens.
21 Go to the other side of the bed.
22 Bring the top linens down over the side of the bed. Straighten all top linens.
23 Tuck in top linens together at the foot of the bed so they are smooth and tight. Miter the corners at the foot of the bed (see Figure 20-12, A, B, and C). Leave the top linens untucked at the sides.
24 Put the pillowcase on the pillow. The zipper, tag, or seam end of the pillow is inserted first. Keep the pillow and pillowcase away from your body and uniform. See Figure 20-16 (pp. 252 and 253) for ways to insert the pillow into the pillowcase. Fold any extra material under the pillow at the open end of the pillowcase.
25 Follow the person's preference and agency practices for finishing the bed. The bed should look neat and wrinkle-free. Linens are not touching the floor. For a neat appearance, the open end of the pillowcase does not face the door. The following methods are common.
  a Method 1—Turn the top hem of the bedspread under the blanket to form a cuff. Turn the top sheet over the bedspread. Hem-stitching is down. The smooth side is up. Place the pillow on the bed. See Figure 20-17, p. 253.
  b Method 2—Fold the top of the bedspread back (enough to fit the pillow in the area). Place the pillow on the bed. Bring the bedspread up over the pillow. Tuck the bedspread under the pillow as in Figure 20-18, p. 253.
  c Method 3—Pull the bedspread up to the head of the mattress. Place the pillow on top. See Figure 20-1.

Post-Procedure

26 Provide for comfort. (See the inside of the back cover.) NOTE: Omit this step if the bed is prepared for a new patient or resident.
27 Attach the call light to the bed. Or place it within the person's reach.
28 Lower the bed to a safe and comfortable level. Follow the care plan. The bed wheels are locked (braked).
29 Raise or lower bed rails. Follow the care plan.

30 Put the towels, washcloth, gown or pajamas, and bath blanket in the bedside stand.
31 Complete a safety check of the room. (See the inside of the back cover.)
32 Follow agency policy for used linens.
33 Practice hand hygiene.

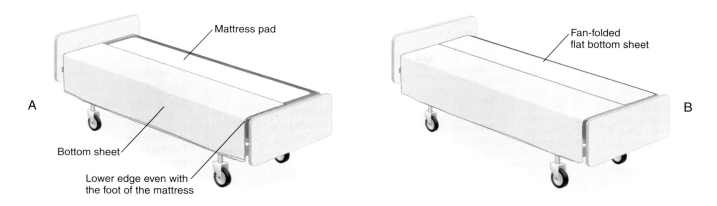

FIGURE 20-11 Applying a flat bottom sheet. A, The bottom sheet is on the bed with the center crease in the middle. The lower edge of the sheet is even with the foot of the mattress. B, The sheet is fan-folded to the other side of the bed.

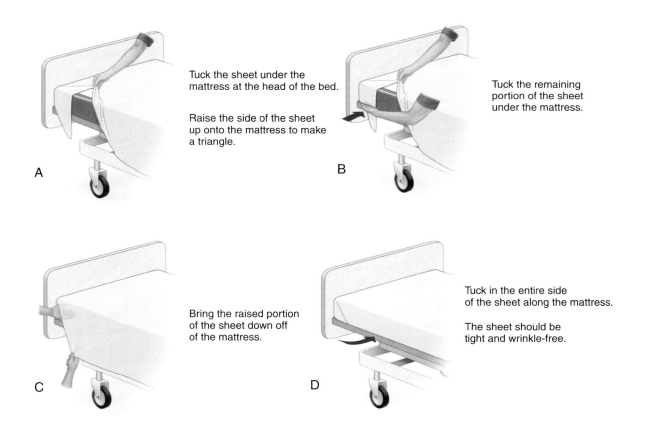

FIGURE 20-12 Making a mitered corner.

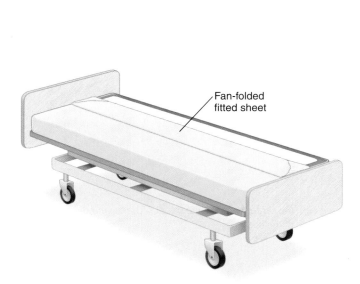

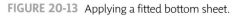

FIGURE 20-13 Applying a fitted bottom sheet.

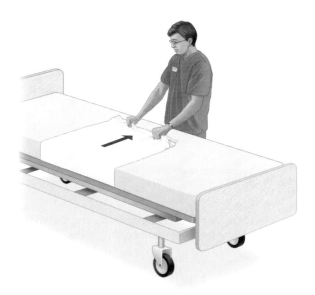

FIGURE 20-14 The drawsheet is pulled tight to remove wrinkles. The drawsheet is tucked in under the sides of the mattress.

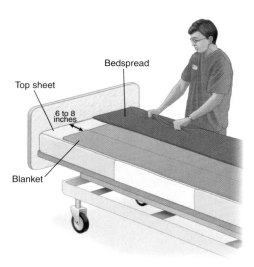

FIGURE 20-15 The bedspread is applied. The top sheet is even with the head of the mattress. The blanket is about 6 to 8 inches from the head of the mattress.

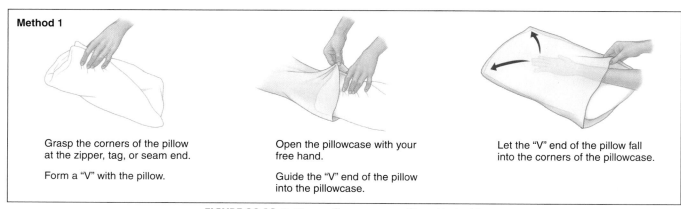

Method 1

Grasp the corners of the pillow at the zipper, tag, or seam end.

Form a "V" with the pillow.

Open the pillowcase with your free hand.

Guide the "V" end of the pillow into the pillowcase.

Let the "V" end of the pillow fall into the corners of the pillowcase.

FIGURE 20-16 Putting a pillowcase on a pillow: Method 1.

Method 2

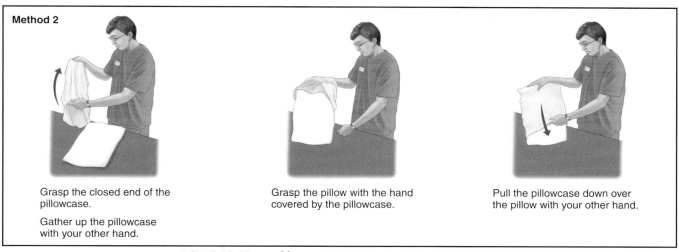

Grasp the closed end of the pillowcase.

Gather up the pillowcase with your other hand.

Grasp the pillow with the hand covered by the pillowcase.

Pull the pillowcase down over the pillow with your other hand.

FIGURE 20-16, cont'd Putting a pillowcase on a pillow: Method 2.

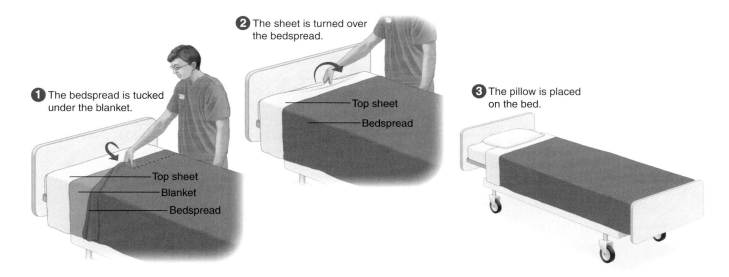

1 The bedspread is tucked under the blanket.

Top sheet
Blanket
Bedspread

2 The sheet is turned over the bedspread.

Top sheet
Bedspread

3 The pillow is placed on the bed.

FIGURE 20-17 Finishing a closed bed by making a cuff with the top linens.

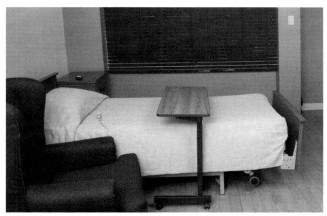

FIGURE 20-18 A closed bed with the pillow under the bedspread. The bedspread is tucked under the pillow.

The Open Bed

A closed bed becomes an open bed by fan-folding the top linens to the foot of the bed (see Fig. 20-2). The person can get into bed with ease. Make this bed for:

* Newly admitted persons arriving by wheelchair
* Persons who are getting ready for bed
* Persons who are out of bed for a short time

⬛ The Occupied Bed

You make an occupied bed when the person stays in bed. The person is rolled to the side and used bottom linens are tucked under the person. Clean bottom linens are put on that side of the bed. Then the person is rolled back onto the clean bottom linens to finish the other side of the bed.

Explain each step to the person before it is done. This is important even if the person cannot respond.

See *Focus on Communication: The Occupied Bed.*
See *Promoting Safety and Comfort: The Occupied Bed.*
See procedure: *Making an Occupied Bed.*

FOCUS ON **COMMUNICATION**

The Occupied Bed

After making an occupied bed, ask about the person's comfort.

* "Are you comfortable?"
* "How can I make you more comfortable?"
* "Are you warm enough?"
* "Do you feel any creases or wrinkles?"
* "Can I adjust your pillow?"
  After making the bed, thank the person for cooperating.

PROMOTING SAFETY AND COMFORT

The Occupied Bed

Safety

The person lies on 1 side and then the other. Protect the person from falling out of bed. If bed rails are used, the far bed rail is up. If bed rails are not used, have a co-worker help you. You work on 1 side of the bed. Your co-worker is on the other side to help turn and position the person and prevent falling.

Keep the person in good alignment. Follow restrictions or limits in the person's movement or position.

Comfort

Cover the person with a bath blanket before removing the top sheet. Do not leave the person uncovered.

Tucked linens create a "bump" in the middle of the bed. For comfort, make the "bump" as low as possible. Do this by fan-folding bottom linens neatly and flatly. Do not let the person's body touch the exposed surface of the mattress.

Adjust the pillow as needed during the procedure. After the procedure, position the person for comfort and as directed by the nurse and the care plan.

Making an Occupied Bed

Quality of Life

* Knock before entering the person's room.
* Address the person by name.
* Introduce yourself by name and title.

* Explain the procedure before starting and during the procedure.
* Protect the person's rights during the procedure.
* Handle the person gently during the procedure.

Pre-Procedure

1 Follow *Delegation Guidelines: Making Beds, p. 249.* See *Promoting Safety and Comfort:*
  a *Making Beds, p. 249*
  b *The Occupied Bed*
2 Ask a co-worker to help you if needed.
3 Practice hand hygiene and get the following supplies.
  • Clean linens (see procedure: *Making a Closed Bed, p. 249*)
  • Bath blanket
  • Gloves
  • Laundry bag
  • Towel, paper towels, or disposable bed protector (as a barrier for clean linens)

4 Arrange items in the person's room. Place linens on a clean surface. First place the barrier between the clean surface and clean linens if required by agency policy.
5 Practice hand hygiene.
6 Identify the person. Check the identification (ID) bracelet against the assignment sheet. Use 2 identifiers (Chapter 11). Also call the person by name.
7 Provide for privacy.
8 Move the call light off of the bed.
9 Raise the bed for body mechanics. Bed rails are up if used. Bed wheels are locked (braked).
10 Lower the head of the bed. It is as flat as possible.

Making an Occupied Bed—cont'd

Procedure

11 Put on gloves if contact with blood or body fluids may occur.
12 Loosen top linens at the foot of the bed.
13 Lower the bed rail near you if up.
14 Fold and remove the bedspread (Fig. 20-19, p. 256). Do the same for the blanket (if used). Place each over the chair or on a clean surface.
15 Cover the person with a bath blanket.
  a Unfold the bath blanket over the top sheet.
  b Have the person hold the bath blanket. If the person is unable, tuck the top part under the person's shoulders.
  c Grasp the top sheet under the bath blanket at the shoulders. Bring the sheet down toward the foot of the bed. Remove the sheet from under the blanket (Fig. 20-20, p. 256).
16 Explain the safety measures you have taken to prevent falling from the bed. Help the person turn onto the side facing away from you. Adjust the pillow for comfort.
17 Loosen bottom linens on the side of the bed near you.
18 Fan-fold bottom linens 1 at a time toward the person (Fig. 20-21, p. 256). If re-using a mattress pad, do not fan-fold it.
19 Remove and discard the gloves. Practice hand hygiene. Put on clean gloves.
20 Place a clean mattress pad on the bed if needed. Unfold it length-wise with the center crease in the middle. Fan-fold the top part toward the person. If re-using a mattress pad, straighten and smooth any wrinkles.
21 Place the bottom sheet on the side of the bed near you. For a flat sheet, see step 12-a in the procedure: *Making a Closed Bed*, p. 249. For a fitted sheet, tuck the corners over the mattress at the head and the foot of the bed on the side near you. Fan-fold the sheet toward the person.
22 *If using a drawsheet* (Fig. 20-22, p. 257):
  a Place the drawsheet on the bed. It is in the middle of the mattress.
  b Open the drawsheet.
  c Fan-fold it toward the person.
  d Tuck in excess fabric at the side of the bed.
23 *If using a waterproof under-pad:*
  a Place the waterproof under-pad on the bed. It is in the middle of the mattress.
  b Fan-fold it toward the person.
24 Explain to the person that there is a "bump" to roll back over. Help the person turn toward you. Adjust the pillow for comfort.
25 Raise the bed rail. Go to the other side and lower the bed rail. (Omit this step if you are working with a co-worker. Your co-worker removes used linens and places clean linens on the other side of the bed.)

26 Loosen and remove the bottom linens (Fig. 20-23, A, p. 257). Remove 1 piece at a time. Place each piece in the laundry bag. (NOTE: If a disposable bed protector is used, discard it in the trash. Do not put it in the laundry bag.)
27 Remove and discard the gloves. Practice hand hygiene.
28 Straighten and smooth the mattress pad if used.
29 Pull the clean bottom sheet toward you and tuck it in. For a flat sheet, make a mitered corner at the top. Tuck the sheet under the mattress from the head to the foot of the bed. For a fitted sheet, tuck the corners over the mattress at the head and the foot of the bed.
30 Pull the drawsheet tightly toward you and tuck it in (Fig. 20-23, B, p. 257).
31 Position the person supine in the center of the bed. Adjust the pillow for comfort.
32 Put the top sheet on the bed. Unfold it length-wise with the center crease in the middle. The large hem is even with the head of the mattress. Hem-stitching is on the outside.
33 Have the person hold the top sheet so you can remove the bath blanket. Or tuck the top sheet under the person's shoulders. Remove the bath blanket. Place it in the laundry bag.
34 Unfold the blanket on the bed if used. The center crease is in the middle and it covers the person. The upper hem is 6 to 8 inches from the head of the mattress.
35 Unfold the bedspread on the bed. The center crease is in the middle and it covers the person. The top hem is even with the head of the mattress.
36 Straighten and smooth top linens.
37 Raise the bed rail. Go to the foot of the bed.
38 Make a 2-inch toe pleat across the foot of the bed (Fig. 20-24, p. 257). The pleat (fold) is about 6 to 8 inches from the foot of the bed. The pleat prevents pressure on the toes from top linens.
39 Tuck in top linens together at the foot of the bed. Avoid removing the toe pleat. Miter the corners at the foot of the bed. Leave the top linens untucked at the sides.
40 Follow the person's preference and agency practices for finishing the bed. If a blanket is used, turn the top hem of the bedspread under the blanket to make a cuff. Bring the top sheet down over the bedspread to form a cuff.
41 Change the pillowcase(s).

Post-Procedure

42 Provide for comfort. (See the inside of the back cover.)
43 Place the call light and other needed items within reach.
44 Lower the bed to a safe and comfortable level. Follow the care plan. The bed wheels are locked (braked).
45 Raise or lower bed rails. Follow the care plan.
46 Put the clean towels, washcloth, gown or pajamas, and bath blanket in the bedside stand.

47 Follow the care plan and the person's preferences for privacy measures to maintain. Leaving the privacy curtain, window coverings, and door open or closed are examples.
48 Complete a safety check of the room. (See the inside of the back cover.)
49 Follow agency policy for used linens.
50 Practice hand hygiene.
51 Report and record your care and observations.

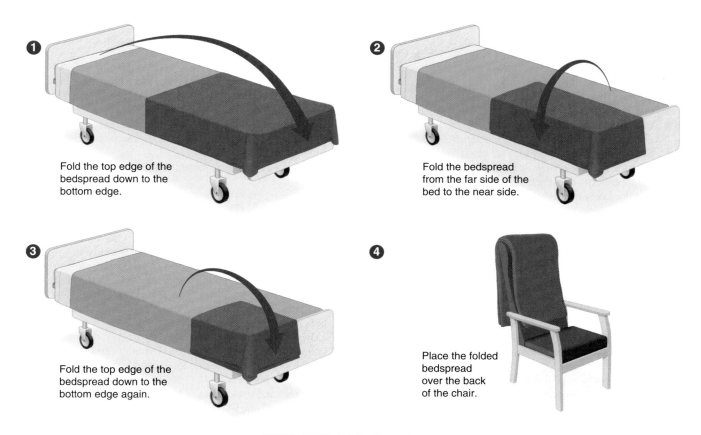

❶ Fold the top edge of the bedspread down to the bottom edge.

❷ Fold the bedspread from the far side of the bed to the near side.

❸ Fold the top edge of the bedspread down to the bottom edge again.

❹ Place the folded bedspread over the back of the chair.

FIGURE 20-19 Folding linens for re-use.

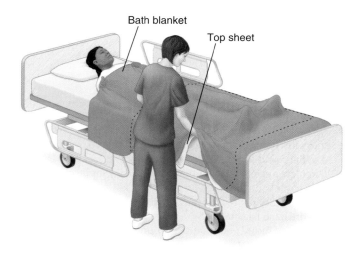

Bath blanket

Top sheet

FIGURE 20-20 The person holds on to the bath blanket. The top sheet is removed from under the bath blanket.

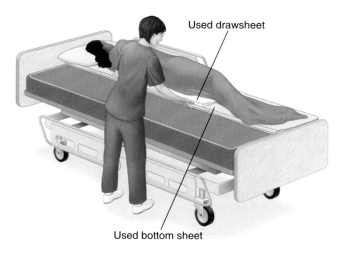

Used drawsheet

Used bottom sheet

FIGURE 20-21 Used bottom linens are tucked under the person.

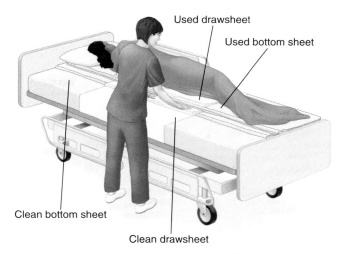

FIGURE 20-22 A clean bottom sheet and drawsheet are on the bed. Both are fan-folded and tucked under the person.

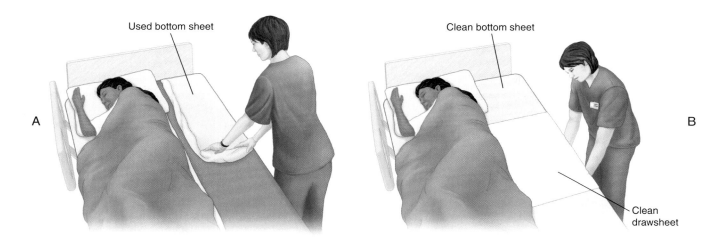

FIGURE 20-23 **A,** The person is turned to the other side. Used linens are removed. (Gloves are removed and hand hygiene is performed before touching clean linens.) **B,** The clean bottom linens are pulled through and tucked in.

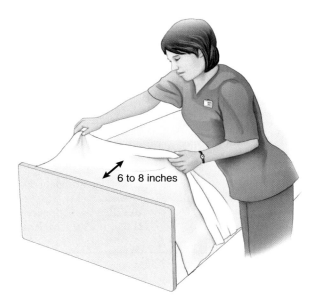

FIGURE 20-24 Making a toe pleat. Pull up on the top linens. Make a 2-inch pleat (fold) across the foot of the bed. The pleat is 6 to 8 inches from the foot of the bed.

The Surgical Bed

The surgical bed also is called a *recovery bed* or *postoperative bed*. Top linens are folded to the side to transfer the person from a stretcher to the bed. These beds are made for persons:

- Returning to their rooms from surgery. A complete linen change is needed.
- Who arrive at the agency by ambulance. A complete linen change is needed if the person:
  - Is a new patient or resident.
  - Is returning to the agency from the hospital.
- Who go by stretcher to treatment or therapy areas. A complete linen change is not needed.
- Using portable tubs (Chapter 22). Because of bathing, a complete linen change is needed.
  See *Promoting Safety and Comfort: The Surgical Bed*.
  See procedure: *Making a Surgical Bed*.

PROMOTING SAFETY AND COMFORT

The Surgical Bed

Safety

See Chapter 18 for stretcher safety. After the transfer, lower the bed to a safe and comfortable level for the person. Bed wheels are locked (braked). Raise or lower bed rails according to the care plan.

Making a Surgical Bed

Pre-Procedure

1 Follow *Delegation Guidelines: Making Beds*, p. 249. **See** *Promoting Safety and Comfort:*
  a *Making Beds*, p. 249
  b *The Surgical Bed*
2 Practice hand hygiene and get the following supplies.
  - Clean linens (see procedure: *Making a Closed Bed*, p. 249)
  - Gloves
  - Laundry bag
  - Equipment requested by the nurse
  - Towel, paper towels, or disposable bed protector (as a barrier for clean linens)

3 Arrange items in the person's room. Place linens on a clean surface. First place the barrier between the clean surface and clean linens if required by agency policy.
4 Practice hand hygiene.
5 Move the call light off of the bed.
6 Raise the bed for body mechanics. Bed rails are down.

Procedure

7 Put on gloves if contact with blood or body fluids may occur.
8 Remove and place the used linens in the laundry bag. Remove gloves. Practice hand hygiene after removing and discarding them.
9 Make a closed bed (see procedure: *Making a Closed Bed*, p. 249). Do not tuck top linens under the mattress.

10 Fold all top linens at the foot of the bed back onto the bed. The fold is even with the edge of the mattress (Fig. 20-25, A).
11 Know on which side of the bed the stretcher will be placed. Fan-fold linens length-wise to the other side of the bed (Fig. 20-25, B).
12 Put a pillowcase on each pillow.
13 Place the pillow(s) on a clean surface.

Post-Procedure

14 Leave the bed in its highest position.
15 Leave both bed rails down.
16 Put the clean towels, washcloth, gown or pajamas, and bath blanket in the bedside stand.
17 Move furniture away from the bed. Allow room for the stretcher and the staff.

18 Do not attach the call light to the bed.
19 Complete a safety check of the room. (See the inside of the back cover.)
20 Follow agency policy for used linens.
21 Practice hand hygiene.

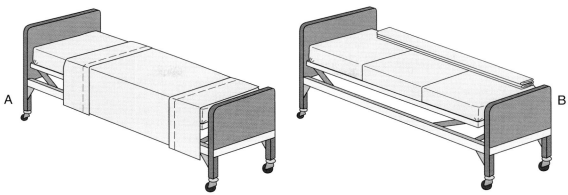

FIGURE 20-25 Surgical bed. **A,** The bottom of the top linens is folded back onto the bed. The fold is even with the edge of the mattress. **B,** Top linens are fan-folded length-wise to the side of the bed.

FOCUS ON P R I D E

The Person, Family, and Yourself

P ersonal and Professional Responsibility

You are responsible for providing a neat and orderly setting. The bed must be clean and well made. If the person stays in bed, straighten and tighten linens as needed. These actions promote comfort and quality of life.

R ights and Respect

Nursing center residents often bring bedspreads, blankets, and so on from home. The items have meaning and value. For example, a resident uses a quilt at night. Made by a family member, the sight and smell of the quilt remind the person of home.

Protect personal items from loss and damage. Handle the person's belongings with care and respect.

I ndependence and Social Interaction

Allow personal choice when possible. For example, the person chooses what time you make the bed. What is best for you may not be best for the person. Consider the person's preferences when planning your day and managing time. The more choices are allowed, the greater the person's sense of control and independence.

D elegation and Teamwork

Making beds with a co-worker is faster, easier, and safer. Make 1 side of the bed while your co-worker makes the other. Always thank your co-worker for helping you. Also, be willing to help others.

E thics and Laws

Leaving a person to lie on wet or soiled linens is neglect. Check persons at risk for wetting or soiling often. This may be from perspiration (sweat), urine, or feces (stools). Change wet or soiled linens as often as needed.

FOCUS ON PRIDE: *Application*

Do you make your bed at home every day? If yes, why? If no, why? Explain why the look and feel of the bed can affect the person's comfort and safety.

Circle the BEST answer.

1 A resident is showering and will be out of bed for the day. You will
   a Make an occupied bed
   b Re-use the linens and make a closed bed
   c Make a closed bed with clean linens
   d Make an open bed with clean linens

2 To transfer a person from a stretcher to the bed, you make
   a A closed bed
   b An open bed
   c An occupied bed
   d A surgical bed

3 When making beds
   a Leave wrinkles in the bottom sheet
   b Check the bed for eyeglasses and other items
   c Shake clean linens to unfold them
   d Take extra linens to another person's room

4 When removing used linens
   a Remove 1 piece at a time
   b Roll all linens together for removal
   c Roll linens toward your body
   d Shake linens to remove crumbs

5 When handling used linens
   a Place them on the floor until you finish making the bed
   b Hold them against your uniform
   c Carry them outside of the room un-bagged
   d Wear gloves to remove linens soiled with urine

6 You have applied a waterproof under-pad correctly if
   a It is in the middle of the mattress
   b The quilted side is down
   c It is under the bottom sheet
   d The corners are mitered

7 A complete linen change is done when
   a The waterproof under-pad is wet
   b The bed is made for a new person
   c The person returns from therapy
   d Linens are loose or wrinkled

8 After making a closed bed
   a Unlock the bed wheels (release the brakes)
   b Leave the bed in the high position
   c Leave used linens in the room
   d Attach the call light to the bed

9 When making an occupied bed
   a Explain that the person will roll over a "bump" of linens
   b Remove the top sheet and leave the person uncovered
   c Lower the far bed rail if working alone
   d Fan-fold bottom linens to the foot of the bed

10 You are making an occupied bed. You just tucked the used linens under the person. Next, you should
   a Have the person roll back onto the uncovered mattress
   b Apply a clean drawsheet before applying a clean bottom sheet
   c Remove gloves and practice hand hygiene before touching clean linens
   d Fold and remove the bath blanket

11 What is the purpose of a toe pleat?
   a It keeps the feet warm.
   b It keeps the feet cool.
   c It prevents pressure on the toes from top linens.
   d It keeps the toes from touching the end of the bed.

12 For a surgical bed
   a Do not secure the bottom linens
   b Fan-fold top linens to the side of the bed
   c Fan-fold top linens to the foot of the bed
   d Do not apply top linens

Answers to Chapter 20 questions are on p. 588.

FOCUS ON **PRACTICE**

Problem Solving

You need to give a person a bath in bed (Chapter 22). The person must remain in bed. Which type of bed will you make? Will you change linens or give the bath first? While changing linens, when will you apply and remove gloves and practice hand hygiene?

CHAPTER 21

Oral Hygiene

- Define the key terms and key abbreviations in this chapter.
- Explain the purposes of oral hygiene.
- Explain why flossing is important.
- Describe the safety measures for giving mouth care to unconscious persons.
- Explain how to care for dentures.
- Identify the observations related to oral hygiene.
- Perform the procedures described in this chapter.
- Explain how to promote PRIDE in the person, the family, and yourself.

KEY TERMS

aspiration Breathing fluid, food, vomitus, or an object into the lungs
denture A removable replacement for missing teeth

hygiene The cleanliness practices that promote health and prevent disease
oral hygiene The practices that promote healthy tissues and structures of the mouth; mouth care

KEY ABBREVIATIONS

ADA   American Dental Association

ID   Identification

The teeth and mucous membranes of the mouth must be kept clean and intact. Otherwise teeth can decay. Microbes can enter the body.

Illness, disease, and some drugs often cause:

- A bad taste in the mouth.
- A whitish coating in the mouth and on the tongue.
- Redness and swelling in the mouth and on the tongue.
- Dry mouth. Dry mouth is common from oxygen, smoking, decreased fluid intake, and anxiety.

STRUCTURE AND FUNCTION OF TEETH

The teeth cut, chop, and grind food into small bits for swallowing and digestion. Normally, adults have 32 permanent teeth. A tooth has 3 main parts (Fig. 21-1).

- The *crown* is the outer part.
- The *neck* is surrounded by *gums (gingivae)*.
- The *root* fits into the bone of the lower or upper jaw.

Teeth are covered with *enamel*. Enamel is a hard, outer coating. Below the enamel is a softer layer called *dentin*. The inner tooth contains nerves and blood vessels.

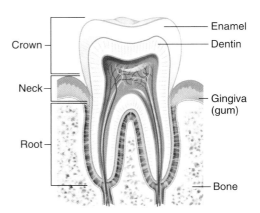

Crown
Neck
Root
Enamel
Dentin
Gingiva (gum)
Bone

FIGURE 21-1 Parts of a tooth.

PURPOSE OF ORAL HYGIENE

Hygiene involves the cleanliness practices that promote health and prevent disease. **Oral hygiene** *(mouth care) relates to the practices that promote healthy tissues and structures of the mouth.* Oral hygiene:

- Keeps the mouth and teeth clean.
- Prevents mouth odors and infections.
- Increases comfort.
- Makes food taste better.
- Reduces the risk for *tooth decay (cavities, dental caries)* and *periodontal disease (gum disease).*
  Plaque and tartar build up from poor oral hygiene.
- *Plaque* is a thin film that sticks to the teeth. It contains saliva, microbes, and other substances.
- *Tartar* is hardened plaque. Tartar builds up at the gum line near the neck of the tooth.

Microbes in plaque produce acids that can damage enamel and cause tooth decay (cavities, dental caries). Brushing and flossing can prevent decay. However, once a cavity forms, a dentist needs to fill it to prevent more damage.

Tartar buildup causes periodontal disease (gum disease). Tissues around the teeth are inflamed. The gums are red and swollen and bleed easily. With severe disease, bone is destroyed and teeth loosen. Tooth loss is common.

The nurse assesses the person's oral care needs. So may the speech-language pathologist and the dietitian.

See *Delegation Guidelines: Purpose of Oral Hygiene.*

See *Promoting Safety and Comfort: Purpose of Oral Hygiene.*

DELEGATION GUIDELINES

Purpose of Oral Hygiene

To assist with oral hygiene, you need this information from the nurse and the care plan.

- The type of oral hygiene to give. See procedures:
  - *Brushing and Flossing the Person's Teeth*
  - *Providing Mouth Care for the Unconscious Person,* p. 266
  - *Providing Denture Care,* p. 268
- If flossing is needed.
- What cleaning agent and equipment to use.
- If you apply lubricant to the lips. If yes, what lubricant to use.
- How often to give oral hygiene.
- How much help the person needs.
- What observations to report and record:
  - Dry, cracked, swollen, or blistered lips
  - Mouth or breath odor
  - Redness, swelling, irritation, sores, or white patches in the mouth or on the tongue
  - Bleeding, swelling, or redness of the gums
  - Painful areas
  - Loose teeth
  - Rough, sharp, or chipped areas on dentures
  - Dentures that fit poorly
- When to report observations.
- What patient or resident concerns to report at once.

PROMOTING SAFETY AND COMFORT

Purpose of Oral Hygiene

Safety

Follow Standard Precautions and the Bloodborne Pathogen Standard. You may have contact with the person's mucous membranes. Gums may bleed during mouth care. Also, the mouth has many microbes. Pathogens spread through sexual contact may be in the mouths of some persons.

Brush gently and carefully. Brushing hard can cause the gums to bleed. Inserting the toothbrush too far can stimulate the gag reflex.

> NOTE: *A task may require more than 1 pair of gloves. Change gloves as needed. Use careful judgment. Remember to practice hand hygiene after removing gloves.*

Comfort

Follow the person's care plan and preferences for how often to perform oral hygiene. The American Dental Association (ADA) recommends brushing for 2 minutes 2 times daily. Some persons need or want oral care more often—after sleep, after meals, and at bedtime. Many people practice oral hygiene before meals. Some persons need mouth care every 2 hours or more often.

FLOSSING

Flossing cleans between the teeth. Flossing removes plaque from areas brushing cannot reach and removes food from between the teeth. It helps prevent periodontal disease and cavities.

Dental floss is commonly used. It is a soft thread used to clean between teeth. Other devices *(interdental cleaners)* may be used. *Inter* means *between.* Small brushes and plastic picks threaded with floss are examples. Some persons use powered air or water flossers to clean between teeth.

The ADA recommends flossing at least once a day. Flossing can be done before or after brushing. The person can choose the best time for thorough flossing—in the morning, after a meal, at bedtime, or when convenient. You need to floss for persons who cannot do so themselves.

EQUIPMENT

A toothbrush, toothpaste, floss or other interdental cleaner, and mouthwash are needed. A toothbrush with soft bristles is best. Using a toothpaste with fluoride helps protect the teeth from decay.

Sponge swabs (p. 265) are used for sore, tender mouths and for unconscious persons. Use sponge swabs with care. Make sure the foam pad is tight on the stick. The person could choke on the foam pad if it comes off.

You also need a kidney basin, water cup, straw, tissues, towels, and gloves. Many persons bring oral hygiene equipment from home. Electric toothbrushes are common.

BRUSHING AND FLOSSING TEETH

Many people perform oral hygiene themselves. Others need help gathering and setting up oral hygiene equipment. You perform oral hygiene for persons who:

- Are very weak.
- Cannot move or use their arms.
- Are too confused to brush their teeth.
  See procedure: *Brushing and Flossing the Person's Teeth.*

Brushing and Flossing the Person's Teeth

Quality of Life

- Knock before entering the person's room.
- Address the person by name.
- Introduce yourself by name and title.

- Explain the procedure before starting and during the procedure.
- Protect the person's rights during the procedure.
- Handle the person gently during the procedure.

Pre-Procedure

1 Follow *Delegation Guidelines: Purpose of Oral Hygiene.* See *Promoting Safety and Comfort: Purpose of Oral Hygiene.*
2 Practice hand hygiene and get the following supplies.
   - Toothbrush with soft bristles
   - Toothpaste
   - Mouthwash (or solution noted on the care plan)
   - Floss or other interdental cleaner (if used)
   - Water cup with cool water
   - Straw
   - Kidney basin
   - Hand towel

   - Towel or paper towels (as a barrier for supplies)
   - Gloves
   - Laundry bag
3 Arrange items in the person's room. Place the barrier (towel, paper towels) on the over-bed table. Arrange items on top.
4 Practice hand hygiene.
5 Identify the person. Check the identification (ID) bracelet against the assignment sheet. Use 2 identifiers (Chapter 11). Also call the person by name.
6 Provide for privacy.
7 Raise the bed for body mechanics. Bed rails are up if used.

Procedure

8 Lower the bed rail near you if up.
9 Assist the person to a sitting position or to a side-lying position near you. (NOTE: Some state competency tests require that the person is at a 60- to 90-degree angle. Other states require a 75- to 90-degree angle.)
10 Place the towel across the chest.
11 Adjust the over-bed table so you can reach it with ease.
12 Practice hand hygiene. Put on the gloves.
13 Hold the toothbrush over the kidney basin. Pour some water over the brush.
14 Apply toothpaste to the toothbrush.
15 Brush the teeth gently with short strokes (Fig. 21-2, p. 264). Brush the inner, outer, and chewing surfaces of upper and lower teeth.
16 Brush the tongue gently (see Fig. 21-2). Also gently brush the roof of the mouth, inside of the cheeks, and gums.
17 Let the person rinse the mouth with water. Hold the kidney basin under the chin (Fig. 21-3, p. 264). Repeat this step as needed.
18 Floss the person's teeth (optional). See Figure 21-4, p. 264.
   a Break off about an 18-inch piece of floss from the dispenser.
   b Wrap most of the floss around one of your middle fingers. Wrap a small amount around the middle finger on the other hand (see Fig. 21-4, A). (As floss is used, unwrap clean floss from the first middle finger. Wrap used floss around the middle finger on the other hand.)

   c Stretch the floss with your thumbs. Hold the floss firmly between your thumbs and index fingers (see Fig. 21-4, B).
   d Start at the back side of an upper back tooth. Work around to the other side of the mouth.
   e Gently insert the floss between the teeth with a rubbing motion. Do not jerk or snap the floss.
   f Gently slide the floss into the space between the gum and the tooth (see Fig. 21-4, C).
   g Rub the floss gently against the side of the tooth. Move away from the gum with slow back-and-forth and up-and-down motions (see Fig. 21-4, D).
   h Use a new section of floss for each tooth. Remember to floss the back side of the last tooth.
   i Floss the lower teeth. Start on one side. Work around to the other side. Remember to floss the back side of the last tooth.
   j Discard the floss.
19 Let the person use mouthwash or other solution. Hold the kidney basin under the chin.
20 Wipe the person's mouth. Remove the towel. Place the towel in the laundry bag.
21 Remove and discard the gloves. Practice hand hygiene.

Post-Procedure

22 Assist with hand hygiene if needed. (See Chapter 14.)
23 Provide for comfort. (See the inside of the back cover.)
24 Place the call light and other needed items within reach.
25 Lower the bed to a safe and comfortable level. Follow the care plan.
26 Raise or lower bed rails. Follow the care plan.
27 Rinse the toothbrush. Clean, rinse, and dry equipment. Use clean, dry paper towels for drying. Return the toothbrush and equipment to their proper place. (Wear gloves.)

28 Clean and dry the over-bed table. Dry with paper towels. Discard the paper towels. Remove and discard the gloves. Practice hand hygiene.
29 Follow the care plan and the person's preferences for privacy measures to maintain. Leaving the privacy curtain, window coverings, and door open or closed are examples.
30 Complete a safety check of the room. (See the inside of the back cover.)
31 Follow agency policy for used linens.
32 Practice hand hygiene.
33 Report and record your care and observations.

Upper teeth   Lower teeth

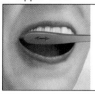 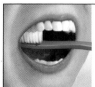 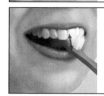 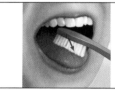

Hold the brush at a 45-degree angle to the gums.
Brush back and forth gently with short strokes.

Brush the inner, outer, and chewing surfaces of the upper and lower teeth.

Tilt the brush to clean the inside of the front teeth.
Brush gently with up-and-down strokes.

Brush the tongue.

FIGURE 21-2 Brushing the teeth and tongue.

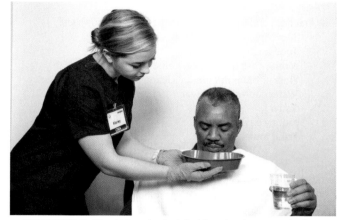

FIGURE 21-3 The kidney basin is held under the person's chin.

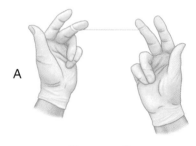

A

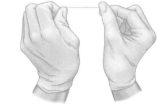

B

Wrap the floss around the middle fingers on both hands.

Hold the floss between your thumbs and index fingers.

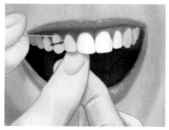

C

Insert the floss between the teeth with a gentle rubbing motion.

Slide the floss into the space between the gum and the tooth.

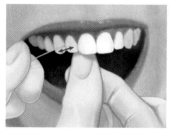

D

Rub the floss gently against the side of the tooth.

Move away from the gum.

FIGURE 21-4 Flossing with dental floss. **A** and **B,** Holding the floss. **C** and **D,** Flossing along the gum line and side of the tooth.

Mouth Care for the Unconscious Person

Unconscious (comatose) persons cannot eat or drink. Some breathe with their mouths open. Many receive oxygen. These factors cause mouth dryness. They also cause crusting on the tongue and mucous membranes. Oral hygiene keeps the mouth clean and moist. It also helps prevent infection.

The care plan states what cleaning agent to use. Apply the cleaning agent with sponge swabs (Fig. 21-5, *A*). To prevent the lips from cracking, apply a lubricant (check the care plan) after cleaning.

Unconscious persons usually cannot swallow. Protect them from choking and aspiration. *Aspiration is breathing fluid, food, vomitus, or an object into the lungs.* It can cause pneumonia and death. To prevent aspiration:

- Position the person on the side with the head turned well to the side (Fig. 21-6). In this position, excess fluid can run out of the mouth.
- Use a small amount of fluid to clean the mouth.
- Do not insert dentures. Unconscious persons do not wear dentures.

Do not use your fingers to keep the person's mouth open. The person can bite down on them. The bite breaks the skin, allowing microbes to enter the body. Infection is a risk. Using a bite block or plastic tongue depressor (bite stick) is a safe way to open the mouth (Fig. 21-5, *B*).

Mouth care is given at least every 2 hours. Follow the nurse's directions and the care plan.

See *Focus on Communication: Mouth Care for the Unconscious Person.*

See *Promoting Safety and Comfort: Mouth Care for the Unconscious Person.*

See procedure: *Providing Mouth Care for the Unconscious Person*, p. 266.

FOCUS ON **COMMUNICATION**
Mouth Care for the Unconscious Person

Unconscious persons cannot speak or respond to you. However, some can hear. Always assume that unconscious persons can hear. Tell the person who you are. Call the person by name. Explain what you are doing step-by-step. Also, tell the person when you are done, when you are leaving, and when you will return.

PROMOTING SAFETY AND COMFORT
Mouth Care for the Unconscious Person

Safety
Use sponge swabs with care. Make sure the sponge pad is tight on the stick. The person could aspirate or choke on the sponge if it comes off the stick.

Press the sponge swab against the side of the cup to squeeze out excess cleaning agent. A small amount of fluid is used to prevent aspiration.

Comfort
Unconscious persons are re-positioned at least every 2 hours. Combine mouth care with skin care, re-positioning, and other comfort measures.

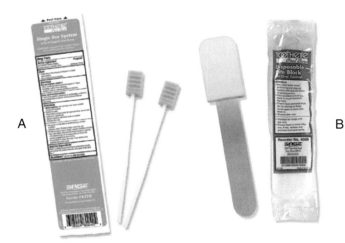

FIGURE 21-5 **A,** Oral sponge swabs. **B,** Bite block. (Courtesy Sage Products, LLC.)

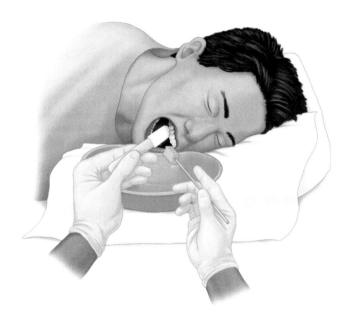

FIGURE 21-6 The unconscious person's head is turned well to the side to prevent aspiration. A bite block keeps the mouth open while cleaning the mouth with swabs.

Providing Mouth Care for the Unconscious Person

Quality of Life

- Knock before entering the person's room.
- Address the person by name.
- Introduce yourself by name and title.

- Explain the procedure before starting and during the procedure.
- Protect the person's rights during the procedure.
- Handle the person gently during the procedure.

Pre-Procedure

1 Follow *Delegation Guidelines: Purpose of Oral Hygiene*, p. 262. See *Promoting Safety and Comfort*:
   a *Purpose of Oral Hygiene*, p. 262
   b *Mouth Care for the Unconscious Person*, p. 265.
2 Practice hand hygiene and get the following supplies.
   - Cleaning agent (check the care plan)
   - Sponge swabs
   - Bite block or plastic tongue depressor
   - Water cup with cool water
   - Hand towel
   - Kidney basin
   - Lip lubricant (check the care plan)
   - Towel or paper towels (as a barrier for supplies)
   - Gloves
   - Laundry bag

3 Arrange items in the person's room. Place the barrier (towel, paper towels) on the over-bed table. Arrange items on top.
4 Practice hand hygiene.
5 Identify the person. Check the ID bracelet against the assignment sheet. Use 2 identifiers (Chapter 11). Also call the person by name.
6 Provide for privacy.
7 Raise the bed for body mechanics. Bed rails are up if used.

Procedure

8 Lower the bed rail near you.
9 Position the person in a side-lying position near you. Turn the person's head well to the side.
10 Place the towel under the person's face and along the chest. This protects the person and bed.
11 Practice hand hygiene. Put on the gloves.
12 Place the kidney basin under the chin.
13 Separate the upper and lower teeth. Use the bite block or plastic tongue depressor. Be gentle. Never use force. If you have problems, ask the nurse for help.
14 Moisten the sponge swabs with the cleaning agent. Squeeze out excess cleaning agent.

15 Clean the mouth.
   a Clean the inner, outer, and chewing surfaces of the upper and lower teeth.
   b Clean the gums and tongue.
   c Swab the roof of the mouth, inside of the cheeks, and the lips.
   d Moisten and squeeze out a clean swab. Swab the mouth to rinse.
   e Place used swabs in the kidney basin.
16 Remove the kidney basin and supplies.
17 Wipe the person's mouth. Remove the towel. Place the towel in the laundry bag.
18 Apply lubricant to the lips.
19 Remove and discard the gloves. Practice hand hygiene.
20 Return the person to a safe and comfortable position.

Post-Procedure

21 Provide for comfort. (See the inside of the back cover.)
22 Place the call light and other needed items within reach.
23 Lower the bed to a safe and comfortable level. Follow the care plan.
24 Raise or lower bed rails. Follow the care plan.
25 Clean, rinse, dry, and return equipment to its proper place. Use clean, dry paper towels for drying. Discard disposable items. (Wear gloves.)
26 Clean and dry the over-bed table. Dry with paper towels. Discard the paper towels. Remove and discard the gloves. Practice hand hygiene.

27 Follow the care plan for privacy measures to maintain. Leaving the privacy curtain, window coverings, and door open or closed are examples.
28 Complete a safety check of the room. (See the inside of the back cover.)
29 Tell the person that you are leaving the room. Say when you will return.
30 Follow agency policy for used linens.
31 Practice hand hygiene.
32 Report and record your care and observations.

DENTURES

A *denture* is a removable replacement for missing teeth (Fig. 21-7). Tooth loss occurs from gum disease, tooth decay, or injury. Often called *false teeth*, complete and partial dentures are common.

* *Complete (full) dentures.* Dentures replace all of the upper or lower teeth.
* *Partial dentures.* The person has some teeth. The partial denture replaces the missing teeth. Natural teeth still need to be brushed and flossed. See procedure: *Brushing and Flossing the Person's Teeth*, p. 263.

Some people do not wear their dentures. Others wear them only for eating. Remind patients and residents not to wrap dentures in tissues or napkins. Otherwise, they are easily discarded.

Denture Care Equipment

For cleaning, you need a denture cleaner, denture cup (see Fig. 21-7), and denture brush or toothbrush. Use only denture cleaning products to avoid damaging dentures. Dentures must be removed for cleaning. Do not use denture cleaning products on dentures while they are still in the mouth.

The manufacturer's instructions tell how to use the cleaning agent and what water temperature to use. Hot water causes warping—dentures lose their shape. When not worn, store them in a denture cup with cool or warm water or a denture soaking solution. Otherwise they can dry out and warp.

A denture adhesive may be used to hold dentures in place and keep food out of the inner part of the denture. The product (paste, cream, powder, pad, or strip) is applied to clean dentures. Follow the manufacturer's instructions for how to apply and the amount to use. Do not use too much adhesive. When cleaning dentures, gently brush to remove the adhesive. Adhesives are not used to fix dentures that fit poorly. Tell the nurse if dentures are loose.

Denture Care

Mouth care is given and dentures are cleaned as often as natural teeth. Dentures are slippery when wet. They easily break or chip if dropped onto a hard surface (floor, sink, counter). Hold them firmly when removing or inserting them (Fig. 21-8). During cleaning, firmly hold them over a sink filled half-way with water. Line the sink with a towel. This prevents the dentures from falling onto a hard surface.

Dentures are removed at bedtime. They are soaked over-night in a denture cleaning solution or water. Rinse the dentures before they are inserted.

If able, the person cleans the dentures. You clean dentures for persons who cannot do so.

See *Promoting Safety and Comfort: Denture Care*.
See procedure: *Providing Denture Care*, p. 268.

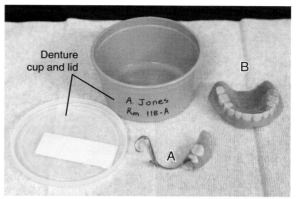

FIGURE 21-7 Dentures. **A,** Partial denture. **B,** Full denture.

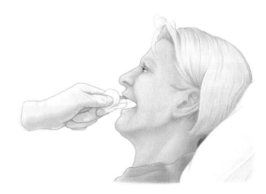

FIGURE 21-8 Removing dentures. Use a piece of gauze to grasp the denture.

PROMOTING SAFETY AND COMFORT

Denture Care

Safety

Dentures are costly. Handle them very carefully. Label the denture cup and lid with the person's name and room and bed number (see Fig. 21-7). Report lost or damaged dentures at once.

Never carry dentures in your hands. Always use a denture cup or kidney basin. You could easily drop the dentures if holding them.

Faucets are contaminated. Use a clean, dry paper towel to turn the faucet on and off and to adjust the faucet. Or use your wrist. If you contaminate your gloves, remove them. Practice hand hygiene. Apply clean gloves.

Never place dentures in or on a contaminated surface. Place dentures in a clean kidney basin or denture cup.

Dentures are rinsed under running water. Do not rinse dentures in the water used to fill the sink. The sink is contaminated.

Providing Denture Care

Quality of Life

- Knock before entering the person's room.
- Address the person by name.
- Introduce yourself by name and title.

- Explain the procedure before starting and during the procedure.
- Protect the person's rights during the procedure.
- Handle the person gently during the procedure.

Pre-Procedure

1 Follow *Delegation Guidelines: Purpose of Oral Hygiene*, p. 262. See *Promoting Safety and Comfort:*
   a *Purpose of Oral Hygiene*, p. 262
   b *Denture Care*, p. 267
2 Practice hand hygiene and get the following supplies.
   - Denture brush or toothbrush (for cleaning dentures)
   - Denture cup and lid labeled with the person's name and room and bed number
   - Denture cleaning agent
   - Denture adhesive as noted in the care plan (if needed)
   - Mouthwash (or other noted solution)
   - Kidney basin
   - 2 hand towels
   - Gauze squares
   - Towels or paper towels (as a barrier for supplies)
   - Gloves
   - Laundry bag

3 Arrange items in the person's room and near the sink.
   a Place a barrier (towel, paper towels) on the over-bed table. Arrange items needed at the bedside on top—gloves, hand towel, gauze squares, kidney basin, mouthwash (or other solution), denture adhesive (if needed).
   b Place a barrier (towel, paper towels) on the counter near the sink. Arrange needed items on top—denture cup and lid, hand towel, denture brush, denture cleaning agent.
4 Practice hand hygiene.
5 Identify the person. Check the ID bracelet against the assignment sheet. Use 2 identifiers (Chapter 11). Also call the person by name.
6 Provide for privacy.

Procedure

7 Place a towel over the person's chest.
8 Practice hand hygiene. Put on gloves.
9 Have the person remove the dentures and place them in the kidney basin.
10 Remove the dentures if the person cannot do so. Use gauze squares for a good grip on the slippery dentures.
   a Grasp the upper denture with your thumb and index finger (see Fig. 21-8). Move it up and down slightly to break the seal. Gently remove the denture. Place it in the kidney basin.
   b Grasp and remove the lower denture with your thumb and index finger. Turn it slightly and lift it out of the person's mouth. Place it in the kidney basin.
11 Take the kidney basin with dentures to the sink.
12 Rinse the denture cup and lid.
13 Line the bottom of the sink with a towel. Do not use paper towels. Fill the sink half-way with water.
14 Rinse each denture under cool or warm running water. Follow agency policy for water temperature.
15 Return dentures to the kidney basin.
16 Apply the denture cleaning agent to the brush.
17 Brush each denture. Brush the inner, outer, and chewing surfaces and all surfaces that touch the gums (Fig. 21-9).
18 Rinse the dentures under running water. Use cool or warm water as directed by the cleaning agent manufacturer.

19 Place dentures in the denture cup. Cover the dentures with cool or warm water. Follow agency policy for water temperature. Close the lid tightly.
20 *If dentures will not be worn,* store them in a safe place. Follow agency policy and the person's preference for where to store dentures. Dentures must be in water or in a denture soaking solution.
21 Clean the kidney basin. Take the kidney basin to the over-bed table. Take the denture cup if dentures will be worn.
22 Have the person use mouthwash (or noted solution). Hold the kidney basin under the chin. Wipe the person's mouth.
23 *If dentures will be worn:*
   a Apply denture adhesive if used. Follow the manufacturer's instructions for how to apply and the amount to use.
   b Have the person insert the dentures. Insert them if the person cannot.
      1) Hold the upper denture firmly with your thumb and index finger. Raise the upper lip with the other hand. Insert the denture. Gently press on the denture with your index finger to make sure it is in place.
      2) Hold the lower denture with your thumb and index finger. Pull the lower lip down slightly. Insert the denture. Gently press down on it to make sure it is in place.
24 Wipe the person's mouth if needed. Remove the towel. Place it in the laundry bag.
25 Remove and discard the gloves. Practice hand hygiene.

Providing Denture Care—cont'd

Post-Procedure

26 Assist with hand hygiene if needed. (See Chapter 14.)
27 Provide for comfort. (See the inside of the back cover.)
28 Place the call light and other needed items within reach.
29 Make sure the bed is at a safe and comfortable level. Follow the care plan.
30 Raise or lower bed rails. Follow the care plan.
31 Drain the sink.
32 Rinse the brushes. Empty and rinse the denture cup if dentures are worn. Clean, rinse, and dry equipment. Use clean, dry paper towels for drying. Return the brushes and equipment to their proper place. Discard disposable items. (Wear gloves.)

33 Clean and dry the over-bed table and counter. Dry with paper towels. Discard the paper towels.
34 Remove the towel from the sink. Squeeze to remove excess water. Place the towel in the laundry bag. Remove and discard the gloves. Practice hand hygiene.
35 Follow the care plan and the person's preferences for privacy measures to maintain. Leaving the privacy curtain, window coverings, and door open or closed are examples.
36 Complete a safety check of the room. (See the inside of the back cover.)
37 Follow agency policy for used linens.
38 Practice hand hygiene.
39 Report and record your care and observations.

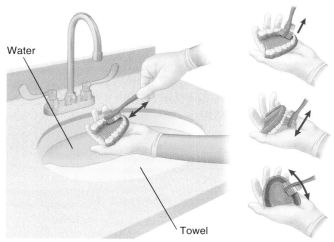

FIGURE 21-9 Cleaning dentures. Hold the dentures over a sink lined with a towel and filled half-way with water. Brush the inner, outer, and chewing surfaces. Brush the surfaces that touch the gums.

REPORTING AND RECORDING

You make many observations while assisting with oral hygiene.

- Dry, cracked, swollen, or blistered lips
- Mouth or breath odor
- Redness, swelling, irritation, sores, or white patches in the mouth or on the tongue
- Bleeding, swelling, or redness of the gums
- Reports of painful areas
- Loose teeth
- Rough, sharp, or chipped areas on dentures
- Loose dentures
- Reports of discomfort from dentures

Report and record your observations and the oral hygiene given. If not recorded, it is assumed that oral hygiene was not given. This can cause serious legal problems. Tell the nurse if the person refuses oral hygiene or if it was not given for another reason.

FOCUS ON P R I D E

The Person, Family, and Yourself

P ersonal and Professional Responsibility

Good oral hygiene helps prevent cavities, periodontal disease, and tooth loss. It also helps prevent breath odors that can be offensive to patients and residents. You have a personal and professional responsibility to practice thorough brushing and flossing.

R ights and Respect

Many people do not like being seen without their dentures. The person has the right to privacy. Allow privacy when the person cleans dentures. If you clean dentures, return them to the person as soon as possible.

I ndependence and Social Interaction

Poor oral hygiene can affect appearance and cause breath odors. When self-esteem is affected, the person may avoid social contact with others. Follow the care plan to meet the person's social needs.

D elegation and Teamwork

Some persons use special equipment for oral care. For example, a person uses a powered water flossing device. Or swabs that connect to suction are used for an unconscious person. (Suction equipment withdraws fluid.) Knowing how to use equipment is part of safe delegation (Chapter 3). Do not perform a task using equipment you are not trained to use or are not comfortable using. Ask the nurse for needed help.

E thics and Laws

Thorough oral hygiene takes time. Follow the person's preferences for when to assist with or perform oral hygiene. Do not neglect oral hygiene.

FOCUS ON PRIDE: *Application*

What are your oral hygiene practices? How do you feel after performing oral hygiene? How can you improve your practices?

REVIEW QUESTIONS

Circle the BEST answer.

1 You perform oral hygiene to
   a Prevent aspiration
   b Keep the mouth dry
   c Prevent mouth odors and infection
   d Remove cavities

2 Which is a sign of periodontal disease?
   a Chapped lips
   b Difficulty swallowing
   c Yellow teeth
   d Red and swollen gums

3 A person's gums bleed. This may be caused by
   a Using a toothbrush with soft bristles
   b Brushing too firmly
   c Inserting dental floss gently
   d Using mouthwash

4 A person should floss
   a Every morning
   b Before meals
   c Before brushing
   d At least once a day

5 You are flossing correctly if you
   a Rub the floss gently against the side of each tooth
   b Only floss the front teeth
   c Rub the floss against the gums firmly
   d Re-use floss

6 When giving mouth care to an unconscious person, you should
   a Replace dentures in the mouth after cleaning
   b Use your fingers to keep the person's mouth open
   c Position the person supine to prevent aspiration
   d Remove excess cleaning agent from the sponge swab

7 How often is mouth care given to an unconscious person?
   a At least every 2 hours
   b At least every 4 hours
   c At least every 8 hours
   d At least twice daily

8 A person has a full upper denture and a partial lower denture. You need to
   a Leave the dentures in the mouth at bedtime
   b Leave the partial denture in the mouth for cleaning
   c Brush and floss the remaining natural teeth
   d Place the upper denture in the sink while cleaning the lower denture

9 When cleaning dentures
   a Rinse the dentures in the water in the sink
   b Carry the dentures in your hands
   c Line the sink with a towel
   d Rinse the dentures in hot water

10 Which statement about denture care is *correct?*
    a Only use denture cleaning products on dentures.
    b Dentures can be stored in a dry denture cup over-night.
    c You do not need to rinse dentures after they soak in a cleaning solution.
    d Dentures do not break or chip easily.

11 A resident tells you that her dentures are loose. You should
    a Call the person's dentist
    b Tell the nurse
    c Line the denture with gauze
    d Apply a thick layer of adhesive

12 Which must you report to the nurse?
    a Clean dentures
    b Moist and intact lips
    c Bleeding gums
    d Food between the teeth

Answers to Chapter 21 questions are on p. 588.

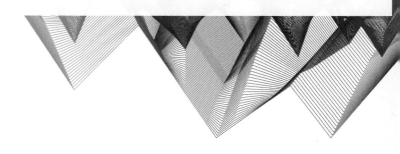

FOCUS ON **PRACTICE**

Problem Solving

Two residents share a bathroom. You are gathering supplies for oral care. Two toothbrushes and tubes of toothpaste are in the bathroom. The items are not labeled. What will you do? How can you be sure that residents use their own equipment?

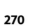

CHAPTER 22

Daily Hygiene and Bathing

OBJECTIVES

- Define the key terms and key abbreviations in this chapter.
- Explain why daily hygiene and bathing are important.
- Describe the care given before and after breakfast, after lunch, and in the evening.
- Describe the rules for bathing.
- Identify safety measures for tub baths and showers.

- Explain why perineal care is important.
- Identify the observations to report and record related to daily hygiene and bathing.
- Perform the procedures described in this chapter.
- Explain how to promote PRIDE in the person, the family, and yourself.

KEY TERMS

bath blanket A covering used for privacy and warmth during bathing, hygiene, and other care measures
circumcised The fold of skin (foreskin) covering the glans of the penis was surgically removed

pericare See "perineal care"
perineal care Cleaning the genital and anal areas; pericare
uncircumcised Foreskin covers the head of the penis

KEY ABBREVIATIONS

C   Centigrade
F   Fahrenheit

ID   Identification

Daily hygiene and bathing practices promote comfort, safety, and health. The skin is the body's first line of defense against disease. Intact skin prevents microbes from entering the body and causing an infection. Besides cleansing, hygiene measures prevent body and breath odors, are relaxing, and increase circulation.

Many factors affect daily hygiene needs—perspiration (sweating), elimination, vomiting, drainage from wounds or body openings, bed rest, and activity. Illness and aging can affect self-care abilities. Culture and personal choice also affect hygiene needs. (See *Caring About Culture: Daily Hygiene and Bathing*, p. 272.) The person's needs and preferences are part of the care plan.

See *Focus on Communication: Daily Hygiene and Bathing*, p. 272.

See *Focus on Older Persons: Daily Hygiene and Bathing*, p. 272.

See *Promoting Safety and Comfort: Daily Hygiene and Bathing*, p. 272.

CARING ABOUT CULTURE

Daily Hygiene and Bathing

Personal hygiene is very important to *East Indian Hindus*. For religious duty, at least 1 bath a day is required. Some believe bathing after a meal is harmful. Another belief is that a cold bath prevents a blood disease. Some believe that eye injuries can occur if bath water is too hot. Hot water can be added to cold water. However, cold water is not added to hot water for a bath. After bathing, the body is carefully dried with a towel.

> *Note: Each person is unique. A person may not follow all of the beliefs and practices of his or her culture. Follow the care plan.*

Modified from Giger JN: *Transcultural nursing: assessment and intervention*, ed 7, St Louis, 2017, Mosby.

FOCUS ON COMMUNICATION

Daily Hygiene and Bathing

During hygiene and bathing procedures, the person must be warm enough. You can ask:
- "Is the room warm enough?"
- "Is the water comfortable?" "Is it too hot?" "Is it too cold?"
- "Are you warm enough?"
- "Is the water starting to cool?"

FOCUS ON OLDER PERSONS

Daily Hygiene and Bathing

Some older persons resist hygiene efforts. Illness, disability, dementia, and personal choice are common reasons. Follow the care plan. Also see Chapter 42.

Bending and reaching are hard for older and disabled persons. Some have weak hand grips. They cannot hold soap or a washcloth. Adaptive (assistive) devices for hygiene promote independence (Fig. 22-1). Let the person do as much as safely possible.

PROMOTING SAFETY AND COMFORT

Daily Hygiene and Bathing

Safety

Hygiene and bathing measures often involve exposing and touching private areas—breasts, perineum, rectum. Sexual abuse has occurred in health care settings. The person may feel threatened or actually be abused. The person needs to be able to call for help. Keep the call light within the person's reach at all times. And always act in a professional manner.

You make observations while assisting with daily hygiene and bathing. The *Delegation Guidelines* in this chapter list the observations to report and record. Also report the following at once.
- Bleeding
- Signs of skin breakdown
- Discharge from the vagina, urinary tract, or rectum
- Unusual odors
- Changes from prior observations

> *Note: A task may require more than 1 pair of gloves. Change gloves as needed. Use careful judgment. Remember to practice hand hygiene after removing gloves.*

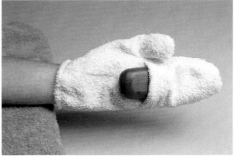
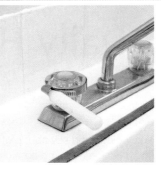
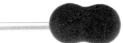

FIGURE 22-1 Adaptive (assistive) devices for hygiene. **A,** A wash mitt holds a bar of soap. **B,** A tap turner makes round knobs easy to turn. **C,** A long-handled sponge is used for hard-to-reach body parts. (Courtesy ElderStore, Alpharetta, Ga.)

DAILY CARE

Most people have hygiene routines and habits. For example, teeth are brushed and the face and hands are washed after sleep. These and other hygiene measures are common before and after meals and at bedtime.

Routine care is given during the day and evening (Box 22-1). You also assist with hygiene as needed. Always protect the right to privacy and to personal choice.

BATHING

Bathing cleans the skin and the genital and anal areas. Microbes, dead skin, perspiration (sweat), and excess oils are removed. A bath is refreshing and relaxing. Circulation is stimulated. Body parts are exercised. Observations are made. You have time to talk to the person.

Complete or partial bed baths, tub baths, or showers are given. The method depends on the person's condition, self-care abilities, and personal choice. In hospitals, bathing is common after breakfast. In nursing centers, bathing is usually before or after breakfast or after the evening meal. The person's choice of bath time is respected when possible.

Bathing frequency is a personal matter. Some people bathe daily. Others bathe 1 or 2 times a week. Some illnesses and dry skin may limit bathing to every 2 or 3 days.

The rules for bed baths, showers, and tub baths are listed in Box 22-2.

See *Focus on Older Persons: Bathing*, p. 274.
See *Delegation Guidelines: Bathing*, p. 274.
See *Promoting Safety and Comfort: Bathing*, p. 275.

BOX 22-1 Daily Care

Before Breakfast (Early Morning Care or AM Care)
- Prepare for breakfast or morning tests.
- Assist with elimination.
- Clean incontinent persons.
- Change wet or soiled linens and garments.
- Assist with washing the face and with hand hygiene.
- Assist with oral hygiene. Insert dentures if worn.
- Assist with dressing and hair care.
- Assist with eyeglasses or contact lenses, hearing aids, and other needed devices.
- Position for breakfast—dining room, bedside chair, or in bed.
- Make beds and straighten units.

After Breakfast (Morning Care)
- Assist with elimination.
- Clean incontinent persons.
- Change wet or soiled linens and garments.
- Assist with washing the face, hand hygiene, oral hygiene, bathing, and perineal care.
- Assist with hair care, shaving, dressing, and undressing.
- Assist with range-of-motion exercises and ambulation.
- Make beds and straighten rooms.

Afternoon Care
- Prepare persons for naps, visitors, or activity programs.
- Assist with elimination.
- Clean incontinent persons.
- Change wet or soiled linens and garments.
- Assist with washing the face, hand hygiene, oral hygiene, and hair care.
- Assist with range-of-motion exercises and ambulation.
- Provide back massages and other comfort measures (Chapter 33).
- Straighten beds and units.

Evening Care (PM Care)
- Prepare for sleep.
- Assist with elimination.
- Clean incontinent persons.
- Change wet or soiled linens and garments.
- Assist with washing the face and with hand hygiene.
- Assist with oral hygiene. Remove dentures if worn.
- Provide back massages and other comfort measures.
- Help with changing into sleepwear.
- Store eyeglasses or contact lenses, hearing aids, and other devices.
- Straighten beds and units.

BOX 22-2 Rules for Bathing

Bathing Method and Time
- Follow the care plan and personal preference for bathing method—bed bath, tub bath, or shower.
- Follow the care plan and personal preference for bathing time.
- Clean the skin any time urine or feces (stools) are present. Bathe areas that had contact with urine or feces. This prevents skin breakdown and odors.

Skin Care Products
- Follow the care plan and personal preference for skin care products.
  - *Bar soaps.* Some bar soaps dry and irritate the skin. This can cause itching, discomfort, and skin injury. Rinse the skin thoroughly to remove all soap.
  - *Body washes and shower gels.* These are gentle on the skin. Many contain a moisturizer or skin softener. Rinse thoroughly after use.
  - *No-rinse cleansers.* Sprays and foams are common. Follow the manufacturer's instructions. Wash and pat dry. No rinsing is needed. Perineal cleansers are for perineal care (p. 284).
  - *Lotions and creams.* These may be applied to the back, elbows, knees, and heels after bathing to protect the skin and prevent skin breakdown.
  - *Powders.* Powders absorb moisture and prevent friction when surfaces rub together. Powder may be applied under the breasts, under the arms, between skin folds, or in the groin area (where a thigh and the abdomen meet). Apply in a thin, even layer after drying the skin well. Excessive amounts cause caking and crusts that irritate the skin.
  - *Deodorants and antiperspirants.* These are applied to the underarms to control body odors and perspiration (sweat). Do not apply to irritated skin.

Safety
- Follow Standard Precautions and the Bloodborne Pathogen Standard.
- Collect needed items before the procedure.
- Use good body mechanics at all times.
- Follow the rules to safely move and transfer the person (Chapters 17 and 18).

Safety—cont'd
- Protect the person from falling.
- Know what water temperature to use. Use the following as a guide for adults. (°F means degrees Fahrenheit and °C means degrees centigrade.)
  - *Bed bath*—usually 110°F to 115°F (43.3°C to 46.1°C)
  - *Tub bath or shower*—usually 105°F (40.5°C)
  - *Perineal care*—usually 105°F to 109°F (40.5°C to 42.7°C)
- Remove hearing aids before bathing. Water damages hearing aids.
- Do not place bar soap in the bath water (basin or tub). Keep bar soap in the soap dish between latherings. This prevents soapy water. It also prevents slipping and falls.

Comfort
- Provide for privacy. Screen the person. Close doors and window coverings—drapes, shades, blinds, shutters, and so on.
- Assist with elimination. Bathing stimulates the need to urinate. Comfort and relaxation increase if the person urinates first.
- Reduce drafts. Close doors and windows.
- Cover the person for privacy and warmth. Use a **bath blanket**—*a covering used for privacy and warmth during bathing, hygiene, and other care measures.*

Independence
- Allow personal choice when possible.
- Encourage the person to help as much as safely possible.

Washing and Drying
- Wash from clean to dirty areas. Use a "head to toe" approach—eyes, face, neck, arms and hands, chest, abdomen, legs and feet, back. Clean the genital and anal areas (perineal area) last (p. 284).
- Rinse the skin thoroughly. You must remove all soap.
- Pat the skin dry to avoid irritating or breaking the skin. Do not rub the skin.
- Dry well under the breasts, between skin folds, in the genital and anal areas, and between the toes. Moisture can collect between skin folds, providing a place for microbes to live and grow. Skin irritation and a rash can occur (Fig. 22-2, p. 274).

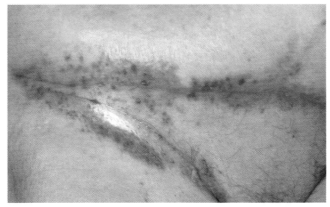

FIGURE 22-2 Moisture can collect between skin folds, causing irritation. Dry between skin folds thoroughly. (From Dinulos JGH: *Habif's clinical dermatology: a color guide to diagnosis and therapy*, ed 7, London, 2021, Elsevier.)

FOCUS ON OLDER PERSONS

Bathing

Aging and soap can dry the skin. Dry skin is easily damaged. Therefore older persons need a complete bed bath, tub bath, or shower only twice a week. They have partial baths on the other days. Some bathe daily without soap. Thorough rinsing is needed for soap. Lotion helps soften the skin.

Bathing procedures can threaten persons with dementia. Confusion can increase. They may fear harm or danger. Some resist care and become agitated and combative. They may shout at you and cry out for help. Remain calm, patient, and soothing. The person may be calmer and less confused or agitated during a certain time of day. Bathing is scheduled for calm times.

The nurse decides the best bathing procedure for the person. The rules in Box 22-2 apply. The care plan also has measures to help the person through the bath. For example:

- Say "cleaned up" or "washed" rather than "shower" or "bath."
- Complete pre-procedure activities. Ready supplies and linens and have everything you need.
- Provide for warmth. Prevent drafts. Have extra towels, an extra bath blanket, or a robe nearby.
- Provide good lighting.
- Draw bath water ahead of time. Test the water temperature and adjust as needed.

- Play soft music to help the person relax.
- Provide for safety.
  - Use a hand-held shower nozzle.
  - Have the person use a shower chair or shower bench.
  - Do not use bath oil. It can make the tub or shower slippery. And it may cause a urinary tract infection.
  - Do not leave the person alone in the tub or shower.
- Tell the person what you are doing step-by-step. Use clear, simple words and sentences.
- Let the person help as much as possible. For example, give the person a washcloth. Say what to wash step-by-step (face, arms, hands). Even if the person does not know what to do, let the person hold the washcloth if safe to do so.
- Put a towel over the shoulders (tub bath) or lap (shower). This helps the person feel less exposed.
- Do not rush the person.
- Use a calm, pleasant voice.
- Distract the person if needed.
- Calm the person.
- Handle the person gently.
- Try a partial bath if a shower or tub bath agitates the person.
- Try the bath later if the person continues to resist care.

DELEGATION GUIDELINES

Bathing

To assist with bathing, you need this information from the nurse and the care plan.

- What bath to give—complete bed bath, partial bath, tub bath, or shower.
- How much help the person needs.
- Activity or position limits.
- What water temperature to use. See Box 22-2.
- What skin care products the person prefers.
- What observations to report and record:
  - The color of the skin, lips, nail beds, and sclera (whites of the eyes)
  - If the skin appears pale, gray-ish, yellow (*jaundice*), or bluish (*cyanotic*)

- The location and description of rashes
- Skin texture—smooth, rough, scaly, flaky, dry, moist
- *Diaphoresis*—profuse (excessive) sweating
- Bruises or open skin areas
- Pale, reddened, or discolored areas, particularly over bony parts
- Drainage or bleeding from wounds or body openings
- Swelling of the feet and legs
- Corns or calluses on the feet (Chapter 35)
- Skin temperature (cold, cool, warm, hot)
- Complaints of pain or discomfort
- When to report observations.
- What patient or resident concerns to report at once.

PROMOTING SAFETY AND COMFORT

Bathing

Safety

Water: Hot water can burn the skin. Measure water temperature according to agency policy. If unsure if the water is too hot, ask the nurse to check it.

Falls and injuries: Protect the person from falls and other injuries. Follow the care plan for bed rail use. Ask a co-worker for help if needed. Make sure bed wheels are locked. When working alone, lower the bed to a safe level before leaving the bedside. Practice the safety measures in Chapters 11 and 12.

Body mechanics: Use good body mechanics to protect yourself from injury (Chapter 16). For the procedure that follows, you work on 1 side of the bed. To avoid straining and reaching, move the person to the side of the bed near you. Or wash 1 side of the body and then move to the other side to finish the bath. If room space allows, wash the side of the body near you (eyes and face, arm, hand, chest, abdomen, leg, foot). Then move the over-bed table with equipment and supplies to the other side of the bed. Finish the bath (arm, hand, leg, foot, back, and perineal care) on that side.

Gloves: Wear gloves when contact with blood or body fluids, mucous membranes, or non-intact skin is likely. Follow Standard Precautions and the Bloodborne Pathogen Standard. (For skills tested in your state, wear gloves as required by your state's competency exam. The procedures in this chapter include glove use.) Remove contaminated gloves and practice hand hygiene before moving to a clean body site or touching clean items or surfaces. Apply clean gloves if needed.

Bathing equipment: Bathing equipment must be clean. A wash basin is used for 1 person. Tubs and showers may be used by many persons. See "Tub Bath and Shower Safety" on p. 281.

Foot care: Ask the nurse if you should clean under the person's toenails. The device used (orangewood stick or nail file) has a sharp tip that could injure the person. Foot injuries can be very serious for some persons. See Chapter 23 for nail care.

Powder: Apply powder with caution. Do not use powders near persons with respiratory disorders. Inhaling powder can irritate the airway and lungs. Before using powder, check with the nurse and the care plan. To safely apply powder:
- Turn away from the person.
- Sprinkle a small amount onto your hand or a cloth. Do not shake or sprinkle powder onto the person.
- Apply the powder in a thin layer.
- Make sure powder does not get on the floor. Powder is slippery and can cause falls.

Bedmaking: For an occupied bed, make the bed after the bath. See Chapter 20.

Comfort

Elimination: Before bathing, let the person meet elimination needs (Chapters 25 and 27). Bathing stimulates the need to urinate. Comfort is greater with an empty bladder. Also bathing is not interrupted.

Warmth: Provide for warmth. Cover the person with a bath blanket. Protect the person from drafts. Make sure the water is warm enough. Cool water causes chilling.

Oral hygiene and grooming: Oral hygiene is common before or after bathing (Chapter 21). Grooming measures often occur with bathing (Chapter 23). Allow personal choice and follow the care plan.

Clothing and sleepwear: If the person prefers, remove clothing or sleepwear after washing the eyes, face, ears, and neck. Removing clothing or sleepwear at this time helps the person feel less exposed and provides more mental comfort with the bath. See Chapter 24 for undressing and dressing.

Perineal care: If able, have the person wash the genital and anal areas. This promotes privacy and helps prevent embarrassment. See "Perineal Care" on p. 284.

The Complete Bed Bath

For a complete bed bath, you wash the person's entire body in bed. Bed baths are usually needed by persons who are:

- Unconscious
- Paralyzed
- In casts or traction
- Weak from illness or surgery
- Unable to bathe themselves

A bed bath is new to some people. Some are embarrassed to have their bodies seen. Some fear exposure. Explain how you give the bath and provide for privacy.

Bath water for bed baths cools rapidly. Heat is lost to the wash basin, over-bed table, washcloth, and your hands. Therefore water temperature for bed baths is usually between 110°F and 115°F (43.3°C and 46.1°C) for adults. Older persons have fragile skin. They need lower water temperatures.

See procedure: *Giving a Complete Bed Bath*, p. 276.

Giving a Complete Bed Bath

Quality of Life

- Knock before entering the person's room.
- Address the person by name.
- Introduce yourself by name and title.

- Explain the procedure before starting and during the procedure.
- Protect the person's rights during the procedure.
- Handle the person gently during the procedure.

Pre-Procedure

1 Follow *Delegation Guidelines: Bathing*, p. 274. See *Promoting Safety and Comfort:*
   a *Daily Hygiene and Bathing*, p. 272
   b *Bathing*, p. 275
2 Practice hand hygiene.
3 Identify the person. Check the identification (ID) bracelet against the assignment sheet. Use 2 identifiers (Chapter 11). Also call the person by name.
4 Collect clean linens. (See procedure: *Making a Closed Bed* in Chapter 20.) Place linens on a clean surface.
5 Get the following supplies.
   - Wash basin
   - Soap or body wash
   - Water thermometer
   - Orangewood stick or nail file
   - Washcloths—1 or more for washing and rinsing (some state competency tests specify a clean, "soap-free" washcloth for rinsing) and at least 4 washcloths for perineal care (p. 284)

   - Towels—at least 1 hand towel, 2 bath towels, a separate towel for perineal care (p. 284)
   - Bath blanket
   - Clothing or sleepwear
   - Lotion and powder
   - Deodorant or antiperspirant
   - Brush and comb
   - Other grooming items as requested
   - Towel or paper towels (as a barrier for supplies)
   - Gloves
   - Laundry bag
6 Place a barrier (towel, paper towels) on the over-bed table. Arrange items on top. Adjust the height as needed.
7 Provide for privacy.
8 Raise the bed for body mechanics. Bed rails are up if used. Lower the bed rail near you if up.

Procedure

9 Practice hand hygiene.
10 Cover the person with a bath blanket. Remove top linens (see procedure: *Making an Occupied Bed* in Chapter 20).
11 Remove clothing or sleepwear. Do not expose the person. Follow agency policy for used clothing or sleepwear. (Wear gloves if clothing is wet or soiled. Practice hand hygiene after removing and discarding gloves.)
12 Fill the wash basin ⅔ (two-thirds) full with water. (Follow the care plan for bed rail use. Raise the rail if used. Lower the bed to a safe level.) Follow the care plan for water temperature. Water temperature is usually 110°F to 115°F (43.3°C to 46.1°C) for adults. Measure water temperature. Use the water thermometer. Or dip your elbow or inner wrist into the basin to test the water.
13 Have the person check the water temperature. Adjust the water temperature as needed.
14 Place the basin on the over-bed table.
15 Raise the bed for body mechanics. Lower the bed rail near you if up.
16 Lower the head of the bed. It is as flat as possible. The person has at least 1 pillow.
17 Practice hand hygiene. Put on gloves.
18 Place a hand towel over the person's chest.
19 Make a mitt with the washcloth (Fig. 22-3, p. 278). Use a mitt for the entire bath. (Note: Some state competency tests require that the corners of the washcloth be contained during bathing. This is one method.)
20 Have the person close the eyes. Wash the eyelids and around the eyes with water. Do not use soap.
   a Clean the far eye. Gently wipe from the inner to the outer aspect of the eye with a corner of the mitt (Fig. 22-4, p. 278).
   b Clean the eye near you. Use a clean part of the washcloth for each stroke.

21 Wash, rinse, and dry the face, ears, and neck.
   a Ask if the person wants soap or body wash used on the face. If so, apply soap or body wash to the washcloth. If not, just use water. Wash the face and ears.
   b Wash the neck using soap or body wash.
   c Rinse all areas. Use a soap-free washcloth.
   d Pat dry with the towel on the chest.
22 Help the person move to the side of the bed near you.
23 Wash, rinse, and dry the far arm.
   a Expose the arm. Place a bath towel length-wise under the arm.
   b Apply soap or body wash to the washcloth.
   c Support the arm with your palm under the person's elbow. The person's forearm rests on your forearm.
   d Wash the arm, shoulder, and underarm. Use long, firm strokes (Fig. 22-5, p. 278).
   e Rinse all areas. Use a soap-free washcloth.
   f Pat dry. Dry well under the underarm.
24 Wash, rinse, and dry the far hand.
   a Method 1—place the basin on the towel. Put the person's hand into the water (Fig. 22-6, p. 278). Have the person exercise the hand and fingers. Wash the hand well. Remove the basin.
   b Method 2—apply soap or body wash to the washcloth. Wash the hand well.
   c Clean under the nails if nail care is done during the bath. Or perform nail care separately (Chapter 23). Use an orangewood stick or nail file.
   d Rinse the hand. Use a soap-free washcloth.
   e Pat dry.
   f Remove the towel under the arm. Cover the arm with the bath blanket.
25 Repeat steps 23 and 24 for the near arm and hand.

Giving a Complete Bed Bath—cont'd

Procedure—cont'd

26 Wash, rinse, and dry the chest.
  a Place a bath towel over the chest cross-wise. Hold the towel in place. Pull the bath blanket from under the towel to the waist.
  b Apply soap or body wash to the washcloth.
  c Lift the towel slightly and wash the chest (Fig. 22-7, p. 278). Do not expose the person.
  d Rinse the chest. Use a soap-free washcloth.
  e Pat dry. Dry well under the breasts.
27 Wash, rinse, and dry the abdomen.
  a Move the towel length-wise over the chest and abdomen. Do not expose the person. Pull the bath blanket down to the pubic area.
  b Apply soap or body wash to the washcloth.
  c Lift the towel slightly and wash the abdomen (Fig. 22-8, p. 278).
  d Rinse the abdomen. Use a soap-free washcloth.
  e Pat dry. Dry well under abdominal skin folds.
28 Pull the bath blanket up to the shoulders. Cover both arms. Remove the towel.
29 Change soapy or cool water as needed. Follow these safety measures.
  a Raise the bed rail if used. Lower the bed to a safe level.
  b Measure bath water temperature as in step 12. Have the person check the water temperature.
  c Raise the bed for body mechanics and lower the bed rail if used when you return.
30 Wash, rinse, and dry the far leg.
  a Uncover the far leg. Do not expose the genital area. Place a towel length-wise under the foot and leg.
  b Apply soap or body wash to a washcloth.
  c Bend the knee and support the leg with your arm. Wash it with long, firm strokes. Wash the skin fold area of the groin.
  d Rinse the leg. Use a soap-free washcloth.
  e Pat dry. Dry the groin area well.
31 Wash, rinse, and dry the far foot.
  a Method 1—place the basin on the towel near the foot. Bend the knee and lift the leg slightly. Slide the basin under the foot. Place the foot in the basin (Fig. 22-9, p. 279). Wash the foot well. Carefully separate the toes. Remove the basin.
  b Method 2—apply soap or body wash to the washcloth. Wash the foot well. Carefully separate the toes.

  c Clean under the nails if instructed to do so and if nail care is done during the bath. Or perform nail care separately (Chapter 23). Use an orangewood stick or nail file.
  d Rinse the foot. Use a soap-free washcloth.
  e Pat dry. Dry well between the toes.
  f Apply lotion to the foot if directed by the nurse and the care plan. Do not apply lotion between the toes.
  g Cover the leg with the bath blanket. Remove the towel.
32 Repeat steps 30 and 31 for the near leg and foot.
33 Change the water. Follow the safety measures in step 29.
34 Wash, rinse, and dry the back and buttocks.
  a Turn the person onto the side away from you. The person is covered with the bath blanket.
  b Uncover the back and buttocks. Do not expose the person. Place a towel length-wise on the bed along the back.
  c Apply soap or body wash to a washcloth.
  d Wash the back. Work from the back of the neck to the lower end of the buttocks. Use long, firm, continuous strokes (Fig. 22-10, p. 279).
  e Rinse the back and buttocks. Use a soap-free washcloth.
  f Pat dry.
35 Place used washcloths and towels in the laundry bag.
36 Turn the person onto the back.
37 Wash, rinse, and dry the genital and anal areas (p. 284).
  a Change the water. Follow the safety measures in step 29. Water temperature for perineal care is lower (usually 105°F to 109°F/40.5°C to 42.7°C).
  b Allow the person to clean the genital and anal areas if able. If the person cannot do so, perform perineal care with clean gloves (p. 284). At least 4 washcloths and a clean towel are needed. Place each washcloth in the laundry bag after 1 use. Washcloths are not re-used for perineal care.
38 Remove and discard the gloves. Practice hand hygiene.
39 Give a back massage (Chapter 33).
40 Apply lotion, powder, and deodorant or antiperspirant as requested. See *Promoting Safety and Comfort: Bathing* (p. 275) for how to safely apply powder.
41 Put clean garments on the person (Chapter 24).
42 Comb and brush the person's hair (Chapter 23).
43 Make the bed (Chapter 20). Remove the bath blanket and place it in the laundry bag.

Post-Procedure

44 Provide for comfort. (See the inside of the back cover.)
45 Place the call light and other needed items within reach.
46 Lower the bed to a safe and comfortable level. Follow the care plan.
47 Raise or lower bed rails. Follow the care plan.
48 Put on clean gloves.
49 Empty, clean, rinse, and dry the wash basin. Use clean, dry paper towels for drying. Return the basin and other supplies to their proper place.
50 Clean and dry the over-bed table. Dry with paper towels. Discard the paper towels.
51 Remove and discard the gloves. Practice hand hygiene.

52 Follow the care plan and the person's preferences for privacy measures to maintain. Leaving the privacy curtain, window coverings, and door open or closed are examples.
53 Complete a safety check of the room. (See the inside of the back cover.)
54 Follow agency policy for used linens.
55 Practice hand hygiene.
56 Report and record your care and observations.

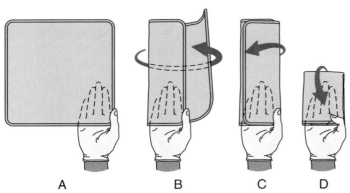

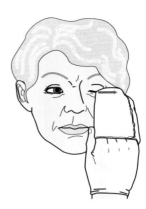

FIGURE 22-3 Making a mitted washcloth. **A,** Grasp the near side of the washcloth with your thumb. **B,** Bring the washcloth around and behind your hand. **C,** Fold the side of the washcloth over your palm as you grasp it with your thumb. **D,** Fold the top of the washcloth down. Tuck it under next to your palm.

FIGURE 22-4 Wash the eyes with a mitted washcloth. Wipe from the inner to the outer aspect of the eye. Use a clean part of the washcloth for each stroke. Use a clean part of the washcloth for the other eye.

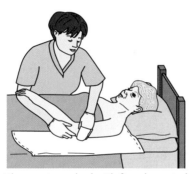

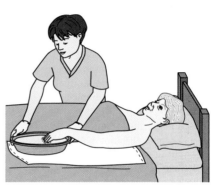

FIGURE 22-5 The arm is washed with firm, long strokes.

FIGURE 22-6 The hand can be washed by placing the wash basin on the bed.

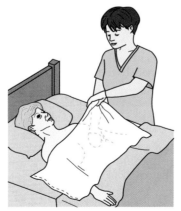

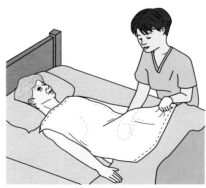

FIGURE 22-7 A bath towel is placed horizontally over the chest area. The towel is lifted slightly to reach under and wash the chest. Breasts are not exposed.

FIGURE 22-8 The bath towel is turned so that it is vertical to cover the chest and abdomen. The towel is lifted slightly to bathe the abdomen. The bath blanket covers the pubic area.

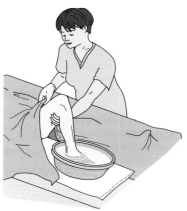

FIGURE 22-9 The foot can be washed by placing it in the wash basin on the bed.

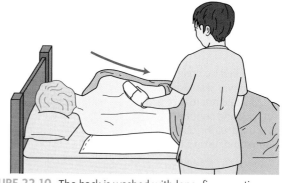

FIGURE 22-10 The back is washed with long, firm, continuous strokes. A towel is placed length-wise on the bed to protect the linens from water. (NOTE: Bed rails are used according to the care plan.)

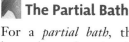 The Partial Bath

For a *partial bath*, the face, hands, underarms, back, buttocks, and perineal area are washed. Bathing prevents odors and discomfort in those areas. Some persons can wash in bed, at the bedside, or at the sink with warm running water (Fig. 22-11). You assist as needed. Most persons need help washing the back. You give partial baths to persons who cannot bathe themselves.

The rules for bathing apply (see Box 22-2). So do the complete bed bath considerations.

See procedure: *Assisting With the Partial Bath.*

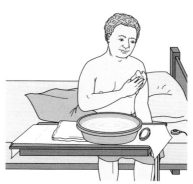

FIGURE 22-11 The person is bathing while sitting on the side of the bed. Needed equipment is within reach.

Assisting With the Partial Bath

Quality of Life

- Knock before entering the person's room.
- Address the person by name.
- Introduce yourself by name and title.

- Explain the procedure before starting and during the procedure.
- Protect the person's rights during the procedure.
- Handle the person gently during the procedure.

Pre-Procedure

1 Follow *Delegation Guidelines: Bathing,* p. 274. See *Promoting Safety and Comfort:*
   a *Daily Hygiene and Bathing,* p. 272
   b *Bathing,* p. 275

2 Follow steps 2 through 7 in procedure: *Giving a Complete Bed Bath,* p. 276. (This procedure explains how to assist with a partial bath in bed.)

Procedure

3 Make sure the bed is in a low position.
4 Practice hand hygiene.
5 Cover the person with a bath blanket. Remove top linens.
6 Fill the wash basin ⅔ (two-thirds) full with water. Water temperature is usually 110°F to 115°F (43.3°C to 46.1°C) or as directed by the nurse. Measure water temperature with the water thermometer. Or test bath water by dipping your elbow or inner wrist into the basin.
7 Have the person check the water temperature. Adjust the water temperature as needed.
8 Place the basin on the over-bed table.
9 Position the person in Fowler's position or sitting at the bedside.

10 Adjust the over-bed table so the person can reach the basin and supplies.
11 Help the person undress. (Wear gloves if clothing is wet or soiled. Practice hand hygiene after removing and discarding gloves.) Use the bath blanket for privacy and warmth.
12 Have the person wash easy-to-reach body parts. Explain that you will wash the back and areas the person cannot reach.
13 Be sure the call light is within reach. Have the person signal when help is needed or bathing is complete.
14 Practice hand hygiene. Then leave the room.
15 Return when the call light is on. Knock before entering. Practice hand hygiene.

Continued

NATCEP VIDEO

Assisting With the Partial Bath—cont'd

Procedure—cont'd

16 Change the bath water. Measure bath water temperature as in step 6.
17 Raise the bed for body mechanics. The far bed rail is up if used.
18 Ask what was washed. Put on gloves. Wash and dry areas the person could not reach. The face, hands, underarms, back, buttocks, and perineal area are washed for the partial bath.
19 Place used washcloths and towels in the laundry bag.
20 Remove and discard the gloves. Practice hand hygiene.

21 Give a back massage (Chapter 33).
22 Apply lotion, powder, and deodorant or antiperspirant as requested.
23 Help the person put on clean garments.
24 Assist with hair care and other grooming needs.
25 Make the bed. Remove the bath blanket and place it in the laundry bag.

Post-Procedure

26 Provide for comfort. (See the inside of the back cover.)
27 Place the call light and other needed items within reach.
28 Lower the bed to a safe and comfortable level. Follow the care plan.
29 Raise or lower bed rails. Follow the care plan.
30 Put on clean gloves.
31 Empty, clean, rinse, and dry the wash basin. Use clean, dry paper towels for drying. Return the basin and supplies to their proper place.
32 Clean and dry the over-bed table. Dry with paper towels. Discard the paper towels.

33 Remove and discard the gloves. Practice hand hygiene.
34 Follow the care plan and the person's preferences for privacy measures to maintain. Leaving the privacy curtain, window coverings, and door open or closed are examples.
35 Complete a safety check of the room. (See the inside of the back cover.)
36 Follow agency policy for used linens.
37 Practice hand hygiene.
38 Report and record your care and observations.

Tub Baths and Showers

Some people like tub baths. Others like showers. Follow the nurse's directions and the care plan for the method used and the amount of help the person needs.

Tub Baths. Tub baths are relaxing. However, a tub bath can make a person feel faint, weak, or tired. These are great risks for persons who were on bed rest. A tub bath lasts no longer than 20 minutes.

To get in and out of the tub, the person may use:
- A tub with a side entry door (Fig. 22-12).
- Bathing lift. The device transports and lifts the person into the tub (Fig. 22-13).
- Mechanical lift (Chapter 18).

Whirlpool tubs have a cleansing action. You wash the upper body. Carefully wash under the breasts and between skin folds. Also wash the perineal area. Pat the person dry with towels after the bath.

Showers. Some people can stand during a shower. Grab bars (safety bars) are used for support. Showers have slip-resistant surfaces. If not, a rubber bath mat is used. Weak or unsteady persons use:
- *Shower chairs.* Water drains through an opening (Fig. 22-14). You may use the chair to transport the person to and from the shower. Or the person transfers to the shower chair in the bathroom or shower room. Lock (brake) the wheels during transfers and during the shower to prevent falls. Shower chairs come in different sizes. Use the correct size.
- *Shower benches.* Some showers contain benches that fold down (Fig. 22-15). The person sits on the bench during the shower.
- *Shower trolleys (portable tubs).* The person has a shower lying down (Fig. 22-16). Lower the sides to transfer the person from the bed to the trolley. Then raise the side rails for transport to the tub or shower room. Use the hand-held nozzle for the shower.

Some shower rooms have 2 or more stations. Provide for privacy. Properly screen and cover the person. Also close doors and shower curtains.

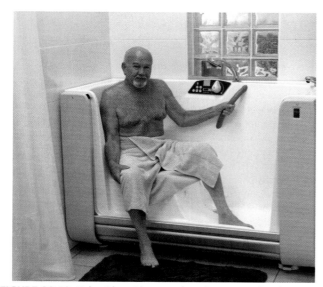

FIGURE 22-12 Tub with a side entry door. (Image used with permission of Arjo Inc.)

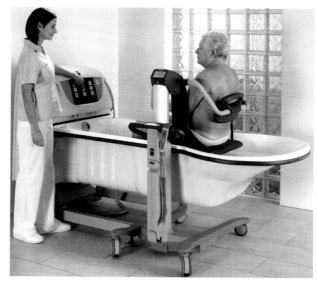

FIGURE 22-13 The lift lowers the person into the tub. (Image used with permission of Arjo Inc.)

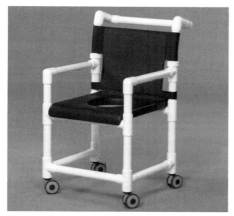

FIGURE 22-14 A shower chair. (Courtesy Innovative Products Unlimited, Niles, Mich.)

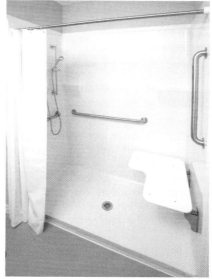

FIGURE 22-15 A shower bench.

Tub Bath and Shower Safety. Falls, burns, and chilling from water are risks during tub baths and showers. Safety is important (Box 22-3, p. 282). The measures in Box 22-2 also apply.

See *Delegation Guidelines: Tub Baths and Showers*, p. 282.

See *Promoting Safety and Comfort: Tub Baths and Showers*, p. 282.

See procedure: *Assisting With a Tub Bath or Shower*, p. 283.

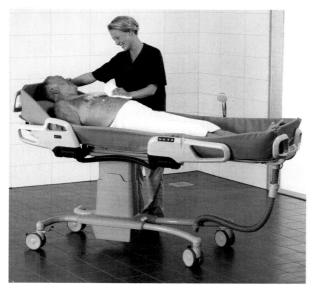

FIGURE 22-16 Shower trolley. The sides are lowered for transfers into and out of the trolley. (Image used with permission of Arjo Inc.)

BOX 22-3 Tub Bath and Shower Safety

Tub Baths and Showers
- Follow agency practices to clean, disinfect, and dry the tub or shower before and after use. Be sure the floor is dry.
- Make sure hand rails, grab bars (safety bars), lifts, and other safety aids are in working order.
- Place a rubber bath mat in the tub or on the shower floor if needed. This is not needed if there are slip-resistant strips or a slip-resistant surface.
- Provide for warmth and privacy. This includes during transport to and from the tub or shower room.
- Place the call light and other needed items within reach. Show how to use the call light.
- Have the person use grab bars (safety bars) to get in and out of the tub or shower.
- Follow the safety measures and transfer procedures for wheelchairs when using wheeled shower chairs. See Chapter 18.
- Know what water temperature to use (usually 105°F/40.5°C).
- Turn cold water on first, then hot water (for a 2-handled faucet). Turn hot water off first, then cold water. This helps prevent burns.
- Keep bar soap in the soap dish between latherings. This helps prevent slipping and falls in tubs and showers. It also prevents soapy tub water.
- Avoid bath oils. They make tub and shower surfaces slippery.
- Do not leave weak or unsteady persons unattended.
- Stay within hearing distance if the person can be left alone. Wait outside the door or shower curtain. You must be nearby if the person calls for you or has an accident.

Tub Baths
- Fill the tub before the person gets into it. For a tub with a side entry door, fill the tub with the person in it. Follow the manufacturer's instructions.
- Monitor water temperature as the tub fills.
- Use the digital display or a water thermometer to measure water temperature.
- Have the person check the water temperature. Adjust as needed.
- Drain the tub before the person gets out of the tub. Cover the person for warmth.

Showers
- Adjust water temperature to prevent chilling and burns.
- Use the digital display when checking water temperature.
- Have the person check the water temperature. Adjust as needed.
- Direct water away from the person when adjusting water temperature and pressure.
- Keep the water spray directed toward the person during the shower. This provides for warmth.
- Do not direct water spray toward the face. This can frighten the person.
- Turn off the shower before the person gets out of the shower.

DELEGATION GUIDELINES
Tub Baths and Showers

Before assisting with a tub bath or shower, you need this information from the nurse and the care plan:
- If the person takes a tub bath or shower
- What water temperature to use (usually 105°F/40.5°C)
- What equipment is needed—bathing lift, mechanical lift, shower chair, shower bench, shower trolley, and so on
- What size shower chair to use (if needed)—standard or bariatric
- How much help the person needs
- If the person can be left alone
- What observations to report and record:
  - Dizziness
  - Light-headedness
  - See *Delegation Guidelines: Bathing*, p. 274
- When to report observations
- What patient or resident concerns to report at once

PROMOTING SAFETY AND COMFORT
Tub Baths and Showers

Safety
Follow the safety measures for transfers (Chapter 18). Follow the care plan for the transfer method and number of staff needed. Remember:
- Slip-resistant footwear is worn for transfers.
- Be sure the floor is dry.
- Have the person use grab bars (safety bars) for support.
- Lock (brake) the wheels on a wheelchair and shower chair.
- Apply a transfer belt (gait belt) over clothing.

Follow the manufacturer's instructions for devices used—tub with a side entry door, bathing lift, mechanical lift, shower chair, and others.

Protect the person from chilling and burns. Remember to measure water temperature. Ask the person if the water is comfortable.

Clean, disinfect, and dry the tub or shower before and after use. This prevents the spread of microbes and infection.

Comfort
Warmth and privacy promote comfort during tub baths and showers.
- Make sure the tub or shower room is warm.
- Provide for privacy. Close the room door. Close window coverings.
- Make sure the water is comfortable for the person.
- Have the person remove clothing or robe and footwear just before getting into the tub or shower. Do not have the person exposed longer than necessary.
- Stay nearby (within hearing distance) if the person can be left alone. Provide as much privacy as possible.

Assisting With a Tub Bath or Shower

Quality of Life

- Knock before entering the person's room.
- Address the person by name.
- Introduce yourself by name and title.

- Explain the procedure before starting and during the procedure.
- Protect the person's rights during the procedure.
- Handle the person gently during the procedure.

Pre-Procedure

1 Follow *Delegation Guidelines:*
 a *Bathing, p. 274*
 b *Tub Baths and Showers*
 See *Promoting Safety and Comfort:*
 a *Daily Hygiene and Bathing, p. 272*
 b *Bathing, p. 275*
 c *Tub Baths and Showers*
2 Reserve the tub or shower room.
3 Practice hand hygiene.
4 Identify the person. Check the ID bracelet against the assignment sheet. Use 2 identifiers (Chapter 11). Also call the person by name.
5 Get the following supplies.
 - Washcloths—at least 1 for bathing or showering and washcloths for perineal care
 - Bath towels—at least 2

- Bath blanket
- Soap or body wash
- Water thermometer (for a tub bath)
- Clothing or sleepwear
- Grooming items as requested
- Robe and slip-resistant footwear
- Rubber bath mat if needed
- Disposable bath mat if needed
- Gloves
- Laundry bag
- Wheelchair, shower chair, and so on as needed

Procedure

6 Place items in the tub or shower room. Use the space provided or a chair.
7 Clean, disinfect, and dry the tub or shower. Use clean, dry paper towels for drying. Be sure the floor is dry. (Wear gloves for this step. Practice hand hygiene after removing and discarding the gloves.)
8 Place a rubber bath mat in the tub or on the shower floor if needed. Do not block the drain.
9 Place the disposable bath mat on the floor in front of the tub or shower if needed.
10 Put the *OCCUPIED* sign on the door.
11 Return to the person's room. Provide for privacy. Practice hand hygiene.
12 Help the person sit on the side of the bed.
13 Help the person put on a robe and slip-resistant footwear. Or the person can leave on clothing.
14 Assist or transport the person to the tub or shower room.
15 Have the person sit on a chair if the person walked to the tub or shower room.
16 Provide for privacy.
17 *For a tub bath:*
 a Fill the tub half-way with warm water (usually 105°F/40.5°C). Follow the care plan for water temperature.
 b Measure water temperature. Use the water thermometer or check the digital display.
 c Have the person check the water temperature. Adjust the water temperature as needed.
18 *For a shower:*
 a Turn on the shower.
 b Adjust water temperature and pressure. Check the digital display. Water temperature is usually 105°F/40.5°C.
 c Have the person check the water temperature. Adjust the water temperature as needed.
19 Help the person undress and remove footwear.

20 Help the person into the tub or shower. Position the shower chair and lock (brake) the wheels.
21 Assist with washing as necessary. Wear gloves.
 a Wash the face, neck, arms, hands, chest, abdomen, legs, feet, back, and buttocks.
 b Provide perineal care if the person is not able. Wear clean gloves and use clean washcloths. Remove and discard gloves. Practice hand hygiene.
 c Follow the care plan and the person's preference for shampooing hair (Chapter 23). Assist with shampooing as needed.
22 Have the person use the call light when done or when help is needed. Remind the person that a tub bath lasts no longer than 20 minutes.
23 Place a towel across the chair.
24 Stay in the room or nearby if the person can be left alone. Check the person at least every 5 minutes.
25 Respond when the person signals for you.
26 Turn off the shower or drain the tub. Cover the person with the bath blanket.
27 Help the person out of the shower or tub and onto the chair.
28 Help the person dry off. Pat gently. Dry well under the breasts, between skin folds, between the toes, and in the perineal area.
29 Place the washcloth and towels in the laundry bag.
30 Apply lotion, powder, and deodorant or antiperspirant as requested.
31 Help the person dress and put on footwear. Place the bath blanket in the laundry bag.
32 Practice hand hygiene.
33 Help the person return to his or her room. Provide for privacy.
34 Assist the person to a chair or into bed.
35 Provide a back massage if the person returns to bed (Chapter 33).
36 Assist with hair care and other grooming needs.

Continued

Assisting With a Tub Bath or Shower—cont'd

Post-Procedure

37 Provide for comfort. (See the inside of the back cover.)
38 Place the call light and other needed items within reach.
39 Raise or lower bed rails. Follow the care plan.
40 Follow the care plan and the person's preferences for privacy measures to maintain. Leaving the privacy curtain, window coverings, and door open or closed are examples.
41 Complete a safety check of the room. (See the inside of the back cover.)
42 Practice hand hygiene. Return to the tub or shower room.

43 Discard disposable items. Return supplies to their proper place.
44 Follow agency policy for used linens.
45 Clean, disinfect, and dry the tub or shower. Dry the tub or shower room floor. Use clean, dry paper towels for drying. Wear gloves. Practice hand hygiene after removing and discarding gloves.
46 Put the *UNOCCUPIED* sign on the door.
47 Report and record your care and observations.

PERINEAL CARE

Perineal care (pericare) involves cleaning the genital and anal areas. These areas provide a warm, moist, and dark place for microbes to grow. Cleaning prevents infection and odors and promotes comfort.

Perineal care is done daily during the bath. It also is done when the area is soiled with urine or feces (stools). Perineal care is very important for persons who:

- Have urinary catheters (Chapter 26).
- Have had rectal or genital surgery.
- Are menstruating (Chapter 9).
- Are incontinent of urine or feces (stools) (Chapters 25 and 27).
- Are uncircumcised (Fig. 22-17). Being *circumcised means that the fold of skin (foreskin) covering the glans of the penis was surgically removed.* Being *uncircumcised means foreskin covers the head of the penis.*

The person does perineal care if able. Otherwise, the nursing staff does so. This procedure can embarrass the person and staff, especially when it involves another gender.

Work from *front to back* or *top to bottom.* The urethral area (front or top) is the cleanest. The anal area (back or bottom) is the dirtiest. Therefore clean from the urethra to the anal area. This prevents spreading bacteria from the anal area to the vagina and urinary system.

The perineal area is delicate and easily injured. Use warm water, not hot. Use washcloths, towelettes, or swabs according to agency policy. Rinse off soap thoroughly. No-rinse perineal cleansers (sprays, foams) are common. These products do not require rinsing. Follow the manufacturer's instructions. Pat the area dry after rinsing. Dry well. This reduces moisture, prevents skin irritation, and promotes comfort.

See *Focus on Communication: Perineal Care.*
See *Delegation Guidelines: Perineal Care.*
See *Promoting Safety and Comfort: Perineal Care.*
See procedure: *Giving Female Perineal Care,* p. 286.
See procedure: *Giving Male Perineal Care,* p. 288.

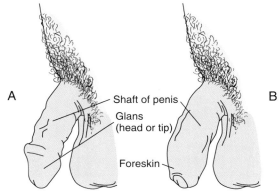

FIGURE 22-17 **A,** Circumcised penis. **B,** Uncircumcised penis.

FOCUS ON **COMMUNICATION**

Perineal Care

Perineal and *perineum* are not common terms. Most people understand *privates, private parts, crotch, genitals,* or *the area between your legs.* Use terms the person understands and that sound professional. Do not use slang or vulgar terms.

Talking to the person about perineal care may be difficult. You may be embarrassed. However, you must explain the procedure. You can say:

- "I'll give you some privacy to finish your bath. Can you reach everything you need? Please call for me if you need help. Here is your call light."
- "I'll give you time to finish your bath. Please wash your genital and rectal areas. Signal for me when you're done or need help."
- "Next I'll clean between your legs. I'll keep you covered with the bath blanket. I'll tell you before I touch you. Please tell me if you feel any pain or discomfort."
- "I'll clean your private parts now. Please let me know if you feel any pain or discomfort."

DELEGATION GUIDELINES

Perineal Care

Before giving perineal care, you need this information from the nurse and the care plan.
- When to give perineal care.
- What terms the person understands—perineum, privates, private parts, crotch, area between the legs, and so on.
- How much help the person needs.
- What water temperature to use—usually 105°F to 109°F (40.5°C to 42.7°C). Water in a basin cools rapidly.
- What cleaning agent to use.

- Any position restrictions or limits.
- What observations to report and record:
  - Odors
  - Redness, swelling, discharge, bleeding, or irritation
  - Complaints of pain, burning, or other discomfort
  - Signs of urinary or fecal incontinence
  - If you cannot retract the foreskin on an uncircumcised penis
- When to report observations.
- What patient or resident concerns to report at once.

PROMOTING SAFETY AND COMFORT

Perineal Care

Safety

Hot water can burn perineal tissues. To prevent burns, measure water temperature according to agency policy. If water seems too hot, ask the nurse to check it.

Contact with body fluids is likely during perineal care. Contact with blood may occur. Follow Standard Precautions and the Bloodborne Pathogen Standard. Wear clean gloves for perineal care.

Persons who are incontinent need perineal care. Waterproof under-pads (Chapter 20) and incontinence products (Chapter 25) are commonly used. Remove wet or soiled items. Place a clean, dry waterproof under-pad under the person before cleaning. See "Applying Incontinence Products" in Chapter 25.

Comfort

Explain how you protect privacy. Close doors and window coverings. Drape (cover) the person with a bath blanket (Fig. 22-18).

Perineal care involves touching the genital and anal areas. The person may prefer someone of the same gender for this care. Or the person may fear sexual assault. Always obtain the person's consent before providing perineal care. For mental comfort, the person may want a family member or another staff member present for the procedure. Ask if the person wants someone present and that person's name. Also keep the call light within the person's reach. If feeling threatened, the person can call for help.

If able, the person performs perineal care. This promotes privacy and helps prevent embarrassment. You need to:
1. Provide clean water. See step 12 in the procedure: *Giving Female Perineal Care*, p. 286.
2. Adjust the over-bed table so the person can reach the wash basin, soap, and towels with ease.
3. Make sure the person understands what to do.
4. Place the call light and other needed items within reach. Have the person signal when finished.
5. Lower the bed to a safe and comfortable level. Follow the care plan.
6. Practice hand hygiene.
7. Leave the room.
8. Answer the call light promptly. Knock before entering the room.
9. Raise the bed for body mechanics.
10. Practice hand hygiene. Put on gloves.
11. Make sure the person has cleaned thoroughly. Assist the person with hand hygiene.
12. Finish the bathing procedure.

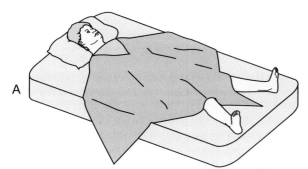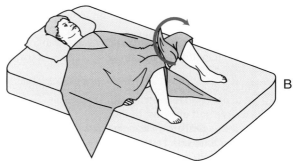

FIGURE 22-18 Draping for perineal care. **A,** Position the bath blanket like a diamond: 1 corner is at the neck, there is a corner at each side, and 1 corner is between the legs. **B,** Wrap the blanket around a leg by bringing the corner around the leg and over the top. Tuck the corner under the hip. Repeat for the other leg.

Giving Female Perineal Care

Quality of Life

- Knock before entering the person's room.
- Address the person by name.
- Introduce yourself by name and title.

- Explain the procedure before starting and during the procedure.
- Protect the person's rights during the procedure.
- Handle the person gently during the procedure.

Pre-Procedure

1 Follow *Delegation Guidelines: Perineal Care*, p. 285. See *Promoting Safety and Comfort*:
   a *Daily Hygiene and Bathing*, p. 272
   b *Perineal Care*, p. 285
2 Practice hand hygiene and get the following supplies.
   - Soap, body wash, or other cleansing agent as directed
   - At least 4 washcloths
   - Bath towel
   - Bath blanket
   - Water thermometer
   - Wash basin
   - Waterproof under-pad

- Gloves
- Laundry bag
- Towel or paper towels (as a barrier for supplies)
3 Place the barrier (towel, paper towels) on the over-bed table. Arrange items on top.
4 Practice hand hygiene.
5 Identify the person. Check the ID bracelet against the assignment sheet. Use 2 identifiers (Chapter 11). Also call the person by name.
6 Provide for privacy.
7 Raise the bed for body mechanics. Bed rails are up if used. Lower the bed rail near you if up.

Procedure

8 Position the person on the back.
9 Cover the person with a bath blanket. Move top linens to the foot of the bed.
10 Drape the person as in Figure 22-18.
11 Raise the bed rail if used. Lower the bed to a safe level.
12 Fill the wash basin. Water temperature is usually 105°F to 109°F (40.5°C to 42.7°C). Follow the care plan for water temperature. Measure water temperature according to agency policy.
13 Have the person check the water temperature. Adjust the water temperature as needed.
14 Place the basin on the over-bed table.
15 Raise the bed for body mechanics. Lower the bed rail if up.
16 Practice hand hygiene. Put on gloves.
17 Place a waterproof under-pad under the buttocks. Have the person raise the hips or turn from side to side. Position the person on the back.
18 Help the person bend the knees and spread the legs. Or help the person spread the legs as much as possible with the knees straight.
19 Fold the corner of the bath blanket between the legs onto the abdomen.
20 Wet the washcloths.
21 Squeeze out water from a washcloth. Make a mitted washcloth. Apply soap, body wash, or other cleansing agent. (Squeeze out water every time you change washcloths. Put used washcloths in the laundry bag. *Do not place used washcloths back in the basin.*)
22 Clean the perineum. Change washcloths as needed.
   a Separate the labia.
   b Clean 1 side of the labia. Clean downward from front to back (top to bottom) with 1 stroke (Fig. 22-19, *A*). Use 1 part of a washcloth.
   c Clean the other side of the labia. Clean downward from front to back (top to bottom) with 1 stroke (Fig. 22-19, *B*). Use a clean part of a washcloth.
   d Clean the vaginal area. Clean downward from front to back (top to bottom) with 1 stroke (Fig. 22-19, *C*). Use a clean part of a washcloth.

23 Rinse the perineum with a clean washcloth. Change washcloths as needed.
   a Separate the labia.
   b Rinse 1 side of the labia. Rinse downward from front to back (top to bottom) with 1 stroke. Use 1 part of a washcloth.
   c Rinse the other side of the labia. Rinse downward from front to back (top to bottom) with 1 stroke. Use a clean part of a washcloth.
   d Rinse the vaginal area. Rinse downward from front to back (top to bottom) with 1 stroke. Use a clean part of a washcloth.
24 Pat dry the perineal area with the towel. Dry from front to back (top to bottom).
25 Fold the blanket back between the legs.
26 Help the person lower the legs and turn onto the side away from you.
27 Apply soap, body wash, or other cleansing agent to a clean mitted washcloth.
28 Clean and rinse the rectal area.
   a Clean from the vagina to the anus with 1 stroke (Fig. 22-20). Use 1 part of the washcloth.
   b Repeat steps 27 and 28-a until the area is clean. Use a clean part of the washcloth for each stroke. Change washcloths as needed.
   c Rinse the rectal area with a clean washcloth. Rinse from the vagina to the anus. Repeat as necessary. Use a clean part of the washcloth for each stroke. Change washcloths as needed.
29 Pat dry the rectal area with the towel. Dry from the vagina to the anus. Place the towel in the laundry bag.
30 Fold and tuck the waterproof under-pad under the person. The wet side is inside. Have the person turn toward you or lay on the back and lift the buttocks. Remove the waterproof under-pad. Place it in the laundry bag. Position the person on the back.
31 Remove and discard the gloves. Practice hand hygiene.
32 Apply clean and dry garments and linens as needed. Remove the bath blanket. Place it in the laundry bag.
33 Position the person for comfort.

Giving Female Perineal Care—cont'd

Post-Procedure

34 Provide for comfort. (See the inside of the back cover.)
35 Place the call light and other needed items within reach.
36 Lower the bed to a safe and comfortable level. Follow the care plan.
37 Raise or lower bed rails. Follow the care plan.
38 Empty, clean, rinse, and dry the wash basin. Use clean, dry paper towels for drying. (Wear gloves.)
39 Return the basin and supplies to their proper place.
40 Clean and dry the over-bed table. Dry with paper towels. Discard the paper towels.

41 Remove and discard the gloves. Practice hand hygiene.
42 Follow the care plan and the person's preferences for privacy measures to maintain. Leaving the privacy curtain, window coverings, and door open or closed are examples.
43 Complete a safety check of the room. (See the inside of the back cover.)
44 Follow agency policy for used linens.
45 Practice hand hygiene.
46 Report and record your care and observations.

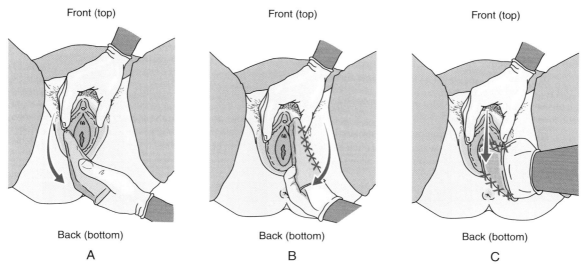

FIGURE 22-19 Cleaning the perineum. **A,** Separate the labia with 1 hand. Use a mitted washcloth to clean 1 side of the labia with a downward stroke. **B,** Clean the other side of the labia with a clean part of the washcloth. Use a downward stroke. **C,** Clean the vaginal area with a clean part of the washcloth. Use a downward stroke. (Note: Used areas of the washcloth are marked with Xs.)

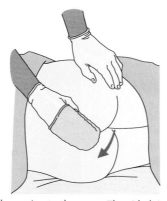

FIGURE 22-20 Clean the rectal area by wiping from the vagina to the anus. The side-lying position allows thorough cleaning of the anal area.

Giving Male Perineal Care

Quality of Life

- Knock before entering the person's room.
- Address the person by name.
- Introduce yourself by name and title.

- Explain the procedure before starting and during the procedure.
- Protect the person's rights during the procedure.
- Handle the person gently during the procedure.

Procedure

1 Follow steps 1 through 17 in procedure: *Giving Female Perineal Care*, p. 286. Drape the person as in Figure 22-18.
2 Fold the corner of the bath blanket between the legs onto the person's abdomen.
3 Wet the washcloths.
4 Squeeze out water from a washcloth. Make a mitted washcloth. Apply soap, body wash, or other cleansing agent. (Squeeze out water every time you change washcloths. Put used washcloths in the laundry bag. *Do not place used washcloths back in the basin.*)
5 Grasp the penis.
6 Retract the foreskin if the person is uncircumcised (Fig. 22-21).
7 Clean the tip. Use a circular motion. Start at the meatus and work outward (Fig. 22-22, A). Repeat as needed. Use a clean part of the washcloth each time.
8 Rinse the tip with another washcloth. Use the same circular motion.
9 Dry the tip (uncircumcised). Return foreskin to its natural position.
10 Clean the shaft of the penis. Use firm downward strokes (Fig. 22-22, B). Use a clean part of a washcloth for each stroke.
11 Rinse the shaft. Use the same downward motion as in step 10. Use a clean part of a washcloth for each stroke.
12 Help the person bend the knees and spread the legs. Or help the person spread the legs as much as possible with the knees straight.
13 Clean the scrotum. Use a clean part of a washcloth.
14 Rinse the scrotum. Use a clean part of a washcloth. Observe for redness and irritation of the skin folds.
15 Pat dry the penis and the scrotum. Use the towel.
16 Fold the bath blanket back between the legs.
17 Help the person lower the legs and turn onto the side away from you.
18 Clean the rectal area. Clean from the scrotum (front or top) to the anus (back or bottom). (See procedure: *Giving Female Perineal Care*, p. 286.) Rinse and dry well. Place used washcloths and the towel in the laundry bag.
19 Fold and tuck the waterproof under-pad under the person. The wet side is inside. Have the person turn toward you or lay on the back and lift the buttocks. Remove the waterproof under-pad. Place it in the laundry bag. Position the person on the back.
20 Remove and discard the gloves. Practice hand hygiene.
21 Apply clean and dry garments and linens as needed. Remove the bath blanket. Place it in the laundry bag.
22 Position the person for comfort.
23 Follow steps 34 through 46 in procedure: *Giving Female Perineal Care*, p. 286.

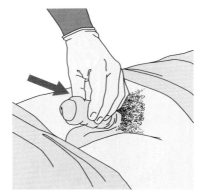

FIGURE 22-21 Retracting foreskin. Pull back the foreskin for perineal care. Return it to the normal position after cleaning, rinsing, and drying the tip of the penis.

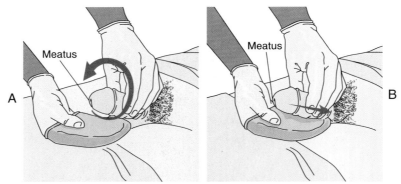

FIGURE 22-22 Cleaning the penis. A, Clean the tip with a circular motion starting at the meatus. B, Clean the shaft with downward strokes.

REPORTING AND RECORDING

You make many observations while assisting with daily hygiene and bathing. See Box 22-4 for a summary of observations to report and record. Report and record the care given. If not recorded, it is assumed that care was not given. Tell the nurse if the person refuses care or if care is not given for another reason.

BOX 22-4 Daily Hygiene and Bathing Observations

Report the Following at Once
- Bleeding
- Signs of skin breakdown
- Discharge from the vagina or urinary tract
- Unusual odors
- Changes from prior observations

Bathing
- The color of the skin, lips, nail beds, and sclera (whites of the eyes)
- If the skin appears pale, gray-ish, yellow (*jaundice*), or bluish *(cyanotic)*
- The location and description of rashes
- Skin texture—smooth, rough, scaly, flaky, dry, moist
- *Diaphoresis*—profuse (excessive) sweating

Bathing—cont'd
- Bruises or open skin areas
- Pale, reddened, or discolored areas, particularly over bony parts
- Drainage or bleeding from wounds or body openings
- Swelling of the feet and legs
- Corns or calluses on the feet (Chapter 35)
- Skin temperature (cold, cool, warm, hot)
- Complaints of pain or discomfort

Perineal Care
- Odors
- Redness, swelling, discharge, bleeding, or irritation
- Complaints of pain, burning, or other discomfort
- Signs of urinary or fecal incontinence
- Foreskin that will not retract on an uncircumcised penis

FOCUS ON   P R I D E

The Person, Family, and Yourself

P ersonal and Professional Responsibility

At first, you may be embarrassed to perform the procedures in this chapter. This improves with practice and experience. Practice perineal care in your classroom on a manikin. Do the full procedure as if it were a real person. Explain each step as you would with a patient or resident. Do not just practice once. Practice until you are comfortable.

R ights and Respect

Patients and residents have the right to choose schedules and routines. They also have the right to refuse care. Some persons refuse if it does not meet their preferences. For example:
- Preferring a bath, a person refuses a shower.
- A patient prefers to bathe at night, not in the morning.
- A male resident prefers perineal care by a male nursing assistant, not a female.

Refusing care for these reasons does not mean the person refuses to be clean. The person may accept if preferences are met. Tell the nurse of any refusal. Adjust as needed to respect the person's preferences.

I ndependence and Social Interaction

Bathing is a personal matter. Allow personal choice for bath time, products used, what to wear, and so on. Encourage self-care to the extent possible. Self-care promotes independence and improves self-esteem.

D elegation and Teamwork

Some agencies have commercial warmers for bath blankets. If a warmer is getting low, fill it. Otherwise, staff find an empty warmer. A co-worker has to fill it and wait for a blanket to heat up.

Avoid having the attitude that "someone else can do it." This shows poor teamwork and work ethics. Take pride in being a helpful and courteous team member.

E thics and Laws

You will perform some tasks often. Bathing is an example. Over time, some staff become less careful with routine tasks. They may forget about dangers. Or they think that nothing bad will happen. This is very unsafe. Always be careful. Harm can result from routine care measures.

FOCUS ON PRIDE: Application

The care measures in this chapter are private and personal. What concerns do you have about performing these procedures? How will you stay calm and professional and ease the person's worries?

Circle the BEST answer.

1   When assisting with daily care, you
    a   Discourage the use of adaptive (assistive) devices
    b   Provide for privacy if there is time
    c   Follow the person's routines and habits
    d   Change soiled linens in the afternoon

2   You are planning for early morning care and morning care. Which should you do *after* breakfast?
    a   Apply eyeglasses and insert hearing aids
    b   Give complete bed baths
    c   Remove sleepwear and dress residents
    d   Provide oral care and insert dentures

3   A person is incontinent. You should plan to
    a   Give perineal care often throughout the day
    b   Give a complete bed bath twice a day
    c   Shower the person once a week
    d   Give a tub bath when the person is soiled

4   To apply powder
    a   Turn the person toward you
    b   Sprinkle a small amount onto your hand
    c   Apply a thick layer of powder
    d   Shake the powder onto the person

5   You are giving a complete bed bath. Which is *correct*?
    a   You use soap to wash the eye from the outer to the inner part.
    b   You keep the person covered with a bath blanket as much as possible.
    c   You continue washing with soapy, cool water.
    d   You use another person's wash basin.

6   When bathing a person
    a   Keep bar soap in the wash basin or tub
    b   Wash from the dirtiest to the cleanest area
    c   Assist with elimination after a bath
    d   Rinse the skin well to remove all soap

7   Water for a complete bed bath is between
    a   100°F and 104°F
    b   105°F and 109°F
    c   110°F and 115°F
    d   120°F and 125°F

8   When drying the person
    a   Dry well between skin folds
    b   Rub the skin dry
    c   Avoid drying between the toes
    d   Allow the person to air dry

9   A person can wash the face, arms, hands, chest, and abdomen. You should
    a   Wash all areas for the person
    b   Leave the other areas unwashed
    c   Allow the person to wash the face and hands
    d   Wash areas the person cannot reach

10 Which is helpful when showering a person with confusion?
    a   Gather supplies after the person is in the shower.
    b   Do not explain what you are doing.
    c   Put a towel over the lap and have the person hold a washcloth.
    d   Work quickly if the person resists.

11 When assisting with a shower in a shower room
    a   Direct the water spray at the person's face
    b   Allow a weak person to stand if you provide support
    c   Go to the person's room to make the bed during the shower
    d   Clean, disinfect, and dry the shower before and after use

12 You are transferring a person to a shower chair in the shower room. Which is *unsafe*?
    a   The floor is wet.
    b   The person has shoes on the feet.
    c   The person holds the grab bar (safety bar).
    d   The shower chair wheels are locked (braked).

13 You are filling a tub for a tub bath. You ask the person to check the water temperature. The person says it is cool. You should
    a   Bathe the person quickly in the cool water
    b   Give a shower instead
    c   Drain the tub fully and refill it
    d   Add warm water and ask if it feels better

14 A person asks you to rinse again at the end of a shower. Which reply is *best*?
    a   "Which areas would you like rinsed?"
    b   "We need to be done. I have other residents to bathe."
    c   "I already rinsed you. Once is good enough."
    d   "I can't. We have used enough water."

15 Water temperature for perineal care is between
    a   100°F and 104°F
    b   105°F and 109°F
    c   110°F and 115°F
    d   120°F and 125°F

16 Which action during perineal care is *correct*?
    a   You rinse and re-use the washcloths.
    b   You do not retract foreskin on an uncircumcised penis.
    c   You wear gloves.
    d   You place washcloths in a sink full of water.

17 These statements are about perineal care. Which is *correct*?
    a   Do not explain the procedure to avoid embarrassment.
    b   The person does perineal care if able.
    c   Clean from the back (bottom) to the front (top).
    d   Draping the person is not needed.

18 You see a rash under a breast during a bath. You should
    a   Ask the nurse to observe the area
    b   Scrub the skin
    c   Apply lotion to the area
    d   Avoid drying the skin

Answers to Chapter 22 questions are on p. 588.

Answers to Chapter 22 questions are on p. 588.

FOCUS ON **PRACTICE**

Problem Solving

A person has abdominal skin folds that are hard for 1 person to lift and clean under alone. The person has redness and itching under the skin folds. The nurse needs to apply a medicated powder to the area after bathing and drying well. Why is it important to dry the area well? How will you plan to provide care using teamwork and communication?

Grooming

Hair care, shaving, and nail and foot care prevent infection and promote comfort. Such measures affect love, belonging, and self-esteem needs.

Grooming measures are matters of personal choice. Hair and nail care preferences vary. Culture also influences grooming practices.

The person performs grooming measures to the extent possible. This promotes independence and quality of life. The person may use adaptive (assistive) devices (Fig. 23-1).

See *Focus on Surveys: Grooming.*

FOCUS ON **SURVEYS**

Grooming

Grooming promotes self-esteem. Therefore surveyors will observe if patients and residents:
- Are groomed according to their wishes.
- Have hair combed and styled.
- Have beards shaved or trimmed.
- Can reach grooming supplies.

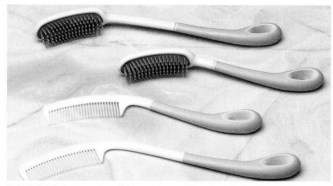

FIGURE 23-1 Long-handled combs and brushes for hair care. (Courtesy North Coast Medical Inc., Morgan Hill, Calif.)

NOTE: *A task may require more than 1 pair of gloves. Change gloves as needed. Use careful judgment. Remember to practice hand hygiene after removing gloves.*

HAIR CARE

The look and feel of hair affect mental well-being. The nursing process reflects the person's culture, personal choice, skin and scalp conditions, health history, and self-care ability. You assist with hair care as needed.

Beauty and barber shops are common in nursing centers. Residents can have their hair shampooed, cut, and styled.

Skin and Scalp Conditions

Skin and scalp conditions include:

- *Alopecia—hair loss.* Hair loss may be complete or partial. Caused by heredity, male pattern baldness occurs with aging. Hair thins in some women with aging. Cancer treatments (radiation therapy to the head and chemotherapy) may cause alopecia in all age-groups.
- *Hirsutism—excessive body hair.* It can occur in men, women, and children. Causes are heredity and abnormal amounts of male hormones.
- *Dandruff—excessive amounts of dry, white flakes from the scalp.* Itching is common. Sometimes eyebrows and ear canals are involved.
- *Pediculosis (lice)—infestation with wingless insects that feed on blood* (Fig. 23-2). *Infestation* means *being in or on a host.* Lice attach their eggs (*nits*) to hair shafts. After hatching, they bite the scalp or skin to feed on blood. About the size of a sesame seed, adult lice are tan to gray-ish white in color. Lice easily spread to others through clothing, head coverings, furniture, beds, towels, bed linens, combs, brushes, and sexual contact. Lice are treated with medicated shampoos, lotions, and creams specific for lice. Thorough bathing is needed. So is washing clothing and linens in hot water. Lice bites cause severe itching.
  - *Pediculosis capitis* ("head lice") is the infestation of the scalp (*capitis*) with lice.
  - *Pediculosis pubis* ("crabs") is the infestation of the pubic (*pubis*) hair with lice.
  - *Pediculosis corporis* is the infestation of the body (*corporis*) with lice.
- *Scabies—a skin disorder caused by a female mite* (Fig. 23-3). A *mite* is a very small spider-like organism. The female mite burrows into the skin and lays eggs. After hatching, the females produce more eggs. Infested with mites, the person has a rash and intense itching. Common sites are between the fingers, the wrists, underarms, thighs, and genital area. Other sites include the breasts, waist, and buttocks. Highly contagious, scabies is transmitted to others by close contact. Special creams are ordered to kill the mites. The person's room is cleaned. Clothing and linens are washed in hot water.

See *Focus on Communication: Skin and Scalp Conditions.*

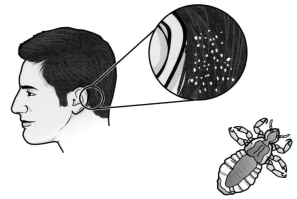

FIGURE 23-2 Head lice. (Redrawn from Medline Plus: *Head lice.* Bethesda, Md., National Institutes of Health.)

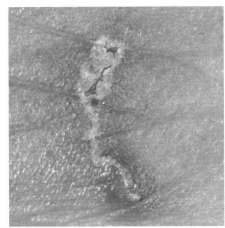

FIGURE 23-3 Scabies. (From Marks JG, Miller JJ: *Lookingbill & Marks' principles of dermatology,* ed 4, St Louis, 2006, Saunders.)

FOCUS ON **COMMUNICATION**
Skin and Scalp Conditions

Some skin or scalp conditions may alarm you. Remain professional. Do not say things that may embarrass the person.

Report an abnormal skin or scalp condition. Describe your observations. For example:

- "There are small red dots on Mr. Olson's right underarm. Would you please look at them?"
- "I saw some small white specks in Ms. Smith's hair. Would you please look at them before I wash her hair?"

Brushing and Combing Hair

The frequency and timing of brushing and combing hair are personal. Brushing and combing hair may be part of early morning care, morning care, or afternoon care (Chapter 22). Some people brush and comb hair before meals, before visitors arrive, and at bedtime.

Encourage patients and residents to do their own hair care. The person chooses how to brush, comb, and style hair. Assist as needed.

Daily brushing and combing prevent matted and tangled hair. So does braiding. You need the person's consent to braid hair. *Never cut the person's hair.*

Special measures are needed for curly, coarse, and dry hair. The person's hair care practices and products are part of the care plan. Let the person guide hair care.

See *Caring About Culture: Brushing and Combing Hair.*

See *Delegation Guidelines: Brushing and Combing Hair.*

See *Promoting Safety and Comfort: Brushing and Combing Hair.*

See procedure: *Brushing and Combing Hair*, p. 294.

CARING ABOUT CULTURE

Brushing and Combing Hair

Small braids (cornrows) are common in some cultural groups. The braids are left intact for shampooing. To undo these braids, the nurse obtains the person's consent.

DELEGATION GUIDELINES

Brushing and Combing Hair

To brush and comb hair, you need this information from the nurse and the care plan.
- How much help the person needs
- What to do for matted or tangled hair
- What to do for curly, coarse, or dry hair
- What hair care products to use
- The person's preferences and routine hair care measures
- What observations to report and record:
  - Scalp sores
  - Flaking
  - Itching
  - Rash
  - Hair falling out in patches; patches of hair loss
  - Very dry or very oily hair
  - Matted or tangled hair
  - The presence of nits or lice
    - Nits (lice eggs attached to hair shafts)—oval and yellow to white in color
    - Lice—about the size of a sesame seed and gray-ish white in color
    - Itching
    - Complaints of a tickling feeling or something moving in the hair
    - Irritability
    - Sores on the head or body caused by scratching
    - Rash
- When to report observations
- What patient or resident concerns to report at once

PROMOTING SAFETY AND COMFORT

Brushing and Combing Hair

Safety

Sharp brush bristles can injure the scalp. So can sharp or broken teeth on a comb. Report concerns about the person's brush or comb.

Wear gloves if the person has scalp sores, nits, lice, or other hair or scalp problems. Follow Standard Precautions and the Bloodborne Pathogen Standard.

Comfort

Protect garments from falling hair with a towel across the back and shoulders. For the person in bed, give hair care before changing linens and the pillowcase. If after a linen change, place a towel across the pillow to collect falling hair.

Brushing and Combing Hair

Quality of Life

- Knock before entering the person's room.
- Address the person by name.
- Introduce yourself by name and title.
- Explain the procedure before starting and during the procedure.
- Protect the person's rights during the procedure.
- Handle the person gently during the procedure.

Pre-Procedure

1 Follow *Delegation Guidelines: Brushing and Combing Hair*, p. 293. **See** *Promoting Safety and Comfort: Brushing and Combing Hair*, p. 293.
2 Practice hand hygiene.
3 Identify the person. Check the identification (ID) bracelet against the assignment sheet. Use 2 identifiers (Chapter 11). Also call the person by name.
4 Ask the person how to style hair.
5 Get the following supplies.
   - Comb and brush
   - Bath towel
   - Other hair care items as requested
   - Laundry bag
6 Arrange items nearby.
7 Provide for privacy.

Procedure

8 Position the person.
   a *In a chair*—Help the person to the chair. The person wears slip-resistant footwear for a transfer. Clothing properly covers the person. Or a robe is applied.
   b *In bed*—Raise the bed for body mechanics. Bed rails are up if used. Lower the bed rail near you. Assist the person to a semi-Fowler's position if allowed.
9 Place a towel across the back and shoulders or across the pillow.
10 Have the person remove eyeglasses if worn. Put them in the eyeglass case. Put the case inside the bedside stand.
11 *Hair that is not matted or tangled.*
   a Use the comb to part the hair.
      1) Part hair down the middle into 2 sides (Fig. 23-4, A).
      2) Divide 1 side into 2 smaller sections (Fig. 23-4, B).
   b Brush 1 of the small sections of hair. Start at the scalp and brush toward the hair ends (Fig. 23-5). Do the same for the other small section of hair. If the person prefers, brush long hair starting at the hair ends.
   c Repeat steps 11, a(2) and b for the other side.
12 *Matted or tangled hair.*
   a Take a small section of hair near the ends.
   b Comb or brush through to the hair ends.
   c Add small sections of hair as you work up to the scalp.
   d Comb or brush through each longer section to the hair ends.
13 Style the hair as the person prefers.
14 Remove the towel. Place it in the laundry bag.
15 Have the person put on eyeglasses if worn.

Post-Procedure

16 Provide for comfort. (See the inside of the back cover.)
17 Place the call light and other needed items within reach.
18 Lower the bed to a safe and comfortable level. Follow the care plan.
19 Raise or lower bed rails. Follow the care plan.
20 Remove hair from the brush or comb. Clean, rinse, dry, and return hair care items to their proper place. Use clean, dry paper towels for drying. Wear gloves for this step. Remove and discard the gloves. Practice hand hygiene.
21 Follow the care plan and the person's preferences for privacy measures to maintain. Leaving the privacy curtain, window coverings, and door open or closed are examples.
22 Complete a safety check of the room. (See the inside of the back cover.)
23 Follow agency policy for used linens.
24 Practice hand hygiene.
25 Report and record your care and observations.

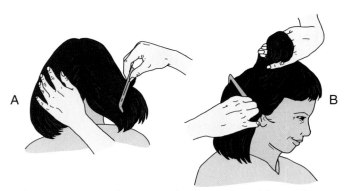

FIGURE 23-4 Parting hair. **A,** Part hair down the middle. Divide it into 2 sides. **B,** Then part 1 side into 2 smaller sections.

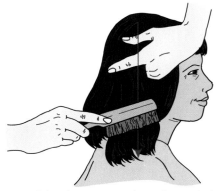

FIGURE 23-5 Brush hair by starting at the scalp. Brush down to the hair ends.

Shampooing

People shampoo 1, 2, or 3 times a week or daily. Hair and scalp condition, hair-style, and personal choice affect frequency.

In nursing centers, shampoos are done on bath days. If done by a hairdresser or barber, do not shampoo hair. Provide a shower cap for the bath or shower.

Shampoo method depends on the person's condition, safety factors, and personal choice. The nurse tells you what method to use.

- *Shampoo during the shower or tub bath.* Use a hand-held nozzle for persons in shower chairs or taking tub baths. Direct a spray of water at the hair.
- *Shampoo at the sink.* The person sits or lies facing away from the sink. A folded towel placed over the sink edge protects the neck. The person's head is tilted back over the sink edge. Or a shampoo tray is used (Fig. 23-6). Use a water pitcher or hand-held nozzle to wet and rinse the hair.
- *Shampoo in bed.* A shampoo basin under the head protects the linens and mattress from water. The device drains into a basin on a chair by the bed (Fig. 23-7). Use a water pitcher to wet and rinse the hair.

Dry and style hair as soon as possible after the shampoo. Women may want hair curled or rolled up before drying. Check with the nurse before doing so.

Shampoo Caps. Commercial shampoo caps have a cleaning agent that does not need rinsing. Some caps also have a conditioner. To use a shampoo cap:

- Warm the package following the manufacturer's instructions.
- Check the temperature. The cap should be warm. Do not use a cap that is too hot.
- Apply the cap to the person's head.
- Massage the hair and scalp gently through the cap. Follow the manufacturer's instructions for how long to massage—usually 1 to 3 minutes. Longer hair may require more time.
- Remove the cap. Do not rinse the hair. Dry the hair with a towel if needed.
- Comb the hair.
    See *Focus on Older Persons: Shampooing.*
    See *Delegation Guidelines: Shampooing*, p. 296.
    See *Promoting Safety and Comfort: Shampooing*, p. 296.
    See procedure: *Shampooing the Person's Hair in Bed*, p. 296.

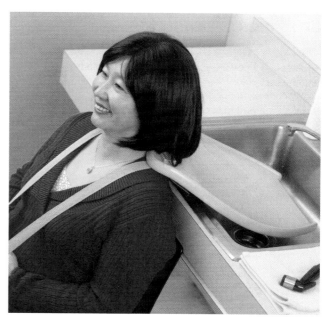

FIGURE 23-6 Shampooing at the sink with a shampoo tray. (Courtesy SP Ableware–Maddak, Wayne, N.J.)

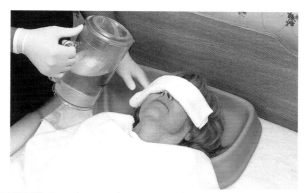

FIGURE 23-7 A shampoo basin is used for a shampoo in bed. Water drains into a collecting basin.

FOCUS ON OLDER PERSONS

Shampooing

Oil gland secretion decreases with aging. Therefore older persons have dry hair. They may shampoo less often than younger adults do.

DELEGATION GUIDELINES
Shampooing

To shampoo a person, you need this information from the nurse and the care plan.
- When to shampoo the person's hair
- What method to use
- What shampoo and conditioner to use
- How to use and store medicated products
- The person's position restrictions or limits
- What water temperature to use—usually 105°F (Fahrenheit) (40.5°C [centigrade])
- If hair is curled or rolled up before drying

- What observations to report and record:
  - Scalp sores
  - Flaking
  - Itching
  - Rash
  - Hair falling out in patches; patches of hair loss
  - Very dry or very oily hair
  - Matted or tangled hair
  - The presence of nits or lice (p. 292)
  - How the person tolerated the procedure
- When to report observations
- What patient or resident concerns to report at once

PROMOTING SAFETY AND COMFORT
Shampooing

Safety

Remove hearing aids before shampooing. Water will damage hearing aids.

Wear gloves if the person has scalp sores, nits, lice, or other hair or scalp problems. Follow Standard Precautions and the Bloodborne Pathogen Standard.

Keep shampoo away from and out of the eyes. Have the person hold a washcloth over the eyes. To rinse, cup your hand at the person's forehead. This keeps soapy water from running down the forehead and into the eyes.

For a shampoo on a stretcher at a sink, see Chapter 18 for stretcher safety. Lock (brake) the wheels. Use the safety straps (if present) and side rails. Keep the far side rail raised during the procedure.

Some people shampoo themselves during a tub bath or shower. Place an extra towel and requested shampoo products within the person's reach. Assist as needed.

Comfort

For a shampoo during the tub bath or shower, the person tips the head back to keep shampoo and water out of the eyes. Support the back of the head with 1 hand. Shampoo with your other hand. Some persons cannot tip their heads back. They lean forward and hold a folded washcloth over the eyes. Support the forehead with 1 hand as you shampoo with the other. Make sure that the person can breathe easily.

Many people have limited range of motion in their necks. They are not shampooed at the sink or on a stretcher.

Shampooing the Person's Hair in Bed

Quality of Life

- Knock before entering the person's room.
- Address the person by name.
- Introduce yourself by name and title.

- Explain the procedure before starting and during the procedure.
- Protect the person's rights during the procedure.
- Handle the person gently during the procedure.

Pre-Procedure

1 Follow *Delegation Guidelines: Shampooing.* See *Promoting Safety and Comfort: Shampooing.*
2 Practice hand hygiene and get the following supplies.
   - 2 bath towels
   - Washcloth
   - Shampoo
   - Hair conditioner (if requested)
   - Water thermometer
   - Water pitcher
   - Shampoo basin
   - Collecting basin
   - Waterproof under-pad
   - Gloves (if needed)

   - Comb and brush
   - Hair dryer
   - Laundry bag
3 Arrange items nearby. Place the collecting basin on a chair by the bed.
4 Practice hand hygiene.
5 Identify the person. Check the ID bracelet against the assignment sheet. Use 2 identifiers (Chapter 11). Also call the person by name.
6 Provide for privacy.
7 Raise the bed for body mechanics. Bed rails are up if used. Lower the bed rail near you if up.

Shampooing the Person's Hair in Bed—cont'd

Procedure

8 Cover the person's chest with a bath towel.
9 Brush and comb the hair to remove tangles.
10 Position the person for a shampoo in bed.
  a Lower the head of the bed. Remove the pillow.
  b Place the waterproof under-pad and shampoo basin under the head and shoulders.
  c Support the head and neck with a folded towel if necessary.
11 Fill the water pitcher. Follow these safety measures.
  a Raise the bed rail if used. Lower the bed to a safe level.
  b Measure water temperature following agency policy. Water temperature is usually 105°F (40.5°C). Have the person check the water temperature. Adjust water temperature as needed.
  c Raise the bed for body mechanics. Lower the bed rail if used when you return.
12 Put on gloves (if needed).
13 Have the person hold a washcloth over the eyes. It should not cover the nose and mouth. (NOTE: A damp washcloth is easier to hold and will not slip. However, your agency may require a dry washcloth.)
14 Use the water pitcher to wet the hair. Ask if the water temperature is comfortable. Adjust as needed.
15 Apply a small amount of shampoo.
16 Work up a lather with both hands. Start at the hairline. Work toward the back of the head.
17 Massage the scalp with your fingertips. Do not scratch the scalp with your fingernails.
18 Rinse the hair until the water runs clear.
19 Repeat steps 15 through 18 as needed.
20 Apply conditioner if used. Follow directions on the container.
21 Squeeze water from the hair.
22 Cover the hair with a bath towel.
23 Remove the shampoo basin, collecting basin, and waterproof under-pad.
24 Dry the person's face with the towel on the chest.
25 Raise the head of the bed.
26 Rub the hair and scalp with the towel. Rub gently. Use the second towel if the first one is wet.
27 Comb the hair to remove tangles.
28 Dry and style hair.
29 Place the towels in the laundry bag. Remove and discard the gloves (if used). Practice hand hygiene after removing and discarding gloves.

Post-Procedure

30 Provide for comfort. (See the inside of the back cover.)
31 Place the call light and other needed items within reach.
32 Lower the bed to a safe and comfortable level. Follow the care plan.
33 Raise or lower bed rails. Follow the care plan.
34 Clean the brush and comb. Clean, rinse, dry, and return equipment to its proper place. Use clean, dry paper towels for drying. Wear gloves for this step. Discard disposable items. Remove and discard the gloves and practice hand hygiene.
35 Follow the care plan and the person's preferences for privacy measures to maintain. Leaving the privacy curtain, window coverings, and door open or closed are examples.
36 Complete a safety check of the room. (See the inside of the back cover.)
37 Follow agency policy for used linens.
38 Practice hand hygiene.
39 Report and record your care and observations.

SHAVING

Shaving is a matter of personal preference. Facial shaving is common among men. Many women shave their legs and underarms. Some women have facial hair. Other hair removal methods include waxing, hair removal products, plucking, and threading.

Electric shavers or safety razors are used (Fig. 23-8). Some persons have their own electric shavers. Or the agency has a shaver. Follow the manufacturer's instructions and agency procedures.

Safety razors (blade razors) have razor blades. They can cause nicks and cuts. Do not use safety razors on persons with healing problems or on those taking anticoagulant drugs. An *anticoagulant* is a drug that prevents or slows down *(anti)* blood clotting *(coagulate)*. Bleeding occurs easily and is hard to stop. A nick or cut can cause serious bleeding. Electric shavers are used.

Follow the rules in Box 23-1 (p. 298) for shaving. If you do not know how to use a person's shaving equipment, ask the nurse for help.

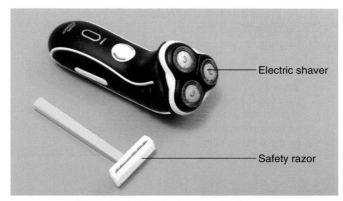

FIGURE 23-8 Electric shaver and safety razor.

See *Focus on Older Persons: Shaving*, p. 298.
See *Delegation Guidelines: Shaving*, p. 298.
See *Promoting Safety and Comfort: Shaving*, p. 298.
See procedure: *Shaving the Person's Face With a Safety Razor*, p. 299.

BOX 23-1 Rules for Shaving

- Use electric shavers for persons taking anticoagulant drugs. Safety razors are not used.
- Protect bed linens and clothing. Place a towel under the part to be shaved. Or place a towel across the person's chest and shoulders to protect clothing.
- Encourage the person to do as much as safely possible.
- Hold the skin taut.
- Do not cut, nick, or irritate the skin. If nicks or cuts occur, apply direct pressure (Chapter 43). Report nicks, cuts, or irritation at once.

Electric Shavers
- Follow the manufacturer's instructions.
- Clean the device before and after use. Open or remove the cutting head. Empty the razor into a wastebasket. If the razor has a cleaning brush, use it to remove hair. Brush gently. Do not tap the razor on the counter or on the side of the wastebasket. This can damage the razor.
- Use on a clean, dry face. Some persons use a pre-electric shave product (oil, lotion, powder) to prevent irritation. (Follow the manufacturer's instructions for a razor that can be used with water.)
- Shave in the correct direction. For a rotary-type shaver (see Fig. 23-8), move the shaver in small circles over the face. Follow the manufacturer's instructions for shaving against or in the direction of hair growth. (NOTE: Some state competency tests require shaving in the direction of hair growth. Follow the manufacturer's instructions and the rules in your state and agency.)
- Shave sensitive areas first if the skin is tender and sensitive. See *Promoting Safety and Comfort: Shaving.* Press lightly. Do not go over the same area many times.
- Charge the device following the manufacturer's instructions.
- Follow safety measures for using electrical equipment (Chapter 11).

Safety Razors
- Soften facial hair before shaving. Apply a warm, moist washcloth or towel to the face for a few minutes.
- Lather the area with shaving cream (shaving gel).
- Shave in the correct direction.
  - *Shaving the face*—shave in the direction of hair growth (Fig. 23-9).
  - *Shaving the underarms*—shave in the direction of hair growth.
  - *Shaving the legs*—shave up from the ankles. This is against hair growth.
- Rinse the razor often to remove hair and lather.
- Rinse the skin thoroughly after shaving. Pat dry.

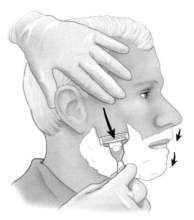

FIGURE 23-9 Shave the face in the direction of hair growth. Use long strokes on the larger areas of the face. Use short strokes around the chin and lips.

DELEGATION GUIDELINES
Shaving

To shave a person, you need this information from the nurse and the care plan.
- What shaver to use—electric or safety
- If the person takes anticoagulant drugs
- When to shave the person
- What facial hair to shave
- If there are tender or sensitive areas on the person's face
- What observations to report and record:
  - Nicks (report at once)
  - Cuts (report at once)
  - Bleeding (report at once)
  - Irritation
- When to report observations
- What patient or resident concerns to report at once

PROMOTING SAFETY AND COMFORT
Shaving

Safety
Safety razors are very sharp. Protect the person and yourself from nicks and cuts. Prevent contact with blood. Wear gloves. Follow Standard Precautions and the Bloodborne Pathogen Standard. Discard used razor blades and disposable shavers in a sharps container. Do not re-cap the razor.

After rinsing a safety razor, wipe it to avoid dripping on the person. To protect yourself from cuts:
- Place a towel or several thicknesses of paper towels on the over-bed table. Do not hold them in your hand.
- Wipe the razor on the towel or paper towels.

Comfort
The neck area below the jaw may be tender and sensitive. Some electric shavers become very warm or hot during use. The heat can irritate the skin. Shave tender areas first while the shaver is cool. Then move to other areas of the face.

Some people apply lotion or after-shave to the skin after shaving. Lotion softens the skin. After-shave closes skin pores. To soften the skin and open pores, apply warmth before shaving (see Box 23-1).

FOCUS ON OLDER PERSONS
Shaving

Older persons with wrinkled skin are at risk for nicks and cuts. Safety razors are not used for them or persons with dementia. Persons with dementia may not understand what you are doing. They may resist care and move suddenly. Serious nicks and cuts can occur. Use electric shavers for these persons.

Shaving the Person's Face With a Safety Razor

Quality of Life

- Knock before entering the person's room.
- Address the person by name.
- Introduce yourself by name and title.
- Explain the procedure before starting and during the procedure.
- Protect the person's rights during the procedure.
- Handle the person gently during the procedure.

Pre-Procedure

1 Follow *Delegation Guidelines: Shaving.* **See** *Promoting Safety and Comfort: Shaving.*
2 Practice hand hygiene and get the following supplies.
  - Wash basin
  - Bath towel
  - Washcloth or hand towel
  - Towel or paper towels (to wipe the razor on)
  - Safety razor
  - Mirror
  - Shaving cream or shaving gel
  - Shaving brush if used
  - After-shave or lotion if used
  - Towel or paper towels (as a barrier for supplies)
  - Gloves
  - Laundry bag
3 Place the barrier (towel, paper towels) on the over-bed table. Arrange supplies on top.
4 Practice hand hygiene.
5 Identify the person. Check the ID bracelet against the assignment sheet. Use 2 identifiers (Chapter 11). Also call the person by name.
6 Provide for privacy.

Procedure

7 Fill the wash basin with warm water.
8 Place the basin on the over-bed table.
9 Raise the bed for body mechanics. Bed rails are up if used. Lower the bed rail near you if up.
10 Assist the person to semi-Fowler's position if allowed or to the supine position.
11 Adjust lighting to clearly see the person's face.
12 Place the towel over the person's chest and shoulders.
13 Adjust the over-bed table for easy reach.
14 Put on gloves.
15 Attach the razor blade to the shaver if necessary.
16 Wash the person's face. Do not dry.
17 Wet the washcloth or hand towel. Wring it out.
18 Apply the washcloth or towel to the face for a few minutes.
19 Apply shaving cream with your hands. If using gel, lather it before applying it. (If needed, change gloves or wipe excess shaving cream from your gloves using a towel or paper towel. Or use a shaving brush to apply lather.)

20 Hold the skin taut with 1 hand.
21 Shave in the direction of hair growth. Use shorter strokes around the chin and lips (see Fig. 23-9).
22 Rinse the razor often. Wipe it on a towel or paper towels.
23 Apply direct pressure to any bleeding areas (Chapter 43).
24 Wash off any remaining lather. Pat dry with the towel on the person's chest.
25 Apply after-shave or lotion if requested. (If there are nicks or cuts, do not apply after-shave or lotion.)
26 Remove the towel. Place the towel and washcloth (or hand towel) in the laundry bag. Remove and discard the gloves. Practice hand hygiene.

Post-Procedure

27 Provide for comfort. (See the inside of the back cover.)
28 Place the call light and other needed items within reach.
29 Lower the bed to a safe and comfortable level. Follow the care plan.
30 Raise or lower bed rails. Follow the care plan.
31 Clean, rinse, dry, and return equipment and supplies to their proper place. Use clean, dry paper towels for drying. Discard the razor blade or disposable razor into the sharps container. Discard other disposable items. Wear gloves.
32 Clean and dry the over-bed table. Dry with paper towels. Discard the paper towels.

33 Remove and discard the gloves. Practice hand hygiene.
34 Follow the care plan and the person's preferences for privacy measures to maintain. Leaving the privacy curtain, window coverings, and door open or closed are examples.
35 Complete a safety check of the room. (See the inside of the back cover.)
36 Follow agency policy for used linens.
37 Practice hand hygiene.
38 Report nicks, cuts, irritation, or bleeding to the nurse at once. Also report and record your care and other observations.

Caring for Mustaches and Beards

Mustaches and beards need daily care. Food and mouth and nose drainage can collect in the whiskers. Daily washing and combing are needed. Ask the person how to groom a mustache or beard. *Never shave or trim a mustache or beard.*

Shaving Legs and Underarms

Shaving legs and underarms varies among cultures. To shave legs and underarms:

- Follow the rules in Box 23-1.
- Collect shaving items with bath items.
- Shave after bathing while the skin is soft.
- Use soap and water, shaving cream (gel), or lotion for the lather. Follow the care plan and the person's preferences.
- Use the kidney basin to rinse the razor. Do not use bath water.

NAIL AND FOOT CARE

Nail and foot care prevents infection, injury, and odors. Hangnails, ingrown nails (nails that grow in at the side), and nails torn away from the skin cause skin breaks. Skin breaks are portals of entry for microbes. Long or broken nails can scratch the skin and snag clothing.

Dirty feet, socks, or stockings harbor microbes and cause odors. Shoes and socks provide a warm, moist place for microbes to grow. Injuries occur from stubbing toes, stepping on sharp objects, or being stepped on. Poorly fitting shoes cause blisters.

Poor circulation prolongs healing. Diabetes and vascular diseases cause poor circulation. Foot injuries or infections are very serious for older persons and those with circulatory disorders.

Nails are easier to clean and trim right after soaking or bathing. Use nail clippers to trim fingernails. *Never use scissors.* Use extreme caution to prevent damage to nearby tissues.

Trimming and clipping toenails can easily cause injuries. *Some agencies do not let nursing assistants cut or trim toenails. Follow agency policy.*

See *Focus on Older Persons: Nail and Foot Care.*
See *Delegation Guidelines: Nail and Foot Care.*
See *Promoting Safety and Comfort: Nail and Foot Care.*
See procedure: *Giving Nail and Foot Care.*

FOCUS ON **OLDER PERSONS**

Nail and Foot Care

Many older persons have thin, fragile skin. Rough, jagged nails can cause skin tears (Chapter 35). Keep nails trimmed and smoothly filed.

Persons with dementia may resist care if they are uncomfortable or do not understand what is happening. Follow the care plan for measures that help the person (Chapter 42). Never use force. These measures may help.

- Provide a calm setting. Soft music can be relaxing.
- Follow the person's habits and routines.
- Have supplies ready before beginning.
- Explain what you are doing step-by-step.
- Talk about something you know the person enjoys.
- Be gentle and respectful.
- Try nail care at another time if the person resists.

DELEGATION GUIDELINES

Nail and Foot Care

To give nail and foot care, you need this information from the nurse and the care plan.

- What water temperature to use (usually 105°F/40.5°C)
- How long to soak fingernails (usually 5 to 10 minutes)
- How long to soak feet (usually 15 to 20 minutes or less)
- If fingernails should be filed but not trimmed
- How to position the person
- What observations to report and record:
  - Dry, reddened, irritated, or callused areas
  - Breaks in the skin
  - Corns (Chapter 35) on top of and between the toes
  - Blisters
  - Very thick nails
  - Loose nails
- When to report observations
- What patient or resident concerns to report at once

PROMOTING SAFETY AND COMFORT

Nail and Foot Care

Safety

To trim fingernails, use nail clippers. Trim straight across (Fig. 23-10). Then file the nails to smooth and round the corners. File in 1 direction. Filing back and forth can weaken the nail.

Some states and agencies do not let nursing assistants cut and trim toenails. A nurse or podiatrist (foot [pod] doctor) cuts toenails and provides foot care for the following persons. *You do not cut or trim the fingernails or toenails for persons who:*

- Have diabetes
- Have poor circulation
- Take drugs that affect blood clotting
- Have nail fungus, very thick nails, or ingrown nails (Chapter 35)

Check between the toes for cracks and sores. If not treated, a serious infection could occur.

The feet are easily burned. Persons with decreased sensation or circulatory problems may not feel hot temperatures.

Do not apply lotion between the toes. Lotion on the feet can be slippery. Slip-resistant footwear is applied before transferring or walking.

Breaks in the skin and bleeding can occur. Some persons do not practice proper hand hygiene after elimination. Some confused persons grab or scratch at under-garments or incontinence products. Feces (stools) may be under the fingernails. Provide frequent hand hygiene for such persons. Wear gloves for nail care. Follow Standard Precautions and the Bloodborne Pathogen Standard.

Comfort

Sometimes you just trim the fingernails. Sometimes you just give foot care. To do both, the person sits at the over-bed table (Fig. 23-11). Provide for warmth and comfort.

Provide for your comfort during nail and foot care. Sit in front of the over-bed table to clean and trim fingernails. For foot care, rest the person's lower leg and foot on your lap. Or position the feet on the floor and kneel on the floor. Lay a towel across your lap or put a disposable waterproof pad (disposable bed protector—Chapter 20) on the floor to protect your uniform. Use good body mechanics. Always support the person's foot and ankle during foot care.

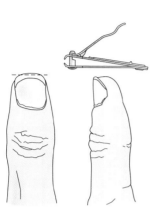

FIGURE 23-10 Trim fingernails straight across. Use nail clippers.

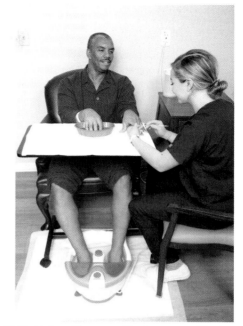

FIGURE 23-11 Nail and foot care. The feet are soaking in a whirlpool foot bath. The fingers are soaking in a kidney basin.

Giving Nail and Foot Care

Quality of Life

- Knock before entering the person's room.
- Address the person by name.
- Introduce yourself by name and title.

- Explain the procedure before starting and during the procedure.
- Protect the person's rights during the procedure.
- Handle the person gently during the procedure.

Pre-Procedure

1 Follow *Delegation Guidelines: Nail and Foot Care.* See *Promoting Safety and Comfort: Nail and Foot Care.*
2 Practice hand hygiene and get the following supplies.
   - Wash basin or whirlpool foot bath
   - Kidney basin
   - Soap
   - Water thermometer
   - Bath towel
   - Washcloth and hand towel (if needed)
   - Nail clippers
   - Orangewood stick
   - Emery board or nail file

   - Lotion for the hands
   - Lotion or petroleum jelly for the feet
   - Towel or paper towels (as a barrier for supplies)
   - Disposable waterproof pad
   - Gloves
   - Laundry bag
3 Place the barrier (towel, paper towels) on the over-bed table. Arrange supplies on top.
4 Practice hand hygiene.
5 Identify the person. Check the ID bracelet against the assignment sheet. Use 2 identifiers (Chapter 11). Also call the person by name.
6 Provide for privacy.

Procedure

7 Assist the person to the bedside chair. Remove footwear and socks or stockings. Place the call light and other needed items within reach.
8 Place the disposable waterproof pad under the feet.
9 Fill the wash basin or whirlpool foot bath ⅔ (two-thirds) full with water. Water temperature is usually 105°F (40.5°C). Measure the temperature with a water thermometer. Test it by dipping your elbow or inner wrist into the basin. Have the person check the water temperature and adjust as needed.
10 Place the basin or foot bath on the disposable waterproof pad.

11 Help the person put the feet into the water. Both bare feet are covered by water.
12 Adjust the over-bed table in front of the person.
13 Fill the kidney basin ⅔ (two-thirds) full with water. See step 9 for water temperature.
14 Place the kidney basin on the over-bed table.
15 Place the person's fingers into the basin. Position the arms for comfort (see Fig. 23-11).
16 Let the fingers soak for 5 to 10 minutes. Let the feet soak for 15 to 20 minutes. Re-warm water as needed.
17 Put on gloves.

Continued

Giving Nail and Foot Care —cont'd

Procedure—cont'd

18 Clean the hands with soap and water if needed or if required by your state's competency exam. Clean between the fingers. Rinse the hands.
19 Remove the kidney basin.
20 Dry the hands and between the fingers thoroughly.
21 Clean under the fingernails with the flat edge of the orangewood stick. Wipe the orangewood stick on a towel or paper towel after each nail.
22 Push cuticles back gently with the orangewood stick or a washcloth if requested by the person.
23 Trim fingernails straight across with the nail clippers (see Fig. 23-10). You may carefully round the corners slightly.
24 File and shape nails with an emery board or nail file. Nails are smooth with no rough edges. Check each nail for smoothness. File as needed. File in 1 direction.
25 Apply lotion to the hands. Warm the lotion first. To warm lotion, rub some between your hands or hold the bottle under warm water.
26 Move the over-bed table to the side. (NOTE: If your agency or state competency test requires clean gloves for foot care, remove and discard gloves. Practice hand hygiene. Put on clean gloves.)
27 Lift a foot out of the water. Support the foot and ankle with 1 hand. With your other hand, wash the foot and between the toes with soap and a washcloth. Return the foot to the water to rinse the foot and between the toes.
28 Repeat step 27 for the other foot.
29 Remove the feet from the water. Dry thoroughly, especially between the toes. Support the foot and ankle as needed.
30 Apply lotion or petroleum jelly to the tops, soles, and heels of the feet. Do not apply between the toes. Warm lotion or petroleum jelly first (see step 25). Remove excess lotion or petroleum jelly with a towel. Support the foot and ankle as needed.
31 Place the used towels and washcloth in the laundry bag. Remove and discard the gloves. Practice hand hygiene.
32 Help the person put on slip-resistant footwear.

Post-Procedure

33 Provide for comfort. (See the inside of the back cover.)
34 Place the call light and other needed items within reach.
35 Raise or lower bed rails. Follow the care plan.
36 Clean, rinse, dry, and return equipment and supplies to their proper place. Use clean, dry paper towels for drying. Discard disposable items. Wear gloves.
37 Clean and dry the over-bed table. Dry with paper towels. Discard the paper towels.
38 Remove and discard the gloves. Practice hand hygiene.
39 Follow the care plan and the person's preferences for privacy measures to maintain. Leaving the privacy curtain, window coverings, and door open or closed are examples.
40 Complete a safety check of the room. (See the inside of the back cover.)
41 Follow agency policy for used linens.
42 Practice hand hygiene.
43 Report and record your care and observations.

FOCUS ON PRIDE

The Person, Family, and Yourself

Personal and Professional Responsibility

Grooming promotes comfort, self-esteem, and body image. Clean hair and nails help mental well-being. So does a clean-shaven face or a well-groomed beard or mustache. Families and visitors notice how patients or residents are groomed. If not groomed well, they may question the quality of care. Grooming is important.

Rights and Respect

Grooming preferences vary. Do not judge the person by your standards or impose your choices on the person. Respect the right to choose. Assist with grooming in a way that improves the person's self-esteem.

Independence and Social Interaction

Some family members want to help with grooming. For example, they want to style the person's hair. Or they want to apply lotion to the person's hands and feet.

With the person's permission, allow family to assist with grooming as much as safely possible. This promotes social interaction. It also involves the family in the person's care.

Delegation and Teamwork

Grooming takes time. You, the person, the nurse, and other team members work together to plan and organize care. For example, a resident had a stroke. Breakfast is at 0800, speech therapy is at 0930, and family visits during lunch. The resident prefers to comb hair, shave, and change clothes after breakfast but before visitors arrive. You plan to assist the resident with grooming after breakfast and before speech therapy.

Do not neglect grooming because of a busy schedule. Plan to meet the person's needs at a time best for the person and the team.

Ethics and Laws

Patients and residents have the right to be free from mistreatment and restraint (Chapter 2). Never force a care measure on a person. If a person resists or refuses care, stop. Do not proceed. Politely ask the person for the reason. Tell the nurse. You, the nurse, and the person can discuss a solution.

FOCUS ON PRIDE: Application

The family may notice when grooming differs from usual. The family may tell you what they expect. Why are their comments important? How can you show that you value their input?

Circle the BEST answer.

1 A person with alopecia has
   a Excessive body hair
   b Dry, white flakes from the scalp
   c An infestation with lice
   d Hair loss

2 Which should you report before giving hair care?
   a Braided hair
   b White specks in the hair
   c Dry hair
   d Dirty hair

3 A person has tangled hair. You should
   a Cut out the tangled sections
   b Comb through small sections starting at the hair ends
   c Brush firmly from the scalp to the hair ends
   d Not brush the hair

4 A person's hair is *not* matted or tangled. When brushing hair, start at
   a The forehead and brush backward
   b The hair ends
   c The scalp
   d The back of the neck and brush forward

5 Brushing keeps the hair
   a Soft and shiny
   b Clean
   c Free of lice
   d Long

6 A person requests a shampoo. You should
   a Shampoo hair during the person's shower
   b Shampoo hair at the sink
   c Shampoo the person in bed
   d Follow the care plan for the shampoo method

7 To keep shampoo out of the eyes during a shower
   a Do not rinse the top of the head
   b Wipe off the shampoo with a washcloth
   c Have the person wear eyeglasses
   d Place a washcloth over the eyes and tip the head back

8 A person is able to shave himself. He needs help setting up and cleaning up. Which should you do?
   a Set up supplies and then clean up supplies after he shaves.
   b Set up supplies, shave him, and clean up supplies.
   c Refuse to set up and clean up supplies because he can shave himself.
   d Set up supplies but tell him to clean up when finished.

9 A resident needs to be shaved. The nurse tells you the resident takes an anticoagulant drug. You need to
   a Use a safety razor and shaving cream
   b Use a safety razor without shaving cream
   c Use the resident's electric shaver
   d Refuse to shave the resident

10 When shaving a person's face with a safety razor
   a Discard the razor in the wastebasket when done
   b Start at the jaw and shave upward
   c Hold the skin taut
   d Shave when the skin is dry

11 A person is nicked during shaving. Your *first* action is to
   a Wash your hands
   b Apply direct pressure
   c Tell the nurse
   d Apply a bandage

12 To trim fingernails, use
   a An emery board
   b Scissors
   c A nail file
   d Nail clippers

13 Which is *correct* when performing nail care?
   a Trim nails straight across and then file them.
   b Trim and file nails before cleaning them.
   c Do not clean under the fingernails.
   d File nails with a firm back-and-forth motion.

14 A person has poor circulation in the legs and feet. You should
   a Trim the person's toenails
   b Use hot water to soak the feet
   c Check the toes for cracks and sores
   d Not perform foot care

15 When giving foot care
   a Dry well between the toes
   b Apply lotion between the toes
   c Do not wash between the toes
   d Do not use soap

Answers to Chapter 23 questions are on p. 588.

FOCUS ON **PRACTICE**

Problem Solving

A resident with dementia has long fingernails. Some are broken and have rough edges. As you begin nail care, the resident resists by pulling away and yelling at you. What do you do? Why is nail care important for this resident? How might you provide care safely?

Dressing and Undressing

Clothing affects comfort and body image. The ability to dress and undress oneself promotes dignity and independence. You will assist patients and residents with dressing needs.

GARMENTS

A *garment is an item of clothing.* Age, gender, culture, comfort, season, and personal preference affect garment choices. An *under-garment is an item of clothing worn next to the skin under clothing.* Bras, undershirts, underwear (underpants, panties, briefs, boxer shorts), and slips are examples. Incontinence products may be worn (Chapter 25).

Hospital patients wear gowns (patient gowns) that open in the back (p. 312). For some examinations and procedures, the opening is in front.

Nursing center residents wear street clothes during the day and sleepwear at bedtime. Resident clothing is labeled with the person's name in a way that respects dignity. For example, labels are inside clothing or shoes. Or a color-coded system is used. Know your agency's policy. Residents must be dressed in their own clothing.

See *Focus on Communication: Garments.*
See *Focus on Surveys: Garments.*

FOCUS ON **SURVEYS**
Garments

Surveyors will observe if residents:
* Are dressed in their own clothes.
* Are dressed in clothing of their choice.
* Are wearing the correct clothing for the time of day.

Changing Garments

In nursing centers, garments are often changed in the morning and at bedtime. They are changed after bathing and when wet or soiled.

In hospitals, the patient changes into a patient gown (p. 312) on admission. The gown is changed daily and as needed. When discharged, the patient changes into his or her own clothing.

The procedures that follow describe how to change garments that:
* *Open in the back.* Patient gowns and bras that fasten in the back are examples.
* *Open in the front.* Shirts with buttons, vests, and coats and jackets are examples.
* *Are pulled over the head (pullover garments).* T-shirts, undershirts, and sweatshirts are examples.

There may be more than 1 method to remove and apply a garment. For example, one person prefers to remove a pullover garment from the head first. Another person needs 1 sleeve removed before bringing the garment over the head. Use the method that is best for the person. Areas of weakness, joint range of motion (Chapter 32), and personal preference are considered.

Health problems can cause weakness or affect function on 1 side of the body. Stroke and hip fracture are examples (Chapter 40). When changing garments, you need to know about areas of weakness.
* The *affected side* *(weak side) is the side of the body with weakness from illness or injury.*
* The *unaffected side* *(strong side) is the side of the body opposite the affected side.*

Some persons dress and undress themselves. Others need help. Allow the person to do as much as is safely possible. This promotes independence. Adaptive (assistive) devices may be used (Fig. 24-1). To assist with dressing and undressing, follow the rules in Box 24-1.

See *Focus on Communication: Changing Garments*, p. 306.
See *Focus on Older Persons: Changing Garments*, p. 306.
See *Delegation Guidelines: Changing Garments*, p. 306.
See *Promoting Safety and Comfort: Changing Garments*, p. 306.
See procedure: *Undressing the Person*, p. 307.
See procedure: *Dressing the Person*, p. 309.

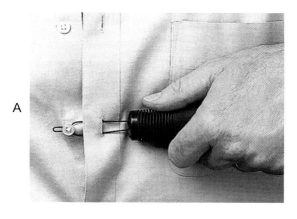

A

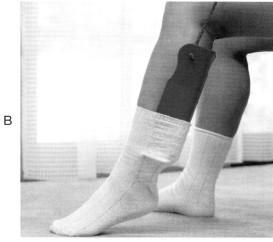

B

FIGURE 24-1 Dressing aids. **A,** A button hook to button and zip clothing. **B,** A sock assist to pull on socks and stockings. (Courtesy North Coast Medical Inc., Morgan Hill, Calif.)

BOX 24-1 Rules for Dressing and Undressing

* Provide for privacy. Do not expose the person.
* Encourage the person to do as much as possible.
* Let the person choose what to wear. Have the person choose the right under-garments.
* Make sure the garments are the person's. (They do not belong to another patient or resident.)
* Make sure garments and footwear are the correct size.
* Consider areas of weakness.
  * Remove clothing from the *unaffected side* (strong side) first.
  * Put clothing on the *affected side* (weak side) first.
* Support the arm or leg to remove or put on a garment.
* Move and handle the body gently. Do not force a joint beyond its range of motion or to the point of pain. See Chapter 32.
* Follow the person's care plan and agency policy for removed garments. The agency or the person's family will launder (wash, dry, and return) the person's clothing. If the family does the laundry, removed clothing is usually kept in the person's room. It is not placed in the agency's hamper for used linens (Chapter 20).

FOCUS ON **COMMUNICATION**

Changing Garments

When changing garments, promote personal choice and independence. You can ask:

- "What would you like to wear today?"
- "There's a concert today. Do you want to wear something special?"
- "Do you need help with your buttons?"
- "Do you need help with your zipper?"

FOCUS ON **OLDER PERSONS**

Changing Garments

Persons with dementia may take longer to dress. Choosing clothing may be hard. Wearing the wrong clothing for the season and wearing clothes that do not match are common. Or they forget to put on a piece of clothing.

Allow the person to do as much as possible. The Alzheimer's and Related Dementias Education and Referral Center (ADEAR) suggests the following.

- Try to assist with dressing at the same time each day. Dressing becomes part of the daily routine.
- Allow extra time. Do not rush the person.
- Let the person choose from 2 or 3 outfits. The family may buy several of the same outfit. Dressing is easier if the person insists on wearing the same thing.
- Choose comfortable, easy to get on and off clothes. Garments with elastic waistbands and Velcro closures are examples. There are no zippers, buttons, hooks, snaps, or other closures.
- Stack clothes in the order they are put on. The person sees 1 item at a time. For example, an under-garment is put on first. The item is on top of the stack.
- Give clear, simple, and step-by-step directions. Give the person 1 item at a time.

DELEGATION GUIDELINES

Changing Garments

To assist with dressing and undressing, you need this information from the nurse and the care plan.

- How much help the person needs
- If the person can sit up and lean forward
- If the person can raise the hips to lift the buttocks off of the bed
- If the person has an affected side (weak side)
- If the person has limited range of motion in any joints
- If certain garments are needed
- What observations to report and record:
  - How much help was given
  - How the person tolerated the procedure
  - Complaints by the person
  - Changes in the person's behavior
- When to report observations
- What patient or resident concerns to report at once

PROMOTING SAFETY AND COMFORT

Changing Garments

Safety

To change garments in bed, you turn the person from side to side. If the person uses bed rails, raise the far bed rail. If bed rails are not used, ask a co-worker to help turn and position the person. This protects the person from falling.

Follow Standard Precautions and the Bloodborne Pathogen Standard. If contact with blood or body fluids is likely, wear gloves. Remove gloves and practice hand hygiene before touching clean garments.

Some persons have limited range of motion in 1 or more joints (Chapter 32). Pain can occur if the affected joint is moved too far. There is stiffness and difficulty moving the joint. Use caution when changing garments. Never force a joint beyond its present range of motion or to the point of pain.

Follow the safety measures for transfers (Chapter 18) and tub baths and showers (Chapter 22) when undressing and dressing in a tub or shower room. Follow the care plan for the transfer method and number of staff needed. Remember these safety measures if the person will stand.

- Slip-resistant footwear is worn for transfers.
- The floor is dry.
- The person uses grab bars (safety bars) for support.
- Wheelchair and shower chair wheels are locked (braked).
- A transfer belt (gait belt) is applied over clothing.

Comfort

Keep the person covered with the bath blanket as much as possible. This provides privacy and warmth.

Check that clothing is applied correctly. For example, the front of the shirt is in front. Adjust clothing for comfort and a neat appearance.

Undressing the Person

Quality of Life

- Knock before entering the person's room.
- Address the person by name.
- Introduce yourself by name and title.
- Explain the procedure before starting and during the procedure.
- Protect the person's rights during the procedure.
- Handle the person gently during the procedure.

Pre-Procedure

1 Follow *Delegation Guidelines: Changing Garments.* See *Promoting Safety and Comfort: Changing Garments.*
2 Ask a co-worker to help turn and position the person if needed.
3 Practice hand hygiene.
4 Identify the person. Check the identification (ID) bracelet against the assignment sheet. Use 2 identifiers (Chapter 11). Also call the person by name.
5 Get the following supplies.
   - Bath blanket
   - Laundry bag
   - Clothing requested by the person
6 Provide for privacy.
7 Raise the bed for body mechanics. Bed rails are up if used.

Procedure

8 Stand on the person's affected (weak) side if the person has one. Lower the bed rail near you if up.
9 Position the person for the procedure. The head of the bed is raised if the person will sit up and lean forward. The head of the bed is flat if the person will turn from side to side.
10 Cover the person with a bath blanket. Fan-fold linens to the foot of the bed. Keep the person covered as much as possible throughout the procedure.
11 Remove garments that open in the back (Fig. 24-2, p. 308).
   a If the person can sit up and lean forward (see Fig. 24-2, A):
      1) Have the person lean forward.
      2) Undo buttons, zippers, ties, snaps, or other closures.
      3) Bring the sides of the garment to the sides of the person.
      4) Have the person sit back.
   b If the person cannot sit up and lean forward (see Fig. 24-2, B):
      1) Turn the person away from you.
      2) Undo buttons, zippers, ties, snaps, or other closures.
      3) Tuck the far side of the garment under the person. Fold the near side onto the chest.
      4) Position the person supine.
   c Slide the garment off of the shoulder and arm on the unaffected (strong) side. Remove the garment from the affected (weak) side.
12 Remove pullover garments (Fig. 24-3, p. 308).
   a Undo any buttons, zippers, ties, snaps, or other closures.
   b Remove the garment from the arm and shoulder on the unaffected (strong) side (see Fig. 24-3, A).
   c Have the person lean forward if able or turn the person toward you to bring the garment up to the neck. Have the person sit back. Or position the person supine.
   d Bring the garment over the head (see Fig. 24-3, B).
   e Remove the garment from the affected (weak) side (see Fig. 24-3, C).

13 Remove garments that open in the front.
   a Undo buttons, zippers, ties, snaps, or other closures.
   b Slide the garment off of the shoulder and arm on the unaffected (strong) side.
   c If the person can sit up and lean forward:
      1) Have the person lean forward.
      2) Bring the garment around the back to the affected (weak) side.
      3) Have the person sit back.
      4) Remove the garment from the affected (weak) side.
   d If the person cannot sit up and lean forward:
      1) Turn the person toward you.
      2) Tuck the removed part of the garment under the person.
      3) Turn the person away from you.
      4) Pull the side of the garment out from under the person. Make sure the person will not lie on it when supine.
      5) Position the person supine.
      6) Remove the garment from the affected (weak) side.
14 Remove pants or slacks.
   a Remove footwear and socks.
   b Position the person supine.
   c Undo buttons, zippers, ties, snaps, or buckles. Remove a belt if worn.
   d If the person can raise the hips to lift the buttocks off of the bed:
      1) Have the person raise the hips.
      2) Bring the pants down over the hips and buttocks.
      3) Have the person lower the hips.
   e If the person cannot raise the hips:
      1) Turn the person toward you.
      2) Slide the pants off of the hip and buttocks on the unaffected (strong) side.
      3) Turn the person away from you.
      4) Slide the pants off of the hip and buttocks on the affected (weak) side.
      5) Position the person supine.
   f Slide the pants down the legs and over the feet.
15 Dress the person. See procedure: *Dressing the Person,* p. 309.

Post-Procedure

16 Provide for comfort. (See the inside of the back cover.)
17 Place the call light and other needed items within reach.
18 Lower the bed to a safe and comfortable level. Follow the care plan.
19 Raise or lower bed rails. Follow the care plan.
20 Follow the care plan and the person's preferences for privacy measures to maintain. Leaving the privacy curtain, window coverings, and door open or closed are examples.
21 Complete a safety check of the room. (See the inside of the back cover.)
22 Follow agency policy for removed clothing and used linens.
23 Practice hand hygiene.
24 Report and record your care and observations.

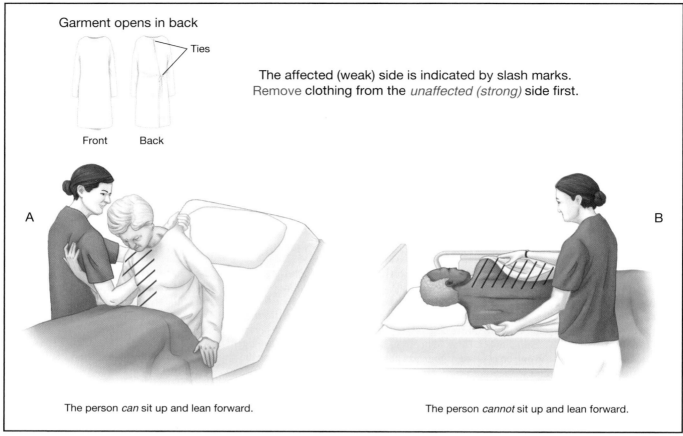

Garment opens in back

Front   Back   Ties

The affected (weak) side is indicated by slash marks.
Remove clothing from the *unaffected (strong)* side first.

A

B

The person *can* sit up and lean forward.

The person *cannot* sit up and lean forward.

FIGURE 24-2 Removing a gown that opens in the back. **A,** The person can sit up and lean forward. The gown is untied and removed. **B,** The person cannot sit up and lean forward. The person is turned to untie and remove the gown.

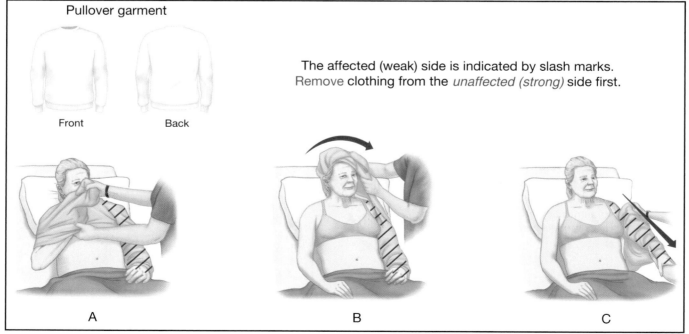

Pullover garment

Front   Back

The affected (weak) side is indicated by slash marks.
Remove clothing from the *unaffected (strong)* side first.

A   B   C

FIGURE 24-3 Removing a pullover shirt. **A,** Remove the shirt from the unaffected (strong) side. **B,** Bring the shirt over the head. **C,** Remove the shirt from the affected (weak) side. (NOTE: Reverse this order when dressing the person. Keep the person covered as much as possible.)

Dressing the Person

NATCEP   VIDEO

Quality of Life

- Knock before entering the person's room.
- Address the person by name.
- Introduce yourself by name and title.
- Explain the procedure before starting and during the procedure.
- Protect the person's rights during the procedure.
- Handle the person gently during the procedure.

Pre-Procedure

1 Follow *Delegation Guidelines: Changing Garments,* p. 306. **See** *Promoting Safety and Comfort: Changing Garments,* p. 306.
2 Ask a co-worker to help turn and position the person if needed.
3 Practice hand hygiene.
4 Identify the person. Check the ID bracelet against the assignment sheet. Use 2 identifiers (Chapter 11). Also call the person by name.
5 Ask what the person would like to wear.
6 Get the following supplies.
   - Bath blanket
   - Laundry bag
   - Clothing requested by the person
7 Provide for privacy.
8 Raise the bed for body mechanics. Bed rails are up if used.

Procedure

9 Stand on the person's affected (weak) side if the person has one. Lower the bed rail near you if up.
10 Position the person for the procedure. The head of the bed is raised if the person will sit up and lean forward. The head of the bed is flat if the person will turn from side to side.
11 Cover the person with a bath blanket. Fan-fold linens to the foot of the bed. Keep the person covered as much as possible throughout the procedure.
12 Undress the person. See procedure: *Undressing the Person,* p. 307.
13 Put on garments that open in the back (Fig. 24-4, p. 310).
   a Slide the correct sleeve of the garment onto the arm and shoulder of the affected (weak) side.
   b Slide the garment's other sleeve onto the arm and shoulder of the unaffected (strong) side.
   c *If the person can sit up and lean forward:*
      1) Have the person lean forward.
      2) Bring the sides of the garment to the back.
      3) Fasten buttons, zippers, ties, snaps, or other closures.
      4) Have the person sit back.
   d *If the person cannot sit up and lean forward:*
      1) Turn the person toward you. Bring the side of the garment around the back (see Fig. 24-4, *A*).
      2) Turn the person away from you. Bring the side of the garment around the back on the other side (see Fig. 24-4, *B*).
      3) Bring the sides of the garment together. Fasten buttons, zippers, ties, snaps, or other closures.
      4) Position the person supine.
14 Put on pullover garments.
   a Slide the correct sleeve of the garment onto the arm and shoulder on the affected (weak) side.
   b Bring the garment over the head.
   c Slide the garment's other sleeve onto the arm and shoulder of the unaffected (strong) side.
   d Bring the garment down.
      1) *If the person can sit up and lean forward,* have the person lean forward. Pull the garment down. Have the person sit back.
      2) *If the person cannot sit up and lean forward:*
         i Turn the person away from you.
         ii Pull the garment down on the affected (weak) side.
         iii Turn the person toward you.
         iv Pull the garment down on the unaffected (strong) side.
         v Position the person supine.
15 Put on garments that open in the front (Fig. 24-5, p. 311).
   a Slide the correct sleeve of the garment onto the arm and shoulder on the affected (weak) side (see Fig. 24-5, *A*).
   b *If the person can sit up and lean forward:*
      1) Have the person lean forward.
      2) Bring the garment around the back to the unaffected (strong) side.
      3) Slide the garment's other sleeve onto the arm and shoulder of the unaffected (strong) side.
      4) Have the person sit back.
   c *If the person cannot sit up and lean forward:*
      1) Turn the person away from you. Bring the garment around the person's back. Tuck the far side of the garment under the person (see Fig. 24-5, *B*).
      2) Turn the person toward you. Bring the garment around the person's unaffected (strong) side (see Fig. 24-5, *C*).
      3) Position the person supine.
      4) Slide the garment onto the arm and shoulder on the unaffected (strong) side (see Fig. 24-5, *D*).
   d Fasten buttons, zippers, ties, snaps, or other closures.
16 Put on pants or slacks (Fig. 24-6, p. 312).
   a Position the person supine.
   b Slide the pants over the feet and up the legs.
   c *If the person can raise the hips to lift the buttocks off of the bed* (see Fig. 24-6, *A*):
      1) Have the person raise the hips.
      2) Bring the pants up over the hips and buttocks.
      3) Have the person lower the hips.
   d *If the person cannot raise the hips* (see Fig. 24-6, *B*):
      1) Turn the person away from you.
      2) Slide the pants over the hip and buttocks on the affected (weak) side.
      3) Turn the person toward you.
      4) Slide the pants over the hip and buttocks on the unaffected (strong) side.
      5) Position the person supine.
   e Fasten buttons, zippers, ties, snaps, a belt buckle, or other closures.
17 Put socks on the person. Socks are up all the way and smooth. See Chapter 35 for how to apply elastic stockings. Apply slip-resistant footwear if the person will get out of bed.
18 Remove the bath blanket. Place it in the laundry bag.
19 Cover the person or help the person out of bed.

Continued

Dressing the Person—cont'd

Post-Procedure

20 Provide for comfort. (See the inside of the back cover.)
21 Place the call light and other needed items within reach.
22 Lower the bed to a safe and comfortable level. Follow the care plan.
23 Raise or lower bed rails. Follow the care plan.
24 Follow the care plan and the person's preferences for privacy measures to maintain. Leaving the privacy curtain, window coverings, and door open or closed are examples.

25 Complete a safety check of the room. (See the inside of the back cover.)
26 Follow agency policy for removed clothing and used linens.
27 Practice hand hygiene.
28 Report and record your care and observations.

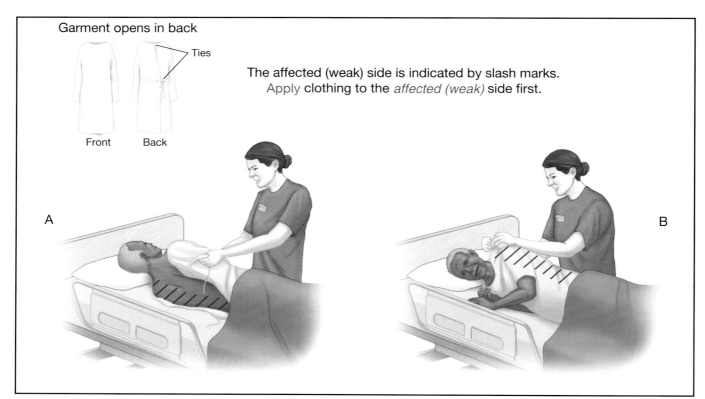

FIGURE 24-4 Applying a gown that opens in the back with the person lying down. A, Turn the person toward you after putting the gown on the arms. Bring the side of the gown to the person's back. B, Turn the person away from you. Bring the other side of the gown to the back and fasten.

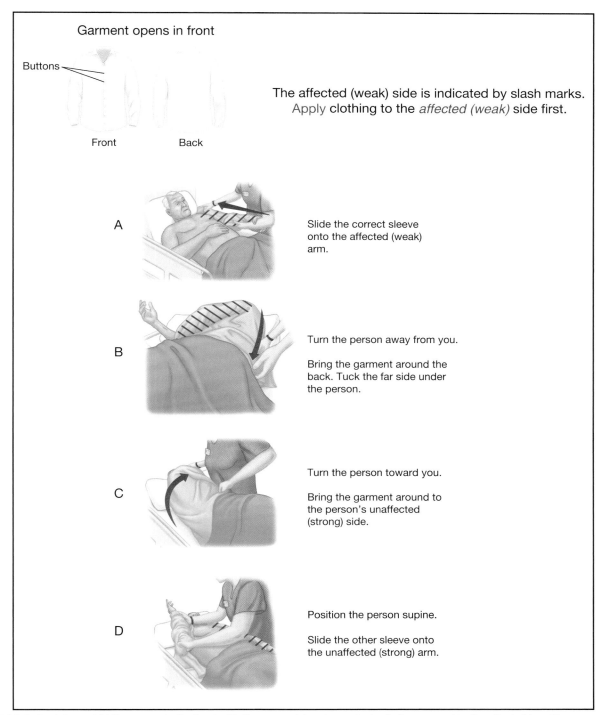

Garment opens in front

Buttons

Front   Back

The affected (weak) side is indicated by slash marks.
Apply clothing to the *affected (weak)* side first.

A Slide the correct sleeve onto the affected (weak) arm.

B Turn the person away from you.

Bring the garment around the back. Tuck the far side under the person.

C Turn the person toward you.

Bring the garment around to the person's unaffected (strong) side.

D Position the person supine.

Slide the other sleeve onto the unaffected (strong) arm.

FIGURE 24-5 Applying a shirt that opens in the front with the person lying down. A, Apply the garment to the affected (weak) arm. B and C, Turn the person to bring the garment around the back to the unaffected (strong) side. D, Position the person supine. Apply the garment to the unaffected (strong) arm. (NOTE: Reverse this order when undressing the person. Keep the person covered as much as possible.)

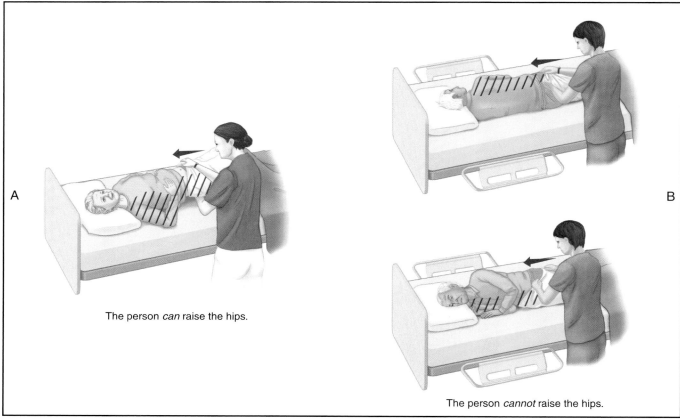

The person *can* raise the hips.

The person *cannot* raise the hips.

FIGURE 24-6 Applying pants. **A,** The person can raise the hips and buttocks off of the bed. The pants are slid over the hips and buttocks. **B,** The person cannot raise the hips. The person is turned to pull the pants up over the hip and buttock on the affected (weak) side and the unaffected (strong) side.

CHANGING PATIENT GOWNS

Patient gowns are designed for comfort and to allow treatment (Fig. 24-7).

- An *intravenous (IV) therapy gown* is used for IV therapy (Chapter 30). The gown opens along the sleeves and closes with ties, snaps, or Velcro.
- A *standard gown* does not open along the sleeves.

For injury or paralysis, remove the gown from the unaffected (strong) arm first. Support the affected (weak) arm while removing the gown. Put the clean gown on the affected (weak) arm first and then on the unaffected (strong) arm.

See *Delegation Guidelines: Changing Patient Gowns.*
See *Promoting Safety and Comfort: Changing Patient Gowns.*
See procedure: *Changing a Standard Patient Gown on a Person With an IV,* p. 314.

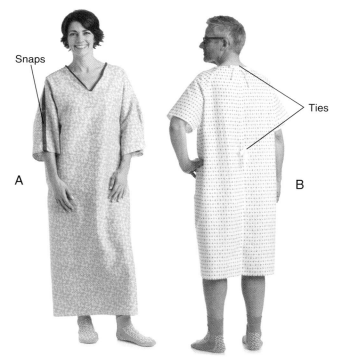

Snaps

Ties

FIGURE 24-7 Patient gowns. **A,** IV therapy gown. Snaps on the sleeves allow for easy changing. **B,** Standard gown. This gown ties at the neck and back. (Courtesy Medline Industries, Inc. © Medline Industries, Inc. 2019.)

DELEGATION GUIDELINES

Changing Patient Gowns

Before changing a gown on a person with an IV, you need this information from the nurse and the care plan.
- Which arm has the IV
- If the person has an IV pump (see *Promoting Safety and Comfort: Changing Patient Gowns*)

PROMOTING SAFETY AND COMFORT

Changing Patient Gowns

Safety

IV pumps control the *flow rate*—how fast fluid enters a vein (Chapter 30). You do not adjust controls on IV pumps. For an IV pump and a standard gown, do not use the following procedure. The nurse handles the arm with the IV.

To change a standard gown, you need to lift the IV bag from the IV pole (Fig. 24-8). Do not disconnect or remove any other parts of the IV set-up. Hold the bag up. Blood can enter the IV tubing if you lower the bag below the IV site. (The *IV site* is where the IV is inserted into the body—usually an arm or hand. The site is covered by a clear dressing.) Moving the IV bag can change the flow rate. Ask the nurse to check the flow rate after you change a gown.

Comfort

Some persons feel exposed when wearing a gown that opens in back. Cover the person for warmth and privacy. A robe or a second gown worn backwards can help the person feel covered. Other gowns over-lap in the back and tie at the side. These gowns provide more privacy. When tied at the side, uncomfortable bows and knots at the back are avoided.

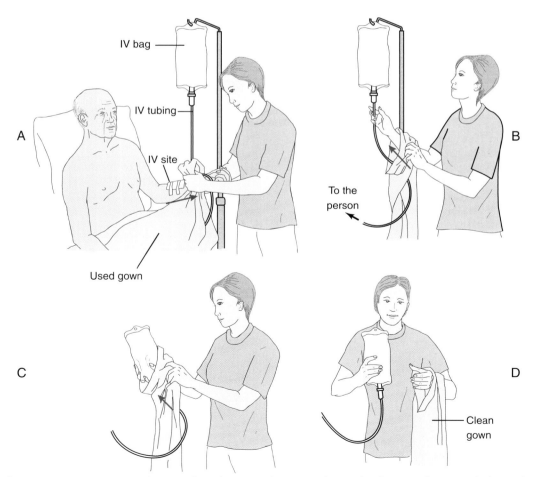

FIGURE 24-8 Changing a gown. **A,** Remove the gown from the arm with no IV. Gather up the sleeve on the arm with the IV. Slip it over the IV site and tubing. Remove it from the arm and hand. **B,** Slip the gathered sleeve along the IV tubing to the bag. **C,** Remove the IV bag from the pole. Pass it through the sleeve. **D,** Slip the gathered sleeve of the clean gown over the IV bag at the shoulder part of the gown.

Changing a Standard Patient Gown on a Person With an IV

Quality of Life

- Knock before entering the person's room.
- Address the person by name.
- Introduce yourself by name and title.
- Explain the procedure before starting and during the procedure.
- Protect the person's rights during the procedure.
- Handle the person gently during the procedure.

Pre-Procedure

1 Follow *Delegation Guidelines:*
   a *Changing Garments*, p. 306
   b *Changing Patient Gowns*, p. 313
   See *Promoting Safety and Comfort:*
   a *Changing Garments*, p. 306
   b *Changing Patient Gowns*, p. 313
2 Practice hand hygiene.
3 Identify the person. Check the ID bracelet against the assignment sheet. Use 2 identifiers (Chapter 11). Also call the person by name.
4 Get the following supplies.
   - Clean gown
   - Bath blanket
   - Laundry bag
5 Provide for privacy.
6 Raise the bed for body mechanics. Bed rails are up if used.

Procedure

7 Lower the bed rail near you if up.
8 Cover the person with the bath blanket. Fan-fold linens to the foot of the bed.
9 Untie the gown. Free parts that the person is lying on.
10 Remove the gown from the arm with *no IV.*
11 Gather up the sleeve of the arm *with the IV.* Slide it over the IV site and tubing. Remove the arm and hand from the sleeve (see Fig. 24-8, *A*).
12 Keep the sleeve gathered. Slide your arm along the tubing to the bag (see Fig. 24-8, *B*).
13 Remove the bag from the pole. Slide the bag and tubing through the sleeve (see Fig. 24-8, *C*). Do not pull on the tubing. Keep the bag above the IV site.
14 Hang the IV bag on the pole.
15 Place the used gown in the laundry bag.
16 Gather the sleeve of the clean gown that will go on the arm with the IV.
17 Remove the bag from the pole. Slip the sleeve over the bag at the shoulder part of the gown (see Fig. 24-8, *D*). Hang the bag.
18 Slide the gathered sleeve over the tubing, hand, arm, and IV site. Then slide it onto the shoulder.
19 Put the other side of the gown on the person. Fasten the gown.
20 Cover the person. Remove and store the bath blanket. Or place it in the laundry bag.

Post-Procedure

21 Provide for comfort. (See the inside of the back cover.)
22 Place the call light and other needed items within reach.
23 Lower the bed to a safe and comfortable level. Follow the care plan.
24 Raise or lower bed rails. Follow the care plan.
25 Follow the care plan and the person's preferences for privacy measures to maintain. Leaving the privacy curtain, window coverings, and door open or closed are examples.
26 Complete a safety check of the room. (See the inside of the back cover.)
27 Follow agency policy for used linens.
28 Practice hand hygiene.
29 Ask the nurse to check the flow rate.
30 Report and record your care and observations.

FOCUS ON P R I D E

The Person, Family, and Yourself

P ersonal and Professional Responsibility

Care measures are not just tasks to be completed. Show that you value the person.
- Be pleasant. Talk with the person.
- Avoid seeming rushed.
- Do a good job. Be thorough and careful.
- Compliment the person after dressing.

R ights and Respect

Appearance affects self-esteem. Garments should be clean, not wrinkled, and comfortable. Matching clothes and clothes for the correct season are worn. If a garment does not fit well, change it. Dress the person in a way that promotes dignity and respect.

I ndependence and Social Interaction

Ask what clothing the person prefers. Ask about comfort and appearance. Also ask if the person wants other items applied. Jewelry is an example. Personal choice promotes independence and quality of life.

D elegation and Teamwork

Some garments are worn as part of the person's treatment. Elastic stockings and binders or compression garments are examples (Chapter 35). You need more information from the nurse and the care plan before applying such garments.

E thics and Laws

Special care measures are needed for persons with confusion or dementia who resist care (Chapter 42). Forcing care and neglecting care are wrong. Patience and problem solving are needed. A co-worker or family member may help with dressing. Or garments are changed at another time. Follow the person's routine. Be kind and gentle.

FOCUS ON PRIDE: *Application*

How does clothing affect your self-image? How will you promote dignity and independence when assisting with dressing and undressing?

REVIEW QUESTIONS

Circle the BEST answer.

1 In long-term care
  a Patient gowns are worn
  b Sleepwear is worn during the day
  c Garments are changed every other day
  d Street clothes are worn during the day

2 For spilled coffee on a shirt, you should
  a Give the person a sweater to cover the spill
  b Clean the shirt with a damp towel
  c Change the shirt at bedtime
  d Change the shirt right away

3 A person has weakness on the right side. Garments are removed
  a From the affected (weak) side first
  b From the unaffected (strong) side first
  c From either side first
  d In the same way they are applied

4 A person has limited range of motion in the left shoulder. Apply the person's shirt
  a To the affected side first
  b To the unaffected side first
  c To either side first
  d In the same way it was removed

5 When dressing
  a Do as much for the person as possible
  b Choose clothing for the person
  c Support the arm or leg
  d Move the person quickly

6 When dressing a person with dementia
  a Choose clothing with buttons
  b Give more than 1 direction at a time
  c Offer many clothing options
  d Follow the person's routine

7 An IV therapy gown
  a Opens at the sleeves
  b Does not have sleeves
  c Must be changed by the nurse
  d Provides less privacy than a standard gown

8 When changing the gown on a person with an IV
  a Hold the IV bag below the IV site
  b Stop the IV pump to change the gown
  c Have the nurse check the flow rate afterward
  d Disconnect the IV to change the gown

Answers to Chapter 24 questions are on p. 588.

FOCUS ON PRACTICE

Problem Solving

Two residents share a room. After dressing the person, you notice that the shirt belongs to the resident's roommate. What will you do? How could this have been prevented?

CHAPTER 25

Urinary Needs

OBJECTIVES

- Define the key terms and key abbreviations in this chapter.
- Describe the rules for normal urination.
- Describe normal urine.
- Identify the observations to report to the nurse.

- Describe urinary incontinence and the care required.
- Describe bladder training methods.
- Perform the procedures described in this chapter.
- Explain how to promote PRIDE in the person, the family, and yourself.

KEY TERMS

dysuria Painful or difficult (*dys*) urination (*uria*); burning on urination

functional incontinence The person has bladder control but cannot use the toilet in time

hematuria Blood (*hemat*) in the urine (*uria*)

mixed incontinence The combination of stress incontinence and urge incontinence

nocturia Frequent urination (*uria*) at night (*noc*)

oliguria Scant amount (*olig*) of urine (*uria*); less than 500 mL in 24 hours

over-flow incontinence Small amounts of urine leak from a full bladder

polyuria Abnormally large amounts (*poly*) of urine (*uria*)

reflex incontinence Urine is lost at predictable intervals when a specific amount of urine is in the bladder

stress incontinence When urine leaks during exercise and certain movements that cause pressure on the bladder

transient incontinence Temporary or occasional incontinence that is reversed when the cause is treated

urge incontinence The loss of urine in response to a sudden, urgent need to void; the person cannot get to a toilet in time

urinary frequency Voiding at frequent intervals

urinary incontinence (UI) The involuntary loss or leakage of urine

urinary retention Not being able to completely empty the bladder

urinary urgency The need to void at once

urination The process of emptying urine from the bladder; voiding

voiding See "urination"

KEY ABBREVIATIONS

BM	Bowel movement
ID	Identification
mL	Milliliter

UI	Urinary incontinence
UTI	Urinary tract infection

Eliminating waste is a physical need. The urinary system removes waste products from the blood. It also maintains the body's water and electrolyte balance.

See *Promoting Safety and Comfort: Urinary Needs.*

PROMOTING SAFETY AND COMFORT

Urinary Needs

Safety

Urinary elimination measures often involve exposing and touching private areas—the perineum and rectum. Sexual abuse has occurred in health care settings. The person may feel threatened or is actually being abused. The person needs to be able to call for help. Keep the call light within the person's reach at all times. Always act in a professional manner.

NORMAL URINATION

The healthy adult produces about 1500 mL (milliliters) or 3 pints of urine a day. Many factors affect urine production—age, disease, the amount and kinds of fluid ingested, salt, body temperature, perspiration (sweating), and some drugs. Some substances increase urine production—coffee, tea, alcohol, and some drugs. A diet high in salt and some drugs cause the body to retain water. When water is retained, less urine is produced.

Urination (voiding) means the process of emptying urine from the bladder. The amount of fluid intake, habits, and available toilet facilities affect frequency. So do activity, work, bladder problems, and illness. People usually void at bedtime, after sleep, and before meals. Some void more often. Voiding at night disturbs sleep.

Some persons need help getting to the bathroom. Others use bedpans, urinals, or commodes. Follow the rules in Box 25-1 and the person's care plan.

See *Focus on Communication: Normal Urination.*

FOCUS ON COMMUNICATION

Normal Urination

Patients and residents may not use the terms "voiding" or "urinating." Do not ask: "Do you need to void?" or "Do you need to urinate?" if the person does not understand these words. Instead, you can ask these questions.
- "Do you need to use the bathroom (toilet)?"
- "Do you need the bedpan (urinal)?"
- "Do you need to pass urine?"
- "Do you need to pass water?"
- "Do you need to pee?"

The word "pee" may offend some persons. Choose words the person understands and uses. Follow the care plan.

BOX 25-1 Rules for Normal Urination

- Practice medical asepsis.
- Follow Standard Precautions. Follow the Bloodborne Pathogen Standard if blood is present.
- Provide fluids as the nurse and care plan direct.
- Follow voiding routines and habits. Check with the nurse and the person's care plan.
- Help the person to the bathroom upon request. Or provide the bedpan, urinal, or commode. The need to void may be urgent.
- Assist the person with urinary needs at regular times. Some people are embarrassed or are too weak to ask for help.
- Help the person assume a normal position for voiding if possible. Women sit or squat. Men stand.
- Warm the bedpan or urinal if time permits. The need may be urgent. (This is important if the item is metal.)
- Cover the person for warmth and privacy.
- Provide for privacy. Pull the privacy curtain around the bed, close room and bathroom doors, and close window coverings.
- Leave the room if the person can be alone. Stay nearby if the person is weak, unsteady, or at risk for falling (Chapter 12). Do not leave persons with dementia alone (Chapter 42).
- Tell the person that running water in the sink, flushing the toilet, or playing music can mask voiding sounds. Voiding with others nearby embarrasses some people.
- Place the call light and toilet paper within reach.
- Allow enough time. Do not rush the person.
- Promote relaxation. Some people like to read.
- Run water slowly in a sink if the person cannot start the urine stream. Hearing the sound of a water stream may help. Or place the person's fingers in warm water.
- Provide perineal care as needed (Chapter 22).
- Assist with hand hygiene after voiding. Provide a wash basin, soap, washcloth, and towel. Some agencies provide hand-wipes.

Observations

Normal urine is pale yellow, straw-colored, or amber (Fig. 25-1, p. 318). It is clear (not cloudy) with no particles. A faint odor is normal. Observe urine for color, clarity, odor, amount (output), particles, and blood.

Ask the nurse to observe urine that looks or smells abnormal. Report these problems.
- *Dysuria—painful or difficult (dys) urination (uria); burning on urination*
- *Hematuria—blood (hemat) in the urine (uria)*
- *Nocturia—frequent urination (uria) at night (noc)*
- *Oliguria—scant amount (olig) of urine (uria); less than 500 mL in 24 hours*
- *Polyuria—abnormally large amounts (poly) of urine (uria)*
- *Urinary frequency—voiding at frequent intervals*
- *Urinary incontinence (UI)—the involuntary loss or leakage of urine*
- *Urinary retention—not being able to completely empty the bladder*
- *Urinary urgency—the need to void at once*

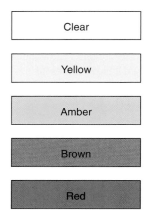

FIGURE 25-1 Color chart for urine. (Redrawn from Weldon, Inc., Fort Worth, Tex.)

VOIDING EQUIPMENT

If the person is unable to use the toilet, other equipment is used for voiding. Bedpans, urinals, and commodes are common.

See *Promoting Safety and Comfort: Voiding Equipment.*

PROMOTING SAFETY AND COMFORT

Voiding Equipment

Safety

Urine is a body fluid. Follow Standard Precautions when handling urinary devices and their contents. This includes bedpans, urinals, commodes, urinary drainage bags (Chapter 26), and incontinence products. Follow the Bloodborne Pathogen Standard if blood is present.

If the device (bedpan, urinal, commode) is new, gloves do not need to be worn when gathering equipment. Apply gloves before helping the person use the device.

When a device is re-used, it is cleaned and disinfected after use. You should still use caution to prevent the transmission of microbes when gathering re-used equipment. Depending on the device and the situation you can:

- Use paper towels or other covering as a barrier when collecting the device. Apply gloves before helping the person use it.
- Apply gloves when gathering equipment. Remove and discard gloves and practice hand hygiene before touching other surfaces (bed controls, bed rails, and so on). Apply clean gloves to help the person use the device.
- Apply gloves when gathering equipment. Keep 1 hand "clean." This hand does not touch the device. Use it to touch other surfaces.

Remove gloves and practice hand hygiene before touching clean items or surfaces. Also use caution to avoid contaminating surfaces in the person's bathroom. A paper towel can be used to turn a faucet on and off.

Patients and residents have their own voiding equipment. Some states and agencies require labeling the device with the person's name and room and bed number. Equipment is not shared among patients and residents.

NOTE: A task may require more than 1 pair of gloves. Change gloves as needed. Use careful judgment. Remember to practice hand hygiene after removing gloves.

Bedpans

Bedpans are used when the person cannot be out of bed. Women use bedpans for voiding and bowel movements (BMs). Men use them for BMs.

A *standard bedpan* is shown in Figure 25-2, *A.* The wide rim at the back goes under the buttocks.

A *fracture pan* has a thin rim. It is only about ½-inch deep at one end (Fig. 25-2, *B*). The smaller end (flat end) goes under the buttocks (Fig. 25-3). The person lies flat. Fracture pans are used:

- By persons with casts
- By persons in traction
- By persons with limited back motion
- By older persons with osteoporosis (fragile bones) or arthritis
- After spinal cord injury or surgery
- After a hip fracture or hip replacement surgery

See *Delegation Guidelines: Bedpans.*
See *Promoting Safety and Comfort: Bedpans.*
See procedure: *Giving the Bedpan.*

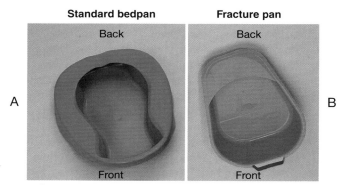

FIGURE 25-2 Bedpans. **A,** Standard bedpan. **B,** Fracture pan.

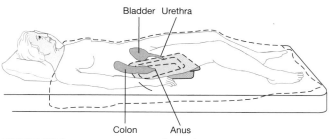

FIGURE 25-3 A person positioned on a fracture pan. The small end (flat end) is under the buttocks.

DELEGATION GUIDELINES
Bedpans

To assist with a bedpan, you need this information from the nurse and the care plan.
- What bedpan to use—standard bedpan or fracture pan
- Position or activity limits
- If the person can raise the hips to place the bedpan
- If you can leave the room or if you need to stay with the person
- If the nurse will observe the results before you flush the contents
- What observations to report and record:
  - Urine color, clarity, and odor
  - Amount
  - Presence of particles
  - Blood in the urine
  - Cloudy urine
  - Complaints of urgency, burning, dysuria, or other problems
  - For bowel movements, see Chapter 27
- When to report observations
- What patient or resident concerns to report at once

PROMOTING SAFETY AND COMFORT
Bedpans

Safety
Remember to raise the bed as needed for good body mechanics. Lower the bed to a safe level before leaving the bedside. Raise or lower the bed rails according to the care plan.

Comfort
Most bedpans are plastic. Metal bedpans are often cold. Warm metal bedpans with warm water and dry them before use. Use clean, dry paper towels for drying.

    The person must not sit on a bedpan for a long time. Bedpans are uncomfortable. They can lead to pressure injuries (Chapter 36).

Giving the Bedpan

Quality of Life

- Knock before entering the person's room.
- Address the person by name.
- Introduce yourself by name and title.

- Explain the procedure before starting and during the procedure.
- Protect the person's rights during the procedure.
- Handle the person gently during the procedure.

Pre-Procedure

1 Follow *Delegation Guidelines: Bedpans.* **See** *Promoting Safety and Comfort:*
  a *Urinary Needs,* p. 317
  b *Voiding Equipment*
  c *Bedpans*
2 Practice hand hygiene.
3 Provide for privacy.
4 Get the following supplies.
- Bedpan
- Bedpan cover (if used)
- Toilet paper
- Waterproof under-pad (if required by agency policy)
- Disposable waterproof pad (as a barrier for the bedpan)
- Bath blanket
- Gloves
- Laundry bag

5 Arrange equipment nearby. Place the bedpan on the chair or bed. Use the disposable waterproof pad as a barrier between the bedpan and the surface.

Procedure

6 Practice hand hygiene.
7 Raise the bed for body mechanics (if the person's needs are not urgent). Lower the bed rail near you if up.
8 Lower the head of the bed. Position the person supine. Or raise the head of the bed slightly for comfort.
9 Cover the person with a bath blanket. Fold the top linens and gown out of the way. Keep the lower body covered.
10 Apply gloves.
11 Place the bedpan (Fig. 25-4, p. 320).
  a *If the person can raise the hips to lift the buttocks off of the bed:*
    1) Have the person flex (bend) the knees and raise the buttocks. The person pushes against the mattress with the feet.
    2) Slide your hand under the lower back. Help raise the buttocks.
    3) If using a waterproof under-pad, place it under the buttocks.
    4) Slide the bedpan under the person (see Fig. 25-4, A).

  b *If the person cannot raise the hips:*
    1) Turn the person to position the waterproof under-pad if needed.
    2) Turn the person onto the side away from you.
    3) Place the bedpan firmly against the buttocks. Push downward on the bedpan and toward the person (see Fig. 25-4, B).
    4) Hold the bedpan securely. Turn the person onto the back.
  c Make sure the bedpan is centered under the person. When the person sits up, the urethra and anus should be over the opening (Fig. 25-5, p. 321).
12 Cover the person with the bath blanket.
13 Remove and discard the gloves. Practice hand hygiene.
14 Raise the head of the bed so the person is in a sitting position (Fowler's position) for a standard bedpan. Or raise the head of the bed to a comfortable level for the person.
15 Check that the person is correctly positioned on the bedpan (see Fig. 25-5).
16 Raise the bed rail if used. Lower the bed.

Continued

Giving the Bedpan—cont'd

Procedure—cont'd

17 Place the toilet paper and call light within reach.
18 Ask the person to signal when done or when help is needed. (NOTE: For some state competency tests, you ask the person to use hand-wipes for hand hygiene after wiping with toilet paper.)
19 Stay with the person as needed. Or leave the room and close the door. (Practice hand hygiene before leaving.) Be respectful. Provide as much privacy as possible.
20 Return when the person signals. Or check on the person every 5 minutes. Knock before entering. Practice hand hygiene.
21 Raise the bed for body mechanics. Lower the bed rail if used. Lower the head of the bed.
22 Apply gloves.
23 Have the person raise the buttocks. Remove the bedpan. Or hold the bedpan and turn the person onto the side away from you. Place the bedpan on the disposable waterproof pad or in the cover (if used).
24 Clean the genital area if the person cannot do so.
  a Clean from the meatus (front or top) to the anus (back or bottom) with toilet paper. Use fresh paper for each wipe. Place used toilet paper in the bedpan.
  b Provide perineal care if needed (Chapter 22).
  c Remove the waterproof under-pad (if used). Place it in the laundry bag.
  d Cover the person with the bath blanket.
  e Remove and discard the gloves. Practice hand hygiene. Apply clean gloves.
25 Lower the person's gown. Cover the person with the top linens. Remove the bath blanket. Place it in the laundry bag.
26 Raise the bed rail if used. Lower the bed.
27 Take the bedpan to the bathroom. Note the color, amount (output), and character of urine or feces (stools). See "Measuring Intake and Output" in Chapter 30.
28 Empty the bedpan contents into the toilet. Rinse the bedpan. Pour the rinse into the toilet and flush.
29 Follow agency procedures to clean and disinfect the bedpan.
30 Return the bedpan to its proper place.
31 Remove and discard the gloves. Practice hand hygiene. Apply clean gloves.
32 Help the person with hand hygiene.
33 Remove and discard the gloves. Practice hand hygiene.

Post-Procedure

34 Provide for comfort. (See the inside of the back cover.)
35 Place the call light and other needed items within reach.
36 Lower the bed to a safe and comfortable level. Follow the care plan.
37 Raise or lower bed rails. Follow the care plan.
38 Discard the disposable waterproof pad. Return the toilet paper to its proper place.
39 Follow the care plan and the person's preferences for privacy measures to maintain. Leaving the privacy curtain, window coverings, and door open or closed are examples.
40 Complete a safety check of the room. (See the inside of the back cover.)
41 Follow agency policy for used linens.
42 Practice hand hygiene.
43 Report and record your care and observations.

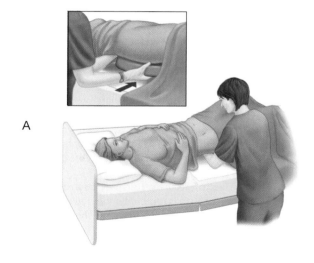
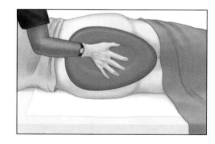
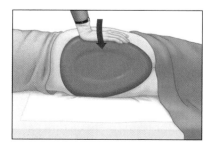

A — The person *can* raise the hips.

B — The person *cannot* raise the hips.

FIGURE 25-4 Placing the bedpan. **A,** Help the person raise the buttocks off of the bed if able. Slide the bedpan under the person. **B,** If the person cannot raise the hips, turn the person to the side. Place the bedpan firmly against the buttocks. Push downward on the bedpan and toward the person. Turn the person onto the back.

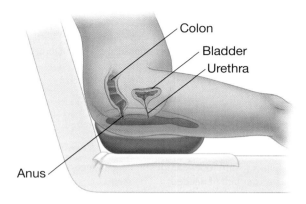

FIGURE 25-5 The person is positioned on the bedpan so the urethra and anus are directly over the opening.

Colon
Bladder
Urethra
Anus

Urinals

Urinals are used for voiding. Plastic urinals designed for men are common (Fig. 25-6, A). They have caps and hook-type handles. Men use urinals when standing (preferred), sitting, or lying in bed. Some men need support when standing. Urinals designed for females are less common (Fig. 25-6, B) but may be used.

After use, the urinal cap is closed to prevent urine spills. Remind the person to use the call light after voiding. The urinal needs to be emptied as soon as possible to prevent spills, slipping, and the growth of microbes.

Do not place urinals on over-bed tables and bedside stands. These are used for eating, as a work surface, and for personal items and supplies. These surfaces must not be contaminated with urine. Follow agency policy for where to place urinals. If the bed has bed rails, the person may hang the urinal on the bed rail.

See *Focus on Communication: Urinals.*
See *Delegation Guidelines: Urinals.*
See *Promoting Safety and Comfort: Urinals.*
See procedure: *Giving the Male Urinal,* p. 322.

FOCUS ON **COMMUNICATION**
Urinals

You may need to assist some men with urinals. Or you may need to stay with the person. For comfort, explain why you must help. You can say:
- "I'll help you use the urinal. I need to stay with you so you don't fall."
- "I'll help you place and remove the urinal so it doesn't spill."

DELEGATION GUIDELINES
Urinals

To assist with urinals, you need this information from the nurse and the care plan.
- How the urinal is used—standing, sitting, or lying in bed.
- If help is needed to place or hold the urinal.
- If the man needs support to stand. If yes, how many staff are needed.
- If you need to stay with the person.
- If the nurse needs to observe the urine.
- What observations to report and record (see *Delegation Guidelines: Bedpans,* p. 319).
- When to report observations.
- What patient or resident concerns to report at once.

PROMOTING SAFETY AND COMFORT
Urinals

Safety
Empty urinals promptly to prevent odors and the spread of microbes. A filled urinal spills easily, causing hazards. Also, it is an unpleasant sight and causes odor. Urinals are cleaned and disinfected after use.

Comfort
For some men, you may need to place the penis in the urinal. This may embarrass the person and you. Act in a professional manner.

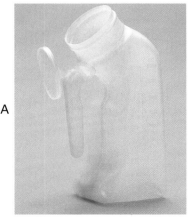
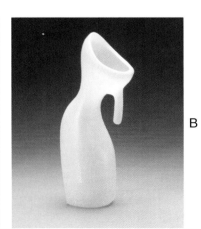

A   B

FIGURE 25-6 Urinals. **A,** Urinal designed for males. **B,** Urinal designed for females. (B, Courtesy Viscot Medical, LLC, East Hanover, N.J.)

Giving the Male Urinal

Quality of Life

- Knock before entering the person's room.
- Address the person by name.
- Introduce yourself by name and title.
- Explain the procedure before starting and during the procedure.
- Protect the person's rights during the procedure.
- Handle the person gently during the procedure.

Pre-Procedure

1 Follow *Delegation Guidelines: Urinals,* p. 321. See *Promoting Safety and Comfort:*
   a *Urinary Needs,* p. 317
   b *Voiding Equipment,* p. 318
   c *Urinals,* p. 321
2 Practice hand hygiene.
3 Provide for privacy.

4 Determine if the man will stand, sit, or lie in bed.
5 Get the following supplies.
   - Urinal
   - Slip-resistant footwear for standing (if needed)
   - Transfer belt (if needed)
   - Gloves

Procedure

6 Practice hand hygiene. Put on gloves.
7 *Standing to use the urinal* (Fig. 25-7, A):
   a Prepare the person to stand. Help the person sit on the side of the bed. Apply slip-resistant footwear. Apply a transfer belt if needed (Chapter 12).
   b Help the person stand. Provide support if the person is unsteady.
   c Give the person the urinal.
8 *Using the urinal in bed* (Fig. 25-7, B):
   a Give the person the urinal.
   b Remind the person to tilt the bottom down to prevent spills.
9 Position the urinal and place the penis in the urinal if the person cannot do so.
10 Remove and discard the gloves if you will leave the person (steps 11 through 15). Practice hand hygiene after removing and discarding gloves.
11 Place the call light within reach. Ask the person to signal when done or when help is needed.

12 Provide for privacy. Cover the person for privacy if in bed.
13 Leave the room and close the door if the person can be left alone. (Practice hand hygiene before leaving.) Be respectful. Provide as much privacy as possible.
14 Return when the person signals. Or check on the person every 5 minutes. Knock before entering.
15 Practice hand hygiene. Put on gloves.
16 Close the urinal cap. Take it to the bathroom.
17 Note the color, amount (output), and clarity of urine.
18 Empty the urinal into the toilet. Rinse the urinal with cold water. Pour rinse into the toilet and flush.
19 Follow agency procedures to clean and disinfect the urinal.
20 Return the urinal to its proper place.
21 Remove and discard the gloves. Practice hand hygiene. Put on clean gloves.
22 Assist with hand hygiene.
23 Remove and discard the gloves. Practice hand hygiene.

Post-Procedure

24 Provide for comfort. (See the inside of the back cover.)
25 Place the call light and other needed items within reach.
26 Raise or lower bed rails. Follow the care plan.
27 Return supplies to their proper place.
28 Follow the care plan and the person's preferences for privacy measures to maintain. Leaving the privacy curtain, window coverings, and door open or closed are examples.

29 Complete a safety check of the room. (See the inside of the back cover.)
30 Follow agency policy for used linens.
31 Practice hand hygiene.
32 Report and record your care and observations.

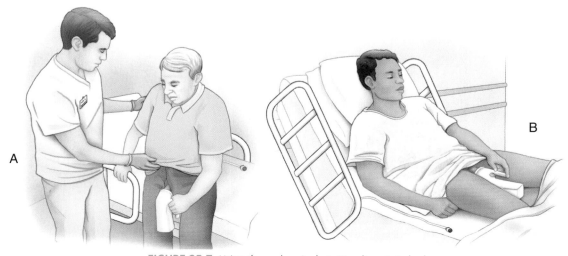

FIGURE 25-7 Using the male urinal. **A,** Standing. **B,** In bed.

Commodes

A commode (bedside commode) is a chair or wheelchair with an opening for a container (Fig. 25-8). Persons unable to walk to the bathroom often use commodes. The commode allows a normal position for elimination. The commode arms and back provide support and help prevent falls.

Some commodes, with the containers removed, are placed over toilets. The person uses the commode arms for support to sit and stand. And the commode serves as a higher toilet seat. If the commode has wheels (see Fig. 25-8, *B*), lock (brake) the wheels after properly positioning the commode over the toilet.

See *Delegation Guidelines: Commodes.*

See *Promoting Safety and Comfort: Commodes.*

See procedure: *Helping the Person to the Commode*, p. 324.

DELEGATION GUIDELINES

Commodes

You need this information from the nurse and care plan when assisting with commode use.

- If the commode is used at the bedside or over the toilet
- How much help the person needs
- If you can leave the room or if you need to stay with the person
- If the nurse needs to observe urine or BMs before you flush the contents
- What observations to report and record (see *Delegation Guidelines: Bedpans*, p. 319)
- When to report observations
- What patient or resident concerns to report at once

PROMOTING SAFETY AND COMFORT

Commodes

Safety

You will transfer the person to and from the commode. Practice safe transfer procedures (Chapter 18). Use the transfer belt. Lock (brake) the wheels. Remove the transfer belt after the transfer. See "Transfer/Gait Belts" in Chapter 12.

Commodes are not shared among patients and residents. When no longer needed, the commode is returned to the supply department for disinfection.

Comfort

After transfer to the commode, cover the person's lap and legs with a bath blanket. This promotes warmth and privacy.

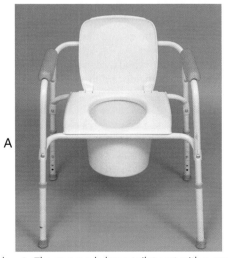
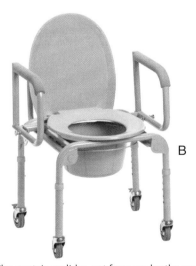

FIGURE 25-8 Commodes. **A,** The commode has a toilet seat with a container. The container slides out from under the seat for emptying. **B,** A commode with wheels. (B, Courtesy drivemedical.com.)

Helping the Person to the Commode

Quality of Life

- Knock before entering the person's room.
- Address the person by name.
- Introduce yourself by name and title.
- Explain the procedure before starting and during the procedure.
- Protect the person's rights during the procedure.
- Handle the person gently during the procedure.

Pre-Procedure

1 Follow *Delegation Guidelines: Commodes, p. 323.* See *Promoting Safety and Comfort:*
  a *Urinary Needs, p. 317*
  b *Voiding Equipment, p. 318*
  c *Commodes, p. 323*
2 Practice hand hygiene.
3 Provide for privacy.

4 Get the following supplies.
  • Commode
  • Toilet paper
  • Bath blanket
  • Transfer belt
  • Slip-resistant footwear
  • Gloves
  • Laundry bag
5 Arrange equipment. Place the commode next to the bed. Check that the wheels are locked (braked).

Procedure

6 Practice hand hygiene.
7 Help the person sit on the side of the bed. Lower the bed rail if used.
8 Help the person put on slip-resistant footwear.
9 Apply the transfer belt.
10 Apply gloves if contact with urine or feces (stools) may occur.
11 Assist the person to the commode. Use the transfer belt. Help the person lower clothing as needed.
12 Remove and discard the gloves if worn and soiled. Practice hand hygiene after removing and discarding gloves.
13 Cover the person's lap and legs with a bath blanket for warmth and privacy. Remove the transfer belt.
14 Place the toilet paper and call light within reach.
15 Ask the person to signal when done or when help is needed. Ask the person to use hand-wipes for hand hygiene after wiping with toilet paper.
16 Stay with the person as needed. Or leave the room and close the door. (Practice hand hygiene before leaving.) Be respectful. Provide as much privacy as possible.
17 Return when the person signals. Or check on the person every 5 minutes. Knock before entering.

18 Practice hand hygiene. Put on gloves.
19 Remove the bath blanket. Place it in the laundry bag.
20 Help the person clean the genital area as needed. Remove and discard the gloves. Practice hand hygiene.
21 Apply the transfer belt. Help the person raise and fasten clothing as needed. Help the person back to bed using the transfer belt. Remove the transfer belt and footwear. Raise the bed rail if used.
22 Put on gloves. Remove and cover the commode container.
23 Take the container to the bathroom.
24 Observe urine and feces (stools) for color, amount (output), and character.
25 Empty the contents into the toilet. Rinse the container. Pour the rinse into the toilet and flush.
26 Follow agency procedures to clean and disinfect the container.
27 Return the container to the commode. Close the lid. Disinfect other parts of the commode if necessary.
28 Remove and discard the gloves. Practice hand hygiene. Put on clean gloves.
29 Assist with hand hygiene.
30 Remove and discard the gloves. Practice hand hygiene.

Post-Procedure

31 Provide for comfort. (See the inside of the back cover.)
32 Place the call light and other needed items within reach.
33 Raise or lower bed rails. Follow the care plan.
34 Return supplies to their proper place.
35 Follow the care plan and the person's preferences for privacy measures to maintain. Leaving the privacy curtain, window coverings, and door open or closed are examples.

36 Complete a safety check of the room. (See the inside of the back cover.)
37 Follow agency policy for used linens.
38 Practice hand hygiene.
39 Report and record your care and observations.

URINARY INCONTINENCE

Persons with urinary incontinence (UI) pass urine without intending to. Older persons are at risk for UI because of urinary tract changes, medical and surgical conditions, and drug therapy. Incontinence is not a normal part of aging.

Types of Urinary Incontinence

UI may be temporary or permanent. Common types of incontinence are:

- *Stress incontinence—urine leaks during exercise and certain movements that cause pressure on the bladder.* Urine loss is small. Often called *dribbling*, it occurs with laughing, sneezing, coughing, lifting, or other activities.
- *Urge incontinence—urine is lost in response to a sudden, urgent need to void. The person cannot get to a toilet in time.* Urinary frequency, urinary urgency, and night-time voiding are common.
- *Mixed incontinence—the person has a combination of stress incontinence and urge incontinence.* Many older women have this type.
- *Over-flow incontinence—small amounts of urine leak from a full bladder.* The person feels like the bladder is not empty. The person dribbles and may have a weak urine stream.
- *Functional incontinence—the person has bladder control but cannot use the toilet in time.* Immobility, restraints, unanswered call lights, no call light within reach, and difficulty removing clothing are causes. Not knowing where to find the bathroom, confusion, and disorientation are other causes.
- *Reflex incontinence—urine is lost at predictable intervals when a specific amount of urine is in the bladder.* The person does not feel the need to void. Nervous system disorders and injuries are common causes.
- *Transient incontinence—temporary or occasional incontinence that is reversed when the cause is treated.* (*Transient* means *for a short time.*)

Incontinence may result from a physical illness or drugs. Some causes can be reversed. Others cannot. If incontinence is a new problem, tell the nurse at once.

Managing Urinary Incontinence

The goals of managing UI are to:
- Prevent urinary tract infections (UTIs).
- Restore as much bladder function as possible.

The person's care plan may include some of the measures listed in Box 25-2. *Good skin care and dry garments and linens are essential.* Promoting normal urinary elimination prevents incontinence in some people (see Box 25-1). Others need bladder training (p. 331). Sometimes catheters are needed (Chapter 26).

BOX 25-2 Urinary Incontinence—Nursing Measures

- Record the person's voidings:
  - Incontinent
  - Successful use of the toilet, bedpan, urinal, or commode
- Record the amount voided (Chapter 30).
- Answer call lights promptly. The need to void may be urgent.
- Promote normal urinary elimination (see Box 25-1).
- Promote normal bowel elimination (Chapter 27).
- Assist with elimination at regular times—after sleep, before and after meals, and at bedtime. Follow the person's routine. Assist promptly when help is requested.
- Encourage pelvic floor muscle exercises as instructed by the nurse (p. 331).
- Follow the person's bladder training program (p. 331).
- Provide a clear path to the bathroom.
- Have the person wear easy-to-remove clothing. UI can occur while dealing with buttons, zippers, other closures, and under-garments.
- Check the person often. Make sure the person is clean and dry.
- Help prevent UTIs.
  - Promote fluid intake as the nurse directs.
  - Have the person wear cotton underwear.
  - Keep the perineal area clean and dry.
  - Clean from front to back (top to bottom) during perineal care (Chapter 22).
- Decrease fluid intake at bedtime.
- Provide good skin care.
- Apply a barrier cream or moisturizer (cream, lotion, paste) to the skin or perineum as directed by the nurse. The application prevents irritation and skin damage.
- Provide dry garments and linens.
- Observe for signs of skin breakdown (Chapters 35 and 36).
- Use incontinence products as the nurse directs. Follow the manufacturer's instructions.
- Do not leave urinals in place to collect urine for persons who are incontinent.
- Keep the perineal area clean and dry (Chapter 22).
  - Protect the person and dry garments and linens from the wet incontinence product.
  - Remove wet incontinence products, garments, and linens.
  - Expose only the perineal area.
  - Use soap (or body wash) and water or a no-rinse product (perineal cleanser). Follow the care plan. For soap (or body wash) and water, use a safe and comfortable water temperature.
  - Dry the perineal area and buttocks.
  - Apply a clean, dry incontinence product and clean, dry garments and linens.
- Follow Standard Precautions. Follow the Bloodborne Pathogen Standard if blood is present.

UI is embarrassing and uncomfortable. Garments are wet and odors develop. Skin irritation, infection, and pressure injuries are risks. Falls are a risk from trying to get to the bathroom quickly. Pride, dignity, and self-esteem are affected. Social isolation, loss of independence, and depression are common. Quality of life suffers.

UI is linked to abuse, mistreatment, and neglect. Frequent care is needed. The person may wet again right after skin care and changing wet garments and linens. Remember, the person does not choose to be incontinent. The person has the right to be free from abuse, mistreatment, and neglect. Kindness, empathy, understanding, and patience are needed.

See *Focus on Surveys: Managing Urinary Incontinence*.
See *Focus on Older Persons: Managing Urinary Incontinence*.

FOCUS ON SURVEYS
Managing Urinary Incontinence

Surveyors observe how incontinence is prevented, improved, or managed. They observe if staff:
- Follow the person's care plan.
- Keep call lights within reach.
- Answer call lights promptly.
- Provide a clear pathway to the bathroom.
- Provide good lighting for voiding.
- Assist with bedpans, urinals, and commodes as needed.
- Assist the person to the bathroom as needed.
- Respond appropriately when incontinence occurs.
- Protect the person's dignity when incontinence occurs.
- Check incontinent persons often.
- Change wet incontinence products and clothing promptly.
- Prevent prolonged exposure of the skin to urine.
- Provide hygiene measures to prevent skin breakdown.

FOCUS ON OLDER PERSONS
Managing Urinary Incontinence

Complications from incontinence pose serious problems for older persons. These include falls, pressure injuries, and UTIs. Hospital or long-term care stays are often necessary.

Persons with dementia may void in the wrong places. Trash cans, planters, and closets are examples. Some persons throw incontinence products on the floor or in the toilet. Others resist staff efforts to stay clean and dry.

Provide safe care. The care plan may include measures recommended by the Alzheimer's Disease and Related Dementias Education and Referral Center (ADEAR).
- Remind the person to go to the bathroom every 2 to 3 hours during the day. Do not wait for the person to ask.
- Show the way or take the person to the bathroom.
- Keep pathways to the bathroom clear.
- Keep the bathroom clutter-free.
- Keep lights on in the pathway and bathroom.
- Have the person wear clothing and under-garments that are easy to remove.
- Post a big sign on the bathroom door that says "Toilet" or "Bathroom."
- Help the person in the bathroom.
- Observe for signs of needing to void. Restlessness and pulling at clothes are examples. Respond promptly.
- Stay calm when the person is incontinent. Give reassurance if the person is upset. (This means to help the person feel less upset and worried.)
- Report incontinence. Report the time, what the person was doing, and other observations. An incontinence pattern may emerge. If so, measures are planned to prevent the problem.
- Prevent incontinence during sleep. Limit the type and amount of fluids in the evening. Follow the care plan.
- Plan ahead for the person leaving the agency. Have the person wear easy-to-remove clothing. Pack extra clothing, incontinence products, and hygiene supplies. Know where to find restrooms.

You may need help to keep the person clean and dry. Ask your co-workers or the nurse for help. Remember, everyone has the right to privacy and safe care. They also have the right to be treated with dignity.

Applying Incontinence Products

Incontinence products help keep the person dry. They usually have 2 layers and a waterproof back. Fluid passes through the top layer. It is absorbed by the bottom layer. Products come in various types and sizes.

Common incontinence products are shown in Figure 25-9. The nurse helps the person select products for his or her needs. To apply them, follow the manufacturer's instructions and agency procedures.

See *Focus on Communication: Applying Incontinence Products.*

See *Delegation Guidelines: Applying Incontinence Products.*

See *Promoting Safety and Comfort: Applying Incontinence Products,* p. 328.

See procedure: *Applying an Incontinence Brief,* p. 328.

FOCUS ON **COMMUNICATION**

Applying Incontinence Products

Incontinence products are often called "adult diapers." The word "diaper" may offend the person or lower self-esteem. Instead, say "brief," "pad," or "underwear." Some persons use the product's brand name. Use a term that promotes dignity and self-esteem.

DELEGATION GUIDELINES

Applying Incontinence Products

To apply an incontinence product, you need this information from the nurse and the care plan.

- What product to use.
- What size to use.
- If a barrier cream is needed. If yes, what cream to use.
- What observations to report and record:
  - Complaints of pain, burning, irritation, or the need to void
  - Signs and symptoms of skin breakdown:
    - Redness, irritation, blisters
    - Complaints of pain, burning, tingling, or itching
  - The amount of urine—small, moderate, large
  - Urine color
  - Blood in the urine
  - Leakage
  - A poor product fit
- When to report observations.
- What patient or resident concerns to report at once.

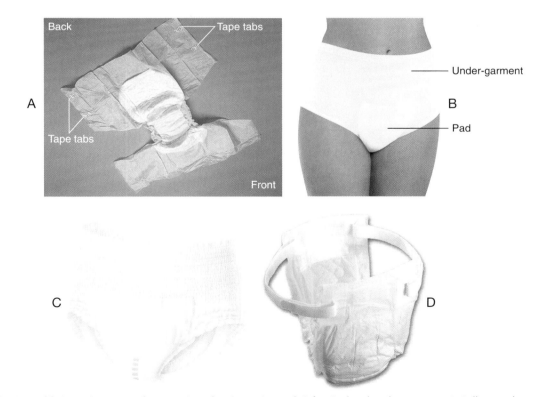

FIGURE 25-9 Disposable incontinence products. A, Complete incontinence brief. B, Pad and under-garment. C, Pull-on underwear. D, Belted under-garment. (B, Courtesy Hartmann USA, Inc., Rock Hill, S.C. C, Courtesy Hartmann Inc., Heidenheim, Germany. D, Courtesy Principle Business Enterprises, Dunbridge, Ohio.)

PROMOTING SAFETY AND COMFORT

Applying Incontinence Products

Safety

To safely apply an incontinence product, follow the manufacturer's instructions. The guidelines in Box 25-3 will help prevent:

- Leakage
- Skin irritation, skin damage, and pressure injuries
- Tearing of the product

Remove the soiled incontinence product from front to back (top to bottom). Apply the new product from front to back (top to bottom). This prevents spreading bacteria from the anal area to the urinary system.

Comfort

For comfort, use the correct size. If the product is too large, urine can leak. If too small, the product will be too tight and uncomfortable.

BOX 25-3 Applying Incontinence Products

- Follow the manufacturer's instructions.
- Use the correct size. The nurse tells you what size to use.
- Note the front and back of the product.
- Position the product correctly.
  - Center the product in the perineal area. For a male, the penis is downward.
  - Position the sides in the groin areas. The *groin* is where a thigh and the abdomen meet.
- Check for proper placement. The product should fit the shape of the body.
- Note the amount of urine (small, moderate, large). Also note how often you change the product. Large amounts of urine may require an extended-wear product.

- Do not let the plastic backing touch the person's skin.
- Provide perineal care after each incontinent episode.
- Do not use the product as a turning or lift sheet.
- Attach the tabs correctly. Some products will tear if you try to unfasten the tape or change the tape's position. Other products have adjustable tabs.
  - Attach the lower tab first. Attach it at a slightly upward angle. Do so for both sides.
  - Attach the upper tab after the lower tab is fastened. Attach it horizontally or at a slightly downward angle. Do so for both sides.

Applying an Incontinence Brief

Quality of Life

- Knock before entering the person's room.
- Address the person by name.
- Introduce yourself by name and title.

- Explain the procedure before starting and during the procedure.
- Protect the person's rights during the procedure.
- Handle the person gently during the procedure.

Pre-Procedure

1 Follow *Delegation Guidelines: Applying Incontinence Products*, p. 327. **See** *Promoting Safety and Comfort:*
   a *Urinary Needs*, p. 317
   b *Voiding Equipment*, p. 318
   c *Applying Incontinence Products*
2 Practice hand hygiene.
3 Provide for privacy.
4 Get the following supplies.
   - Incontinence brief
   - Barrier cream or moisturizer as directed by the nurse
   - Soap, body wash, or perineal cleanser
   - Items for perineal care (Chapter 22)
   - Waterproof under-pad
   - Bath blanket
   - Towel or paper towels (as a barrier for supplies)
   - Plastic trash bag
   - Gloves
   - Laundry bag

5 Place the barrier (towel, paper towels) on the over-bed table. Arrange items on top.
6 Practice hand hygiene.
7 Identify the person. Check the identification (ID) bracelet against the assignment sheet. Use 2 identifiers (Chapter 11). Also call the person by name.
8 Mark the date, time, and your initials on the new product.
9 Fill the wash basin and place it on the over-bed table. Water temperature is usually 105°F to 109°F (Fahrenheit) (40.5°C to 42.7°C [centigrade]). Measure water temperature according to agency policy. Have the person check the water temperature. Adjust as needed.
10 Raise the bed for body mechanics. Bed rails are up if used. Lower the bed rail near you if up.

Applying an Incontinence Brief—cont'd

Procedure

11 Position the person on the back. Lower the head of the bed. The bed is as flat as possible.
12 Practice hand hygiene. Put on gloves.
13 Cover the person with a bath blanket. Lower top linens to the foot of the bed. If linens are wet, remove them and place them in the laundry bag.
14 Place a waterproof under-pad under the buttocks. Have the person raise the buttocks off of the bed. Or turn the person from side to side. Position the person supine.
15 Lower pants or slacks if worn. Remove any wet garments. Follow agency policy for removed clothing.
16 Fold back part of the bath blanket. Raise the person's gown if worn. Keep the person covered as much as possible.
17 Have the person spread the legs.
18 Remove the used brief (Fig. 25-10, p. 330).
  a Loosen all of the tabs on the brief. Tuck the far side of the back panel under the person.
  b Observe the urine. Estimate the amount (small, medium, large). Observe for urine color and blood.
  c Roll the front of the product toward the back (bottom) (see Fig. 25-10, A).
  d Have the person turn onto the side away from you. Continue rolling the product from front to back (see Fig. 25-10, B).
  e Remove the brief.
19 Place the used brief in the trash bag. Tie or seal the bag and set it aside.
20 Position the person supine.
21 Perform perineal care (Chapter 22) wearing clean gloves. Clean all areas that had contact with urine. Wash, rinse, and dry the skin fold areas of the groin. Apply the barrier cream or moisturizer.
22 Remove the waterproof under-pad. Place it in the laundry bag.
23 Remove and discard the gloves. Practice hand hygiene. Put on clean gloves.

24 Apply the new brief (Fig. 25-11, p. 330).
  a Unfold the brief. Unfold any side panels.
  b Have the person turn onto the side away from you.
  c Fold the brief length-wise along the center.
  d Insert the brief between the legs from front to back (see Fig. 25-11, A).
  e Unfold and spread the back panel to cover the buttocks (see Fig. 25-11, B).
  f Position the person supine.
  g Unfold and spread the front panel (see Fig. 25-11, C).
  h Check the brief's alignment. The brief is centered in the perineal area and positioned high in the groin areas. The buttocks are covered. The brief fits the shape of the body. For a man, the penis is downward.
  i Over-lap the back side panels over the front side panels.
25 Secure the brief (Fig. 25-12, p. 330).
  a Pull the lower tab forward on the side near you. Attach it at a slightly upward angle. Do the same for the other side.
  b Pull the upper tab forward on the side near you. Attach it horizontally or at a slightly downward angle. Do the same for the other side.
26 Smooth out all wrinkles and folds.
27 Ask about comfort. Ask if the product feels too loose or too tight. Check for wrinkles or creases. Make sure the product does not rub or irritate the groin. Adjust the product as needed.
28 Raise or put on pants or slacks if worn. Or lower the person's gown.
29 Position the person for comfort. Cover the person. Remove the bath blanket. Place it in the laundry bag.
30 Remove and discard the gloves. Practice hand hygiene.

Post-Procedure

31 Provide for comfort. (See the inside of the back cover.)
32 Place the call light and other needed items within reach.
33 Lower the bed to a safe and comfortable level. Follow the care plan.
34 Raise or lower bed rails. Follow the care plan.
35 Empty, clean, rinse, and dry the wash basin. Use clean, dry paper towels for drying. (Wear gloves.)
36 Return the basin and supplies to their proper place.
37 Clean and dry the over-bed table. Dry with paper towels. Discard the paper towels.

38 Remove and discard the gloves. Practice hand hygiene.
39 Follow the care plan and the person's preferences for privacy measures to maintain. Leaving the privacy curtain, window coverings, and door open or closed are examples.
40 Complete a safety check of the room. (See the inside of the back cover.)
41 Follow agency policy for used linens.
42 Practice hand hygiene.
43 Report and record your care and observations.

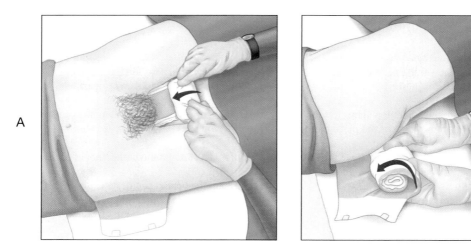

FIGURE 25-10   Removing a used incontinence brief. **A,** Roll the front of the brief toward the back. (NOTE: The far side of the back panel is tucked under the person.) **B,** Turn the person. Continue rolling the used brief from front to back.

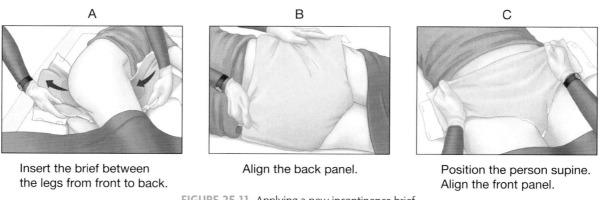

Insert the brief between the legs from front to back.

Align the back panel.

Position the person supine. Align the front panel.

FIGURE 25-11   Applying a new incontinence brief.

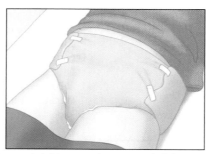

FIGURE 25-12   Securing an incontinence brief. Lower tabs are at a slightly upward angle. Upper tabs are horizontal.

BLADDER TRAINING

Bladder training may help with incontinence. Control of urination is the goal. Bladder control promotes comfort and quality of life. It also increases self-esteem. Successful bladder training may take several weeks.

These methods may be used to help the person gain control of urination.

- *Pelvic floor muscle exercises (Kegel exercises).* The person is taught to contract pelvic muscles as if trying to stop a urine stream. The person contracts the muscles for about 3 to 5 seconds, relaxes, and contracts again. This is done 5 to 10 times. The exercises are done 3 to 4 times daily.
- *Bladder re-training (bladder rehabilitation).* The goal is to increase the time between the urge to void and voiding. The person is taught to:
  - Urinate following a schedule rather than the urge to void.
  - Resist the urge to urinate if it is not yet time to void.
  - Slowly increase the time between voids.

Some methods rely more on staff than the person. Such methods may be helpful for persons with confusion or dementia.

- *Scheduled (timed) voiding.* Voiding is scheduled at regular times to match the person's voiding habits. Staff assist the person to void at scheduled times—every 2 hours during the day is common.
- *Prompted voiding.* The person learns to recognize the need to void and ask for help or void without help. Staff monitor, prompt, and provide positive feedback at regular times based on the person's voiding habits.
  - *Monitoring*—staff ask about the need to void. Staff also may ask if the person feels wet or dry. The person is checked for incontinence and cleaned if needed.
  - *Prompting*—staff ask the person to void. The person is never forced to try to void.
  - *Positive feedback*—staff encourage correct awareness of being wet or dry and normal urination. Staff use positive words. Negative feedback is not given.

For persons preparing to stop the use of a urinary catheter (Chapter 26), the catheter may be clamped (pinched closed). This allows the bladder to fill. The catheter is unclamped (released) at scheduled times to empty the bladder. A bladder training method may be used after catheter removal.

FOCUS ON P R I D E

The Person, Family, and Yourself

P ersonal and Professional Responsibility

Some persons easily talk about urinary elimination. Others are shy or embarrassed. Note the person's verbal and nonverbal communication (Chapter 6). Watch for discomfort with words or topics. Be professional and speak with confidence. This puts the person at ease.

R ights and Respect

Illness and aging affect voiding in private. Respect the right to privacy. Allow as much privacy as safely possible. If you must stay in the room, stand just outside the bathroom door in case the person needs you. Or stand on the other side of the privacy curtain if safe to do so. Follow the nurse's directions and the care plan.

Flush toilets and empty urinals, bedpans, and commodes promptly. The person has the right to a neat and clean setting. Do your best to promote comfort, dignity, and respect when assisting with elimination needs.

I ndependence and Social Interaction

Some persons can meet their own voiding needs. Others need some help but can be left alone to void. For persons needing some help, check on them often. Make sure the call light is within reach. Respond promptly.

D elegation and Teamwork

Accurate reporting and recording are important parts of delegation. See "Observations" on p. 317. Changes in urination may require changes in care. Report urinary problems and abnormal urine to the nurse. If unsure what to report or record, ask the nurse.

E thics and Laws

Negligence occurs when a person does not act in a reasonable and careful manner and the person or the person's property is harmed (Chapter 4). The error is not intentional, but the negligent person is responsible. For example, a patient is left on a bedpan for hours. A pressure injury results.

To prevent mistakes and errors:
- Be careful and focused. Avoid distractions.
- Remind the person to use the call light if you do not return promptly.
- Use reminders. This is important when you are busy. For example, set a timer on your watch or write yourself a note.

Take pride in developing good habits that promote safety and quality of care.

FOCUS ON PRIDE: *Application*

How does incontinence affect the person's dignity? How can it be prevented? Explain how your words and actions promote dignity when a person is incontinent.

REVIEW QUESTIONS

Circle the BEST answer.

1 Which is abnormal?
   a Clear, amber urine
   b Urine with a faint odor
   c Cloudy urine with particles
   d Urine output of 1500 mL in 24 hours

2 Which prevents normal elimination?
   a Helping the person assume a normal position for voiding
   b Providing privacy
   c Helping the person to the bathroom as soon as requested
   d Staying with the person who uses a bedpan

3 Which definition is *correct?*
   a Dysuria means painful or difficult urination.
   b Oliguria means a large amount of urine.
   c Urinary retention means the need to void at once.
   d Urinary incontinence means the inability to void.

4 The person using a standard bedpan is in
   a Fowler's position
   b The supine position
   c The prone position
   d The side-lying position

5 To use a fracture pan
   a The person is in Fowler's position
   b The smaller end (flat end) is under the buttocks
   c The nurse must position the pan
   d The pan can be left in place for a long time

6 After using the urinal, the person should
   a Put it on the bedside stand
   b Use the call light
   c Put it on the over-bed table
   d Empty it

7 After a person uses a commode, you should
   a Empty, rinse, clean, and disinfect the commode
   b Return the commode to the supply area
   c Get a new container
   d Get a new commode

8 Urinary incontinence
   a Cannot be treated
   b Does not have mental or social effects
   c Is a normal part of aging
   d Requires good skin care

9 Which is a cause of functional incontinence?
   a A nervous system disorder
   b Sneezing
   c Unanswered call light
   d UTI

10 A resident with dementia is restless and pulling at the pants. What should you do *first?*
   a Distract the person with an activity.
   b Help the person to the bathroom.
   c Play calming music.
   d Take the person for a walk.

11 When applying an incontinence product
   a Make sure the product is loose in the groin area
   b Remove the old product from back to front
   c Apply the new product from front to back
   d Use the product to turn and position the person

12 The goal of bladder training is to
   a Control the amount voided daily
   b Promote voiding at times best for staff
   c Allow the person to walk to the bathroom
   d Gain control of urination

13 Bladder re-training involves
   a Resisting the urge to void
   b Voiding every time the urge is felt
   c Negative feedback when incontinence occurs
   d Frequent voiding throughout the day and night

14 A person is incontinent. Which statement promotes dignity?
   a "You are doing this on purpose."
   b "Why didn't you ask for help like I told you to?"
   c "I will help you get clean and dry."
   d "This is the last time I am going to clean you today."

Answers to Chapter 25 questions are on p. 588.

FOCUS ON **PRACTICE**

Problem Solving

You assist a patient onto the commode. The person is unsteady and cannot be left alone. The person says: "I can't go if you stand here." What do you do? How will you provide privacy and safe care?

CHAPTER 26

Urinary Catheters

OBJECTIVES

- Define the key terms and key abbreviations in this chapter.
- Explain why urinary catheters are used.
- Describe 3 types of urinary catheters.
- Explain the purpose and rules for catheter care.
- Describe 2 urine drainage systems.
- Explain how to re-connect a catheter and drainage tubing.
- Explain how to apply a condom catheter.
- Perform the procedures described in this chapter.
- Explain how to promote PRIDE in the person, the family, and yourself.

KEY TERMS

catheter A tube used to drain or inject fluid through a body opening
catheterization The process of inserting a catheter
condom catheter A soft sheath that slides over the penis and is used to drain urine

indwelling catheter A catheter left in the bladder so urine drains constantly into a drainage bag; retention or Foley catheter
straight catheter A catheter that drains the bladder and then is removed

KEY ABBREVIATIONS

BM   Bowel movement
CAUTI   Catheter-associated urinary tract infection
ID   Identification

IV   Intravenous
mL   Milliliter
UTI   Urinary tract infection

A *catheter is a tube used to drain or inject fluid through a body opening. A urinary catheter drains urine. Catheterization is the process of inserting a catheter.* With proper training, guidance, and assistance, some states and agencies let nursing assistants insert and remove urinary catheters.

See *Focus on Surveys: Urinary Catheters.*

See *Promoting Safety and Comfort: Urinary Catheters,* p. 334.

FOCUS ON **SURVEYS**

Urinary Catheters

Surveys are done to check the quality of treatments and services. The surveyor may ask you about:
- Your training about handling catheters, catheter tubing, drainage bags, catheter care, urinary tract infections (UTIs), catheter-related injuries, dislodgment (moving out of place), and skin breakdown
- What observations to report, when to report them, and to whom you should report
  Answer questions the best you can. If you do not know an answer, tell the surveyor who you would ask or where you would find the answer.

PROMOTING SAFETY AND COMFORT

Urinary Catheters

Safety

Urinary catheter procedures often involve exposing and touching the perineum. Sexual abuse has occurred in health care settings. The person may feel threatened or is actually being abused. The person needs to be able to call for help. Keep the call light within the person's reach at all times. Always act in a professional manner.

Urine is a body fluid. Follow Standard Precautions for the procedures in this chapter. Follow the Bloodborne Pathogen Standard if blood is present.

NOTE: *A task may require more than 1 pair of gloves. Change gloves as needed. Use careful judgment. Remember to practice hand hygiene after removing gloves.*

CATHETERS

There are different types of catheters.

- A *straight catheter* drains the bladder and then is removed.
- An ***indwelling catheter*** *(retention or Foley catheter) is left in the bladder. Urine drains constantly into a drainage bag.* A balloon by the tip is inflated with sterile water after the catheter is inserted. The balloon prevents the catheter from coming out of the bladder (Fig. 26-1). Tubing connects the catheter to a urine drainage bag. See Figure 26-2 for parts of an indwelling catheter and urine drainage system.
- Used for men, a *condom catheter* is a soft sheath that slides over the penis. This type is not inserted into the bladder. See "Condom Catheters" on p. 340.

Purposes of Catheters

Catheters are used:

- To keep the bladder empty before, during, and after surgery.
- To promote comfort. Some people cannot use the toilet, bedpan, urinal, or commode. For them, catheters can promote comfort and prevent incontinence.
- To protect wounds and pressure injuries from contact with urine.
- For hourly urine output measurements.
- To collect sterile urine specimens.
- To measure the amount of urine in the bladder after the person voids (*residual urine).*

Catheters do not treat the cause of incontinence. They are a last resort for incontinence.

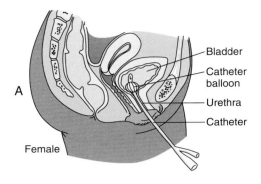
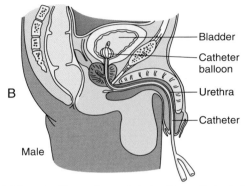

FIGURE 26-1 Indwelling catheter. **A,** Indwelling catheter in the female bladder. The inflated balloon at the tip prevents the catheter from slipping out through the urethra. **B,** Indwelling catheter with the balloon inflated in the male bladder.

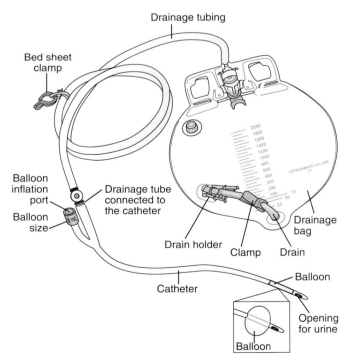

FIGURE 26-2 Parts of an indwelling catheter and urine drainage system.

Catheter-Associated UTIs

The urinary system is sterile. Infection can occur if microbes enter. Catheters create a high risk for UTIs. A *catheter-associated urinary tract infection (CAUTI)* occurs when microbes enter the urinary tract through the catheter and cause an infection. Microbes travel up the catheter into the bladder and kidneys. CAUTIs can cause severe illness and death. Proper catheter care can reduce the risk of a CAUTI.

CATHETER CARE

You will care for persons with indwelling catheters. Follow the rules in Box 26-1 to promote safety and comfort.

See *Delegation Guidelines: Catheter Care*, p. 336.
See *Promoting Safety and Comfort: Catheter Care*, p. 336.
See procedure: *Giving Catheter Care*, p. 337.

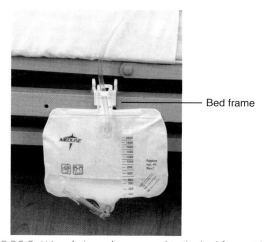

FIGURE 26-3 Urine drainage bag secured to the bed frame. The bag does not touch the floor.

BOX 26-1 Indwelling Catheter Care

Preventing Infection
- Follow the rules of medical asepsis.
- Follow Standard Precautions. Follow the Bloodborne Pathogen Standard if blood is present.
- Encourage fluid intake as directed by the nurse and care plan.

The Drainage System
- Allow urine to flow freely through the catheter and drainage tube. Tubing should not have kinks. The person should not lie on the tubing.
- Keep the catheter connected to the drainage tube. Follow the measures on p. 338 if the catheter and drainage tube are disconnected.
- Keep the drainage tube and bag below the bladder. This prevents urine from flowing backward into the bladder. For a bed or chair transfer, keep the drainage bag lower than the bladder. Secure the drainage bag to the bed frame or chair after the transfer. See Figure 26-3.
- Move the drainage bag to the other side of the bed for turning and re-positioning on the other side.
- Hang the bag from the bed frame, lower part of the chair or wheelchair, or lower part of the IV (intravenous) pole.
- *Do not hang the drainage bag on a bed rail.* The bag is higher than the bladder when the bed rail is raised.
- Position tubing so it will not get tangled in wheelchair wheels.
- Hold the bag lower than the bladder when the person walks.
- Do not let the drainage bag touch or rest on the floor. This can contaminate the system.
- Position drainage tubing in a straight line or coil it on the bed. Secure it to the bottom linens (Fig. 26-4, p. 336). Follow the nurse's directions and agency policy. Use a clip, bed sheet clamp, or other device as the nurse directs. Tubing must not loop below the drainage bag.

The Catheter
- Secure the catheter as the nurse directs.
  - Females: to the thigh (see Fig. 26-4, A).
  - Males:
    - To the thigh (see Fig. 26-4, B).
    - To the lower abdomen. This site may be used for long-term catheter use. The drainage bag remains below the bladder. Drainage is not affected.

The Catheter—cont'd
- Use a tube holder, tape, leg band, or other device to secure the catheter to the thigh or abdomen (Fig. 26-5, p. 336). The nurse tells you what to use. Securing the catheter prevents excess movement and friction at the insertion site (meatus). Catheter movement and friction can damage the meatus.
- Check for leaks. Check the connections to the drainage tube and the drainage bag. Report any leaks at once.
- Provide perineal care and catheter care according to the care plan—daily, twice a day, after bowel movements (BMs), or when vaginal discharge is present. (See procedure: *Giving Catheter Care*, p. 337.)

Measuring Urine (Output)
- Empty the drainage bag and measure urine:
  - At the end of the shift
  - To change to and from a leg bag and a standard drainage bag (p. 338)
  - When the bag is becoming full
  - Before measuring the person's weight (Chapter 31)
- Report an increase or decrease in urine amount.
- Provide a measuring container (graduate) for each person. This prevents the spread of microbes from 1 person to another.
- Do not let the drain on the drainage bag touch any surface.
- See procedure: *Emptying a Urine Drainage Bag*, p. 339.

Observations
- Report complaints at once—pain, burning, the need to void, or irritation. Also report the color, clarity, and odor of urine and the presence of particles or blood.
- Observe for signs and symptoms of a UTI. Report the following at once.
  - Fever.
  - Chills.
  - Flank pain or tenderness. The flank area is in the back between the ribs and the hip.
  - Change in the urine—blood, foul smell, particles, cloudiness, *oliguria* (scant [small] amount of urine).
  - Change in mental or functional status—confusion, decreased appetite, falls, decreased activity, tiredness, and so on.
  - Urine leakage around the catheter.

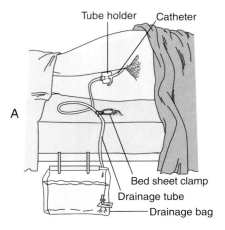

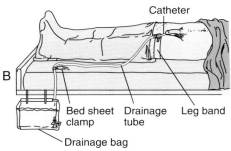

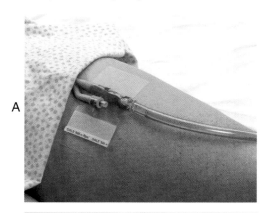

FIGURE 26-4 Securing catheters. **A,** The catheter is secured to the woman's thigh with a tube holder. The drainage tube is coiled on the bed and secured to bottom linens with a bed sheet clamp. **B,** The catheter is secured to the man's thigh with a leg band. Drainage tubing is in a straight line and secured to bottom linens with a bed sheet clamp. The drainage bag is at the foot of the bed.

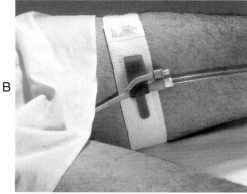

FIGURE 26-5 Catheter securing devices. **A,** Tube holder. **B,** Leg band. (© 2013–2016 Dale Medical Products, Inc. All rights reserved.)

DELEGATION GUIDELINES
Catheter Care

Before performing catheter care, you need this information from the nurse and the care plan.

- When to give catheter care—daily, twice a day, after BMs, or because of vaginal discharge
- What water temperature to use for perineal care
- Where to secure the catheter—which thigh (sites are rotated to prevent skin breakdown) or the lower abdomen (for some males)
- How to secure the catheter—tube holder, leg band, tape, or other device
- How to position the drainage tubing—straight line or coiled on the bed
- Where to secure the drainage tubing and hang the drainage bag—bed, chair, or wheelchair
- How to secure drainage tubing—clip, bed sheet clamp, or other device
- What observations to report and record:
  - Complaints of pain, burning, irritation, or the need to void (report at once)
  - Crusting, abnormal drainage, or secretions
  - The color, clarity, and odor of urine
  - Particles in the urine
  - Blood in the urine (report at once)
  - Cloudy urine
  - Urine leaking at the insertion site
  - Drainage system leaks
- When to report observations
- What patient or resident concerns to report at once

PROMOTING SAFETY AND COMFORT
Catheter Care

Safety
In some agencies, perineal care (Chapter 22) is sufficient hygiene for indwelling catheters. The procedure that follows is not used. Follow agency policy and the care plan when a person has a catheter.

When giving catheter care, clean, rinse, and dry the catheter from the meatus down at least 4 inches. Move in 1 direction (away from the meatus). If needed, repeat with a clean area of the washcloth (towel) or a clean washcloth (towel).

Comfort
The catheter must not pull at the insertion site. This causes discomfort and irritation. Hold the catheter securely during catheter care. Then properly secure the catheter. Make sure the tubing is not under the person. Besides blocking urine flow, lying on the tubing is uncomfortable. It can also cause skin breakdown.

Giving Catheter Care

Quality of Life

- Knock before entering the person's room.
- Address the person by name.
- Introduce yourself by name and title.

- Explain the procedure before starting and during the procedure.
- Protect the person's rights during the procedure.
- Handle the person gently during the procedure.

Pre-Procedure

1 Follow *Delegation Guidelines:*
  a *Perineal Care* (Chapter 22)
  b *Catheter Care*
  See *Promoting Safety and Comfort:*
  a *Perineal Care* (Chapter 22)
  b *Urinary Catheters*, p. 334
  c *Catheter Care*
2 Practice hand hygiene and get the following supplies.
  - Items for perineal care (Chapter 22)
  - At least 2 washcloths and 1 towel for catheter care
  - Bath blanket
  - Towel or paper towels (as a barrier for supplies)
  - Gloves
  - Laundry bag

3 Place the barrier (towel, paper towels) on the over-bed table. Arrange items on top.
4 Practice hand hygiene.
5 Identify the person. Check the identification (ID) bracelet against the assignment sheet. Use 2 identifiers (Chapter 11). Also call the person by name.
6 Fill the wash basin and place it on the over-bed table. Water temperature is about 105°F to 109°F (Fahrenheit) (40.5°C to 42.7°C [centigrade]). Measure water temperature according to agency policy. Have the person check the water temperature and adjust as needed.
7 Provide for privacy.
8 Raise the bed for body mechanics. Bed rails are up if used. Lower the bed rail near you if up.

Procedure

9 Cover the person with a bath blanket. Fan-fold top linens to the foot of the bed.
10 Position and drape the person for perineal care (Chapter 22).
11 Practice hand hygiene. Put on gloves.
12 Place the waterproof under-pad under the buttocks. To do so, have the person raise the buttocks off of the bed. Or turn the person from side to side.
13 Fold back the bath blanket to expose the perineal area.
14 Check the drainage tubing. Make sure it is not kinked and that urine can flow freely.
15 Separate the labia (female). In an uncircumcised male, retract the foreskin (Chapter 22). Check for crusts, abnormal drainage, or secretions.
16 Give perineal care (Chapter 22). Keep the foreskin of the uncircumcised male retracted until step 19.
17 Clean, rinse, and dry the catheter.
  a Apply soap, body wash, or other cleansing agent to a clean, wet washcloth.
  b Hold the catheter at the meatus (Fig. 26-6, p. 338). Do so for all of step 17.
  c Clean the catheter from the meatus down the catheter at least 4 inches. Clean downward, away from the meatus with 1 stroke. See Figure 26-6. Do not tug or pull on the catheter. Repeat as needed with a clean area of the washcloth. Use another clean washcloth if needed.

  d Wet a clean, soap-free washcloth.
  e Rinse from the meatus down the catheter at least 4 inches. Rinse downward, away from the meatus with 1 stroke. Do not tug or pull on the catheter. Repeat as needed with a clean area of the washcloth. Use another clean washcloth if needed.
  f Dry from the meatus down the catheter at least 4 inches. Do not tug or pull on the catheter.
18 Pat dry the perineal area. Dry from front to back (top to bottom).
19 Return the foreskin (uncircumcised male) to its natural position.
20 Secure the catheter. Position the tubing in a straight line or coiled on the bed. Follow the nurse's directions. Secure the tubing to the bottom linens (see Fig. 26-4).
21 Cover the person with the bath blanket. Remove the waterproof under-pad. Place it in the laundry bag.
22 Remove and discard the gloves. Practice hand hygiene.
23 Cover the person. Remove the bath blanket. Place it in the laundry bag.

Post-Procedure

24 Provide for comfort. (See the inside of the back cover.)
25 Place the call light and other needed items within reach.
26 Lower the bed to a safe and comfortable level. Follow the care plan.
27 Raise or lower bed rails. Follow the care plan.
28 Clean, rinse, dry, and return equipment to its proper place. Use clean, dry paper towels for drying. Discard disposable items. (Wear gloves for this step.)
29 Clean and dry the over-bed table. Dry with paper towels. Discard the paper towels.

30 Remove and discard the gloves. Practice hand hygiene.
31 Follow the care plan and the person's preferences for privacy measures to maintain. Leaving the privacy curtain, window coverings, and door open or closed are examples.
32 Complete a safety check of the room. (See the inside of the back cover.)
33 Follow agency policy for used linens.
34 Practice hand hygiene.
35 Report and record your care and observations.

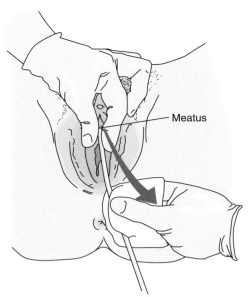

FIGURE 26-6 Cleaning the catheter. Hold the catheter at the meatus. Start at the meatus. Clean downward, away from the meatus. Clean at least 4 inches of the catheter.

URINE DRAINAGE SYSTEMS

A closed drainage system is used for indwelling catheters. Only urine should enter the system. See Box 26-1 to prevent infection and for proper care of the drainage system.

There are 2 types of urine drainage bags.

- *Standard drainage bags* usually hold at least 2000 mL (milliliters) of urine (see Fig. 26-3).
- *Leg bags* attach to the thigh or calf with elastic bands or Velcro (p. 340). Leg bags hold less than 1000 mL of urine.

Drainage systems can become disconnected. If that happens, tell the nurse at once. Do not touch the ends of the catheter or tubing. Box 26-2 describes how to re-connect the catheter and tubing.

A graduate (measuring container for fluid) is used when emptying drainage bags. You will learn how to measure liquids using a graduate in Chapter 30.

See *Delegation Guidelines: Urine Drainage Systems.*

See *Promoting Safety and Comfort: Urine Drainage Systems.*

See procedure: *Emptying a Urine Drainage Bag.*

BOX 26-2 Re-Connecting a Catheter and Drainage Tube

1 Practice hand hygiene. Put on gloves.
2 Wipe the end of the drainage tube with an antiseptic wipe.
3 Wipe the end of the catheter with another antiseptic wipe.
4 Do not put the ends down. Do not touch the ends after you clean them.
5 Connect the drainage tubing to the catheter.
6 Discard the wipes following agency policy.
7 Remove the gloves. Practice hand hygiene.

DELEGATION GUIDELINES
Urine Drainage Systems

Before emptying a urine drainage bag, you need this information from the nurse and the care plan.

- When to empty the urine drainage bag
- If the person uses a leg bag
- What leg bag straps to use—elastic or Velcro
- When to switch a standard drainage bag and leg bag
- If you should clean or discard the drainage bag
- What observations to report and record:
  - The amount of urine measured (Chapter 30)
  - The color, clarity, and odor of urine
  - Particles in the urine
  - Blood in the urine
  - Cloudy urine
  - Complaints of pain, burning, irritation, or the need to void
  - Drainage system leaks
- When to report observations
- What patient or resident concerns to report at once

PROMOTING SAFETY AND COMFORT
Urine Drainage Systems

Safety

Urine drains from the bladder through the catheter and into the drainage bag. Gravity allows urine to drain. *Gravity* is a natural force that pulls things downward. Always keep the drainage bag below bladder level. This allows urine to flow downward from the force of gravity.

Leg bags hold less urine than standard drainage bags. Check leg bags often. Empty the leg bag if it is becoming half full. Measure, report, and record the amount of urine.

Comfort

Urine in a drainage bag embarrasses some people. Visitors can see the urine. To promote mental comfort, have visitors sit on the side away from the drainage bag. Try to empty the bag before visitors arrive. Measure, report, and record the amount of urine.

Some agencies have drainage bag holders. The drainage bag is placed inside the holder. The holder promotes privacy.

Emptying a Urine Drainage Bag

Quality of Life

- Knock before entering the person's room.
- Address the person by name.
- Introduce yourself by name and title.

- Explain the procedure before starting and during the procedure.
- Protect the person's rights during the procedure.
- Handle the person gently during the procedure.

Pre-Procedure

1 Follow *Delegation Guidelines: Urine Drainage Systems.* See *Promoting Safety and Comfort:*
   a *Urinary Catheters,* p. 334
   b *Urine Drainage Systems*
2 Practice hand hygiene and get the following supplies.
   - Graduate (measuring container)
   - Gloves
   - Paper towels or a disposable waterproof pad
   - Antiseptic wipe

3 Arrange items in the person's room.
4 Practice hand hygiene.
5 Identify the person. Check the ID bracelet against the assignment sheet. Use 2 identifiers (Chapter 11). Also call the person by name.
6 Provide for privacy.

Procedure

7 Put on gloves.
8 Place a paper towel or disposable waterproof pad on the floor. Place the graduate on top of it.
9 Place the graduate under the drainage bag.
10 Open the clamp on the drain.
11 Let all urine drain into the graduate. The drain does not touch the graduate (Fig. 26-7).
12 Clean the end of the drain with an antiseptic wipe. Discard the wipe following agency policy.
13 Clamp and position the drain in the holder (Fig. 26-8).

14 Measure urine. See procedure: *Measuring Intake and Output* in Chapter 30.
15 Remove and discard the paper towel or disposable waterproof pad.
16 Empty the graduate into the toilet. Rinse the graduate. Empty the rinse into the toilet and flush.
17 Follow agency procedures to clean and disinfect the graduate.
18 Return the graduate to its proper place.
19 Remove and discard the gloves. Practice hand hygiene.
20 Record the time and amount of urine on the intake and output (I&O) record (Chapter 30).

Post-Procedure

21 Provide for comfort. (See the inside of the back cover.)
22 Place the call light and other needed items within reach.
23 Follow the care plan and the person's preferences for privacy measures to maintain. Leaving the privacy curtain, window coverings, and door open or closed are examples.

24 Complete a safety check of the room. (See the inside of the back cover.)
25 Practice hand hygiene.
26 Report and record your care and observations.

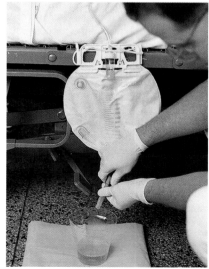

FIGURE 26-7 The clamp on the drainage bag is opened. The drain is directed into the graduate. The drain does not touch the inside of the graduate. (From Potter PA, Perry AG, Stockert PA, Hall AM: *Fundamentals of nursing,* ed 10, St Louis, 2021, Elsevier.)

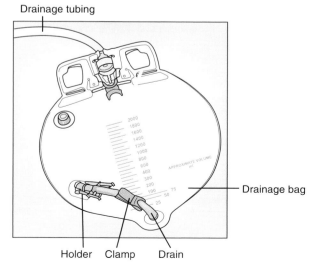

FIGURE 26-8 The clamp is closed and positioned in the holder on the drainage bag.

Condom Catheters

Condom catheters may be used for incontinent men. They also are called *external catheters*, *Texas catheters*, and *urinary sheaths*. A **condom catheter** *is a soft sheath that slides over the penis and is used to drain urine.* Tubing connects the condom catheter to the drainage bag. Many men prefer leg bags (Fig. 26-9).

Condom catheters are changed daily after perineal care. Thoroughly wash and dry the penis before applying the catheter.

Condom catheters come in different sizes and styles. The nurse measures the person for the correct size. The catheter is either self-adhesive or non-adhesive.

- *Self-adhesive catheters* have adhesive inside the catheter. The adhesive secures the catheter to the penis.
- *Non-adhesive catheters* require an adhesive strip or other securing method provided by the manufacturer. *If an adhesive strip is used, do not apply it completely around the penis in a circle. Apply the adhesive strip in a spiral* (see Fig. 26-9). This allows blood flow to the penis. *Do not use other types of tape.* They do not expand. Blood flow to the penis will be cut off, injuring the penis.

Follow the manufacturer's instructions for how to secure the catheter. The procedure that follows is used as a guide.

See *Delegation Guidelines: Condom Catheters.*
See *Promoting Safety and Comfort: Condom Catheters.*
See procedure: *Applying a Condom Catheter.*

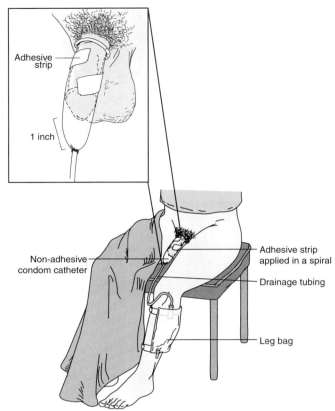

FIGURE 26-9 Condom catheter attached to a leg bag. A 1-inch space is between the penis and the end of the catheter. Elastic tape is applied in a *spiral* to secure a non-adhesive condom catheter to the penis.

DELEGATION GUIDELINES
Condom Catheters

To remove or apply a condom catheter, you need this information from the nurse and the care plan.
- What type of condom catheter to use—self-adhesive or non-adhesive
- What size condom catheter to use
- When to remove the catheter and apply a new one
- If a leg bag or standard drainage bag is used
- What leg bag straps to use—elastic or Velcro
- What water temperature to use for perineal care
- What observations to report and record:
  - Reddened or open areas on the penis
  - Swelling of the penis
  - Color, clarity, and odor of urine
  - Particles in the urine
  - Blood in the urine
  - Cloudy urine
- When to report observations
- What patient or resident concerns to report at once

PROMOTING SAFETY AND COMFORT
Condom Catheters

Safety

Do not apply a condom catheter if the penis is red, irritated, or shows signs of skin breakdown. Report your observations at once.

If you do not know how to use your agency's condom catheters, have the nurse show you the correct application. Then ask the nurse to observe you applying the catheter.

Blood must flow to the penis. If an adhesive strip is needed, use what is packaged with the catheter. Apply it in a spiral.

Comfort

To apply a condom catheter, you need to touch and handle the penis. This can embarrass the person. Explain the procedure. Provide privacy. Keep the person covered as much as possible. Act in a professional manner.

The penis may begin to become erect when touched. Cover the person. Allow time for the penis to return to its relaxed state. Give reassurance that this is a normal response. If needed, allow privacy and say when you will return. Or ask the person to signal for you to finish the procedure. Provide for safety. Place the urinal and call light in reach. Knock before entering the room.

Applying a Condom Catheter

Quality of Life

- Knock before entering the person's room.
- Address the person by name.
- Introduce yourself by name and title.
- Explain the procedure before starting and during the procedure.
- Protect the person's rights during the procedure.
- Handle the person gently during the procedure.

Pre-Procedure

1 Follow *Delegation Guidelines:*
   a *Perineal Care* (Chapter 22)
   b *Condom Catheters*
   See *Promoting Safety and Comfort:*
   a *Perineal Care* (Chapter 22)
   b *Urinary Catheters,* p. 334
   c *Condom Catheters*
2 Practice hand hygiene and get the following supplies.
   - Condom catheter (with adhesive strip if needed)
   - Standard drainage bag or leg bag
   - Cap for the drainage bag
   - Basin of warm water (See step 6 in the procedure: *Giving Catheter Care,* p. 337.)
   - Soap, body wash, or other cleansing agent
   - Towel and washcloths
   - Bath blanket

   - Waterproof under-pad
   - Towel or paper towels (as a barrier for supplies)
   - Gloves
   - Laundry bag
   - Supplies for emptying the drainage bag (See procedure: *Emptying a Urine Drainage Bag,* p. 339.)

3 Place the barrier (towel, paper towels) on the over-bed table. Arrange items on top.
4 Practice hand hygiene.
5 Identify the person. Check the ID bracelet against the assignment sheet. Use 2 identifiers (Chapter 11). Also call the person by name.
6 Provide for privacy.
7 Raise the bed for body mechanics. Bed rails are up if used. Lower the bed rail near you if up.

Procedure

8 Cover the person with a bath blanket. Lower top linens.
9 Position and drape the person for perineal care (Chapter 22).
10 Practice hand hygiene. Put on gloves.
11 Position the waterproof under-pad under the person. Have the person raise the buttocks off of the bed. Or turn the person from side to side.
12 Secure the standard drainage bag to the bed frame. Or have a leg bag ready. Close the drain.
13 Fold back the bath blanket to expose the genital area. Keep the person covered as much as possible.
14 Remove the used condom catheter.
   a *For a catheter with a single-sided adhesive strip (outside)—* remove the adhesive strip.
   b *For a self-adhesive catheter—* if needed, wet a washcloth with warm water. Apply it to the penis for a few minutes. This helps release the adhesive.
   c Roll the sheath off of the penis.
   d *For a catheter with a double-sided adhesive strip (inside)—* remove the adhesive strip after rolling the sheath off of the penis.
15 Disconnect the used drainage tubing from the condom catheter. Cap the drainage tube.
16 Discard the condom catheter and adhesive strip (if used).
17 Provide perineal care (Chapter 22). Be sure the penis is dried well. For an uncircumcised male, the foreskin is returned to its natural position before the new condom catheter is applied.
18 Observe the penis for reddened areas, skin breakdown, and irritation. If present, do not apply a new catheter. Call for the nurse.
19 Remove and discard the gloves. Practice hand hygiene. Put on clean gloves.

20 Apply the new condom catheter. Follow the manufacturer's instructions.
   a Grasp the penis.
   b *For a catheter with a double-sided adhesive strip (inside):*
      1) Remove the paper liner from 1 side of the adhesive strip.
      2) Apply the adhesive strip in a spiral on the penis. Begin just behind the penis head. Do not apply the adhesive strip completely around the penis.
      3) Remove the paper liner from the other side of the adhesive strip.
      4) Roll the condom onto the penis. Follow the manufacturer's instructions for the amount of space to leave between the catheter and the penis tip. A 1-inch space is common.
      5) Gently press the condom to the adhesive strip on the penis.
   c *For a catheter with a single-sided adhesive strip (outside):*
      1) Roll the condom onto the penis. Follow the manufacturer's instructions for the amount of space to leave between the catheter and the penis tip. A 1-inch space is common.
      2) Remove the paper liner from the adhesive strip.
      3) Apply the adhesive strip in a spiral over the condom catheter (see Fig. 26-9). Begin at the penis head. Do not apply the adhesive strip completely around the penis.
   d *For a self-adhesive catheter:*
      1) Roll the condom onto the penis. Follow the manufacturer's instructions for the amount of space to leave between the catheter and the penis tip.
      2) Gently press the condom to the penis. Follow the manufacturer's instructions for the amount of time to hold. About 1 minute is common.

Continued

Applying a Condom Catheter—cont'd

Procedure—cont'd

21 Make sure the penis tip does not touch the condom. Make sure the condom is not twisted.
22 Connect the condom catheter to the new drainage tubing. Secure excess tubing on the bed. Or attach a leg bag.

23 Cover the person with the bath blanket. Remove the waterproof under-pad. Place it in the laundry bag.
24 Remove and discard the gloves. Practice hand hygiene.
25 Cover the person. Remove the bath blanket. Place it in the laundry bag.

Post-Procedure

26 Provide for comfort. (See the inside of the back cover.)
27 Place the call light and other needed items within reach.
28 Lower the bed to a safe and comfortable level. Follow the care plan.
29 Raise or lower bed rails. Follow the care plan.
30 Empty, clean, rinse, and dry the wash basin and other equipment. Use clean, dry paper towels for drying. Return items to their proper place. (Wear gloves.)
31 Clean and dry the over-bed table. Dry with paper towels. Discard the paper towels.
32 Empty the used drainage bag. See procedure: *Emptying a Urine Drainage Bag*, p. 339. Measure and record the urine amount (Chapter 30). Follow agency procedures to clean and store or discard the drainage bag.

33 Remove and discard the gloves. Practice hand hygiene.
34 Follow the care plan and the person's preferences for privacy measures to maintain. Leaving the privacy curtain, window coverings, and door open or closed are examples.
35 Complete a safety check of the room. (See the inside of the back cover.)
36 Follow agency policy for used linens.
37 Practice hand hygiene.
38 Report and record your care and observations.

FOCUS ON P R I D E

The Person, Family, and Yourself

P ersonal and Professional Responsibility

With urinary catheters, the risk of UTIs is high. How you give care can lower the risk of UTI. Do you:
- Prevent urine from flowing back into the bladder when moving the drainage bag?
- Use a clean area of the washcloth for each stroke during catheter care?
- Keep the drain from touching the graduate or other surface?
- Use a clean, separate graduate to empty each person's drainage bag?

R ights and Respect

Respect the right to privacy. Simple actions make a difference. For example, knock before entering a room. Before any procedure, explain how you will provide privacy. This is very important for procedures that involve exposing and touching private areas.

I ndependence and Social Interaction

Urinary catheters are short-term or long-term. Some persons manage their own catheters. The nurse teaches the person to provide catheter care. You:
- Give encouragement. Be kind, patient, and professional.
- Reinforce the nurse's instructions.
- Tell the nurse if the person has questions or if you think more teaching is needed.

D elegation and Teamwork

Tasks become more complex as more care equipment is needed. For example, you need to transfer a person from the chair to bed. The person has a urinary catheter. You must:
- Keep the catheter and drainage tube free of kinks.
- Keep the drainage bag below bladder level.
- Avoid resting the bag on the floor.
- Make sure the person is not lying on the drainage tube.

E thics and Laws

With more training, some states and agencies allow nursing assistants to remove or insert indwelling catheters. Others do not. Follow state and agency rules. Never perform a task outside your role limits.

FOCUS ON PRIDE: Application

How might needing a urinary catheter affect the person mentally? How can you promote mental comfort?

Circle the BEST answer.

1 Urinary catheters are used
   a To prevent urinary tract infections
   b To treat the cause of incontinence
   c To keep the bladder empty for surgery
   d For staff convenience with incontinent persons

2 A person has a catheter. Which is *safe*?
   a Keeping the drainage bag above the bladder level
   b Taping a leak at the connection site
   c Attaching the drainage bag to the bed rail
   d Removing a kink from the drainage tubing

3 A person has a catheter. Which is *correct*?
   a Report pain, burning, or irritation at once.
   b Allow the tubing to hang below the drainage bag.
   c Empty the drainage bag once daily.
   d Use the same graduate for all persons.

4 A person has a catheter. You are going to turn the person from the left to the right side. What should you do with the drainage bag?
   a Move it to the right side.
   b Keep it on the left side.
   c Hang it from an IV pole.
   d Remove it.

5 For a female, the catheter is secured to
   a The abdomen
   b The gown with a safety pin
   c The thigh with a tube holder
   d The bottom linens with tape

6 For catheter care
   a Clean from the drainage tube connection up the catheter at least 4 inches
   b Clean from the meatus down the catheter at least 4 inches
   c Pull on the catheter to make sure it is secure
   d Clamp the catheter to prevent leaking

7 Which statement about drainage systems is *true*?
   a A leg bag holds about 2000 mL.
   b A standard drainage bag holds less than a leg bag.
   c A closed drainage system means the drain cannot be opened.
   d Microbes in the drainage system can cause a UTI.

8 A drainage system becomes disconnected. You need
   a A new drainage bag and paper towels
   b A graduate and a new catheter
   c Gloves and antiseptic wipes
   d A waterproof under-pad and a catheter clamp

9 When emptying a standard drainage bag
   a Do not let the drain touch the graduate
   b Gloves are not needed
   c Clamp the catheter
   d Disconnect the catheter and drainage bag

10 A condom catheter requires an adhesive strip to secure it to the penis. Apply the adhesive strip
   a Completely around the penis
   b To the thigh
   c To the abdomen
   d In a spiral

Answers to Chapter 26 questions are on p. 588.

FOCUS ON **PRACTICE**

Problem Solving

A patient with a urinary catheter tells you: "I feel like I have to pee, and I feel pressure down there." The patient points to the lower abdomen. There is no urine in the drainage bag. Is this normal? What do you do?

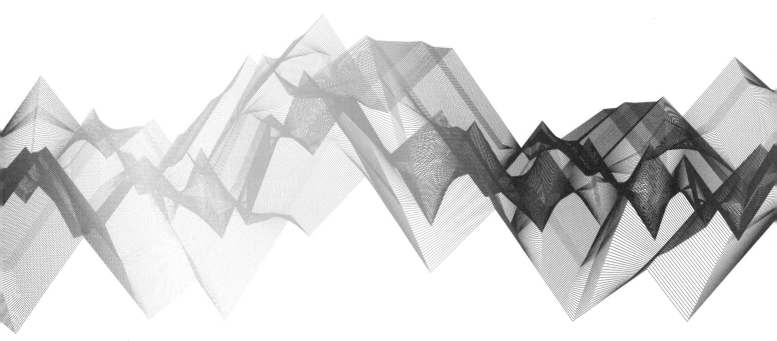

CHAPTER 27

Bowel Needs

Bowel elimination is a basic physical need. Wastes are excreted from the gastro-intestinal (GI) system (Chapter 9). Normal bowel elimination is important.

Problems easily occur. You assist patients and residents to meet bowel needs.

See *Delegation Guidelines: Bowel Needs.*
See *Promoting Safety and Comfort: Bowel Needs.*

Your state and agency may not allow you to perform the procedure and some of the care measures in this chapter. Before performing a procedure, make sure that:

- Your state allows you to perform the procedure.
- The procedure is in your job description.
- You have the necessary education and training.
- You review the procedure with a nurse.
- A nurse is available to answer questions and to guide and assist you as needed.

PROMOTING SAFETY AND COMFORT

Bowel Needs

Safety

Assisting with bowel needs may involve exposing and touching the rectum, a private area. And you may have to give perineal care. Sexual abuse has occurred in health care settings. The person may feel threatened or is actually being abused. The person needs to be able to call for help. Always keep the call light within the person's reach. And always act in a professional manner.

Contact with feces (stools) is likely when assisting with bowel needs. Follow Standard Precautions. Follow the Bloodborne Pathogen Standard if blood is present.

NOTE: *A task may require more than 1 pair of gloves. Change gloves as needed. Use careful judgment. Remember to practice hand hygiene after removing gloves.*

NORMAL BOWEL ELIMINATION

Bowel movements (BMs) vary from person to person. Frequency varies—daily, 2 to 3 times a day, every 2 to 3 days. Time of day also varies.

To assist with bowel elimination, you need to know these terms.

- *Defecation* (bowel movement) *is the process of excreting feces from the rectum through the anus.*
- *Feces* (stool or stools) *refers to the semi-solid mass of waste products in the colon that is expelled through the anus.*
- *Stool* (stools) *refers to excreted feces.*
   See *Focus on Communication: Normal Bowel Elimination.*

FOCUS ON COMMUNICATION

Normal Bowel Elimination

The term *bowel movement* and the abbreviation *BM* are commonly used. For some people, *poop* is a common word. For others, it is embarrassing. In this chapter, *stool* or *stools* refers to excreted feces. The word *feces* may be less familiar to patients and residents. Use a term the person understands and uses. Be professional.

Observations

Carefully observe stools. Ask the nurse to observe abnormal stools. Report and record the following.

- Color (Fig. 27-1)—normally brown. Beets, tomato juice or soup, red Jell-O, and foods with red food coloring can cause red-colored stools. Green vegetables can cause green stools. Diseases and infection can cause clay-colored or white, pale, orange-colored, or green-colored stools. Some drugs can cause dark stools.
- Amount—small, medium, large. Liquid (watery) stools are measured in milliliters (mL). See "Intake and Output" in Chapter 30.
- Presence of mucus—usually none. Disease and infection can cause stools with mucus.
- Signs of bleeding—bleeding in the stomach and small intestine causes *black, tarry stools* (**melena**). Bleeding in the lower colon and rectum causes red-colored stools.
- Odor—usually a normal odor caused by bacteria in the intestines. Certain foods and drugs can cause odors.
- Shape and consistency (Fig. 27-2, p. 346)—normally soft, formed, moist, and shaped like the rectum.
- The time the person had a BM.
- Number and frequency of BMs.
- Complaints of pain or discomfort.
   See *Focus on Communication: Observations*, p. 346.

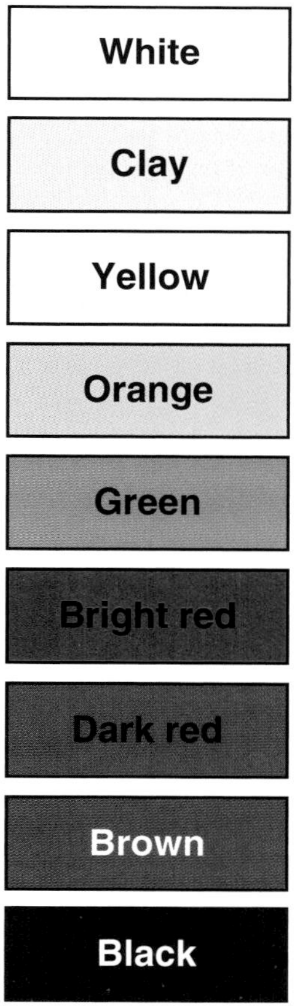

White

Clay

Yellow

Orange

Green

Bright red

Dark red

Brown

Black

FIGURE 27-1 Color chart for stools.

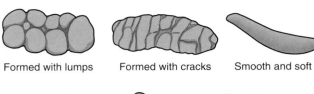

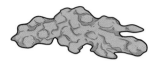

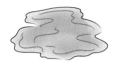

Formed with lumps Formed with cracks Smooth and soft

Small hard lumps Small soft lumps

Loose and unformed Watery

FIGURE 27-2 Stool shapes and consistencies.

FOCUS ON **COMMUNICATION**

Observations

Many patients and residents tend to their own bowel needs. Information is needed for the person's record and the nursing process. To ask about BMs, you can say:

- "Did you have a BM today?"
- "Please tell me about your BM."
- "When did you have a BM?"
- "What was the amount?"
- "Were the stools soft or hard?"
- "Were the stools formed or loose?"
- "What was the color?"
- "Did you have bleeding, pain, or problems having a BM?"
- "Did you pass any gas?"
- "Do you need to pass more gas?"
- "Do you need help cleaning yourself?"

FACTORS AFFECTING BMs

These factors affect BM frequency, consistency, color, and odor. Normal, regular elimination is a goal of the nursing process.

- *Privacy.* Lack of privacy can prevent a BM despite the urge. Odors and sounds are embarrassing. Some people ignore the urge when people are present.
- *Habits.* After breakfast is a common time for a BM. Being relaxed, not tense, is helpful. To relax, some people drink a hot beverage, read, or take a walk.
- *Diet—high-fiber foods.* High-fiber foods leave a residue, creating bulk to prevent constipation. Fruits, vegetables, and whole-grain cereals and breads are high in fiber. Intake of such foods may be poor. Digestion problems and chewing difficulties (loss of teeth, poorly fitting dentures) are causes. Bran may be added to cereal, prunes, or prune juice.

- *Diet—other foods.* Milk and milk products may cause constipation or diarrhea. Chocolate and other foods cause similar reactions. Spicy foods can irritate the intestines, causing frequent BMs or diarrhea. Gas-forming foods stimulate *peristalsis*—the alternating contraction and relaxation of intestinal muscles that move feces through the intestines. Such foods include onions, beans, cabbage, cauliflower, radishes, and cucumbers.
- *Fluids.* Feces contain water. Stool consistency depends on how much water is absorbed by the colon. Feces harden and dry when large amounts of water are absorbed or from poor fluid intake or vomiting. Hard, dry feces move slowly through the colon, leading to constipation. Drinking 6 to 8 glasses of water daily promotes normal BMs. Warm fluids—coffee, tea, hot cider, warm water—increase peristalsis.
- *Activity.* Exercise and activity maintain muscle tone and stimulate peristalsis. Constipation may result from inactivity or bed rest.
- *Drugs.* Drugs can cause or prevent constipation or diarrhea. Other drugs have diarrhea or constipation as side effects.
- *Disability.* Some people have a BM whenever feces enter the rectum. They have no control. A bowel training program is needed (p. 348).
- *Aging.* Age affects bowel elimination. See *Focus on Older Persons: Factors Affecting BMs.*

FOCUS ON **OLDER PERSONS**

Factors Affecting BMs

Aging causes GI changes. Feces pass through the intestines more slowly. Constipation is a risk. Some older persons lose bowel control.

Many older persons are very concerned if they do not have a BM every day. The nurse instructs about normal elimination.

Safety and Comfort

The care plan has measures to meet bowel needs. It may involve diet, fluids, and exercise. The measures in Box 27-1 promote safety and comfort.

See *Focus on Communication: Safety and Comfort.*

FOCUS ON **COMMUNICATION**

Safety and Comfort

Odors and sounds are common with BMs. Control your verbal and nonverbal responses. Be professional. Do not laugh at or make fun of a person. Your words and actions must promote comfort, dignity, and self-esteem.

BOX 27-1 Safety and Comfort for Bowel Needs

- Assist the person promptly. BM needs may be urgent.
- Practice medical asepsis.
- Follow Standard Precautions. Follow the Bloodborne Pathogen Standard if blood is present.
- Provide for privacy.
  - Ask visitors to leave the room.
  - Close doors, privacy curtains, and window coverings.
- Help the person to the toilet or commode. Or provide the bedpan.
- Wheel the person into the bathroom on the commode if possible. This provides privacy. Remove the container and position the commode over the toilet. Then lock (brake) the commode wheels.
- Warm the bedpan (if used). This is important if the bedpan is metal.
- Position the person in a sitting or squatting position.
- Cover the person for warmth and privacy.
- Allow enough time for a BM.
- Place the call light and toilet paper within reach.
- Leave the room if the person can be alone. Check on the person at least every 5 minutes.
- Stay nearby if the person is weak or unsteady.
- Be sure the person is wiped and cleaned well. Provide perineal care as needed.
- Flush stools promptly. This reduces odors and prevents the spread of microbes.
- Assist the person with hand hygiene after elimination.
- Follow the care plan for fecal incontinence.

COMMON PROBLEMS

Common problems include constipation, fecal impaction, diarrhea, fecal incontinence, and flatulence.

Constipation

When feces move slowly through the bowel, more water is absorbed. Constipation can occur. *Constipation is the passage of a hard, dry stool.* The person strains to have a BM. Stools are large or marble-sized. Large stools cause pain as they pass through the anus.

Common causes of constipation include:
- A low-fiber diet
- Ignoring the urge to have a BM
- Decreased fluid intake
- Inactivity
- Drugs
- Aging
- Certain diseases

Diet changes, fluids, and activity prevent or relieve constipation. The doctor may order 1 or more of the following.
- Stool softeners—drugs that soften feces
- Laxatives—drugs that promote bowel elimination
- Suppositories (p. 348)
- Enemas (p. 349)

Fecal Impaction

A *fecal impaction is the prolonged retention and buildup of feces in the rectum.* Feces are hard or putty-like. Fecal impaction results from un-relieved constipation. The person cannot have a BM. More water is absorbed from the already hard feces. Liquid feces pass around the hardened fecal mass in the rectum and seep from the anus.

Signs and symptoms of fecal impaction include:
- Trying many times to have a BM
- Abdominal discomfort
- Abdominal distention (swelling)
- Nausea
- Cramping
- Rectal pain
- Poor appetite (especially older persons)
- Confusion (especially older persons)
- Fever (especially older persons)

Fecal impaction is a serious problem. It must be prevented. Follow agency policy for recording BMs. Report large stools or difficulty passing stools. Also tell the nurse if the person is concerned about constipation.

Diarrhea

Diarrhea is the frequent passage of liquid stools. Feces move through the intestines rapidly. This reduces the time for fluid absorption. The need for a BM is urgent. Some people cannot get to a bathroom in time. Abdominal cramping, nausea, and vomiting may occur.

Causes of diarrhea include infections, some drugs, irritating foods, and microbes in food and water. Diet and drugs are ordered to reduce peristalsis. You need to:
- Assist with elimination needs promptly.
- Dispose of stools promptly. This prevents odors and the spread of microbes.
- Give good skin care. Liquid stools irritate the skin. So does frequent wiping with toilet paper. Skin breakdown and pressure injuries are risks.

Dehydration is a risk from fluid loss. *Dehydration is a decrease in the amount of water in the body.* See Chapter 30.

Microbes can cause diarrhea. Preventing their spread is important. Always follow Standard Precautions when in contact with stools.

See *Focus on Older Persons: Diarrhea.*
See *Promoting Safety and Comfort: Diarrhea*, p. 348.

FOCUS ON **OLDER PERSONS**

Diarrhea

Older persons are at risk for dehydration. The amount of body water decreases with aging. Many diseases affect body fluids. So do many drugs. Report signs of diarrhea at once. Ask the nurse to observe the stool. Death is a risk when dehydration is not recognized and treated.

PROMOTING SAFETY AND COMFORT

Diarrhea

Safety

The need for a BM is urgent when the person has diarrhea. Answer call lights promptly. Some people cannot get to a bathroom in time. Soiling results. Assist the person with hygiene needs and garment changes as needed. Be patient and kind. The person cannot control BMs.

Clostridioides difficile (Clostridium difficile [C. difficile]) is a microbe that causes diarrhea and intestinal infections. Commonly called *C. diff*, it can cause death. Persons at risk are older, are ill, or have prolonged use of antibiotics. Older persons in hospitals and nursing centers are at high risk. Signs and symptoms include:

- Watery diarrhea
- Fever
- Loss of appetite
- Nausea
- Abdominal pain or tenderness

The microbe is found in feces. A person becomes infected by touching items or surfaces contaminated with expelled feces and when touching the mouth or mucous membranes. *C. diff* can be found on bed linens, bed rails, toilets, bathroom fixtures, sinks, care supplies and equipment, walker handles, cart handles, bedside and over-bed tables, phones, TV remotes, personal electronics (computers, tablets, music players), and so on. You can spread the microbe if your contaminated hands or gloves:

- Touch a person
- Contaminate surfaces

Standard Precautions and Contact Precautions are required (Chapter 15). Wear a gown and gloves when entering the person's room and giving care. Practice good hand-washing. Alcohol-based hand sanitizers are not as effective against *C. difficile* as soap and water. Care items and surfaces are disinfected with a bleach solution.

Fecal Incontinence

Fecal incontinence is the inability to control the passage of feces and flatus through the anus. Causes include:

- Intestinal diseases.
- Nervous system diseases and injuries.
- Fecal impaction or diarrhea.
- Some drugs.
- Chronic illness.
- Aging.
- Mental health disorders or dementia (Chapters 41 and 42). The person may not recognize needing to or having a BM.
- Unanswered call lights.
- Not getting to the bathroom in time. The person may have mobility problems or may walk slowly. The bathroom may be too far away or in use.
- Problems removing clothes.
- Not finding the bathroom in a new setting.

Fecal incontinence has emotional effects. Frustration, embarrassment, anger, and humiliation are common. The person may need:

- Bowel training
- Help with elimination after meals and every 2 to 3 hours
- Incontinence products (Chapter 25) to keep garments and linens clean
- Good skin care
  See *Focus on Older Persons: Fecal Incontinence.*

FOCUS ON OLDER PERSONS

Fecal Incontinence

Persons with dementia may smear stools on themselves, furniture, and walls. Some are not aware of having BMs. Some resist care. Follow the care plan. The measures for urinary incontinence (Chapter 25) may be part of the care plan for fecal incontinence. Be patient. Ask for help from co-workers. Talk to the nurse if you have problems keeping the person clean.

Flatulence

Gas and air are normally in the stomach and intestines. They are expelled through the mouth (burping, belching, eructating) and anus. *Gas or air passed through the anus is called **flatus**. **Flatulence** is the excessive formation of gas or air in the stomach and intestines.* Causes include:

- Swallowing air while eating and drinking
- Bacterial action in the intestines
- Gas-forming foods (p. 346)
- Constipation
- Certain digestive disorders
- Bowel and abdominal surgeries
- Drugs that decrease peristalsis

If flatus is not expelled, the intestines swell or enlarge *(distend)* from the pressure of gases. Abdominal cramping or pain, shortness of breath, and a swollen abdomen *(bloating)* occur. Exercise, walking, moving in bed, and the left side-lying position help to expel flatus. Enemas and drugs may be ordered to relieve flatulence.

BOWEL TRAINING

Bowel training has 2 goals.

- To gain control of BMs.
- To develop a regular pattern of elimination. Fecal impaction, constipation, and fecal incontinence are prevented.

Meals, especially breakfast, stimulate peristalsis and the urge for a BM. The person's usual time for a BM is noted on the care plan. So is toilet, commode, or bedpan use. The care plan includes a high-fiber diet, increased fluids, warm fluids, activity, and privacy. Follow the person's care plan for bowel training.

The doctor may order a suppository to stimulate a BM. A *suppository is a cone-shaped, solid drug that is inserted into a body opening. It melts at body temperature.* A nurse inserts a rectal suppository into the rectum (Fig. 27-3). A BM occurs about 30 minutes later.

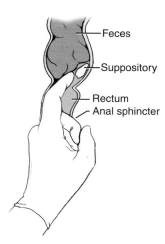

FIGURE 27-3   The suppository is inserted along the rectal wall. (Modified from Williams P: *deWit's fundamental concepts and skills for nursing*, ed 6, St Louis, 2022, Elsevier.)

ENEMAS

An *enema is the introduction of fluid into the rectum and lower colon.* Enemas are ordered to:

- Remove feces.
- Relieve constipation, fecal impaction, or flatulence.
- Clean the bowel of feces before certain surgeries and diagnostic procedures.

Safety and comfort measures for bowel needs are practiced when giving enemas (see Box 27-1).

The enema ordered depends on the purpose—cleansing, constipation, fecal impaction, or flatulence.

- *Tap water enema*—is obtained from a faucet.
- *Saline enema*—a solution of salt and water. For adults, 1 or 2 teaspoons of table salt are added to 500 to 1000 mL (milliliters) of tap water.
- *Soapsuds enema (SSE)*—for adults, 3 to 5 mL of castile soap is added to 500 to 1000 mL of tap water.
- *Small-volume enema*—the enema solution is in a bottle and ready to give.
- *Oil-retention enema*—contains oil to soften feces and lubricate the rectum. Most are ready-to-use.

See *Promoting Safety and Comfort: Enemas.*

PROMOTING SAFETY AND COMFORT

Enemas

Safety

Enemas are usually safe procedures. Many people give themselves enemas at home. However, enemas are dangerous for older persons and those with certain heart and kidney diseases.

Comfort

The nurse may ask you to assist with enemas. Or you may be asked to give a small-volume enema. Before an enema, make sure that the bathroom is ready for use. Or have the bedpan or commode ready. Always keep a bedpan nearby in case the enema solution and stools are expelled. You promote mental comfort when the person knows the bathroom, commode, or bedpan is ready.

The person should retain the solution for as long as possible. Provide for a comfortable left semi-prone or left side-lying position. When comfortable, it is easier to tolerate the procedure.

The Cleansing Enema

Cleansing enemas clean the bowel of feces and flatus. They relieve constipation and fecal impaction. They are given before certain surgeries and diagnostic procedures.

A tap water, saline, or soapsuds enema is ordered. An *enemas until clear* order means that enemas are given until the return solution is clear and free of stools. Agency policy may allow repeating enemas 2 or 3 times. You may be asked to assist the nurse with cleansing enemas.

The Small-Volume Enema

Small-volume enemas irritate and distend the rectum to cause a BM. They are ordered for constipation or when the bowel does not need complete cleansing.

The solution is usually given at room temperature. To give the enema, insert the lubricated tip 2 inches into the rectum for an adult. Gently squeeze and roll up the plastic container from the bottom. Do not release pressure on the bottle. Otherwise, solution is drawn from the rectum back into the bottle. Follow the rules for giving a small-volume enema in Box 27-2.

See *Delegation Guidelines: The Small-Volume Enema.*
See procedure: *Giving a Small-Volume Enema*, p. 350.

BOX 27-2   Giving a Small-Volume Enema

- Have the person void first. This increases comfort during the procedure.
- Position the person as the nurse directs. The left semi-prone or left side-lying position is preferred.
- Stop insertion if there is resistance, the person complains of pain, or bleeding occurs.
- Have the person retain the solution until there is an urge to have a BM. This usually takes 1 to 5 minutes or as long as 10 minutes.
- Keep the person in the left semi-prone or left side-lying position to help retain the enema. Cover the person for warmth.
- Make sure the bathroom will be vacant when the person needs to have a BM. Make sure that another person will not use the bathroom. If the person uses the bedpan or commode, have the device ready.
- Ask the nurse to observe the enema results.

DELEGATION GUIDELINES

The Small-Volume Enema

If giving an enema to an adult is delegated to you, make sure the conditions in *Delegation Guidelines: Bowel Needs* (p. 345) are met. If those conditions are met, you need this information from the nurse.

- When to give the enema
- What position to use—left semi-prone or left side-lying position
- How far to insert the enema tip—usually 2 inches for adults
- How long the person should try to retain the solution
- What observations to report and record:
  - The amount of solution given
  - Bleeding or resistance when inserting the enema tip
  - How long the person retained the enema solution
  - Color, amount, consistency, shape, and odor of stools
  - Complaints of cramping, pain, or discomfort
  - Complaints of nausea or weakness
  - How the person tolerated the procedure
- When to report observations
- What patient or resident concerns to report at once

Giving a Small-Volume Enema

Quality of Life

- Knock before entering the person's room.
- Address the person by name.
- Introduce yourself by name and title.

- Explain the procedure before starting and during the procedure.
- Protect the person's rights during the procedure.
- Handle the person gently during the procedure.

Pre-Procedure

1 Follow *Delegation Guidelines:*
  a *Bowel Needs,* p. 345
  b *The Small-Volume Enema,* p. 349
  See *Promoting Safety and Comfort:*
  a *Bowel Needs,* p. 345
  b *Enemas,* p. 349
2 Practice hand hygiene and get the following supplies.
  - Small-volume enema
  - Commode or bedpan (and disposable waterproof pad)
  - Toilet paper
  - Slip-resistant footwear (if needed)
  - Robe (if needed)

  - Bath blanket
  - Waterproof under-pad
  - Gloves
  - Laundry bag
3 Arrange items in the person's room.
4 Practice hand hygiene.
5 Identify the person. Check the identification (ID) bracelet against the assignment sheet. Use 2 identifiers (Chapter 11). Also call the person by name.
6 Provide for privacy.
7 Raise the bed for body mechanics. Bed rails are up if used. Lower the bed rail near you if up.

Procedure

8 Cover the person with a bath blanket. Fan-fold top linens to the foot of the bed.
9 Practice hand hygiene. Put on gloves.
10 Place the waterproof under-pad under the buttocks.
11 Position the person in the left semi-prone or left side-lying position.
12 Have the bedpan nearby. Use the disposable waterproof pad as a barrier.
13 Expose the anal area.
14 Remove the cap from the enema tip.
15 Separate the buttocks to see the anus.
16 Ask the person to take a deep breath through the mouth.
17 Insert the enema tip 2 inches into the adult's rectum (Fig. 27-4). Do this as the person exhales. Insert the tip gently. Stop if the person complains of pain, you feel resistance, or bleeding occurs.
18 Squeeze and roll up the container gently. Release pressure on the bottle after you remove the tip from the rectum.
19 Put the container into the box, tip first. Discard the container and box.
20 Remove and discard the gloves. Practice hand hygiene.
21 Have the person maintain the left semi-prone or left side-lying position. Be sure the person is comfortable. Cover the person with the bath blanket.
22 Assist the person to the bathroom or commode when the person has the urge to have a BM. Or help the person onto the bedpan and raise the head of the bed.

23 Follow these privacy and safety measures.
  - Be sure the person's clothing properly covers the person or apply a robe when up.
  - Apply slip-resistant footwear if the person will stand.
  - Be sure the bed is at a low level that is safe and comfortable.
  - Raise or lower bed rails according to the care plan.
  - Wear gloves as needed. Practice hand hygiene after removing and discarding gloves.
24 Place the call light and toilet paper within reach. Remind the person not to flush the toilet if used.
25 Stay with the person as needed. Or leave the room and close the door. (Practice hand hygiene before leaving.) Be respectful. Provide as much privacy as possible.
26 Return when the person signals. Or check on the person every 5 minutes. Knock before entering.
27 Practice hand hygiene. Put on gloves.
28 Assist with wiping and perineal care (Chapter 22) as needed. Remove and discard the gloves. Practice hand hygiene. Put on clean gloves.
29 Cover or transfer the person as needed. Remove the waterproof under-pad and bath blanket. Put them in the laundry bag.
30 Observe enema results for amount, color, consistency, shape, and odor. Call the nurse to observe the results.
31 Empty and rinse equipment into the toilet as needed. (Wait for the nurse to observe the results before flushing.)
32 Follow agency procedures to clean and disinfect equipment. Return equipment to its proper place.
33 Remove and discard the gloves. Practice hand hygiene. Put on clean gloves.
34 Assist with hand hygiene. Remove and discard the gloves. Practice hand hygiene.

Post-Procedure

35 Provide for comfort. (See the inside of the back cover.)
36 Place the call light and other needed items within reach.
37 Lower the bed to a safe and comfortable level. Follow the care plan.
38 Raise or lower bed rails. Follow the care plan.
39 Follow the care plan and the person's preferences for privacy measures to maintain. Leaving the privacy curtain, window coverings, and door open or closed are examples.

40 Complete a safety check of the room. (See the inside of the back cover.)
41 Follow agency policy for used linens and used supplies.
42 Practice hand hygiene.
43 Report and record your care and observations.

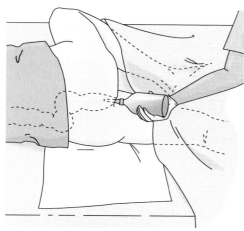

FIGURE 27-4 The small-volume enema tip is inserted 2 inches into the rectum.

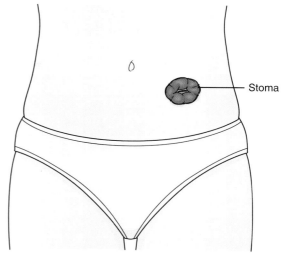

FIGURE 27-5 A stoma on the surface of the body.

The Oil-Retention Enema

Oil-retention enemas relieve constipation and fecal impaction. The oil softens feces and lubricates the rectum so feces pass with ease. Depending on the type, the oil-retention enema may act quickly. For others, the oil is retained for 30 minutes to 1 to 3 hours. Most oil-retention enemas are ready-to-use.

Giving an oil-retention enema is like giving a small-volume enema. After an oil-retention enema is given:

- Leave the person in the left semi-prone or left side-lying position. Cover the person for warmth.
- Instruct the person to retain the enema until the urge to have a BM is felt.
- Place extra waterproof under-pads on the bed if needed.
- Check the person often.
  See *Promoting Safety and Comfort: The Oil-Retention Enema.*

PROMOTING SAFETY AND COMFORT

The Oil-Retention Enema

Safety

An oil-retention enema may be retained for at least 30 minutes. Leave the room after giving the enema. Check on the person often. Say when you will return. Remind the person to signal if help is needed. Report any problems at once.

THE PERSON WITH AN OSTOMY

Sometimes part of the intestines is removed surgically. Cancer, bowel disease, and trauma (stab or bullet wounds) are common reasons. An ostomy is sometimes necessary. An *ostomy is a surgically created opening that connects an internal organ to the body's surface. The surgically created opening seen on the body's surface is called a* **stoma** (Fig. 27-5). An ostomy pouch is worn over the stoma to collect stools and flatus.

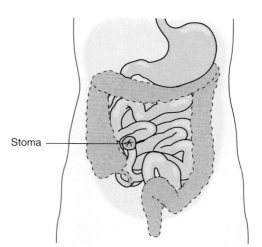

FIGURE 27-6 An ileostomy. The entire large intestine is removed. *Shading* shows the part of the bowel surgically removed.

Ileostomy

An *ileostomy is a surgically created opening* (stomy) *between the ileum (small intestine* [ileo]*) and the body's surface.* Part of the ileum is brought out onto the body's surface and a stoma is made. The entire colon is removed (Fig. 27-6).

Liquid stools drain constantly from an ileostomy. Water is not absorbed because the colon was removed. Feces in the small intestine contain digestive juices that are very irritating to the skin. The ostomy pouch must fit well. Stools must not touch the skin. Good skin care is required.

Colostomy

A *colostomy is a surgically created opening* (stomy) *between the colon* (colo) *and the body's surface.* Part of the colon is brought out onto the body's surface and a stoma is made. Feces and flatus pass through the stoma instead of the anus.

With a permanent colostomy, the diseased part of the colon is removed. A temporary colostomy gives the diseased or injured bowel time to heal. After healing, the bowel is surgically re-connected.

The colostomy site depends on the site of disease or injury (Fig. 27-7). Stool consistency—liquid to formed—depends on the colostomy site. The more colon remaining to absorb water, the more solid and formed the stool. If the colostomy is near the end of the colon, stools are formed.

Stools irritate the skin. Skin care prevents skin breakdown around the stoma. The skin is washed and dried. A skin barrier applied around the stoma prevents stools from having contact with the skin. The skin barrier is part of the pouch or a separate device.

Ostomy Pouches

A plastic ostomy pouch with an adhesive back is applied to the skin. Some pouches are secured to ostomy belts. See Figure 27-8. The pouch bulges when stools or flatus pass into it. An outlet (drain) is opened to empty the pouch of stools or to release flatus.

The pouch is changed every 2 to 7 days and when it leaks. Frequent pouch changes can damage the skin. Pouches are not flushed down the toilet.

Odors are prevented by:
* Using odor-free pouches.
* Performing good hygiene.
* Emptying the pouch.
* Avoiding gas-forming foods.
* Putting deodorants into the pouch.

The person wears normal clothes. Tight garments can prevent feces from entering the pouch. Also, bulging from stools and flatus can be seen with tight clothes.

Peristalsis decreases during sleep and increases after eating and drinking. After sleep, the stoma is less likely to expel feces. If the person showers or bathes with the pouch off, it is best done before breakfast. Showers and baths are delayed for 1 to 2 hours after a new pouch is applied. This gives adhesive time to seal to the skin.

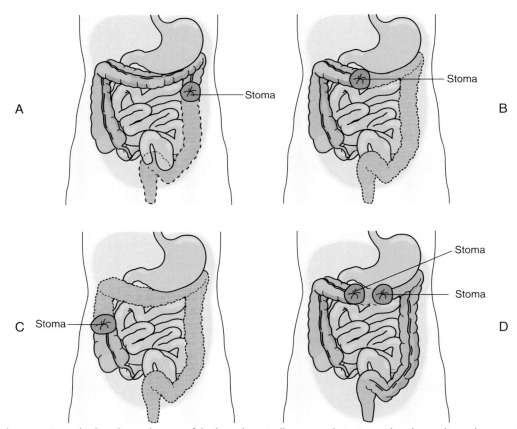

FIGURE 27-7 Colostomy sites. *Shading* shows the part of the bowel surgically removed. **A,** Sigmoid or descending colostomy. **B,** Transverse colostomy. **C,** Ascending colostomy. **D,** Double-barrel colostomy has 2 stomas. One allows for the excretion of feces. The other is for drugs to help the bowel heal. This type is usually temporary.

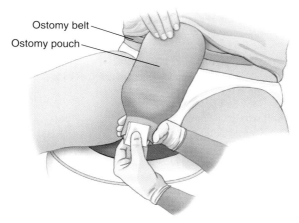

Ostomy belt
Ostomy pouch

FIGURE 27-8 An ostomy pouch secured to an ostomy belt. The pouch is emptied by directing it into the toilet and opening the outlet. The outlet is cleaned before it is closed.

Emptying Ostomy Pouches. An ostomy pouch is emptied when it is about one-third (⅓) to one-half (½) full with stools or flatus. Depending on the person, ostomy type, and ostomy location, pouches are usually emptied 2 to 6 times a day. Because ileostomies constantly drain liquid feces, ileostomy pouches are emptied more often than colostomy pouches.

Pouches are emptied into the toilet (see Fig. 27-8) or a bedpan. Before emptying, toilet paper is placed in the toilet to prevent splashing. The outlet is wiped with toilet paper or a pre-moistened wipe after emptying (see Fig. 27-8). The pouch is closed with a clip, clamp, or other closure (Fig. 27-9).

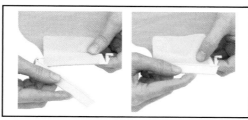

FIGURE 27-9 A clamp is used to close the ostomy pouch. (Courtesy Hollister Incorporated, Libertyville, Ill.)

FOCUS ON P R I D E

The Person, Family, and Yourself

P ersonal and Professional Responsibility

Skin care needs after bowel elimination vary. Some persons are independent. Others require help with wiping and hand hygiene. If the person is soiled, provide perineal care. For persons with diarrhea or fecal incontinence, more frequent care is needed.

Follow the person's care plan. Give care as often as needed with a helpful attitude. Allow as much independence as possible.

R ights and Respect

Bowel needs require privacy. Some persons are embarrassed to have a BM in a strange setting. To promote comfort and privacy:
- Ask others to leave the room.
- Close doors, privacy curtains, and window coverings.
- Turn on water or music to mask sounds.
- Cover the person.
- Allow enough time. Place the call light nearby. Ask the person to call if help is needed.
- Knock before entering the room. Tell the person who you are. Ask if you can enter before opening the door completely.
- Use an agency-approved spray for odors.

I ndependence and Social Interaction

Some persons have had ostomies for a long time. They may have special routines or care measures. When you assist, ask what they prefer. To promote independence, allow personal choice and control as much as safely possible.

D elegation and Teamwork

The nurse may delegate a task that you have not done before. Giving an enema is an example. Never attempt a task that you are not comfortable doing. Make sure your state and agency allow you to perform the procedure. If those conditions are met, you can politely say: "I'm sorry, but I have not done that task before. I am not comfortable doing it on my own. Would you please show me how it is done?"

Guidance and assistance are part of the nurse's role in delegation. The nurse needs to know your comfort level with tasks. Never be ashamed to ask for guidance and assistance.

E thics and Laws

All persons must be protected from abuse, mistreatment, and neglect. Examples include:
- Leaving a person sitting or lying in urine or stools
- Leaving a person on a toilet, commode, or bedpan for a long time
- Telling a person to void or have a BM in bed

Federal and state laws require the reporting and investigating of abuse, mistreatment, and neglect. Protect the person and yourself. Check patients or residents often. Be careful and focused. Always treat the person with dignity.

FOCUS ON PRIDE: *Application*

You are asked to do an unfamiliar task. Do you seek help? Do you try to do it alone? Does asking for help bother you?

Circle the BEST answer.

1 Which is *true*?
   a A person must have a BM every day.
   b Stools are normally brown, soft, and formed.
   c Diarrhea occurs when feces move slowly through the bowel.
   d Constipation occurs when feces move quickly through the bowel.

2 Which should you ask the nurse to observe?
   a A black and tarry stool
   b The person's first BM of the day
   c Stool with an odor
   d A formed stool

3 A person is worried about constipation. You should
   a Decrease the person's fluid intake
   b Help the person to the bathroom every hour
   c Tell the person not to worry
   d Report the concern to the nurse

4 The prolonged retention and buildup of feces in the rectum is called
   a Constipation
   b Fecal impaction
   c Diarrhea
   d Fecal incontinence

5 These measures promote normal BMs. Which is outside your role limits?
   a Provide oral fluids according to the care plan.
   b Assist with activity according to the care plan.
   c Give drugs to control diarrhea.
   d Provide privacy for bowel elimination.

6 Dehydration is a risk from
   a Fecal impaction
   b Flatulence
   c Constipation
   d Diarrhea

7 A person has *C. difficile*. You should
   a Disinfect care items with soap and water
   b Use an alcohol-based hand sanitizer for hand hygiene
   c Wear a gown and gloves when giving care
   d Refuse to care for the person

8 Bowel training is aimed at
   a Bowel control and regular elimination
   b Ostomy control
   c Promoting toilet use
   d Preventing bleeding

9 You are preparing a person for an enema. You need to position the person in the
   a High-Fowler's position
   b Left semi-prone position
   c Fowler's position
   d Supine position

10 A small-volume enema is retained
   a For 2 minutes
   b At least 10 to 20 minutes
   c At least 30 minutes
   d Until the urge to have a BM is felt

11 A person has an ileostomy. Which is *normal*?
   a Stools are liquid and drain constantly into the pouch.
   b Stools are small hard lumps that pass every 2 to 4 hours.
   c Stools are large and formed and pass every 1 to 2 days.
   d The person has pain when stools pass.

12 When emptying an ostomy pouch, you should
   a Wait until the pouch is full to empty it
   b Wipe the outlet clean after emptying the pouch
   c Remove the pouch to empty it
   d Empty the contents into the wastebasket

Answers to Chapter 27 questions are on p. 588.

Answers to Chapter 27 questions are on p. 588.

FOCUS ON **PRACTICE**

Problem Solving

You respond to a resident's call light. The resident needs to have a BM urgently. The bathroom is occupied by the roommate. What do you do?

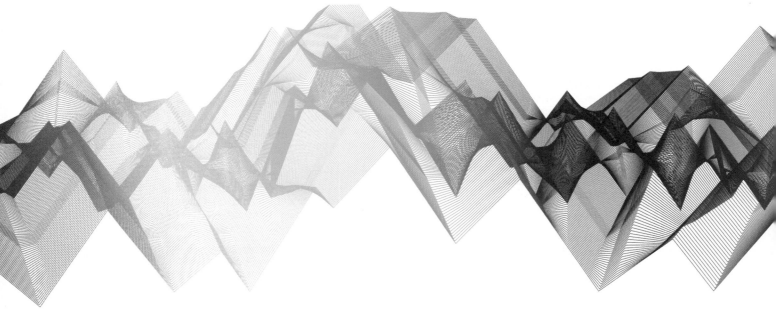

CHAPTER 28

Nutrition

OBJECTIVES

- Define the key terms and key abbreviations in this chapter.
- Explain the purpose and use of the MyPlate symbol.
- Describe the functions and sources of nutrients.
- Explain how to read and use food labels.
- Describe the special diets and between-meal snacks.
- Explain how to assist with measuring food intake.
- Explain how to promote PRIDE in the person, the family, and yourself.

KEY TERMS

calorie The fuel or energy value of food
cholesterol A soft, waxy substance found in the bloodstream and all body cells
dysphagia Difficulty *(dys)* swallowing *(phagia)*

nutrient A substance that is ingested, digested, absorbed, and used by the body
nutrition The processes involved in the ingestion, digestion, absorption, and use of food and fluids by the body

KEY ABBREVIATIONS

FDA	Food and Drug Administration		**mg**	Milligram
GI	Gastro-intestinal		**oz**	Ounce
HHS	U.S. Department of Health & Human Services		**USDA**	United States Department of Agriculture

Food is a basic need. The person's diet affects physical and mental well-being and function. A poor diet and poor eating habits:

- Increase the risk for disease and infection.
- Cause chronic illnesses to become worse.
- Cause healing problems.
- Increase the risk for accidents and injuries.

Many factors affect dietary needs and practices. Culture, finances, age, illness, food allergies, weight and height, physical activity, and personal choice are examples. The health team includes these and other factors in planning the person's nutrition needs.

NOTE: Federal agencies often issue and revise nutrition-related guidelines. Dietary Guidelines for Americans (p. 356), Physical Activity Guidelines for Americans (p. 356), MyPlate (p. 356), and food labels (p. 358) are examples. The Internet provides access to the most current information.

BASIC NUTRITION

Nutrition is the processes involved in the ingestion, digestion, absorption, and use of food and fluids by the body. Foods and fluids contain nutrients. A *nutrient is a substance that is ingested, digested, absorbed, and used by the body.* Nutrients are grouped into fats, proteins, carbohydrates, vitamins, minerals, and water. See "Nutrients" on p. 358.

Fats, proteins, and carbohydrates provide fuel for energy. A *calorie is the fuel or energy value of food.*

- 1 gram of fat—9 calories
- 1 gram of protein—4 calories
- 1 gram of carbohydrate—4 calories

A well-balanced diet and correct calorie intake are needed for growth, healing, and body function. A high-fat, high-calorie diet causes weight gain and obesity. A low-calorie diet promotes weight loss.

Dietary and Activity Guidelines

Dietary Guidelines for Americans are issued every 5 years by the U.S. Department of Agriculture (USDA) and the U.S. Department of Health & Human Services (HHS). The guidelines help promote health, reduce the risk of chronic diseases, and meet nutrient needs. For the most current dietary guidelines, search the Internet for *Dietary Guidelines for Americans.*

The HHS also issues *Physical Activity Guidelines for Americans.* These guidelines are used along with the dietary guidelines to promote health. For the most current activity guidelines, search the Internet for *Physical Activity Guidelines for Americans.*

Physical Activity. The HHS recommends that adults do at least 1 of the following weekly.

- 2 hours and 30 minutes of moderate-intensity physical activity
- 1 hour and 15 minutes of vigorous-intensity physical activity

Activities should be *aerobic.* Aerobic activities make the heart beat faster. To determine if an activity is moderate or vigorous, a person can try talking while being active.

- An activity is *moderate-intensity* if breathing is harder than normal but the person can still have a conversation.
- An activity is *vigorous-intensity* if the person can say only a few words before needing to take a breath.

Adults also should do muscle-strengthening activities at least 2 days a week. Push-ups, sit-ups, and weight-lifting are examples.

See *Focus on Older Persons: Physical Activity.*

> ## FOCUS ON **OLDER PERSONS**
> ### Physical Activity
> Physical activity can help older persons maintain strength and independence. Activity also can help manage many health problems, including diabetes and high blood pressure (Chapter 40). Exercises that maintain or improve balance are helpful for persons at risk for falls.

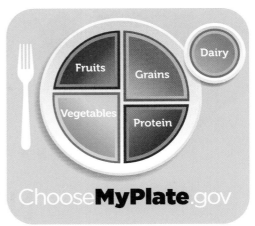

FIGURE 28-1 The MyPlate symbol. (Courtesy U.S. Department of Agriculture, Center for Nutrition and Policy Promotion.)

MyPlate. The MyPlate symbol (Fig. 28-1) encourages healthy eating from 5 food groups. Issued by the USDA, MyPlate is based on the *Dietary Guidelines for Americans.* MyPlate helps people:

- Learn how much to eat from each food group.
- Look at their eating routine and make choices that are rich in nutrients.
- Develop a healthy eating routine that can improve current and future health.
- Eat a variety of grains, vegetables, fruits, dairy foods, and protein foods. Added sugars, saturated fat (p. 358), and sodium are limited.

Food Groups

The 5 food groups are:

- Grains group
- Vegetable group
- Fruit group
- Dairy group
- Protein foods group

The amount needed from each food group depends on age, biological sex, height and weight, and physical activity. See Table 28-1 for food sources, general recommendations for daily servings and serving sizes for adults, and health benefits.

TABLE 28-1 Food Groups

Food Sources	Daily Servings and Serving Sizes	Health Benefits
Grains - Grains are foods made from wheat, rice, oats, cornmeal, barley, or other cereal grains. Bread, pasta, oatmeal, breakfast cereals, tortillas, and grits are examples. - *Whole grains* have the entire grain kernel. Whole-wheat flour, bulgur (cracked wheat), oatmeal, whole-grain cornmeal, and brown rice are examples. - *Refined grains* are processed to remove parts of the grain kernel. White flour, white bread, and white rice are examples. They have less dietary fiber than whole grains.	**Daily Servings** - Adult women: 5 to 8 ounces (oz) with at least 3 to 4 oz from whole grains - Adult men: 6 to 10 oz with at least 3 to 5 oz from whole grains **Serving Sizes** - 1 oz = 1 slice of bread - 1 oz = 1 cup breakfast cereal - 1 oz = ½ cup cooked rice, oatmeal, or pasta	- May lower cholesterol (p. 358) and may reduce the risk of heart disease, including heart attack and stroke. - May help digestion and prevent constipation. (Fiber is important for proper bowel function.) - May help with weight management. - May prevent certain birth defects. - Contain dietary fiber, several B vitamins (thiamin, riboflavin, niacin, folate [folic acid]), and minerals (iron, magnesium, and selenium).

TABLE 28-1 Food Groups—cont'd

Food Sources	Daily Servings and Serving Sizes	Health Benefits
Vegetables • Vegetables can be raw, cooked, fresh, frozen, canned, dried, or juiced. • *Dark green vegetables*—broccoli, collard greens, dark green leafy lettuce, kale, mustard greens, romaine lettuce, spinach, turnip greens, watercress. • *Red and orange vegetables*—acorn, butternut, and hubbard squashes; carrots; pumpkin; red and orange peppers; sweet potatoes; tomatoes; tomato juice. • *Beans, peas, and lentils*—black beans, black-eyed peas, garbanzo beans (chickpeas), kidney beans, pinto beans, split peas, lentils. • *Starchy vegetables*—corn, green peas, hominy, potatoes. • *Other vegetables*—avocado, bean sprouts, cabbage, cauliflower, celery, cucumbers, green beans, green peppers, iceberg (head) lettuce, mushrooms, onions, summer squash, zucchini.	**Daily Servings** • Adult women: 2 to 3 cups • Adult men: 2½ to 4 cups **Serving Sizes** • 1 cup = 1 cup raw or cooked vegetables or vegetable juice • 1 cup = 2 cups raw leafy greens	• May lower cholesterol and may reduce the risk of heart disease, including heart attack and stroke. • May protect against certain cancers. • May help lower calorie intake. Most vegetables are low in fat and calories. • May prevent certain birth defects. • Contain potassium, dietary fiber, folate (folic acid), and vitamins A and C.
Fruits • Any fruit or 100% fruit juice counts as part of the fruit group. • Fruits may be fresh, frozen, canned, or dried. They may be whole, cut up, pureed, or cooked. • Avoid fruits canned in syrup. Syrup contains added sugar. Choose fruits canned in 100% fruit juice or water.	**Daily Servings** • Adult women: 1½ to 2 cups • Adult men: 2 to 2½ cups **Serving Sizes** • 1 cup = 1 cup fruit • 1 cup = 1 cup fruit juice • 1 cup = ½ cup dried fruit	• May lower cholesterol and may reduce the risk of heart disease, including heart attack and stroke. • May protect against certain cancers. • May help bowel function. • May help lower fat and calorie intake. Most fruits are low in fat and calories. • Contain no cholesterol. • Are low in sodium (salt). • Contain potassium, dietary fiber, vitamin C, and folate (folic acid).
Dairy • All fluid milk products are part of the dairy group. So are many foods made from milk. Yogurt and cheese are examples. • Low-fat or fat-free choices are best. • Cream, cream cheese, and butter are not in this group.	**Daily Servings** • Adult women: 3 cups • Adult men: 3 cups **Serving Sizes** • 1 cup = 1 cup milk, yogurt, or soy milk • 1 cup = 1½ oz natural cheese • 1 cup = 1 oz processed cheese	• Help build bones and teeth and maintain bone mass. This may reduce the risk of osteoporosis. • May reduce the risk of high blood pressure. • Contain calcium, potassium, vitamin D, and protein.

Protein Foods
• All foods made from meat, poultry, seafood, eggs, processed soy products, nuts, and seeds are protein foods.
• Beans, peas, and lentils are in this group and the vegetable group.
• Some protein foods are high in saturated fat (p. 358). For healthy choices, remember:
  ◦ Choose lean or low-fat meat and poultry.
  ◦ Limit foods high in saturated fat. Fatty cuts of beef, pork, and lamb; regular (75% to 85% lean) ground beef; regular sausages, hot dogs, and bacon are examples.
  ◦ Seafood like salmon, trout, and anchovies contain healthy fats.
  ◦ Processed meats (ham, sausage, hot dogs, luncheon and deli meats) have added sodium (salt).
  ◦ Vary the kinds of protein foods eaten. Include seafood, nuts, seeds, and soy products throughout the week.
	Daily Servings
	• Adult women: 5 to 6½ oz
	• Adult men: 5½ to 7 oz
	
	Serving Sizes
	• 1 oz = 1 oz lean meat, poultry, or fish
	• 1 oz = 1 egg
	• 1 oz = 1 tablespoon peanut butter
	• 1 oz = ¼ cup cooked beans
	• 1 oz = ½ oz nuts or seeds
		• Contain nutrients needed for health and body maintenance—protein, B vitamins (niacin, thiamin, riboflavin, and B_6), vitamin E, iron, zinc, and magnesium.
		• Proteins (p. 358) are building blocks needed for body structure and function.

Modified from U.S. Department of Agriculture: *Eat Healthy.*

Nutrients

No food or food group has every essential nutrient. A well-balanced diet ensures an adequate intake of essential nutrients.

- *Protein*—the most important nutrient, protein is needed for tissue growth and repair. Sources include meat, fish, poultry, eggs, milk and milk products, cereals, beans, peas, and nuts.
- *Carbohydrates*—provide energy and fiber for bowel elimination. Sources are fruits, vegetables, breads, cereals, and sugar.
  - *Dietary fiber (fiber)*—fiber is not digested. It provides the bulky part of chyme for elimination. Good sources include whole grains, fruits, vegetables, beans and peas, and nuts and seeds.
  - *Sugars*—are broken down by the body into glucose. Glucose is used for energy.
- *Fats*—provide energy. They add flavor and help the body use certain vitamins. Unneeded dietary fat is stored as body fat *(adipose tissue)*. See "Fats and Oils."
- *Vitamins*—are needed for certain body functions. The body stores vitamins A, D, E, and K. Vitamins C and the B complex vitamins are not stored. They must be ingested daily. The lack of a certain vitamin results in illness.
- *Minerals*—are needed for bone and tooth formation, nerve and muscle function, fluid balance, and other body processes. Foods containing calcium help prevent musculo-skeletal changes.
- *Water*—is needed for all body processes (Chapter 30).

Fats and Oils

Solid fats are solid at room temperature. Butter, beef fat (tallow, suet), chicken fat, pork fat (lard), stick margarine, and shortening are examples. Desserts and baked goods, many cheeses, and whole milk also contain solid fats. Solid fats contain more unhealthy fats called saturated fats and *trans* fats. (No longer recognized as safe, the major source of artificial *trans* fat in the U.S. food supply was removed as of June 2018.)

Saturated fats affect cholesterol levels. *Cholesterol is a soft, waxy substance found in the bloodstream and all body cells.* When certain cholesterol levels are high, the risk for heart disease increases. Eating less saturated fat can improve cholesterol and lower the risk for heart disease.

Oils are liquid fats. Oils come from plants and fish. Oils are not a food group, but they do provide nutrients (unsaturated fats and vitamin E). Oils (including vegetable oils [canola, corn, olive] and oils in foods such as seafood and nuts) are part of a healthy diet.

Food Labels

Food labels are used to make informed food choices for a healthy diet (Fig. 28-2). Food labels contain information about:

- *Serving size and the number of servings in each package.* Nutrition information on the label is based on 1 serving. The serving size is not a recommendation of how much to eat or drink.
- *Calories.* The number of calories in 1 serving. The number of servings eaten determines the number of calories eaten.
- *Nutrients.* The U.S. Food and Drug Administration (FDA) recommends eating:
  - Less saturated fat, sodium, and added sugars
  - More dietary fiber, vitamin D, calcium, iron, and potassium
- *Percent Daily Value (%DV).* The %DV shows how much of a nutrient is in 1 serving of the food. The %DV helps you decide if a food is high or low in a nutrient. The value is based on a 2000-calorie daily diet. According to the FDA, a 5% DV is low. A DV of 20% or more is high.

See *Focus on Math: Food Labels.*

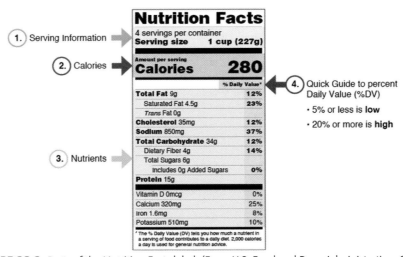

FIGURE 28-2 Parts of the Nutrition Facts label. (From U.S. Food and Drug Administration, 2020.)

FOCUS ON MATH
Food Labels

The nutrition information on a food label is based on 1 serving. When reading a label, note the serving size amount. The number of calories and nutrients listed is based on that amount. If less is eaten, less calories and nutrients are consumed. If more is eaten, more calories and nutrients are consumed.

See the table below for how to calculate the number of calories, total fat, and sodium for different serving amounts of the food label shown in Figure 28-2.

	Calories	Total Fat	Sodium
1 Serving = 1 cup	280 calories	9 grams	850 milligrams
1/2 Serving = 1/2 cup (divide by 2)	140 calories	4½ grams	425 milligrams
2 Servings = 2 cups (multiply by 2)	560 calories	18 grams	1700 milligrams

SPECIAL DIETS

Doctors may order special diets (Table 28-2).
- For a nutritional deficiency or a disease
- For weight gain or loss
- To remove or decrease certain substances in the diet

Persons with diseases of the heart, kidneys, gallbladder, pancreas, liver, stomach, or intestines often need special diets. High-protein diets are needed to heal wounds and pressure injuries. Adding bran to the diet provides fiber for bowel elimination.

The sodium-controlled diet is often ordered (p. 361). So is a diabetes meal plan (p. 362). Persons with swallowing problems may need a dysphagia diet (p. 362 and Chapter 29). *Regular diet (general diet)* means there are no dietary limits or restrictions.

Surgery and some tests, procedures, and treatments require that nothing is eaten. The person has an NPO order. *NPO* stands for *nil per os*—nothing by mouth (Chapter 29).

The health team considers the need for dietary changes, personal choices, religion, culture, and eating problems. They also consider food allergies and intolerances (sensitivities) (Chapter 29). The nurse and dietitian teach the person and family about the diet.

TABLE 28-2 Special Diets

Diet	Use	Foods Allowed/Restricted
Clear liquid—foods liquid at room temperature and clear or able to see through; non-irritating; non–gas forming; leave a small amount of residue	After surgery; for acute illness, infection, nausea, and vomiting; and to prepare for GI (gastro-intestinal) exams	Water, tea, and coffee (*without milk or cream*); carbonated drinks; gelatin; fruit juices *without pulp* (apple, grape, cranberry); fat-free broth; hard candy, sugar, and Popsicles; *may need to avoid liquids with red coloring*
Full liquid—foods liquid at room temperature	Advance from clear-liquid diet after surgery; for stomach irritation, fever, nausea, and vomiting; for persons unable to chew, swallow, or digest solid foods	Foods on the clear-liquid diet; custard; eggnog; strained soups; strained fruit and vegetable juices; milk and milk-shakes; cooked cereals; plain ice cream and sherbet; plain pudding; yogurt
Mechanical soft—semi-solid foods that are easily digested	Advance from full-liquid diet; chewing problems, GI disorders, and infections	All liquids; eggs (*not fried*); broiled, baked, or roasted meat, fish, or poultry that is chopped or shredded; mild cheeses (American, Swiss, cheddar, cream, cottage); strained fruit juices; refined bread (*no crust*) and crackers; cooked cereal; cooked or pureed vegetables; cooked or canned fruit *without skin or seeds*; plain pudding; plain cakes and soft cookies *without fruit or nuts*
Fiber- and residue-restricted—foods that leave a small amount of residue in the colon	Diseases of the colon and diarrhea	Coffee, tea, milk, carbonated drinks, strained fruit and vegetable juices; refined bread and crackers; creamed and refined cereal; rice; cottage and cream cheese; eggs (*not fried*); plain puddings and cakes; gelatin; custard; sherbet and ice cream; canned or cooked fruit *without skin or seeds*; potatoes (*not fried*); strained cooked vegetables; plain pasta; *no raw fruits or vegetables*

Continued

TABLE 28-2 Special Diets—cont'd

Diet	Use	Foods Allowed/Restricted
High-fiber—foods that increase residue and fiber in the colon to stimulate peristalsis	Constipation and GI disorders	All fruits and vegetables, whole-wheat bread, whole-grain cereals, whole-grain rice, beans, and nuts are promoted; other foods (dairy, meat) are allowed but are not high-fiber
Bland—foods that are non-irritating and low in roughage; foods served at moderate temperatures; no strong spices or condiments	Ulcers, gallbladder disorders, and some intestinal disorders; after abdominal surgery	Lean meats; white bread; creamed and refined cereals; cream or cottage cheese; gelatin; plain puddings, cakes, and cookies; eggs *(not fried)*; butter and cream; canned fruits and vegetables *without skin and seeds;* strained fruit juices; potatoes *(not fried);* pastas and rice; strained or soft cooked carrots, peas, beets, spinach, squash, and asparagus tips; creamed soups from allowed vegetables; *no fried or spicy foods*
High-calorie—3000 to 4000 calories daily; includes 3 full meals and between-meal snacks	Weight gain and some thyroid problems	Dietary increases in all foods; large portions of regular diet with 3 between-meal snacks
Calorie-controlled—adequate nutrients while controlling calories to promote weight loss and reduce body fat	Weight loss	Foods low in fats and carbohydrates and lean meats; *avoid butter, cream, rice, gravies, salad oils, noodles, cakes, pastries, carbonated and alcoholic drinks, candy, potato chips, and similar foods*
High-iron—foods high in iron	Anemia; after blood loss; for women during the reproductive years	Liver and other organ meats; lean meats; egg yolks; shellfish; dried fruits; dried beans; green leafy vegetables; lima beans; peanut butter; enriched breads and cereals
Fat-controlled (low cholesterol)—foods low in fat and prepared without adding fat	Heart, gallbladder, and liver diseases; disorders of fat digestion; diseases of the pancreas	Skim milk (fat-free) or buttermilk; cottage cheese *(no other cheeses allowed);* gelatin; sherbet; fruit; lean meat, poultry, and fish (baked, broiled, or roasted); fat-free broth; soups made with skim milk (fat-free); margarine; rice, pasta, breads, and cereals; vegetables; potatoes
High-protein—aids and promotes tissue healing	Burns, high fever, infection, and some liver diseases	Meat, milk, eggs, cheese, fish, poultry; breads and cereals; green leafy vegetables
Sodium-controlled—a certain amount of sodium is allowed	Heart disease, fluid retention, liver diseases, and some kidney diseases	Fruits and vegetables and unsalted butter are allowed; *adding salt at the table is not allowed; highly salted foods and foods high in sodium are not allowed; the use of salt during cooking may be restricted*
Gluten-free—foods without the gluten protein	Celiac disease	Beans; seeds; nuts; eggs; meats, fish, and poultry *(without breading, batter, or marinade);* fruits and vegetables; most dairy foods; gluten-free grains and starches (arrowroot, corn, cornmeal, hominy, flax, millet, rice, soy, and tapioca); gluten-free flours (rice, soy, corn, potato, bean); *no foods containing wheat, barley, triticale, or rye*
Lactose-free—foods without lactose (a sugar in milk and milk products)	Lactose intolerance	Lactose-free or lactose-reduced milk and milk products; vegetables, fruits, and breads and cereals not prepared with milk or milk products; plain meat, fish, poultry, and eggs; avoid *regular milk and milk products (yogurt, cheese);* avoid *boxed, canned, frozen, packaged, or prepared foods containing milk or milk products*
Diabetes meal plan—food and fluids are balanced with physical activity and drugs to manage blood glucose levels (Chapter 40)	Diabetes	Determined by nutritional and energy requirements and drugs to treat diabetes; *limit fried foods, foods high in fat and sodium, foods and drinks with added sugars;* sugar substitutes are allowed

The Sodium-Controlled Diet

According to the American Heart Association (AHA), the average amount of sodium in the daily diet is greater than 3400 mg (milligrams). Lowering sodium (commonly called salt) in the diet reduces the risk of high blood pressure, heart disease, and stroke. For most adults, the AHA recommends limiting sodium intake to no more than 2300 mg a day. The AHA says that no more than 1500 mg daily is a better goal.

With too much sodium, the body retains (holds) water. Tissues swell. There is excess fluid in the blood vessels. The heart works harder. With heart disease, the extra workload can cause serious problems or death.

Sodium control lowers the amount of sodium in the body. Less water is retained. Less water in the tissues and blood vessels reduces the heart's workload.

The doctor orders the amount of sodium allowed. Sodium-controlled diets involve:

- Omitting high-sodium foods (Box 28-1)
- Not adding salt to food at the table
- Limiting the amount of salt used in cooking
- Diet planning

BOX 28-1 High-Sodium Foods

Grains
- Baked goods—biscuits, muffins, cakes, cookies, pies, pastries, sweet rolls, donuts, and so on
- Breads and rolls
- Cereals—cold, instant hot
- Noodle mixes
- Pancakes
- Salted snack foods—pretzels, corn chips, popcorn, crackers, chips, and so on
- Stuffing mixes
- Waffles

Vegetables
- Canned vegetables
- Olives
- Pickles and other pickled vegetables
- Relish
- Sauerkraut
- Tomato sauce or paste
- Vegetable juices—tomato, V8, Bloody Mary mixes
- Vegetables with sauces, creams, or seasonings

Fruits
- None—fruits are not high in sodium

Dairy Group
- Buttermilk
- Cheese
- Commercial dips made with sour cream

Protein Foods
- Bacon and Canadian bacon
- Canned meats and fish—chicken, tuna, salmon, anchovies, sardines
- Caviar
- Chipped, dried, and corned beef and other meats
- Deli meats—turkey, ham, bologna, salami, pastrami, and so on

Protein Foods—cont'd
- Dried fish
- Ham
- Herring
- Hot dogs (frankfurters)
- Liverwurst
- Lox and smoked salmon
- Mackerel
- Pepperoni
- Salt pork
- Sausages
- Scrapple
- Shellfish—shrimp, crab, clams, oysters, scallops, lobster

Other
- Asian foods—Chinese, Japanese, East Indian, Thai, Vietnamese
- Baking soda and baking powder
- Catsup (ketchup)
- Cocoa mixes
- Commercially prepared dinners—frozen, canned, boxed, and so on
- Mayonnaise
- Mexican foods
- Mustard
- Pasta dishes—lasagna, manicotti, ravioli
- Peanut butter
- Pizzas
- Pot pies
- Salad dressings
- Salted nuts or seeds
- Sauces—soy, teriyaki, Worcestershire, steak, barbecue, pasta, chili, cocktail
- Seasoning salts—garlic, onion, celery, meat tenderizers, monosodium glutamate (MSG), and so on
- Soups—canned, packaged, instant, dried, bouillon

Diabetes Meal Plan

Diabetes is a chronic illness in which the body cannot produce or use insulin properly (Chapter 40). The pancreas produces and secretes insulin. Insulin lets the body use sugar. Without enough insulin, sugar builds up in the bloodstream. It is not used by cells for energy. Treatment usually involves insulin or other drugs, diet, and exercise.

A meal plan for healthy eating is developed. It often involves:

- Food preferences (likes, eating habits, meal times, culture, and life-style). Food amounts and preparation methods may be restricted.
- Portion control. Healthy foods from each food group are eaten. The person's meal plan states the amounts allowed from each group.
- Carbohydrate counting (carb counting). The person keeps track of the amount of carbohydrates eaten each day.
- Eating meals and snacks at regular times. The person may need to eat at regular times to maintain a certain blood glucose (blood sugar) level.

Serve meals and snacks on time. Always check what was eaten. Report what the person did and did not eat. A between-meal snack makes up for what was not eaten. The nurse tells you what to provide. The amount of insulin given depends on food intake and physical activity. Report changes in the person's eating habits.

The Dysphagia Diet

Dysphagia means difficulty (dys) *swallowing* (phagia). Breathing food and fluids into the lungs *(aspiration)* is a risk. Food thickness and texture are changed to ease swallowing. Liquids are often thickened to meet the person's needs. See "Dysphagia" in Chapter 29.

Between-Meal Snacks

Many special diets involve between-meal snacks. Snacks provide extra nutrients. Common snacks are crackers, milk, juice, a milk-shake, cake, wafers, a sandwich, gelatin, and custard.

FOOD INTAKE

Food intake is measured in different ways. Follow agency policy for the method used.

- *Percentage of food eaten.* Food intake ranges from 0 to 100 percent (%). Some agencies record the percent of the whole meal tray. Others record the percent of each food item eaten. See Figure 28-3.
- *Calorie counts.* Note what the person ate and how much. For example, a chicken breast, rice, beans, fruit salad, and pudding were served. The person ate all the chicken, half the rice, and the fruit salad. The beans and pudding were not eaten. Note these on the flow sheet. A nurse or dietitian converts these portions into calories.

See *Focus on Math: Food Intake.*
See *Focus on Communication: Food Intake.*

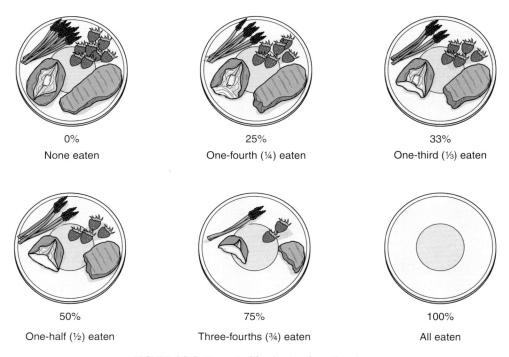

| 0% | 25% | 33% |
| None eaten | One-fourth (¼) eaten | One-third (⅓) eaten |

| 50% | 75% | 100% |
| One-half (½) eaten | Three-fourths (¾) eaten | All eaten |

FIGURE 28-3 Percent of food eaten from the plate.

FOCUS ON MATH
Food Intake

To measure food intake, you need to understand percents. Percents measure parts of a whole (Fig. 28-4). The "whole" is written as 100%.

To measure food intake, compare the food left to that served. Depending on agency policy and the food type, *estimate* or *calculate* food intake. To estimate, record the approximate amount of food eaten. See Figure 28-3. *To calculate:*

1 Subtract the amount left from the amount served. (This is the amount the person ate.)
2 Divide the number from step 1 by the amount served (the number of pieces making up the whole).
3 Multiply the number from step 2 by 100 for a percent. (*Percent means out of 100.*)

For example, 8 apple slices were served; 2 remain on the plate.

8 slices − 2 slices = 6 slices
The person ate 6 apple slices; 8 were served.
6 slices (number eaten) ÷ 8 slices (number served) = 0.75
0.75 × 100 = 75%
75% of the apple slices were eaten.

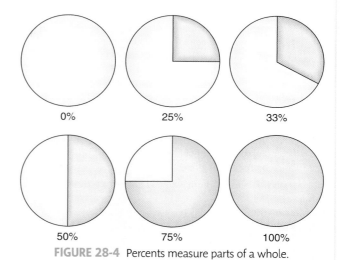
FIGURE 28-4 Percents measure parts of a whole.

FOCUS ON COMMUNICATION
Food Intake

The person may not eat everything served. You need to ask why and tell the nurse. You can say:
- "Did your food taste okay?"
- "Was there anything wrong with your food?"
- "Was there something you didn't like?"
- "Was your food too hot or too cold?"
- "Would you like something else?"
- "Weren't you hungry?"

FOCUS ON P R I D E
The Person, Family, and Yourself

P ersonal and Professional Responsibility

Your nutrition choices matter. The food and drinks you choose regularly over time make up your eating pattern. Healthy patterns and regular physical activity promote health. You need to be healthy in order to care for others.

R ights and Respect

People often comment about food likes and dislikes. People have the right to express what they prefer. Do not say the person is complaining or being picky. Learning the person's likes and dislikes can improve nutrition. It also shows interest and concern for the person.

I ndependence and Social Interaction

Physical activity can be a social experience. Walking with a friend, riding bicycles as a family, or golfing with others are examples. Regular physical activity has long-term health benefits. Choose activities you enjoy.

D elegation and Teamwork

Measuring food intake takes practice. You may have questions. Do not guess. Ask for help. During your training, ask your instructor. At work, ask the nurse or dietary staff.

E thics and Laws

Each person is different. A person may have a special diet or food allergy (Chapter 29). You must know what each person can and cannot have. Know each person's needs. Protect the person from harm. If unsure, ask the nurse.

FOCUS ON PRIDE: Application

Consider your life-style choices. Do you try to eat a healthy diet? What do you do for regular physical activity? What goals do you have? Even small changes can improve health.

Circle the BEST answer.

1 Nutrition is
   a Fats, proteins, carbohydrates, vitamins, and minerals
   b The processes involved in the ingestion, digestion, absorption, and use of food and fluids by the body
   c The amount of food eaten
   d The balance between calories taken in and used by the body

2 Which is healthy?
   a Limiting nutrient-rich foods
   b Eating from all 5 food groups
   c Increasing the amount of high-sodium foods
   d Eating more refined grains

3 A person wants to eat more whole grains. Which choice is *best*?
   a Brown rice
   b White bread
   c White rice
   d Pasta made with white flour

4 Which would meet an adult male's daily dairy needs?
   a 1 slice of bread, 1 cup of cheese, and ½ oz of nuts
   b 2 cups of milk and 1 cup of cooked rice
   c 1 cup of milk, 1 cup of yogurt, and 1½ oz of cheese
   d 2 tablespoons of peanut butter and 1 egg

5 In which food group does saturated fat need to be considered?
   a Grains
   b Vegetables
   c Fruit
   d Protein foods

6 Protein is needed for
   a Tissue growth and repair
   b Fiber for bowel elimination
   c Fluid balance
   d Improved food taste

7 Which foods provide the *most* protein?
   a Butter and cream
   b Tomatoes and potatoes
   c Meats and fish
   d Corn and lettuce

8 A person needs more fiber to promote bowel elimination. Which choice is *best*?
   a Refined grains
   b Fruits and vegetables
   c Meats
   d Dairy foods

9 These statements are about fats and oils. Which is *true*?
   a Vegetable oils and oils in fish and nuts are healthy choices.
   b Butter, beef fat, and chicken fat are healthy choices.
   c Saturated fats do not affect heart disease risk.
   d Oils are a food group.

10 The serving information on a food label tells you
   a The serving size and number of servings in the package
   b How much you should eat of the product
   c How the product needs to be stored before serving
   d How to cook and serve the product

11 These statements are about special diets. Which is *true*?
   a A person on a full liquid diet can have rice and bread.
   b Meats on a mechanical soft diet are chopped or shredded.
   c A person on a gluten-free diet can have whole-wheat bread.
   d A lactose-free diet can include milk products.

12 The sodium-controlled diet involves
   a Omitting high-sodium foods
   b Adding salt to food at the table
   c Using 3000 mg of salt in cooking
   d A sodium-intake flow sheet

13 Diabetes meal planning involves
   a Changing the thickness of foods
   b Eating larger food portions
   c Controlling sodium
   d Eating at regular times

14 A dysphagia diet is used for persons with
   a High blood pressure
   b Nausea
   c Difficulty swallowing
   d A decreased appetite

15 A resident eats half of the food on the meal tray. Food intake for this meal is
   a 25%
   b 33%
   c 50%
   d 75%

Answers to Chapter 28 questions are on p. 588.

FOCUS ON **PRACTICE**

Problem Solving

A resident with diabetes has an order for a diabetes meal plan. You serve the person coffee. The person says: "I like it sweetened." The agency has sugar packets and sugar substitute packets available. What will you do? What will you do if you do not know what the person can have?

CHAPTER 29

Meeting Nutrition Needs

OBJECTIVES

- Define the key terms and key abbreviations in this chapter.
- Describe the factors that affect eating and nutrition.
- Identify the signs and symptoms of dysphagia and aspiration.
- Identify the safety measures to prevent aspiration.
- Describe CMS requirements for the food served.

- Explain how to assist with nutrition needs.
- Explain how to assist with enteral nutrition.
- Identify the precautions to prevent regurgitation and aspiration from tube feedings.
- Perform the procedures described in this chapter.
- Explain how to promote PRIDE in the person, the family, and yourself.

KEY TERMS

anorexia The loss of appetite
aspiration Breathing fluid, food, vomitus, or an object into the lungs
dysphagia Difficulty *(dys)* swallowing *(phagia)*
enteral nutrition Giving nutrients into the gastro-intestinal (GI) tract *(enteral)* through a feeding tube

gavage The process of giving a tube feeding
regurgitation The backward flow of stomach contents into the mouth

KEY ABBREVIATIONS

CMS	Centers for Medicare & Medicaid Services
GI	Gastro-intestinal
ID	Identification

NG	Naso-gastric
NPO	Nothing by mouth

A team approach is needed to meet a person's nutrition needs. The person, nursing team, doctor, dietitian, speech therapist, and occupational therapist are involved. So is the family if necessary. The person's likes, dislikes, and life-long habits are part of the care plan.

You help meet nutritional needs by preparing patients and residents for meals and serving meal trays. When necessary, you may need to feed a person.

See *Focus on Surveys: Meeting Nutrition Needs.*

> **FOCUS ON SURVEYS**
> Meeting Nutrition Needs
>
> The health team develops a care plan to meet the person's nutrition needs. Surveyors may ask you:
> - How food and fluid intake are observed and reported (Chapters 28 and 30).
> - How eating ability is observed and reported.
> - About the measures to prevent or meet changes in nutrition needs. Snacks and frequent meals are examples.
> - About the goals for nutrition in the care plan.

FACTORS AFFECTING EATING AND NUTRITION

Many factors affect eating and nutrition. They begin in childhood and continue throughout life.

Culture and Religion

Culture influences dietary practices, food choices, and food preparation. Frying, baking, smoking, or roasting food and eating raw food are some cultural practices. So is using sauces, herbs, and spices.

Selecting, preparing, and eating food often involve religion. For example, certain foods are not allowed. Or only certain foods or no foods are eaten during a *fast*. A person may follow all, some, or none of the dietary practices of his or her faith. Respect the person's religious practices.

See *Caring About Culture: Food Practices.*

CARING ABOUT CULTURE

Food Practices

Rice, corn, and beans are protein sources in *Mexico*. In the *Philippines*, rice is a main food. And fish, vegetables, and native fruits are preferred. In *China*, a meal of rice with meat, fish, and vegetables is common. High sodium content is from using soy sauce and dried and preserved foods.

Note: *Each person is unique. A person may not follow all of the beliefs and practices of his or her culture. Follow the care plan.*

Modified from D'Avanzo CE: *Pocket guide to cultural health assessment,* ed 4, St Louis, 2008, Mosby.

Personal Choice and Finances

Food likes and dislikes are influenced by foods served in the home. Food choices depend on how food looks, how it is prepared, its smell, and ingredients. Usually food likes change with age and social experiences. Personal choice may involve a vegetarian diet. The focus is on plants for food—fruits, vegetables, dried beans and peas, grains, seeds, and nuts.

People with limited incomes often buy cheaper carbohydrate foods. Their diets often lack protein and certain vitamins and minerals.

Appetite and Body Reactions

Appetite relates to the desire for food. *Loss of appetite (anorexia)* can occur. Causes include illness, drugs, anxiety, pain, and depression. Unpleasant sights, thoughts, and smells are other causes.

Food allergies cause an immune response. The person may react with a rash, swelling, or itching. Some reactions are life-threatening (Chapter 43). Foods that cause allergic reactions are avoided.

A *food intolerance (food sensitivity)* occurs when there are problems digesting certain foods. There are negative body reactions. But the immune system is not activated. Nausea, vomiting, diarrhea, indigestion, gas, or headaches may occur. Some reactions can be treated or prevented.

Aging

Many gastro-intestinal (GI) changes occur with aging. Taste and smell dull. Appetite decreases. Secretion of digestive juices decreases. Fried and fatty foods may cause indigestion.

Some people avoid the high-fiber foods needed for bowel elimination—apricots, celery, and fruits and vegetables with skins and seeds. High-fiber foods are hard to chew and can irritate the intestines.

Foods providing soft bulk are often ordered for chewing problems or constipation. Whole-grain cereals and cooked fruits and vegetables are examples.

Calorie needs are lower. Energy and activity levels are lower. Foods that contain calcium help prevent musculoskeletal changes. Protein is needed for tissue growth and repair. Because of cost, diets may lack high-protein foods.

Illness and Disability

Appetite often decreases during illness and recovery from injuries. However, nutrition needs increase. The body must fight infection, heal tissue, and replace lost blood cells. Nutrients lost through vomiting and diarrhea need to be replaced.

Drugs can cause appetite loss, confusion, nausea, constipation, impaired taste, or changes in GI function. They can cause inflammation of the mouth, throat, esophagus, and stomach.

Disease or injury can affect the hands, wrists, and arms. Adaptive equipment (assistive devices) let the person eat independently (Fig. 29-1). The speech therapist and occupational therapist teach the person how to use them. Make sure each person has needed devices.

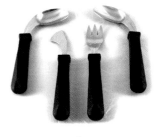
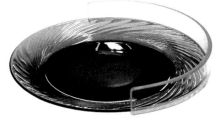
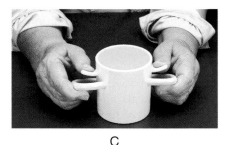

A   B   C

FIGURE 29-1 Adaptive equipment (assistive devices) for eating. **A,** Eating utensils have tapered and angled handles. The knife cuts with slicing and rocking motions. **B,** The plate guard helps keep food on the plate. **C,** The thumb grips on the cup help prevent spilling. (Images courtesy Elderstore, Alpharetta, Ga.)

Chewing and Swallowing Problems

Mouth, teeth, and gum problems can affect chewing. Examples include oral pain, dry or sore mouth, gum disease (Chapter 21), dental problems, and dentures that fit poorly. Broken, decayed, or missing teeth also affect chewing (especially meats).

Stroke; pain; confusion; dry mouth; and diseases of the mouth, throat, and esophagus can affect swallowing. See "Dysphagia."

DYSPHAGIA

Dysphagia means difficulty (dys) *swallowing* (phagia). A *slow swallow* means the person has difficulty getting enough food and fluids for good nutrition and fluid balance. An *unsafe swallow* means that food enters the airway (aspiration). *Aspiration is breathing fluid, food, vomitus, or an object into the lungs.*

When feeding a person with dysphagia, you must:

- Know the signs and symptoms of dysphagia (Box 29-1).
- Feed the person according to the care plan.
- Follow the person's ordered diet. A dysphagia diet is common. Food and fluid thicknesses are changed to meet the person's needs (see Box 29-1).
- Follow aspiration precautions (see Box 29-1) and the care plan.
- Report changes in how the person eats.
- Report signs and symptoms of aspiration at once (see Box 29-1).

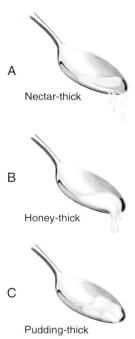

A
Nectar-thick

B
Honey-thick

C
Pudding-thick

FIGURE 29-2   A, Nectar-thick liquid. **B,** Honey-thick liquid. **C,** Pudding-thick (spoon-thick) liquid.

BOX 29-1 Dysphagia

Dysphagia Signs and Symptoms

- Avoids foods that need chewing.
- Avoids foods with certain textures and temperatures.
- Tires during a meal.
- Has food spill out of the mouth while eating.
- "Pockets" or "squirrels" food in the cheeks. This means that food remains or is hidden in the mouth.
- Eats slowly, especially solid foods.
- Complains that food will not go down or that food is stuck.
- Coughs or chokes before, during, or after swallowing.
- Regurgitates food after eating (p. 374).
- Spits out food suddenly and almost violently.
- Has food come up through the nose.
- Has hoarseness—especially after eating.
- Makes gurgling sounds while talking or breathing after swallowing.
- Has a runny nose, sneezes, or has excessive drooling.
- Complains of frequent heartburn.
- Has a decreased appetite.

Dysphagia Diet

- The doctor, speech therapist, occupational therapist, dietitian, and nurse choose food and liquid thicknesses.
- Food thickness and texture are changed to ease swallowing.
  - *Mechanical soft*—foods have a moist, soft texture. Meats are chopped, blended, or ground. Vegetables are cooked well.
  - *Pureed*—foods have a smooth, uniform texture and hold their shape on a spoon. Foods are "pudding-like" and have no lumps.

Dysphagia Diet—cont'd

- Liquids are thickened as needed (Fig. 29-2).
  - *Nectar-thick liquid*—mildly thick. The liquid coats and drips off of a spoon. It can flow through a straw.
  - *Honey-thick liquid*—moderately thick. The liquid flows off of a spoon like honey. The person can drink it from a cup.
  - *Pudding-thick (spoon-thick) liquid*—extremely thick. The liquid stays on a spoon in a soft mound. It can be sipped or served with a spoon.

Aspiration Precautions

- Help the person with meals and snacks. Follow the care plan.
- Position the person upright as the nurse and care plan direct. The person remains upright for at least 1 hour after eating.
- Support the upper back, shoulders, and neck with a pillow.
- Follow the care plan for straw use. A straw may not be allowed.
- Check the person's mouth after eating for pocketing. Check inside the cheeks, under the tongue, and on the roof of the mouth. Remove any food (p. 370).
- Provide mouth care after eating.
- Observe for signs and symptoms of aspiration. Report the following at once.
  - Choking
  - Coughing
  - Difficulty breathing during or after meals or snacks
  - Abnormal breathing or respiratory sounds
- Report and record your observations.

NUTRITION AND FOOD REQUIREMENTS

The Centers for Medicare & Medicaid Services (CMS) requires that the health team assess the person's nutrition status and factors affecting eating and nutrition. The CMS has requirements for the food served in nursing centers.

- Each person's nutrition needs are met.
- The person's religious and cultural needs and preferences are met.
- The person's diet is well balanced. It is nourishing and tastes good. Food is well seasoned. It is not too salty or too sweet.
- Food is appetizing. It has an appealing aroma (smell) and is attractive.
- Hot food is served hot. Cold food is served cold.
- Food is served promptly. If not, hot food cools and cold food warms.
- Food is prepared to meet each person's needs. Special diets are followed (Chapter 28). Food is cut, ground, chopped, or pureed to meet the person's individual needs.
- Other foods are offered if the food served is refused. The substituted food must have a similar nutritional value to the first foods served.
- Each person receives at least 3 meals a day. A bedtime snack is offered.
- The center provides needed adaptive equipment (assistive devices) and utensils (see Fig. 29-1). They promote independence. Make sure the person has needed equipment.

Dining Programs

Nursing center dining programs vary. These are examples.

- *Social dining.* A table seats 4 to 6 residents (Fig. 29-3). Food items are selected from a daily menu. Food is served as in a restaurant. Residents feed themselves if able. Staff help with feeding as needed.
- *Low-stimulation dining.* Distractions are prevented. The health team decides where each person should sit.
- *Restaurant-style menus.* Food is selected from a menu to allow more food choices. The person is served as in a restaurant.
- *Open dining.* A buffet is open for several hours. Residents can eat any time while the buffet is open.

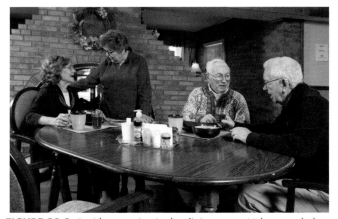

FIGURE 29-3 Residents eating in the dining room. Volunteers help as needed.

PREPARING FOR MEALS

Preparing patients and residents for meals promotes comfort. To promote comfort:

- Provide oral hygiene. Make sure dentures are in place.
- Make sure eyeglasses and hearing aids are in place.
- Assist with elimination needs.
- Make sure incontinent persons are clean and dry.
- Position the person in a comfortable, upright position.
- Reduce or remove unpleasant odors, sights, and sounds. See Chapter 19.
- Follow the care plan for pain-relief measures. See Chapter 33.
- Assist the person with hand hygiene.
  See *Delegation Guidelines: Preparing for Meals.*
  See *Promoting Safety and Comfort: Preparing for Meals.*
  See procedure: *Preparing the Person for a Meal.*

DELEGATION GUIDELINES
Preparing for Meals

To prepare a person for a meal, you need this information from the nurse and the care plan.

- How much help the person needs
- Where the person will eat—room or dining room
- What the person uses for elimination—toilet, commode, bedpan, or urinal
- What type of oral hygiene to give
- If the person wears dentures
- If the person wears eyeglasses or hearing aids
- How to position the person—in bed, a chair, or wheelchair
- If the person needs help to the dining room
- If the person uses a wheelchair, walker, or cane
- When to report observations
- What patient or resident concerns to report at once

PROMOTING SAFETY AND COMFORT
Preparing for Meals

Safety

Before meals, the person needs to eliminate and have oral hygiene and hand hygiene. Follow the practices of medical asepsis and Standard Precautions. Also follow them to clean equipment and the room.

> NOTE: *This task may require more than 1 pair of gloves. Change gloves as needed. Use careful judgment. Remember to practice hand hygiene after removing gloves.*

Preparing the Person for a Meal

Quality of Life

- Knock before entering the person's room.
- Address the person by name.
- Introduce yourself by name and title.
- Explain the procedure before starting and during the procedure.
- Protect the person's rights during the procedure.
- Handle the person gently during the procedure.

Pre-Procedure

1 Follow *Delegation Guidelines: Preparing for Meals.* See *Promoting Safety and Comfort: Preparing for Meals.*
2 Practice hand hygiene and get the following supplies.
  - Supplies for oral hygiene (Chapter 21)
  - Supplies for elimination (Chapter 25)
  - Supplies for hand hygiene—hand-wipes or soap, water, washcloth, and towel
  - Supplies for a transfer if needed (Chapter 18)
  - Gloves

3 Arrange items in the person's room.
4 Practice hand hygiene.
5 Identify the person. Check the identification (ID) bracelet against the assignment sheet. Use 2 identifiers (Chapter 11). Also call the person by name.
6 Provide for privacy.

Procedure

7 Make sure eyeglasses and hearing aids are in place.
8 Assist with oral hygiene as needed. Make sure dentures are in place. Wear gloves and practice hand hygiene after removing and discarding them.
9 Assist with elimination as needed. Make sure the person is clean and dry if incontinent. Wear gloves and practice hand hygiene after removing and discarding them.
10 Assist with hand hygiene. Wear gloves and practice hand hygiene after removing and discarding them.

11 *For the person who will eat in bed:*
  a Raise the head of the bed to a comfortable position—Fowler's (45 to 60 degrees) or high-Fowler's (60 to 90 degrees). (NOTE: Some state competency tests require at least 45 degrees, others require 75 to 90 degrees.)
  b Remove items from the over-bed table. Clean the table.
  c Adjust the over-bed table in front of the person.
12 *For the person who will sit in a chair:*
  a Position the person in a chair or wheelchair.
  b Remove items from the over-bed table. Clean the table.
  c Adjust the over-bed table in front of the person.
13 *For the person who eats in the dining room,* assist the person to the dining room.

Post-Procedure

14 Provide for comfort. (See the inside of the back cover.)
15 Place the call light and other needed items within reach.
16 Clean and disinfect equipment as needed. Return equipment to its proper place. Wear gloves and practice hand hygiene after removing and discarding them.
17 Straighten the room. Eliminate unpleasant noise, odors, or equipment.

18 Follow the care plan and the person's preferences for privacy measures to maintain. Leaving the privacy curtain, window coverings, and door open or closed are examples.
19 Complete a safety check of the room. (See the inside of the back cover.)
20 Practice hand hygiene.
21 Report and record your care and observations.

SERVING MEALS

Food is served in covered containers to keep foods at the correct temperature. Hot food is kept hot. Cold food is kept cold. Uncover food just before the person eats. Uncovered food changes temperature quickly.

Prepare persons for meals before food is served. If they are ready to eat, you can serve meals promptly. Food is kept at the correct temperature.

Serve meals in the assigned order. In nursing centers, residents seated at tables are served at the same time.

If food is not served within 15 minutes, re-check food temperatures. Follow agency policy. If not at the correct temperature, get fresh food. Temperature guides and food thermometers are in dining rooms and in nursing unit kitchens. Some agencies allow re-heating in microwave ovens.

Snacks are served upon arrival on the nursing unit. Provide needed utensils, a straw, and a napkin. Follow the same considerations and procedures for serving meals and feeding the person (p. 371).

See *Delegation Guidelines: Serving Meals,* p. 370.
See *Promoting Safety and Comfort: Serving Meals,* p. 370.
See procedure: *Serving Meal Trays,* p. 370.

DELEGATION GUIDELINES

Serving Meals

To serve meal trays, you need this information from the nurse and the care plan.

- The person's food allergies or intolerances (if any)
- What adaptive equipment (assistive devices) are needed
- If the person needs help opening cartons, cutting food, buttering bread, and so on
- If the person's food intake (Chapter 28) and fluid intake (Chapter 30) are measured
- When to report observations
- What patient or resident concerns to report at once

PROMOTING SAFETY AND COMFORT

Serving Meals

Safety

Always check food temperature after re-heating. Food that is too hot can cause burns.

After eating, check the person's mouth for food (pocketing). Remove any food. Follow these safety measures.

- Use sponge swabs (Chapter 21) as needed. Wear gloves. Practice hand hygiene after removing and discarding them.
- Have the person tip the chin downward (toward the chest) to prevent aspiration.
- Call for the nurse if you cannot remove food easily.

Comfort

Check the person's position when serving a meal. The position may have changed after the person was prepared to eat. Provide other comfort measures as needed. See the inside of the back cover.

Serving Meal Trays

Quality of Life

- Knock before entering the person's room.
- Address the person by name.
- Introduce yourself by name and title.

- Explain the procedure before starting and during the procedure.
- Protect the person's rights during the procedure.
- Handle the person gently during the procedure.

Pre-Procedure

1 Follow *Delegation Guidelines: Serving Meals.* See *Promoting Safety and Comfort: Serving Meals.*
2 Practice hand hygiene.

3 Prepare the person for the meal if not already done. See procedure: *Preparing the Person for a Meal,* p. 369.

Procedure

4 Check items on the tray with the dietary card. Make sure the tray is complete and has needed adaptive equipment (assistive devices).
5 Identify the person. Check the ID bracelet against the dietary card. Use 2 identifiers (Chapter 11). Also call the person by name.
6 Place the tray within the person's reach. Adjust the over-bed table as needed.
7 Remove food covers. Open cartons, cut food into bite-sized pieces, butter bread, and so on as needed. Season food as the person prefers and as the care plan allows.
8 Place the napkin, adaptive equipment (assistive devices), and eating utensils within reach. Help the person apply the clothes protector (towel, napkin) if needed.
9 Place the call light within reach.

10 Do the following when the person is done eating.
  a Measure and record fluid intake if ordered (Chapter 30).
  b Note the amount and type of foods eaten (Chapter 28).
  c Check for and remove any food in the mouth (pocketing). See *Promoting Safety and Comfort: Serving Meals.*
  d Remove the item used to protect clothing (clothes protector, towel, napkin). Follow agency policy for used linens. Discard a disposable napkin.
  e Remove the tray.
  f Clean spills. Clean and dry the over-bed table if used. Dry with paper towels. Discard the paper towels.
  g Change any soiled clothing. Follow agency policy for removed clothing.
  h Assist with oral hygiene and hand hygiene. Provide for privacy. Wear gloves. Practice hand hygiene after removing and discarding gloves.
  i Help the person return to bed if needed.

Post-Procedure

11 Provide for comfort. (See the inside of the back cover.)
12 Place the call light and other needed items within reach.
13 Raise or lower bed rails. Follow the care plan.
14 Complete a safety check of the room. (See the inside of the back cover.)
15 Follow the care plan and the person's preferences for privacy measures to maintain. Leaving the privacy curtain, window coverings, and door open or closed are examples.

16 Follow agency policy for used linens.
17 Practice hand hygiene.
18 Report and record your care and observations.

FEEDING THE PERSON

Weakness, paralysis, casts, confusion, and other limits can make self-feeding impossible. These persons are fed.

Serve food and fluids in the order the person prefers. Offer fluids during the meal. Fluids help the person chew and swallow.

Use teaspoons to feed the person. They are safer than forks. The teaspoon should be only one-third (⅓) full (Fig. 29-4). This portion is chewed and swallowed easily. Some people need smaller portions. Follow the care plan.

Persons who need to be fed may feel angry or embarrassed. Some are depressed, resentful, or refuse to eat. Let them do what they can. Some can handle "finger foods" (bread, cookies, crackers). If strong enough, let them hold milk or juice cups (never hot drinks). Follow ordered activity limits. Provide support. Encourage them to try, even if food is spilled.

Visually impaired persons often recognize foods from their aromas. Describe what is on the plate and what you are offering. For persons who feed themselves, describe foods and fluids and their place on the plate. Use the numbers on a clock for the location of foods (Fig. 29-5).

Many people pray before eating. Allow time and privacy for prayer. This shows respect and caring.

Meals provide social contact with others. Talk with the person. Allow time to chew and swallow. Sit facing the person. Sitting is more relaxing. It shows that you have time. You can also see how well the person is eating and watch for swallowing problems.

See *Focus on Older Persons: Feeding the Person.*
See *Focus on Surveys: Feeding the Person.*
See *Delegation Guidelines: Feeding the Person,* p. 372.
See *Promoting Safety and Comfort: Feeding the Person,* p. 372.
See procedure: *Feeding the Person,* p. 372.

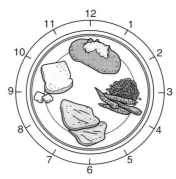

FIGURE 29-5 The numbers on a clock are used to help a visually impaired person locate food.

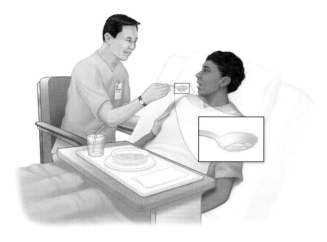

FIGURE 29-4 A spoon is used to feed the person. The spoon is one-third (⅓) full.

FOCUS ON **OLDER PERSONS**

Feeding the Person

Persons with dementia may become distracted during meals. Some do not sit long enough to eat. Others forget how to use eating utensils. Some persons resist efforts to help them eat. A confused person may throw or spit food.

These measures may be helpful for persons with dementia. Follow the person's care plan.
- Keep meal times and the setting consistent.
- Provide a calm, quiet setting. Limit noise and distractions. This helps the person focus.
- Limit the number of food choices.
- Offer several small meals during the day instead of larger ones.
- Use straws or cups with lids. These make drinking easier.
- Provide finger foods if the person has problems with utensils. A bowl may be easier to use than a plate.
- Provide healthy snacks. Keep snacks where the person can see them.

Be patient. Tell the nurse if you feel upset or impatient. The person has the right to be treated with dignity and respect.

FOCUS ON **SURVEYS**

Feeding the Person

Surveyors focus on nutritional needs. They observe if staff:
- Provide help with eating.
- Encourage the person to eat.
- Help the person use adaptive equipment (assistive devices).
- Feed the person if necessary.

DELEGATION GUIDELINES

Feeding the Person

Before feeding a person, you need this information from the nurse and the care plan.

- The person's food allergies or intolerances (if any)
- Why the person needs help
- How much help the person needs
- How to position the person
- If the person can manage finger foods
- The person's activity limits
- The person's dietary restrictions
- Feeding portion size—⅓ teaspoonful or less
- Needed safety measures if the person has dysphagia
- If the person can use a straw
- What observations to report and record:
  - The amount and kind of food eaten
  - Complaints of nausea or dysphagia
  - Signs and symptoms of dysphagia
  - Signs and symptoms of aspiration
- When to report observations
- What patient or resident concerns to report at once

PROMOTING SAFETY AND COMFORT

Feeding the Person

Safety

Check food temperature. Very hot foods and fluids can burn the person.

Prevent aspiration. Check the person's mouth before offering more food or fluids. The mouth must be empty between bites and swallows.

The person must be alert enough to eat. Health problems, drug side effects, and fatigue can affect level of consciousness. *Do not try to feed a person who is drowsy.* Tell the nurse right away.

Some training programs do not allow students to feed residents in their rooms without staff or the instructor present. Some training programs only allow students to assist with feeding in the dining area. Follow the rules for your training program.

Comfort

The person will eat better if not rushed. Sit to show that you have time. Standing communicates being in a hurry.

Wipe the person's hands, face, and mouth as needed during the meal. Use the napkin or a wet washcloth. Then dry the person with a towel.

Feeding the Person

Quality of Life

- Knock before entering the person's room.
- Address the person by name.
- Introduce yourself by name and title.

- Explain the procedure before starting and during the procedure.
- Protect the person's rights during the procedure.
- Handle the person gently during the procedure.

Pre-Procedure

1 Follow *Delegation Guidelines: Feeding the Person.* See *Promoting Safety and Comfort:*
   a *Serving Meals, p. 370*
   b *Feeding the Person*
2 Practice hand hygiene.

3 Position the person in a comfortable position for eating—sitting in a chair or in Fowler's (45 to 60 degrees) or high-Fowler's (60 to 90 degrees). (NOTE: Some state competency tests require at least 45 degrees, others require 75 to 90 degrees.)
4 Get the tray. Place the tray on the over-bed table or dining table where the person can reach it.

Procedure

5 Check items on the tray with the dietary card. Make sure the tray is complete.
6 Identify the person. Check the ID bracelet against the dietary card. Use 2 identifiers (Chapter 11). Also call the person by name.
7 Drape a napkin across the person's chest and underneath the chin. Or apply a clothes protector or towel.
8 Clean the person's hands. (NOTE: Some state competency tests require soap and water. Others allow hand sanitizer or a hand-wipe.)
9 Tell the person what foods and fluids are on the tray.
10 Prepare food for eating. Cut food into bite-sized pieces. Season food as the person prefers and as the care plan allows.
11 Place the chair where you can sit comfortably. Sit facing the person at eye level.
12 Serve foods in the order the person prefers. Identify foods as you serve them. Alternate between solid and liquid foods. Use a spoon for safety (see Fig. 29-4). Allow enough time to chew and swallow. Do not rush the person.

13 Offer fluids (water, coffee, milk, juice, tea, or other fluid) frequently. (NOTE: Some state competency tests require that a drink is offered for at least every 2 to 3 bites of food.)
14 Check the person's mouth before offering more food or fluids. Make sure the mouth is empty between bites and swallows. Ask if the person is ready for the next bite or drink.
15 Use straws (if allowed) for liquids if the person cannot drink out of a glass or cup. Have 1 straw for each liquid. Provide short straws for weak persons. Follow the care plan for using straws.
16 Wipe the person's hands, face, and mouth as needed during the meal. Use the napkin or a hand-wipe.
17 Follow the care plan if the person has dysphagia. (Some persons with dysphagia do not use straws.) Give thickened liquid with a spoon if needed.
18 Talk with the person in a pleasant manner.
19 Encourage the person to eat as much as possible.

Feeding the Person—cont'd

Procedure—cont'd

20 Wipe the person's mouth with a napkin or a hand-wipe when finished. Discard the napkin or hand-wipe.
21 Note how much and which foods were eaten (Chapter 28).
22 Measure and record fluid intake if ordered (Chapter 30).
23 Remove the item used to protect clothing (clothes protector, towel, napkin). Follow agency policy for used linens. Discard a disposable napkin.

24 Remove the tray.
25 Take the person to his or her room (if in a dining area). Clean and dry the over-bed table (if used in the person's room). Dry with paper towels. Discard the paper towels.
26 Assist with oral hygiene and hand hygiene. Provide for privacy. Wear gloves. Practice hand hygiene after removing and discarding gloves.

Post-Procedure

27 Provide for comfort. (See the inside of the back cover.)
28 Place the call light and other needed items within reach.
29 Raise or lower bed rails. Follow the care plan.
30 Complete a safety check of the room. (See the inside of the back cover.)

31 Follow the care plan and the person's preferences for privacy measures to maintain. Leaving the privacy curtain, window coverings, and door open or closed are examples.
32 Return the food tray to the food cart.
33 Practice hand hygiene.
34 Report and record your care and observations.

ASSISTING WITH SPECIAL NEEDS

Some persons cannot eat or drink because of illness, surgery, or injury. They may have chewing, swallowing, or other eating problems. Others cannot eat enough to meet their nutritional needs. Nutritional support may be ordered to meet food and fluid needs.

See *Delegation Guidelines: Assisting With Special Needs.*

DELEGATION GUIDELINES

Assisting With Special Needs

Your state and agency may not allow you to assist with some care measures or procedures involving nutritional support. Before assisting, make sure that:
• Your state allows you to perform the task.
• The task is in your job description.
• You have the necessary education and training.
• You know how to use the agency's equipment and supplies.
• You review the agency's procedure.
• You review the task with the nurse.
• A nurse is available to guide and assist you as needed.
• An RN (registered nurse) has identified and labeled all tubes, catheters, and needles.

Enteral Nutrition

Some persons require enteral nutrition. *Enteral nutrition is giving nutrients into the gastro-intestinal (GI) tract (enteral) through a feeding tube.* These feeding tubes are common.
• *Naso-gastric (NG) tube.* A feeding tube is inserted through the nose (*naso*) into the stomach (*gastro*) (Fig. 29-6).
• *Gastrostomy tube.* A feeding tube is inserted through a surgically created opening (*stomy*) in the stomach (*gastro*) (Fig. 29-7).

Receiving nutrients through a tube (tube feeding) replaces or supplements (adds to) normal nutrition. *Gavage is the process of giving a tube feeding* (Fig. 29-8, p. 374).

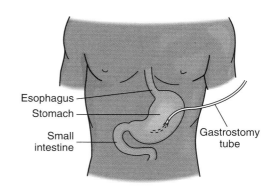

FIGURE 29-6 A naso-gastric (NG) tube is inserted through the nose and esophagus and into the stomach.

FIGURE 29-7 A gastrostomy tube.

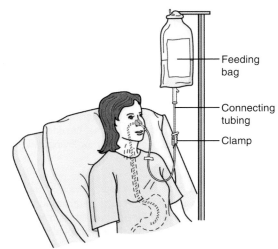

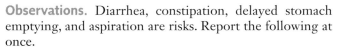

FIGURE 29-8 A tube feeding is given. (NOTE: The feeding tube is secured to the person's nose and shirt.)

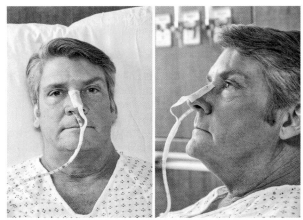

FIGURE 29-9 The feeding tube is secured to the nose. (From Perry AG, Potter PA, Ostendorf WR: *Nursing interventions & clinical skills*, ed 7, St Louis, 2020, Elsevier.)

Observations. Diarrhea, constipation, delayed stomach emptying, and aspiration are risks. Report the following at once.
- Nausea
- Discomfort during the feeding
- Vomiting
- Distended (enlarged and swollen) abdomen
- Coughing
- Complaints of indigestion or heartburn
- Redness, irritation, swelling, drainage, odor, or pain at the tube's insertion site
- Fever
- Signs and symptoms of respiratory distress (Chapter 37)
- Increased pulse rate
- Complaints of flatulence (Chapter 27)
- Diarrhea (Chapter 27)

Regurgitation and Aspiration. Aspiration is a major risk from tube feedings. It can cause pneumonia and death. Aspiration can occur:
- *During insertion.* An NG tube can slip into the airway. An x-ray is taken after insertion to check tube placement.
- *From the tube moving out of place.* Coughing, sneezing, vomiting, suctioning (the process of withdrawing or sucking up fluids), and poor positioning are common causes. A tube can move from the stomach into the esophagus and then into the airway. The RN checks tube placement before a feeding. *You never check feeding tube placement.*
- *From regurgitation.* **Regurgitation** *is the backward flow of stomach contents into the mouth.* Delayed stomach emptying and over-feeding are common causes.

Preventing Regurgitation and Aspiration. To help prevent regurgitation and aspiration:
- Position the person in Fowler's or semi-Fowler's position during feedings. Follow the care plan and the nurse's directions.
- Maintain Fowler's or semi-Fowler's position after feedings. Do so for 1 to 2 hours after a feeding or at all times. This allows formula to move through the GI tract. Follow the care plan and the nurse's directions.
- Avoid the left side-lying position. It prevents the stomach from emptying into the small intestine.

Comfort Measures. Persons with feeding tubes usually are not allowed to eat or drink. The abbreviation *NPO* means *nothing by mouth*. Dry mouth, dry lips, and sore throat cause discomfort. Sometimes hard candy or gum is allowed. These measures are common every 2 hours while the person is awake.
- Oral hygiene
- Lubricant for the lips
- Mouth rinses

Feeding tubes can irritate and cause pressure on the nose. These measures are common.
- Clean the nose and nostrils every 4 to 8 hours.
- Secure the tube to the nose (Fig. 29-9). Use tape or a tube holder. Tube holders have foam cushions that prevent pressure on the nose. Re-taping is not needed. Re-taping irritates the nose.
- Secure the tube to the person's garment at the shoulder area (see Fig. 29-8). Do 1 of the following according to agency policy.
  - Loop a rubber band around the tube. Then pin the rubber band to the garment with a safety pin.
  - Tape the tube to the garment.

FOCUS ON P R I D E

The Person, Family, and Yourself

P ersonal and Professional Responsibility

The person's care plan includes food allergies and intolerances and any special dietary needs. These are often listed on the dietary card delivered with the meal tray. You are responsible for following each person's care plan. Check the meal tray and dietary card carefully. If you have a question, ask the nurse.

R ights and Respect

The person has the right to refuse a food or drink because of personal preference. If refused, a substitute (alternative) should be offered.

I ndependence and Social Interaction

You can help make meal time pleasant. Smile and greet each person as you serve food. Ask if help is needed. Talk with the person as you prepare food. When feeding, focus on the person. Meal time should be as pleasant as possible.

D elegation and Teamwork

Meals are a busy time. Teamwork is important. Staff work together to help residents to the dining area and serve food promptly. Staff must make sure everyone is served and nutrition needs are met. Have a helpful attitude.

E thics and Laws

A person's nutrition needs can change. Poor appetite, decreased food intake, and weight loss signal a change. The health team must address changes in nutrition needs. Neglect can result from unmet needs. Tell the nurse about any changes or concerns.

FOCUS ON PRIDE: *Application*

How do sights, sounds, smells, and personal preferences affect meal time? How can you help make it pleasant?

REVIEW QUESTIONS

Circle the BEST answer.

1 These statements are about factors affecting eating and nutrition. Which is *true*?
   a Culture and religion do not affect dietary practices.
   b Negative body reactions affect food choices.
   c Less nutrients are needed during illness and recovery.
   d Food appearance and smell are not important factors.

2 Persons with dysphagia
   a Are fed in the semi-Fowler's position
   b Have a regular diet
   c Are fed according to the care plan
   d Eat alone in their rooms

3 A person coughs and drools while eating. You should
   a Give the person a drink
   b Puree the person's food
   c Give mouth care and continue feeding
   d Tell the nurse

4 A person requires pudding-thick liquid. This liquid should be
   a Mildly thick and able to flow through a straw
   b Moderately thick and flow off of a spoon
   c Moderately thick with lumps
   d Extremely thick and mound on a spoon

5 Nursing centers must
   a Serve food promptly
   b Serve 2 meals a day
   c Serve food at room temperature to avoid burns
   d Serve food under-seasoned to lower sodium intake

6 A resident refuses to eat pork. The person
   a Should be offered a different item of similar nutritional value
   b Cannot refuse menu items without a special diet order
   c Should have the family bring a meal when pork is served
   d Needs to try foods before refusing them

Continued

7 Which promotes comfort and preparation for a meal?
   a The urinal is nearby and contains urine.
   b The incontinent person is clean and dry.
   c Dentures are in the denture cup in the bathroom.
   d The person used the bathroom without hand hygiene afterward.

8 A person needs help opening cartons and cutting food. You should
   a Ask dietary staff to help the person
   b Tell the person you do not have time
   c Assist the person as needed
   d Refuse to help to promote independence

9 A person is served a meal tray. Which is a problem?
   a The food was served in a covered container.
   b The tray contains adaptive equipment (assistive devices).
   c The dietary card lists "strawberries" as an allergy. Pears were served.
   d The dietary card lists "pureed diet." A whole pork chop was served.

10 You are assisting with feeding in the dining room. A person is drowsy and will not drink from a straw. You should
   a Yell to awaken the person
   b Tell the nurse right away
   c Try to give the person bites of food
   d Go feed someone else

11 When feeding a person
   a Ask in what order the person likes foods served
   b Use a fork
   c Stand facing the person
   d Talk with your co-workers

12 After feeding a person
   a Leave the person's clothing protector in place
   b Use your fingers to remove food left in the mouth
   c Clean the person's face and hands
   d Position the person supine if aspiration is a risk

13 Which position prevents regurgitation after a tube feeding?
   a Fowler's or semi-Fowler's position
   b The supine position
   c The left or right side-lying position
   d The prone position

14 A person with a feeding tube is NPO. Which should you question?
   a Provide oral hygiene.
   b Provide mouth rinses.
   c Give clear liquids.
   d Apply lubricant to the lips.

15 A person has an NG tube. To prevent nasal irritation
   a Clean the tube every 8 hours
   b Replace the tape on the nose every 4 hours
   c Remove the tube every 4 hours
   d Secure the tube to the person's gown

Answers to Chapter 29 questions are on p. 588.

FOCUS ON PRACTICE

Problem Solving

After receiving a breakfast tray, a resident says: "I didn't ask for eggs this morning." You check the dietary card and notice the tray is for another person. What will you do? Why is this a problem?

CHAPTER 30

Fluid Needs

OBJECTIVES

- Define the key terms and key abbreviations in this chapter.
- Describe adult fluid requirements.
- Identify the causes and signs and symptoms of dehydration.
- Explain how to assist with special fluid orders.
- Explain the purpose of intake and output records.
- Identify what to count as fluid intake and output.
- Explain how to assist with fluid needs.
- Explain how to provide drinking water.
- Explain how to assist with IV therapy.
- Perform the procedures described in this chapter.
- Explain how to promote PRIDE in the person, the family, and yourself.

KEY TERMS

dehydration A decrease in the amount of water in the body
edema The swelling of body tissues with water
flow rate The number of drops per minute (gtt/min) or milliliters per hour (mL/hr)

graduate A measuring container for fluid
intake The amount of fluid taken in; input
intravenous (IV) therapy Giving fluids through a tube inserted into a vein; IV and IV infusion
output The amount of fluid lost

KEY ABBREVIATIONS

gtt	Drops
gtt/min	Drops per minute
ID	Identification
I&O	Intake and output
IV	Intravenous

mL	Milliliter
mL/hr	Milliliters per hour
NPO	*Nil per os;* nothing by mouth
oz	Ounce

Water is needed to live. Death can result from too much or too little water. You will help meet fluid needs. Measuring intake and output and providing drinking water are examples.

Some persons need intravenous (IV) therapy to meet fluid needs. You must understand your role limits and how to safely assist with IV therapy.

FLUID BALANCE

Water is ingested through fluids and foods. Water is normally lost through urine and feces (stools). It is also lost through the skin (perspiration) and the lungs (expiration).

The words *hydrated* and *hydration* relate to normal fluid balance. When a person is hydrated, the body has enough water to function normally. For normal hydration, fluid intake must roughly equal output.

- **Intake** *(input) is the amount of fluid taken in.*
- **Output** *is the amount of fluid lost.*

Edema occurs when fluid intake exceeds fluid output. *Edema is the swelling of body tissues with water.* It is common in people with heart, kidney, and liver diseases. Edema often occurs in the legs, ankles, and feet (Fig. 30-1). *Pulmonary edema* is a severe form of edema affecting the lungs (Chapter 40).

Dehydration occurs when output exceeds intake. *Dehydration is a decrease in the amount of water in the body.* Common causes and signs and symptoms of dehydration are listed in Box 30-1.

See *Focus on Older Persons: Fluid Balance.*

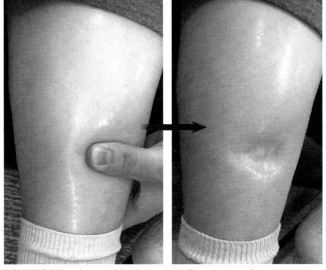

FIGURE 30-1 Edema in the lower leg. The nurse applies pressure to the body part to check for edema. (Courtesy Kellie White.)

BOX 30-1 Dehydration

Common Causes
- Bleeding
- Diarrhea
- Drug therapy
- Fever
- Fluid intake: poor
- Fluid restriction
- Fluids: refusing
- Function problems: difficulty drinking, reaching fluids, communicating fluid needs
- Level of consciousness: altered
- Sweating (perspiration): excess *(diaphoresis)*
- Urine production: increased
- Vomiting

Signs and Symptoms
- Blood pressure: low
- Confusion, delirium (Chapter 42)
- Dark yellow or amber colored urine
- Dizziness, feeling light-headed
- Dry, cool skin
- Dry mouth, coated tongue
- Fatigue
- Headache
- Irritability
- Muscle cramps
- *Oliguria*—scant (small) amount of urine
- Postural hypotension (Chapter 32)
- Poor *skin turgor*—when pinched and released, skin slowly returns to its normal position
- Pulse: fast
- Respirations: fast
- Shock (Chapter 43)
- Thirst
- Unconsciousness

FOCUS ON OLDER PERSONS

Fluid Balance

The amount of body water decreases as people age. In older persons, the thirst sensation decreases. They need water but may not feel thirsty. Offer water often.

Older persons are at risk for diseases affecting fluid balance. They commonly take drugs that affect fluid balance. Dehydration and edema are risks. Some persons have special fluid orders.

Persons with dementia are at higher risk for dehydration (Chapter 42). In early dementia, the person may not remember to drink fluids regularly. As dementia progresses, the person may have trouble turning on a faucet or filling a cup. In the late stage, communicating needs is severely impaired. Follow the care plan to meet the person's needs. Observe closely for signs and symptoms of dehydration.

Normal Fluid Requirements

An adult needs 1500 mL (milliliters) of fluid daily to survive. About 2000 to 2500 mL are needed for normal fluid balance. Fluid requirements increase with hot weather, exercise, fever, illness, and excess fluid losses.

SPECIAL FLUID ORDERS

The person may need a special fluid order to meet fluid needs. The order is part of the person's care plan. The nurse teaches the person and family what the person is allowed to have. Common fluid orders are listed in Table 30-1.

TABLE 30-1   Common Fluid Orders

Fluid Order	Description	Some Uses	Care Measures
Encourage fluids	The person drinks an increased amount of fluid.	Dehydration, urinary tract infections, kidney stones	• Follow the care plan for the amount. • Keep a variety of fluids within the person's reach. • Offer fluids often and help the person drink if not able to do so alone.
Restrict fluids	Fluids are limited to a certain amount.	Edema, kidney failure, heart failure	• Follow the care plan for the amount allowed. • Offer fluids in small amounts and in small containers. • Remove the water mug or keep it out of sight. • Provide frequent oral hygiene to keep the mouth moist.
Nothing by mouth (NPO)	The person cannot eat or drink anything. NPO stands for *nil per os*—nothing *(nil)* by *(per)* mouth *(os)*.	Before and after surgery, before some laboratory tests and diagnostic procedures, to treat certain illnesses	• Post an NPO sign above the bed or at the room door. Follow agency policy. • Remove the water mug from the room. • Provide frequent oral hygiene. The person must not swallow any fluid. • Follow the nurse's directions for how long the person will be NPO. The person is NPO for 6 to 12 hours before surgery and for some tests and procedures.
Thickened liquids	Water and all fluids are thickened by the dietary department.	Difficulty swallowing *(dysphagia)*	• Serve thickened liquids as directed by the nurse and the care plan. Thickened commercial fluids are used. Or the dietary department thickens fluids. • Follow agency policy for how to record intake for thickened liquids. • See "Dysphagia" in Chapter 29.

INTAKE AND OUTPUT

An intake and output (I&O) record monitors the amounts of fluid taken into (intake) and fluid leaving (output) the body. You will measure and record I&O.

• *Intake.* All oral fluids are measured and recorded—water, milk, coffee, tea, juices, soups, and soft drinks. So are foods that melt at room temperature—ice cream, sherbet, custard, gelatin, and Popsicles. The nurse measures and records intravenous (IV) fluids (p. 384) and tube feedings (Chapter 29).
• *Output.* Urine, vomitus, diarrhea, and wound drainage amounts are measured and recorded. Output from an ostomy (Chapter 27) and drainage from suction are also included as output. (*Suction* means *to withdraw fluid.* Fluid suctioned from the stomach through a naso-gastric [NG] tube is an example.)

I&O records are used to plan and evaluate treatment. They also are kept for special fluid orders.

Measuring Intake and Output

Intake and output are measured in milliliters (mL). See Box 30-2 for amounts to know.

You must know the serving sizes of bowls, dishes, cups, pitchers, mugs, glasses, and other containers. This information may be on the I&O record (Fig. 30-2, p. 380). Or the serving size is on the container.

A measuring container for fluid is called a **graduate.** Like a measuring cup, the graduate is marked in ounces (oz) and milliliters (mL). For an accurate measurement, place the device on a flat surface and read it at eye level (Fig. 30-3, p. 380). Separate graduates are used for intake and for output.

The amount measured is recorded in the correct column on the I&O record (see Fig. 30-2). Amounts are totaled at the end of the shift and 24-hour day. The totals are entered into the person's medical record.

The urinal, commode, bedpan, or specimen pan (Chapter 34) is used to void. Remind the person not to void in the toilet. Urine voided into the toilet cannot be measured. Also remind the person to put toilet paper into the wastebasket.

See *Focus on Math: Measuring Intake and Output*, p. 381.
See *Delegation Guidelines: Measuring Intake and Output*, p. 382.
See *Promoting Safety and Comfort: Measuring Intake and Output*, p. 382.
See procedure: *Measuring Intake and Output*, p. 382.

BOX 30-2 I&O Measures

1 cubic centimeter (cc) = 1 mL
1 teaspoon = 5 mL
1 tablespoon = 15 mL
1 oz = 30 mL

1 cup = 240 mL
1 pint = about 500 mL
1 quart = about 1000 mL
1 liter (L) = 1000 mL

FLUID INTAKE AND OUTPUT FLOW SHEET
DATE *Oct 12*

RECORD TOTALS IN PATIENT'S MEDICAL RECORD		DIET/FLUID ORDERS *Regular*	
Water glass	240 mL	Gelatin	120 mL
Juice glass	120 mL	Ice cream	90 mL
Milk carton	240 mL	Broth/strained soup	180 mL
Coffee cup	240 mL	Styrofoam cup	180 mL
Soft drink can	360 mL	Water mug	1000 mL
Tea glass	180 mL	Ice chips	½ amount of mL in cup

		INTAKE				OUTPUT		
TIME	ORAL	TYPE & AMOUNT	TIME	IV	ENTERAL	TIME	SOURCE	AMOUNT
	FLUIDS					2330	Void	225 mL
						0545	Void	325 mL
0645	MUG/OTHER	Water 200 mL						
		8-HOUR SUB-TOTAL			200 mL	**8-HOUR SUB-TOTAL**		550 mL
0830	BREAKFAST	Coffee 240 mL Milk 160 mL				0750	Void	200 mL
						0930	Void	225 mL
						1145	Void	250 mL
						1330	Void	200 mL
1015	SNACK	Juice 120 mL						
1230	LUNCH	Soft drink 240 mL Ice cream 90 mL Soup 90 mL						
	SNACK							
1450	MUG/OTHER	Water 300 mL						
		8-HOUR SUB-TOTAL			1240 mL	**8-HOUR SUB-TOTAL**		875 mL
1740	DINNER	Tea 180 mL Soft drink 100 mL				1505	Void	275 mL
						1655	Void	150 mL
						2010	Void	150 mL
						2115	Vomitus	100 mL
1930	SNACK	Gelatin 120 mL						
2230	MUG/OTHER	Water 325 mL						
		8-HOUR SUB-TOTAL			725 mL	**8-HOUR SUB-TOTAL**		675 mL
		24-HOUR TOTAL			2165 mL	**24-HOUR TOTAL**		2100 mL

(Left margin time blocks: 2300-0700, 0700-1500, 1500-2300)

FIGURE 30-2 A sample intake and output (I&O) record.

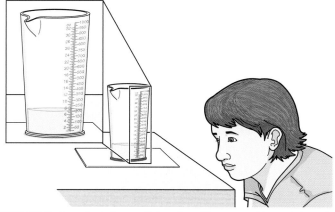

FIGURE 30-3 A graduate is on a flat surface. The amount is read at eye level.

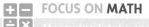

FOCUS ON MATH

Measuring Intake and Output

To measure I&O, you must accurately read and calculate measurements.

Reading Measuring Containers

Measuring containers (graduates, urinals, and specimen pans) are marked in mL (milliliters) and oz (ounces). The container may not have all lines labeled. To calculate unlabeled measurements (Fig. 30-4):

1 Choose the labeled line above the fluid level and the labeled line below it.

400 mL and 300 mL

2 Subtract these 2 numbers. The result is called the *difference.*

400 mL − 300 mL = 100 mL

3 Count the number of spaces between the 2 labeled lines in step 1.

4 spaces

4 Divide the difference in step 2 by the number of spaces.

100 mL ÷ 4 spaces = 25 mL
Each line increases by 25 mL.

NOTE: Some state competency tests instruct to round up to the nearest 25 mL if the fluid level is between measurement lines. To *round up* means to choose the higher value.

Converting Ounces to Milliliters

In health care settings, intake is measured in mL (milliliters). Some containers show the serving amount in oz (ounces). You need to convert (change) the serving amount from oz to mL. One oz equals 30 mL (1 oz = 30 mL). To convert, multiply the number of oz by 30. For example:

A *coffee cup holds 8 oz. Multiply 8 oz by 30 (the number of mL in each oz). The 8 oz coffee cup equals 240 mL.*

8 oz × 30 mL/oz = 240 mL
(mL/oz is read as "milliliters per ounce")
8 oz equals 240 mL.

Measuring Intake

To measure intake, subtract the amount of liquid left (remaining amount) from the full amount of liquid served (full serving amount).

1 Check the full serving amount. This is found on the container or on the I&O record.
2 Measure the amount of liquid left in the container. Use a graduate.
3 Subtract the amount in step 2 from the amount in step 1. For example:

A *person was served a 120 mL glass of juice. You pour the liquid left in the glass into a graduate. You measure 90 mL in the graduate and calculate the intake amount.*

120 mL (amount served) − 90 mL (amount left) =
30 mL (intake amount)

The person drank 30 mL of juice.

For total intake for a meal, measure the intake for each liquid served. Add the intake amounts from each liquid together. For example:

A *person drank all of a cup of coffee (240 mL) and 30 mL of juice.*

Liquid	Amount Served	Amount Left	Intake Amount
Coffee	240 mL	0 mL	240 mL
Juice	120 mL	90 mL	30 mL
		Total Intake	240 mL + 30 mL = 270 mL

The total intake for this meal was 270 mL.

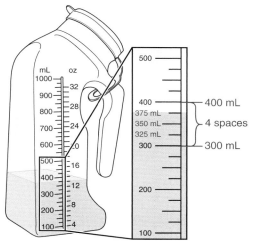

400 mL − 300 mL = 100 mL
100 mL ÷ 4 = 25 mL
Each line increases by 25 mL.

FIGURE 30-4 Calculating unlabeled measurements. Divide the difference between 2 labeled lines by the number of spaces between the 2 lines. Each line on this urinal increases by 25 mL. The measurements between 300 mL and 400 mL are 325 mL, 350 mL, and 375 mL.

Measuring Output

For output, measure the amount of liquid in the measuring device (graduate, urinal, specimen pan). See "Reading Measuring Containers" if you need to calculate an unlabeled measurement on the device.

Totaling I&O for a Shift

A shift total (sub-total) is calculated at the end of the shift. See Figure 30-2. The intake amounts during the shift are added together. The output amounts during the shift are added together. For example:

- Intake for a shift—during your shift a person drank 220 mL at breakfast, 390 mL at lunch, 90 mL as a snack, and 400 mL of water. The total intake for your shift is 1100 mL.

220 mL + 390 mL + 90 mL + 400 mL = 1100mL

- Output for a shift—a person voided 3 times during your shift. The amounts were 200 mL, 250 mL, and 100 mL. The total output for your shift is 550 mL.

200 mL + 250 mL + 100 mL = 550 mL

Totaling 24-Hour I&O

Intake and output amounts are totaled at the end of the 24-hour day. See Figure 30-2. The intake amounts for the full day are added together. The output amounts for the full day are added together. For example:

- 24-hour intake—a person drank 125 mL during the first shift, 1100 mL during the second shift, and 600 mL during the third shift. The total 24-hour intake amount is 1825 mL.

125 mL + 1100 mL + 600 mL = 1825 mL

- 24-hour output—a person voided 450 mL during the first shift, 550 mL during the second shift, and 800 mL during the third shift. The total 24-hour output amount is 1800 mL.

450 mL + 550 mL + 800 mL = 1800 mL

DELEGATION GUIDELINES

Measuring Intake and Output

When measuring I&O, you need this information from the nurse and the care plan.

- If the person has a special fluid order (p. 378)
- When to report measurements—hourly or end-of-shift
- What the person uses for voiding—urinal, bedpan, commode, or specimen pan (Chapters 25 and 34)
- If the person has a catheter (Chapter 26)
- What patient or resident concerns to report at once

PROMOTING SAFETY AND COMFORT

Measuring Intake and Output

Safety

Urine, vomitus, diarrhea, and wound drainage are body fluids. Follow Standard Precautions when measuring output. Follow the Bloodborne Pathogen Standard if blood is present. Follow agency procedures to disinfect the graduate and device used for output collection after use.

Remember to use separate graduates for intake and output.

Note: A task may require more than 1 pair of gloves. Change gloves as needed. Use careful judgment. Remember to practice hand hygiene after removing gloves.

Comfort

Promptly measure and empty the contents of urinals, bedpans, commodes, specimen pans, and kidney basins. This helps prevent or reduce odors. Odors can disturb the person.

Measuring Intake and Output

Quality of Life

- Knock before entering the person's room.
- Address the person by name.
- Introduce yourself by name and title.

- Explain the procedure before starting and during the procedure.
- Protect the person's rights during the procedure.
- Handle the person gently during the procedure.

Pre-Procedure

1 Follow *Delegation Guidelines: Measuring Intake and Output.* See *Promoting Safety and Comfort: Measuring Intake and Output.*
2 Practice hand hygiene and get the following supplies.
  - I&O record
  - 2 graduates:
    - A graduate for intake
    - A graduate for output
  - Needed supplies for urinary or bowel elimination (Chapters 25, 26, and 27)

  - Gloves
  - Paper towels or a disposable waterproof pad
3 Arrange items in the person's room.
4 Practice hand hygiene.
5 Identify the person. Check the identification (ID) bracelet against the I&O record. Use 2 identifiers (Chapter 11). Also call the person by name.
6 Provide for privacy.

Procedure

7 Put on gloves.
8 Measure intake.
  a Pour liquid remaining in the container into the graduate used to measure intake. Avoid spills and splashes on the outside of the graduate.
  b Place the graduate on a flat surface. Measure the amount at eye level (see Fig. 30-3).
  c Check the serving amount on the I&O record. Or check the serving size of each container.
  d Subtract the remaining amount from the full serving amount. Note the amount. (For example, a cup holds 240 mL. The amount in the graduate is 50 mL. 240 mL – 50 mL = 190 mL.)
  e Pour fluid in the graduate back into the container.
  f Repeat steps 8, a–e for each liquid.
  g Add the amounts from each liquid together.
  h Record the time and amount on the I&O record.
  i Empty, clean, rinse, and dry the graduate. Use clean, dry paper towels for drying. Return the graduate to its proper place.

9 Assist with elimination if needed. Measure output.
  a Pour the fluid into the graduate used to measure output. Avoid spills and splashes on the outside of the graduate.
  b Place the device on a paper towel (or disposable waterproof pad) on a flat surface. Measure the amount at eye level.
  c Dispose of fluid in the toilet. Avoid splashes.
  d Rinse the graduate. Pour the rinse into the toilet and flush. Follow agency procedures for cleaning and disinfection. Return the graduate to its proper place.
  e Rinse the voiding receptacle or other container. Pour the rinse into the toilet and flush. Follow agency procedures for cleaning and disinfection. Return the item to its proper place.
  f Remove and discard the gloves. Practice hand hygiene.
  g Record the output amount on the person's I&O record.

Post-Procedure

10 Provide for comfort. (See the inside of the back cover.)
11 Place the call light and other needed items within reach.
12 Follow the care plan and the person's preferences for privacy measures to maintain. Leaving the privacy curtain, window coverings, and door open or closed are examples.

13 Complete a safety check of the room. (See the inside of the back cover.)
14 Practice hand hygiene.
15 Report and record your care and observations.

PROVIDING DRINKING WATER

You normally provide fresh drinking water each shift and when the person's water mug (cup, pitcher) is empty (Fig. 30-5). Follow the care plan and the nurse's instructions for persons with special fluid orders (p. 378).

- Fluid restriction—the person is not given more than the limited amount.
- NPO—the person is not given fluids.
- Thickened liquids—the person must be given liquids of a certain thickness (Chapter 29).

Some agencies do not use the following procedure. Instead, each mug is filled as needed. You take the mug to an ice and water dispenser. Fill the mug with ice first. Then add water. Follow the agency's procedure for providing fresh drinking water.

See *Focus on Communication: Providing Drinking Water.*
See *Delegation Guidelines: Providing Drinking Water.*
See *Promoting Safety and Comfort: Providing Drinking Water.*
See procedure: *Providing Drinking Water.*

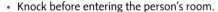

FIGURE 30-5 Water mug with straw. The mug is marked in ounces (oz) and milliliters (mL).

FOCUS ON COMMUNICATION
Providing Drinking Water

People vary about ice in their water. Ask what the person prefers. You can say:
- "Would you like ice in your water?"
- "How much ice do you prefer in your water?"
- "Do you like more ice or more water?"
  Also ask where to place the mug. Be sure the person can reach it.

DELEGATION GUIDELINES
Providing Drinking Water

To provide drinking water, you need this information from the nurse and the care plan.
- The person's fluid orders
- How much ice to add
- If the person uses a straw

PROMOTING SAFETY AND COMFORT
Providing Drinking Water

Safety
Water mugs can spread microbes. To prevent the spread of microbes:
- Label the mug with the person's name and room and bed number.
- Do not touch the rim or inside of the mug or lid.
- Do not let the ice scoop touch the mug, lid, or straw.
- Place the ice scoop in the scoop holder or on a towel for the scoop. Do not place it in the ice container or dispenser.
- Keep the ice chest closed when not in use.
- Make sure the mug is clean. Also check for cracks and chips. Provide a new mug as needed.
- Practice hand hygiene between each mug. This prevents the spread of microbes from 1 person's mug to another person's mug.

Providing Drinking Water

Quality of Life
- Knock before entering the person's room.
- Address the person by name.
- Introduce yourself by name and title.
- Explain the procedure before starting and during the procedure.
- Protect the person's rights during the procedure.
- Handle the person gently during the procedure.

Pre-Procedure
1 Follow *Delegation Guidelines: Providing Drinking Water.*
  See *Promoting Safety and Comfort: Providing Drinking Water.*
2 Obtain a list of special fluid orders from the nurse. Or use your assignment sheet.
3 Practice hand hygiene and get the following supplies.
  - Cart
  - Ice chest filled with ice
  - Cover for the ice chest
  - Scoop
  - Paper towels
  - Water mugs
  - Water pitcher filled with cold water (optional depending on agency procedure)
  - Towel for the scoop (if there is no scoop holder)
4 Cover the cart with paper towels. Arrange equipment on top of the paper towels.

Continued

Providing Drinking Water—cont'd

Procedure

5   Take the cart to the person's room door. Do not take the cart into the room.
6   Check the person's fluid orders. Use the list from the nurse or your assignment sheet.
7   Practice hand hygiene.
8   Identify the person. Check the ID bracelet against the fluid orders sheet or your assignment sheet. Use 2 identifiers (Chapter 11). Also call the person by name.
9   Take the mug from the over-bed table. Empty it into the room sink or bathroom sink.

10 Determine if a new mug is needed.
11 Use the scoop to fill the mug with ice (Fig. 30-6). Do not let the scoop touch the mug, lid, or straw.
12 Place the ice scoop in the scoop holder or on a clean towel.
13 Fill the mug with water. Get water from the room sink or bathroom sink or the water pitcher on the cart.
14 Place the mug on the over-bed table.
15 Make sure the mug is within the person's reach.

Post-Procedure

16 Provide for comfort. (See the inside of the back cover.)
17 Place the call light and other needed items within reach.
18 Complete a safety check of the room. (See the inside of the back cover.)

19 Practice hand hygiene.
20 Repeat steps 5 through 19 for each person.

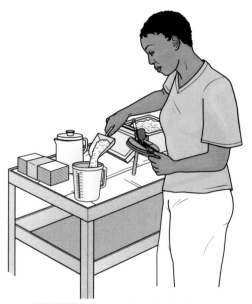

FIGURE 30-6 Providing drinking water.

IV THERAPY

Intravenous (IV) therapy (IV, IV infusion) is giving fluids through a tube inserted into a vein. See Figure 30-7 for the basic equipment used.

- The fluid to be infused (put into the body) is in a plastic bag—*IV bag.*
- A needle is inserted into a vein. Usually, the needle retracts (is removed) and a small, flexible tube called a *catheter (cannula)* is left in the vein (*venous catheter, intravenous cannula*) (see Fig. 30-7).
- *Infusion tubing (IV tube)* connects the catheter (cannula) to the IV bag.
  - Fluid drips from the bag into a *drip chamber.*
  - A *clamp* is used to start, stop, or regulate (change) how fast the fluid flows (flow rate).
- The IV bag hangs from an IV pole (IV standard) or ceiling hook.

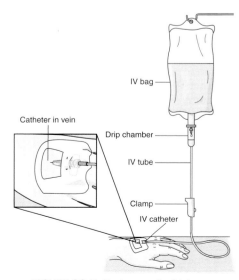

Catheter in vein

IV bag
Drip chamber
IV tube
Clamp
IV catheter

FIGURE 30-7 Equipment for IV therapy.

Flow Rate

The doctor orders the amount of fluid to give *(infuse)* and the amount of time to give it in. With this information, the RN (registered nurse) figures the flow rate. The ***flow rate*** *is the number of drops per minute (gtt/min) or milliliters per hour (mL/hr).* The abbreviation *gtt* means *drops.* The Latin word *guttae* means *drops.*

An electronic pump is often used (Fig. 30-8). The flow rate is displayed in mL/hr. An alarm sounds if something is wrong. Tell the nurse at once if you hear an alarm. If a pump is not used, the RN sets the clamp for the flow rate. *Never adjust any controls on IV pumps or change the position of the clamp.*

See *Focus on Math: Flow Rate.*

See *Promoting Safety and Comfort: Flow Rate.*

 FOCUS ON **MATH**

Flow Rate

Counting Drops per Minute

You can check the flow rate when a pump is not used. The nurse tells you the number of drops per minute (gtt/min). Use a watch. Count the number of drops that fall in the drip chamber in 1 minute (60 seconds). See Figure 30-9. Tell the nurse at once if:

- No fluid is dripping.
- The rate is too fast or too slow.
- The bag is empty or close to being empty.

For example: The nurse tells you the number of drops per minute is to be 25 gtt/min. You count 31 gtt/min.

31 gtt/min (rate counted) is greater than 25 gtt/min (correct rate).

The rate is too fast. You tell the nurse.

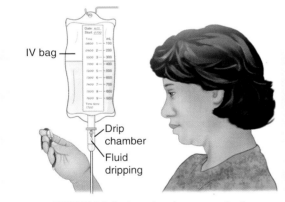

FIGURE 30-9 Counting drops per minute.

PROMOTING SAFETY AND COMFORT

Flow Rate

Safety

The person can suffer serious harm if the flow rate is too fast or too slow. Flow rate changes can occur from:

- Position changes
- Kinked tubes
- Lying on the tube

Never change the position of the clamp or adjust any controls on infusion pumps. Tell the nurse at once about a problem with the flow rate.

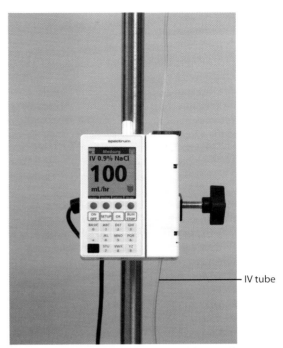

FIGURE 30-8 Electronic IV pump. (Modified from Williams PA: *Fundamental concepts and skills for nursing,* ed 5, St Louis, 2018, Elsevier.)

Assisting With IV Therapy

You help meet the safety, hygiene, and activity needs of persons with IVs. Follow the safety measures in Box 30-3 (p. 386). Report any sign or symptom listed in Box 30-3 at once.

You never start or maintain IV therapy. Nor do you regulate the flow rate or change IV bags. You never give blood or IV drugs.

See *Focus on Communication: Assisting With IV Therapy.*

FOCUS ON **COMMUNICATION**

Assisting With IV Therapy

For an IV in the arm, arm position can affect fluid flow. You may need to remind the person:

- To position the arm a certain way
- About position limits

For example, a bent arm causes the fluid flow to stop. You can say: "Please keep your arm straight. The fluid will not flow through your IV when your arm is bent."

BOX 30-3 IV Therapy

Safety Measures
- Follow Standard Precautions and the Bloodborne Pathogen Standard.
- Keep the IV site clean and dry. Follow the nurse's instructions for protecting the site during showering or bathing. You may need to apply a plastic bag, plastic wrap, or glove to the site.
- Do not move the catheter. Correct position must be maintained. If the catheter is moved, it may come out of the vein. Then fluid flows into tissues *(infiltration)*. Or the flow stops.
- Follow the safety measures for restraints (Chapter 13) when the person's movements are limited. The nurse may splint the extremity to prevent movement. Or the nurse may apply a protective device to prevent the catheter from moving. Restraints are a last resort.
- Protect the IV bag, tubing, and catheter when the person walks. Portable IV poles (IV standards) are used.
- Plan moving and transfer procedures to avoid pulling on the IV site. Allow enough slack in the tubing. Move the IV pole (IV standard) as needed. The catheter can move from pressure on the tube.
- Know if you need the nurse's help during garment changes. Plan ahead and communicate needs.
  - IV therapy gown—You can change the gown. The snaps (ties, Velcro) along the sleeves are unfastened and fastened for gown changes.
  - Standard gown—You can change the gown if an electronic pump is not used. See Chapter 24. If a pump is used, the nurse handles the arm with the IV.

Safety Measures—cont'd
- Tell the nurse if an IV pump alarm sounds. This may mean:
  - There is air in the tubing.
  - The infusion is done.
  - The pump's battery is low.
  - Fluid flow is blocked. Kinks in the tubing and closed clamps are common reasons.

Signs and Symptoms of Complications
- Report the following at once.
  - Local—at the IV site
    - Bleeding
    - Blood backing up into the IV tube
    - Puffiness or swelling
    - Pale or reddened skin
    - Complaints of pain at or above the IV site
    - Hot or cold skin near the site
  - Systemic—involving the whole body
    - *Fever* (elevated body temperature)
    - Itching
    - Changes in blood pressure: increase or decrease
    - Pulse rate greater than 100 beats per minute
    - Irregular pulse
    - *Cyanosis* (bluish color)
    - Confusion or changes in mental function
    - Loss of consciousness
    - Difficulty breathing or shortness of breath
    - Decreasing or no urine output
    - Chest pain
    - Nausea

FOCUS ON PRIDE

The Person, Family, and Yourself

P ersonal and Professional Responsibility

An *attentive* person is careful, alert, and thorough. These qualities are important when assisting with fluid needs. Follow each person's fluid order. Measure and record I&O correctly. Watch for signs and symptoms of dehydration. Report problems at once.

R ights and Respect

Patients and residents may complain about orders and treatments. For example, a resident does not like thickened liquids. Or a patient has an order to encourage fluids. The person is tired of being reminded to drink. Do not ignore complaints. They communicate needs. Listen and show respect.

I ndependence and Social Interaction

An IV in the arm can limit hand and arm movement. You may need to assist with hygiene, grooming, food and fluid, or activity needs. Assist only to the extent needed. The person should do as much as safely possible.

D elegation and Teamwork

Some skills require math. Measuring I&O is an example. Math is hard for some persons. You may need extra practice. Tell your instructor. On the job, ask the nurse if you have a question. Do not be embarrassed to ask for help.

E thics and Laws

When you hear an IV pump alarm (sound), tell the nurse. Do so even if not assigned to the person. You do not adjust controls on IV pumps. Working within your role limits protects the person from harm and yourself from losing your ability to work as a nursing assistant.

FOCUS ON PRIDE: Application

A person with an order to restrict fluids complains of thirst. How can you meet the person's needs?

Circle the BEST answer.

1. Which is a source of fluid loss?
   a. Edema
   b. Hydration
   c. Perspiration
   d. IV therapy

2. A person with diarrhea has scant, dark yellow urine. This is a sign of
   a. Normal hydration
   b. Edema
   c. Infection
   d. Dehydration

3. A person has edema. Which should you question?
   a. Encourage fluids.
   b. Restrict fluids.
   c. Provide frequent oral hygiene.
   d. Monitor I&O.

4. A person is NPO. You should
   a. Provide a variety of fluids
   b. Remove the water mug from the room
   c. Offer fluids in small amounts and in small containers
   d. Remove oral hygiene equipment from the room

5. Which are counted as fluid intake?
   a. Broths and ice cream
   b. Sauces and melted cheese
   c. Thick stews and mashed potatoes
   d. Butter and syrup

6. A person drank all of an 8-oz carton of milk. How many mL of fluid would you chart on the I&O record?
   a. 8 mL
   b. 60 mL
   c. 120 mL
   d. 240 mL

7. A person was served 240 mL of coffee and 120 mL of juice. You measure 50 mL of coffee and 60 mL of juice left. What do you chart for intake on the I&O record?
   a. 110 mL
   b. 250 mL
   c. 360 mL
   d. 470 mL

8. When measuring output
   a. Convert measurements to ounces
   b. Use the same graduate you used for intake
   c. Place the graduate on a flat surface and read it at eye level
   d. Gloves are not needed

9. During your shift a patient vomited twice—125 mL and 75 mL. The patient had diarrhea once—50 mL. You empty 500 mL from the urine drainage bag. What is the total shift output amount?
   a. 200 mL
   b. 250 mL
   c. 500 mL
   d. 750 mL

10. Before providing fresh drinking water, you need to know the person's
    a. Food intake
    b. Fluid orders
    c. Diet
    d. Preferred beverages

11. Which prevents contamination when passing drinking water?
    a. Labeling the mug with the person's name
    b. Keeping the ice chest open when not in use
    c. Leaving the ice scoop in the ice container
    d. Touching the mug with the ice scoop

12. The IV flow rate is
    a. The number of gtt/hr
    b. The amount of fluid given in 1 minute
    c. The number of gtt/min or mL/hr
    d. The amount of fluid in the IV bag

13. What is the *correct* way to check an IV flow rate?
    a. Count the drops in 30 seconds. Multiply the number by 2.
    b. Count the drops for 1 minute.
    c. Check if the fluid is dripping.
    d. Measure the amount of fluid.

14. You note that the IV bag is almost empty. You should
    a. Clamp the IV tubing
    b. Tell the nurse
    c. Remove the IV
    d. Adjust the flow rate

15. You see swelling around an IV site. You should
    a. Tell the nurse
    b. Move the IV catheter
    c. Remove the IV
    d. Clamp the IV tubing

Answers to Chapter 30 questions are on p. 588.

FOCUS ON **PRACTICE**

Problem Solving

A person has an IV controlled with an electronic pump. The person is wearing a standard gown. You need to bathe the person, change the gown, and transfer the person from the bed to the wheelchair. What do you need to plan for and communicate?

CHAPTER 31

Measurements

OBJECTIVES

- Define the key terms and key abbreviations in this chapter.
- Explain why vital signs are measured.
- List the factors affecting vital signs.
- Identify the normal ranges for each temperature site.
- Explain when to use each temperature site.
- Explain how to use thermometers.
- Identify the pulse sites.

- Describe a normal pulse and normal respirations.
- Describe the practices for measuring blood pressure.
- Identify the normal ranges for blood pressure.
- Explain how to prepare the person for weight and height measurements.
- Perform the procedures described in this chapter.
- Explain how to promote PRIDE in the person, the family, and yourself.

KEY TERMS

afebrile Without *(a)* a fever *(febrile)*

blood pressure (BP) The amount of force exerted against the walls of an artery by the blood

body temperature The amount of heat in the body that is a balance between the amount of heat produced and the amount lost by the body

bradycardia A slow *(brady)* heart rate *(cardia)*; less than 60 beats per minute

diastolic pressure The pressure in the arteries when the heart is at rest

febrile With a fever

fever Elevated body temperature

hypertension High blood pressure

hypotension Low blood pressure

pulse The beat of the heart felt at an artery as a wave of blood passes through the artery

pulse rate The number of heartbeats or pulses in 1 minute

respiration Breathing air into *(inhalation)* and out of *(exhalation)* the lungs

stethoscope An instrument used to listen to the sounds produced by the heart, lungs, and other body organs

systolic pressure The pressure in the arteries when the heart contracts

tachycardia A rapid *(tachy)* heart rate *(cardia)*; more than 100 beats per minute

thermometer A device used to measure *(meter)* temperature *(thermo)*

vital signs Temperature, pulse, respirations, and blood pressure; pulse oximetry and pain are included in some agencies

KEY ABBREVIATIONS

BP	Blood pressure	IV	Intravenous
C	Centigrade	mm	Millimeter
F	Fahrenheit	mm Hg	Millimeters of mercury
Hg	Mercury	TPR	Temperature, pulse, and respirations
ID	Identification		

Measurements are used for the nursing process. They help the nurse plan for and evaluate care. You will assist by measuring vital signs, weight, and height. Food intake (Chapter 28), fluid intake and output (Chapter 30), and pulse oximetry (Chapter 37) are other measurements. You will also collect information about the person's pain (Chapter 33).

VITAL SIGNS

Vital signs reflect the function of 3 body processes—regulation of body temperature, breathing, and heart function. The *vital signs of body function are:*

- *Temperature*
- *Pulse*
- *Respirations*
- *Blood pressure*
- *Pulse oximetry (in some agencies)*
- *Pain (in some agencies)*

Vital signs are often called TPR (temperature, pulse, and respirations) and BP (blood pressure). See "Pulse Oximetry" (p. 406 and Chapter 37) and "Pain" (p. 406 and Chapter 33).

A person's vital signs vary within certain limits. Box 31-1 lists factors that affect vital signs.

Vital signs detect even minor changes in normal body function. They tell about treatment response. They often signal life-threatening events.

You must accurately measure, record, and report vital signs. If unsure of your measurements, ask the nurse for help. Unless otherwise ordered, take vital signs with the person at rest—lying or sitting. Report the following at once.

- Any vital sign that is changed from a prior measurement. The nurse tells you what change is important.
- An abnormal vital sign (a vital sign above or below the normal range).
  See *Focus on Older Persons: Vital Signs.*
  See *Focus on Communication: Vital Signs.*

FOCUS ON OLDER PERSONS

Vital Signs

When measuring vital signs, the person with dementia may move, hit at you, or grab equipment. This is not safe for the person or you. Two staff members may be needed. One tries to calm and distract the person. The other measures the vital signs.

Try the procedure when the person is calmer. Or take the respirations and pulse at one time. Then take the temperature and blood pressure later.

Approach the person calmly. Use a soothing voice. Explain what you will do. Do not rush. Follow the care plan for the best way to calm and distract the person. If you cannot measure vital signs, tell the nurse.

FOCUS ON COMMUNICATION

Vital Signs

Some persons like to know their vital signs. If agency policy allows, tell the person the measurements. With the person's consent, you can tell family members if they ask. This information is private and confidential. Roommates and visitors must not hear what you say. For greater privacy, write the measurements for the person.

A measurement may be abnormal. Or you are not able to feel a pulse or hear a blood pressure. Do not alarm the person. You can say:

- "I have a question about your blood pressure. I'll ask the nurse to take it."
- "It was difficult to hear your blood pressure. I need to try to take it again."
- "Your pulse is a little slow (fast). I'll have the nurse check it."
- "Your temperature is higher than normal. I'll use another thermometer and have the nurse check you."

Body Temperature

Body temperature is the amount of heat in the body. It is a balance between the amount of heat produced and the amount lost by the body. Heat is produced as cells use nutrients for energy. It is lost through the skin, breathing, urine, and feces (stools). Body temperature is fairly stable. It is lower in the morning and higher in the afternoon and evening. See Box 31-1 for factors that can affect body temperature.

You use thermometers to measure temperature. A *thermometer is a device used to measure* (meter) *temperature* (thermo). Thermometers have Fahrenheit (F) or centigrade (C) scales. Use the degrees symbol (°) to record temperatures.

Temperature Sites. Temperature sites are listed in Box 31-2, p. 390. Each site has a normal range (Table 31-1, p. 390). Always report temperatures above or below the normal range.

Fever means an elevated body temperature. Fever is the body's response to infection. The body raises the temperature in an attempt to kill invading microbes. These terms are used to describe the person.

- *Febrile—with a fever.* (The Latin word *febris* means *fever.*)
- *Afebrile—without* (a) *a fever* (febrile).
  See *Focus on Older Persons: Temperature Sites,* p. 390.
  See *Focus on Communication: Temperature Sites,* p. 390.
  See *Promoting Safety and Comfort: Temperature Sites,* p. 390.

BOX 31-1 Factors Affecting Vital Signs			
• Activity, exercise	• Biological sex (male, female)	• Pain	• Weather
• Age	• Drugs	• Sleep	• Weight
• Anger	• Eating	• Smoking	
• Anxiety, fear	• Illness	• Stress	

BOX 31-2 Temperature Sites

Oral Site (Mouth)

Oral temperatures are *not* taken if the person:
- Is under 4 or 5 years of age
- Is unconscious
- Has had surgery or an injury to the face, neck, nose, or mouth
- Is receiving oxygen
- Breathes through the mouth
- Has a naso-gastric tube
- Is restless, confused, or disoriented
- Is paralyzed on 1 side of the body
- Has a sore mouth
- Has a convulsive (seizure) disorder

Rectal Site (Rectum)

The rectal site is used for infants and children under 3 years old. Rectal temperatures are taken when the oral site cannot be used. Rectal temperatures are *not* taken if the person:
- Has diarrhea
- Has a rectal disorder or injury
- Has heart disease
- Had rectal surgery
- Is confused or agitated

Axillary Site (Underarm)

The axillary site is less reliable than other sites. It is used when other sites cannot be used. Do *not* use this site right after bathing.

Tympanic Membrane Site (Ear)

The site has fewer microbes than the mouth or rectum. The risk of spreading infection is reduced. The route is comfortable and non-invasive. Too much earwax can cause an incorrect measurement. This site is *not* used if the person has:
- An ear disorder
- Ear drainage

Temporal Artery Site (Forehead)

Body temperature is measured at the temporal artery in the forehead. The site is non-invasive.

FOCUS ON OLDER PERSONS

Temperature Sites

Older persons may not respond to infection with a fever. Monitor closely for other signs and symptoms of infection (Chapter 14).

Tympanic membrane and temporal artery sites are used for persons who are confused and resist care. Oral and rectal sites are unsafe. The person may move, resist care, or bite down on the thermometer. This can injure the mouth, teeth, or rectum.

FOCUS ON COMMUNICATION

Temperature Sites

Some persons have difficulty keeping an oral thermometer in place correctly. The rectal site can be uncomfortable. The axillary site has a longer measurement time than the other sites. To promote comfort, talk the person through the procedure. You can say:
- "I'm almost done. Are you doing okay?"
- "The thermometer is working. Please hold it still under your tongue a little longer."

PROMOTING SAFETY AND COMFORT

Temperature Sites

Safety

Rectal temperatures are dangerous for persons with heart disease. The thermometer can stimulate the vagus nerve and slow the heart rate to dangerous levels.

Thermometer Types. There are different types of thermometers. See Table 31-2. Electronic thermometers display the temperature on the front of the device. Follow the manufacturer's instructions and agency procedures to use, clean, and store thermometers.

See *Promoting Safety and Comfort: Thermometer Types.*

PROMOTING SAFETY AND COMFORT

Thermometer Types

Safety

Mercury-glass thermometers are not common today. Safer chemicals have replaced mercury. However, do not assume that a glass thermometer has a mercury-free mixture. If a thermometer breaks, tell the nurse at once. Do not touch the substance. Do not let the person do so. Follow agency procedures for handling hazardous materials. See Chapter 11.

TABLE 31-1 Normal Body Temperatures

Site	Baseline	Normal Range
Oral	98.6°F (37.0°C)	97.6°F to 99.6°F (36.5°C to 37.5°C)
Rectal	99.6°F (37.5°C)	98.6°F to 100.6°F (37.0°C to 38.1°C)
Axillary	97.6°F (36.5°C)	96.6°F to 98.6°F (35.9°C to 37.0°C)
Tympanic membrane	98.6°F (37.0°C)	98.6°F (37.0°C)
Temporal artery	99.6°F (37.5°C)	99.6°F (37.5°C)

TABLE 31-2 Thermometer Types

Thermometer Type	Description	Guidelines for Use
Standard electronic thermometer (Fig. 31-1, *A*, p. 392)	• Battery operated. • The *probe* is inserted at the measurement site. • Measures temperature in 4 to 15 seconds. **Measurement sites:** • Oral • Rectal • Axillary	• Oral and axillary probes are *blue*. • Rectal probes are *red*. • *Probe covers* are disposable sheaths used to prevent the spread of infection. • Apply a new cover for each use. Discard after use.
Tympanic membrane thermometer (Fig. 31-1, *B*, p. 392)	• Battery operated. • Measures temperature in 1 to 3 seconds. **Measurement site:** • Tympanic membrane (ear)	• Do not use if there is ear drainage. • Probe covers are used. Discard after use. • Gently insert the covered probe into the ear.
Temporal artery thermometer (Fig. 31-1, *C*, p. 392)	• Battery operated. • Measures temperature in 3 to 4 seconds. **Measurement site:** • Temporal artery (forehead)	• Probe covers prevent the spread of infection. Discard after use. • Use the exposed side of the head. Do not use the side covered by hair, a dressing, a hat, or other covering. Do not use the side that was on a pillow.
Non-contact infrared thermometer (Fig. 31-1, *D*, p. 392)	• Battery operated. • There is no contact between the person and the device. • Measures surface (skin) temperature and calculates body temperature. Best used for screening, abnormal temperatures should be measured with another thermometer type. • Most measure temperature within 1 second. **Measurement site:** • Forehead (common)	• No contact prevents the spread of infection. • Use in a draft-free area that is out of direct sunlight and not near a heat source. • Room temperature and humidity may affect temperature readings. • Be sure the forehead is clean, dry, and exposed. Coverings (headbands, hats), hair, and sweat can affect measurements. • Hold the thermometer straight in front of the forehead. Follow the manufacturer's instructions for the angle and distance from the forehead. • Do not touch the sensor area.
Digital thermometer (Fig. 31-1, *E*, p. 392)	• Small and battery operated. • Measures temperature in 6 to 60 seconds. **Measurement sites:** • Oral • Rectal • Axillary	• Probe covers prevent the spread of infection. Discard after use.
Glass thermometer (Fig. 31-1, *F*, p. 392)	• A hollow glass tube filled with a substance that expands and rises in the tube when heated. When cooled, the substance moves back down the tube. • Measurement times vary by site. **Measurement sites:** • Oral • Rectal • Axillary	• The *stem* part is held. The *tip* is inserted at the measurement site. ◦ Oral and axillary thermometers have a *blue* stem. They may have long and slender, stubby, or pear-shaped tips. ◦ Rectal thermometers have a *red* stem and a stubby tip. • Problems with use include: ◦ Long measurement times—oral 2 to 3 minutes, rectal 2 minutes, axillary 5 to 10 minutes. ◦ They break easily and can injure the measurement site. ◦ Mercury thermometers are hazardous. See *Promoting Safety and Comfort: Thermometer Types.* • See "Using a Glass Thermometer" (p. 394) and "Reading a Glass Thermometer" (p. 395).

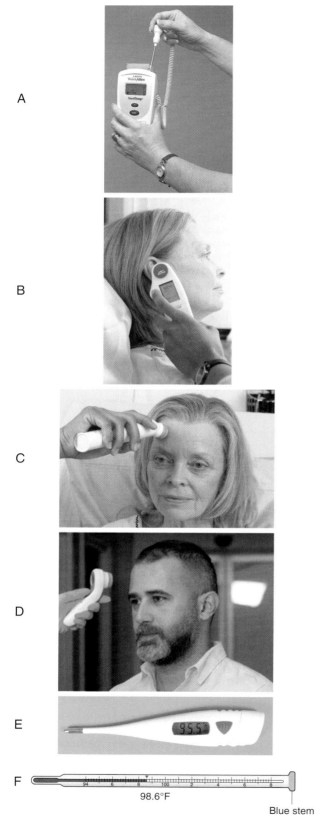

FIGURE 31-1 Thermometer types. **A,** Standard electronic thermometer. **B,** Tympanic membrane thermometer. **C,** Temporal artery thermometer. **D,** Non-contact infrared thermometer. **E,** Digital thermometer. **F,** Glass thermometer with a blue stem (for oral or axillary temperatures). (D, Modified from U.S. Food and Drug Administration, 2020.)

Taking Temperatures. The nurse and care plan tell you:
- When to take the person's temperature
- What site to use
- What thermometer to use

There are many types of electronic thermometers. Follow the manufacturer's instructions. The procedure that follows is used as a guide.

See *Delegation Guidelines: Taking Temperatures.*

See *Promoting Safety and Comfort: Taking Temperatures.*

See procedure: *Taking a Temperature With an Electronic Thermometer.*

DELEGATION GUIDELINES
Taking Temperatures

Before taking temperatures, you need this information from the nurse and the care plan.
- What site to use for each person—oral, rectal, axillary, tympanic membrane, or temporal artery
- What thermometer to use for each person
- How long to leave a glass thermometer in place
- When to take temperatures
- Which persons are at risk for a fever
- What observations to report and record
- When to report observations
- What patient or resident concerns to report at once:
  - A temperature changed from a past measurement
  - A temperature above or below the normal range for the site used

---

PROMOTING SAFETY AND COMFORT
Taking Temperatures

Safety

Probe covers (sheaths) are used on thermometers to prevent the spread of microbes from person to person. Or dedicated equipment is used (Chapter 15)—patients and residents have their own thermometers. Follow Standard Precautions when taking temperatures. Follow the Bloodborne Pathogen Standard if blood is present. Wear gloves if contact with blood or body fluids is likely.

With rectal temperatures, gloved hands may have contact with feces (stools). Plan ahead to avoid contaminating other items (such as your note pad, assignment sheet, or pen). You can:
- Note the measurement with an unsoiled, gloved hand and then finish the procedure.
- Use the thermometer's "recall" or "memory" function if it has one. This shows the last temperature measured. Finish the procedure. Remove gloves and practice hand hygiene. Then view the measurement again to note accurately.
- Remove soiled gloves and practice hand hygiene. Note the measurement. Apply clean gloves to wipe the person and complete the procedure.

NOTE: A task may require more than 1 pair of gloves. Change gloves as needed. Use careful judgment. Remember to practice hand hygiene after removing gloves.

Comfort

Do not leave a thermometer in place longer than needed. This affects comfort.

Taking a Temperature With an Electronic Thermometer

Quality of Life

- Knock before entering the person's room.
- Address the person by name.
- Introduce yourself by name and title.
- Explain the procedure before starting and during the procedure.
- Protect the person's rights during the procedure.
- Handle the person gently during the procedure.

Pre-Procedure

1 Follow *Delegation Guidelines: Taking Temperatures.* See *Promoting Safety and Comfort: Taking Temperatures.*
2 For an oral temperature, ask the person not to eat, drink, smoke, or chew gum for at least 15 to 20 minutes before the measurement or as required by agency policy.
3 Practice hand hygiene and get the following supplies.
   - Thermometer—standard electronic, tympanic membrane, or temporal artery
   - Probe for a standard electronic thermometer:
     - Blue—oral or axillary
     - Red—rectal
   - Probe covers
   - Toilet paper and lubricant as directed by the nurse (rectal temperature)
   - Towel and laundry bag (axillary temperature)
   - Gloves as needed
4 Plug the probe into the thermometer if using a standard electronic thermometer.
5 Arrange items in the person's room if needed.
6 Practice hand hygiene.
7 Identify the person. Check the identification (ID) bracelet against the assignment sheet. Use 2 identifiers (Chapter 11). Also call the person by name.
8 Provide for privacy.

Procedure

9 Position the person.
   a *For an oral, axillary, tympanic membrane, or temporal artery temperature*—Have the person sit or lie down.
   b *For a rectal temperature*—Assist the person into a semi-prone or side-lying position.
10 Put on gloves if contact with blood or body fluids is likely.
11 Insert the probe into a probe cover.
12 *For an oral temperature:*
   a Have the person open the mouth and raise the tongue.
   b Place the covered probe at the base of the tongue and to 1 side (Fig. 31-2, p. 394).
   c Have the person lower the tongue and close the mouth.
   d Start the thermometer if needed. Hold the probe in place until the thermometer indicates the temperature is measured. A tone or a flashing or steady light is common.
13 *For a rectal temperature:*
   a Lubricate the end of the covered probe.
   b Expose the anal area.
   c Raise the upper buttock (Fig. 31-3, p. 394).
   d Insert the probe ½ inch into the rectum.
   e Start the thermometer if needed. Hold the probe in place until the thermometer indicates the temperature is measured. A tone or a flashing or steady light is common.
14 *For an axillary temperature:*
   a Help the person remove an arm from the gown. Do not expose the person.
   b Dry the axilla with the towel.
   c Place the covered probe in the center of the axilla (Fig. 31-4, p. 394).
   d Place the person's arm over the chest.
   e Start the thermometer if needed. Hold the probe in place until the thermometer indicates the temperature is measured. A tone or a flashing or steady light is common.

15 *For a tympanic membrane temperature:*
   a Have the person turn the head so the ear is in front of you.
   b Pull up and back on the adult's ear to straighten the ear canal (Fig. 31-5, p. 394).
   c Insert the covered probe gently.
   d Start the thermometer if needed. Hold the probe in place until the thermometer indicates the temperature is measured. A tone or a flashing or steady light is common.
16 *For a temporal artery temperature:*
   a Place the device in the center of the forehead.
   b Press the scan button.
   c Slide the device right or left across the temporal artery (p. 396) (see Fig. 31-1, C). Use the side of the head that is exposed. Keep the thermometer flat on the forehead and in contact with the skin.
   d Release the scan button when the thermometer reaches the hairline.
17 Remove the probe from the site. Read the temperature on the display.
18 Press the eject button to discard the cover.
19 Note the person's name, temperature, and temperature site on your note pad or assignment sheet.
20 Return the probe to the holder.
21 Help the person put the gown back on (axillary temperature). For a rectal temperature:
   a Wipe the anal area with toilet paper to remove lubricant.
   b Cover the person.
   c Dispose of used toilet paper.
   d Remove and discard the gloves. Practice hand hygiene.

Post-Procedure

22 Provide for comfort. (See the inside of the back cover.)
23 Place the call light and other needed items within reach.
24 Follow the care plan and the person's preferences for privacy measures to maintain. Leaving the privacy curtain, window coverings, and door open or closed are examples.
25 Complete a safety check of the room. (See the inside of the back cover.)
26 Practice hand hygiene.
27 Return the thermometer to the charging unit. Follow agency policy for disinfection.
28 Report and record the temperature. Note the temperature site. Report an abnormal temperature at once.

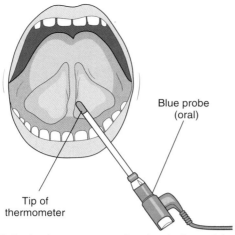

FIGURE 31-2 The thermometer is placed at the base of the tongue (under the tongue) and to 1 side.

Tip of thermometer

Blue probe (oral)

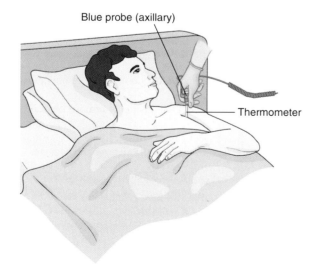

Red probe (rectal)

FIGURE 31-3 The rectal temperature is taken with the person in a side-lying position. The buttock is raised to expose the anus.

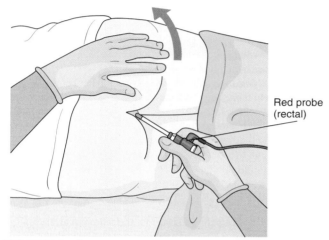

Blue probe (axillary)

Thermometer

FIGURE 31-4 The thermometer is in the center of the axilla and the person's arm is over the chest.

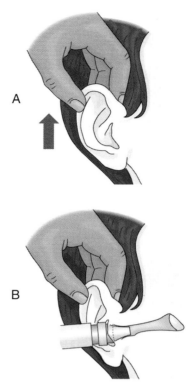

A

B

FIGURE 31-5 Tympanic membrane thermometer. **A,** The adult's ear is pulled up and back. **B,** The probe is inserted into the ear canal.

Using a Glass Thermometer. Glass thermometers are not commonly used in health care settings. You may be taught how to use them in your training program. To use a glass thermometer:

1 Rinse the thermometer under cold, running water if it was soaking in a disinfectant. Do not use hot water. The substance inside can expand and break the thermometer. Dry the thermometer from the stem to the tip with tissues.

2 Check for breaks, cracks, or chips. Discard it following agency policy if it is broken, cracked, or chipped.

3 Shake down the thermometer below the lowest number. Hold the device by the stem. Stand away from walls, tables, and other hard surfaces. Flex and snap your wrist until the substance is below 94°F or 34°C (Fig. 31-6).

4 Insert it into a plastic cover if used (Fig. 31-7).

5 Insert the thermometer at the measurement site. See Table 31-2 for the measurement times for each site.

6 After use, remove the plastic cover and read the thermometer. See "Reading a Glass Thermometer." Record the temperature.

7 Shake down the thermometer again. Clean, disinfect, and store the thermometer following agency policy.

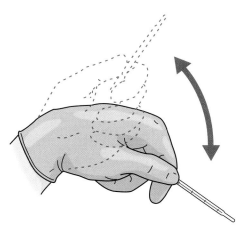

FIGURE 31-6 The wrist is snapped to shake down the thermometer. This moves the substance down the tube.

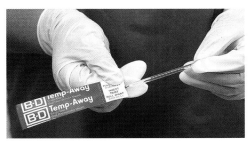

FIGURE 31-7 The thermometer is inserted into a plastic cover.

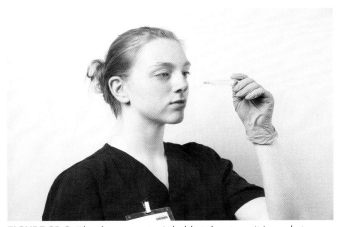

FIGURE 31-8 The thermometer is held at the stem. It is read at eye level.

Reading a Glass Thermometer. Do the following to read a glass thermometer.

1 Hold it at the stem. Bring it to eye level (Fig. 31-8).
2 Turn it until you can see the numbers and the long and short lines.
3 Turn it back and forth slowly until you can see the silver or red line.
4 Read from the tip toward the stem.
5 Read the nearest degree (long line) to the left of the silver or red line.
6 Read the nearest tenth of a degree (short line)—an even number on a Fahrenheit thermometer.
   See *Focus on Math: Reading a Glass Thermometer.*

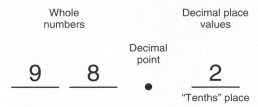

FOCUS ON MATH

Reading a Glass Thermometer

To read a thermometer, you must understand whole numbers and decimals. Whole numbers are 0, 1, 2, 3, and so on. They are to the *left* of the decimal point. The numbers to the *right* of the decimal point (decimal place values) are part of a whole number. See Figure 31-9.

The first decimal place value is the "tenths" place. It is read as 1-tenth, 2-tenths, 3-tenths, and so on to 9-tenths. Thermometers are read to the "tenths" place (1 number past the decimal point).

Whole numbers		Decimal point	Decimal place values
9	8	•	2
			"Tenths" place

FIGURE 31-9 Values used to read thermometers.

To read a glass thermometer (Fig. 31-10):
1 Read the nearest long line to the left of the silver or red line.
   • Fahrenheit—Each long line is 1 degree from 94°F to 108°F.
   • Centigrade—Each long line is 1 degree from 34°C to 42°C.
2 Read the nearest tenth of a degree (short line).
   • Fahrenheit—Each short line is 0.2 (2-tenths) of a degree (2-tenths, 4-tenths, 6-tenths, and 8-tenths).
   • Centigrade—Each short line is 0.1 (1-tenth) of a degree (1-tenth, 2-tenths, 3-tenths, and so on to 9-tenths).

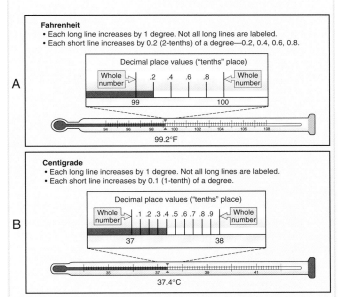

FIGURE 31-10 Reading thermometers. **A,** Fahrenheit thermometer. This thermometer is read as "ninety-nine point two degrees Fahrenheit." **B,** Centigrade thermometer. This thermometer is read as "thirty-seven point four degrees centigrade."

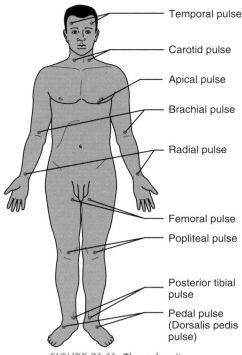

FIGURE 31-11 The pulse sites.

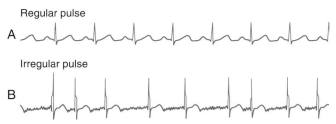

FIGURE 31-12 A, The electrocardiogram shows a regular pulse. The beats occur at regular intervals. (NOTE: Each tall spike is a beat.) B, These beats are at irregular intervals.

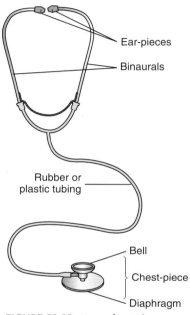

FIGURE 31-13 Parts of a stethoscope.

Pulse

The *pulse is the beat of the heart felt at an artery as a wave of blood passes through the artery.* A pulse occurs when the heart beats.

The temporal, carotid, brachial, radial, femoral, popliteal, posterior tibial, and dorsalis pedis (pedal) pulses are on each side of the body (Fig. 31-11). The radial pulse is used most often. It is easy to reach and find. The person is not exposed.

The apical pulse is over the tip (apex) of the heart. This pulse is taken with a stethoscope. See "Using a Stethoscope."

Pulse Rate. The *pulse rate is the number of heartbeats or pulses in 1 minute.* Pulse rate is affected by the factors in Box 31-1. Some drugs increase the pulse rate. Other drugs slow the pulse.

The adult pulse rate is normally between 60 and 100 beats per minute. A rate of less than 60 or more than 100 is abnormal. Report abnormal pulses at once.
* *Tachycardia is a rapid* (tachy) *heart rate* (cardia). *The heart rate is more than 100 beats per minute.*
* *Bradycardia is a slow* (brady) *heart rate* (cardia). *The heart rate is less than 60 beats per minute.*

Pulse Rhythm and Force. The pulse *rhythm* should be in a regular pattern. The pause between beats is the same. An irregular pulse is when the beats are not evenly spaced or beats are skipped (Fig. 31-12).

Force relates to pulse strength. A forceful pulse is easy to feel. It is described as *strong, full,* or *bounding.* Hard-to-feel pulses are described as *weak, thready,* or *feeble.*

Using a Stethoscope. A *stethoscope is an instrument used to listen to the sounds produced by the heart, lungs, and other body organs* (Fig. 31-13). You use it to hear apical pulses and for blood pressures (p. 401). See Box 31-3 for how to use a stethoscope.

See *Focus on Communication: Using a Stethoscope.*
See *Promoting Safety and Comfort: Using a Stethoscope.*

BOX 31-3 Using a Stethoscope

* Wipe the ear-pieces and chest-piece with antiseptic wipes before and after use. See Figure 31-13 for the parts of a stethoscope.
* Place the ear-piece tips in your ears. The bend of the tips points forward. Ear-pieces should fit snugly to block out noises. They should not cause ear pain or discomfort.
* Tap the diaphragm gently. You should hear the tapping. If not, turn the chest-piece at the tubing. Gently tap the diaphragm again. Proceed if you hear the tapping sound. Check with the nurse if you do not hear the tapping.
* Place the diaphragm over the pulse site. Hold it in place as in Figure 31-14.
* Prevent noise. Do not let anything touch the tubing. Ask the person to be silent. Make sure the room is quiet.

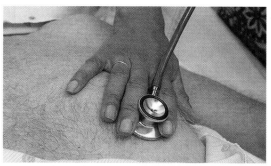

FIGURE 31-14 The stethoscope is held in place with the fingertips of the index and middle fingers.

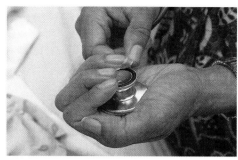

FIGURE 31-15 The diaphragm of the stethoscope is warmed in the palm of the hand.

FOCUS ON COMMUNICATION

Using a Stethoscope

Hearing through the stethoscope is hard when the person talks. Politely ask the person to be silent. Explain the procedure. Tell the person when and for how long to be silent. You can say:

I am going to check your pulse with a stethoscope. It is hard to hear your heart beat when you talk. Please do not talk when my stethoscope is on your chest. It will take about 1 minute.

The person may forget and begin talking. You can politely say: "This will only take 1 minute. Please stay quiet until I say that I'm done." Thank the person when you are done.

PROMOTING SAFETY AND COMFORT

Using a Stethoscope

Safety

Stethoscopes are in contact with many persons and staff. You must prevent infection. Wipe the ear-pieces and chest-piece with antiseptic wipes before and after use.

For Transmission-Based Precautions, dedicated equipment is kept in the room (Chapter 15). Equipment that must be shared is disinfected after use.

Comfort

Stethoscope diaphragms tend to be cold. Warm the diaphragm in your hand before putting it on the person (Fig. 31-15). Cold diaphragms can startle the person.

Taking Pulses. You will take radial and apical pulses. You must count, report, and record accurately.

The radial pulse is used for routine vital signs. Place the first 2 or 3 fingertips against the radial artery. The radial artery is on the thumb side of the wrist (Fig. 31-16). Follow agency policy for how long to count. The following is common.

- Regular pulse—Count the pulse for 30 seconds. Multiply by 2 for the number of pulses in 1 minute.
- Irregular pulse—Count the pulse for 1 minute.

The apical pulse is located 2 to 3 inches left of the sternum (Fig. 31-17, p. 398). Use a stethoscope and count the pulse for 1 minute. The heartbeat normally sounds like a *lub-dub*. Count each *lub-dub* as 1 beat. Do not count the *lub* as 1 beat and the *dub* as another.

Apical pulses are taken on persons who:
- Have heart disease.
- Have irregular heart rhythms.
- Take drugs that affect the heart.

(NOTE: State competency tests require the use of a watch with a second [sweep] hand when taking pulses.)

See *Focus on Math: Taking Pulses*, p. 398.
See *Delegation Guidelines: Taking Pulses*, p. 398.
See *Promoting Safety and Comfort: Taking Pulses*, p. 398.
See procedure: *Taking a Radial Pulse*, p. 399.
See procedure: *Taking an Apical Pulse*, p. 399.

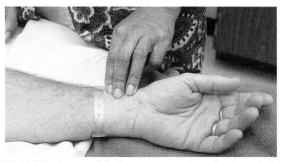

FIGURE 31-16 The 3 middle fingers are used to take the radial pulse.

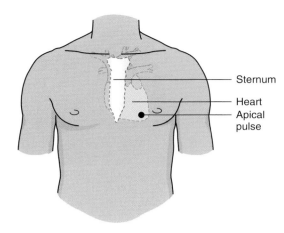

- Sternum
- Heart
- Apical pulse

FIGURE 31-17 The apical pulse is located 2 to 3 inches to the left of the sternum (breastbone).

 FOCUS ON MATH
Taking Pulses

To count a pulse, use a watch with a second (sweep) hand. Start counting when the second (sweep) hand is at the 12, 3, 6, or 9 position. When counting a pulse for 30 seconds, do 1 of the following. See Figure 31-18.

- When starting at 12, count until position 6.
- When starting at 3, count until position 9.
- When starting at 6, count until position 12.
- When starting at 9, count until position 3.
  For a 60-second pulse, count until the second (sweep) hand is back at the start position—12, 3, 6, or 9.

Radial Pulses
Pulse rate is measured in beats per minute. When you measure a regular pulse for 30 seconds, multiply the number by 2. This gives the number of beats per minute (60 seconds). For example: *You count 36 beats in 30 seconds. For the number of beats per minute, multiply 36 by 2.*

36 beats × 2 = 72 beats

The pulse is 72 beats per minute.

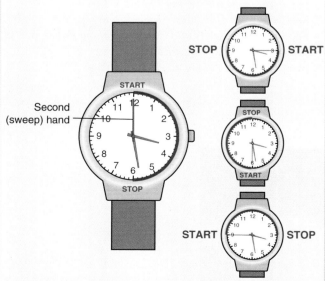

FIGURE 31-18 Using a watch with a second (sweep) hand to count for 30 seconds.

DELEGATION GUIDELINES
Taking Pulses

Before taking a pulse, you need this information from the nurse and the care plan.
- What pulse to take for each person—radial or apical
- When to take the pulse
- What other vital signs to measure
- How long to count the pulse—30 seconds or 1 minute
- If the nurse has concerns about certain patients or residents
- What observations to report and record:
  - The pulse site
  - The pulse rate—report a pulse rate less than 60 *(bradycardia)* or more than 100 *(tachycardia)* beats per minute at once
  - If the pulse is regular or irregular
  - Pulse force—strong (full, bounding) or weak (thready, feeble)
- When to report the pulse rate
- What patient or resident concerns to report at once

PROMOTING SAFETY AND COMFORT
Taking Pulses

Safety
Use your first 2 or 3 fingertips to take a pulse. Do not use your thumb. You could mistake the pulse in your thumb for the person's pulse. Reporting and recording the wrong pulse rate can harm the person.

Comfort
Position the person's arm so it is supported. Do not let the arm dangle.

Taking a Radial Pulse

Quality of Life

- Knock before entering the person's room.
- Address the person by name.
- Introduce yourself by name and title.
- Explain the procedure before starting and during the procedure.
- Protect the person's rights during the procedure.
- Handle the person gently during the procedure.

Pre-Procedure

1 Follow *Delegation Guidelines: Taking Pulses.* See *Promoting Safety and Comfort: Taking Pulses.*
2 Practice hand hygiene.
3 Identify the person. Check the ID bracelet against the assignment sheet. Use 2 identifiers (Chapter 11). Also call the person by name.
4 Provide for privacy.

Procedure

5 Have the person sit or lie down.
6 Locate the radial pulse on the thumb side of the person's wrist. Use your first 2 or 3 middle fingertips (see Fig. 31-16).
7 Note if the pulse is strong or weak and regular or irregular.
8 Count the pulse for 30 seconds. Multiply the number of beats by 2 for the number of pulses in 60 seconds (1 minute). This is the pulse rate. For example:
- You count 45 beats in 30 seconds.
- Multiply 45 beats by 2.
- 45 beats × 2 = 90 beats per minute.
9 Count the pulse for 1 minute if:
- Directed by the nurse and the care plan.
- Required by agency policy.
- The pulse was irregular.
- Required for your state competency test.
10 Note the following on your note pad or assignment sheet.
a The person's name
b Pulse rate
c Pulse strength
d If the pulse was regular or irregular

Post-Procedure

11 Provide for comfort. (See the inside of the back cover.)
12 Place the call light and other needed items within reach.
13 Follow the care plan and the person's preferences for privacy measures to maintain. Leaving the privacy curtain, window coverings, and door open or closed are examples.
14 Complete a safety check of the room. (See the inside of the back cover.)
15 Practice hand hygiene.
16 Report and record the pulse rate and your observations. Report an abnormal pulse at once.

Taking an Apical Pulse

Quality of Life

- Knock before entering the person's room.
- Address the person by name.
- Introduce yourself by name and title.
- Explain the procedure before starting and during the procedure.
- Protect the person's rights during the procedure.
- Handle the person gently during the procedure.

Pre-Procedure

1 Follow *Delegation Guidelines: Taking Pulses.* See *Promoting Safety and Comfort: Using a Stethoscope,* p. 397.
2 Practice hand hygiene and get the following supplies.
- Stethoscope
- Antiseptic wipes
3 Practice hand hygiene.
4 Identify the person. Check the ID bracelet against the assignment sheet. Use 2 identifiers (Chapter 11). Also call the person by name.
5 Provide for privacy.

Procedure

6 Clean the stethoscope ear-pieces and chest-piece with an antiseptic wipe. Discard the wipe.
7 Have the person sit or lie down.
8 Expose the upper part of the left chest. Expose a woman's breasts only to the extent necessary.
9 Warm the diaphragm in your palm.
10 Place the stethoscope ear-pieces in your ears. The bend of the tips points forward.
11 Find the apical pulse. Place the diaphragm 2 to 3 inches to the left of the breastbone (see Fig. 31-17).
12 Count the pulse for 1 minute. (Count each lub-dub as 1 beat.) Note if it was regular or irregular.
13 Cover the person. Remove the stethoscope ear-pieces from your ears.
14 Note the person's name and pulse rate on your note pad or assignment sheet. Note if the pulse was regular or irregular.

Continued

Taking an Apical Pulse—cont'd

Post-Procedure

15 Provide for comfort. (See the inside of the back cover.)
16 Place the call light and other needed items within reach.
17 Follow the care plan and the person's preferences for privacy measures to maintain. Leaving the privacy curtain, window coverings, and door open or closed are examples.
18 Complete a safety check of the room. (See the inside of the back cover.)

19 Clean the stethoscope ear-pieces and chest-piece with an antiseptic wipe. Discard the wipe.
20 Practice hand hygiene.
21 Return the stethoscope to its proper place.
22 Report and record your observations. Record the pulse rate with *Ap* for apical. Report an abnormal pulse at once.

Respirations

Respiration means breathing air into (inhalation) *and out of* (exhalation) *the lungs.* Each respiration involves:
* 1 inhalation—The chest rises. Air enters the lungs.
* 1 exhalation—The chest falls. Air leaves the lungs.

The healthy adult has 12 to 20 respirations per minute. See Box 31-1 for the factors affecting vital signs. Heart and respiratory diseases often increase the respiratory rate.

Respirations are normally quiet, effortless, and regular. Both sides of the chest rise and fall equally. See Chapter 37 for abnormal respiratory patterns.

Counting Respirations. Count respirations when the person is at rest. Position the person so you can see the chest rise and fall. To some extent, a person can control the rate and depth of breathing. People tend to change their breathing patterns when they know their respirations are being counted. Therefore do not tell the person that you are counting them.

Count respirations right after taking a pulse. Keep your fingers or stethoscope over the pulse site. The person assumes you are taking the pulse. To count respirations, watch the chest rise and fall. Count chest rises for 30 seconds. Multiply the number by 2 for the number of respirations in 1 minute. If you note an abnormal pattern, count respirations for 1 minute.

(NOTE: State competency tests require the use of a watch with a second [sweep] hand when counting respirations.)

See *Focus on Math: Counting Respirations.*
See *Delegation Guidelines: Counting Respirations.*
See procedure: *Counting Respirations.*

FOCUS ON MATH
Counting Respirations

Respirations are measured in breaths per minute. When you count regular respirations for 30 seconds, multiply the number by 2. This gives the number of respirations per minute (60 seconds). For example: *You count 8 breaths in 30 seconds. For the number of breaths per minute, multiply 8 by 2.*

$$8 \text{ breaths} \times 2 = 16 \text{ breaths}$$
The respiratory rate is 16 breaths per minute.

Like when taking pulses, you use a watch with a second (sweep) hand to count respirations. See *Focus on Math: Taking Pulses* (p. 398) for how to use a second (sweep) hand.

DELEGATION GUIDELINES
Counting Respirations

Before counting respirations, you need this information from the nurse and the care plan.
* How long to count respirations for each person—30 seconds or 1 minute
* When to count respirations
* If the nurse has concerns about certain patients or residents
* What other vital signs to measure
* What observations to report and record:
  * The respiratory rate
  * Equality and depth of respirations
  * If the respirations were regular or irregular
  * If the person has pain or difficulty breathing
  * Any respiratory noises
  * An abnormal respiratory pattern (Chapter 37)
* When to report observations
* What patient or resident concerns to report at once

Counting Respirations

Procedure

1 Follow *Delegation Guidelines: Counting Respirations.*
2 Count respirations after taking the pulse. (Do this if the person tends to change the breathing pattern when being watched.) Keep your fingers or stethoscope over the pulse site.
3 Do not tell the person you are counting respirations.
4 Count chest rises. Each rise and fall of the chest is 1 respiration.
5 Note the following.
   • If respirations are regular
   • If both sides of the chest rise equally
   • The depth of respirations
   • If the person has any pain or difficulty breathing
   • An abnormal respiratory pattern

6 Count respirations for 30 seconds. Multiply the number by 2 for the number of respirations in 60 seconds (1 minute). This is the respiratory rate. For example:
   • You count 9 breaths in 30 seconds.
   • Multiply 9 breaths by 2.
   • 9 breaths × 2 = 18 breaths per minute.
7 Count respirations for 1 minute if:
   • Directed by the nurse and the care plan.
   • Required by agency policy.
   • They are abnormal or irregular.
   • Required for your state competency test.
8 Note the person's name, respiratory rate, and other observations on your note pad or assignment sheet.

Post-Procedure

9 Provide for comfort. (See the inside of the back cover.)
10 Place the call light and other needed items within reach.
11 Follow the care plan and the person's preferences for privacy measures to maintain. Leaving the privacy curtain, window coverings, and door open or closed are examples.

12 Complete a safety check of the room. (See the inside of the back cover.)
13 Practice hand hygiene.
14 Report and record the respiratory rate and your observations. Report abnormal respirations at once.

Blood Pressure

Blood pressure (BP) is the amount of force exerted against the walls of an artery by the blood. BP is controlled by:
• The force of heart contractions
• The amount of blood pumped with each heartbeat
• How easily the blood flows through the blood vessels

Systole is the period of heart muscle contraction. The heart is pumping blood. *Diastole* is the period of heart muscle relaxation. The heart is at rest.

You measure systolic and diastolic pressures. The *systolic pressure is the pressure in the arteries when the heart contracts.* It is the higher pressure. The *diastolic pressure is the pressure in the arteries when the heart is at rest.* It is the lower pressure.

BP is measured in millimeters (mm) of mercury (Hg). The systolic pressure is recorded over the diastolic pressure. For example, a systolic pressure of 120 mm Hg (millimeters of mercury) and a diastolic pressure of 80 mm Hg are written as 120/80 mm Hg. This is read as "120 over 80 millimeters of mercury."

Normal and Abnormal Blood Pressures. BP can change from minute to minute. BP has normal ranges.
• *Systolic pressure*—90 mm Hg or higher but lower than 120 mm Hg
• *Diastolic pressure*—60 mm Hg or higher but lower than 80 mm Hg

Treatment is indicated for *hypertension (high blood pressure)* and *hypotension (low blood pressure).* Blood pressure is high when:
• The systolic pressure is 140 mm Hg or higher.
• The diastolic pressure is 90 mm Hg or higher.

When heart disease risk factors are present, a systolic pressure of 130 mm Hg or higher or a diastolic pressure of 80 mm Hg or higher may be considered hypertension. See Chapter 40.

Some people normally have low blood pressures. However, hypotension can signal a life-threatening problem. Blood pressure is low when:
• The systolic pressure is below 90 mm Hg.
• The diastolic pressure is below 60 mm Hg.

Report a systolic measurement at or above 120 mm Hg or below 90 mm Hg. Report a diastolic measurement at or above 80 mm Hg or below 60 mm Hg.

See *Focus on Communication: Normal and Abnormal Blood Pressures.*

FOCUS ON COMMUNICATION

Normal and Abnormal Blood Pressures

If agency policy allows, you can tell the person the BP. If the BP is abnormal, the person may worry and say: "That is higher (lower) than normal for me." Be calm and professional. You can say: "Yes, it was a little high (low). I will tell your nurse."

Report abnormal blood pressures to the nurse. You must report some concerns at once. For example, a BP is 82/58 and the person is dizzy. You help the person lie down and press the call light to report your concern. You identify yourself and say: "Please have the nurse come to room 216 right away." When the nurse arrives, you say: "I measured the BP at 82/58 with the complaint of dizziness. How can I help?"

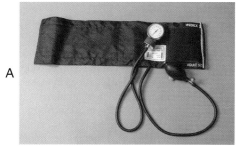
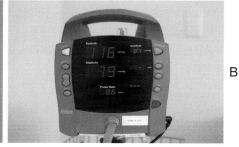

A

B

FIGURE 31-19 Blood pressure equipment. **A,** Aneroid manometer and cuff. **B,** Electronic manometer.

Blood Pressure Equipment. A *sphygmomanometer* has a cuff and a measuring device for measuring blood pressure. *Sphygmo* means *pulse*. A device for measuring pressure is called a *manometer*. These types are common:

- The *aneroid type* is a manual device with a round dial and a needle that points to the numbers (Fig. 31-19, *A*). (*Manual* relates to *being operated by hand*.)
- The *electronic type* shows the systolic and diastolic pressures and the pulse rate (Fig. 31-19, *B*).

You wrap the blood pressure cuff around the upper arm. Tubing connects the cuff to the manometer. When inflated (filled with air), the cuff causes pressure over the brachial artery. BP is measured as the cuff deflates (air is released).

- *Aneroid type.* A tube connects the cuff to a small, hand-held bulb. See Figure 31-20. To use the aneroid type:
  1 Hold the bulb with the air-release valve up.
  2 Turn the air-release valve clockwise (to the right) to close the valve.
  3 Squeeze the bulb. Squeezing the bulb inflates the cuff. (If you hear air leaking out and the cuff is not filling with air, the valve is not closed.)
  4 Turn the valve counter-clockwise (to the left) to deflate the cuff. Only turn the valve slightly. Turning the valve too much will cause the cuff to deflate too quickly.
  5 Use a stethoscope to listen over the brachial artery as the cuff slowly deflates. Blood flowing through the arteries produces sounds.
     - The first sound heard is the systolic pressure.
     - The last sound heard is the diastolic pressure.
- *Electronic type.* No stethoscope is needed. A button is pressed to inflate the cuff. The cuff deflates automatically. The BP is displayed. Follow the manufacturer's instructions.

See *Promoting Safety and Comfort: Blood Pressure Equipment.*

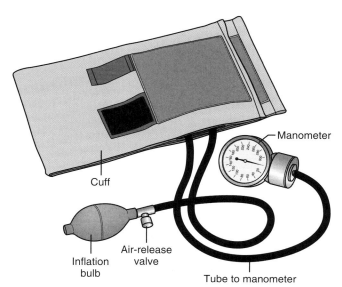

Manometer

Cuff

Air-release valve

Inflation bulb

Tube to manometer

FIGURE 31-20 Parts of an aneroid sphygmomanometer.

PROMOTING SAFETY AND COMFORT

Blood Pressure Equipment

Safety

Manometers containing mercury are being phased out of health care (Fig. 31-21). Some agencies may still use them. Handle mercury manometers carefully. If one breaks, call for the nurse at once. Do not touch the mercury. Do not let the person touch it. The agency follows special procedures for handling hazardous substances. See Chapter 11.

Comfort

Inflate the cuff only to the extent necessary. (See procedure: *Measuring Blood Pressure With an Aneroid Manometer,* p. 404.) The inflated cuff causes discomfort. The higher the inflation, the greater the discomfort.

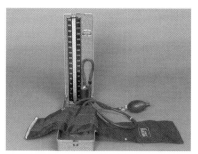

FIGURE 31-21   A mercury manometer.

Measuring Blood Pressure. You measure blood pressure in the brachial artery. Correct cuff size, cuff placement, and arm position are needed for an accurate measurement. Box 31-4 lists the guidelines for measuring blood pressure.

See *Focus on Math: Measuring Blood Pressure,* p. 404.

See *Delegation Guidelines: Measuring Blood Pressure,* p. 404.

See procedure: *Measuring Blood Pressure With an Aneroid Manometer,* p. 404.

See procedure: *Measuring Blood Pressure With an Electronic Manometer,* p. 406.

BOX 31-4 Measuring Blood Pressure—Guidelines

- Do not take BP on an arm:
  - With an IV (intravenous) infusion
  - With an arm cast
  - With a dialysis access site
  - On the side of breast surgery
  - That is injured
- Ask the nurse if unsure of which arm to use.
- Let the person rest for 10 to 20 minutes before measuring BP.
- Measure BP with the person sitting or lying. Sometimes BP is measured in the standing position.
- Position the arm at the level of the heart. Support the arm with the palm up.
- Apply the cuff to the bare upper arm. Clothing can affect the measurement.
- Make sure the cuff is snug. A loose cuff causes a wrong reading.
- Use a larger cuff if the person has a large arm. Use a small cuff for a very small arm. Ask the nurse what size to use. Also check the care plan.
- Ask the person to be still during the measurement. Electronic BP manometers measure BP using sensors. Movement can affect accuracy.
- Ask the nurse for help if you have trouble measuring a BP. Frequent measurements at the same site can block blood flow and cause injury.

Aneroid Type
- Make sure the room is quiet. Talking, TV, music, and sounds from the hallway can affect hearing through a stethoscope.
- Have the manometer where you can clearly see it.
- Place the diaphragm of the stethoscope firmly over the brachial artery. The entire diaphragm has contact with the skin.
- Use 1 of the following methods as directed by your instructor or the nurse. Methods 1 and 2 use the pulse as a guide for how much to inflate the cuff and at what point to listen for the systolic pressure. The systolic reading should be near the point where the pulse stops (Method 1) or returns (Method 2).

Aneroid Type—cont'd
- *Method 1—Feel for the pulse to stop.*
  1. Find the radial pulse.
  2. Inflate the cuff until you cannot feel the pulse. Note this point.
  3. Inflate the cuff 30 mm Hg beyond where you last felt the pulse.
  4. Deflate the cuff slowly and listen with the stethoscope over the brachial artery.
- *Method 2—Feel for the pulse to stop. Check that the pulse returns at this point.*
  1. Find the radial pulse.
  2. Inflate the cuff until you cannot feel the pulse. Note this point.
  3. Inflate the cuff 30 mm Hg beyond where you last felt the pulse.
  4. Deflate the cuff slowly. Note the point where you feel the pulse.
  5. Wait 30 seconds.
  6. Inflate the cuff again, 30 mm Hg beyond where you felt the pulse return.
  7. Deflate the cuff slowly and listen with the stethoscope over the brachial artery.
- *Method 3—Inflate the cuff beyond the usual systolic pressure.*
  1. Inflate the cuff 160 mm Hg to 180 mm Hg.
  2. Deflate the cuff completely if you hear a blood pressure sound right away when listening with the stethoscope over the brachial artery.
  3. Re-inflate the cuff to 200 mm Hg if needed.
  4. Deflate the cuff slowly and listen with the stethoscope over the brachial artery.
- Measure the systolic and diastolic pressures.
  - The first sound is the systolic pressure.
  - The point where the sound disappears (the last sound heard) is the diastolic pressure.
- Take the BP again if you are not sure of accuracy. Wait 30 to 60 seconds to repeat the measurement. Do not repeat the measurement multiple times using the same arm. Ask the nurse to take the BP if you are unsure of the measurement.
- Tell the nurse at once if you cannot hear the blood pressure.

FOCUS ON MATH
Measuring Blood Pressure

Aneroid manometers have long and short lines (Fig. 31-22).
- Long lines mark 10 mm Hg values.
- Short lines mark 2 mm Hg values (2, 4, 6, and 8).
  Read the manometer as the cuff deflates. The needle is dropping.
- If the needle is at a long line, note this value. Long line values end in 0. For example: 70, 80, 90, 100, 110, 120, and so on.
- If the needle is between 2 long lines:
  - Note the value of the long line below the needle.
  - Note the short line. Count up from the long line below by even numbers. Short line values end with 2, 4, 6, or 8. See Figure 31-22.

  For example: *The needle is at the 3rd short line between 90 and 100. Count up by even numbers from 90. Line 1 is 92. Line 2 is 94. Line 3 is 96. The value is 96.*

  If needed, round up to the nearest 2 mm Hg. When you *round up*, you choose the higher value. For example: *The needle is between 82 and 80. Report and record the value as 82 mm Hg.*

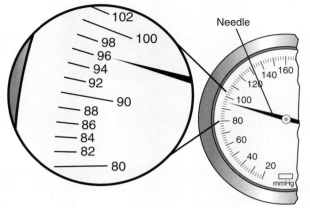

FIGURE 31-22 Reading the aneroid manometer. Long lines mark 10 mm Hg values. Short lines mark 2 mm Hg values.

DELEGATION GUIDELINES
Measuring Blood Pressure

Before measuring BP, you need this information from the nurse and the care plan.
- When to measure BP
- What sphygmomanometer to use (p. 402)
- What arm to use
- The person's normal blood pressure range
- If the nurse has concerns about certain patients or residents
- If the person needs to be lying down, sitting, or standing
- What size cuff to use—regular, child-sized, extra-large
- What observations to report and record
- When to report the BP measurement
- What patient or resident concerns to report at once

Measuring Blood Pressure With an Aneroid Manometer

Quality of Life

- Knock before entering the person's room.
- Address the person by name.
- Introduce yourself by name and title.
- Explain the procedure before starting and during the procedure.
- Protect the person's rights during the procedure.
- Handle the person gently during the procedure.

Pre-Procedure

1 Follow *Delegation Guidelines: Measuring Blood Pressure.* See *Promoting Safety and Comfort:*
   a *Using a Stethoscope*, p. 397
   b *Blood Pressure Equipment*, p. 402
2 Practice hand hygiene and get the following supplies.
   - Aneroid sphygmomanometer
   - Stethoscope
   - Antiseptic wipes
3 Practice hand hygiene.
4 Identify the person. Check the ID bracelet against the assignment sheet. Use 2 identifiers (Chapter 11). Also call the person by name.
5 Provide for privacy.

Procedure

6 Have the person sit or lie down.
7 Position the person's arm level with the heart. The palm is up.
8 Clean the stethoscope ear-pieces and chest-piece with an antiseptic wipe. Warm the diaphragm in your palm. Discard the wipe.
9 Stand no more than 3 feet away from the manometer.
10 Expose the upper arm.
11 Squeeze the cuff to expel (remove) any air. Close the valve on the bulb.
12 Find the brachial artery at the inner aspect of the elbow. (The brachial artery is on the little finger side of the arm.) Use your fingertips.
13 Locate the arrow on the cuff (Fig. 31-23, *A*). Align the arrow with the brachial artery (Fig. 31-23, *B*). Wrap the cuff around the upper arm at least 1 inch above the elbow. It is even and snug.

Measuring Blood Pressure With an Aneroid Manometer—cont'd

Procedure—cont'd

14 Use Method 1 or 2 if directed by your instructor or the nurse. See Box 31-4. These methods guide how much to inflate the cuff and at what point to listen for the systolic pressure. This procedure uses Method 3.
15 Place the stethoscope ear-pieces in your ears. Place the stethoscope's diaphragm over the brachial artery (Fig. 31-23, C). Do not place it under the cuff.
16 Inflate the cuff 160 mm Hg to 180 mm Hg. Deflate the cuff if you hear a blood pressure sound. Re-inflate the cuff to 200 mm Hg if needed.
17 Deflate the cuff at an even rate of 2 to 4 millimeters per second. Slowly turn the valve counter-clockwise to deflate the cuff. If the manometer needle (see Fig. 31-22) stops dropping and the cuff is not deflating, you need to turn the valve more.

18 Note the point where you hear the first sound (Fig. 31-24, A). This is the systolic reading.
19 Continue to deflate the cuff. Note the point where the sound disappears (the last sound heard). This is the diastolic reading (Fig. 31-24, B).
20 Deflate the cuff completely. Remove the cuff. Remove the stethoscope ear-pieces from your ears.
21 Note the person's name and BP on your note pad or assignment sheet. The BP in Figure 31-24 is written as 130/84 mm Hg.
22 Return the cuff to the case or wall holder.

Post-Procedure

23 Provide for comfort. (See the inside of the back cover.)
24 Place the call light and other needed items within reach.
25 Follow the care plan and the person's preferences for privacy measures to maintain. Leaving the privacy curtain, window coverings, and door open or closed are examples.
26 Complete a safety check of the room. (See the inside of the back cover.)

27 Clean the stethoscope ear-pieces and chest-piece with an antiseptic wipe. Discard the wipe.
28 Practice hand hygiene.
29 Return equipment to its proper place. Follow agency policy for disinfection.
30 Report and record the BP. Note which arm was used. Report an abnormal BP at once.

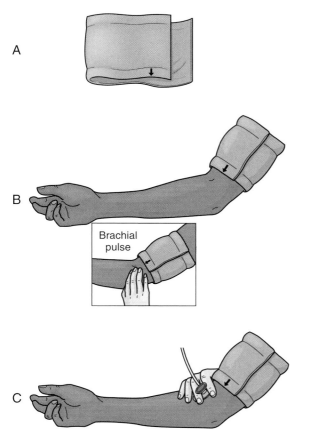

FIGURE 31-23 Measuring blood pressure. A, The arrow is used for correct cuff alignment. B, The cuff is placed so the arrow is aligned with the brachial artery. C, The diaphragm of the stethoscope is over the brachial artery.

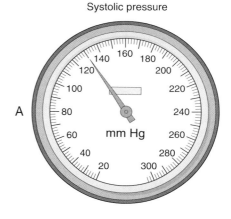
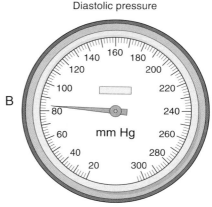

FIGURE 31-24 Manometer readings. A, This manometer is at 130 mm Hg for a systolic pressure. B, This manometer is at 84 mm Hg for a diastolic pressure. (NOTE: Both pressures are above the normal range.)

Measuring Blood Pressure With an Electronic Manometer

Quality of Life

- Knock before entering the person's room.
- Address the person by name.
- Introduce yourself by name and title.

- Explain the procedure before starting and during the procedure.
- Protect the person's rights during the procedure.
- Handle the person gently during the procedure.

Pre-Procedure

1 Follow *Delegation Guidelines: Measuring Blood Pressure*, p. 404.
2 Practice hand hygiene and get the following supplies.
   - Electronic BP manometer
   - BP cuff for use with the device (in the correct size for the person)
3 Practice hand hygiene.

4 Identify the person. Check the ID bracelet against the assignment sheet. Use 2 identifiers (Chapter 11). Also call the person by name.
5 Provide for privacy.

Procedure

6 Have the person sit or lie down.
7 Position the arm level with the heart.
8 Expose the upper arm. The palm is up.
9 Squeeze the cuff to expel (remove) any air.
10 Turn on the electronic BP manometer.
11 Connect the cuff to the manometer's connection tubing.
12 Find the brachial artery at the inner aspect of the elbow. (The brachial artery is on the little finger side of the arm.) Use your fingertips.
13 Locate the arrow on the cuff. Align the arrow with the brachial artery. Wrap the cuff around the upper arm at least 1 inch above the elbow. It is even and snug.

14 Press the start button on the device. Leave the cuff in place while the device measures the BP. Ask the person to be still.
15 Remove the cuff after the BP is measured. The BP is displayed on the device.
16 Note the person's name and BP on your note pad or assignment sheet.
17 Follow agency policy for where to store the cuff (in the person's room or with the BP manometer).

Post-Procedure

18 Provide for comfort. (See the inside of the back cover.)
19 Place the call light and other needed items within reach.
20 Follow the care plan and the person's preferences for privacy measures to maintain. Leaving the privacy curtain, window coverings, and door open or closed are examples.
21 Complete a safety check of the room. (See the inside of the back cover.)

22 Practice hand hygiene.
23 Return the equipment to its proper place. Follow agency policy for disinfection.
24 Report and record the BP. Note which arm was used. Report an abnormal BP at once.

PULSE OXIMETRY

Pulse oximetry measures the oxygen level in the blood. This is often measured with temperature, pulse, respirations, and blood pressure. It may be a vital sign in some agencies. See "Pulse Oximetry" in Chapter 37.

PAIN

Pain is a warning sign from the body. It signals tissue damage. Therefore many agencies consider it to be a vital sign. See "Pain" in Chapter 33.

WEIGHT AND HEIGHT

Weight and height are measured on admission to the agency. Then the person is weighed daily, weekly, or monthly. This is done to measure weight gain or loss.

A standing scale (Fig. 31-25) is used for persons able to stand and walk. Wheelchair scales (Fig. 31-26) are also common. Chair, bed, and lift scales may also be used for persons who cannot stand. To measure weight and height, follow the guidelines in Box 31-5.

See *Focus on Communication: Weight and Height.*
See *Focus on Math: Weight and Height*, p. 408.
See *Delegation Guidelines: Weight and Height*, p. 409.
See procedure: *Measuring Weight and Height With a Standing Scale*, p. 409.

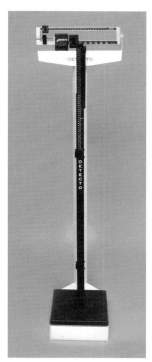

FIGURE 31-25 A standing scale. (NOTE: This is a balance scale.)

BOX 31-5 Measuring Weight and Height

- Follow the manufacturer's instructions for the scale used.
- Practice safety measures to prevent falls. See Chapter 12.
- Have the person wear a patient gown or sleepwear only. Clothes add weight. Footwear adds to the weight and height measurements.
- Protect the person from chilling and drafts. See Chapter 19.
- Have the person void before being weighed. A full bladder adds weight.
- Provide a dry incontinence product if needed. A wet product adds weight.
- Weigh the person at the same time of day. Before breakfast is the best time. Food and fluids add weight.
- Use the same scale for daily, weekly, and monthly weights. Scales weigh differently.
- Balance the scale at zero (0) before weighing the person.
  - For a balance scale (see Fig. 31-25), move the weights to zero.
  - For a digital scale (see Fig. 31-26), press the "Zero" or "Tare" button with nothing on the scale if the scale needs to be balanced at zero (0).

FOCUS ON **COMMUNICATION**

Weight and Height

Some agencies use pounds (lb) for weight. Others use kilograms (kg) (2.2 lb = 1 kg). For height, some agencies use feet (ft) and inches (in). Others only use inches.

Ask the nurse what measurements to use. Follow agency policy for reporting and recording weight and height.

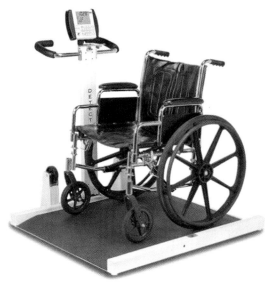

FIGURE 31-26 A wheelchair scale. (NOTE: This is a digital scale.) (Courtesy Detecto.)

To use a wheelchair scale:

1. Weigh the person's wheelchair while the person is in bed or in a chair. Note the wheelchair's weight.

2. Weigh the person while seated in the wheelchair.

3. Subtract the weight of the wheelchair (weight from step 1) from the weight of the person in the wheelchair (weight from step 2). This is the person's weight.

FOCUS ON MATH
Weight and Height

Weight—Reading the Scale

Standing scales (balance scales) have 2 bars with measurements (Fig. 31-27).

- The lower bar is divided into 50 pound (lb) values.
- The upper bar has long and short lines.
  - Long lines are 1 lb values.
  - Short lines are ¼, ½, and ¾ lb values.

The lower and upper bar values are added for the weight. For example: *The lower bar is at 100 lb and the upper bar is at 34 lb. The person's weight is 134 lb.*

$$100 \text{ lb} + 34 \text{ lb} = 134 \text{ lb}$$

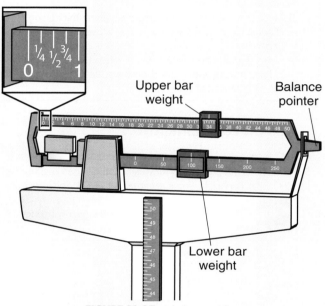

Upper bar weight

Balance pointer

Lower bar weight

FIGURE 31-27 A balance scale.

Height—Reading the Height Rod

The height rod has 2 sections—upper and lower. Raise or lower the upper section to adjust to the person's height. If the person is taller than the lower section, read the height at the movable part of the height rod.

The rod is marked with 1 inch (in) and ¼ inch values (¼, ½, ¾). Read height to the nearest ¼ inch. The numbers on the lower section increase moving *up* the rod. The numbers on the upper section increase moving *down* the rod. See Figure 31-28.

Height—Converting Inches Into Feet and Inches

There are 12 inches (in) in 1 foot (ft) (1 ft = 12 in). To convert inches into feet and inches, divide the number of inches by 12. If it does not divide evenly by 12, the number left over is the number of inches. For example: *Convert 64 inches into feet and inches.*

$$
\begin{array}{r}
5 \text{ Number of feet} \\
12 \text{ Inches per foot } \overline{\smash{)}\ 64 \text{ Inches}} \\
-60 \\
\hline
4 \text{ Number of inches}
\end{array}
$$

64 inches = 5 ft 4 in

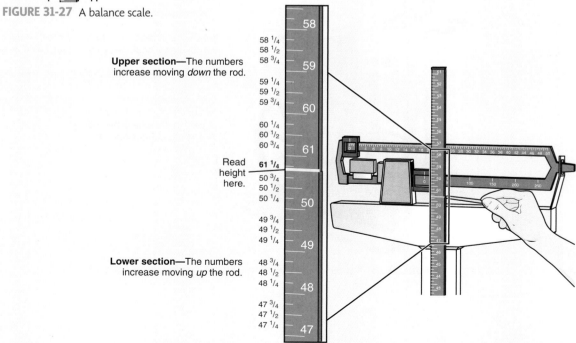

Upper section—The numbers increase moving *down* the rod.

58
58 ¼
58 ½
58 ¾
59
59 ¼
59 ½
59 ¾
60
60 ¼
60 ½
60 ¾
61

Read height here. → **61 ¼**

50 ¾
50 ½
50 ¼
50
49 ¾
49 ½
49 ¼
49

Lower section—The numbers increase moving *up* the rod.

48 ¾
48 ½
48 ¼
48
47 ¾
47 ½
47 ¼
47

FIGURE 31-28 Height is read at the movable part of the height rod. (NOTE: The movable part of the height rod is marked with a yellow line.) This height rod measures 61¼ inches (5 feet 1¼ inches).

DELEGATION GUIDELINES

Weight and Height

To measure weight and height, you need this information from the nurse and the care plan.
- When to measure weight and height
- What scale to use
- When to report the measurements
- What patient or resident concerns to report at once

Measuring Weight and Height With a Standing Scale

Quality of Life

- Knock before entering the person's room.
- Address the person by name.
- Introduce yourself by name and title.

- Explain the procedure before starting and during the procedure.
- Protect the person's rights during the procedure.
- Handle the person gently during the procedure.

Pre-Procedure

1 Follow *Delegation Guidelines: Weight and Height.*
2 Ask the person to void.
3 Practice hand hygiene.
4 Bring the scale and paper towels to the person's room if the person is not assisted to the area where the scale is kept. Or gather items as needed for ambulation (walking) to the scale (Chapter 32). (Be sure the person is covered for warmth and privacy.)

5 Practice hand hygiene.
6 Identify the person. Check the ID bracelet against the assignment sheet. Use 2 identifiers (Chapter 11). Also call the person by name.
7 Provide for privacy.

Procedure

8 Place the paper towels on the scale platform.
9 Raise the height rod.
10 Move the weights to zero (0). The pointer is in the middle.
11 Have the person remove footwear. Assist as needed. The person wears only a gown or sleepwear. (NOTE: For some state competency tests, shoes are worn.)
12 Help the person stand in the center of the scale. Arms are at the sides. The person does not hold on to anyone or any thing. See Figure 31-29, p. 410.
13 Move the lower and upper weights until the balance pointer is in the middle (see Fig. 31-27).
14 Note the weight on your note pad or assignment sheet.

15 Ask the person to stand very straight.
16 Lower the height rod until it rests on the person's head (Fig. 31-30, p. 410).
17 Read the height at the movable part of the height rod. Record the height in inches (or in feet and inches) to the nearest ¼ inch. See Figure 31-28.
18 Note the height on your note pad or assignment sheet.
19 Raise the height rod. Help the person step off of the scale.
20 Help put on slip-resistant footwear if the person will be up. Or help the person back to bed.
21 Lower the height rod. Adjust the weights to zero (0) if this is your agency's policy.

Post-Procedure

22 Provide for comfort. (See the inside of the back cover.)
23 Place the call light and other needed items within reach.
24 Raise or lower bed rails. Follow the care plan.
25 Follow the care plan and the person's preferences for privacy measures to maintain. Leaving the privacy curtain, window coverings, and door open or closed are examples.

26 Complete a safety check of the room. (See the inside of the back cover.)
27 Discard the paper towels.
28 Practice hand hygiene.
29 Return the scale to its proper place if it was moved.
30 Report and record the measurements.

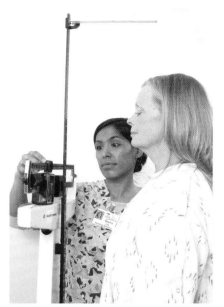

FIGURE 31-29 The person is weighed.

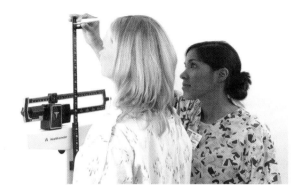

FIGURE 31-30 The height rod rests on the person's head.

FOCUS ON P R I D E

The Person, Family, and Yourself

P ersonal and Professional Responsibility

You must know the normal ranges for vital signs. For an adult:
- Oral temperature—98.6°F (37.0°C). See Table 31-1 for normal temperatures at other sites.
- Pulse—60 to 100 beats per minute.
- Respirations—12 to 20 breaths per minute.
- Blood pressure—90/60 mm Hg or higher but lower than 120/80 mm Hg.

Learning to measure vital signs takes practice. Do not be upset if you struggle at first. Plan when and what you will practice. Use class time wisely. Tell your instructor if you need more practice. Never be ashamed to ask for more practice time. Practice builds confidence.

R ights and Respect

The nurse may ask you to re-take a measurement. Or the nurse may re-check the measurement. Do not be offended. Show respect. Avoid negative thoughts or statements about the nurse or yourself. It does not mean the nurse does not trust you or that you have done something wrong. The nurse checks the measurements for safe care.

I ndependence and Social Interaction

Personal choice promotes independence. The person may prefer a certain arm for pulses and blood pressures. If safe to do so, use the arm the person prefers. Unless directed otherwise, let the person choose to sit or lie when vital signs are measured.

D elegation and Teamwork

You may care for persons needing Transmission-Based Precautions (Chapter 15). You must prevent the spread of infection from equipment. Some agencies have isolation carts or kits with equipment for vital signs. The equipment is left in the person's room. Do not use your own stethoscope or bring other equipment into the room. If equipment must be brought in, disinfect it after use. Special disinfectants may be needed. Follow agency policy to protect others from infection.

E thics and Laws

Measurements must be accurate. Tell the nurse if you are unsure of any measurement. For example, you cannot feel a pulse or hear a blood pressure. Never make up a measurement. Reporting or recording false measurements is wrong. The person can be harmed. Take pride in doing the right thing by honest reporting and recording.

FOCUS ON PRIDE: *Application*

Plan to practice measurements at school and at home. Practice on classmates, family, and friends. Who will you practice with? What will you practice most at school? What can you practice at home?

Circle the BEST answer.

1 Which should you report at once?
   a An oral temperature of 98.4°F
   b A rectal temperature of 101.6°F
   c An axillary temperature of 97.6°F
   d An oral temperature of 97.8°F

2 A rectal temperature is taken when the person
   a Is unconscious
   b Has heart disease
   c Is confused
   d Has diarrhea

3 To use an electronic thermometer
   a Shake down the thermometer before each use
   b Leave the thermometer in place for 2 minutes
   c Cover the probe with a probe cover
   d Use the blue probe for a rectal temperature

4 Which is usually used to take an adult's pulse?
   a The radial pulse
   b The apical pulse
   c The carotid pulse
   d The brachial pulse

5 For an adult, which pulse do you report at once?
   a A regular pulse at 64 beats per minute
   b A strong pulse at 78 beats per minute
   c A regular pulse at 90 beats per minute
   d An irregular pulse at 124 beats per minute

6 You count a regular pulse for 30 seconds. Which is *true*?
   a Divide the number of beats by 2 for the pulse rate.
   b If you count 44 beats, record a pulse rate of 44.
   c If you count 44 beats, record a pulse rate of 88.
   d Ask the nurse to check a regular pulse.

7 Which statement about measuring respirations is *true*?
   a Count the rise and fall of the chest as 2 respirations.
   b Count an abnormal pattern for 30 seconds.
   c A rate of 14 is abnormal for an adult.
   d Respirations are normally quiet.

8 Respirations are usually counted
   a After taking the temperature
   b After activity
   c After taking the pulse
   d After taking the blood pressure

9 Which adult blood pressure is normal?
   a 80/54 mm Hg
   b 140/90 mm Hg
   c 112/78 mm Hg
   d 130/82 mm Hg

10 When measuring BP
   a Apply the cuff to the bare upper arm
   b Use the arm with an IV infusion
   c Make sure the cuff is loose
   d Place the stethoscope under the cuff

11 You apply the BP cuff to the person's arm. You place the stethoscope over the brachial artery. What do you do next?
   a Listen for the pulse with the cuff deflated.
   b Inflate the cuff as much as possible.
   c Listen for sounds as you inflate the cuff.
   d Inflate the cuff and listen for sounds as you deflate the cuff.

12 When measuring BP, you hear the first sound at 116. You should
   a Re-check the measurement because it is abnormal
   b Record the pulse as 116 beats per minute
   c Record 116 as the top number (the systolic pressure)
   d Record 116 as the bottom number (the diastolic pressure)

13 When taking a BP, you hear the last sound at the 1st short line above 70. You record the
   a Systolic pressure as 70
   b Diastolic pressure as 71
   c Systolic pressure as 72
   d Diastolic pressure as 72

14 You are not sure you heard a BP correctly. You should
   a Record what you think you heard
   b Measure the BP again after 60 seconds
   c Repeat the BP using the bell part of the stethoscope
   d Ask another nursing assistant to take the BP

15 When using electronic BP equipment, you need
   a A stethoscope and antiseptic wipes
   b A BP cuff that connects to the device
   c An inflation bulb with an air-release valve
   d The nurse to operate the equipment

16 You are going to measure weight with a standing scale. Which should you correct before weighing the person?
   a The person is wearing a heavy coat.
   b The scale is balanced at zero (0).
   c There is a paper towel on the scale platform.
   d The person is in the center of the scale with arms at the sides.

17 When measuring height with a standing scale
   a Balance the height rod at zero (0)
   b Be sure footwear is worn
   c Read the height at the movable part of the rod
   d Record height to the nearest inch

18 What is 68 inches in feet and inches?
   a 4 ft 0 in
   b 5 ft 6 in
   c 5 ft 8 in
   d 6 ft 8 in

Answers to Chapter 31 questions are on p. 588.

FOCUS ON PRACTICE

Problem Solving

A person's pulse is 110. The respiratory rate is 24. The oral temperature is 100.8°F. You think you heard the BP at 86/52. You are unsure of the measurement. What will you do? Are any of the vital signs abnormal? What must you do?

CHAPTER 32

Exercise and Activity Needs

Exercise and activity are important for every body system. Illness, surgery, injury, pain, and aging can cause weakness and some activity limits.

You help promote exercise and activity in all persons to the extent possible. The care plan and your assignment sheet include the person's activity level and needed exercises.

See *Focus on Older Persons: Exercise and Activity Needs.*

> ### FOCUS ON **OLDER PERSONS**
> #### *Exercise and Activity Needs*
>
> Persons with dementia may resist exercise and activity. They may fear harm, become agitated or combative, or cry out for help. Do not force the person to exercise or take part in activities. Stay calm and ask the nurse for help. Follow the care plan.

MOBILITY AND IMMOBILITY

*Mobility refers to a person's ability to move. **Immobility** is the inability to move.* Immobility (inactivity), whether mild or severe, affects every body system and mental well-being. ***Deconditioning** is the loss of muscle strength from inactivity.* When not active, deconditioning can occur quickly. See "Complications From Immobility."

Bed Rest

***Bed rest** means restricting a person to bed and limiting activity for health reasons.* Bed rest is ordered for a health problem or because of a change in the person's condition. Common reasons are to:

- Reduce oxygen needs.
- Reduce pain.
- Reduce swelling.
- Promote healing.
  These types of bed rest are common.
- *Strict (complete) bed rest.* Everything is done for the person. All activities of daily living (ADL) are done in bed.
- *Bed rest.* The person performs some ADL. Self-feeding, oral hygiene, bathing, shaving, and hair care are often allowed.
- *Bed rest with commode privileges.* The commode is used at the bedside for elimination.
- *Bed rest with bathroom privileges (bed rest with BRP).* The bathroom is used for elimination.

Bed rest definitions vary among agencies. Follow the person's care plan and your assignment sheet for the activities allowed. Ask the nurse if you have questions about a person's activity limits.

Complications From Immobility

Immobility can cause serious complications. Pressure injuries, constipation, and fecal impaction can result. Urinary tract infections and renal calculi (kidney stones) can occur. So can blood clots (thrombi) and pneumonia (inflammation and infection of the lung).

The musculo-skeletal system is affected too. For normal movement, you must help prevent the following.

- A ***contracture** is decreased motion and stiffness of a joint caused by shortening* (contracting) *of a muscle.* The contracted muscle is fixed into position, is deformed, and cannot stretch (Fig. 32-1). Common sites are the fingers, wrists, elbows, toes, ankles, knees, and hips. They can also occur in the neck and spine. The site is deformed and stiff.
- *Atrophy is the decrease in size or the wasting away of tissue.* Tissues shrink in size. *Muscle atrophy* is a decrease in size or a wasting away of muscle (Fig. 32-2).

***Postural hypotension** (orthostatic hypotension) is abnormally low* (hypo) *blood pressure when the person suddenly stands up* (postural). When moving from lying to sitting to standing, the blood pressure drops. The person becomes dizzy, weak, and has spots before the eyes. *Syncope* (fainting) can occur (Chapter 43).

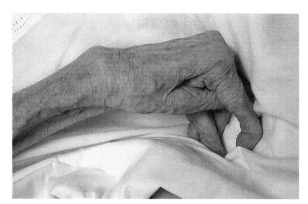

FIGURE 32-1 A contracture.

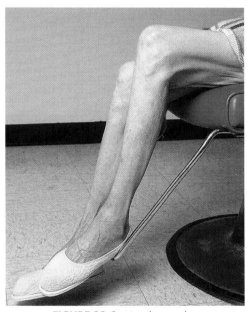

FIGURE 32-2 Muscle atrophy.

Preventing Complications

Good nursing care can prevent complications from immobility. Exercise helps prevent contractures, muscle atrophy, and other complications from immobility. Some exercise occurs with ADL. Range-of-motion exercises (p. 414) promote joint mobility. Weight-bearing exercises are needed to gain muscle strength. See "Ambulation" on p. 421.

Good alignment and frequent position changes are important measures. Devices may be used to support body parts and maintain proper position. See "Positioning Devices" on p. 418.

Increasing mobility to the extent possible is a goal. The person progresses in stages from:

1. Supine to Fowler's position
2. Fowler's position to sitting on the side of the bed
3. Sitting on the side of the bed to standing
4. Standing to walking or sitting in a chair

The person's care plan includes needed care measures to prevent complications and promote mobility.

See *Promoting Safety and Comfort: Preventing Complications,* p. 414.

PROMOTING SAFETY AND COMFORT
Preventing Complications

Safety

Slowly changing positions is key to preventing postural hypotension. Give the person time to adjust to 1 position (supine, Fowler's position, sitting, standing) before moving to the next. Ask about weakness, dizziness, or spots before the eyes. Return the person to the previous position if any occur. For example, the person is dizzy while standing. Help the person sit.

Measure vital signs. While the person is lying down, measure blood pressure, pulse, respirations, and pulse oximetry (Chapters 31 and 37). Measure vital signs in other positions (sitting, standing) as directed by the nurse.

Report and record the person's vital signs and symptoms. Call for the nurse at once if you have concerns about the person's condition.

RANGE-OF-MOTION EXERCISES

*The movement of a joint to the extent possible without causing pain is the **range of motion (ROM)** of the joint. Range-of-motion exercises involve moving the joints through their complete range of motion* (Box 32-1). *Depending on the person's abilities, ROM exercises are active, passive, or active-assistive.*

- *Active* ROM exercises—are done by the person.
- *Passive* ROM (PROM) exercises—you move the joints through their range of motion.
- *Active-assistive* ROM exercises—the person does the exercises with some help.

See *Focus on Surveys: Range-of-Motion Exercises.*
See *Delegation Guidelines: Range-of-Motion Exercises.*
See *Promoting Safety and Comfort: Range-of-Motion Exercises.*
See procedure: *Performing Range-of-Motion Exercises.*

BOX 32-1 Range-of-Motion Exercises

Joint Movements
- **Abduction**—*moving a body part away from the mid-line of the body*
- **Adduction**—*moving a body part toward the mid-line of the body*
- **Opposition**—*touching an opposite finger with the thumb*
- **Flexion**—*bending a body part*
- **Extension**—*straightening a body part*
- **Hyperextension**—*excessive straightening of a body part*
- **Dorsiflexion**—*bending the toes and foot up at the ankle*
- **Plantar flexion**—*bending the foot down at the ankle*
- **Rotation**—*turning the joint*
- **Internal rotation**—*turning the joint inward*
- **External rotation**—*turning the joint outward*
- **Pronation**—*turning the joint downward*
- **Supination**—*turning the joint upward*

Safety and Comfort Measures
- Cover the person with a bath blanket for warmth and privacy.
- Exercise only the joints the nurse tells you to exercise.
- Use good body mechanics.
- Expose only the body part being exercised.
- Support the part being exercised at all times.
- Move the joint slowly, smoothly, and gently.
- Do not force a joint beyond its present range of motion or to the point of pain. As each joint is exercised, ask if the person:
    - Feels that the joint cannot move any farther.
    - Feels pain or discomfort in the joint.
    - Needs to stop or rest.
- Observe for signs of pain (Chapter 33). Restlessness and grimacing are examples.
- Stop if you meet resistance or suspect pain. Tell the nurse.

FOCUS ON **SURVEYS**
Range-of-Motion Exercises

ROM exercises are part of the person's care plan. They are usually done at least 2 times a day. Persons on bed rest need more frequent ROM exercises. The goal may be 1 of the following.
- Increase range of motion.
- Prevent loss or further decreases in range of motion. Surveyors may observe you performing ROM activities.

DELEGATION GUIDELINES
Range-of-Motion Exercises

When delegated ROM exercises, you need this information from the nurse and the care plan.
- If ROM exercises are active, passive, or active-assistive
- Which joints to exercise
- What ROM exercises to do (see Box 32-1)
- When to do the exercises
- How many times to repeat each exercise
- What observations to report and record:
    - The time the exercises were performed
    - The joints exercised and the exercises performed
    - The number of times the exercises were performed on each joint
    - Complaints of pain or signs of stiffness or spasm; specify the joint or body part involved
    - The degree to which the person took part in the exercises
    - When to report observations
- What patient or resident concerns to report at once

PROMOTING SAFETY AND COMFORT
Range-of-Motion Exercises

Safety

ROM exercises can cause pain and injury if not done correctly. Practice the safety measures in Box 32-1. Remind the person to tell you about any pain during the procedure.

ROM exercises to the neck can cause serious injury if not done correctly. Some agencies give nursing assistants special training before doing such exercises. Other agencies do not let nursing assistants do them. Know your agency's policy. Perform ROM exercises to the neck only if allowed by your agency, if you received needed training, and if the nurse instructs you to do so. In some agencies, only physical therapists do neck exercises.

Comfort

To promote physical comfort during ROM exercises, see Box 32-1. Provide privacy to promote mental comfort.

Performing Range-of-Motion Exercises

Quality of Life

- Knock before entering the person's room.
- Address the person by name.
- Introduce yourself by name and title.

- Explain the procedure before starting and during the procedure.
- Protect the person's rights during the procedure.
- Handle the person gently during the procedure.

Pre-Procedure

1 Follow *Delegation Guidelines: Range-of-Motion Exercises.* See *Promoting Safety and Comfort: Range-of-Motion Exercises.*
2 Practice hand hygiene.
3 Identify the person. Check the identification (ID) bracelet against the assignment sheet. Use 2 identifiers (Chapter 11). Also call the person by name.

4 Get a bath blanket.
5 Provide for privacy.
6 Raise the bed for body mechanics. Bed rails are up if used. Lower the bed rail near you if up.

Procedure

7 Position the person supine.
8 Cover the person with the bath blanket. Fan-fold top linens to the foot of the bed.
9 Exercise the neck *if allowed by your agency and if the nurse instructs you to do so* (Fig. 32-3, p. 416).
  a Place your hands over the ears to support the head. Support the jaw with your fingers.
  b Flexion—bring the head forward. The chin touches the chest.
  c Extension—straighten the head.
  d Hyperextension—bring the head backward until the chin points up.
  e Rotation—turn the head from side to side.
  f Lateral flexion—move the head to the right and to the left.
  g Repeat flexion, extension, hyperextension, rotation, and lateral flexion 5 times—or the number of times stated on the care plan.
10 Exercise the shoulder (Fig. 32-4, p. 416).
  a Support the wrist with 1 hand. Support the elbow with the other hand.
  b Flexion—raise the arm straight up in front and over the head.
  c Extension—bring the arm down.
  d Hyperextension—move the arm behind the body. (Do this if the person is in a straight-backed chair or is standing.)
  e Abduction—move the straight arm away from the side of the body.
  f Adduction—move the straight arm to the side of the body.
  g Internal rotation—bend the elbow. Place it at the same level as the shoulder. Move the forearm and hand so the fingers point down.
  h External rotation—move the forearm and hand so the fingers point up.
  i Repeat flexion, extension, hyperextension, abduction, adduction, and internal and external rotation 5 times—or the number of times stated on the care plan.
11 Exercise the elbow (Fig. 32-5, p. 416).
  a Support the wrist with 1 hand. Support the elbow with your other hand.
  b Flexion—bend the arm so the same-side shoulder is touched.
  c Extension—straighten the arm.
  d Repeat flexion and extension 5 times—or the number of times stated on the care plan.

12 Exercise the forearm (Fig. 32-6, p. 416).
  a Continue to support the wrist and elbow.
  b Pronation—turn the hand so the palm is down.
  c Supination—turn the hand so the palm is up.
  d Repeat pronation and supination 5 times—or the number of times stated on the care plan.
13 Exercise the wrist (Fig. 32-7, p. 417).
  a Support the wrist with both of your hands.
  b Flexion—bend the hand down.
  c Extension—straighten the hand.
  d Hyperextension—bend the hand back.
  e Radial flexion (deviation)—turn the hand toward the thumb.
  f Ulnar flexion (deviation)—turn the hand toward the little finger.
  g Repeat flexion, extension, hyperextension, radial flexion (deviation), and ulnar flexion (deviation) 5 times—or the number of times stated on the care plan.
14 Exercise the thumb (Fig. 32-8, p. 417).
  a Support the person's hand with 1 hand. Support the thumb with your other hand.
  b Abduction—move the thumb out from the inner part of the index finger.
  c Adduction—move the thumb back next to the index finger.
  d Opposition—touch each fingertip with the thumb.
  e Flexion—bend the thumb into the hand.
  f Extension—move the thumb out to the side of the fingers.
  g Repeat abduction, adduction, opposition, flexion, and extension 5 times—or the number of times stated on the care plan.
15 Exercise the fingers (Fig. 32-9, p. 417).
  a Abduction—spread the fingers apart.
  b Adduction—bring the fingers together.
  c Flexion—make a fist.
  d Extension—straighten the fingers so the fingers, hand, and arm are straight.
  e Repeat abduction, adduction, flexion, and extension 5 times—or the number of times stated on the care plan.

Continued

Performing Range-of-Motion Exercises—cont'd

Procedure—cont'd

16 Exercise the hip (Fig. 32-10).
   a Support the leg. Place 1 hand under the knee. Place your other hand under the ankle.
   b Flexion—raise the leg.
   c Extension—straighten the leg.
   d Hyperextension—move the leg behind the body. (Do this if the person is standing.)
   e Abduction—move the leg away from the body.
   f Adduction—move the leg toward the other leg.
   g Internal rotation—turn the leg inward.
   h External rotation—turn the leg outward.
   i Repeat flexion, extension, hyperextension, abduction, adduction, and internal and external rotation 5 times—or the number of times stated on the care plan.

17 Exercise the knee (Fig. 32-11).
   a Support the knee. Place 1 hand under the knee. Place your other hand under the ankle.
   b Flexion—bend the knee.
   c Extension—straighten the knee.
   d Repeat flexion and extension 5 times—or the number of times stated on the care plan.

18 Exercise the ankle (Fig. 32-12).
   a Support the foot and ankle. Place 1 hand under the foot. Place your other hand under the ankle.
   b Dorsiflexion—pull the foot upward. Push down on the heel at the same time.
   c Plantar flexion—turn the foot down. Or point the toes.
   d Repeat dorsiflexion and plantar flexion 5 times—or the number of times stated on the care plan.

19 Exercise the foot (Fig. 32-13).
   a Continue to support the foot and ankle.
   b Pronation—turn the outside of the foot up and the inside down.
   c Supination—turn the inside of the foot up and the outside down.
   d Repeat pronation and supination 5 times—or the number of times stated on the care plan.

20 Exercise the toes (Fig. 32-14).
   a Flexion—curl the toes.
   b Extension—straighten the toes.
   c Abduction—spread the toes.
   d Adduction—put the toes together.
   e Repeat flexion, extension, abduction, and adduction 5 times—or the number of times stated on the care plan.

21 Cover the leg. Raise the bed rail if used.
22 Go to the other side. Lower the bed rail near you if up.
23 Repeat steps 10 through 20. Cover the leg when done.

Post-Procedure

24 Provide for comfort. (See the inside of the back cover.)
25 Cover the person with the top linens. Remove the bath blanket.
26 Place the call light and other needed items within reach.
27 Lower the bed to a safe and comfortable level. Follow the care plan.
28 Raise or lower bed rails. Follow the care plan.
29 Fold and return the bath blanket to its proper place. Or follow agency policy for used linens.
30 Follow the care plan and the person's preferences for privacy measures to maintain. Leaving the privacy curtain, window coverings, and door open or closed are examples.
31 Complete a safety check of the room. (See the inside of the back cover.)
32 Practice hand hygiene.
33 Report and record your care and observations.

Flexion   Extension   Hyperextension   Rotation   Lateral flexion

FIGURE 32-3 Range-of-motion exercises for the neck.

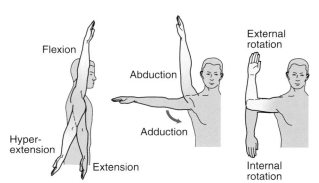
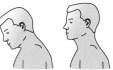

Flexion
Abduction
External rotation
Adduction
Hyper-extension
Extension
Internal rotation

FIGURE 32-4 Range-of-motion exercises for the shoulder.

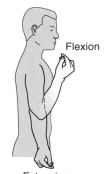

Flexion
Extension

FIGURE 32-5 Range-of-motion exercises for the elbow.

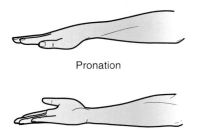

Pronation
Supination

FIGURE 32-6 Range-of-motion exercises for the forearm.

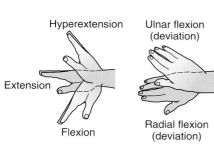

FIGURE 32-7 Range-of-motion exercises for the wrist.

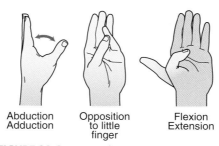

FIGURE 32-8 Range-of-motion exercises for the thumb.

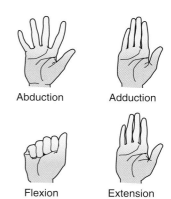

FIGURE 32-9 Range-of-motion exercises for the fingers.

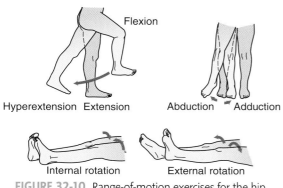

FIGURE 32-10 Range-of-motion exercises for the hip.

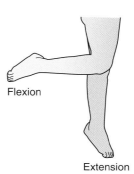

FIGURE 32-11 Range-of-motion exercises for the knee.

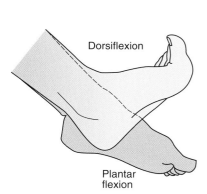

FIGURE 32-12 Range-of-motion exercises for the ankle.

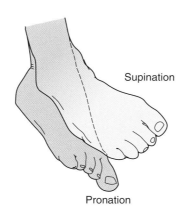

FIGURE 32-13 Range-of-motion exercises for the foot.

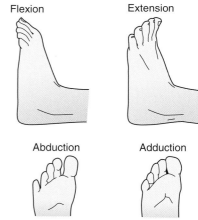

FIGURE 32-14 Range-of-motion exercises for the toes.

POSITIONING DEVICES

Body alignment and positioning were discussed in Chapter 16. Positioning (supportive) devices are used to maintain a certain position. See Table 32-1.

An **orthotic** *is a device used to support a muscle, promote a certain motion, or correct a deformity.* (Ortho *means* to straighten.) Paralysis and muscle weakness are common reasons for orthotic devices. Braces and ankle-foot orthoses (AFOs) are examples (see Table 32-1).

Keep the skin and bony points in contact with positioning devices clean and dry. This prevents skin breakdown. Report redness or signs of skin breakdown at once. Also report complaints of pain or discomfort. The care plan tells you when to use positioning devices.

Table 32-1	**Positioning Devices**	
Device	Description	Example
Foot-board	• Prevents plantar flexion that can lead to footdrop. **Footdrop** *is when the foot falls down at the ankle (permanent plantar flexion).* • The soles of the feet are flush against the foot-board. • Foot-boards also serve as bed cradles by keeping top linens off of the feet and toes.	
Bed cradle	• Keeps the weight of top linens off of the feet and toes. Heavy top linens can cause footdrop and pressure injuries (Chapter 36).	
Trochanter roll	• Prevents the hips and legs from turning outward (external rotation). • A bath blanket or bath towel is folded to the desired length and rolled up tightly. The flat end is placed under the person from the hip to the knee. The roll is tucked alongside the body.	
Hip abduction wedge	• Keeps the hips abducted (apart). • The wedge is placed between the person's legs. The device is common after hip replacement surgery.	

Table 32-1   Positioning Devices—cont'd

Device	Description	Example
Hand roll (hand grip)	• Prevents contractures of the thumb, fingers, and wrist.	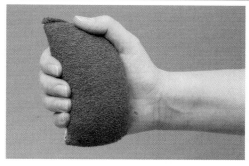
Finger cushion	• Prevents contractures of the thumb, fingers, and wrist. The fingers are separated.	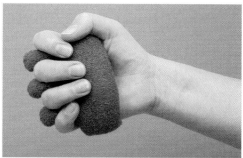
Splint	• Keeps elbows, wrists, thumbs, fingers, ankles, or knees in the normal position. • They are usually secured in place with Velcro.	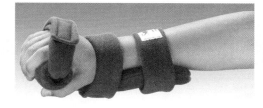
Brace	• Supports a weak body part. Prevents or corrects deformities or prevents joint movement. • Applied over the ankle, knee, or back.	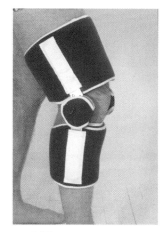
Ankle-foot orthosis (AFO)	• Provides support and alignment to the ankle and foot. Used for footdrop, an AFO is common after a stroke. • Worn with a sock and shoe and secured with a Velcro strap.	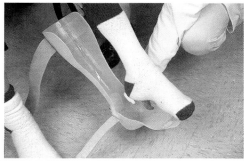

Splint image courtesy Ongoing Care Solutions, Inc., Pinellas Park, Fla. Knee brace image courtesy AliMed, Inc., Dedham, Mass.

WALKING AIDS

Some people are weak and unsteady and need help walking. Canes and walkers are common for safety. Sometimes crutches are needed. Orthotic devices (p. 418) may also be used. A physical therapist (PT) teaches the person how to use needed devices.

Canes

Canes are used for weakness on 1 side of the body. They help provide balance and support. Single-tip and 4-point (quad) canes are common (Fig. 32-15).

A cane is held on the strong side (unaffected side) of the body. For example, if the left leg is weak, the cane is held in the right hand. The grip is level with the hip. The tip is positioned about 6 to 10 inches to the side of the strong foot.

When walking:

1 The cane is moved forward along with the weak leg. It is even with the weak leg (Fig. 32-16, *A*).
2 The cane is left in place as the strong leg is moved forward past the cane and the weak leg (Fig. 32-16, *B*). See *Promoting Safety and Comfort: Canes.*

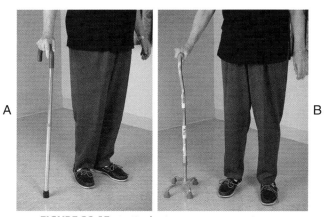

FIGURE 32-15 **A,** Single-tip cane. **B,** Four-point cane.

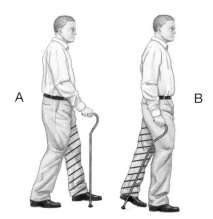

FIGURE 32-16 Walking with a cane. **A,** The cane is moved forward along with the weak leg. The cane is even with the weak leg. **B,** The cane is left in place. The strong leg is moved forward past the cane and the weak leg. (*NOTE: The weak leg is indicated by slash marks.*)

PROMOTING SAFETY AND COMFORT

Canes

Safety

Check that the person's cane is within reach and will not fall to the floor when not in use. A 4-point (quad) cane will stand freely. A single-tip cane needs to be securely propped in place. Otherwise, it will fall to the floor. The person can fall trying to reach the cane.

Cane handles are touched often. Microbes can live and grow on handles. Follow agency procedures for routine cleaning and disinfecting of surfaces touched often. Also, help the person with hand hygiene before using a cane if the person's hands may be contaminated. This includes after elimination and after contact with blood or body fluids.

Walkers

A walker gives more support than a cane. Wheeled walkers have wheels on the front legs and rubber tips on the back legs (Fig. 32-17). Rubber tips on the back legs prevent the walker from moving while the person is standing. To walk, the person pushes the walker about 6 to 8 inches in front of the feet.

Walker accessories are common. Baskets, pouches, and trays can attach to the walker for needed items. This allows more independence. The hands are free to grip the walker. Gliders or walker tennis balls are also common. Placed on the rear legs, they allow the walker to slide more easily on carpets and other surfaces. See Figure 32-18.

See *Promoting Safety and Comfort: Walkers.*

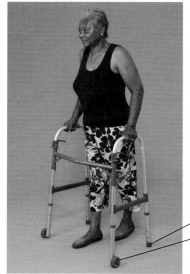

— Rubber tip
— Wheel on the outside of the walker

FIGURE 32-17 Wheeled walker.

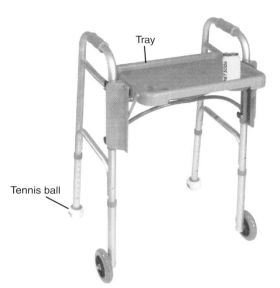

FIGURE 32-18 This walker has a tray and walker tennis balls on the rear legs. (Courtesy Drivemedical.com.)

PROMOTING SAFETY AND COMFORT

Walkers

Safety

Wheels are usually on the outside of the walker (see Fig. 32-17). With wheels on the outside, the walker is too wide for some doorways. Moving the wheels to the inside of the walker reduces the width. The person can go through narrower doorways.

Walkers vary in design. Some walkers have brakes and seats. The person sits to rest. Never push the walker when the person is seated.

Like canes, walker handles are touched often. They need to be cleaned and disinfected regularly. See *Promoting Safety and Comfort: Canes.*

Crutches

Crutches are used when the person cannot use 1 leg or when 1 or both legs need to gain strength. Injury, surgery, and deformity are some reasons for needing crutches. The need may be temporary or permanent.

Falls are a risk. Follow these safety measures.

- Check the crutch tips. They must not be worn down, torn, or wet. Replace worn or torn crutch tips. Dry wet tips with a towel or paper towels.
- Check crutches for flaws. Check wooden crutches for cracks and metal crutches for bends.
- Tighten all bolts.
- Have the person wear street shoes. They must be flat and have slip-resistant soles.
- Make sure clothes fit well. Loose clothes may get caught between the crutches and underarms. Loose clothes and long skirts can hang forward and block the person's view of the feet and crutch tips.
- Practice safety measures to prevent falls (Chapter 12).
- Keep crutches within the person's reach. Put them by the person's chair or against a wall.

AMBULATION

Ambulation is the act of walking. To walk, contractures and muscle atrophy must be prevented. After bed rest, activity increases in stages. First the person sits upright. Next the person stands. Then the person walks a few steps. Distance increases as the person gains strength.

Follow the care plan when helping a person walk (Fig. 32-19). Use a gait (transfer) belt (Chapter 12). Hand rails or a cane or walker provide support. Check the person for postural hypotension (p. 413).

See *Focus on Communication: Ambulation.*
See *Delegation Guidelines: Ambulation,* p. 422.
See *Promoting Safety and Comfort: Ambulation,* p. 422.
See procedure: *Assisting With Ambulation,* p. 422.

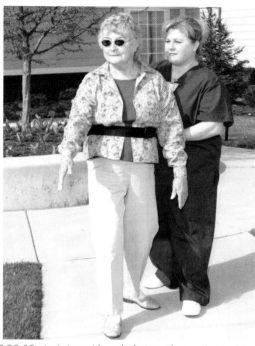

FIGURE 32-19 Assisting with ambulation. The nursing assistant walks at the person's side and slightly behind her. A gait belt is used for safety.

FOCUS ON COMMUNICATION

Ambulation

Before ambulating, explain the activity. This promotes comfort and reduces fear. Explain:

- How far to walk
- What adaptive (assistive) devices are used
- That you will use a gait belt
- How you will assist
- What the person is to report to you
- How you will help if the person begins to fall
  For example, you can say:

I am going to help you walk from your bed to the doorway and back. This belt helps support you while you walk. I will be at your side holding the belt at all times. Tell me right away if you feel unsteady, dizzy, weak, or faint. Also tell me if you feel any pain or discomfort. If you begin to fall, I will use the belt to pull you close to me and gently lower you to the floor. Do you have any questions?

DELEGATION GUIDELINES
Ambulation

Before helping with ambulation, you need this information from the nurse and the care plan.
- How much help the person needs
- If the person wears an orthotic device
- If the person uses a cane, walker, or crutches
- Areas of weakness—right arm or leg, left arm or leg
- How far to walk the person
- What observations to report and record:
  - How well the person tolerated the activity
  - Shuffling, sliding, limping, or walking on tip-toes
  - Balance problems
  - Complaints of pain or discomfort
  - Complaints of postural hypotension—weakness, dizziness, spots before the eyes, feeling faint
  - The distance walked
- When to report observations
- What patient or resident concerns to report at once

PROMOTING SAFETY AND COMFORT
Ambulation

Safety
Practice the safety measures to prevent falls (Chapter 12). Use a gait belt to help the person stand and during ambulation.

If a walker is used, remind the person not to pull on the walker to stand. The walker can tip. The person pushes on the mattress or the chair's armrests to stand (Chapter 18).

Remind the person to walk normally. Encourage the person to stand erect (upright) with the head up and the back straight. Discourage shuffling, sliding, and walking on tip-toes.

Comfort
The fear of falling affects mental comfort. Explain the purpose of the gait belt. Also explain how you will help if the person starts to fall (Chapter 12).

Assisting With Ambulation

Quality of Life

- Knock before entering the person's room.
- Address the person by name.
- Introduce yourself by name and title.
- Explain the procedure before starting and during the procedure.
- Protect the person's rights during the procedure.
- Handle the person gently during the procedure.

Pre-Procedure

1 Follow *Delegation Guidelines: Ambulation.* See *Promoting Safety and Comfort: Ambulation.*
2 Practice hand hygiene and get the following supplies.
   - Slip-resistant footwear
   - Paper towel or towel to protect bottom linens (if needed)
   - Gait (transfer) belt
   - Walker or cane (if needed)
3 Arrange items in the person's room.
4 Practice hand hygiene.
5 Identify the person. Check the ID bracelet against the assignment sheet. Use 2 identifiers (Chapter 11). Also call the person by name.
6 Provide for privacy.

Procedure

7 Adjust the bed to a safe and comfortable level for a transfer. Follow the care plan. Lock (brake) the bed wheels.
8 Fan-fold top linens to the foot of the bed.
9 Place the paper towel or towel under the person's feet to protect bottom linens. Put footwear on the person. Or apply footwear when the person is seated on the side of the bed (step 10).
10 Help the person sit on the side of the bed. (See procedure: *Sitting on the Side of the Bed [Dangling]* in Chapter 17.)
11 Make sure the person's feet are flat on the floor.
12 Make sure the person is properly dressed.
13 Apply the gait belt at the waist over clothing. (See procedure: *Using a Transfer/Gait Belt* in Chapter 12.)
14 Position the walker (if used) in front of the person. Or have the person hold the cane (if used) on the strong side.
15 Help the person stand. (See procedure: *Transferring the Person to a Chair or Wheelchair* in Chapter 18.) Grasp the gait belt at each side.
16 Stand at the weak side while the person gains balance. Hold the belt at the side and back. Grasp the handles or grasp the belt from underneath. Hands are in an upward position (upward grasp).
17 Encourage the person to stand erect (upright) with the head up and the back straight.
18 *Positioning a walker or cane:*
   a Walker—the walker is 6 to 8 inches in front of the person.
   b Cane—the cane is held on the strong side. The tip is 6 to 10 inches to the side of the strong foot.
19 Help the person walk. Walk to the side and slightly behind the person on the person's weak side. Provide support with the gait belt (see Fig. 32-19). Have the person use the hand rail on the strong side (unless using a walker or cane).
20 *For a walker or cane:*
   a Walker—with both hands, the person pushes the walker 6 to 8 inches in front of the feet.
   b Cane:
      1) The cane (on the strong side) is moved forward along with the weak leg. It is even with the weak leg (see Fig. 32-16, A).
      2) The strong leg is moved forward past the cane and the weak leg (see Fig. 32-16, B).

Assisting With Ambulation—cont'd

Procedure—cont'd

21 Encourage the person to walk normally. The heel strikes the floor first. Discourage shuffling, sliding, or walking on tip-toes.
22 Walk the ordered distance if the person tolerates the activity. Do not rush the person.
23 Help the person return to bed. Remove the gait belt. (See procedure: *Transferring the Person From a Chair or Wheelchair to Bed* in Chapter 18.)

24 Remove the shoes. Remove the paper towel or towel over the bottom sheet (if used). Discard the paper towel or follow agency policy for used linens.
25 Lower the head of the bed. Help the person to the center of the bed.

Post-Procedure

26 Provide for comfort. (See the inside of the back cover.)
27 Place the call light and other needed items within reach.
28 Raise or lower bed rails. Follow the care plan.
29 Return the shoes to their proper place.
30 Follow the care plan and the person's preferences for privacy measures to maintain. Leaving the privacy curtain, window coverings, and door open or closed are examples.

31 Complete a safety check of the room. (See the inside of the back cover.)
32 Practice hand hygiene.
33 Report and record your care and observations.

FOCUS ON P R I D E

The Person, Family, and Yourself

P ersonal and Professional Responsibility

Exercise and activity promote normal function of all body systems. Good conditioning has long-term effects. To promote activity, exercise, and well-being, you can:
- Encourage the person to be as active as possible.
- Resist the urge to do things that the person can safely do alone or with some help.
- Focus on the person's abilities.
- Give praise when the person is doing well, making progress, or gave a good effort.

R ights and Respect

Garments must provide privacy during exercise and activity. When ambulating, the person's gown must not be open in the back. During ROM exercises, cover the person with a bath blanket. Expose only the body part being exercised. Protect the right to privacy. Privacy promotes dignity and mental comfort.

I ndependence and Social Interaction

Nursing center activity programs promote physical, mental, and social well-being. Joints and muscles are exercised. Circulation is stimulated. Social interaction is mentally stimulating.

Bingo, movies, dances, exercise groups, shopping and museum trips, concerts, and guest speakers are common. Residents may tell you about favorite pastimes. Listen with interest. Suggest options that they may like. Allow personal choice to promote independence.

D elegation and Teamwork

To meet goals, all staff must follow the person's care plan. Progress slows or stops when only some staff follow the plan. For example, a person is to walk to and from the dining room at meal times. To save time, some staff push the person to the dining room in a wheelchair. Deconditioning results. All staff must do their part for the person's well-being.

E thics and Laws

You can lose your ability to work as a nursing assistant for handling persons in ways that cause harm. Work carefully. Move patients and residents in a way that shows you care for their comfort, safety, and well-being.

FOCUS ON PRIDE: *Application*

How can you encourage independence and self-worth in persons needing help with exercise and activity?

Circle the BEST answer.

1 The purpose of bed rest is to
   a Prevent postural hypotension
   b Reduce pain and promote healing
   c Prevent pressure injuries, constipation, and blood clots
   d Cause contractures and muscle atrophy

2 A contracture is
   a The loss of muscle strength from inactivity
   b A decrease in the size of a muscle
   c A blood clot in the muscle
   d Decreased motion and stiffness of a joint

3 Which statement about complications from immobility is *true*?
   a ROM exercises and frequent position changes can prevent complications.
   b Complications of immobility are minor.
   c It takes a long time for deconditioning to occur.
   d Complications cannot be prevented.

4 You sit a person up at the side of the bed to transfer to the commode. The person says: "I feel faint." What should you do?
   a Transfer the person to the commode.
   b Lay the person down in bed.
   c Have the person sit on the side of the bed longer.
   d Leave to get the nurse.

5 Before beginning passive range-of-motion (PROM) exercises, you need to explain that
   a The person will move the joints alone
   b You will uncover the person to prevent sweating
   c The person should tell you if there is pain
   d The goal is to push past points of resistance

6 When performing PROM exercises, which may cause injury?
   a Supporting the part being exercised
   b Moving the joint slowly, smoothly, and gently
   c Forcing the joint through its full range of motion
   d Exercising only the joints indicated by the nurse

7 Flexion involves
   a Bending the body part
   b Straightening the body part
   c Moving the body part toward the body
   d Moving the body part away from the body

8 Turning the joint downward is called
   a Dorsiflexion
   b Rotation
   c Supination
   d Pronation

9 Which prevents the hip from turning outward?
   a A cane
   b A foot-board
   c A trochanter roll
   d A knee brace

10 A person uses a finger cushion to prevent finger contractures. Which is *correct*?
    a Clean and dry the skin under the device before use.
    b Follow agency policies for restraint use while using the device.
    c Force the fingers to extend when placing the device.
    d Only use the device when the person has hand pain.

11 Which helps prevent permanent plantar flexion (footdrop)?
    a An abduction wedge
    b A foot-board
    c A trochanter roll
    d Crutches

12 A hip abduction wedge
    a Keeps the legs apart
    b Keeps the legs together
    c Keeps the legs crossed
    d Raises both legs

13 A person wears an ankle-foot orthosis (AFO). Which is *correct*?
    a Remind the person that a shoe is not worn with the device.
    b Remove the person's sock before application.
    c Check for redness on areas in contact with the AFO.
    d Do not remove the orthosis for bathing.

14 A person is using a cane. Which needs to be corrected?
    a The person moves the cane along with the weak leg.
    b The grip is level with the hip.
    c The cane's tip is about 10 inches to the side of the foot.
    d The person is holding the cane on the weak side.

15 Which provides the most support for walking?
    a Single-tip cane
    b Four-point (quad) cane
    c A knee brace
    d Walker

16 Which describes proper use of a wheeled walker?
    a The person pulls on the walker handles to stand.
    b The walker is pushed 6 to 8 inches in front of the feet.
    c The person's back is hunched (bent over) during use.
    d The walker is not used to walk short distances.

17 When assisting with ambulation
    a Grasp the top of the gait belt with 1 hand
    b Have the person walk without footwear
    c Remind the person not to shuffle the feet
    d Walk on the person's strong side

18 What should you say to promote normal walking?
    a "Keep your back straight and your head up."
    b "Look down at your feet so you don't trip."
    c "Slide your feet if it is hard to lift them."
    d "You need to walk faster."

Answers to Chapter 32 questions are on p. 588.

FOCUS ON **PRACTICE**

Problem Solving

You are assisting a resident to ambulate in the hallway with a walker and gait belt. The resident says: "I feel dizzy." No chair is nearby. A wheelchair is at the nurses' station at the end of the hallway. What will you do? How might planning and teamwork help in this situation?

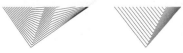

CHAPTER 33

Comfort and Rest Needs

OBJECTIVES

- Define the key terms and key abbreviation in this chapter.
- Explain why comfort, rest, and sleep are important.
- Explain why pain is personal.
- Identify the factors affecting pain and the different types of pain.
- List the signs and symptoms of pain.
- List the nursing measures for comfort and pain relief.
- Explain the purposes of a back massage.

- Explain why meeting basic needs promotes rest.
- Identify when rest is needed.
- Describe the factors affecting sleep.
- List the nursing measures that promote rest and sleep.
- Perform the procedure described in this chapter.
- Explain how to promote PRIDE in the person, the family, and yourself.

KEY TERMS

acute pain Pain that is sharp or severe; felt suddenly from injury, disease, trauma, or surgery
chronic pain Pain that continues for a long time (longer than 12 weeks, occurs off and on, or is persistent [constant])
comfort A state of well-being; the person has no physical or emotional pain and is calm and at ease
discomfort See "pain"
insomnia A chronic condition in which the person cannot sleep or stay asleep all night

pain To ache, hurt, or be sore; discomfort
rest To be calm, at ease, and relaxed with no anxiety or stress
sleep apnea Pauses (a) in breathing (pnea) that occur during sleep
sleep deprivation The amount and quality of sleep are not adequate, causing reduced function and alertness
sleepwalking When the person leaves the bed and walks about while sleeping

KEY ABBREVIATION

ID   Identification

Comfort and rest are needed for well-being. The whole person (physical, emotional, social, and spiritual) is affected by comfort and rest. When problems occur, quality of life is affected.

Rest and sleep restore energy. Pain, illness, and injury increase the need for rest and sleep. The body needs more energy for healing, repair, and daily functions.

COMFORT

Comfort is a state of well-being. The person has no physical or emotional pain and is calm and at ease. Age, illness, and activity affect comfort. So do temperature, ventilation, noise, odors, and lighting (Chapter 19). Pain is a major factor affecting comfort.

See *Focus on Communication: Comfort*, p. 426.

FOCUS ON COMMUNICATION

Comfort

Do not assume the person is comfortable. For example, you can ask the following.

- "Are you comfortable?"
- "Are you warm enough?"
- "Do you need another blanket?"
- "Do you need another pillow?"
- "Should I adjust your pillow?"

Communication can promote mental comfort. It provides reassurance that needs will be met. You can say: "I want you to be comfortable. Please tell me how I can help you be more comfortable." Follow through with meeting the person's comfort needs. See "Comfort Measures" on p. 428.

Pain

Pain (discomfort) means to ache, hurt, or be sore. Pain is a warning sign from the body. Often considered to be a vital sign (Chapter 31), it signals tissue damage. Pain often causes the person to seek health care.

Pain is subjective (Chapter 7). That means you cannot see, hear, touch or feel, or smell another person's pain or discomfort. You must rely on what the person says. If a person reports pain (discomfort), the person has pain (discomfort).

Pain is personal. That is, pain differs for each person. What *hurts* to one person may *ache* or be *sore* to another person. Many factors affect pain and the person's response to pain. See Box 33-1.

You must believe what patients and residents tell you about their pain. Report complaints of pain to the nurse for the nursing process.

BOX 33-1 Factors Affecting Pain

Past and current experiences. One's experiences and those of others help in learning about pain and what to expect. Pain severity, its cause, how long it lasted, and pain relief affect the person's current response to pain.

Anxiety. Anxiety relates to feelings of fear, dread, worry, and concern. The person is uneasy and tense. Pain can cause anxiety, which makes pain worse. Helping the person understand the cause of pain and what to expect helps to reduce anxiety and lessen pain.

Rest and sleep needs. Such needs increase with illness and injury. Pain seems worse when rest and sleep are affected.

Attention. Pain seems worse when it is the person's main focus. Pain seems worse when there are no distractions—TV, visitors, activity, and so on. Especially at night when unable to sleep, the person has time to think about pain.

Support from others. Dealing with pain is often easier when family and friends offer comfort and support. Touch, encouragement, or being available or nearby helps the person deal with pain. Facing pain alone is hard.

Personal and family duties. Some people try to ignore or deny pain because of a job, school, or caring for children, a partner, or parents.

The meaning of pain. Pain can have different meanings. For example, pain can:

- Be a sign of weakness.
- Signal the need for tests and treatment.
- Bring pleasure, such as the pain of childbirth.
- Be useful. For example, the person does not have to work or can avoid certain people.
- Lead to doting and pampering. The person likes the attention.

Culture. Culture affects pain responses. In some cultures, the person in pain is stoic. To be *stoic* means *to show no reaction to joy, sorrow, pleasure, or pain.* Strong verbal and nonverbal pain reactions are seen in other cultures. See *Caring About Culture: Pain.*

Illness. Some diseases affect pain sensations. The person may not feel pain. If pain is not felt, the person does not know to seek health care. Disease or injury may go undetected.

Age. See *Focus on Older Persons: Pain.*

CARING ABOUT CULTURE

Pain

Some people of *Mexico* and the *Philippines* may appear stoic in reaction to pain. In the *Philippines,* some people view pain as the will of God and believe that God will give strength to bear the pain.

In *Vietnam,* pain may be severe before some people request pain-relief measures. In *China,* showing emotion may be viewed as a weakness of character. If so, pain is often suppressed.

Non-English-speaking persons may have problems describing pain in English. The agency uses interpreters to communicate with the person.

NOTE: *Each person is unique. A person may not follow all of the beliefs and practices of his or her culture. Follow the care plan.*

Modified from D'Avanzo CE: *Pocket guide to cultural health assessment,* ed 4, St Louis, 2008, Mosby.

FOCUS ON OLDER PERSONS

Pain

Some older persons have many painful health problems. Chronic (long-term) pain may mask new pain. Or new pain is ignored. They may think it involves a known problem. Or pain is denied or ignored because of what it may mean.

Thinking and reasoning are affected in some older persons. Some cannot tell you about pain. Behavior changes can signal pain. For example:

- An older person has increased confusion, restlessness, and loss of appetite.
- A person who normally moans and groans becomes quiet and withdrawn.
- A friendly and outgoing person becomes agitated and aggressive.
- A person who is normally quiet becomes restless and cries easily.

Always report behavior changes. All persons have the right to correct pain management. The nurse does a pain assessment when behavior changes.

Types of Pain.

Doctors use the type of pain for diagnosing. Nurses use the type for the nursing process. Pain can signal a new problem. Or it may be an ongoing symptom.

Acute pain is sharp or severe. It is felt suddenly from injury, disease, trauma, or surgery. Acute pain signals a new injury or a life-threatening event. There is tissue damage. Acute pain lasts a short time and lessens with healing.

Chronic pain continues for a long time (longer than 12 weeks, occurs off and on, or is persistent [constant]). Chronic pain is often a symptom of an ongoing health problem. Arthritis is an example. Sometimes healing has occurred. There is no longer tissue damage, but pain remains.

Sometimes pain is felt in other areas or is sensed in areas no longer present. *Radiating pain* is felt at the site of tissue damage and spreads to other areas. For example, low back pain can radiate to the buttocks and legs. Gallbladder disease can cause pain in the right upper abdomen, the back, and the right shoulder (Fig. 33-1). *Phantom pain* seems to come from a body part that is no longer there. For example, a person with an amputated leg may still sense leg pain.

Signs and Symptoms.

Promptly report any information you collect about pain. Write down what the person says. Use the person's exact words to report and record. The nurse needs the following information.

- *Location.* Where is the pain? Ask the person to point to the area. Ask the person if the pain is anywhere else and to point to those areas.
- *Onset and duration.* When did the pain start? How long has it lasted?
- *Intensity.* Is the pain mild, moderate, or severe? Have the person rate the pain on a scale of 0 to 10, with 10 as the most severe (Fig. 33-2). Or use the *Wong-Baker FACES® Pain Rating Scale* (Fig. 33-3). To use the scale, explain that each face shows how a person feels. Read the description for each face. Ask which face best matches how the person feels.
- *Description.* Have the person describe the pain or discomfort. *Aching, burning, cramping, dull, sharp,* and *throbbing* are examples. *Pressure, soreness,* and *tenderness* are others.
- *Factors causing pain.* These are called *precipitating factors.* To *precipitate* means *to cause.* Such factors include moving or turning in bed, coughing or deep breathing, and exercise. Ask what the person was doing before the pain started and when it started.
- *Factors affecting pain.* Ask what makes the pain better and what makes it worse.
- *Vital signs.* Measure pulse, respirations, and blood pressure (Chapter 31). Vital signs often increase with acute pain. They may be normal with chronic pain.
- *Other signs and symptoms.* Does the person have other symptoms—dizziness, nausea, vomiting, weakness, numbness or tingling, or others? Box 33-2 (p. 428) lists the signs and symptoms that often occur with pain.
See *Focus on Surveys: Signs and Symptoms,* p. 428.
See *Focus on Communication: Signs and Symptoms,* p. 428.

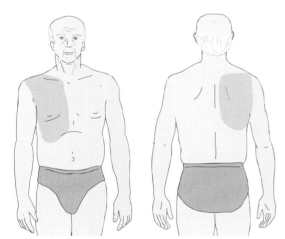

FIGURE 33-1 Gallbladder pain may radiate (spread) to the right upper abdomen, the back, and the right shoulder.

Ask the person to rate the pain on a scale of 0 to 10.										
No pain										Worst pain imaginable
0	1	2	3	4	5	6	7	8	9	10

FIGURE 33-2 Pain rating scale. (Modified from Williams P: *deWit's fundamental concepts and skills for nursing,* ed 5, St Louis, 2018, Elsevier.)

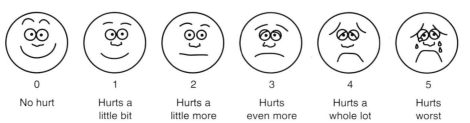

0	1	2	3	4	5
No hurt	Hurts a little bit	Hurts a little more	Hurts even more	Hurts a whole lot	Hurts worst

FIGURE 33-3 Wong-Baker FACES® Pain Rating Scale. (Modified from Hockenberry MJ et al.: *Wong's nursing care of infants and children,* ed 10, St Louis, 2015, Mosby.)

BOX 33-2 Pain—Signs and Symptoms

Body Responses
- Appetite: changes in
- Dizziness
- Nausea; vomiting
- Numbness; tingling
- Skin: pale *(pallor)*
- Sleep: difficulty with
- Sweating *(diaphoresis)*
- Vital signs (pulse, respirations, and blood pressure): increased
- Weakness
- Weight loss

Behaviors
- Clenching the jaw
- Crying
- Frowning
- Gait: changes in; limping
- Gasping
- Grimacing
- Groaning; grunting; moaning
- Holding the affected body part (splinting; guarding)
- Irritability
- Mood: changes in; depressed
- Pacing
- Positioning: maintaining 1 position; refusing to move; frequent position changes
- Pulling away when touched
- Quietness
- Resisting care
- Restlessness
- Rubbing a body part or area
- Screaming
- Speech: slow or rapid; loud or quiet
- Whimpering

FOCUS ON SURVEYS

Signs and Symptoms

Pain interferes with well-being—function, mobility, mood, sleep, and quality of life. The agency must:
- Recognize when a person has pain.
- Identify when pain might occur.
- Evaluate pain and its causes.
- Manage or prevent pain.
  You may be the first to observe signs and symptoms of pain. You must recognize and report a change in the person's behavior and function. You follow the care plan for pain-relief measures. Therefore a surveyor may ask you about pain. Examples are:
- What are the signs and symptoms of pain?
- How do you ask a person to rate the intensity of pain?
- What factors can cause pain or make it worse?
- When and how do you report observations about pain?
- How do you assist the nurse with pain-relief measures? (See "Comfort Measures.")

FOCUS ON COMMUNICATION

Signs and Symptoms

A person may use words like "hurt" or "discomfort" instead of "pain." Use words that the person uses.
   Some persons have trouble rating pain intensity on a 0 to 10 scale. Instead, ask if the pain is mild, moderate, or severe.

Comfort Measures

The nurse uses the nursing process to promote comfort and relieve pain. The care plan may include the measures in Box 33-3. Sometimes distraction, relaxation, and guided imagery are needed. If asked to assist, the nurse tells you what to do.

- *Distraction*—the person's attention is focused on something unrelated to pain. Music, games, singing, praying, TV, and needlework can distract attention.
- *Relaxation*—the person is free from mental and physical stress. The person is taught to breathe deeply and slowly and to contract and relax muscle groups. A comfortable position and a quiet room are important.
- *Guided imagery*—involves creating and focusing on a relaxing image. The person is coached to relax and focus on a pleasant scene. A calm, soft voice is used to help the person focus. Soft music, a blanket for warmth, and a darkened room may help.

Nurses give ordered pain-relief drugs. Such drugs can cause postural hypotension (Chapter 32), drowsiness, dizziness, and coordination problems. Protect the person from injury and falls. Follow the care plan for needed safety measures.

BOX 33-3 Comfort Measures

- Position the person in good alignment. Use pillows for support.
- Keep bed linens clean, dry, tight, and wrinkle-free.
- Make sure the person is not lying on tubes.
- Assist with elimination needs.
- Adjust the room temperature to meet the person's needs.
- Provide blankets for warmth and to prevent chilling.
- Use correct moving and turning procedures.
- Wait 30 minutes after pain-relief drugs are given to give care or start activities.
- Give a back massage.
- Provide soft music to distract the person.
- Talk softly and gently.
- Use touch to provide comfort.
- Allow family and friends at the bedside as requested by the person.
- Avoid sudden or jarring movements of the bed or chair.
- Handle the person gently.
- Practice safety measures if the person takes strong pain-relief drugs or sedatives.
  - Keep the bed in a low position that is safe and comfortable for the person. Follow the care plan.
  - Raise bed rails as directed. Follow the care plan.
  - Check on the person every 10 to 15 minutes.
  - Provide help when the person needs to stand and walk. Use a transfer/gait belt (Chapter 12).
- Apply warm or cold applications as directed by the nurse (Chapter 35).
- Provide a calm, quiet, darkened setting.

The Back Massage. The back massage (back rub) can promote comfort and help relieve pain. It relaxes muscles and stimulates circulation. Good times for back massages are after re-positioning, after baths or showers, and with evening care. Back massages last 3 to 5 minutes. Observe the skin before the massage. Look for breaks in the skin, bruises, reddened areas, and other signs of skin breakdown.

Lotion reduces friction during the massage and softens the skin. Warm the lotion before applying it. Do 1 of the following.

- Rub some lotion between your hands.
- Place the bottle in the bath water.
- Hold the bottle under warm water.

Use firm strokes. Keep your hands in contact with the person's skin. After the massage, apply lotion to the elbows, knees, and heels. Those bony areas are at risk for skin breakdown.

See *Delegation Guidelines: The Back Massage.*
See *Promoting Safety and Comfort: The Back Massage.*
See procedure: *Giving a Back Massage.*

DELEGATION GUIDELINES
The Back Massage

Before giving a back massage, you need this information from the nurse and the care plan.

- If the person can have a back massage. See *Promoting Safety and Comfort: The Back Massage.*
- How to position the person.
- If the person has position limits. If yes, what are they?
- When to give a back massage.
- If the person needs back massages often for comfort and to relax.
- What observations to report and record:
  - Breaks in the skin
  - Bruising
  - Reddened areas
  - Signs of skin breakdown
- When to report observations.
- What patient or resident concerns to report at once.

PROMOTING SAFETY AND COMFORT
The Back Massage

Safety

Back massages can harm persons with certain heart diseases, back injuries and surgeries, skin diseases, and lung disorders. Check with the nurse and the care plan before giving back massages.

Do not massage reddened bony areas. Reddened areas signal skin breakdown and pressure injuries. Massage can cause more tissue damage.

Wear gloves if the person's skin is not intact. Do not massage areas of non-intact skin. Always follow Standard Precautions and the Bloodborne Pathogen Standard.

Comfort

The prone position is best for a massage. The side-lying position is often used. Older and disabled persons usually find the side-lying position more comfortable.

Giving a Back Massage

Quality of Life

- Knock before entering the person's room.
- Address the person by name.
- Introduce yourself by name and title.
- Explain the procedure before starting and during the procedure.
- Protect the person's rights during the procedure.
- Handle the person gently during the procedure.

Pre-Procedure

1 Follow *Delegation Guidelines: The Back Massage.* See *Promoting Safety and Comfort: The Back Massage.*
2 Practice hand hygiene and get the following supplies.
  - Bath blanket
  - Bath towel
  - Lotion
  - Laundry bag
3 Arrange items in the person's room.
4 Practice hand hygiene.
5 Identify the person. Check the identification (ID) bracelet against the assignment sheet. Use 2 identifiers (Chapter 11). Also call the person by name.
6 Provide for privacy.
7 Raise the bed for body mechanics. Bed rails are up if used. Lower the bed rail near you if up.

Procedure

8 Position the person in the prone or side-lying position. The back is toward you.
9 Cover the person with a bath blanket. Expose the back, shoulders, and upper arms.
10 Lay the towel on the bed along the back. Do this if the person is in a side-lying position.
11 Warm the lotion.
12 Explain that the lotion may feel cool and wet.
13 Apply lotion to the lower back area.
14 Stroke up from the lower back to the shoulders. Then stroke down over the upper arms. Stroke up the upper arms, across the shoulders, and down the back (Fig. 33-4, p. 430). Use firm strokes. Keep your hands in contact with the person's skin.
15 Repeat step 14 for at least 3 minutes.

Continued

Giving a Back Massage—cont'd

Procedure—cont'd

16 Knead the back (Fig. 33-5).
  a Grasp the skin between your thumb and fingers.
  b Knead half of the back. Start at the lower back and move up to the shoulder. Then knead down from the shoulder to the lower back.
  c Repeat on the other half of the back.
17 Apply lotion to bony areas. Use circular motions with the tips of your index and middle fingers. *(Do not massage reddened bony areas.)*

18 Use fast movements to stimulate. Use slow movements to relax the person.
19 Stroke with long, firm movements to end the massage. Tell the person when you are finishing.
20 Straighten and secure clothing or sleepwear.
21 Cover the person. Remove the towel and bath blanket. Place them in the laundry bag.
22 Practice hand hygiene.

Post-Procedure

23 Provide for comfort. (See the inside of the back cover.)
24 Place the call light and other needed items within reach.
25 Lower the bed to a safe and comfortable level. Follow the care plan.
26 Raise or lower bed rails. Follow the care plan.
27 Return lotion to its proper place.
28 Follow the care plan and the person's preferences for privacy measures to maintain. Leaving the privacy curtain, window coverings, and door open or closed are examples.

29 Complete a safety check of the room. (See the inside of the back cover.)
30 Practice hand hygiene.
31 Follow agency policy for used linens.
32 Report and record your care and observations.

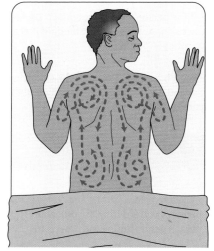

FIGURE 33-4 The person is in the prone position for a back massage. Stroke upward from the lower back to the shoulders, down over the upper arms, back up the upper arms, across the shoulders, and down to the lower back.

FIGURE 33-5 Knead by picking up tissue between the thumb and fingers.

REST

Rest means to be calm, at ease, and relaxed with no anxiety or stress. Rest may involve no activity. Or the person does calming and relaxing things. Some people garden, bake, golf, walk, or do woodworking. Distraction, relaxation, and guided imagery also promote rest. So does a back massage.

A person is more relaxed when basic needs are met. Meet food, fluid, and elimination needs before times of rest. The person needs to feel safe, secure, and comfortable. Proper positioning and good alignment are important. Provide a quiet and clean setting. Keep the call light within reach. It is comforting to know how to get help if needed.

Plan and organize care for uninterrupted rest. Ill or injured persons need to rest often. Some persons need rest before or after a procedure. Some like to rest after meals. Health care routines usually allow for afternoon rest. Be aware of the person's limits. Allow rest when needed.

SLEEP

Sleep is a basic need. The mind and body rest. The body saves energy. Body functions slow. Vital signs are lower than when awake. Tissue healing and repair occur. Sleep lowers stress, tension, and anxiety. It refreshes and renews the person. The person regains energy and mental alertness. The person thinks and functions better after sleep.

Factors Affecting Sleep

Many factors affect the amount and quality of sleep.

- *Illness.* Illness increases the need for sleep. Pain, nausea, vomiting, coughing, difficulty breathing, diarrhea, frequent voiding, and itching can interfere with sleep. So can treatments and therapies and being awakened for treatments or drugs. Care devices can cause uncomfortable positions.
- *Nutrition.* Sleep needs increase with weight gain and decrease with weight loss. Drinks and foods with caffeine (coffee, tea, colas, chocolate) prevent sleep. The protein *tryptophan* tends to help sleep. It is found in protein sources—milk, cheese, red meat, fish, poultry, and peanuts.
- *Exercise.* Exercise helps people sleep well. For some, exercising close to bedtime causes wakefulness. For them, exercise earlier in the day is best.
- *Sleep setting.* The bed, pillows, noises, temperature, lighting, and a sleeping partner are part of the person's sleep setting. Any change in the usual setting can interfere with sleep.
- *Drugs and other substances.* Sleeping pills promote sleep. Drugs for anxiety, depression, and pain may cause sleep. Some drugs cause nightmares and frequent voiding. Alcohol can interfere with sleep. A stimulant, caffeine prevents sleep. Caffeine is found in some drugs and some drinks and foods. See "Nutrition" above.
- *Life-style changes.* Life-style relates to a person's daily routines and way of living. The person has usual sleep and wake times. Work, school, play, social events, and travel are some factors affecting the person's sleep-wake times.
- *Emotional problems.* Fear, worry, depression, and anxiety affect sleep. Causes include problems with health, money, work, family, and relationships.
- *Age.* Sleep needs vary for each age-group. The amount needed normally decreases with age.
  See *Focus on Older Persons: Factors Affecting Sleep.*

Sleep Disorders

Sleep disorders involve repeated sleep problems. The amount and quality of sleep are affected. Physical and behavioral problems may result.

- *Insomnia is a chronic condition in which the person cannot sleep or stay asleep all night.*
- *Sleep deprivation is when the amount and quality of sleep are not adequate, causing reduced function and alertness.* Sleep is interrupted.
- *Sleepwalking is when the person leaves the bed and walks about while sleeping.* The person is not aware of sleepwalking and has no memory of the event. The event lasts 3 to 4 minutes or longer. Protect the person from injury. Falls are a risk. Awaken a sleepwalker gently. The person is easily startled. Guide the person back to bed.
- *Sleep apnea is when pauses in breathing occur during sleep.* Apnea is the *lack or absence* (a) of *breathing* (pnea). Pauses last a few seconds to over a minute and can occur many times during sleep. The most common cause is blockage of the airway from relaxed muscles and tissues. See Chapter 37.

Promoting Sleep

The nurse assesses the person's sleep patterns. Report any complaints about sleep. Also report any physical or behavioral problems resulting from sleep disorders. Decreased attention span, fatigue, irritability, mood changes, memory problems, and day-time sleepiness are common.

Measures are planned to promote sleep (Box 33-4, p. 432). The person is involved in care planning. The person chooses when to nap or go to bed. The person chooses the measures that promote comfort, rest, and sleep. Follow the care plan and the person's wishes.

FOCUS ON OLDER PERSONS

Factors Affecting Sleep

Older adults need about 7 to 9 hours of sleep each night. Some older persons also nap during the day. Plan care for uninterrupted naps.

Sleep problems are common with Alzheimer's disease and other dementias. Night-time wandering is common. Restlessness and confusion often increase at night. This increases the risk of falls. Night-time wandering in a safe and supervised setting is allowed for some persons. Others need to be quietly and calmly directed back to their rooms. Measures to promote sleep are tried. See "Promoting Sleep" and Chapter 42. Follow the care plan.

BOX 33-4 Promoting Sleep

- Plan care for uninterrupted rest.
- Encourage the person to avoid business or family matters before bedtime.
- Allow a flexible bedtime. Bedtime is when the person is tired, not a certain time.
- Provide a comfortable room temperature.
- Let the person take a warm bath or shower.
- Provide a bedtime snack.
- Avoid caffeine (coffee, tea, colas, chocolate).
- Avoid alcoholic beverages.
- Have the person void (urinate) before going to bed.
- Make sure incontinent persons are clean and dry.
- Follow bedtime rituals and routines.
- Have the person wear loose-fitting sleepwear.
- Provide for extra warmth (blankets, socks) as needed.
- Make sure linens are clean, dry, and wrinkle-free.
- Position the person in good alignment and in a comfortable position.
- Support body parts as ordered.
- Give a back massage.
- Provide measures to relieve pain.
- Let the person read, listen to music, or watch TV.
- Assist with relaxation exercises as ordered.
- Sit and talk with the person.
- Reduce noise.
- Darken the room—close window coverings and the privacy curtain. Shut off or dim lights.
- Dim lights in hallways and the nursing unit.

FOCUS ON PRIDE

The Person, Family, and Yourself

P ersonal and Professional Responsibility

Unmanaged pain decreases quality of life. You have an important role in assisting with pain relief. You talk with patients and residents and listen to their needs. Report signs and symptoms of pain. Report what the person said and what you observed. The nurse uses this information to assess, plan, and evaluate pain relief.

R ights and Respect

Your care can either promote comfort and relaxation or cause stress, discomfort, and worry. For example:
- Are you prompt to meet needs?
- Do you ask about the person's preferences?
- Do you communicate in a respectful way?
- Do you allow time for rest?
- Do you leave the person's room clean, neat, and safe?

Take pride in providing care in a way that protects the right to quality of life.

I ndependence and Social Interaction

A person's emotional, spiritual, and social needs affect comfort. Visits or calls from friends and family can be comforting. Reading cards or letters may be relaxing and restful. For some, religious ceremonies or rituals promote peace and healing. Allow time and privacy for such needs.

D elegation and Teamwork

The health team coordinates care and therapies with pain-relief measures and rest periods. It is common to wait 30 minutes after a pain-relief drug is given to perform procedures and provide care. The nurse tells you how long to wait. The person is allowed to rest after tiring activities, procedures, and therapies. Planning and communication are needed for effective teamwork and quality care.

E thics and Laws

Questioning what the person says about pain can be harmful. For example, a person rates headache pain as 7 on the 0 to 10 pain rating scale. The person is working a crossword puzzle and listening to music. When you have a headache, you need to rest in a dark, quiet room. You doubt the person and decide not to tell the nurse.

The person really had a bad headache. The person was using the crossword puzzle and music as distractions. Because you did not report the pain, the person did not receive pain-relief measures.

Ignoring a person's pain is wrong. Reporting a different pain rating is wrong. Avoid making judgments about the person's pain. Accurate reporting is needed for proper pain management.

FOCUS ON PRIDE: Application

Family and visitors often provide comfort. How will you welcome the person's visitors? How will you show you value them and their time with the person?

Circle the BEST answer.

1 Which statement about pain is *true*?
   a Pain is a warning sign from the body.
   b Age and culture do not affect pain responses.
   c Pain experiences are the same for each person.
   d Pain can be measured with equipment.

2 A person is restless and complains of pain. You should
   a Rate the intensity based on the person's behavior
   b Give a pain-relief drug and tell the nurse
   c Tell the nurse only if you think the person has pain
   d Report the person's exact words

3 A person has had knee pain on and off for several years. This type of pain is
   a Acute pain
   b Chronic pain
   c Radiating pain
   d Not important

4 Moving causes a person pain. The nurse gave a pain-relief drug. When should you give care that involves moving the person?
   a Right before the drug is given
   b Right after the drug is given
   c 30 minutes after the drug is given
   d When you have time

5 A drug was given for pain relief. The nurse said the drug can cause drowsiness and dizziness. To promote safety
   a Keep the bed in the raised position
   b Quickly change positions to avoid dizziness
   c Check on the person every 2 hours
   d Provide help if the person needs to get up

6 Which measure promotes comfort and pain relief?
   a Providing a blanket
   b Speaking loudly
   c Keeping bright lights on in the room
   d Asking about comfort every 5 minutes

7 When giving a back massage
   a Massage for 15 to 20 minutes
   b Warm the lotion before applying it
   c Massage reddened areas
   d Position the person in Fowler's position

8 Which shows that you understand how basic needs affect rest?
   a You leave the call light out of the person's reach.
   b You let an alarm sound for 5 minutes before responding.
   c You help the person to the bathroom before rest.
   d You lay the person down on wet, wrinkled linens.

9 A person tires easily. You are giving morning care. When should the person rest?
   a After you complete morning care
   b After the bath and before hair care
   c After you make the bed
   d When the person needs to

10 Which statement about sleep is *true*?
   a Sleep increases stress, tension, and anxiety.
   b Persons with dementia usually sleep well at night.
   c The body does not heal during sleep.
   d Sleep deprivation can affect functioning.

11 Which can prevent sleep?
   a Cheese
   b Chocolate
   c Milk
   d Beef

12 Which measure before bedtime promotes sleep?
   a Following the person's routines
   b Asking the person about family matters
   c Providing hot tea
   d Leaving the hallway light on

Answers to Chapter 33 questions are on p. 588.

FOCUS ON **PRACTICE**

Problem Solving

Prioritize the following comfort needs. Which would you do first, second, third, and last? Explain your reasons for the order.

- Provide a blanket.
- Report chest pain that began suddenly.
- Help a person who received a pain-relief drug 1 hour ago to the bathroom.
- Provide a back massage before bedtime.

CHAPTER 34

Collecting Specimens

OBJECTIVES

- Define the key terms and key abbreviations in this chapter.
- Explain why specimens are collected.
- Explain the rules for collecting specimens.
- Describe the different types of urine specimens.
- Describe 5 urine tests.
- Explain how to use reagent strips.

- Describe how to collect a stool specimen.
- Describe how to collect a sputum specimen.
- Explain how blood glucose is tested.
- Perform the procedures described in this chapter.
- Explain how to promote PRIDE in the person, the family, and yourself.

KEY TERMS

acetone See "ketone"
glucometer A device for measuring *(meter)* blood glucose *(gluco)*; glucose meter
glucosuria Sugar *(glucose)* in the urine *(uria)*
hematuria Blood *(hemat)* in the urine *(uria)*
hemoptysis Bloody *(hemo)* sputum *(ptysis* means *to spit)*

ketone A substance appearing in urine from the rapid breakdown of fat for energy; acetone, ketone body
ketone body See "ketone"
melena A black, tarry stool
sputum Mucus from the respiratory system that is expectorated (expelled) through the mouth

KEY ABBREVIATIONS

APRN	Advanced practice registered nurse		mL	Milliliter
BM	Bowel movement		oz	Ounce
ID	Identification		U/A; UA	Urinalysis
I&O	Intake and output			

Specimens *(samples)* are collected and tested to prevent, detect, and treat disease. Some specimens are tested at the bedside. Most are tested in the laboratory. All laboratory specimens require *requisition slips* with identifying information and the test ordered. The specimen container is labeled following agency policy. To collect specimens, follow the rules in Box 34-1.

See *Promoting Safety and Comfort: Collecting Specimens.*

BOX 34-1 Collecting Specimens

- Follow the rules for medical asepsis.
- Follow Standard Precautions and the Bloodborne Pathogen Standard.
- Use a clean container for each specimen.
- Use the correct container.
- Do not touch the inside of the container or the inside of the lid.
- Identify the person. Check the identification (ID) bracelet against the laboratory requisition slip or assignment sheet. Compare all information. Ask the person to state his or her first and last name and birthdate.
- Label the container in the person's presence. Provide clear, accurate information.
- Collect the specimen at the correct time.
- Ask a female needing a urine specimen if she is having a menstrual period. Tell the nurse. Menstruating may cause blood to be in the urine specimen.
- Ask the person not to have a bowel movement (BM) when collecting a urine specimen. Urine specimens must not contain stools.
- Ask the person to void before collecting a stool specimen. Stool specimens must not contain urine.
- Have the person put toilet paper in the toilet or in a disposable bag. Discard following agency policy. Urine and stool specimens must not contain toilet paper.
- Secure the lid on the specimen container tightly.
- Place the specimen container in a plastic bag with a *BIOHAZARD* label. Do not let the container touch the outside of the bag.
- Seal the bag containing the specimen securely.
- Take the specimen and requisition slip to the laboratory or storage area.

PROMOTING SAFETY AND COMFORT

Collecting Specimens

Safety

Correct identification is important when collecting and testing specimens. To identify the person, check the ID bracelet against all information on the requisition slip. The following identifying practices are also common.

- The person states or spells his or her first and last name.
- The person states his or her birthdate.
- The person identifies who ordered the test. For example, the person gives the name of the doctor or advanced practice registered nurse (APRN).

Blood and body fluids (including secretions and excretions) may contain microbes and blood. This includes urine, stool, and sputum specimens. Follow Standard Precautions when collecting, testing, and handling specimens. Follow the Bloodborne Pathogen Standard if blood is present.

NOTE: A task may require more than 1 pair of gloves. Change gloves as needed. Use careful judgment. Remember to practice hand hygiene after removing gloves.

URINE SPECIMENS

Urine specimens are collected for urine tests. Follow the rules in Box 34-1.

See *Delegation Guidelines: Urine Specimens.*
See *Promoting Safety and Comfort: Urine Specimens.*

DELEGATION GUIDELINES

Urine Specimens

To collect a urine specimen, you need this information from the nurse and the care plan.

- Voiding device—bedpan, urinal, commode, or toilet with a specimen pan
- The type of specimen needed
- What time to collect the specimen
- What special measures are needed
- If you need to test the specimen (p. 439)
- If measuring intake and output (I&O) is ordered (Chapter 30)
- What observations to report and record:
  - Problems obtaining the specimen
  - Color, clarity, and odor of urine
  - Blood in the urine
  - Particles in the urine
  - Complaints of pain, burning, urgency, difficulty voiding, or other problems
  - The time the specimen was collected
- When to report observations
- What patient or resident concerns to report at once

PROMOTING SAFETY AND COMFORT

Urine Specimens

Comfort

Clear specimen containers show urine. This may embarrass some people. Cloudy urine specimen containers are common.

 ### The Random Urine Specimen

The random urine specimen is used for a routine urinalysis (U/A; UA). No special measures are needed. It is collected any time in a 24-hour period. Many people collect the specimen themselves. Weak and very ill persons need help.

See procedure: *Collecting a Random Urine Specimen,* p. 436.

Collecting a Random Urine Specimen

Quality of Life

- Knock before entering the person's room.
- Address the person by name.
- Introduce yourself by name and title.

- Explain the procedure before starting and during the procedure.
- Protect the person's rights during the procedure.
- Handle the person gently during the procedure.

Pre-Procedure

1 Follow *Delegation Guidelines: Urine Specimens*, p. 435. **See** *Promoting Safety and Comfort:*
  a *Collecting Specimens*, p. 435
  b *Urine Specimens*, p. 435
2 Practice hand hygiene and get the following supplies.
- Laboratory requisition slip
- Specimen container and lid
- Voiding device (clean, un-used)—bedpan and cover (if used), urinal, commode, or specimen pan (Fig. 34-1)
- Graduate to measure output
- Specimen label

- Disposable bag (if needed)
- Plastic bag with a *BIOHAZARD* label
- Gloves
3 Arrange items in the person's room (bathroom). Open the plastic bag.
4 Practice hand hygiene.
5 Identify the person. Check the ID bracelet against the requisition slip. Compare all information. Also call the person by name. Ask the person to state his or her first and last name and birthdate.
6 Label the specimen container in the person's presence.
7 Provide for privacy.

Procedure

8 Put on gloves.
9 Place the specimen pan on the toilet or commode container if used (see Fig. 34-1).
10 Ask the person to urinate into the voiding device. Have the person put toilet paper into the toilet. Or provide a disposable bag and follow agency policy for disposal. Toilet paper is not put in the bedpan or specimen pan.
11 Take the voiding device to the bathroom if a bedpan, urinal, or commode was used.
12 Pour about 120 mL (milliliters) (4 oz [ounces]) into the specimen container.

13 Secure the lid on the specimen container tightly. Put the container in the plastic bag. Do not let the container touch the outside of the bag.
14 Measure urine if I&O are ordered. Include the specimen amount.
15 Dispose of excess urine in the toilet. Avoid splashes. Rinse equipment. Pour the rinse into the toilet and flush. Follow agency procedures for cleaning and disinfection. Return equipment to its proper place.
16 Remove and discard the gloves. Practice hand hygiene. Put on clean gloves.
17 Seal the bag containing the specimen container.
18 Assist with hand hygiene. Remove and discard the gloves. Practice hand hygiene.

Post-Procedure

19 Provide for comfort. (See the inside of the back cover.)
20 Place the call light and other needed items within reach.
21 Raise or lower bed rails. Follow the care plan.
22 Follow the care plan and the person's preferences for privacy measures to maintain. Leaving the privacy curtain, window coverings, and door open or closed are examples.
23 Complete a safety check of the room. (See the inside of the back cover.)

24 Practice hand hygiene.
25 Take the specimen and requisition slip to the laboratory or storage area. Wear gloves if that is agency policy.
26 Remove and discard the gloves (if worn). Practice hand hygiene.
27 Report and record your care and observations.

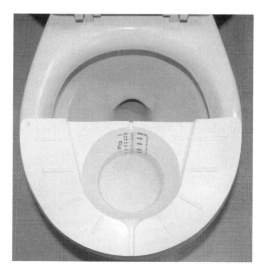

FIGURE 34-1 The specimen pan is at the front of the toilet on the toilet rim for a urine specimen. (NOTE: The toilet seat is lowered over the specimen pan for voiding.)

The Midstream Specimen

The midstream specimen is also called a *clean-voided specimen* or *clean-catch specimen*. The perineal area is cleaned first to reduce the number of microbes in the urethral area. The person starts to void into a device. Then the person stops the urine stream. A sterile specimen container is positioned. The person voids into the container until the specimen is obtained.

Stopping and starting the urine stream is hard for many people. You may need to position and hold the specimen container after the person starts to void (Fig. 34-2).

See *Focus on Communication: The Midstream Specimen.*

See procedure: *Collecting a Midstream Specimen.*

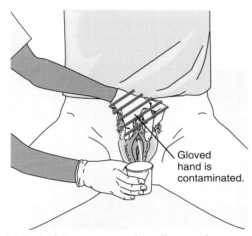

FIGURE 34-2 The labia are separated to collect a midstream specimen.

Gloved hand is contaminated.

FOCUS ON **COMMUNICATION**

The Midstream Specimen

Some persons can collect the midstream specimen without help. To explain the procedure, use words the person understands. Show the supplies and how to use them. Also, ask if the person has questions. For example:

I need to collect a midstream urine specimen. This means I need urine from the middle of your urine stream. First, wipe well with this towelette (show the towelette) from the front to back. The specimen goes in this cup (show the specimen cup). Please do not touch the inside of the cup. Start urinating and then stop. Position the cup to catch urine and start urinating again. If you cannot stop the stream, position the cup during the middle of the stream. I need at least this much urine if possible (point to the measurement on the cup). Remove the cup when it is about that full. Finish urinating. Secure the lid on the cup. Please do not touch the inside of the lid. I will take the specimen when you are done.

Then ask if the person has questions. Make sure the person understands what to do. You can say: "Please tell me what you will do so I know that you understand."

Collecting a Midstream Specimen

Quality of Life

- Knock before entering the person's room.
- Address the person by name.
- Introduce yourself by name and title.

- Explain the procedure before starting and during the procedure.
- Protect the person's rights during the procedure.
- Handle the person gently during the procedure.

Pre-Procedure

1 Follow *Delegation Guidelines: Urine Specimens*, p. 435. See *Promoting Safety and Comfort:*
   a *Collecting Specimens*, p. 435
   b *Urine Specimens*, p. 435
2 Practice hand hygiene and get the following supplies.
   - Laboratory requisition slip
   - Midstream specimen kit—specimen container, label, towelettes, sterile gloves
   - Voiding device—bedpan and cover (if used), urinal, commode, or specimen pan if needed
   - Graduate to measure output
   - Supplies for perineal care (Chapter 22)
   - Plastic bag with a *BIOHAZARD* label

   - Sterile gloves (if not part of the specimen kit and required by agency policy)
   - Disposable gloves
   - Paper towels
3 Arrange items in the person's room (bathroom). Open the plastic bag.
4 Practice hand hygiene.
5 Identify the person. Check the ID bracelet against the requisition slip. Compare all information. Also call the person by name. Ask the person to state his or her first and last name and birthdate.
6 Provide for privacy.

Procedure

7 Practice hand hygiene. Put on gloves.
8 Provide perineal care (Chapter 22). Remove and discard the gloves. Practice hand hygiene.

9 Open the specimen kit.
10 Put on gloves. Apply sterile gloves if required by agency policy.
11 Open the packet of towelettes.

Continued

Collecting a Midstream Specimen—cont'd

Procedure—cont'd

12 Open the specimen container. Do not touch the inside of the container or lid. The inside is sterile. Set the lid down with the inside up.

13 *For a female*—clean the perineal area with towelettes.
   a Spread the labia with your thumb and index finger. Use your non-dominant hand. (This hand is now contaminated. It must not touch anything sterile.)
   b Clean down the urethral area from front to back (top to bottom). Use a clean towelette for each stroke. Discard towelettes after use.
   c Keep the labia separated to collect the specimen (steps 15 through 18).

14 *For a male*—clean the penis with towelettes.
   a Hold the penis with your non-dominant hand. (This hand is now contaminated. It must not touch anything sterile.)
   b Clean the penis starting at the meatus. (Retract the foreskin if the male is uncircumcised.) Clean in a circular motion. Start at the center and work outward. Discard towelettes after use.
   c Hold the penis (and keep the foreskin retracted in the uncircumcised male) until the specimen is collected (steps 15 through 18).

15 Have the person void into a device.

16 Pass the specimen container into the urine stream. Keep the labia separated (see Fig. 34-2) or the foreskin retracted.

17 Collect about 30 to 90 mL (1 to 3 oz) of urine. (Some agencies require 90 to 120 mL [3 to 4 oz]. Follow agency procedures for the amount to collect.)

18 Remove the specimen container. Set it on a paper towel.

19 Release the labia or penis. (Release the foreskin of the uncircumcised male.) Let the person finish voiding into the device.

20 Remove and discard soiled gloves. Practice hand hygiene. Put on clean gloves.

21 Secure the lid on the specimen container tightly. Touch only the outside of the container and lid. Wipe the outside of the container. Discard used paper towels. Label the specimen container in the person's presence. Place the container in the plastic bag. The container must not touch the outside of the bag.

22 Provide toilet paper when the person is done voiding.

23 Take the voiding device to the bathroom if a bedpan, urinal, or commode was used.

24 Measure urine if I&O are ordered. Include the specimen amount.

25 Dispose of excess urine in the toilet. Avoid splashes. Rinse equipment. Pour the rinse into the toilet and flush. Follow agency procedures for cleaning and disinfection. Return equipment to its proper place.

26 Remove and discard the gloves. Practice hand hygiene. Put on clean gloves.

27 Seal the bag containing the specimen container.

28 Assist with hand hygiene. Remove and discard the gloves. Practice hand hygiene.

Post-Procedure

29 Provide for comfort. (See the inside of the back cover.)

30 Place the call light and other needed items within reach.

31 Raise or lower the bed rails. Follow the care plan.

32 Follow the care plan and the person's preferences for privacy measures to maintain. Leaving the privacy curtain, window coverings, and door open or closed are examples.

33 Complete a safety check of the room. (See the inside of the back cover.)

34 Practice hand hygiene.

35 Take the specimen and requisition slip to the laboratory or storage area. Wear gloves if that is agency policy.

36 Remove and discard the gloves (if worn). Practice hand hygiene.

37 Report and record your care and observations.

Urinary Catheter Specimens

A straight catheter (Chapter 26) may be needed to collect a specimen. A nurse inserts the catheter into the bladder and removes it after collecting the specimen. You may need to collect supplies or help position the person. Assist as the nurse directs.

A urine specimen can be collected from an indwelling catheter (Chapter 26). Urine in the drainage bag is not used. The port on the drainage tubing is used to collect the specimen. The nurse:

1 Clamps the drainage tubing so fresh urine can collect in the catheter.
2 Cleans the port.
3 Connects a syringe to the port (Fig. 34-3).
4 Aspirates (draws up) urine into the syringe.
5 Unclamps the drainage tubing.

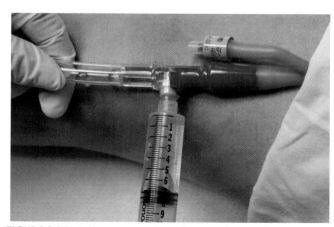

FIGURE 34-3 Collecting a specimen from a urinary catheter. A syringe is connected to the port on the drainage tubing. (From Perry AG, Potter PA, Ostendorf WR: *Nursing interventions & clinical skills*, ed 7, St Louis, 2020, Elsevier.)

The 24-Hour Urine Specimen

All urine voided during 24 hours is collected for a 24-hour urine specimen. To prevent microbe growth, the urine is chilled on ice or refrigerated. A preservative may be added to the collection container.

The person voids to start the test with an empty bladder. Discard this voiding. Save *all voidings* for the next 24 hours. The person and staff must clearly understand the procedure and the test period. This test is re-started if:

- A voiding was not saved.
- Toilet paper was discarded into the specimen.
- The specimen contains stools.

Testing Urine

The doctor or APRN orders the type and frequency of urine tests. Random urine specimens are needed. Reagent (test) strips are used for various urine tests. See Figure 34-4.

The nurse may have you do these simple tests.

- *Testing for pH*—Urine pH measures if urine is acidic or alkaline. Changes in normal pH (4.6 to 8.0) occur from illness, food, and drugs.
- *Testing for blood*—Injury and disease can cause hematuria. *Hematuria means blood* (hemat) *in the urine* (uria). Sometimes blood is seen in the urine. At other times it is unseen *(occult)*.
- *Testing for glucose and ketones*—In diabetes, the pancreas does not secrete enough insulin (Chapter 40). The body needs insulin to use sugar for energy. If not used, sugar builds up in the blood. Some sugar appears in the urine. *Glucosuria means sugar* (glucose) *in the urine* (uria). Diabetes may cause ketones in the urine. *Ketones (ketone bodies, acetone) are substances appearing in urine from the rapid breakdown of fat for energy.* The body uses fat for energy if it cannot use sugar. Tests for glucose and ketones are usually done 4 times a day—30 minutes before meals and at bedtime. Test results are used for drug and diet decisions.
- *Testing for infection*—The presence of certain white blood cells can signal a urinary tract infection.
- *Testing for protein*—Protein in the urine can signal kidney and other diseases.
  See *Delegation Guidelines: Testing Urine.*
  See *Promoting Safety and Comfort: Testing Urine.*
  See procedure: *Testing Urine With Reagent Strips*, p. 440.

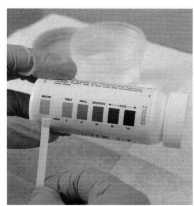

To use a reagent (test) strip:

- Do not touch the test area on the strip.
- Dip the strip into urine.
- Compare the strip with the color chart on the bottle.

FIGURE 34-4 Reagent (test) strips have sections that change color when reacting with urine.

DELEGATION GUIDELINES
Testing Urine

If testing urine is delegated to you, you need this information from the nurse and the care plan.

- What test is needed
- What equipment and reagent strips to use
- When to test urine
- Instructions for the test ordered
- If the nurse will observe test results
- What observations to report and record:
  - The time you collected and tested the specimen
  - Test results
  - Problems obtaining the specimen
  - Color, clarity, and odor of urine
  - Blood or particles in the urine
  - Complaints of pain, burning, urgency, difficulty voiding, or other problems
- When to report test results and observations
- What patient or resident concerns to report at once

PROMOTING SAFETY AND COMFORT
Testing Urine

Safety

Accuracy is important. Promptly report results. Ordered drugs may depend on the results.

When using reagent (test) strips:

- Check the color of the strips. Do not use discolored strips.
- Check the expiration date on the bottle. Do not use the strips if the date has passed.
- Follow the manufacturer's instructions for an accurate result. Test results are used for diagnosis and treatment. A wrong result can cause serious harm.

Testing Urine With Reagent Strips

Quality of Life

- Knock before entering the person's room.
- Address the person by name.
- Introduce yourself by name and title.

- Explain the procedure before starting and during the procedure.
- Protect the person's rights during the procedure.
- Handle the person gently during the procedure.

Pre-Procedure

1 Follow *Delegation Guidelines: Testing Urine*, p. 439. See *Promoting Safety and Comfort:*
   a *Collecting Specimens*, p. 435
   b *Testing Urine*, p. 439
2 Practice hand hygiene and get the following supplies.
   - Reagent (test) strips for the ordered test
   - Equipment for the urine specimen (see procedure: *Collecting a Random Urine Specimen*, p. 436)
   - Gloves

3 Arrange items in the person's room (bathroom).
4 Practice hand hygiene.
5 Identify the person. Check the ID bracelet against the assignment sheet. Use 2 identifiers (Chapter 11). Also call the person by name. Ask the person to state his or her first and last name and birthdate.
6 Provide for privacy.

Procedure

7 Put on gloves.
8 Collect the urine specimen. See procedure: *Collecting a Random Urine Specimen*, p. 436.
9 Remove a strip from the bottle. Put the cap tightly on the bottle at once.
10 Dip the strip test area into the urine.
11 Remove the strip after the correct amount of time. See the manufacturer's instructions.
12 Tap the strip gently against the urine container. This removes excess urine.

13 Wait the required amount of time. See the manufacturer's instructions.
14 Compare the strip with the color chart on the bottle (see Fig. 34-4). Read the results.
15 Discard disposable items.
16 Dispose of urine in the toilet. Avoid splashes. Rinse equipment. Pour the rinse into the toilet and flush. Follow agency procedures for cleaning and disinfection. Return equipment to its proper place.
17 Remove and discard the gloves. Practice hand hygiene.

Post-Procedure

18 Provide for comfort. (See the inside of the back cover.)
19 Place the call light and other needed items within reach.
20 Raise or lower bed rails. Follow the care plan.
21 Follow the care plan and the person's preferences for privacy measures to maintain. Leaving the privacy curtain, window coverings, and door open or closed are examples.

22 Complete a safety check of the room. (See the inside of the back cover.)
23 Practice hand hygiene.
24 Report and record the test results and other observations.

STOOL SPECIMENS

Stools are studied for abnormal contents. Fat, microbes, worms, and blood are examples. Blood in stools can be:

- Visible. Bleeding from low in the bowels can cause red stools. Bleeding in the stomach or upper gastro-intestinal tract can cause *black, tarry stools called* **melena**.
- Unseen *(occult)*. *Occult* means *hidden or not seen*. Occult blood tests are used to screen for colon cancer and other digestive disorders.

Urine must not contaminate the stool specimen. The person uses 1 device for voiding and another for a BM. Some tests require a warm stool. The specimen is taken at once to the laboratory or storage area. Follow the rules in Box 34-1.

See *Focus on Communication: Stool Specimens*.
See *Delegation Guidelines: Stool Specimens*.
See *Promoting Safety and Comfort: Stool Specimens*.
See procedure: *Collecting a Stool Specimen*.

FOCUS ON COMMUNICATION

Stool Specimens

Before you begin, explain what the person needs to do and what you will do. Show the equipment and supplies and how to use them. For example:

I need to collect a specimen from a bowel movement. I'm going to place the specimen pan (show specimen pan) at the back of the toilet. Urinate into the toilet. Your bowel movement collects in the specimen pan. Please put toilet paper in the toilet, not in the specimen pan. After your bowel movement, put your call light on right away. I'll collect the specimen in this container (show the specimen container).

Then ask if the person has questions. If you do not know the answer, tell the nurse. Make sure the person understands what to do. You can say: "Please tell me what you will do so I know that you understand."

DELEGATION GUIDELINES
Stool Specimens

Before collecting a stool specimen, you need this information from the nurse.
- What time to collect the specimen
- What equipment and special measures are needed
- If the nurse wants to observe the stool
- What observations to report and record:
  - The time you collected the specimen
  - Problems obtaining the specimen
  - Color, amount, consistency, and odor of stools
  - Complaints of pain or discomfort
- When to report observations
- What patient or resident concerns to report at once

PROMOTING SAFETY AND COMFORT
Stool Specimens

Comfort
Stools normally have an odor. A person may be embarrassed that you need a specimen. Complete the task quickly and carefully. Act in a professional manner.

Collecting a Stool Specimen

Quality of Life

- Knock before entering the person's room.
- Address the person by name.
- Introduce yourself by name and title.
- Explain the procedure before starting and during the procedure.
- Protect the person's rights during the procedure.
- Handle the person gently during the procedure.

Pre-Procedure

1 Follow *Delegation Guidelines: Stool Specimens*. See *Promoting Safety and Comfort:*
  a *Collecting Specimens*, p. 435
  b *Stool Specimens*
2 Practice hand hygiene and get the following supplies.
  - Laboratory requisition slip
  - Device to collect the BM (clean, un-used)—bedpan and cover (if used) or specimen pan
  - Device for voiding if the person will void—bedpan and cover (if used), commode, urinal, or specimen pan
  - Stool specimen container and lid
  - Specimen label
  - Tongue blades
  - Disposable bag
  - Plastic bag with a *BIOHAZARD* label
  - Toilet paper
  - Gloves
3 Arrange items in the person's room (bathroom). Open the plastic bag.
4 Practice hand hygiene.
5 Identify the person. Check the ID bracelet against the requisition slip. Compare all information. Also call the person by name. Ask the person to state his or her first and last name and birthdate.
6 Label the specimen container in the person's presence.
7 Provide for privacy.

Procedure

8 Put on gloves.
9 Have the person void. Provide the voiding device if not using the bathroom. Empty the device into the toilet. Avoid splashes. Rinse the device. Pour the rinse into the toilet and flush. Follow agency procedures for cleaning and disinfection. Return the device to its proper place.
10 Put the specimen pan on the back of the toilet or commode if used (Fig. 34-5, p. 442). Or provide the bedpan.
11 Ask the person not to put toilet paper into the bedpan, commode, or specimen pan. Have the person put toilet paper in the toilet. Or provide a disposable bag and follow agency policy for disposal.
12 Remove and discard the gloves. Practice hand hygiene.
13 Place the call light and toilet paper within reach. Provide for safety. Practice hand hygiene and leave the room if the person can be left alone.
14 Return when the person signals. Or check on the person every 5 minutes. Knock before entering.
15 Practice hand hygiene. Put on clean gloves.
16 Assist the person off the toilet or commode (if used). Or remove the bedpan (if used). Assist with wiping and perineal care as needed.
17 Remove and discard soiled gloves. Practice hand hygiene. Put on clean gloves.
18 Note the color, amount, consistency, and odor of stools.
19 Collect the specimen.
  a Use a tongue blade to place about 2 tablespoons of stool in the specimen container (Fig. 34-6, p. 442). Take the sample from:
    - The middle of a formed stool
    - Areas of pus, mucus, or blood and watery areas
    - The middle and both ends of a hard stool
  b Secure the lid on the specimen container tightly.
  c Place the container in the plastic bag. Do not let the container touch the outside of the bag.
  d Wrap the tongue blade in toilet paper. Discard it in the disposable bag.
20 Dispose of excess stool in the toilet. Avoid splashes. Rinse equipment. Pour the rinse into the toilet and flush. Follow agency procedures for cleaning and disinfection. Return equipment to its proper place.
21 Remove and discard the gloves. Practice hand hygiene. Put on clean gloves.
22 Seal the bag containing the specimen container.
23 Assist with hand hygiene. Remove and discard the gloves. Practice hand hygiene.

Continued

Collecting a Stool Specimen—cont'd

Post-Procedure

24 Provide for comfort. (See the inside of the back cover.)
25 Place the call light and other needed items within reach.
26 Raise or lower bed rails. Follow the care plan.
27 Follow the care plan and the person's preferences for privacy measures to maintain. Leaving the privacy curtain, window coverings, and door open or closed are examples.
28 Complete a safety check of the room. (See the inside of the back cover.)

29 Practice hand hygiene.
30 Take the specimen and requisition slip to the laboratory or storage area. Wear gloves if that is agency policy.
31 Remove and discard the gloves (if worn). Practice hand hygiene.
32 Report and record your care and observations.

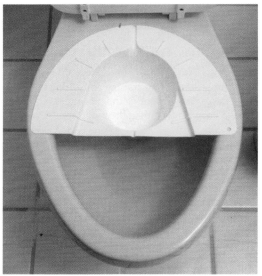

FIGURE 34-5 The specimen pan is placed at the back of the toilet for a stool specimen. (NOTE: The toilet seat is lowered over the specimen pan for the BM.)

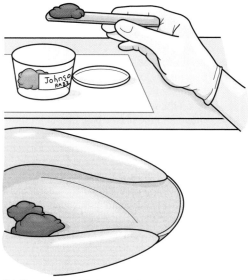

FIGURE 34-6 A tongue blade is used to transfer a small amount of stool from the bedpan to the specimen container.

SPUTUM SPECIMENS

Respiratory disorders cause the lungs, bronchi, and trachea to secrete mucus. *Mucus from the respiratory system is called **sputum** when expectorated (expelled) through the mouth.* Sputum specimens are studied for blood, microbes, and abnormal cells.

Sputum is not saliva. Saliva ("spit") is a thin, clear liquid produced by the salivary glands in the mouth. Sputum is coughed up from the bronchi and trachea. This can be painful and hard to do. Collecting a specimen is easier in the morning. Secretions collect in the trachea and bronchi during sleep. They are coughed up on awakening.

Follow the rules in Box 34-1. Also have the person rinse the mouth with water. Rinsing decreases saliva and removes food particles. Mouthwash is not used. It destroys some of the microbes in the mouth.

See *Delegation Guidelines: Sputum Specimens.*
See *Promoting Safety and Comfort: Sputum Specimens.*
See procedure: *Collecting a Sputum Specimen.*

DELEGATION GUIDELINES

Sputum Specimens

To collect a sputum specimen, you need this information from the nurse.

- When to collect the specimen
- The amount needed—usually 1 to 2 teaspoons
- If the person uses the bathroom
- If the person can hold the sputum container
- If you need to wear a mask or respirator or other personal protective equipment (see *Promoting Safety and Comfort: Sputum Specimens*)
- What observations to report and record:
  - The time the specimen was collected
  - The amount collected
  - How easily the person raised the sputum
  - Sputum color—clear, white, yellow, green, brown, or red
  - Sputum odor—none or foul odor
  - Sputum consistency—thick, watery, or frothy (with bubbles or foam)
  - *Hemoptysis*—bloody (*hemo*) sputum (*ptysis* means to spit)
  - If the person could not produce sputum
  - Any other observations
- When to report observations
- What patient or resident concerns to report at once

PROMOTING SAFETY AND COMFORT
Sputum Specimens

Safety

Always use Standard Precautions. Follow Transmission-Based Precautions as directed by the nurse. A mask is worn for Droplet Precautions. A respirator is worn for Airborne Precautions. See Chapter 15.

Comfort

The procedure can embarrass the person. Coughing and expectorating sounds can disturb others. Also, sputum is not pleasant to look at. Privacy is important. Some sputum specimen containers are cloudy to hide the contents. Covering a clear container with a paper towel may be helpful.

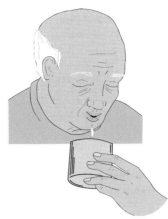

FIGURE 34-7 The person expectorates (spits) into the center of the specimen container.

Collecting a Sputum Specimen

Quality of Life

- Knock before entering the person's room.
- Address the person by name.
- Introduce yourself by name and title.
- Explain the procedure before starting and during the procedure.
- Protect the person's rights during the procedure.
- Handle the person gently during the procedure.

Pre-Procedure

1 Follow *Delegation Guidelines: Sputum Specimens.* See *Promoting Safety and Comfort:*
   a *Collecting Specimens,* p. 435
   b *Sputum Specimens*
2 Practice hand hygiene and get the following supplies.
   - Laboratory requisition slip
   - Sputum specimen container and lid
   - Specimen label
   - Plastic bag with a *BIOHAZARD* label
   - Tissues
   - Gloves
3 Arrange items in the person's room (bathroom). Open the plastic bag.
4 Practice hand hygiene.
5 Identify the person. Check the ID bracelet against the requisition slip. Compare all information. Also call the person by name. Ask the person to state his or her first and last name and birthdate.
6 Label the specimen container in the person's presence.
7 Provide for privacy. If able, the person uses the bathroom for the procedure.

Procedure

8 Put on gloves.
9 Have the person rinse the mouth with clear water.
10 Have the person hold the container. Only the outside is touched.
11 Have the person cover the mouth and nose with tissues when coughing. Follow agency policy for used tissues.
12 Have the person take 2 or 3 breaths and cough up the sputum.
13 Have the person expectorate (spit) directly into the container (Fig. 34-7). Sputum must not touch the outside of the container.
14 Collect 1 to 2 teaspoons of sputum.
15 Secure the lid on the specimen container tightly.
16 Place the container in the plastic bag. Do not let the container touch the outside of the bag.
17 Remove and discard the gloves. Practice hand hygiene. Put on clean gloves.
18 Seal the bag containing the specimen container.
19 Assist with hand hygiene. Remove and discard the gloves. Practice hand hygiene.

Post-Procedure

20 Provide for comfort. (See the inside of the back cover.)
21 Place the call light and other needed items within reach.
22 Raise or lower bed rails. Follow the care plan.
23 Follow the care plan and the person's preferences for privacy measures to maintain. Leaving the privacy curtain, window coverings, and door open or closed are examples.
24 Complete a safety check of the room. (See the inside of the back cover.)
25 Practice hand hygiene.
26 Take the specimen and the requisition slip to the laboratory or storage area. Wear gloves if that is agency policy.
27 Remove and discard the gloves (if worn). Practice hand hygiene.
28 Report and record your care and observations.

BLOOD GLUCOSE TESTING

Blood glucose testing (Fig. 34-8) is used for persons with diabetes. The skin is punctured. A drop of blood is collected and tested. Measurements before meals and at bedtime are common. Results are used to regulate drugs and diet.

Some states and agencies allow nursing assistants to perform blood glucose testing. If allowed, make sure that:

- You have the necessary training.
- You know how to use the agency's equipment.
- You review the procedure with a nurse.
- The nurse is available to answer questions and to guide and assist you as needed.

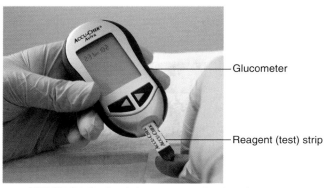

Glucometer

Reagent (test) strip

FIGURE 34-8 Blood glucose is tested with a glucometer.

Blood Glucose Testing Equipment

To perform a blood glucose test, the following supplies are needed.

- *Gloves and antiseptic wipes.* Gloves are worn. The skin puncture site is cleaned with an antiseptic wipe. The side of a fingertip is a common site. The puncture site is not touched after it is cleaned.
- *A sterile, disposable lancet.* A lancet is a short, pointed blade. It is used to puncture the skin to obtain the blood sample. The blade is discarded in the sharps container after use.
- *A glucometer* (see Fig. 34-8). A **glucometer** *(glucose meter) is a device for measuring* (meter) *blood glucose* (gluco). The test result (a number) is displayed on the front of the device.
- *A bottle of reagent strips (test strips).* A strip is inserted into the glucometer. A drop of blood is applied to the reagent (test) strip. See Figure 34-8.
- *Gauze squares.* Pressure is applied with gauze squares over the puncture site until bleeding stops.

FOCUS ON P R I D E

The Person, Family, and Yourself

P ersonal and Professional Responsibility

You must collect specimens on the right person. Otherwise, one or both persons could be harmed. Before collecting a specimen, carefully identify the person.

In some agencies, collection information is written on the specimen container. Collection date and time and the collector's name or initials are examples. Follow agency policy to properly collect and label specimens.

R ights and Respect

Specimen collection can be embarrassing. To respect the right to privacy:

- Politely ask visitors to leave the room.
- Close doors, privacy curtains, and window coverings.
- Leave the room if it is safe to do so. If you cannot leave, tell the person why.

I ndependence and Social Interaction

Some persons can collect their own specimens. Doing so promotes independence and reduces embarrassment.

Explain the procedure and show the person the container. Tell the person where you are placing the container. When ready to collect the specimen, the person knows where to find the container.

D elegation and Teamwork

Before taking a specimen to the laboratory, tell the nurse and your co-workers. Ask if other staff need specimens delivered. Doing so saves staff time. This also prevents having too many staff members off the unit at the same time. Return from the laboratory promptly.

E thics and Laws

If you did not collect a specimen correctly, do not send it to the laboratory. Tell the nurse. Then collect the specimen at the next opportunity. Test results must be accurate for correct diagnosis and treatment. Take pride in honestly reporting mistakes.

FOCUS ON PRIDE: *Application*

What mistakes could occur in specimen collection? What can you do to prevent such mistakes? Explain why failing to report a mistake can be harmful.

Circle the BEST answer.

1 Which specimen was collected *correctly*?
   a A stool specimen that contains urine
   b A urine specimen that contains toilet paper
   c A sputum specimen with a label and requisition slip
   d A urine specimen with a loose lid

2 A random urine specimen is collected
   a After sleep
   b Before meals
   c After meals
   d Any time

3 Perineal care is given before
   a Collecting a random urine specimen
   b Collecting a midstream urine specimen
   c Testing a urine specimen for ketones
   d Collecting a stool specimen

4 To collect a midstream specimen on a female
   a Spread the labia to expose the urethral area
   b Clean the urethral area from back to front
   c Collect urine at the start of the urine stream
   d Collect about 10 mL of urine

5 You discard a voiding 12 hours after the start of a 24-hour urine specimen. You should
   a Tell the nurse so the test can be re-started
   b Send the specimen collected over 12 hours to the laboratory
   c Not report the missed void so the 24-hour specimen is done on time
   d Ask the nurse to extend the collection time by 1 hour

6 Urine is tested for glucose
   a To measure the pH
   b To check for blood
   c To check for sugar
   d To check for infection

7 You are testing urine using reagent strips. Which is *correct*?
   a Obtain a 24-hour urine specimen for testing.
   b Touch the test area to make sure it is secure.
   c Use the reagent strips if the expiration date has passed.
   d Compare the strip with the color chart on the bottle.

8 A stool appears black and tarry. This is
   a Occult blood
   b Hematuria
   c Melena
   d Normal feces

9 A person has a BM in a bedpan. Part of the stool is red and watery. When collecting a sample, you should
   a Avoid the red, watery part
   b Collect from the red, watery part
   c Take the bedpan to the laboratory
   d Flush the stool and collect a different sample later

10 The best time to collect a sputum specimen is
   a On awakening
   b After meals
   c At bedtime
   d After oral hygiene

11 A sputum specimen is needed. Have the person
   a Use mouthwash
   b Rinse the mouth with clear water
   c Brush the teeth
   d Remove dentures

12 In your agency, nurses measure blood glucose. You can
   a Gather the needed supplies and clean up after the test
   b Perform the test if you know how
   c Puncture the site and have the nurse use the glucometer
   d Teach the person how to check his or her own blood glucose

Answers to Chapter 34 questions are on p. 588.

FOCUS ON PRACTICE

Problem Solving

A midstream urine specimen is ordered. You give the patient the specimen cup and pack of towelettes and ask: "Do you know what to do?" The patient says: "Yes, I've done this before." You tell the patient to leave the specimen in the bathroom and signal for you when done.

You return and notice the towelettes are unopened. What do you do? Should you send the specimen to the laboratory? How could this have been prevented?

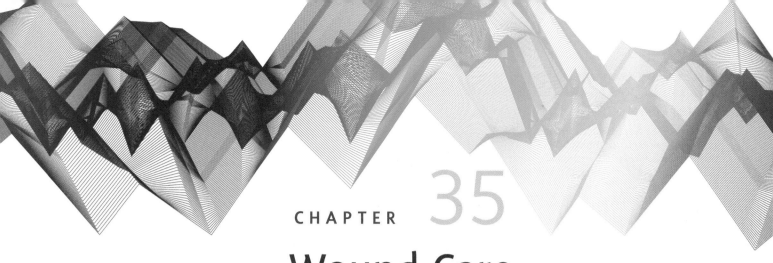

CHAPTER 35

Wound Care

OBJECTIVES

- Define the key terms and key abbreviations in this chapter.
- Describe skin tears and circulatory ulcers and the persons at risk.
- Explain how to help prevent skin tears and circulatory ulcers.
- Describe foot care for persons with diabetes.
- Explain the purposes of elastic stockings and elastic bandages.

- Explain the purposes of wound dressings.
- Explain the rules for applying dressings.
- Describe what to observe about wounds.
- Explain the purpose, effects, and complications of heat and cold applications.
- Describe the rules for applying heat and cold.
- Perform the procedures described in this chapter.
- Explain how to promote PRIDE in the person, the family, and yourself.

KEY TERMS

constrict To narrow
dilate To expand or open wider
skin tear A break or rip in the outer layers of the skin; the epidermis (top skin layer) separates from the underlying tissues

ulcer A shallow or deep crater-like sore of the skin or mucous membrane
wound A break in the skin or mucous membrane

KEY ABBREVIATIONS

AE	Anti-embolism; anti-embolic
C	Centigrade
F	Fahrenheit

ID	Identification
PPE	Personal protective equipment

A *wound* is a break in the skin or mucous membrane. Wounds commonly result from:

- Surgery
- *Trauma*—an accident or violent act that injures the skin, mucous membranes, bones, and organs
- Unrelieved pressure or friction (Chapter 36)
- Decreased blood flow through arteries or veins
- Nerve damage

Wounds are portals of entry for microbes. Infection is a major threat. Wound care includes preventing infection and further injury to the wound and nearby tissues.

See *Delegation Guidelines: Wound Care.*
See *Promoting Safety and Comfort: Wound Care.*

DELEGATION GUIDELINES
Wound Care

Your state and agency may not allow you to perform some of the procedures in this chapter. Before performing a procedure, make sure that:
- Your state allows you to perform the procedure.
- The procedure is in your job description.
- You have the necessary education and training.
- You review the procedure with a nurse.
- A nurse is available to answer questions and to guide and assist you as needed.

PROMOTING SAFETY AND COMFORT
Wound Care

Safety

Wound care may involve contact with blood, body fluids, and non-intact skin. Follow Standard Precautions and the Bloodborne Pathogen Standard. Wear personal protective equipment (PPE) as needed. Gloves, gowns, masks, and eye protection are necessary when splashes and splatters are likely.

NOTE: *A task may require more than 1 pair of gloves. Change gloves as needed. Use careful judgment. Remember to practice hand hygiene after removing gloves.*

SKIN TEARS

A *skin tear is a break or rip in the outer layers of the skin* (Fig. 35-1). *The epidermis (top skin layer) separates from the underlying tissues* (Chapter 9). The hands, arms, and lower legs are common sites for skin tears. Skin tears are caused by:
- Friction, shearing (Chapter 17), pulling, or pressure on the skin.
- Falls or bumping a hard surface. Beds, bed rails, chairs, wheelchair parts, walkers, and tables are dangers.
- Holding an arm or leg too tight.
- Removing tape or adhesives.
- Bathing, dressing, and other tasks.
- Pulling buttons and zippers across fragile skin.
- Jewelry—yours or the person's. Rings, watches, and bracelets are examples.
- Long or jagged fingernails (yours or the person's) and long or jagged toenails.

Skin tears are painful. They are portals of entry for microbes. Infection is a risk. Tell the nurse at once if you cause or find a skin tear. To prevent skin tears, follow the care plan and the measures in Box 35-1.

See *Focus on Older Persons: Skin Tears.*

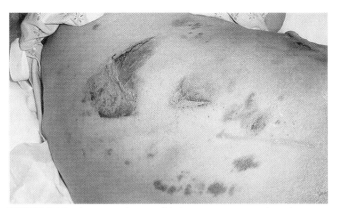

FIGURE 35-1 Skin tear. The top skin layer is torn away. (Used with permission from Rosemary Kohr, RN, PhD, ACNP (cert), www.lhsc.on.ca/wound, Rosemary.Kohr@Lhasa.on.ca.)

BOX 35-1 Preventing Skin Tears

- Follow the care plan and safety rules to:
  - Move, turn, position, or transfer the person.
    - Prevent shearing and friction.
    - Use an assist device to move and turn the person in bed.
    - Use pillows to support arms and legs.
  - Bathe the person.
  - Keep the skin moisturized and apply lotion.
  - Offer fluids.
- Keep your fingernails short and smoothly filed.
- Keep the person's fingernails short and smoothly filed. Report long, tough, or jagged toenails.
- Do not wear rings with large or raised stones. Do not wear bracelets.
- Be patient and calm when the person is confused, agitated, or resists care.
- Dress and undress the person carefully. The person wears soft clothes with long sleeves and long pants.
- Apply arm or leg protectors as ordered.
- Provide a safe setting.
  - Pad bed rails and wheelchair arms, footplates, and leg supports.
  - Provide good lighting so the person can see. The person must avoid bumping into furniture, walls, and equipment.
  - Provide a safe area for wandering (Chapter 42).
- Remove tape carefully. To remove tape, hold the skin down and gently pull the tape ends toward the wound.
- Do not apply adhesive tape (p. 453).

FOCUS ON OLDER PERSONS
Skin Tears

Thin and fragile skin is common in older persons. Slight pressure can cause a skin tear. Persons who are confused may resist care. They often move quickly and without warning. Or they pull away during care. Some try to hit or kick. These sudden movements can cause skin tears.

Never force care on a person. Chapter 42 describes how to care for persons who are confused and resist care. Always follow the care plan.

CIRCULATORY ULCERS

An *ulcer* *is a shallow or deep crater-like sore of the skin or mucous membrane. Circulatory ulcers (vascular ulcers)* are open sores on the lower legs or feet. They are caused by decreased blood flow through the arteries or veins. These wounds are hard to heal. Infection and gangrene can develop. *Gangrene* is a condition in which there is death of tissue.

Circulatory ulcers include:

- *Venous ulcers (stasis ulcers)* are open sores on the lower legs or feet caused by poor venous blood flow (Fig. 35-2, *A*). *Stasis* means *stopped or slowed fluid flow.* Leg veins do not return blood to the heart normally. Blood collects in the veins. The buildup of fluid and increased pressure prevent oxygen and nutrients from getting to tissues. The heels and inner part of the ankles are common sites. A dull, aching pain is common.
- *Arterial ulcers (ischemic ulcers)* are open wounds on the lower legs or feet caused by poor arterial blood flow (Fig. 35-2, *B*). *Ischemic* means *reduced blood flow to a body part.* Poor blood flow causes cell death and tissue damage. Arterial ulcers are found between the toes, on top of the toes, and on the outer side of the ankle. These wounds can be painful. Lowering the legs may help relieve pain.
- *Diabetic foot ulcers* are open wounds on the foot caused by complications from diabetes (Fig. 35-2, *C*). Diabetes (Chapter 40) can affect the nerves and blood vessels. With nerve damage, the person can lose sensation in a foot or leg. The person may not feel pain, heat, or cold. When blood vessels are affected, blood flow decreases. Tissues and cells do not get needed oxygen and nutrients. Sores heal poorly. Infection and tissue death (gangrene) are risks. Sometimes the affected part must be amputated.

Prevention and Treatment

Check the person's feet and legs daily. Report any sign of a problem at once. You must help prevent skin breakdown on the legs and feet. Follow the care plan to prevent and treat circulatory ulcers (Box 35-2). Diabetes foot care can prevent foot problems that cause diabetic foot ulcers (Box 35-3). The doctor orders drugs and treatments as needed.

Persons at risk need professional foot care. *You do not cut the toenails of persons with diseases affecting circulation.*

BOX 35-2 Preventing Circulatory Ulcers

- Remind the person not to sit with the legs crossed.
- Re-position the person according to the care plan—at least every 2 hours.
- Do not use elastic or rubber band–type garters to hold socks or hose in place.
- Apply elastic stockings or elastic bandages as directed (p. 450 and p. 452).
- Do not dress the person in tight clothes.
- Provide good skin care daily and as needed. Keep the feet clean and dry. Clean and dry between the toes.
- Report toenails in need of trimming and filing.
- Do not scrub or rub the skin during bathing and drying.
- Keep linens clean, dry, and wrinkle-free.
- Avoid injury to the legs and feet.
- Make sure shoes fit well.
- Keep pressure off of the heels and other bony areas. Use pillows or other devices as directed.
- Check the person's legs and feet. Report skin breaks or changes in skin color.
- Do not massage over pressure points (Chapter 36). *Never rub or massage reddened areas.*
- Use protective devices as directed.
- Follow the care plan for walking and exercises.

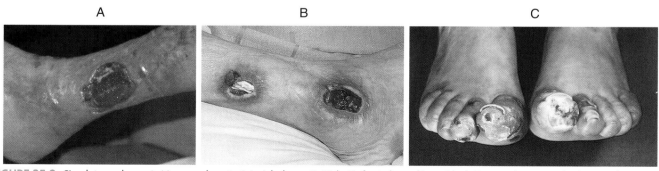

FIGURE 35-2 Circulatory ulcers. **A,** Venous ulcer. **B,** Arterial ulcers. **C,** Diabetic foot ulcers. (From Black JM, Hawks JH: *Medical-surgical nursing: clinical management for positive outcomes,* ed 8, St Louis, 2009, Saunders.)

BOX 35-3 Diabetes Foot Care

Common Problems

- *Corns and calluses* (Fig. 35-3, A). These are thick layers of skin caused by too much rubbing or pressure on the same spot.
- *Blisters* (Fig. 35-3, B). These form when shoes rub on the same spot.
- *Ingrown toenails* (Fig. 35-3, C). An edge of a toenail grows into the skin.
- *Bunions* (Fig. 35-3, D). A bunion is a bump on the outside edge of the big toe. The big toe slants toward the small toes.
- *Plantar warts* (Fig. 35-3, E). *Plantar* means *sole*. Plantar warts occur on the soles (bottoms) of the feet.
- *Hammer toes* (Fig. 35-3, F). One or more toes are flexed.
- *Dry and cracked skin* (Fig. 35-3, G). The dry skin can crack, causing portals of entry for microbes. Infection can occur.
- *Athlete's foot* (Fig. 35-3, H). This is a fungus causing itching, burning, redness, and cracked skin between the toes and on the soles of the feet.
- *Fungal infection of the toenails* (Fig. 35-3, I). The toenails become thick and hard to cut. They may be yellow, brown, or black.

Observations

- Check the feet daily for:
  - Cuts
  - Sores
  - Blisters
  - Redness
  - Calluses
  - Infected toenails
  - Ingrown toenails
  - Blood, pus, or watery drainage
  - Warm skin

Care Measures

- Wash the feet daily in warm water with mild soap.
  - Do not use hot water.
  - Test the water temperature with your elbow or use a water thermometer. Because burns are a risk, water temperature should be 90°F to 95°F (Fahrenheit) (32.2°C to 35°C [centigrade]).
  - Do not soak the feet in water. The skin could dry out.
  - Dry the feet well, especially between the toes.
- Apply a thin layer of talcum powder or cornstarch between the toes. This keeps the skin between the toes dry.
- Apply a thin layer of lotion, cream, or petroleum jelly on the tops and bottoms of the feet (not between the toes). Do so after washing and drying to keep the skin soft and smooth.
- Have the person wear closed-toed shoes and clean socks, stockings, or nylons. This prevents blisters and sores.
  - Socks, stockings, and nylons do not have holes or seams.
  - Lightly padded socks are best.
  - Tight socks or knee-high stockings are avoided.
  - Athletic and walking shoes are best. They have laces, Velcro, or buckles for easy adjustment.
  - Open-toed shoes, sandals, flip-flops, pointy shoes, and high-heels are not worn.
  - Vinyl and plastic shoes are not worn. They do not stretch and do not allow air movement inside the shoes.
- Check shoes for sharp edges or objects in the shoes. Make sure the lining is smooth.
- Do not allow the person to walk barefoot.
- Provide socks at night for cold feet.
- Promote blood flow to the feet. Have the person:
  - Elevate the feet when sitting.
  - Wiggle the toes for 5 minutes 2 or 3 times a day.
  - Move the ankles up and down and in and out.
  - Avoid crossing the legs.
- Do not trim or cut toenails or cut corns or calluses or try to smooth them. Professional foot care is needed.

Modified from National Institute of Diabetes and Digestive and Kidney Diseases: *Diabetes and foot problems*, January 2017.

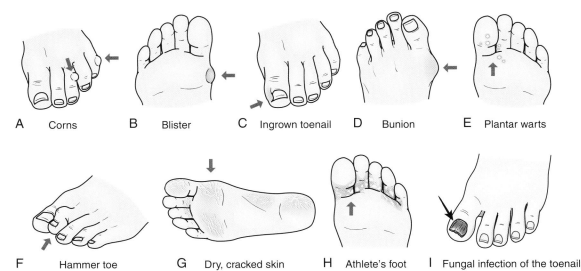

| A Corns | B Blister | C Ingrown toenail | D Bunion | E Plantar warts |

| F Hammer toe | G Dry, cracked skin | H Athlete's foot | I Fungal infection of the toenail |

FIGURE 35-3 Foot problems common with diabetes. (Redrawn from National Institute of Diabetes and Digestive and Kidney Diseases: *Prevent diabetes problems: keep your feet healthy*, NIH Publication No. 14-4282, Bethesda, Md, February 2014, U.S. Department of Health and Human Services.)

Elastic Stockings. Elastic stockings put pressure on the veins. This promotes venous blood return to the heart. Leg swelling is reduced. Stockings also help prevent blood clots (*thrombi*) in leg veins. A blood clot is called a *thrombus*.

If blood flow is sluggish, blood clots may form. They can form in the deep leg veins in the lower legs or thighs (Fig. 35-4, *A*). A blood clot (*thrombus*) can break loose and travel through the bloodstream. It then becomes an *embolus*—a blood clot that travels through the vascular system until it lodges in a blood vessel (Fig. 35-4, *B*). An embolus from a vein lodges in the lungs (*pulmonary embolism*) and can cause severe respiratory problems and death. Report chest pain or shortness of breath at once.

Persons at risk for thrombi include those who:
- Have heart, circulatory, or lymphatic disorders.
- Are on bed rest.
- Are older.
- Are pregnant.
- Have had surgery.
The type of stockings used depends on their purpose.
- *Anti-embolism or anti-embolic (AE) stockings* are used to prevent blood clots. These may also be called TED hose (*TED* stands for *thrombo-embolic deterrent* or *thrombo-embolic disease*). Common after surgery, these stockings are not usually used long-term.
- *Compression stockings* may be used long-term. They improve blood flow in the legs and prevent leg swelling. Compression stockings are available in different pressures (light to strong) and lengths (knee-high to thigh-high).

The person usually has 2 pairs of stockings. Wash 1 pair while the other pair is worn. Wash them by hand with a mild soap. Hang them to dry.

See *Delegation Guidelines: Elastic Stockings.*
See *Promoting Safety and Comfort: Elastic Stockings.*
See procedure: *Applying Elastic Stockings.*

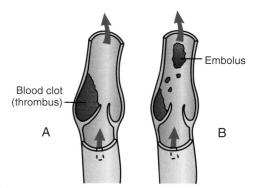

FIGURE 35-4 **A,** A blood clot is attached to the wall of a vein. The *arrows* show the direction of blood flow. **B,** Part of the thrombus breaks off and becomes an embolus. The embolus travels through the vascular system until it lodges in a distant vessel.

DELEGATION GUIDELINES
Elastic Stockings

To apply elastic stockings, you need this information from the nurse and the care plan.
- What type of stockings to use
- What size to use—small, medium, large, or extra-large
- What length to use—knee-high or thigh-high
- When to remove them and for how long—for bathing, some are removed overnight
- What observations to report and record:
  - The size and length of stockings applied
  - When you applied the stockings
  - Skin color and temperature
  - Leg and foot swelling
  - Skin tears, wounds, or signs of skin breakdown
  - Complaints of pain, tingling, or numbness
  - When you removed the stockings and for how long
  - When you re-applied the stockings
  - When you washed the stockings
- When to report observations
- What patient or resident concerns to report at once

PROMOTING SAFETY AND COMFORT
Elastic Stockings

Safety
Some stockings have a toe opening. The opening is used to check circulation, skin color, and skin temperature in the toes. Apply the stocking so the toe opening is over the top of the toes or under the toes. Follow the manufacturer's instructions.

Stockings must not have twists, creases, or wrinkles. Twists can affect circulation. So can stockings that roll up, bunch up, or have the toe opening wrapped around the toes. Creases and wrinkles can cause skin breakdown. Do not fold the top of the stocking down.

Loose stockings do not exert pressure on the veins. Stockings that are too tight can affect circulation. Tell the nurse if the stockings are too loose or too tight.

Comfort
Apply stockings before the person gets out of bed. Legs can swell from sitting or standing. Stockings are hard to put on swollen legs. The person is in bed while stockings are off. This prevents the legs from swelling.

Be sure the legs are dried well before applying stockings. Damp skin from water or lotion makes application hard. Powder may be applied as directed by the nurse.

Gently handle and move the person's foot and leg. Do not force the joints (toes, foot, ankle, knee, and hip) beyond their range of motion or to the point of pain.

Applying Elastic Stockings

Quality of Life

- Knock before entering the person's room.
- Address the person by name.
- Introduce yourself by name and title.
- Explain the procedure before starting and during the procedure.
- Protect the person's rights during the procedure.
- Handle the person gently during the procedure.

Pre-Procedure

1 Follow *Delegation Guidelines: Elastic Stockings.*
   See *Promoting Safety and Comfort: Elastic Stockings.*
2 Practice hand hygiene and get the following supplies.
   - Elastic stockings in the correct size and length
   - Bath blanket (if needed)
3 Identify the person. Check the identification (ID) bracelet against the assignment sheet. Use 2 identifiers (Chapter 11). Also call the person by name.
4 Provide for privacy.
5 Raise the bed for body mechanics. Bed rails are up if used. Lower the bed rail near you if up.

Procedure

6 Position the person supine.
7 Fan-fold top linens to the foot of the bed. If needed, use a bath blanket to cover the person.
8 Gather or turn the stocking inside out down to the heel.
9 Slip the foot of the stocking over the toes, foot, and heel (Fig. 35-5, A). Properly position the heel pocket on the heel. The toe opening is over or under the toes. Follow the manufacturer's instructions.
10 Grasp the stocking top. Roll or pull the stocking up the leg. It turns right side out as it is rolled or pulled up.
11 Adjust the stocking as needed. Make sure the stocking does not cause pressure on the toes.
12 Remove twists, creases, or wrinkles. Make sure the stocking is even, snug, smooth, and wrinkle-free (Fig. 35-5, B).
13 Repeat steps 8 through 12 for the other leg.
14 Cover the person. Remove the bath blanket (if used). Fold and return the bath blanket to its proper place. Or follow agency policy for used linens.

Post-Procedure

15 Provide for comfort. (See the inside of the back cover.)
16 Place the call light and other needed items within reach.
17 Lower the bed to a safe and comfortable level. Follow the care plan.
18 Raise or lower bed rails. Follow the care plan.
19 Follow the care plan and the person's preferences for privacy measures to maintain. Leaving the privacy curtain, window coverings, and door open or closed are examples.
20 Complete a safety check of the room. (See the inside of the back cover.)
21 Practice hand hygiene.
22 Report and record your care and observations.

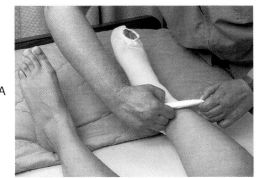
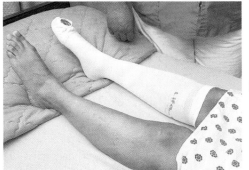

FIGURE 35-5 Applying elastic stockings. **A,** The stocking is slipped over the toes, foot, and heel. **B,** The stocking turns right side out as it is pulled up over the leg. The heel is positioned in the heel pocket of the stocking.

Elastic Bandages. Elastic bandages have the same purposes as elastic stockings. They also provide support and reduce swelling from injuries. Another use is to hold dressings in place. They are applied to arms and legs. To apply bandages:

* Use the correct size—length and width.
* Position the person in good alignment.
* Face the person during the procedure.
* Start at the lower (*distal*) part of the extremity. Work upward to the top (*proximal*) part. See Figure 35-6.
* Expose the fingers or toes if possible. This allows circulation checks.
* Apply the bandage with firm, even pressure.
* Check the color and temperature of the extremity every hour.
* Re-apply a loose or wrinkled bandage.
* Replace a moist or soiled bandage.
  See *Focus on Communication: Elastic Bandages.*
  See *Delegation Guidelines: Elastic Bandages.*
  See *Promoting Safety and Comfort: Elastic Bandages.*
  See procedure: *Applying an Elastic Bandage.*

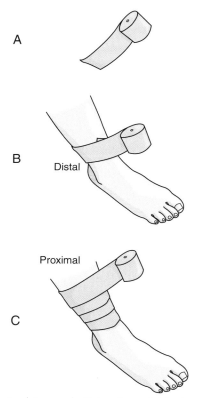

FIGURE 35-6 Applying an elastic bandage. **A,** The bandage roll is up. The loose end is at the bottom. **B,** The bandage is applied to the lower (*distal*) and smallest part with 2 circular turns. **C,** The bandage is applied with spiral turns in an upward (*proximal*) direction.

FOCUS ON COMMUNICATION

Elastic Bandages

Elastic bandages should promote comfort. To check for comfort, ask:

* "Does the bandage feel too tight?"
* "Do you feel pain, itching, or numbness?" If yes: "What do you feel?" "Where do you feel it?"

DELEGATION GUIDELINES

Elastic Bandages

To apply elastic bandages, you need this information from the nurse and the care plan.

* Where to apply the bandage
* What width and length to use
* When to remove the bandage and for how long
* What observations to report and record:
  * The width and length applied
  * When you applied the bandage
  * Skin color and temperature
  * Swelling of the part
  * Skin tears, wounds, or signs of skin breakdown
  * Complaints of pain, itching, tingling, or numbness
  * A wet or soiled bandage
  * When you removed the bandage and for how long
  * When you re-applied the bandage
* When to report observations
* What patient or resident concerns to report at once

PROMOTING SAFETY AND COMFORT

Elastic Bandages

Safety

Elastic bandages must be firm and snug but not tight. A tight bandage can affect circulation.

Manufacturers supply bandages with hook and loop, clip, tape, or Velcro closures. Metal or plastic clips can injure the skin if they are loose, fall off, or cause pressure. Check the clips often for correct placement.

Some agencies do not allow nursing assistants to apply elastic bandages. Know your agency's policy.

Comfort

A tight bandage can cause pain and discomfort. If the person complains of pain, tingling, or numbness, remove the bandage. Tell the nurse at once.

Applying an Elastic Bandage

Quality of Life

- Knock before entering the person's room.
- Address the person by name.
- Introduce yourself by name and title.

- Explain the procedure before starting and during the procedure.
- Protect the person's rights during the procedure.
- Handle the person gently during the procedure.

Pre-Procedure

1 Follow *Delegation Guidelines: Elastic Bandages.* **See** *Promoting Safety and Comfort: Elastic Bandages.*
2 Practice hand hygiene and get an elastic bandage with closures as directed by the nurse.
3 Identify the person. Check the ID bracelet against the assignment sheet. Use 2 identifiers (Chapter 11). Also call the person by name.

4 Provide for privacy.
5 Raise the bed for body mechanics. Bed rails are up if used. Lower the bed rail near you if up.

Procedure

6 Help the person to a comfortable position in good alignment. Expose the part to bandage.
7 Make sure the area is clean and dry.
8 Hold the bandage with the roll up. The loose end is on the bottom (see Fig. 35-6, A).
9 Apply the bandage to the lower (*distal*) and smallest part of the wrist, foot, ankle, or knee (see Fig. 35-6, B).
10 Make 2 circular turns around the part.
11 Make over-lapping spiral turns in an upward (*proximal*) direction. Each turn over-laps ½ to ¾ (one-half to three-fourths) of the previous turn (see Fig. 35-6, C). Each over-lap is equal.

12 Apply the bandage smoothly with firm, even pressure. It is not tight.
13 End the bandage with 2 circular turns.
14 Secure the bandage with the manufacturer's closure. Clips are not under the body part.
15 Check the fingers or toes for coldness or *cyanosis* (bluish color). Ask about pain, itching, numbness, or tingling. Remove the bandage if any are noted. Report your observations.

Post-Procedure

16 Provide for comfort. (See the inside of the back cover.)
17 Place the call light and other needed items within reach.
18 Lower the bed to a safe and comfortable level. Follow the care plan.
19 Raise or lower bed rails. Follow the care plan.
20 Follow the care plan and the person's preferences for privacy measures to maintain. Leaving the privacy curtain, window coverings, and door open or closed are examples.

21 Complete a safety check of the room. (See the inside of the back cover.)
22 Practice hand hygiene.
23 Report and record your care and observations.

DRESSINGS

Wound dressings have many functions. They:
- Protect wounds from injury and microbes.
- Absorb drainage.
- Remove dead tissue.
- Promote comfort.
- Cover unsightly wounds.
- Provide a moist environment for wound healing.
- Apply pressure (pressure dressings) to help control bleeding.

Securing Dressings

Dressings must be secured over wounds. Microbes can enter the wound and drainage can escape if the dressing is dislodged. Tape and Montgomery straps (p. 454) secure dressings. Binders (p. 456) hold dressings in place.

Tape. Adhesive, paper, plastic, cloth, and elastic tapes are common. Adhesive tape sticks well. However, adhesive problems include:
- It is hard to remove from the skin.
- It can irritate the skin.
- Skin tears or abrasions can occur when tape is removed.
- Adhesive tape allergies are common.

Paper, plastic, and cloth tapes usually do not cause allergic reactions. Elastic tape allows movement of the body part.

Tape comes in different widths—½, ¾, 1, 2, and 3 inch widths are common. Taping methods vary. Taping the top, middle, and bottom; taping the edges; and fully covering the dressing with tape are 3 methods. Tape should extend beyond the sides of the dressing (Fig. 35-7, p. 454). *Do not apply tape to circle the entire body part. If swelling occurs, circulation to the part is impaired.*

See *Focus on Communication: Tape,* p. 454.

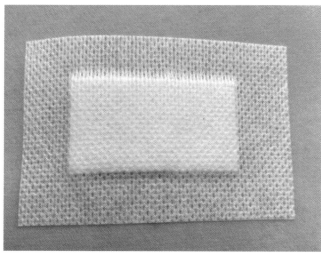

FIGURE 35-7 The tape extends beyond the sides of the dressing.

Montgomery Straps. Montgomery straps (Fig. 35-8) are used for large dressings and frequent dressing changes. A Montgomery strap has a tape strip and cloth tie. With the dressing in place, the tape strips are placed on both sides of the dressing. Then the straps are secured over the dressing.

The straps are undone for the dressing change. The tape strips stay in place. They are removed if soiled. Montgomery straps protect the skin from frequent tape application and removal.

Applying Dressings

Some agencies let you apply dry, non-sterile dressings to simple wounds. Follow the rules in Box 35-4.

See *Delegation Guidelines: Applying Dressings.*
See *Promoting Safety and Comfort: Applying Dressings.*
See procedure: *Applying a Dry, Non-Sterile Dressing.*

BOX 35-4 Applying Dressings

- Let pain-relief drugs take effect, usually 30 minutes. The dressing change can cause discomfort. The nurse gives the drug and tells you how long to wait.
- Meet fluid and elimination needs before you begin.
- Collect equipment and supplies before you begin.
- Do not bend or reach over your work area.
- Control your nonverbal communication. Wound odors, appearance, and drainage may be unpleasant. Do not communicate your thoughts or reaction to the person.
- Remove soiled dressings so the person cannot see the soiled side. The drainage and its color may upset the person.
- Do not force the person to look at the wound. A wound can affect body image and self-esteem. The nurse helps the person deal with the wound.
- Remove tape by gently pulling the tape ends toward the wound.
- Remove dressings gently. They may stick to the wound or surrounding skin. If the dressing sticks, the nurse may have you wet the dressing with a saline solution. A wet dressing is easier to remove.
- Clean the wound with saline as directed by the nurse (Fig. 35-9).
- Touch only the outer edges of new dressings.
- Report and record your observations. See *Delegation Guidelines: Applying Dressings.*

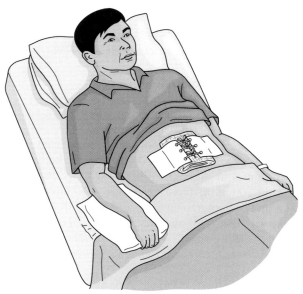

FIGURE 35-8 Montgomery straps.

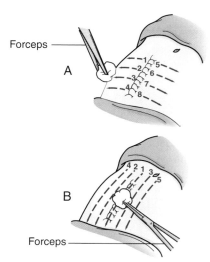

FIGURE 35-9 Cleaning a wound. **A,** Start at the wound and stroke out to the surrounding skin. Use new gauze for each stroke. **B,** Clean the wound from the top to the bottom. Start at the wound. Then clean the surrounding areas. Use new gauze for each stroke. (From Potter PA, Perry AG, Stockert PA, Hall AM: *Fundamentals of nursing,* ed 10, St Louis, 2021, Elsevier.)

DELEGATION GUIDELINES

Applying Dressings

When applying a dressing is delegated to you, you need this information from the nurse.

- When to change the dressing
- When a pain-relief drug will take effect
- What to do if the dressing sticks to the wound
- How to clean the wound
- What dressings to use
- How to secure the dressing—tape or Montgomery straps
- If tape is used, what kind and size to use
- What observations to report and record:
  - Supplies used to dress the wound and secure the dressing
  - A red or swollen wound
  - An area around the wound that is warm to touch
  - If wound edges are closed or separated
  - A wound that has broken open *(dehiscence)*
  - Drainage appearance—clear, bloody, or watery and blood-tinged; thick and green, yellow, or brown
  - The amount of drainage
  - Wound or drainage odor
  - Intactness and color of surrounding tissues
  - Possible dressing contamination—urine, feces, other body fluids, dislodged dressing
  - Pain
  - Fever
- When to report observations
- What patient or resident concerns to report at once

PROMOTING SAFETY AND COMFORT

Applying Dressings

Safety

Tape removal can cause skin tears in persons with thin, fragile skin. Use extreme care to remove tape. Do not apply tape to irritated, injured, or non-intact skin. Tape can further damage the skin.

Dressings containing blood are biohazardous waste (Chapter 14). Follow the Bloodborne Pathogen Standard and agency policy to dispose of soiled dressings.

Comfort

Wounds and dressing changes can cause discomfort or pain. Allow time for a pain-relief drug to take effect before a dressing change. Gently apply and remove tape and dressings.

The person may not report discomfort from a dressing. You should ask:

- "Is the dressing comfortable?"
- "Does the tape cause pain or itching?"

Applying a Dry, Non-Sterile Dressing

Quality of Life

- Knock before entering the person's room.
- Address the person by name.
- Introduce yourself by name and title.
- Explain the procedure before starting and during the procedure.
- Protect the person's rights during the procedure.
- Handle the person gently during the procedure.

Pre-Procedure

1 Follow *Delegation Guidelines:*
  a *Wound Care*, p. 447
  b *Applying Dressings*
  See *Promoting Safety and Comfort:*
  a *Wound Care*, p. 447
  b *Applying Dressings*
2 Practice hand hygiene and get the following supplies.
  - Gloves
  - PPE (personal protective equipment) as needed
  - Tape or Montgomery straps
  - Dressings as directed by the nurse
  - 4 × 4 gauze
  - Saline solution as directed by the nurse
  - Cleaning solution as directed by the nurse

- Adhesive remover
- Dressing set with scissors and forceps
- Plastic bag
- Bath blanket
3 Arrange your work area. You should not have to reach over or turn your back on your work area.
4 Practice hand hygiene.
5 Identify the person. Check the ID bracelet against the assignment sheet. Use 2 identifiers (Chapter 11). Also call the person by name.
6 Provide for privacy.
7 Raise the bed for body mechanics. Bed rails are up if used. Lower the bed rail near you if up.

Procedure

8 Help the person to a comfortable position.
9 Cover the person with a bath blanket. Fan-fold top linens to the foot of the bed.
10 Expose the affected body part.
11 Make a cuff on the plastic bag. Place the bag within reach.
12 Practice hand hygiene.

Continued

Applying a Dry, Non-Sterile Dressing—cont'd

Procedure—cont'd

13 Don needed PPE. Put on gloves.
14 Remove tape or undo Montgomery straps.
   a *Tape:* Hold the skin down. Gently pull the tape toward the wound. Apply adhesive remover during removal if needed. Follow the manufacturer's instructions.
   b *Montgomery straps:* Undo the straps. Fold the straps away from the wound.
15 Remove any adhesive from the skin. Follow the manufacturer's instructions for adhesive remover use. Clean away from the wound.
16 Remove dressings with a gloved hand or with forceps. Start with the top dressing and remove each layer. Keep the soiled side away from the person's sight. Put dressings in the plastic bag. They must not touch the outside of the bag.
17 Remove the dressing over the wound very gently. It may stick to the wound. If directed by the nurse, moisten the dressing with saline if it sticks to the wound. Discard the dressing as in step 16.

18 Observe the wound and wound drainage.
19 Remove the gloves. Put them in the bag. Practice hand hygiene.
20 Open the new dressings.
21 Put on clean gloves.
22 Clean the wound with saline or other solution as directed by the nurse. See Figure 35-9.
23 Apply dressings as directed by the nurse. Touch only the outer edges of the dressing. Do not touch the part that will have contact with the wound.
24 Secure the dressings. Use tape or Montgomery straps.
25 Remove the gloves. Put them in the bag.
26 Remove and discard PPE.
27 Practice hand hygiene.
28 Cover the person. Remove the bath blanket. Fold and return the bath blanket to its proper place. Or follow agency policy for used linens.

Post-Procedure

29 Provide for comfort. (See the inside of the back cover.)
30 Place the call light and other needed items within reach.
31 Lower the bed to a safe and comfortable level. Follow the care plan.
32 Raise or lower bed rails. Follow the care plan.
33 Return equipment and supplies to their proper place. Leave extra dressings and tape in the room.
34 Discard used supplies in the bag. Tie the bag closed. Discard the bag following agency policy. Follow the Bloodborne Pathogen Standard. (Wear gloves for this step.)

35 Clean and dry your work area. Dry with paper towels. Discard the paper towels.
36 Remove and discard the gloves. Practice hand hygiene.
37 Follow the care plan and the person's preferences for privacy measures to maintain. Leaving the privacy curtain, window coverings, and door open or closed are examples.
38 Complete a safety check of the room. (See the inside of the back cover.)
39 Practice hand hygiene.
40 Report and record your care and observations.

BINDERS AND COMPRESSION GARMENTS

Binders are wide bands of elastic fabric. They support wounds and hold dressings in place. They also prevent or reduce swelling, promote comfort, and prevent injury. These binders are common.

- *Abdominal binder*—provides abdominal support and holds dressings in place (Fig. 35-10). The top part is at the waist. The lower part is over the hips. Binders are secured in place with Velcro or with hook and loop closures.
- *Breast binder*—supports the breasts after surgery (Fig. 35-11). It is secured in place with Velcro or padded zippers.

Compression garments are made of a tight, stretchy fabric (Fig. 35-12). Common after plastic surgery, they help:

- Reduce swelling.
- Prevent fluid buildup at the surgical site.
- Hold the skin against the body.
- Achieve the desired shape.

Box 35-5 lists the rules for applying binders and compression garments.

See *Focus on Communication: Binders and Compression Garments.*

See *Promoting Safety and Comfort: Binders and Compression Garments.*

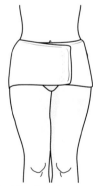

FIGURE 35-10 Abdominal binder. The top part is at the waist. The lower part is over the hips.

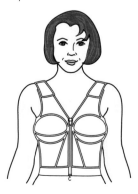

FIGURE 35-11 Breast binder.

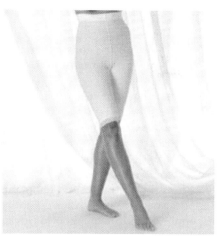

FIGURE 35-12 Compression garment. (Courtesy Rainey Compression Essentials, Atlanta, Ga.)

BOX 35-5 Binders and Compression Garments

- Follow the manufacturer's instructions.
- Position the person in good alignment.
- Apply the device for firm, even pressure over the area.
- Apply the device so it is snug. It must not interfere with breathing or circulation.
- Re-apply the device if it is out of position or causes discomfort.
- Change the device if moist or soiled. This prevents the growth of microbes.
- Tell the nurse at once if the person's breathing changes.
- Check the skin under and around the device. Tell the nurse at once if there is redness, irritation, or other signs of a skin problem.

FOCUS ON **COMMUNICATION**

Binders and Compression Garments

The person may not tell you about pain or discomfort. You need to ask:
- "Is the binder (garment) too tight or too loose?"
- "Does the binder (garment) cause pain?"
- "Do you feel pressure from the binder (garment)?" If yes: "Where? Please show me."

PROMOTING SAFETY AND COMFORT

Binders and Compression Garments

Safety

Apply binders and compression garments properly. Doing so helps prevent discomfort, skin irritation, and circulatory and respiratory problems. Correct application is needed for safety and for the device to work properly.

Comfort

A binder or compression garment should promote comfort. Tell the nurse if the device causes pain or discomfort.

HEAT AND COLD APPLICATIONS

Heat and cold applications:
- Promote healing.
- Promote comfort.
- Reduce tissue swelling.

Heat Applications

Heat applications can be applied to almost any body part. They are used for musculo-skeletal injuries or problems (sprains, arthritis). Heat:
- Relieves pain.
- Relaxes muscles.
- Promotes healing.
- Reduces tissue swelling.
- Decreases joint stiffness.

When heat is applied to the skin, blood vessels in the area dilate. ***Dilate*** *means to expand or open wider* (Fig. 35-13). Blood flow increases. Excess fluid is removed from the area faster. The skin is red and warm.

Complications of Heat. High temperatures can cause burns. Report pain, excess redness, and blisters at once. Also observe for pale skin. When heat is applied too long, blood vessels ***constrict*** *(narrow)* (see Fig. 35-13). Blood flow decreases. Tissues receive less oxygen. Tissue damage occurs. The skin is pale.

Older and fair-skinned persons have fragile skin that is easily burned. Persons with problems sensing heat and pain also are at risk. Nervous system damage, altered awareness, diabetes, and circulatory disorders can affect sensation. So can confusion and some drugs.

Metal implants pose risks. Metal conducts heat. Deep tissues can be burned. Pacemakers (cardiac devices) and some joint replacements are made of metal. Do not apply heat to an implant area.

Heat is not applied to a pregnant woman's abdomen. The heat can affect fetal growth.

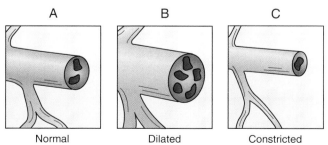

A	B	C
Normal	Dilated	Constricted

FIGURE 35-13 A, A blood vessel under normal conditions. **B,** Dilated blood vessel. **C,** Constricted blood vessel.

Cold Applications

Cold applications are often used to treat sprains and fractures. Cold applications:

* Reduce pain.
* Prevent swelling.
* Decrease circulation and bleeding.
* Cool the body when fever is present.

Cold has the opposite effect of heat. When cold is applied to the skin, blood vessels constrict (see Fig. 35-13). Blood flow decreases.

Cold is useful right after an injury. Decreased blood flow reduces bleeding. Less fluid collects in the tissues. Cold numbs the skin. This helps reduce or relieve pain in the part.

Complications of Cold. Complications of cold applications include pain, burns, blisters, and poor circulation. Burns and blisters occur from intense cold. They also occur from dry cold in direct contact with the skin.

When cold is applied for a long time, blood vessels dilate. Blood flow increases. Prolonged application of cold has the same effect as heat applications.

Older and fair-skinned persons have fragile skin. They are at great risk for complications. So are persons with sensory impairments.

Moist and Dry Applications

Applications are moist or dry.

* *Moist applications*—water has contact with the skin.
* *Dry applications*—water does not have contact with the skin.

Moist applications have greater and faster effects than dry applications. To prevent injury:

* *Moist heat applications* have lower (cooler) temperatures than *dry heat applications*.
* *Moist cold applications* have higher (warmer) temperatures than *dry cold applications*.

Dry applications stay at the desired temperature longer than moist applications. However, they do not penetrate as well as moist applications. Since higher or lower temperatures are needed for the desired effect, complications are still a risk.

Table 35-1 describes the different types of moist and dry heat and cold applications.

TABLE 35-1 **Heat and Cold Application Types**		
Type	Description	Example
Hot or cold compress	• Moist heat or cold application, depending on the water temperature. • A *compress* is a soft pad applied over a body area. It is usually made of cloth. • The compress is placed in water, wrung out, applied to the area, and covered to maintain the desired temperature longer.	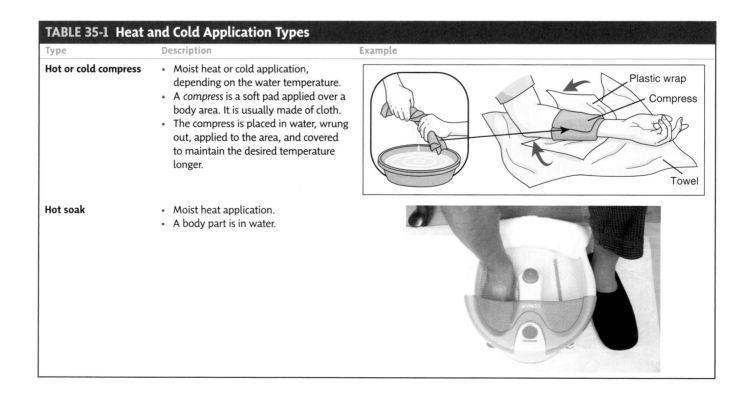
Hot soak	• Moist heat application. • A body part is in water.	

TABLE 35-1 Heat and Cold Application Types—cont'd

Type	Description	Example
Sitz bath	• Moist heat application. • The perineal and rectal areas are immersed in warm or hot water. (*Sitz* means *seat* in German.) • A disposable sitz bath is used over a toilet seat.	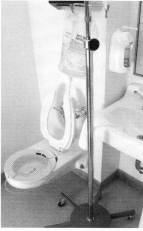
Aquathermia pad (Aqua-K, K-Pad)	• Dry heat application. • A therapy pad is connected to hoses on an electric heating unit. • The unit is filled with distilled water. Heated water is circulated through the hose to tubes inside the pad and back to the heating unit.	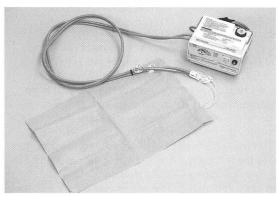
Hot or cold pack	• Moist or dry heat or cold application, depending on the type. • A commercial pack is applied. Some packs are disposable (single-use). Others are re-usable. • Packs are activated following the manufacturer's instructions. Striking, kneading, or squeezing the pack before use is common. • Re-usable cold packs are stored in the freezer.	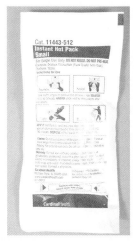
Ice bag	• Dry cold application. • The bag is filled with crushed ice or ice chips and closed. • Bags, collars, and gloves are different types.	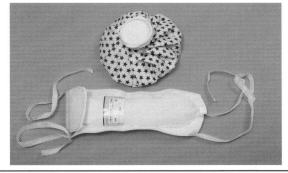

Applying Heat and Cold

Protect the person from injury during heat and cold applications. Follow the rules in Box 35-6. See Table 35-2 for heat and cold temperature ranges.

See *Delegation Guidelines: Applying Heat and Cold.*
See *Promoting Safety and Comfort: Applying Heat and Cold.*
See procedure: *Applying Heat and Cold Applications.*

BOX 35-6 Applying Heat and Cold

- Know how to use the equipment. Follow the manufacturer's instructions for commercial devices.
- Measure the temperature of moist applications. Follow agency policy or use a water thermometer.
- Follow agency policies for safe temperature ranges. See Table 35-2.
- Do not apply *very hot* (above 106°F or 41.1°C) applications. Tissue damage can occur. A nurse applies *very hot* applications.
- Ask the nurse what temperature to use.
  - Heat—cooler temperatures for persons at risk.
  - Cold—warmer temperatures for persons at risk.
- Have the nurse show you the application site.
- Cover dry heat or cold applications before applying them. Use a flannel cover, towel, or other cover as directed.
- Provide for privacy. Properly screen and drape the person. Expose only the body part involved.
- Maintain comfort and body alignment during the procedure.
- Observe the skin every 5 minutes during the procedure. See *Delegation Guidelines: Applying Heat and Cold.*
- Do not let the person change the temperature of the application.
- Know how long to leave the application in place. Heat and cold are applied no longer than 15 to 20 minutes.
- Follow the rules for electrical safety when using electrical appliances for heat. See Chapter 11.
- Tell the person to notify you at once if:
  - The application feels too hot or too cold.
  - The person feels pain, numbness, or burning.
  - The person feels weak, faint, or drowsy.
- Place the call light within the person's reach.
- Complete a safety check before leaving the room. (See the inside of the back cover.)
- Clean and dry re-usable equipment after use. Follow agency procedures. Discard disposable equipment.

TABLE 35-2 Heat and Cold Temperature Ranges

Temperature	Fahrenheit (F) Range	Centigrade (C) Range
Hot	99°F to 106°F	37°C to 41°C
Warm	93°F to 98°F	34°C to 37°C
Tepid	80°F to 92°F	26°C to 34°C
Cool	65°F to 79°F	18°C to 26°C
Cold	50°F to 64°F	10°C to 18°C

Modified from Perry AG, Potter PA, Ostendorf WR: *Nursing interventions & clinical skills,* ed 7, St Louis, 2020, Mosby.

DELEGATION GUIDELINES
Applying Heat and Cold

To apply heat or cold, you need this information from the nurse and the care plan.
- What application to apply
- How to cover the application
- What temperature to use (see Table 35-2)
- The application site
- How long to leave the application in place
- What observations to report and record:
  - Complaints of pain or discomfort, numbness, or burning
  - Excess redness
  - Blisters
  - Pale, white, or gray skin
  - *Cyanosis*—bluish *(cyano)* color
  - Shivering
  - Rapid pulse, weakness, faintness, and drowsiness (sitz bath)
  - Time, site, and length of application
- When to report observations
- What patient or resident concerns to report at once

PROMOTING SAFETY AND COMFORT
Applying Heat and Cold

Safety
Keep the call light within reach. Check the person every 5 minutes. Also follow these safety measures.
- *Sitz bath.* Blood flow increases to the perineum and rectum. Therefore less blood flows to other areas. Observe for signs of weakness, fainting, or fatigue. Also protect the person from injury, chills, and burns.
- *Aquathermia pad:*
  - Follow electrical safety measures (Chapter 11).
  - Check the device for damage or flaws.
  - Follow the manufacturer's instructions.
  - Place the heating unit on an even, uncluttered surface. This prevents it from being knocked over or knocked off the surface.
  - Check the hoses for kinks or bubbles. Water must flow freely.
  - Place the pad in a flannel cover. The flannel absorbs perspiration at the application site. (Some agencies use towels or pillowcases.)
  - Secure the pad in place with ties, tape, or rolled gauze. Do not use pins. They can puncture the pad and cause leaks.
  - Do not place the pad under a body part. Heat cannot escape. Burns can result if heat cannot escape.
  - Give the temperature setting key to the nurse. This prevents anyone from changing the temperature. The temperature is usually set at 105°F (40.5°C) with a key.
- *Commercial hot and cold packs.* Read warning labels. Follow the manufacturer's instructions.
  Some persons have medicated patches or ointments applied to the skin. Do not apply heat over such areas.

Comfort
Cold applications can cause chills and shivering. Provide for warmth. Use bath blankets or other blankets as needed.

Applying Heat and Cold Applications

- Knock before entering the person's room.
- Address the person by name.
- Introduce yourself by name and title.

- Explain the procedure before starting and during the procedure.
- Protect the person's rights during the procedure.
- Handle the person gently during the procedure.

Pre-Procedure

1 Follow *Delegation Guidelines:*
  a *Wound Care,* p. 447
  b *Applying Heat and Cold*
  See *Promoting Safety and Comfort: Applying Heat and Cold.*
2 Practice hand hygiene and get the following supplies.
  - *For a hot compress:*
    - Basin
    - Water thermometer
    - Small towel, washcloth, or gauze squares
    - Plastic wrap or aquathermia pad
    - Ties, tape, or rolled gauze
    - Bath towel
    - Waterproof under-pad
  - *For a hot soak:*
    - Water basin or arm or foot bath
    - Water thermometer
    - Waterproof under-pad
    - Bath blanket
    - Towel
  - *For a sitz bath:*
    - Disposable sitz bath
    - Water thermometer
    - 2 bath blankets, bath towels, and a clean gown

  - *For an aquathermia pad:*
    - Aquathermia pad and heating unit
    - Distilled water
    - Flannel cover or other cover as directed
    - Ties, tape, or rolled gauze
  - *For a hot or cold pack:*
    - Commercial pack
    - Pack cover
    - Ties, tape, or rolled gauze (if needed)
    - Waterproof under-pad
  - *For an ice bag, ice collar, or ice glove:*
    - Ice bag, collar, or glove
    - Crushed ice
    - Flannel cover or other cover as directed
    - Paper towels
  - *For a cold compress:*
    - Large basin with ice
    - Small basin with cold water
    - Gauze squares, washcloths, or small towels
    - Waterproof under-pad
3 Arrange items in the person's room.
4 Practice hand hygiene.
5 Identify the person. Check the ID bracelet against the assignment sheet. Use 2 identifiers (Chapter 11). Also call the person by name.
6 Provide for privacy.

Procedure

7 Position the person for the procedure.
8 Place the waterproof under-pad (if needed) under the body part.
9 *For a hot compress:*
  a Fill the basin ½ to ⅔ (one-half to two-thirds) full with hot water as directed. Measure water temperature.
  b Place the compress in the water and wring out.
  c Apply the compress over the area. Note the time.
  d Cover the compress as directed. Do 1 of the following.
    1) Apply plastic wrap and then a bath towel. Secure the towel in place with ties, tape, or rolled gauze.
    2) Apply an aquathermia pad.
10 *For a hot soak:*
  a Fill the container ½ (one-half) full with hot water. Measure water temperature.
  b Place the part into the water. Pad the edge of the container with a towel. Note the time.
  c Cover the person with a bath blanket for warmth.
11 *For a sitz bath:*
  a Place the sitz bath on the toilet seat.
  b Fill the sitz bath ⅔ (two-thirds) full with water. Measure water temperature.
  c Secure the gown above the waist.
  d Help the person sit on the sitz bath. Note the time.
  e Provide for warmth. Place a bath blanket around the shoulders. Place the other over the legs.
  f Stay with the person if the person is weak or unsteady.

12 *For an aquathermia pad:*
  a Fill the heating unit to the fill line with distilled water.
  b Open any hose clamps. Follow the manufacturer's instructions to fill the connecting hoses and pad with water and remove air. Be sure there are no kinks in the hoses or the pad.
  c Set the temperature as the nurse directs (usually 105°F/40.5°C). Remove the key.
  d Place the pad in the cover.
  e Set the heating unit on the bedside stand. Keep the pad and connecting hoses level with the unit.
  f Plug in the unit. Let water warm to the desired temperature.
  g Apply the pad to the part. Note the time.
  h Secure the pad in place with ties, tape, or rolled gauze.
13 *For a hot or cold pack:*
  a Squeeze, knead, or strike the pack as directed by the manufacturer.
  b Place the pack in the cover.
  c Apply the pack. Note the time.
  d Secure the pack in place with ties, tape, or rolled gauze. Some packs are secured with Velcro straps.

Continued

Applying Heat and Cold Applications—cont'd

Procedure—cont'd

14 *For an ice bag, collar, or glove:*
   a Fill the device with water. Put in the stopper. Turn the device upside down to check for leaks.
   b Empty the device.
   c Fill the device ½ to ⅔ (one-half to two-thirds) full with crushed ice or ice chips.
   d Remove excess air. Bend, twist, or squeeze the device. Or press it against a firm surface.
   e Place the cap or stopper on securely.
   f Dry the device with paper towels.
   g Place the device in the cover.
   h Apply the device. Note the time.
   i Secure the device with ties, tape, or rolled gauze.

15 *For a cold compress:*
   a Place the small basin with cold water into the large basin with ice.
   b Place the compresses into the cold water.
   c Wring out a compress.
   d Apply the compress to the part. Note the time.
16 Place the call light and other needed items within reach. Maintain privacy measures as needed and as the person prefers.
17 Raise or lower bed rails. Follow the care plan.
18 Do the following every 5 minutes.
   a Check the person for signs and symptoms of complications (see *Delegation Guidelines: Applying Heat and Cold,* p. 460). Remove the application if any occur. Tell the nurse at once.
   b Check the application for cooling (hot application) or warming (cold application).
19 Remove the application after 15 to 20 minutes.

Post-Procedure

20 Provide for comfort. (See the inside of the back cover.)
21 Place the call light and other needed items within reach.
22 Raise or lower bed rails. Follow the care plan.
23 Follow agency procedures for cleaning and drying re-usable items. Return items to their proper place. Discard disposable items. Follow agency policy for used linens. Follow Standard Precautions. Remove and discard gloves (if worn). Practice hand hygiene.

24 Follow the care plan and the person's preferences for privacy measures to maintain. Leaving the privacy curtain, window coverings, and door open or closed are examples.
25 Complete a safety check of the room. (See the inside of the back cover.)
26 Practice hand hygiene.
27 Report and record your care and observations.

FOCUS ON P R I D E

The Person, Family, and Yourself

P ersonal and Professional Responsibility

As a nursing assistant, you have responsibilities for wound care. For example, if you are careless during a transfer, you can cause a skin tear. If you rush during a bath, you may not notice a wound between skin folds. If you do not apply shoes properly, a foot ulcer can develop.

How you provide care affects the person's health, safety, and quality of life. Take pride in working safely and carefully.

R ights and Respect

A person may have questions about the reasons for care. Avoid pat answers like: "It's to help you get better" or "The doctor (nurse) says you need it." The person has the right to be informed. Ask the nurse to explain reasons for care. Wait until questions are answered before performing the care measure.

I ndependence and Social Interaction

Patients and residents can plan if they know what will happen. For example, a person wants to make a phone call before a hot compress. Or a person wants a hot soak done before visitors arrive. You promote independence when you involve the person in planning.

D elegation and Teamwork

Wound care can be painful and tiring. To promote comfort and rest:
- Plan care with the nurse. Ask when pain-relief drugs will be given and will take effect. Allow rest periods before and after care.
- Be prepared. Leaving to get supplies causes delays. Care and procedures take longer than planned.
- Assist the nurse as instructed. You may need to position the person or raise a body part while the nurse changes a dressing. Teamwork reduces the amount of energy the person must use.

E thics and Laws

Agency practices vary for charging supplies. Ethical practice involves honestly following agency rules. Not charging supplies correctly costs the nursing unit and agency money. Taking supplies home for your own use is unethical. This is stealing. Take pride in following agency rules and being an honest and reliable member of the nursing team.

FOCUS ON PRIDE: *Application*

Providing comfort is an important part of every task. What special considerations are needed for wound care? How will you know if you have met the person's comfort needs?

Circle the BEST answer.

1 Which can cause skin tears?
   a Keeping your nails trimmed and smooth
   b Dressing the person in soft clothing
   c Wearing rings
   d Padding wheelchair footplates

2 A person is at risk for circulatory ulcers. Which measure should you question?
   a Report toenails in need of trimming.
   b Hold socks in place with elastic garters.
   c Check the legs and feet carefully during skin care.
   d Re-position the person every hour.

3 A person has diabetes. When providing foot care
   a Dry well between the toes
   b Apply lotion between the toes
   c Trim the toenails
   d Use hot water

4 Elastic stockings
   a Hold dressings in place
   b Slow blood flow
   c Prevent pressure injuries
   d Prevent blood clots

5 Elastic stockings are applied
   a When the person is standing
   b Before the person gets out of bed
   c After breakfast
   d For 30 minutes and then removed

6 The purpose of an elastic bandage is to
   a Prevent infection
   b Absorb drainage
   c Provide moisture for wound healing
   d Reduce swelling

7 When applying an elastic bandage
   a Position the part in good alignment
   b Cover the fingers or toes if possible
   c Apply it from the large to small part of the extremity
   d Apply it from the upper to lower part of the extremity

8 Dressings
   a Protect the wound from injury and microbes
   b Prevent drainage
   c Provide a dry environment for healing
   d Support the wound and reduce swelling

9 To secure a dressing, apply tape
   a Around the entire body part
   b In an X pattern over the dressing
   c So it extends beyond the sides of the dressing
   d Loosely

10 To remove tape
   a Pull it away from the wound
   b Pull it toward the wound
   c Use forceps
   d Use a saline solution

11 An abdominal binder is used to
   a Prevent blood clots
   b Prevent wound infection
   c Provide support and hold dressings in place
   d Decrease swelling and circulation

12 The *greatest* threat from heat applications is
   a Infection
   b Burns
   c Chilling
   d Skin tears

13 A nurse asks you to apply a hot pack. Which should you question?
   a Check that the pack's temperature is at least 110°F (43.3°C).
   b Place the pack in a cover.
   c Secure the pack in place with ties.
   d Check the person for complications every 5 minutes.

14 When using an aquathermia pad
   a Do not cover the pad
   b Place the pad under the person
   c Check for kinks in the hoses
   d Secure the pad in place with pins

15 Which signals a complication of a cold application?
   a Cool skin
   b Cyanosis
   c Decreased swelling
   d Fever

16 Moist cold compresses are left in place no longer than
   a 20 minutes
   b 30 minutes
   c 45 minutes
   d 60 minutes

Answers to Chapter 35 questions are on p. 588.

FOCUS ON PRACTICE

Problem Solving

An older resident has thin, fragile skin. You notice a new skin tear on the person's arm. What do you do? How can you prevent skin tears?

CHAPTER 36

Pressure Injuries

OBJECTIVES

- Define the key terms and key abbreviations in this chapter.
- Describe the causes and risk factors for pressure injuries.
- Identify the persons at risk for pressure injuries.
- Identify the sites for pressure injuries.

- Describe the stages of pressure injuries.
- Explain how to prevent pressure injuries.
- Identify the complications from pressure injuries.
- Explain how to promote PRIDE in the person, the family, and yourself.

KEY TERMS

bony prominence An area where the bone sticks out or projects from the flat surface of the body; pressure point
intact skin Normal skin and skin layers without damage or breaks
pressure injury Localized damage to the skin and underlying soft tissue; the injury is usually over a bony prominence or related to a medical or other device and results from pressure or pressure in combination with shear

pressure point See "bony prominence"
shear When layers of the skin rub against each other; when the skin remains in place and underlying tissues move and stretch, tearing underlying capillaries and blood vessels and causing tissue damage
ulcer A shallow or deep crater-like sore of the skin or mucous membrane

KEY ABBREVIATIONS

CMS   Centers for Medicare & Medicaid Services

NPIAP   National Pressure Injury Advisory Panel

The National Pressure Injury Advisory Panel (NPIAP) defines *pressure injury* (Fig. 36-1) *as:*
- *Localized damage to the skin and underlying soft tissue.*
- *The injury is usually over a bony prominence or related to a medical or other device.*
- *The injury results from pressure or pressure in combination with shear.*

A **bony prominence (pressure point)** *is an area where the bone sticks out or projects from the flat surface of the body.* The back of the head, shoulder blades, elbows, hips, spine, sacrum, knees, ankles, heels, and toes are bony prominences (Fig. 36-2).

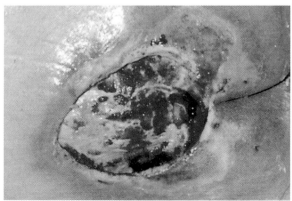

FIGURE 36-1 A pressure injury. (From Ostomy Wound Management, *Proceedings from the November National V.A.C.® 51[2A, supp]: 7S, Feb 2005, HMP Communications. Used with permission.)*

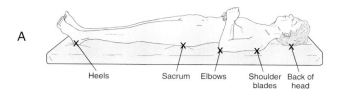

A — Heels, Sacrum, Elbows, Shoulder blades, Back of head

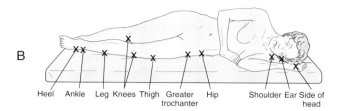

B — Heel, Ankle, Leg, Knees, Thigh, Greater trochanter, Hip, Shoulder, Ear, Side of head

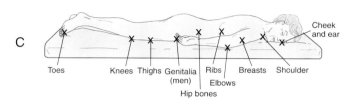

C — Toes, Knees, Thighs, Genitalia (men), Hip bones, Ribs, Elbows, Breasts, Shoulder, Cheek and ear

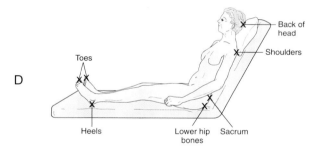

D — Back of head, Shoulders, Toes, Heels, Lower hip bones, Sacrum

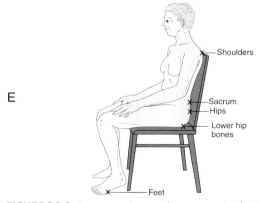

E — Shoulders, Sacrum, Hips, Lower hip bones, Feet

FIGURE 36-2 Bony prominences (pressure points). **A,** The supine position. **B,** The lateral position. **C,** The prone position. **D,** Fowler's position. **E,** Sitting position.

Healthy Skin – Lightly Pigmented

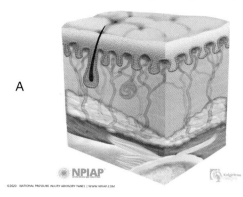

A

Healthy Skin – Darkly Pigmented

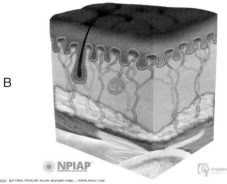

B

FIGURE 36-3 Intact skin. **A,** Healthy skin with light pigment. **B,** Healthy skin with dark pigment. (Note: Pigment gives color to the skin.) (Used with permission from the National Pressure Injury Advisory Panel [NPIAP]. Copyright 2020 NPIAP.)

Pressure injuries result from intense or prolonged pressure and shear. *Shear is when layers of the skin rub against each other. Or shear is when the skin remains in place and underlying tissues move and stretch, tearing underlying capillaries and blood vessels. Tissue damage occurs.*

Possibly painful, a pressure injury may involve intact skin or an open ulcer.

- *Intact skin is normal skin and skin layers without damage or breaks* (Fig. 36-3).
- An *ulcer is a shallow or deep crater-like sore of the skin or mucous membrane* (see Fig. 36-1).

Some agencies and organizations use the term *pressure ulcer.* The term *bedsore* is commonly used by patients, residents, and families. Pressure injury, pressure ulcer, and bedsore essentially mean the same thing.

RISK FACTORS

Pressure and shearing are the major causes of pressure injuries. Unrelieved pressure squeezes tiny blood vessels. For example, pressure occurs when the skin over a bony area is squeezed between hard surfaces (Fig. 36-4). The bone is 1 hard surface. The other is usually the mattress or seat of a chair. Squeezing or pressure prevents blood flow to the skin and underlying tissues. Oxygen and nutrients cannot get to the cells. Skin and tissues die.

Shear occurs when the person slides down in the bed or chair. Blood vessels and tissues are damaged. Blood flow to the area is reduced.

See Box 36-1 for pressure injury risk factors. Agencies must identify persons at risk for pressure injuries. The health team assesses the person's physical and mental health. A person's risk may increase during an illness, from condition changes, because of injury or surgery, or from medical devices. The person's care plan must include measures to reduce or remove risk factors. See "Persons at Risk."

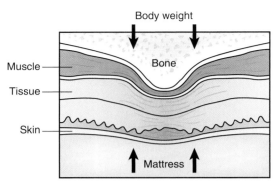

FIGURE 36-4 Tissue under pressure. The skin is squeezed between 2 hard surfaces—the bone and the mattress. (Redrawn from Agency for Healthcare Research and Quality: *Understanding your body: what are pressure ulcers?* Rockville, Md, November 2007, U.S. Department of Health and Human Services.)

PERSONS AT RISK

Persons at risk for pressure injuries are those who:
- Are *bedfast* (confined to bed) or *chairfast* (confined to a chair).
- Need some or total help moving.
- Are agitated, have muscle spasms, or have involuntary muscle movements causing friction against surfaces.
- Are incontinent of urine or feces.
- Are exposed to moisture—urine, feces, wound drainage, sweat, or saliva.
- Have poor nutrition or poor fluid balance.
- Have limited awareness.
- Have problems sensing pain or pressure.
- Have circulatory problems.
- Are obese, have weight loss, or are very thin.
- Have medical devices.
- Have an existing or healed pressure injury.
  See *Focus on Older Persons: Persons at Risk*.

BOX 36-1 Pressure Injury Risk Factors

- Aging and age-related skin changes
- Skin breakdown (changes or damage to skin) and non-intact skin
- Dry skin
- Fragile and weak capillaries
- General thinning of the skin
- Loss of the fatty layer under the skin
- Decreased sensation to touch, heat, and cold
- Decreased mobility
- Limited activity: for example, sitting in a chair or lying in bed most or all of the day
- Chronic diseases (diabetes, high blood pressure)
- Diseases that decrease circulation and oxygen to tissues; poor circulation to an area
- Fever
- Poor nutrition
- Poor hydration
- Incontinence: urinary, fecal
- Moisture in dark body areas: skin folds, under breasts, perineal area
- Pressure on bony parts (pressure points)
- Poor fingernail and toenail care
- Friction (rubbing of 1 surface against another) and shearing
- *Edema* (the swelling of body tissues with water)

FOCUS ON **OLDER PERSONS**

Persons at Risk

Older persons have thin, fragile skin that is easily injured. Some have chronic diseases affecting mobility, nutrition, circulation, and awareness.

The Centers for Medicare & Medicaid Services (CMS) requires that nursing centers identify persons at risk for pressure injuries. A person can develop a pressure injury within 2 to 6 hours after the onset of pressure.

PRESSURE INJURY SITES

Pressure injuries usually occur over bony prominences (pressure points). These areas bear the body's weight in certain positions (see Fig. 36-2). Pressure from body weight can reduce the blood supply to the skin. The sacrum and heels are common sites for pressure injuries.

Medical device–related pressure injuries can develop at sites where devices are used for diagnostic or treatment purposes. For example, eyeglasses can cause pressure and friction on the ears. Oxygen tubing (Chapter 37) can cause pressure on the nose, face, and ears. Pressure can occur on an ear from the mattress when in a side-lying position. Tubes, casts, braces, and other devices can cause pressure on hands, arms, legs, and feet. Pressure can occur on the buttocks from bedpans.

Mucosal membrane pressure injuries are found in mucous membranes where a medical device is used. A urinary catheter can cause pressure and friction on the meatus. A feeding tube can cause pressure in the nose.

Pressure injuries can occur where skin has contact with skin. Common sites are between abdominal folds, the legs, the buttocks, the thighs, and under the breasts.

PRESSURE INJURY STAGES

Understanding the following terms will help you as you study the different pressure injury stages.

- *Erythema* means *red* or *redness*.
- *Blanch* means *to become white*.
  - *Blanchable*—When pressure is applied to the skin, blood is pressed away. This causes the skin to become white or pale (Fig. 36-5). When pressure is relieved, the skin returns to its normal color.
  - *Non-blanchable*—The skin does not become white or pale when pressure is applied and removed (see Fig. 36-5).
- *Slough* is dead tissue that is shed from the skin. It is usually light colored, soft, and moist. It may be stringy at times. See Figure 36-6.
- *Eschar* is thick, leathery dead tissue that may be loose or adhered to the skin. It is often black or brown. See Figure 36-7.

Pressure injuries range from reddened intact skin to tissue loss with bone exposure. For pressure injury stages, see Figure 36-8 (pp. 468-469).

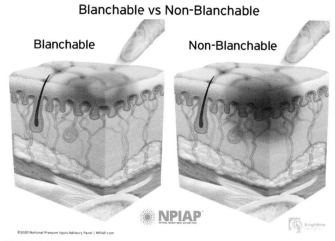

FIGURE 36-5 Blanchable and non-blanchable skin. (Used with permission from the National Pressure Injury Advisory Panel [NPIAP]. Copyright 2020 NPIAP.)

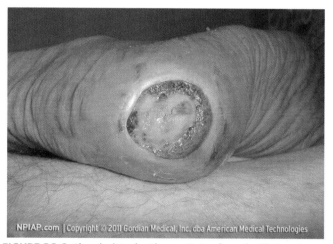

FIGURE 36-6 Slough. (Used with permission from the National Pressure Injury Advisory Panel [NPIAP]. Copyright 2020 NPIAP.)

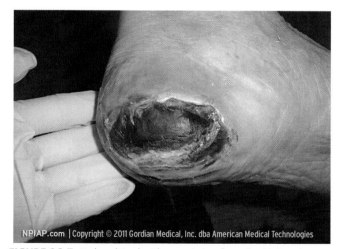

FIGURE 36-7 Eschar. (Used with permission from the National Pressure Injury Advisory Panel [NPIAP]. Copyright 2020 NPIAP.)

Stage and Description	Drawing	Example

Stage 1 Pressure Injury

Non-blanchable erythema of intact skin

Intact skin has a reddened area that is non-blanchable.

Stage 1 Pressure Injury – Lightly Pigmented

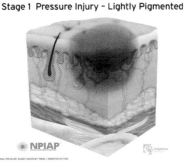

Stage 1 Pressure Injury – Darkly Pigmented

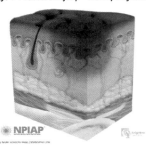

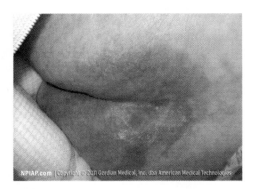

NOTE: *NPIAP defines a Stage 1 pressure injury as intact skin with a localized area of non-blanchable erythema, which may appear differently in darkly pigmented skin. Presence of blanchable erythema or changes in sensation, temperature, or firmness may precede visual changes. Color changes do not include purple or maroon discoloration; these may indicate deep tissue pressure injury.*

Stage 2 Pressure Injury

Partial-thickness skin loss with exposed dermis

The wound is pink or red and moist. It may involve a broken or intact blister. Fat and deeper tissues are not visible.

Stage 2 Pressure Injury

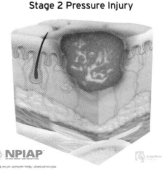

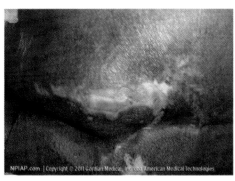

NOTE: *NPIAP defines a Stage 2 pressure injury as partial-thickness loss of skin with exposed dermis. The wound bed is viable, pink or red, moist, and may also present as an intact or ruptured serum-filled blister. Adipose (fat) is not visible and deeper tissues are not visible. Granulation tissue, slough and eschar are not present. These injuries commonly result from adverse microclimate and shear in the skin over the pelvis and shear in the heel. This stage should not be used to describe moisture associated skin damage (MASD) including incontinence associated dermatitis (IAD), intertriginous dermatitis (ITD), medical adhesive related skin injury (MARSI), or traumatic wounds (skin tears, burns, abrasions).*

Stage 3 Pressure Injury

Full-thickness skin loss

The skin is gone. Fat can be seen in the ulcer. Slough, eschar, or both may be present.

Stage 3 Pressure Injury

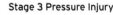
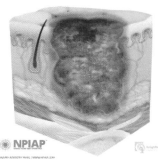

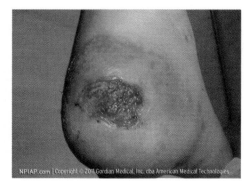

NOTE: *NPIAP defines a Stage 3 pressure injury as full-thickness loss of skin, in which adipose (fat) is visible in the ulcer and granulation tissue and epibole (rolled wound edges) are often present. Slough and/or eschar may be visible. The depth of tissue damage varies by anatomical location; areas of significant adiposity can develop deep wounds. Undermining and tunneling may occur. Fascia, muscle, tendon, ligament, cartilage and/or bone are not exposed. If slough or eschar obscures the extent of tissue loss this is an Unstageable Pressure Injury.*

FIGURE 36-8 Pressure injury stages. (Illustrations, photos, and definitions used with permission from the National Pressure Injury Advisory Panel [NPIAP]. Copyright 2020 NPIAP.)

Stage and Description	Drawing	Example

Stage 4 Pressure Injury

Full-thickness skin and tissue loss

The skin is gone. Muscle, tendon, ligament, cartilage, or bone is exposed. Slough, eschar, or both may be present.

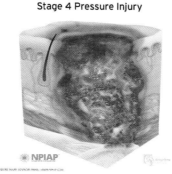

Stage 4 Pressure Injury

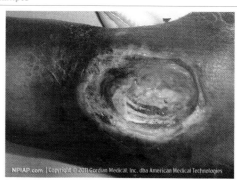

NOTE: *NPIAP defines a Stage 4 pressure injury as full-thickness skin and tissue loss with exposed or directly palpable fascia, muscle, tendon, ligament, cartilage or bone in the ulcer. Slough and/or eschar may be visible. Epibole (rolled edges), undermining and/or tunneling often occur. Depth varies by anatomical location. If slough or eschar obscures the extent of tissue loss this is an Unstageable Pressure Injury.*

Unstageable Pressure Injury

Obscured full-thickness skin and tissue loss

There is skin and tissue loss. The extent of tissue damage cannot be seen because of slough or eschar. (*Obscure* means *not plain or clear.*) When slough or eschar is removed, the injury can be seen.

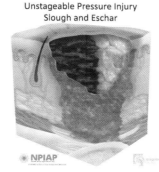

Unstageable Pressure Injury
Slough and Eschar

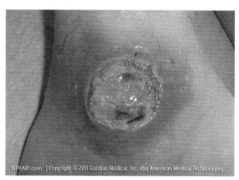

NOTE: *NPIAP defines an Unstageable Pressure Injury as full-thickness skin and tissue loss in which the extent of tissue damage within the ulcer cannot be confirmed because it is obscured by slough or eschar. If slough or eschar is removed, a Stage 3 or Stage 4 pressure injury will be revealed. Stable eschar (i.e. dry, adherent, intact without erythema or fluctuance) on the heel or ischemic limb should not be softened or removed.*

Deep Tissue Pressure Injury

Persistent non-blanchable deep red, maroon, or purple discoloration

Intact or non-intact skin is deep red, maroon, or purple and remains non-blanchable. The wound is dark or is a blood-filled blister.

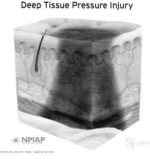

Deep Tissue Pressure Injury

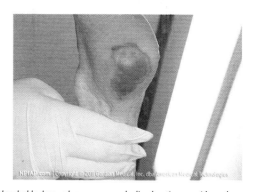

NOTE: *NPIAP defines a deep tissue pressure injury as intact or non-intact skin with localized area of persistent non-blanchable deep red, maroon, purple discoloration or epidermal separation revealing a dark wound bed or blood filled blister. Pain and temperature change often precede skin color changes. Discoloration may appear differently in darkly pigmented skin. This injury results from intense and/or prolonged pressure and shear forces at the bone-muscle interface. The wound may evolve rapidly to reveal the actual extent of tissue injury, or may resolve without tissue loss. If necrotic tissue, subcutaneous tissue, granulation tissue, fascia, muscle or other underlying structures are visible, this indicates a full thickness pressure injury (Unstageable, Stage 3 or Stage 4). Do not use DTPI to describe vascular, traumatic, neuropathic, or dermatologic conditions.*

FIGURE 36-8, cont'd

Observations

Inspect the skin every time you give care. This includes during or after transfers, re-positioning, bathing, and elimination procedures. Pay close attention to bony prominences. Also observe areas where skin has contact with skin. If needed, have help to lift the body part to look for skin changes. Check sites that have contact with medical devices.

Report areas of redness, skin color changes, blisters, or skin or tissue loss. The nurse needs to assess the site. If needed, help the nurse turn or position the person to assess the area.

See *Focus on Communication: Observations*, p. 470.

PREVENTION AND TREATMENT

Preventing pressure injuries is much easier than trying to heal them. Pressure injury prevention involves:
- Identifying persons at risk. The health team assesses the person's risk factors and skin condition.
- Prevention measures for those at risk. Good nursing care, cleanliness, and skin care are essential. Managing moisture, good nutrition and fluid balance, and relieving pressure also are key measures. Box 36-2 lists common measures used to prevent skin damage and pressure injuries. Always follow the person's care plan.

Some agencies use symbols or colored stickers as pressure injury alerts. Placed on the person's door or medical record, the alerts remind the staff that the person is at risk.

See *Focus on Surveys: Prevention and Treatment.*

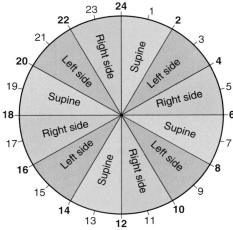

FIGURE 36-9 Turn clock. The clock shows the times to turn the person and to what position.

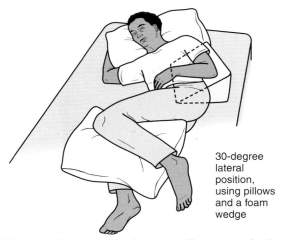

30-degree lateral position, using pillows and a foam wedge

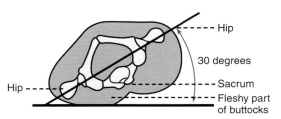

FIGURE 36-10 The 30-degree lateral position. Pillows are under the head, shoulder, and leg. This position inclines (lifts up) the hip to avoid pressure on the hip. The person does not lie on the hip as in the side-lying position.

BOX 36-2 Preventing Pressure Injuries

Moving and Positioning

- Follow the person's re-positioning schedule (Fig. 36-9). Re-position bedfast persons at least every 1 to 2 hours. Re-position chairfast persons at least every hour. Some persons are re-positioned every 15 minutes.
- Remind persons sitting in recliners, chairs, or wheelchairs to shift positions at least every 15 minutes.
- Position the person according to the care plan. Use pillows for support as directed. The 30-degree lateral position is recommended (Fig. 36-10).
- Do not position the person:
  - On a pressure injury
  - On a reddened area
  - On tubes or other medical devices
- Do not leave a person on a bedpan longer than needed.
- Do not let the person sit on donut-shaped cushions.
- Prevent shearing and friction during moving and transfer procedures. Do not drag the person. Use assist devices as directed. See Chapters 17 and 18.
- Use slow, gradual turns and movements when re-positioning persons who are critically ill.
- Prevent shearing. Do not raise the head of the bed more than 30 degrees. Follow the care plan for:
  - When to raise the head of the bed
  - How far to raise the head of the bed
  - How long (in minutes) to raise the head of the bed
- Use pillows, foam wedges, or other devices to prevent bony areas from contact with bony areas and firm surfaces. The ankles, knees, hips, and sacrum are examples.
- Keep the heels and ankles off of the bed. Use pillows or other devices as directed. Place the pillows or devices under the lower legs from mid-calf to the ankles.
- Use protective devices as directed (p. 472).
- Support the feet properly when the person is sitting upright in a chair or wheelchair. Use a footstool if the person's feet do not touch the floor when sitting in a chair. The body slides forward when the feet do not touch the floor. For the person in a wheelchair, position the feet on the footrests.

Skin Care

- Inspect the skin every time you give care. See "Observations." Report any concern at once.
- Follow the person's bathing schedule. Some persons do not need a bath or shower every day.
- Do not use hot water to bathe or clean the skin. Hot water can irritate the skin.
- Use a cleansing agent as directed. Soap can dry and irritate the skin.
- Provide good skin care.
  - The skin is clean and dry after bathing.
  - The skin is free of moisture from a bath or shower and from urine, feces (stools), perspiration, wound drainage, and other secretions.
  - Skin under the breasts, in the groin area, and under abdominal folds is clean and dry.

Skin Care—cont'd

- Prevent skin exposure to moisture.
  - Check persons who are at risk for moisture exposure often.
  - For persons who are incontinent of urine or feces (stools):
    - Follow measures to prevent incontinence.
    - Provide good skin care and change linens and garments at the time of soiling.
    - Use incontinence products as directed.
    - Apply an ointment or moisture barrier. Follow the care plan.
  - For persons who perspire heavily or have wound drainage, provide good skin care. Change linens and garments as needed.
- Apply moisturizer to dry areas—hands, elbows, hips, ankles, heels, and so on. The nurse tells you what to use and what areas need attention.
- Give a back massage when re-positioning the person. Do not massage bony areas.
- Do not massage over pressure points. *Never rub or massage reddened areas.*
- Keep linens clean, dry, and wrinkle-free.
- Make sure the bed or chair is free of objects. Crumbs, pins, pencils, pens, and coins are examples.
- Do not irritate the skin. Avoid scrubbing or vigorous rubbing when bathing or drying the person.
- Use pillows and blankets to prevent skin from being in contact with skin.
- Make sure clothes do not increase the risk for pressure injuries.
  - Avoid seams, buttons, or zippers that press against the skin.
  - Avoid tight clothes.
  - Keep clothes from bunching up or wrinkling.
- Make sure socks and shoes are in good repair. Socks should not have holes, wrinkles, or creases. Make sure there is nothing in the shoes before the person puts them on.
- Do not apply heat or cold (Chapter 35) directly on a pressure injury.
- See Chapter 35 for diabetes foot care.

Medical Devices

- Use the correct device in the correct size. Follow the care plan.
- Apply and secure the device correctly. Follow the manufacturer's directions.
- Move or re-position the device according to the care plan.
- Check the skin under a medical device for edema and signs of a pressure injury.
- Protect the skin under the device as directed by the nurse.
- Do not position the person on top of a medical device.
- Ask about the person's comfort. Tell the nurse if the device is causing discomfort or is too loose or too tight.

Protective Devices

Wound care products, drugs, treatments, dressings, and equipment are ordered to promote healing. Support surfaces relieve or reduce pressure. Such surfaces include foam, air, alternating air, gel, or water mattresses.

Protective devices are often used to prevent and treat skin breakdown and pressure injuries. These devices are common.

- *Bed cradle.* A bed cradle is a metal frame placed on the bed and over the person (Chapter 32). Top linens are brought over the cradle to prevent pressure on the legs, feet, and toes.
- *Heel elevators.* These raise the heels and feet off of the bed (Fig. 36-11). They prevent pressure. Some also prevent footdrop (Chapter 32).
- *Elbow and heel protectors.* These devices are made of foam padding, pressure-relieving gel, sheepskin, or other cushioning materials. They fit the shape of elbows and heels (Fig. 36-12).
- *Gel- or fluid-filled pads and cushions.* These devices have a pressure-relieving gel or fluid (Fig. 36-13). They are used for chairs and wheelchairs to prevent pressure. If the outer case is vinyl, the device may be placed in a fabric cover to protect the skin.
- *Special beds.* Some beds have air flowing through the mattress. An *alternating pressure mattress* (Fig. 36-14) has many tubes that fill and release air at certain times. This changes where pressure is placed on the body. Some beds rotate from side to side. Alignment stays the same. Pressure points change as the bed rotates. They are useful for persons with spinal cord injuries. Follow the manufacturer's instructions and the nurse's directions for linens to use on special beds.
- *Other equipment.* Pillows, trochanter rolls, foot-boards, and other positioning devices may be used (Chapter 32). They maintain good alignment.

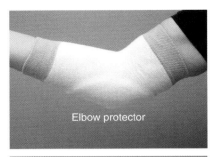
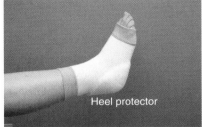

FIGURE 36-12 Elbow and heel protectors.

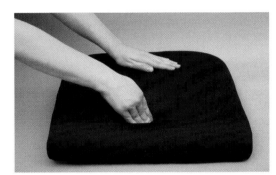

FIGURE 36-13 Gel cushion.

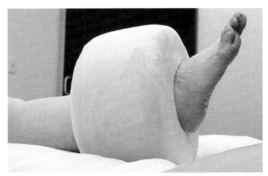

FIGURE 36-11 Heel elevator.

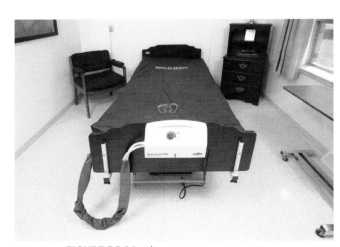

FIGURE 36-14 Alternating pressure mattress.

COMPLICATIONS

Infection is the most common complication of pressure injuries. A wound is *infected* when bacteria invade the tissues around or in the pressure injury. The person has signs and symptoms of infection (Chapter 14). Pain and delayed healing may signal an infection.

Osteomyelitis is a risk if the pressure injury is over a bony prominence. The risk is great if the wound is not healing. *Osteomyelitis* means inflammation *(itis)* of the bone *(osteo)* and bone marrow *(myel)*. Pain is severe. Treatment includes bed rest and antibiotics. Careful and gentle positioning is needed. Surgery may be done to remove dead bone and tissue.

Pressure injuries can cause pain. Pain management is important. Pain may affect movement and activity. Immobility is a risk factor for pressure injuries. And it may delay healing of an existing pressure injury.

FOCUS ON P R I D E

The Person, Family, and Yourself

P ersonal and Professional Responsibility

You have an important role in preventing and treating pressure injuries. Your attitude and quality of work affect the person. If you take your role seriously and believe you have a positive impact, the person benefits. If you are careless and lack concern for the person's well-being, harm can result.

You are an important part of the nursing team. Take pride in your role. Work to the best of your ability.

R ights and Respect

You have the right and responsibility to speak for patients and residents. This is called being an *advocate* (Chapter 2). You may be the first to notice a pressure injury. Reporting your observations can prevent further harm and result in prompt actions to promote healing. Take pride in being a voice for your patients and residents.

I ndependence and Social Interaction

Pressure injury healing can take a long time. As time passes, loneliness and depression can occur. Physical needs are great. Do not neglect mental and social needs. Be kind. Show compassion. Take time to listen. Give care in a way that improves quality of life.

D elegation and Teamwork

You must be thorough and accurate when completing, reporting, and recording care measures. The following example shows how poor communication, negligence, and false recording can cause harm.

A nursing assistant did not report placing a resident on the bedpan at 2250 (10:50 PM). The next shift began at 2300 (11:00 PM). Several hours later, the resident was still on the bedpan. A pressure injury had developed. The resident's care plan included re-positioning every 2 hours. While the chart showed that the person had been re-positioned, it really had not been done.

You must be careful and honest. Report and record when you complete a task. Give needed information to on-coming staff. Never report or record something you did not do. Also, do not report or record before completing a task.

E thics and Laws

Agencies must have a plan to predict, prevent, and treat pressure injuries early. Assessments are done on admission and regularly. The agency must take action to address risks.

Know your agency's policies and procedures for identifying those at risk for pressure injuries. Follow the measures in Box 36-2 and the care plan to do your part to prevent pressure injuries.

FOCUS ON PRIDE: *Application*

Describe the physical, mental, and social effects a pressure injury can have. How can you help meet the person's needs?

Circle the BEST answer.

1 A pressure injury is
   a An open wound
   b A localized injury to the skin and underlying tissue
   c A bony prominence
   d Dead tissue

2 Unrelieved pressure is a problem because it
   a Dilates (widens) blood vessels
   b Prevents pain sensation
   c Causes edema (swelling)
   d Prevents blood flow

3 A person is in Fowler's position. This places pressure on
   a The knees and ankles
   b The ribs and breasts
   c The cheek and ear
   d The sacrum and heels

4 Which contributes to the development of pressure injuries?
   a Shear
   b Slough
   c Eschar
   d Skin blanching

5 A person is bedfast (confined to bed). This person has
   a No risk of pressure injury
   b A low risk of pressure injury
   c An average risk of pressure injury
   d A high risk of pressure injury

6 Which is a risk factor for pressure injuries?
   a Balanced diet
   b Intact skin
   c Incontinence
   d Increased circulation

7 In a light-skinned person, a Stage 1 Pressure Injury has
   a A blister
   b A reddened area
   c Drainage
   d A bruise

8 You are giving a bed bath. Why do you inspect the sacrum and heels?
   a The person cannot see these areas.
   b You are responsible for assessing the skin.
   c These are common sites for pressure injuries.
   d The skin is most fragile in these areas.

9 A person requires oxygen therapy. The person says the tubing rubs the ears. You should
   a Ask the nurse how to protect the skin under the tubing
   b Tape the tubing in place to prevent movement
   c Tell the person that pressure injuries cannot occur on the ears
   d Have the person remove the tubing if it feels uncomfortable

10 Which pressure injury prevention measure should you question?
   a Re-position the person every 2 hours.
   b Scrub the skin during bathing.
   c Apply lotion to dry areas.
   d Keep linens clean, dry, and wrinkle-free.

11 You should position the person
   a On an existing pressure injury
   b On a reddened area
   c On tubes or other medical devices
   d Using assist devices

12 What is the preferred position for preventing pressure injuries?
   a 30-degree lateral position
   b Fowler's position
   c Prone position
   d Supine position

13 Which keeps the heels and ankles off of the bed?
   a A bed cradle
   b Pillows
   c An alternating pressure mattress
   d Trochanter rolls

14 A person in a chair should shift position at least every
   a 15 minutes
   b 30 minutes
   c Hour
   d 2 hours

15 You show you understand pressure injury prevention measures when you
   a Keep the head of the bed raised higher than 45 degrees
   b Inspect the person's skin every time you give care
   c Give a bath every day with soap and hot water
   d Rub bony areas firmly during a back massage

16 To prevent skin damage from moisture
   a Avoid using lotion on dry areas
   b Check incontinent persons every 4 hours
   c Dry under the breasts and in the groin area well
   d Change linens once daily for persons who perspire heavily

17 You see a reddened area on the person's skin. What should you do?
   a Rub the area.
   b Apply a moisturizer.
   c Apply a moisture barrier.
   d Tell the nurse.

18 You assist the nurse with pressure injuries by
   a Assessing pressure injury risk factors
   b Diagnosing pressure injury stages
   c Performing pressure injury prevention measures
   d Deciding how to treat pressure injuries

Answers to Chapter 36 questions are on p. 588.

FOCUS ON **PRACTICE**

Problem Solving

A resident at risk for pressure injuries complains when awakened for care. You and a co-worker enter the room for re-positioning. The person is asleep. What will you do? What is the risk of waiting to re-position? How can you provide safe, quality care that avoids causing frustration?

CHAPTER 37

Oxygen Needs

OBJECTIVES

- Define the key terms and key abbreviations in this chapter.
- Describe hypoxia and abnormal respirations.
- Identify the signs and symptoms of altered respiratory function.
- Describe pulse oximetry.

- Explain the measures to meet oxygen needs.
- Describe 3 devices used to give oxygen.
- Explain how to safely assist with oxygen therapy.
- Perform the procedures described in this chapter.
- Explain how to promote PRIDE in the person, the family, and yourself.

KEY TERMS

apnea The lack or absence (a) of breathing (pnea)
bradypnea Slow (brady) breathing (pnea); respirations are fewer than 12 per minute
Cheyne-Stokes respirations Respirations gradually increase in rate and depth and then become shallow and slow; breathing may stop (apnea) for 10 to 20 seconds
cyanosis Bluish color (cyano) to the skin, lips, mucous membranes, and nail beds
dyspnea Difficult, labored, or painful (dys) breathing (pnea)
hyperventilation Breathing (ventilation) is rapid (hyper) and deeper than normal
hypoventilation Breathing (ventilation) is slow (hypo), shallow, and sometimes irregular

hypoxia Cells do not have enough (hypo) oxygen (oxia)
Kussmaul respirations Very deep and rapid respirations
orthopnea Breathing (pnea) deeply and comfortably only when sitting (ortho)
orthopneic position Sitting up (ortho) and leaning over a table to breathe (pneic)
oxygen concentration The amount (percent [%]) of hemoglobin containing oxygen
pulse oximetry Measures (metry) the oxygen (oxi) concentration in arterial blood
tachypnea Rapid (tachy) breathing (pnea); respirations are more than 20 per minute

KEY ABBREVIATIONS

CO_2	Carbon dioxide
CPAP	Continuous positive airway pressure
ID	Identification

L/min	Liters per minute
O_2	Oxygen
SpO_2	Saturation of peripheral oxygen (oxygen concentration)

Oxygen is a gas. It has no taste, odor, or color. It is a basic need required for life. Death occurs within minutes if breathing stops. Brain and other organ damage can occur without enough oxygen. Illness, surgery, and injuries affect the amount of oxygen in the body.

To assist with oxygen needs, you need to be able to recognize altered respiratory function. You may help with tests, measurements, and measures to meet oxygen needs. You must also know your role in assisting with oxygen therapy.

ALTERED RESPIRATORY FUNCTION

Respiratory function involves 3 processes. Respiratory function is altered if even 1 process is affected.

- Air moves into and out of the lungs.
- Oxygen (O_2) and carbon dioxide (CO_2) are exchanged between the alveoli and capillaries.
- The blood carries O_2 to the cells and removes CO_2 from them.

Hypoxia means that cells do not have enough (hypo) *oxygen* (oxia). Cells cannot function properly. The brain is very sensitive to inadequate O_2. Restlessness, dizziness, and disorientation are early signs. Report the signs and symptoms of altered respiratory function in Box 37-1 at once.

Hypoxia threatens life. All organs need O_2 to function. Oxygen is given (p. 481). The cause of hypoxia is treated.

BOX 37-1 Altered Respiratory Function

- Restlessness
- Dizziness
- Disorientation and confusion
- Behavior and personality changes
- Concentrating and following directions: problems with
- Anxiety and apprehension
- Fatigue
- Agitation
- Pulse rate: increased
- Respirations:
  - Increased rate and depth
  - Breathing pattern: abnormal
  - Shortness of breath or complaints of being "winded" or "short-winded"
  - Noisy, wheezing, wet-sounding, *stridor* (a loud, high-pitched sound from airway blockage)
- Sitting position—upright, leaning forward, hunched over a table
- *Cyanosis—bluish color* (cyano) *to the skin, lips, mucous membranes, and nail beds*
- Cough (note type, frequency, and time of day)
  - Dry and hacking
  - Harsh and barking
  - Productive (produces sputum) or non-productive
- Sputum (mucus from the respiratory system)
  - Color—clear, white, yellow, green, brown, or red
  - Odor—none or foul odor
  - Consistency—thick, watery, or frothy (with bubbles or foam)
  - *Hemoptysis—bloody* (hemo) *sputum (ptysis means to spit);* note if the sputum is bright red, dark red, blood-tinged, or streaked with blood
- Chest pain (note location)
  - Constant or comes and goes
  - Person's description—stabbing, knife-like, aching
  - What makes it worse—movement, coughing, yawning, sneezing, sighing, deep breathing, position
- Vital signs: changes in

Abnormal Respirations

Adults normally breathe 12 to 20 times per minute. Normal respirations are quiet, effortless, and regular. Both sides of the chest rise and fall equally. These breathing patterns are abnormal (Fig. 37-1).

- *Tachypnea—rapid* (tachy) *breathing* (pnea). *Respirations are more than 20 per minute.*
- *Bradypnea—slow* (brady) *breathing* (pnea). *Respirations are fewer than 12 per minute.*
- *Apnea—the lack or absence* (a) *of breathing* (pnea).
- *Hypoventilation—breathing* (ventilation) *is slow* (hypo), *shallow, and sometimes irregular.*
- *Hyperventilation—breathing* (ventilation) *is rapid* (hyper) *and deeper than normal.*
- *Dyspnea—difficult, labored, or painful* (dys) *breathing* (pnea).
- *Cheyne-Stokes respirations—respirations gradually increase in rate and depth and then become shallow and slow. Breathing may stop* (apnea) *for 10 to 20 seconds.*
- *Orthopnea—breathing* (pnea) *deeply and comfortably only when sitting* (ortho).
- *Kussmaul respirations—very deep and rapid respirations.*

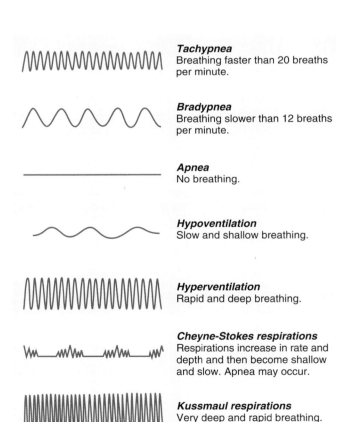

Tachypnea
Breathing faster than 20 breaths per minute.

Bradypnea
Breathing slower than 12 breaths per minute.

Apnea
No breathing.

Hypoventilation
Slow and shallow breathing.

Hyperventilation
Rapid and deep breathing.

Cheyne-Stokes respirations
Respirations increase in rate and depth and then become shallow and slow. Apnea may occur.

Kussmaul respirations
Very deep and rapid breathing.

FIGURE 37-1 Some abnormal breathing patterns.

RESPIRATORY TESTS

Various tests may be ordered to detect lung changes. A chest x-ray is an example. You may be involved in pulse oximetry and the collection of sputum specimens (Chapter 34). Assist with other tests as directed by the nurse.

Pulse Oximetry

Pulse oximetry measures (metry) *the oxygen* (oxi) *concentration in arterial blood.* **Oxygen concentration** *is the amount (percent [%]) of hemoglobin containing O_2.* An agency may use 1 of these terms.

- *Pulse oximetry* or *pulse ox.*
- *O_2 saturation* or *O_2 sat.*
- *SpO_2* (saturation of peripheral oxygen). *Saturation* means to be *filled.* Peripheral relates to the *surface.* SpO_2 measures the amount of hemoglobin near the surface of the skin that is filled with oxygen.

The normal oxygen concentration range is between 95% and 100%. For example, if 97% of all hemoglobin carries O_2, tissues get enough oxygen. If only 90% contains O_2, tissues do not get enough oxygen.

A *pulse oximeter* is used to measure oxygen concentration. A sensor attaches to a finger, toe, earlobe, nose, or forehead (Fig. 37-2). Good blood flow to the site is needed. Avoid swollen sites and sites with skin breaks. Bright light, nail polish, non-natural nails, and movements affect measurements. For a good sensor site:

- Place a towel over the sensor to block bright lights.
- Remove nail polish or use another site.
- Do not use finger sites with non-natural nails.
- Use the earlobe if there is finger movement from shivering, seizures, or tremors.
- Do not measure blood pressure on the side of a finger site. Blood pressure cuffs affect blood flow.

The pulse oximeter shows the pulse rate along with the oxygen concentration (see Fig. 37-2, *A*). Oxygen concentration is often measured with vital signs (see Fig. 37-2, *B*). Report and record measurements according to agency policy.

See *Delegation Guidelines: Pulse Oximetry.*
See *Promoting Safety and Comfort: Pulse Oximetry,* p. 478.
See procedure: *Using a Pulse Oximeter,* p. 478.

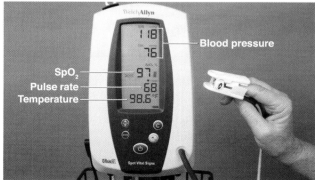

FIGURE 37-2 Pulse oximetry. **A,** A pulse oximetry sensor is attached to a finger. The device displays the O_2 concentration (SpO_2) and pulse. **B,** O_2 concentration (SpO_2) is often measured with vital signs.

DELEGATION GUIDELINES
Pulse Oximetry

To assist with pulse oximetry, you need this information from the nurse and the care plan.
- Reason for the measurement: routine, continuous monitoring, or condition change
- What site to use
- How to use the equipment
- What sensor to use
- What tape to use (if needed)
- The person's normal SpO_2 range
- Alarm limits for SpO_2 and pulse rate (if set)
- When to do the measurement
- What pulse site to use: apical or radial
- How often to check the site for continuous monitoring (usually at least every 2 hours)
- What observations to report and record:
  - The date and time
  - The SpO_2 and display pulse rate (see Fig. 37-2)
  - Apical or radial pulse rate
  - What the person was doing at the time
  - Oxygen flow rate (p. 483) and the device used (p. 482)
- When to report observations
- What patient or resident concerns to report at once:
  - An SpO_2 below the alarm limit (usually 95%)
  - A pulse rate above or below the alarm limit
  - The signs and symptoms listed in Box 37-1

PROMOTING SAFETY AND COMFORT
Pulse Oximetry

Safety

The person's condition can change quickly. Pulse oximetry does not lessen the need for good observation. Observe for signs and symptoms of altered respiratory function (see Box 37-1).

Comfort

A clip-on sensor feels like a clothespin. It should not hurt or cause discomfort. Ask the person to tell you at once if it causes pain, discomfort, or too much pressure. Change the sensor site as directed by the nurse.

Using a Pulse Oximeter

Quality of Life

- Knock before entering the person's room.
- Address the person by name.
- Introduce yourself by name and title.
- Explain the procedure before starting and during the procedure.
- Protect the person's rights during the procedure.
- Handle the person gently during the procedure.

Pre-Procedure

1 Follow *Delegation Guidelines: Pulse Oximetry*, p. 477. See *Promoting Safety and Comfort: Pulse Oximetry*.
2 Practice hand hygiene and get the following supplies.
   - Oximeter
   - Sensor (if not part of the device)
   - Tape (if needed)
   - Alcohol wipe
3 Arrange your work area.
4 Practice hand hygiene.
5 Identify the person. Check the identification (ID) bracelet against your assignment sheet. Use 2 identifiers (Chapter 11). Also call the person by name.
6 Provide for privacy.

Procedure

7 Provide for comfort.
8 Select and clean the site with an alcohol wipe. Discard the wipe. If measuring blood pressure, use 1 arm for blood pressure and a site on the other arm for pulse oximetry.
9 Clip or tape the sensor to the site. If needed, connect the sensor to the oximeter.
10 Turn on the oximeter.
11 *For continuous monitoring:*
   a Set the high and low alarm limits for SpO$_2$ and pulse rate.
   b Turn on audio and visual alarms.
12 Check the apical or radial pulse with the pulse on the display. The pulse rates should be about the same. Note both pulses on your assignment sheet.
13 Read the SpO$_2$ on the display. Note the value on the flow sheet and your assignment sheet.
14 Leave the sensor in place for continuous monitoring. Otherwise, turn off the device and remove the sensor.

Post-Procedure

15 Provide for comfort. (See the inside of the back cover.)
16 Place the call light and other needed items within reach.
17 Follow the care plan and the person's preferences for privacy measures to maintain. Leaving the privacy curtain, window coverings, and door open or closed are examples.
18 Complete a safety check of the room. (See the inside of the back cover.)
19 Practice hand hygiene.
20 Return the device to its proper place (unless monitoring is continuous). Follow agency policy for disinfection.
21 Report and record the SpO$_2$, the pulse rates, and your other observations.

MEETING OXYGEN NEEDS

Air must move deep into the lungs to alveoli where O$_2$ and CO$_2$ are exchanged. Disease, injury, and surgery can prevent air from reaching the alveoli. Pain, immobility, and some drugs interfere with deep breathing and coughing. Therefore secretions collect in the airway and lungs. Microbes can grow in the secretions. Infection is a threat.

See *Focus on Communication: Meeting Oxygen Needs*.

FOCUS ON COMMUNICATION
Meeting Oxygen Needs

The questions you ask the person assist the nurse with the nursing process. For example:
- "Do you need more pillows?"
- "Do you want the head of your bed raised more?"
- "How often are you coughing?"
- "Are you coughing anything up?"
- "Are you coughing up mucus? Please use a tissue to cough up mucus. Clean your hands and use your call light. The nurse will observe the mucus."

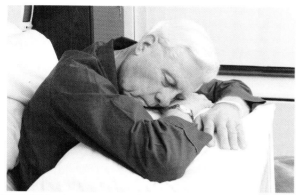

FIGURE 37-3 The person is in the orthopneic position. A pillow is on the over-bed table for comfort.

Positioning

Breathing is usually easier in the semi-Fowler's and Fowler's positions. Persons with difficulty breathing often prefer the *orthopneic position—sitting up* (ortho) *and leaning over a table to breathe* (pneic). Place a pillow on the table to increase comfort (Fig. 37-3).

If the person must lie flat for a procedure, raise the head of the bed as soon as possible. Raise it at once if the person has difficulty breathing.

Position changes are needed at least every 2 hours. Follow the care plan.

Deep Breathing and Coughing

Deep breathing moves air into most parts of the lungs. Coughing removes mucus. Deep-breathing and coughing exercises are done after surgery or injury and during bed rest. The exercises are painful after surgery or injury. Breaking an incision open while coughing is a fear.

Deep breathing and coughing are usually done every 1 to 2 hours while awake.

See *Focus on Communication: Deep Breathing and Coughing.*

See *Delegation Guidelines: Deep Breathing and Coughing.*

See *Promoting Safety and Comfort: Deep Breathing and Coughing.*

See procedure: *Assisting With Deep-Breathing and Coughing Exercises.*

FOCUS ON COMMUNICATION
Deep Breathing and Coughing

To encourage cough etiquette (Chapter 15), you can say:

Please cover your nose and mouth with tissues when coughing. I'll put these tissues where you can reach them. Here is a waste container for your used tissues. Where would you like it? Also, please wash your hands after coughing. Let me know if you need help.

DELEGATION GUIDELINES
Deep Breathing and Coughing

To assist with deep-breathing and coughing exercises, you need this information from the nurse and the care plan.
- When to do them and how often
- How many deep breaths and coughs are needed
- What observations to report and record:
  - The number of deep breaths and coughs
  - How the person tolerated the procedure
- When to report observations
- What patient or resident concerns to report at once

PROMOTING SAFETY AND COMFORT
Deep Breathing and Coughing

Safety
Respiratory hygiene and cough etiquette are needed for a productive cough (Chapter 15). The person needs to:
- Cover the nose and mouth to cough or sneeze.
- Use tissues to contain respiratory secretions.
- Dispose of tissues in the nearest waste container after use.
- Wash the hands after coughing, sneezing, or contact with respiratory secretions.

While the person is covering the nose and mouth, you need to splint a chest or abdominal incision with your hands or a pillow. See step 8, b in procedure: *Assisting With Deep-Breathing and Coughing Exercises.* Wear gloves to splint the incision.

Assisting With Deep-Breathing and Coughing Exercises

Quality of Life

- Knock before entering the person's room.
- Address the person by name.
- Introduce yourself by name and title.

- Explain the procedure before starting and during the procedure.
- Protect the person's rights during the procedure.
- Handle the person gently during the procedure.

Pre-Procedure

1 Follow *Delegation Guidelines: Deep Breathing and Coughing.* See *Promoting Safety and Comfort: Deep Breathing and Coughing.*
2 Practice hand hygiene.
3 Identify the person. Check the ID bracelet against the assignment sheet. Use 2 identifiers (Chapter 11). Also call the person by name.

4 Provide for privacy.
5 Raise the bed for body mechanics. Bed rails are up if used. Lower the bed rail near you if up.

Continued

Assisting With Deep-Breathing and Coughing Exercises—cont'd

Procedure

6 Help the person to a comfortable sitting position.
- Sitting on the side of the bed
- Semi-Fowler's
- Fowler's

7 *For deep breathing:*
   a Have the person place the hands over the rib cage (Fig. 37-4).
   b Have the person inhale through the nose and breathe as deeply as possible (Fig. 37-5).
   c Ask the person to hold the breath for 2 to 3 seconds.
   d Ask the person to exhale slowly through pursed lips (see Fig. 37-5). Have the person exhale until the ribs move as far down as possible.
   e Repeat this step 4 more times. Have the person take normal breaths as needed before each deep breath.

8 *For coughing:*
   a *If the person does not have a productive cough:* Have the person place both hands over the chest or abdominal incision. One hand is on top of the other (Fig. 37-6, A). Or the person holds a pillow or folded towel over the chest or abdominal incision (Fig. 37-6, B).
   b *If the person has a productive cough:*
      1) Have the person practice cough etiquette.
      2) Splint the chest or abdominal incision with your hands or a pillow. Wear gloves.
   c Have the person take in a deep breath as in step 7.
   d Ask the person to cough strongly 2 times with the mouth open.

9 Assist with hand hygiene. Wear gloves. Remove and discard gloves. Practice hand hygiene.

Post-Procedure

10 Provide for comfort. (See the inside of the back cover.)
11 Place the call light and other needed items within reach.
12 Lower the bed to a safe and comfortable level. Raise or lower bed rails. Follow the care plan.
13 Follow the care plan and the person's preferences for privacy measures to maintain. Leaving the privacy curtain, window coverings, and door open or closed are examples.
14 Complete a safety check of the room. (See the inside of the back cover.)
15 Practice hand hygiene.
16 Report and record your care and observations.

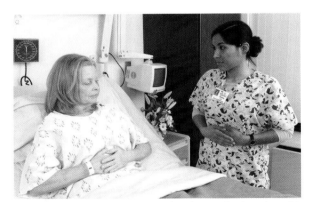

FIGURE 37-4 The hands are over the rib cage for deep breathing.

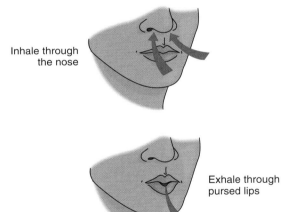

FIGURE 37-5 The person inhales through the nose and exhales through pursed lips during the deep-breathing exercise.

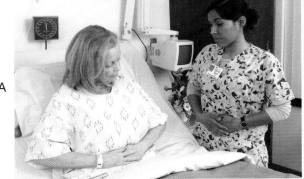

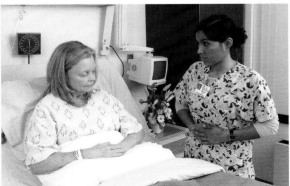

FIGURE 37-6 The incision is supported for the coughing exercise. A, The hands are over the incision. B, A pillow is held over the incision.

ASSISTING WITH OXYGEN THERAPY

Disease, injury, and surgery often affect breathing and oxygen needs. Oxygen therapy is ordered when the amount of O_2 in the blood is less than normal (*hypoxemia*). Oxygen is needed constantly or for symptom relief—chest pain or shortness of breath. Persons with respiratory diseases may have enough oxygen at rest. With mild exercise or activity, they become short of breath. Oxygen therapy helps relieve shortness of breath.

Oxygen is treated as a drug. The doctor orders when to give O_2, the amount, and the device to use. Harm can result from too much or not enough oxygen. *You do not give oxygen.* The nurse and respiratory therapist start and maintain oxygen therapy. You help provide safe care.

Oxygen Sources

Oxygen is supplied as follows.

- *Wall outlet.* O_2 is piped into each person's unit (Fig. 37-7).
- *Oxygen tank.* Portable oxygen tanks are used for emergencies, for transfers, and by persons who walk or use wheelchairs (Fig. 37-8). A gauge tells how much O_2 is left (Fig. 37-9).
- *Liquid oxygen system.* A portable unit is filled from a stationary unit (Fig. 37-10, p. 482). Depending on unit size and the flow rate (p. 483), the portable unit has enough O_2 for about 8 to 20 hours of use. A dial shows the amount of O_2 in the unit. Follow the manufacturer's instructions to check the amount.
- *Oxygen concentrator.* The machine removes oxygen from the air (Fig. 37-11, p. 482). A power source is needed. An oxygen tank is needed for power failures and mobility.

See *Promoting Safety and Comfort: Oxygen Sources.*

PROMOTING SAFETY AND COMFORT

Oxygen Sources

Safety

Liquid oxygen is very cold. If touched, it can freeze the skin. Tampering with equipment is unsafe and could damage the equipment. Follow agency procedures and the manufacturer's instructions for liquid oxygen.

Many activities increase the need for O_2. These include moving in bed, transfer procedures, and walking. Do not remove the person's O_2. If needed, ask the nurse for longer tubing. Or ask the nurse to change to a portable oxygen tank.

Oxygen tanks and liquid oxygen systems contain a certain amount of O_2. When the O_2 level is low, a new tank is needed or the liquid oxygen system is refilled. Check the O_2 level often. Report a low O_2 level at once.

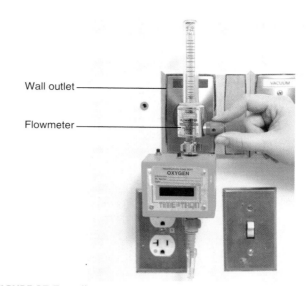

FIGURE 37-7 Wall oxygen outlet. The flowmeter is used to set the oxygen flow rate.

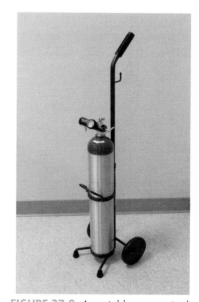

FIGURE 37-8 A portable oxygen tank.

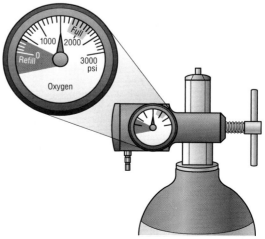

FIGURE 37-9 The gauge shows the amount of oxygen in the tank.

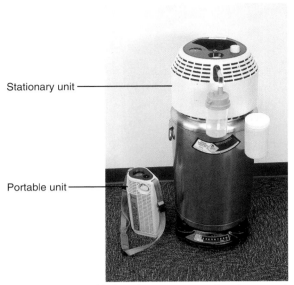

FIGURE 37-10 A portable liquid oxygen unit and stationary unit. (Modified from Perry AG, Potter PA, Ostendorf WR, Laplante N: *Clinical nursing skills & techniques*, ed 10, St Louis, 2022, Mosby.)

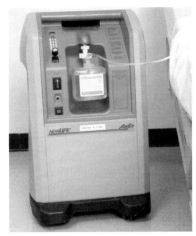

FIGURE 37-11 Oxygen concentrator.

Oxygen Devices

Different devices may be ordered for giving O_2. The type used depends on the person's oxygen needs. See Table 37-1 for 3 types of devices used to deliver oxygen.

TABLE 37-1 Types of Oxygen Devices			
Device	**Description**	**Care Considerations**	**Example**
Nasal cannula	• Prongs are inserted into the nostrils. The prong openings face downward. • Tubing goes behind the ears and under the chin.	• Allows for eating and drinking. • Tight prongs can irritate the nose. • Pressure on the ears and cheekbones can occur.	Prong openings face downward
Simple face mask	• A mask covers the nose and mouth. • An elastic strap goes around the head to secure the device. • Small holes (vents) in the sides of the mask allow CO_2 to escape when exhaling. Vents also allow room air into the mask when inhaling.	• Talking and eating are hard to do with a mask. For eating, the nurse changes the mask to a cannula. • Moisture can build up under the mask. Keep the face clean and dry to prevent irritation. • Vomiting while wearing a mask can cause aspiration.	Vents
Non-rebreather mask	• The mask has a reservoir bag for O_2. • Exhaled air leaves through holes (vents) in the mask. Vent covers do not allow room air into the mask. • Only O_2 from the bag is inhaled. Exhaled air and room air are not inhaled.	• The reservoir bag must not totally deflate (collapse) when inhaling. Suffocation can occur if there is not enough air in the bag. • These masks are used for emergency situations. The person is not left alone when in use.	Adjustable nose clip, Strap, Mask, Vent cover, O_2 tubing, Reservoir bag

Oxygen Flow Rates

The *flow rate* is the amount of oxygen given. It is measured in liters per minute (L/min). The ordered flow rate may be ½ (one-half) to 15 liters of O_2 per minute. The nurse or respiratory therapist sets the flow rate with a flowmeter (see Fig. 37-7).

The nurse and care plan tell you the person's flow rate. Always check the flow rate. Tell the nurse at once if it is too high or too low. A nurse or respiratory therapist will adjust the flow rate. Some states and agencies let nursing assistants adjust O_2 flow rates. Know your agency's policy.

Oxygen Safety

You assist the nurse with oxygen therapy. *You do not give oxygen. You do not adjust the flow rate unless allowed by your state and agency.* However, you must give safe care. Follow the rules in Box 37-2. Also follow the rules for fire and the use of oxygen (Chapter 11).

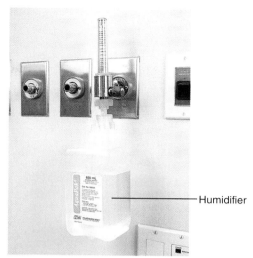

FIGURE 37-12 Oxygen set-up with a humidifier. — Humidifier

BOX 37-2 Oxygen Safety

- Do not remove the oxygen device.
- Make sure the device is secure but not tight.
- Check areas where oxygen devices contact the skin. Pressure injuries can develop where medical devices cause pressure on the skin. Report any sign of a pressure injury at once (Chapter 36). Check for irritation or skin changes:
  - Behind the ears
  - Under the nose (cannula)
  - Around the face (mask)
  - On the cheekbones
- Keep the face clean and dry when a mask is used.
- Do not shut off the O_2 flow unless there is a fire. *Turn off the O_2 flow if there is a fire. Remove the oxygen device.*
- Do not adjust the flow rate unless allowed by your state and agency.
- Tell the nurse at once if a:
  - Flow rate is too high or too low.
  - Humidifier is not bubbling (Fig. 37-12). Humidified (moist) oxygen prevents drying of the airway's mucous membranes. Bubbling means that moisture (water vapor) is being produced.
- Maintain an adequate water level in a humidifier.
- Secure tubing in place. Tape, clamp, or pin it to the person's garment following agency policy. Do not puncture the tubing.
- Make sure there are no kinks in the tubing.
- Make sure the person does not lie on any part of the tubing.
- Make sure an oxygen tank is secure in its holder.
- Report signs and symptoms of altered respiratory function or abnormal breathing patterns at once. See p. 476.
- Follow the care plan for oral hygiene.
- Make sure the oxygen device is clean and free of mucus.
- See "Fire and Oxygen" in Chapter 11.

DEVICES FOR SLEEP APNEA

Sleep apnea is a sleep disorder that causes pauses in breathing during sleep (Chapter 33). The most common cause is blockage of the airway. During sleep, muscles in the throat relax and soft tissues collapse, closing the airway.

Persons with sleep apnea may use a device to keep the airway open.

- *Continuous positive airway pressure (CPAP).* A mask that covers the nose or the nose and mouth is attached to a pump (Fig. 37-13, p. 484). Air pressure is forced through the mask to keep the airway open. The same amount of pressure goes through the mask when the person inhales and exhales.
- *Bilevel positive airway pressure (BiPAP).* This works like a CPAP except more pressure is given when breathing in. Less pressure is given when breathing out. The change in pressure is more comfortable for some persons.

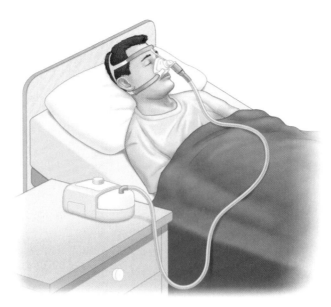

FIGURE 37-13   A continuous positive airway pressure (CPAP) device used for sleep apnea.

FOCUS ON P R I D E

The Person, Family, and Yourself

P ersonal and Professional Responsibility

A person may say: "I'm not getting enough air." Yet the person seems to be breathing comfortably. You cannot feel what the person feels. Trust what the person tells you.

If the person uses oxygen therapy, you can check the oxygen set-up.
- Is the O₂ turned on and at the correct flow rate?
- Is there enough O₂ remaining in a portable oxygen tank or liquid oxygen unit?
- Is the tubing connected to the O₂ source?
- Are there any kinks in the tubing?
- Is the oxygen device (nasal cannula or mask) properly in place?
  Do not dismiss what the person tells you. If you do not find a problem or you cannot correct the problem, tell the nurse at once.

R ights and Respect

People have the right to a safe setting. Smoking is not allowed where oxygen is used and stored. *NO SMOKING* signs are common in rooms and hallways. You may need to remind the person or visitors not to smoke. Be polite and respectful. Show the person where smoking is allowed.

I ndependence and Social Interaction

Needing long-term oxygen therapy changes a person's life. Portable oxygen sources increase independence. Small oxygen tanks and portable liquid oxygen units are examples. Such devices allow freedom and promote quality of life.

D elegation and Teamwork

If asked to give oxygen or adjust a flow rate, politely refuse. Refusing to perform a task is your right and duty when the task is beyond the legal limits of your role. Do not ignore the request. Tell the nurse that you can assist. Gathering supplies is an example. Or ask if you can help with a different task.

E thics and Laws

Performing tasks that you are not trained to do can cause harm. You can lose your job and your ability to work as a nursing assistant. Take pride in following the limits of your role and providing safe care.

FOCUS ON PRIDE: *Application*

What are the limits to your role when assisting with oxygen therapy? Why are such limits important? Explain the value of your role. How do you help the nurse and patient or resident?

Circle the BEST answer.

1 Hypoxia is
   a Not enough oxygen in the blood
   b The amount of hemoglobin that contains oxygen
   c Not enough oxygen in the cells
   d The lack of carbon dioxide

2 An early sign of altered respiratory function is
   a Cyanosis
   b Increased pulse
   c Restlessness
   d Dyspnea

3 A person breathes deeply and comfortably only while sitting. This is called
   a Apnea
   b Orthopnea
   c Bradypnea
   d Kussmaul respirations

4 Tachypnea means that respirations are
   a Slow
   b Rapid
   c Absent
   d Difficult or painful

5 Which should you report to the nurse at once?
   a A respiratory rate of 18 per minute
   b An SpO_2 of 97%
   c Bubbling in a humidifier
   d Dyspnea

6 A person's SpO_2 is 98%. Which is *true*?
   a The pulse oximeter is wrong.
   b The pulse is 98 beats per minute.
   c The measurement is within the normal range.
   d The person has hypoxia.

7 A person has non-natural nails. Which is another pulse oximetry sensor site?
   a The wrist
   b The chest
   c The upper arm
   d An earlobe

8 You are assisting with deep breathing and coughing. You need to explain the procedure again if the person
   a Inhales through pursed lips
   b Sits in a comfortable position
   c Inhales deeply through the nose
   d Holds a pillow over an incision

9 A person has a productive cough. You remind the person to
   a Use an oxygen mask
   b Cover the nose and mouth when coughing
   c Cough and deep breathe twice daily
   d Inhale through the mouth

10 Liquid oxygen can freeze the skin.
    a True
    b False

11 Oxygen flow rate is measured in
    a mm Hg
    b mL/hr
    c L/min
    d SpO_2

12 When assisting with oxygen therapy, you can
    a Turn the oxygen on and off
    b Start the oxygen
    c Decide what device to use
    d Keep connecting tubing secure and free of kinks

13 A person complains of pressure on the ears from nasal cannula tubing. You should
    a Check for irritation and tell the nurse
    b Change the cannula to a mask
    c Remove the device
    d Explain that the pressure is normal

14 A person is receiving O_2. Which should you question?
    a Provide oral hygiene.
    b Use a portable tank for walking.
    c Turn off the O_2 before measuring SpO_2.
    d Secure tubing in place.

15 A CPAP device is used
    a For sleep apnea
    b To measure oxygen concentration
    c To promote coughing
    d For portable oxygen therapy

Answers to Chapter 37 questions are on p. 588.

FOCUS ON **PRACTICE**

Problem Solving

A person is receiving oxygen therapy by nasal cannula. The oxygen tubing will not reach from the wall oxygen outlet to the bathroom. The person removes the nasal cannula and walks to the bathroom. The person becomes short of breath and uses the call light in the bathroom to call for help. You respond. What will you do? How could this have been prevented?

CHAPTER 38

Rehabilitation Needs

OBJECTIVES

- Define the key terms and key abbreviations in this chapter.
- Describe how rehabilitation involves the whole person.
- Identify the complications to prevent.
- Identify the common reactions to rehabilitation.

- Explain your role in rehabilitation.
- List the common rehabilitation programs and services.
- Explain how to promote PRIDE in the person, the family, and yourself.

KEY TERMS

activities of daily living (ADL) The activities usually done during a normal day in a person's life
disability Any lost, absent, or impaired physical or mental function
prosthesis An artificial replacement for a missing body part
rehabilitation The process of restoring a person's highest possible level of physical, psychological, social, and economic function

restorative aide A nursing assistant with special training in restorative nursing and rehabilitation skills
restorative nursing care Care that helps persons regain health and strength for safe and independent living

KEY ABBREVIATIONS

ADL   Activities of daily living

ROM   Range-of-motion

Disease, injury, and surgery can affect body function. Often more than 1 function is lost.

A *disability is any lost, absent, or impaired physical or mental function.* Causes are acute or chronic.

- An *acute problem* has a short course with complete recovery. A fracture (broken bone) is an example.
- A *chronic problem* has a long course. The problem is controlled—not cured—with treatment. Arthritis and paralysis are chronic health problems.

Disabilities can affect eating, bathing, dressing, walking, and work ability. The degree of disability affects how much function is possible. The person may depend totally or in part on others for basic needs.

Rehabilitation is the process of restoring a person's highest possible level of physical, psychological, social, and economic function. Physical, occupational, and speech-language therapists are among the health team members involved (Chapter 1). The goals of rehabilitation are to:

- Prevent or reduce the degree of disability.
- Improve abilities for the highest level of independence. Self-care or returning to work may be a goal. If improved function is not possible, the goal is to prevent further loss of function for the best possible quality of life.
- Help the person adjust to the disability.

Some persons return home after rehabilitation. The process may continue in home or community settings.

See *Focus on Older Persons: Rehabilitation Needs.*

486

RESTORATIVE NURSING

Some patients and residents need more care after their rehabilitation program ends. *Restorative nursing care is care that helps persons regain health and strength for safe and independent living.* Restorative nursing measures promote:

- Healing
- Self-care
- Elimination
- Positioning
- Mobility
- Communication
- Cognitive function

Rehabilitation and restorative nursing may occur at the same time. For example, a person needs physical therapy for rehabilitation after joint replacement surgery. The person also needs restorative nursing care to help with walking and to promote healing of the surgical incision. Both rehabilitation and restorative nursing focus on the whole person.

Restorative Aides

Some agencies have restorative aides. A *restorative aide is a nursing assistant with special training in restorative nursing and rehabilitation skills.* These aides assist the nursing and health teams as needed. Required training varies among states. If there are no state requirements, the agency provides needed training.

THE WHOLE PERSON

Health problems and disabilities affect the whole person. Physical, psychological, social, and economic effects occur. The person learns to adjust to the changes. Abilities—what the person can do—are stressed.

See *Focus on Older Persons: The Whole Person.*

Physical Aspects

Rehabilitation starts when the person first seeks health care. Complications are prevented from bed rest, a long illness, surgery, or injury. Complications can cause further disability. Bowel and bladder problems are prevented. So are contractures and pressure injuries. Good alignment, turning and re-positioning, range-of-motion (ROM) exercises, and positioning devices are needed (Chapters 16, 17, and 32). Good skin care also prevents pressure injuries (Chapters 22 and 36).

Elimination. Some persons need bladder training (Chapter 25). The method depends on the person's problems, abilities, and needs. Some need bowel training (Chapter 27). Bowel control and regular elimination are goals. Fecal impaction, constipation, and fecal incontinence are prevented.

Self-Care. Self-care is a major goal. *Activities of daily living (ADL) are the activities usually done during a normal day in a person's life.* ADL include bathing, oral hygiene, dressing, eating, elimination, and moving about. The health team evaluates the person's ADL abilities and the need for self-help devices.

Sometimes the hands, wrists, and arms are affected. Adaptive (assistive) devices are often changed, made, or bought for the person's needs.

- Eating devices include glass holders, plate guards, and silverware with curved handles or cuffs (Chapter 29). Some devices attach to splints (Fig. 38-1).
- Electric toothbrushes have back-and-forth brushing motions for oral hygiene.
- Adaptive (assistive) devices for hygiene and grooming promote independence (Chapters 22 and 23).

Adaptive (assistive) devices are useful for cooking, dressing (Chapter 24), writing, phone calls, and other tasks. Some are shown in Figure 38-2, p. 488.

See *Focus on Surveys: Self-Care,* p. 488.

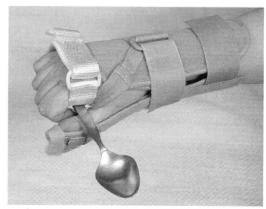

FIGURE 38-1 Eating device attached to a splint.

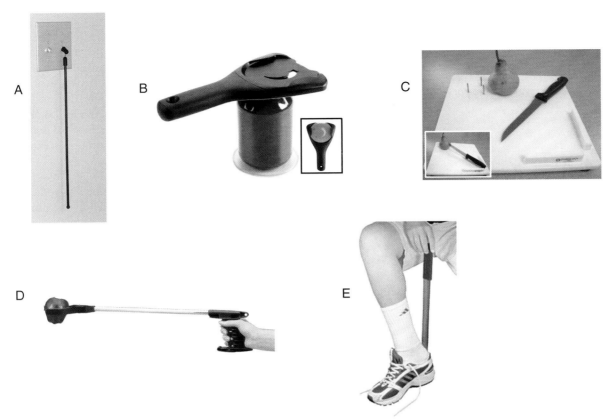

FIGURE 38-2 **A,** Light switch extender. **B,** Jar opener. **C,** Cutting board. **D,** Reacher. **E,** Shoehorn. (A and C, Courtesy Parsons ADL, Inc. Tottenham, Ontario. B, Courtesy OXO International, Inc., New York, N.Y. D and E, Images provided by Performance Health.)

Nutrition. Difficulty swallowing *(dysphagia)* may occur after a stroke. The person may need a dysphagia diet (Chapter 29). If possible, the person learns exercises to improve swallowing. Persons who cannot swallow need enteral nutrition (Chapter 29).

Mobility. The person may need to learn how to move in bed. Or the person may need crutches or a walker, cane, or brace (Chapter 32). Physical and occupational therapies are common for musculo-skeletal and nervous system problems. Some people need wheelchairs. If possible, they learn wheelchair transfers. Such transfers include to and from the bed, toilet, bathtub, sofa, and chair and in and out of vehicles (Fig. 38-3).

An amputation also affects mobility. A ***prosthesis*** *is an artificial replacement for a missing body part.* The person learns how to use the artificial arm or leg (Chapter 40). The goal is for the device to be like the missing body part in function and appearance.

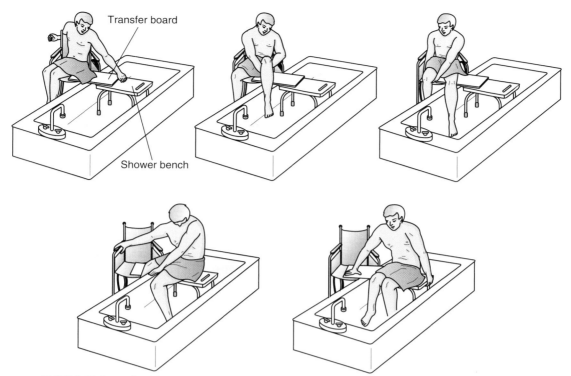

FIGURE 38-3 A wheelchair to tub transfer. A transfer board (sliding board) and shower bench are used.

Communication

Aphasia (Chapter 39) may occur from a stroke. *Aphasia* is the total or partial loss (*a*) of the ability to use or understand language (*phasia*). It results from damage to parts of the brain responsible for language and speech. Speech therapy and communication devices are helpful (Chapters 6 and 39).

See *Focus on Communication: Communication.*

FOCUS ON **COMMUNICATION**

Communication

Persons with speech disorders may need other communication methods. Pictures, reading, writing, facial expressions, and gestures are examples. All health team members and the family use the same method with the person. Changing methods can cause confusion and delay progress.

Psychological and Social Aspects

A disability can affect function and appearance. Self-esteem and relationships may change. Feelings of being unwhole, useless, unattractive, unclean, or undesirable can occur. Some persons become depressed or angry.

Some persons deny the disability. Others expect that therapy will quickly correct the problem. Some think therapy time alone is enough to make progress. The nurse and therapist help the person with expectations, goals, and a plan of care.

A good attitude and motivation are important. While the person understands safety limits, the focus is on abilities and strengths. Progress may be slow. Learning a new task is a reminder of the disability.

Remind persons of their progress. Give support, reassurance, and encouragement. Psychological and social needs are part of the care plan. Spiritual support helps some persons.

See *Focus on Communication: Psychological and Social Aspects.*

FOCUS ON **COMMUNICATION**

Psychological and Social Aspects

Emotional needs are great during rehabilitation. Good communication and support provide encouragement.
- Listen to the person.
- Show concern, not pity.
- Focus on what the person can do. Point out even slight progress.
- Be polite but firm. Do not let the person control you.
- Do not shout at or insult the person. Such behaviors are abuse and mistreatment.
- Do not argue with the person.
- Tell the nurse about problems. The person may need other support measures.

Economic Aspects

Some persons return to their jobs. Those who cannot do so are assessed for work skills, work history, interests, and talents. A job skill may be restored or a new one learned. The goal is gainful employment. Help is given finding a job.

THE PERSON'S SETTING

The setting must be safe and meet the person's needs (Chapter 19). Needed changes are made. For example, the over-bed table, bedside stand, call light, and other needed items are moved to the person's strong (unaffected) side. If unable to use the call light, another communication aid is used. The rehabilitation team helps the person and family plan for needed changes at home.

THE REHABILITATION TEAM

Rehabilitation is a team effort. The person is the key team member. The person, family, doctor, and nursing and health teams set goals and plan care. The focus is to regain function and independence.

The team meets often to discuss the person's progress. The rehabilitation plan is changed as needed. The person and family attend the meetings when possible. Families provide support and encouragement. Often they help with home care.

Your Role

You help promote the person's independence. Preventing decline in function also is a goal. The many procedures, care measures, and rules in this book apply. Safety, communication, legal, and ethical aspects apply. So do the measures in Box 38-1.

See *Focus on Communication: Your Role.*

REHABILITATION PROGRAMS

Common rehabilitation programs include:

- *Cardiac rehabilitation*—for heart disorders
- *Brain injury rehabilitation*—for nervous system disorders, including traumatic brain injury
- *Spinal cord rehabilitation*—for spinal cord injuries
- *Stroke rehabilitation*—after a stroke
- *Respiratory rehabilitation*—for respiratory system disorders such as chronic obstructive pulmonary disease, after lung surgery, and for respiratory complications from other health problems
- *Orthopedic rehabilitation*—for fractures, joint replacement surgery, and other musculo-skeletal problems
- *Amputee rehabilitation*—for amputation of a limb
- *Hearing, speech, and vision rehabilitation*—for persons who are hard of hearing or deaf, have speech problems, are blind, or have severe vision problems
- *Drug and alcohol treatment*—for persons addicted to drugs or alcohol
- *Behavioral health treatment*—for those with mental health disorders
- *Rehabilitation for complex medical and surgical conditions*—wound care, diabetes, and burns are examples

After hospital care, the person may transfer to a nursing center or rehabilitation agency. Home care agencies, adult day-care centers, and assisted living residences may also provide rehabilitation services (Chapter 1).

BOX 38-1 Assisting With Rehabilitation Needs

Physical Needs

- Follow the care plan and the nurse's instructions.
- Follow the person's daily routine.
- Provide for safety.
- Report early signs and symptoms of complications. They include pressure injuries, contractures, and bowel and bladder problems.
- Keep the person in good alignment.
- Turn and re-position the person as directed.
- Use safe transfer methods.
- Practice measures to prevent pressure injuries.
- Perform ROM exercises as instructed.
- Remember that muscles will atrophy if not used. Contractures can also develop.
- Know how to use and apply adaptive (assistive) devices.
- Provide and apply needed adaptive (assistive) devices.

Psychological and Social Needs

- Protect the person's rights. Privacy and personal choice are very important.
- Encourage performing ADL to the extent possible.
- Allow time to complete tasks. Do not rush the person.
- Give praise for even a little progress.
- Provide emotional support and reassurance.
- Try to understand and appreciate the person's situation, feelings, and concerns.
- Do not pity the person or give sympathy.
- Provide for spiritual needs.
- Practice the methods developed by the rehabilitation team. You will better assist the person.
- Practice the task that the person must do. This helps you guide and direct the person.
- Stress what the person can do. Focus on abilities and strengths, not on disabilities and weaknesses.
- Have a hopeful outlook.

FOCUS ON COMMUNICATION

Your Role

The nurse or therapist teaches the person and family about measures to gain function and independence. If the person or family needs more teaching, tell the nurse.

You may need to guide and direct the person during care. Listen to how the nurse or therapist guides and directs the person. Use those words. Hearing the same thing helps the person learn and remember what to do.

QUALITY OF LIFE

Successful rehabilitation improves quality of life. A hopeful and winning outlook is needed. The more the person can do alone, the better the person's quality of life. See *Focus on PRIDE: The Person, Family, and Yourself* for ways to promote independence.

To promote quality of life:
- Protect the right to privacy.
- Encourage personal choice.
- Protect the right to be free from abuse and mistreatment.
- Encourage activities.
- Provide a safe setting.
- Show patience, understanding, and sensitivity.

FOCUS ON P R I D E

The Person, Family, and Yourself

P ersonal and Professional Responsibility

Often nursing assistants are promoted to restorative aide positions. Professional behaviors are highly valued for promotions. Patience, kindness, and good communication skills are needed. Staff with a positive attitude, good work ethics, and excellent job performance are considered first.

Becoming a restorative aide allows you to advance as a nursing assistant. Seek out learning opportunities and practice positive work habits. Take pride in continuing to learn, improve, and grow as a nursing assistant.

R ights and Respect

Rehabilitation is challenging for the person, the family, and the nursing staff. No matter how difficult the situation, the person's rights are always protected. See Chapter 2.

Losing patience can cause frustration. Unkind remarks and actions toward the person are not allowed. Protect the person from abuse and mistreatment. Treat the person with dignity and respect.

I ndependence and Social Interaction

Quality of life improves the more the person can do independently. To promote independence:
- Stress the person's abilities and strengths.
- Let the person choose activities of interest.
- Remain patient. Do not rush the person.
- Promote self-care. Know what the person can do. Resist the urge to do those things for the person.
- Provide limited help if the person needs only some help.
- Offer encouragement and support.
- Have the person use adaptive (assistive) devices as needed.
- Encourage personal choice. Personal choice allows control.

D elegation and Teamwork

Disability affects the whole person. The person may be overwhelmed, sad, angry, or discouraged. Such feelings can be hard to control. Outbursts may occur.

The person does not choose loss of function. If the person's emotional responses upset you, think how the person must feel. You must:
- Show patience, understanding, sensitivity, and respect.
- Be calm and act in a professional manner.
- Control your words and actions.

The nurse can suggest ways to help you control or express your feelings. You may need to assist with other persons for a while. Take pride in being a part of a strong, supportive team.

E thics and Laws

The person may not want to practice rehabilitation procedures or methods. The person may want you to give care instead. To make progress, the person needs to follow the rehabilitation plan. Do not let the person control you. Report any problems to the nurse.

FOCUS ON PRIDE: *Application*

Do you know someone with a disability? How does the disability affect the whole person? How does it affect the person's family?

Circle the BEST answer.

1 Which statement about rehabilitation is *true*?
  a Only chronic problems require rehabilitation.
  b Rehabilitation for older persons is usually fast-paced.
  c You do not need to know how to use the person's adaptive (assistive) devices.
  d Personal preferences are considered in the rehabilitation plan.

2 Rehabilitation and restorative nursing care focus on
  a What the person cannot do
  b Self-care
  c The whole person
  d Mobility and communication

3 Rehabilitation involves preventing
  a Angry feelings
  b Contractures and pressure injuries
  c The use of adaptive (assistive) devices
  d Nursing center care

4 You are helping a person dress. The person is supposed to practice using a shoehorn to put on shoes. Which comment is *best*?
  a "If I put your shoes on you, we will finish faster."
  b "You are doing well. Let me know if you need help tying."
  c "It is so sad that you cannot put your shoes on anymore."
  d "You should be able to do this without the shoehorn."

5 A person has weakness on the right side. ADL are
  a Done by the person to the extent possible
  b Done by you
  c Delayed until the right side can be used
  d Supervised by a therapist

6 Which shows you understand the psychological effects of rehabilitation?
  a You laugh when the person makes mistakes.
  b You talk about the person's weaknesses more than strengths.
  c You convey hopefulness and talk about what the person can do.
  d You argue with the person about the best way to do a task.

7 To provide emotional support during rehabilitation
  a Remind residents of their limits
  b Give sympathy and show pity
  c Talk about your feelings
  d Listen and give praise

8 A person is not allowed food until exercises are done. This is abuse and mistreatment.
  a True
  b False

9 During therapy, a person wants music played. You should
  a Explain that music is not allowed
  b Choose some music
  c Ask the person to choose some music
  d Ask a therapist to choose some music

10 A person's right side is weak. You move the call light to the left side. You promote quality of life by
  a Encouraging self-care
  b Allowing personal choice
  c Providing for safety
  d Taking part in activities

Answers to Chapter 38 questions are on p. 588.

FOCUS ON **PRACTICE**

Problem Solving

A person's care plan includes long-handled devices for dressing and bathing. During the bath, you provide a long-handled sponge. The person says: "I don't feel like using that today. Will you wash my feet for me?" What will you say and do? How will your response affect the person's progress?

CHAPTER 39

Hearing, Speech, and Vision Problems

OBJECTIVES

- Define the key terms and key abbreviations in this chapter.
- Describe the common ear, speech, and eye disorders.
- Describe how to communicate with persons who have hearing loss.
- Explain the purpose of a hearing aid.
- Describe how to care for hearing aids.

- Explain how to communicate with persons who have speech disorders.
- Explain how to assist persons who are visually impaired or blind.
- Perform the procedure described in this chapter.
- Explain how to promote PRIDE in the person, the family, and yourself.

KEY TERMS

aphasia The total or partial loss *(a)* of the ability to use or understand language *(phasia)*
blindness The absence of sight
braille A touch reading and writing system that uses raised dots for each letter of the alphabet; the first 10 letters also represent the numbers 0 through 9
deafness Hearing loss in which it is impossible for the person to understand speech through hearing alone

hearing loss Not being able to hear the range of sounds associated with normal hearing
low vision Vision loss that cannot be corrected with eyeglasses, contact lenses, drugs, or surgery; vision loss interferes with every-day activities
tinnitus A ringing, roaring, hissing, or buzzing sound in the ears or head
vertigo Dizziness

KEY ABBREVIATIONS

AMD   Age-related macular degeneration

ASL   American Sign Language

Hearing, speech, and vision are important for self-care, work, most activities, and safety and security needs. Hearing, speech, and vision disorders occur in all age-groups. Common causes are birth defects, injuries, infections, diseases, and aging.

HEARING DISORDERS

The ear functions in hearing and balance. Hearing is needed for clear speech, responding to others, safety, and awareness of surroundings.

Meniere's Disease

Meniere's disease involves the inner ear. Fluid buildup in the inner ear causes swelling and pressure. Usually 1 ear is affected. Symptoms are sudden. They include:
- *Vertigo—dizziness*
- *Tinnitus—a ringing, roaring, hissing, or buzzing sound in the ears or head*
- Hearing loss
- Feeling of fullness or pressure in the ear

493

An attack usually involves vertigo, tinnitus, and hearing loss. Vertigo causes whirling and spinning sensations. The dizziness causes severe nausea and vomiting. An episode can last 20 minutes or 2 to 24 hours.

Drugs and a low-salt diet may decrease fluid in the inner ear. Smoking, caffeine, and alcohol are avoided. Safety is needed during vertigo.

- Have the person lie down.
- Prevent falls. Assist with walking and use bed rails according to the care plan.
- Have the person keep the head still and focus on an object that does not move. The person avoids turning the head. Do not move around while talking with the person.
- Avoid sudden movements. The person moves slowly.
- Prevent flashing lights (such as from TV) and bright lights.

Hearing Loss

Hearing loss is not being able to hear the range of sounds associated with normal hearing. Losses are mild to deafness. *Deafness is hearing loss in which it is impossible for the person to understand speech through hearing alone.*

Causes include damage to the outer, middle, or inner ear or to the acoustic nerve (Chapter 9). Aging and exposure to loud noises are risk factors. See Box 39-1 for some signs and symptoms of hearing loss.

Hearing is needed for clear speech. Pronouncing words and voice volume depend on hearing yourself. Hearing loss may result in slurred speech or pronouncing words wrong. Some people have monotone speech or drop word endings. It may be hard to understand the person. Do not assume or pretend that you understand. Serious problems can result. See "Speech Disorders" on p. 496.

See *Focus on Communication: Hearing Loss.*

BOX 39-1 Hearing Loss—Signs and Symptoms

- Problems:
  - Hearing on the phone
  - Hearing with background noise or in noisy areas
  - Following conversations when 2 or more people are speaking
  - Understanding women and children
- Straining to understand a conversation
- Hearing voices as mumbled or slurred
- Misunderstanding what others say
- Answering questions or responding inappropriately
- Asking others to repeat themselves
- Speaking too loudly
- Leaning forward to hear
- Turning and cupping the better ear toward the speaker
- Turning up the TV, radio, music, or other sound sources so loud that others complain

---

FOCUS ON COMMUNICATION

Hearing Loss

The National Association of the Deaf (NAD) uses the terms *deaf* and *hard of hearing* to describe persons with hearing loss. Do not use the terms *deaf and dumb, deaf-mute,* or *hearing-impaired.* Such terms may offend persons who are hard of hearing.

Communication. Persons with hearing loss may wear hearing aids or lip-read (speech-read). They watch facial expressions, gestures, and body language. American Sign Language (ASL) uses signs made with the hands and other movements such as facial expressions, gestures, and postures (Fig. 39-1).

Some people have *hearing dogs.* The dog alerts the person to sounds. Phones, doorbells, smoke alarms, alarm clocks, babies' cries, sirens, and on-coming cars are examples.

See Box 39-2 for measures to promote hearing and communication.

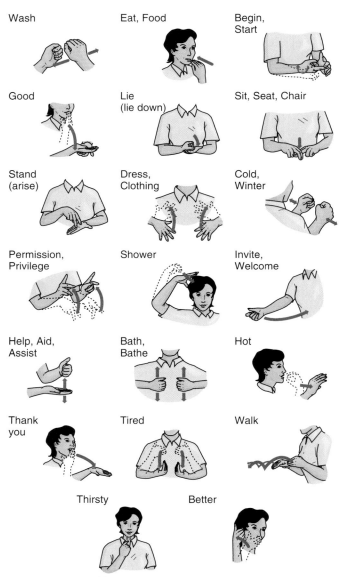

FIGURE 39-1 American Sign Language examples.

BOX 39-2 Measures to Promote Hearing

The Setting
- Reduce or eliminate background noises. Turn off radios, music players, TVs, air conditioners, fans, and so on.
- Provide a quiet place to talk. Avoid areas with loud sound.
- Have the person sit where able to hear best.

The Person
- Make sure the person's hearing aid is turned on, working, and properly placed in or behind the ear.
- Have the person wear needed eyeglasses or contact lenses. The person needs to see your face to lip-read (speech-read).

You
- Gain attention. Alert the person to your presence. Raise an arm or hand or lightly touch the person's hand, arm, or shoulder. Do not startle or approach the person from behind.
- Position yourself at the person's level. Sit if the person is sitting. Stand if the person is standing.
- Face the person when speaking. Do not turn or walk away while you are talking. Do not talk from the doorway or another room.
- Have light shine on your face. Shadows and glares affect the ability to see your face clearly.
- Maintain eye contact with the person.
- Speak clearly, distinctly, and at a normal rate. Do not talk too fast or too slow.
- Speak in a normal tone of voice. Do not shout or mumble.
- State the person's name before starting a conversation. This gains the person's attention and focus.
- Adjust the pitch of your voice as needed. Ask if the person can hear you better.
  - If no hearing aid, lower the pitch. Higher-pitched voices can be harder to hear than lower-pitched voices.
  - If a hearing aid is worn, raise the pitch slightly.
- Do not cover your mouth, smoke, eat, or chew gum while talking. Mouth movements are affected.
- Keep your hands away from your face.
- Stand or sit on the side of the better ear.
- State the topic of conversation first.
- Say when you are changing the subject. State the new topic.
- Use short sentences and simple words.
- Pause between sentences. Ensure understanding before speaking again.
- Use gestures and facial expressions as useful clues.
- Write out important names, words, numbers, addresses, appointments, and so on.
- Re-phrase if the person does not seem to understand. Do not repeat the same words again and again.
- Keep conversations and discussions short. This avoids tiring the person.
- Be alert to messages sent by your facial expressions, gestures, and body language.
- Be alert to the person's nonverbal communication. For example, watch for puzzled looks and expressions of anger, frustration, excitement, fatigue, and so on.

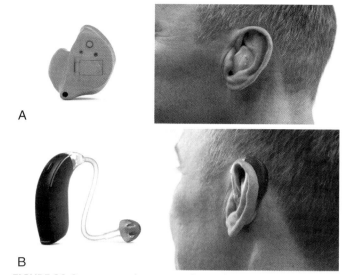

FIGURE 39-2 Hearing aids. **A,** An in-the-ear hearing aid. **B,** A behind-the-ear hearing aid. (Courtesy GN Hearing/ReSound.)

BOX 39-3 Hearing Aids—Care Measures

- Hold and handle hearing aids gently. This includes when removing, inserting, or cleaning the device and when inserting batteries.
- Do the following if a hearing aid does not seem to work properly.
  - Check if the hearing aid is *on*. The device has an *on* and *off* switch or function.
  - Check the battery position.
  - Insert a new battery if needed. Use the correct battery size.
  - Clean the hearing aid. Follow the manufacturer's instructions.
- Hold the hearing aid over a soft cloth or soft surface to change the battery or to clean the device.
- Clean the hearing aid according to the manufacturer's instructions. Wiping with a soft, dry cloth is a common cleaning method.
- Do not expose the hearing aid to heat or extreme cold.
- Have the person remove the hearing aid before using a hair dryer, hair spray, spray perfumes, shaving lotions, or powders.
- Protect the hearing aid from water. The person does not wear a hearing aid during a bath or shower or when shampooing the hair.
- Check meal trays and bed linens for hearing aids. The person may have removed the hearing aid and set it aside.
- Remove and turn off the hearing aid at bedtime. This saves battery life. Remove the battery if the person prefers.
- Place the hearing aid in its storage case when not worn. Place the storage case in the top drawer of the bedside stand.

Hearing Aids. *Hearing aids* make sounds louder. They do not correct, restore, or cure hearing problems. The person hears better because the device makes sounds louder. Background noise and speech are louder. Some types can reduce background noise. The measures in Box 39-2 apply.

Two common types of hearing aids are in-the-ear and behind-the-ear (Fig. 39-2). Hearing aids are costly. Protect them from damage. The care measures in Box 39-3 are general. Follow the manufacturer's instructions and the nurse's directions for how to insert, remove, and care for the person's hearing aid.

SPEECH DISORDERS

Speech disorders affect oral communication. Hearing loss and brain injury are common causes. These problems are common.

- *Aphasia.* See "Aphasia."
- *Apraxia of speech. Apraxia* means not (*a*) to act, do, or perform (*praxia*). The brain is unable to direct the movements needed for normal sound production. The person understands and knows what to say. However, the person cannot use speech muscles to make words for understandable speech.
- *Dysarthria. Dysarthria* means difficult or poor (*dys*) speech (*arthria*). The muscles used for speech are weak. Slurred, soft, slow, or hoarse speech can occur.

To communicate with a person with a speech disorder, practice the measures in Box 39-4. A speech-language pathologist can help the person:

- Use remaining abilities.
- Restore or improve language abilities to the extent possible.
- Learn communication methods.
- Strengthen speech muscles.

BOX 39-4 Communicating With Persons With Speech Disorders

The Person
- Have the person repeat or re-phrase statements as needed.
- Have the person write down key words or the message.
- Have the person point, gesture, or draw key words.

You
- Follow the care plan for a consistent approach.
- Provide a calm, quiet setting. Turn off the TV, radio, music, and other distractions.
- Include the person in conversations.
- Listen and give the person your full attention.
- Use short, simple sentences.
- Repeat yourself as needed.
- Repeat what the person has said. Ask if you understood correctly.
- Write down key words as needed.
- Speak in a normal tone. Do not talk in a babyish or child-like way.
- Ask questions to which you know the answers. This helps you learn how the person speaks.
- Allow the person enough time to talk.
- Determine the topic being discussed. This helps you understand main points. Watch lip movements.
- Watch facial expressions, gestures, and body language. They give clues about what is being said.
- Do not correct the person's speech.
- Be patient and kind. Emotional needs are great. Frustration, depression, and anger are common.

Aphasia

Aphasia is the total or partial loss (a) *of the ability to use or understand language* (phasia). Parts of the brain responsible for language are damaged. Stroke, head injury, brain infections, dementia, and brain tumors are common causes.

Expressive aphasia (Broca's aphasia) relates to difficulty expressing or sending out thoughts through speech or writing. The person knows what to say but has problems speaking or writing. The person usually can understand others. The person may:

- Omit small words such as "is," "and," "of," and "the."
- Speak in 1-word or short sentences (less than 4 words). For example, the person says "2 cup table" to mean "There are 2 cups on the table."
- Put words in the wrong order. The person may say "room bath" for "bathroom."
- Think one thing but say another. The person may want food but asks for a book.
- Call people the wrong names.
- Make up words.
- Produce sounds and no words.

Receptive aphasia (Wernicke's aphasia) is difficulty understanding language. The person has trouble understanding what is said or written. The person may speak using long sentences with no meaning. The person says unnecessary words and uses made-up words. The person is often unaware of mistakes.

Some people have both expressive and receptive aphasia. *Global aphasia (mixed aphasia)* involves difficulty expressing or sending out thoughts and difficulty understanding language. The person has problems speaking and understanding language.

EYE DISORDERS

Vision problems range from mild loss to complete blindness. *Blindness is the absence of sight.* Vision loss is sudden or gradual. One or both eyes are affected.

Cataracts

A cataract is clouding of the lens. The normal lens is clear. *Cataract* comes from the Greek word for *waterfall.* Trying to see is like looking through a waterfall. Cataracts can occur in 1 or both eyes. Signs and symptoms include:

- Cloudy, blurry, or dimmed vision (Fig. 39-3, *A* and *B*).
- Colors seem faded and brownish. Blues and purples are hard to see.
- Sensitivity to light and glares.
- Poor vision at night.
- Halos around lights.
- Double vision in the affected eye.

Surgery is the only treatment. Surgery is done when the cataract affects daily activities. The lens is replaced with a plastic lens. Vision improves after surgery. See Box 39-5 for care measures after cataract surgery.

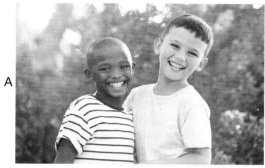
Normal Vision

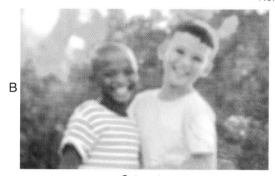
Cataracts

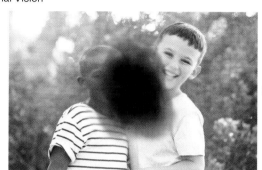
Age-Related Macular Degeneration

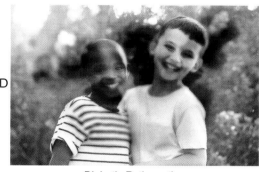
Diabetic Retinopathy

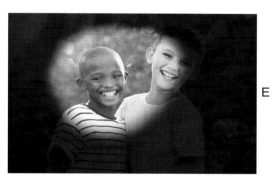
Glaucoma

FIGURE 39-3 Vision loss with eye disorders. **A,** Normal vision. **B,** Vision loss from cataracts. **C,** Vision loss from macular degeneration. **D,** Vision loss from diabetic retinopathy. **E,** Vision loss from glaucoma. (From National Eye Institute, National Institutes of Health.)

BOX 39-5 Cataract Surgery—Post-Operative Care

- Have the person wear ordered eyeglasses or eye shield as directed. If ordered, the shield is worn for sleep, including naps.
- Follow measures for persons who are blind or visually impaired when an eye shield is worn (p. 498). There may be vision loss in the other eye.
- Remind the person not to rub or press the affected eye.
- Do not bump the eye.
- Place the over-bed table and bedside stand on the un-operative side.
- Place the call light and needed items within reach.
- Report eye drainage or complaints of pain at once.
- Remind the person not to bend, stoop, or lift heavy things. Avoid coughing, sneezing, and vomiting if possible.

Age-Related Macular Degeneration

Age-related macular degeneration (AMD) is common in people age 50 and older. AMD affects the macula of the eye (Chapter 9). The macula contains cells that are sensitive to light, color, and the fine detail needed for central vision.

AMD causes blurring of central vision. *Central vision* is what you see "straight-ahead." It is needed to read, write, drive, cook, and see faces and for fine detail. Over time, blind spots (blank spots) occur in the center of vision (see Fig. 39-3, *A* and *C*).

Onset is gradual and painless. For advanced AMD, no treatment can prevent vision loss. Eye injections and laser treatments may stop or slow the disease progress.

Diabetic Retinopathy

In diabetic retinopathy, blood vessels in the retina are damaged. A complication of diabetes, it is a leading cause of blindness. Usually both eyes are affected.

Vision blurs and the person may see dark "floating" spots or streaks (see Fig. 39-3, *A* and *D*). Often there are no early warning signs.

The person needs to control diabetes, blood pressure, and cholesterol. Eye injections, laser treatments, or eye surgery may be used to prevent worsening vision.

Glaucoma

With glaucoma, fluid builds up in the eye, causing pressure on the optic nerve. The optic nerve is damaged. Vision loss with eventual blindness occurs.

Glaucoma can affect 1 or both eyes. Onset is sudden or gradual. Peripheral vision (side vision) is lost. The person sees through a "tunnel" (see Fig. 39-3, *A* and *E*), has blurred vision, and sees halos around lights.

Glaucoma has no cure. Prior damage cannot be reversed. Drugs, laser treatments, or surgery may be used to control glaucoma and prevent further damage to the optic nerve.

Low Vision

Low vision is vision loss that cannot be corrected with eyeglasses, contact lenses, drugs, or surgery. The vision loss interferes with every-day activities. While wearing eyeglasses or contact lenses, the person has problems:
- Recognizing faces of family and friends
- Doing tasks that require close vision—reading, cooking, sewing, and so on
- Picking out and matching clothing colors
- Reading signs (traffic, stores)
- Doing things because lighting seems dimmer
- Seeing a TV or computer screen clearly

The person learns to use visual and adaptive (assistive) devices. Examples include:
- Prescription reading glasses
- Large-print reading materials
- Hand-held, stand (mounted), or video magnifiers
- Audio tapes
- Electronic reading machines
- Computers with large print and speech systems
- Phones, clocks, and watches with large numbers and that talk
- Lighting that can be adjusted

Impaired Vision and Blindness

Some people are totally blind. Others sense some light but have no usable vision. Others have some usable vision but cannot read newsprint. A person who is legally blind sees at 20 feet what a person with normal vision sees at 200 feet.

Loss of sight is serious. Adjustments can be hard and long. Special education and rehabilitation programs help the person adjust to the vision loss and learn to be independent. The goal is to be as active as possible and have quality of life.

Braille. *Braille is a touch reading and writing system that uses raised dots for each letter of the alphabet* (Fig. 39-4). *The first 10 letters also represent the numbers 0 through 9.* Braille is read by moving the hands from left to right along each line of braille.

Special devices allow computer access—keyboards, displays, and printers. A "braille display" lets the person read the information. Braille printers produce printouts in braille.

Mobility. Persons who are blind or visually impaired learn to move about using a long cane or a guide dog. Both are used world-wide.
- Long canes are white or silver-gray with red tips. Do not interfere with the arm holding the cane. The person stores the cane when not in use. If you store the cane, ask the person where to place it.
- A guide dog sees for a person. The dog responds to the master's commands. Commands are disobeyed to avoid danger. For example, the guide dog disobeys a command to cross the street if a car is coming. Do not pet, feed, or distract a guide dog. Such actions can place the person in danger.

Meeting Needs. The person's care plan includes measures to meet the person's needs. Safety measures are included. Follow the practices in Box 39-6 according to the care plan.

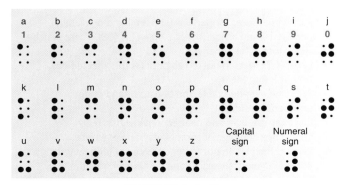

FIGURE 39-4 Braille.

BOX 39-6 Caring for Persons Who Are Blind or Visually Impaired

The Setting

- Report worn or loose carpeting and other flooring. Also report throw rugs, plastic runners, and furniture with wheels.
- Keep furniture, equipment, electrical cords, and other items out of areas where the person will walk.
- Keep chairs pushed in under the table or desk.
- Keep room doors fully open or fully closed.
- Keep drawers and cabinet, cupboard, and closet doors fully closed.
- Report burnt-out light bulbs.
- Provide preferred lighting. Tell the person if lights are on or off.
- Adjust window coverings to prevent glares. Sunny days and bright, snowy days cause glares.
- Keep the call light and TV, light, and other controls within reach.
- Use night-lights in the person's room, bathroom, and hallway.
- Practice safety measures to prevent falls (Chapter 12).
- Orient the person to the room. Describe the layout. Include the location and purpose of furniture and equipment.
- Let the person touch and find furniture and equipment.
- Do not re-arrange furniture and equipment.
- Use colors and contrast. Solid, bright colors (red, orange, yellow) are best. Avoid pastels, patterns, prints, designs, and stripes. Light against dark provides contrast. For example, use a white plate with a dark placemat.
- Provide the same meal-time setting. Arrange things in the same way for each meal.
  - Have the person sit in good light.
  - Arrange the place setting.
    - The knife and spoon are to the right of the plate.
    - The fork and napkin are to the left of the plate.
    - The glass or cup is to the right of the plate if the person is right-handed. It is to the left of the plate if left-handed.
  - Arrange dishes, seasonings, and condiments in a straight line or in a semi-circle just beyond the place setting.
  - Explain the location of food and beverages. Use the face of a clock (Chapter 29). Or guide the person's hand to each item on the tray or place setting.
  - Cut meat, open containers, and perform other tasks as needed.
- Complete a safety check before leaving the room. (See the inside of the back cover.)

The Person

- Have the person wear comfortable shoes that fit correctly.
- Have the person use hand and stair railings and grab (safety) bars.
- Assist with walking as needed. Offer to guide and help the person. Respect the person's answer. If help is accepted:
  - Offer your arm. State which arm is offered. Tap the back of your hand against the person's hand.
  - Have the person hold on to your arm just above the elbow. Do not grab the person's arm.
  - Walk at a normal pace. Walk 1 step ahead of the person. Stand next to the person at the top and bottom of stairs and when crossing streets.
  - Never push, pull, or guide the person in front of you.
  - Pause to change direction, step up, or step down.
  - Warn of stairs, elevators, escalators, doors, turns, furniture, and other obstructions. State if steps are up or down.
  - Have the person hold on to a railing, the wall, or a strong surface if you need to step away. Tell the person that you are leaving and what to hold on to.

The Person —cont'd

- Guide the person to a seat by placing your guiding arm on the seat. The person moves a hand down your arm to the seat.
- Let the person do as much as possible. Do not do things that the person can do.
- Provide visual and adaptive (assistive) devices. Follow the care plan.

You

- Identify yourself when you enter the room. Give your name, title, and reason for being there. Do not touch the person before the person is aware of your presence.
- Ask how much the person can see. Do not assume the person is totally blind or has some vision.
- Identify others. Say where each person is and what the person is doing.
- Offer to help. Simply say: "May I help you?" Respect the person's answer.
- Leave the person's belongings where you found them. Do not move or re-arrange things. If you must move things, tell the person what you moved and where.

Communication

- Face the person when speaking. Speak slowly and clearly.
- Use a normal tone of voice. Do not shout or speak loudly.
- Address the person by name. This shows that you are directing a comment or question to the person.
- Speak directly to the person. Do not talk just to others who are present.
- Feel free to use words such as "see," "look," "read," or "watch TV." You can use "blind" and "visually impaired." However, it is respectful to refer to the person first. You also can use colors, sizes, shapes, patterns, designs, and so on.
- Describe people, places, and things thoroughly. Do not leave out a detail because you do not think it is important.
- Warn of dangers. Give a calm and clear warning. You can say "wait" first. Then describe the danger. For example: "Wait, there is ice on the sidewalk."
- Greet the person by name when the person enters a room. This alerts the person to your presence. Say who you are. Also identify others in the room.
- Listen to the person. Give verbal cues that you are listening. Say: "yes," "okay," "I see," "tell me more," "I don't understand," and so on.
- Answer questions. Provide specific and descriptive responses.
- Give step-by-step explanations as you give care. Say when the procedure is over.
- Give specific directions.
  - Say: "right behind you," "on your left," or "in front of you." Avoid phrases like "over here" or "over there."
  - Tell the distance. For example: "three steps in front of you" or "at the end of the hallway by the nurses' station."
  - Give landmarks if possible. Sounds and scents can serve as "landmarks." "By the kitchen" is an example.
- Tell the person when you are leaving the room or the area. If appropriate, state where you are going. For example: "I'm going to go into your bathroom now."
- Tell the person when you are ending a conversation. For example: "Thank you for sharing stories about your children."

Corrective Lenses

Eyeglasses and contact lenses correct many vision problems.

- *Eyeglasses*—Eyeglasses are worn for reading, for seeing at a distance, or for all activities. Eyeglass lenses are hardened glass or plastic. Clean them daily and as needed. Wash glass lenses with warm water. Dry them with a lens cloth or cotton cloth. Plastic lenses scratch easily. Use special cleaning solutions and cloths.
- *Contact lenses*—Contact lenses fit on the eye. There are hard and soft contacts. Contact lenses are usually only worn while awake. Some can be worn day and night for up to 30 days. Contacts are removed, cleaned, and stored according to the manufacturer's instructions. Depending on the type, they are discarded daily, weekly, or monthly. Report and record the following.
- Eye redness or irritation
- Eye drainage
- Eye pain or discomfort
- Blurred or fuzzy vision
  See *Delegation Guidelines: Corrective Lenses.*
  See *Promoting Safety and Comfort: Corrective Lenses.*
  See procedure: *Caring for Eyeglasses.*

DELEGATION GUIDELINES
Corrective Lenses

Cleaning eyeglasses is a routine care measure. Do not wait until the nurse tells you to clean them. Clean them daily and as needed.

To clean eyeglasses, find out if you need a special cleaning solution. Then follow the manufacturer's instructions.

PROMOTING SAFETY AND COMFORT
Corrective Lenses

Safety
Dirty eyeglasses can cause signs and symptoms of a vision problem. The person may worry about a problem when you simply need to clean the eyeglasses.

Eyeglasses are costly. Protect them from loss or damage. When not worn, put them in their case. Place the case in the top drawer of the bedside stand.

Some agencies let nursing assistants remove and insert contact lenses. Others do not. If allowed to insert and remove contacts, follow agency procedures.

Caring for Eyeglasses

Quality of Life
- Knock before entering the person's room.
- Address the person by name.
- Introduce yourself by name and title.
- Explain the procedure before starting and during the procedure.
- Protect the person's rights during the procedure.
- Handle the person gently during the procedure.

Pre-Procedure
1 Follow *Delegation Guidelines: Corrective Lenses.* **See** *Promoting Safety and Comfort: Corrective Lenses.*
2 Practice hand hygiene and get the following supplies.
   - Eyeglass case
   - Cleaning solution or warm water
   - Disposable lens cloth or cotton cloth

Procedure
3 Remove the eyeglasses.
   a Hold the frames in front of the ears (Fig. 39-5, A).
   b Lift the frames from the ears. Bring the eyeglasses down away from the face (Fig. 39-5, B).
4 Clean the lenses with a cleaning solution or warm water. Clean in a circular motion. Dry the lenses with the cloth.
5 *For the person not wearing eyeglasses:*
   a Open the eyeglass case.
   b Fold the glasses. Put them in the case. Do not touch the clean lenses.
   c Place the case in the top drawer of the bedside stand.
6 *For the person wearing eyeglasses:*
   a Hold the frames at each side. Place them over the ears.
   b Adjust the eyeglasses so the nose-piece rests on the nose.
   c Return the case to the top drawer of the bedside stand.

Post-Procedure
7 Provide for comfort. (See the inside of the back cover.)
8 Place the call light and other needed items within reach.
9 Return the cleaning solution to its proper place.
10 Discard a disposable cloth.
11 Complete a safety check of the room. (See the inside of the back cover.)
12 Practice hand hygiene.
13 Report and record your care and observations.

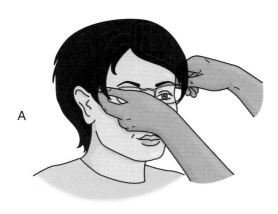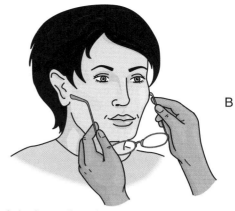

FIGURE 39-5 Removing eyeglasses. **A,** Hold the frames in front of the ears. **B,** Lift the frames from the ears. Bring the glasses down away from the face.

FOCUS ON P R I D E

The Person, Family, and Yourself

P ersonal and Professional Responsibility

Hearing aids, contact lenses, and eyeglasses are costly to repair or replace. Protect devices from loss or damage. If a device is lost or damaged, tell the nurse. Take pride in being responsible and honest.

R ights and Respect

Many persons with hearing, speech, and vision problems have overcome great challenges. They take pride in how they have adapted. They deserve to be treated with dignity and respect. Do not pity the person. Treat the person like an adult, not like a child. Focus on the person's abilities, not disabilities.

Always refer to the person first. Then state the disability if needed. For example, a nurse says: "Please take Mrs. Jones a warm blanket. She is blind, so remember to knock and introduce yourself before entering the room. She will place the blanket as she prefers."

I ndependence and Social Interaction

Adjusting to a hearing, speech, or vision problem is often long and hard. Take time to listen. Be patient, understanding, and sensitive to the person's needs and feelings. Allow the person to be in control to the extent possible. This helps promote independence to improve quality of life.

D elegation and Teamwork

Hearing loss requires changes in communication. Communication measures are part of the care plan. A consistent approach is needed. The health team uses the same methods to communicate with the person. Follow the care plan.

E thics and Laws

The *Americans With Disabilities Act (ADA) of 1990* protects the rights of persons with disabilities. It includes persons with limited hearing, speech, and vision. The ADA covers rights such as employment, access to services and places, and the use of communication devices.

To comply with the ADA, agencies often provide:
- Braille on signs for areas with public access. Lobbies, restrooms, elevators, and cafeterias are examples.
- Communication devices for hearing or speech problems. For example, a device with a keyboard and screen is connected to a phone line. The device is used instead of a phone.
- Sign language interpreters.
- Information in large print and braille.

Ask about your agency's resources. Offer to help. If not sure how to help, ask the nurse. Take pride in helping others.

FOCUS ON PRIDE: *Application*

Hearing, speech, and vision problems do not affect intelligence. Some behaviors insult the person. Treating the person like a child and talking to others but not the person are examples. What are other examples? Identify ways to show dignity and respect.

REVIEW QUESTIONS

Circle the BEST answer.

1. Care of the person with Meniere's disease includes
   a. Wearing a hearing aid
   b. Preventing falls from vertigo
   c. Speech therapy
   d. Treating infection

2. When talking to a person with hearing loss
   a. Shout
   b. Change the subject if the person does not seem to understand
   c. Avoid using gestures and facial expressions
   d. Use short sentences and simple words

3. A hearing aid
   a. Corrects a hearing problem
   b. Makes sounds louder
   c. Makes speech clearer
   d. Removes background noise

4. A hearing aid does not seem to be working. Your *first* action is to
   a. See if it is turned on
   b. Wash it with soap and water
   c. Have it repaired
   d. Remove the batteries

5. A person wears hearing aids. Which care measure is *correct*?
   a. Leave the hearing aids in while showering.
   b. Leave the hearing aids in while styling hair with a hair dryer and hair spray.
   c. Hold the hearing aids over a sink when cleaning them.
   d. Store the hearing aids in their case when not worn.

6. A person has aphasia. You know that
   a. The person cannot hear
   b. Mouth and face muscles are affected
   c. The person has a language disorder
   d. The person cannot speak

7. A person with receptive aphasia
   a. Has trouble understanding speech and writing
   b. Is aware of mistakes in speech
   c. Speaks in phrases or short sentences
   d. Has trouble hearing sounds

8. A person has a speech disorder. You should
   a. Correct the person's speech
   b. Discourage the writing of words
   c. Leave the TV on while talking
   d. Ask the person to repeat as needed

9. A person with a cataract
   a. Has cloudy, blurry, or dim vision
   b. Loses central vision
   c. Has eye pain
   d. Is blind

10. A person had cataract surgery. Which would you question?
    a. Remind the person not to bend or lift heavy objects.
    b. Let the person rub the eye.
    c. Place the over-bed table on the un-operative side.
    d. Leave an eye shield on during naps.

11. A person has AMD. Which is *true*?
    a. There is a blind spot in the center of vision.
    b. Lost vision can be restored with surgery.
    c. Peripheral (side) vision is lost.
    d. Vision is blurry with spots.

12. Braille involves
    a. A long cane for walking
    b. Raised dots arranged for letters of the alphabet
    c. A guide dog
    d. Corrective lenses

13. Which are dangers for persons who are blind or visually impaired?
    a. Closed drawers
    b. Doors that are fully open
    c. Equipment in hallways
    d. Night-lights

14. A person is visually impaired. You should
    a. Move furniture to provide variety
    b. Avoid words such as "see" and "look"
    c. Assume that the person has no sight
    d. Provide a consistent meal-time setting

15. A person is blind. To give directions you can say
    a. "Over there"
    b. "Right here"
    c. "Across the room"
    d. "On your left"

16. When eyeglasses are not worn they should be
    a. Soaked in a cleaning solution
    b. Taken to the nurses' station
    c. Put in the eyeglass case
    d. Placed in the bathroom

Answers to Chapter 39 questions are on p. 588.

FOCUS ON **PRACTICE**

Problem Solving

A resident asks for help completing the weekly menu. You are to read each option and mark the choices. Hard of hearing, the resident struggles to hear you. You repeat the meal options many times. What will you do? How can you promote hearing and communication?

CHAPTER 40

Common Health Problems

OBJECTIVES

- Define the key terms and key abbreviations in this chapter.
- Describe cancer and how it is treated.
- Describe musculo-skeletal and nervous system disorders and the care required.
- Describe cardiovascular and respiratory disorders and the care required.
- Describe digestive, urinary, and reproductive disorders and the care required.
- Describe endocrine, immune system, and skin disorders and the care required.
- Explain how to promote PRIDE in the person, the family, and yourself.

KEY TERMS

arthritis Joint *(arthr)* inflammation *(itis)*
arthroplasty The surgical replacement *(plasty)* of a joint *(arthro)*
benign tumor A tumor that does not spread to other body parts
cancer See "malignant tumor"
emesis See "vomitus"
fracture A broken bone
hemiplegia Paralysis *(plegia)* on 1 side *(hemi)* of the body
hyperglycemia High *(hyper)* sugar *(glyc)* in the blood *(emia)*
hypertension High blood pressure
hypoglycemia Low *(hypo)* sugar *(glyc)* in the blood *(emia)*

malignant tumor A tumor that invades and destroys nearby tissues and can spread to other body parts; cancer
metastasis The spread of cancer to other body parts
paralysis Loss of muscle function
paraplegia Paralysis in the legs and lower trunk
pneumonia Inflammation and infection of lung tissue
quadriplegia Paralysis in the arms, legs, and trunk; tetraplegia
tumor A new growth of abnormal cells that is benign or malignant
vomitus The food and fluids expelled from the stomach through the mouth; emesis

KEY ABBREVIATIONS

AIDS	Acquired immunodeficiency syndrome	IV	Intravenous
ALS	Amyotrophic lateral sclerosis	MI	Myocardial infarction
BPH	Benign prostatic hyperplasia	mm Hg	Millimeters of mercury
CAD	Coronary artery disease	MS	Multiple sclerosis
CKD	Chronic kidney disease	O_2	Oxygen
CO_2	Carbon dioxide	RA	Rheumatoid arthritis
COPD	Chronic obstructive pulmonary disease	ROM	Range-of-motion
CVA	Cerebrovascular accident	STD	Sexually transmitted disease
ESRD	End-stage renal disease	STI	Sexually transmitted infection
HBV	Hepatitis B virus	TB	Tuberculosis
HIV	Human immunodeficiency virus	TIA	Transient ischemic attack
IBD	Inflammatory bowel disease	UTI	Urinary tract infection

Understanding common health problems gives meaning to the required care. The nurse gives you more information as needed. See Chapter 9 for more information on body structure and function.

CANCER

Cells reproduce for tissue growth and repair. Cells divide in an orderly way. Sometimes cell division and growth are out of control. A mass or clump of cells develops. This *new growth of abnormal cells is called a* **tumor.** *Tumors are benign or malignant* (Fig. 40-1).

- *Benign tumors do not spread to other body parts.* They can grow to a large size but rarely threaten life. They usually do not grow back when removed.
- *Malignant tumors (cancer) invade and destroy nearby tissues. They can spread to other body parts.* They may be life-threatening. Sometimes they grow back after removal.

    Metastasis is the spread of cancer to other body parts (Fig. 40-2). If not treated and controlled, cancer cells break off the tumor and travel to other body parts. New tumors grow at those sites.

Risk Factors

Cancer is the second leading cause of death in the United States. The National Cancer Institute describes these risk factors.

- *Age.* Advancing age is the most important risk factor. However, cancer can occur at any age.
- *Tobacco.* This includes using tobacco (smoking, snuff, and chewing tobacco) and being around tobacco (second-hand smoke). This risk can be avoided.
- *Radiation.* Sources are sun light, x-rays, and radon gas that forms in the soil and some rocks.
- *Infections.* Certain viruses and bacteria increase the risk of cancers—cervix, penis, vagina, anus, nose and throat, lung, liver, lymphoma, leukemia, Kaposi's sarcoma (associated with acquired immunodeficiency syndrome [AIDS], p. 525), stomach.
- *Immuno-suppressive drugs.* Such drugs are often used for organ transplant patients to prevent rejection of the transplant. They lower the body's ability to stop cancer from forming.
- *Alcohol.* Alcohol is linked to the increased risk of cancers of the mouth, throat, esophagus, larynx, liver, and breast.
- *Hormones.* The female hormones estrogen and progesterone are known to increase the risk of breast and uterine cancers.
- *Diet and obesity.* A healthy diet, physical activity, and a healthy weight may reduce the risk of some cancers. Obesity is linked to post-menopausal breast cancer and cancers of the colon, rectum, uterus, esophagus, kidney, pancreas, and gallbladder.
- *Environment.* Air pollution, second-hand smoke, and asbestos are linked to lung cancer. Drinking water with large amounts of arsenic is linked to skin, bladder, and lung cancers.

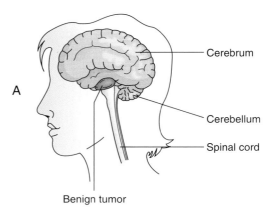

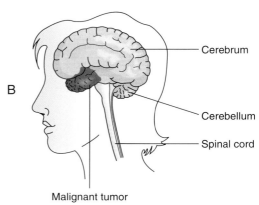

FIGURE 40-1 Tumors. **A,** A benign tumor grows within a local area. **B,** A malignant tumor invades other tissues.

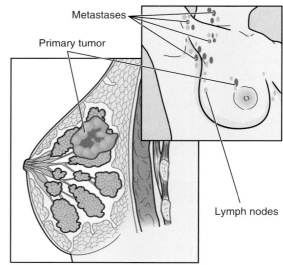

FIGURE 40-2 A tumor in the breast has metastasized to the lymph nodes.

Cancer Signs and Symptoms

Cancer can occur almost anywhere. Box 40-1 lists some signs and symptoms of cancer. Cancer may not cause pain. Waiting for pain as a symptom can delay diagnosis and treatment. If detected early, cancer can be treated and controlled.

BOX 40-1 Cancer—Signs and Symptoms

- Breast changes
  - Lump or firm feeling in the breast or under the arm
  - Nipple changes or discharge
  - Itchy, red, scaly, dimpled, or puckered skin
- Bladder changes
  - Trouble urinating
  - Pain with urination
  - *Hematuria*—blood in the urine
- Bleeding or bruising for no known reason
- Bowel changes
  - Blood in the stools
  - Changes in bowel habits
- Cough or hoarseness that does not go away
- Eating problems
  - Pain after eating (heartburn or indigestion that does not go away)
  - Abdominal pain
  - Trouble swallowing
  - Nausea and vomiting
  - Changes in appetite
- Fatigue (severe and lasting)
- Fever or night sweats for no known reason
- Mouth changes
  - A white or red patch on the tongue or in the mouth
  - Bleeding, pain, or numbness in the lip or mouth
- Neurological problems
  - Headaches
  - Seizures
  - Vision changes
  - Hearing changes
  - Facial drooping
- Skin changes
  - A skin-colored lump that bleeds or turns scaly
  - A new mole or a change in an existing mole
  - A sore that does not heal
  - *Jaundice*—yellowish skin and eyes
- Swelling or lumps on any body part
- Weight gain or loss for no known reason

Modified from National Cancer Institute: *Symptoms of cancer*, updated May 16, 2019.

Treatment

Treatment depends on the tumor type, its site and size, and if it has spread. The treatment goal may be to:

- Cure the cancer.
- Control the disease.
- Reduce symptoms.

Common treatments are surgery, radiation therapy, and chemotherapy.

- *Surgery* removes tumors.
- *Radiation therapy (radiotherapy)* kills cancer cells. X-ray beams are aimed at the tumor. Sometimes radioactive material is implanted in or near the tumor. Cancer cells and normal cells receive radiation. Healthy cells are damaged. Skin changes occur at the treatment site—dryness, itching, swelling, peeling, redness, blistering, hair loss. Special skin care measures are ordered. Extra rest is needed for fatigue. Discomfort, nausea, vomiting, diarrhea, and loss of appetite *(anorexia)* are other side effects.
- *Chemotherapy* involves drugs that kill cancer cells. Cancer cells and normal cells are affected. Side effects include fatigue, hair loss *(alopecia)*, poor appetite, nausea, vomiting, diarrhea, and *stomatitis*—inflammation *(itis)* of the mouth *(stomat)*. Bleeding and infection are risks from decreased blood cell production. Emotional changes and changes in thinking and memory can occur.

The Person's Needs

Persons with cancer have many needs. They include:
- Pain relief or control
- Rest and exercise
- Fluids and nutrition
- Preventing skin breakdown
- Preventing constipation or diarrhea
- Dealing with treatment side effects
- Psychological, social, and spiritual needs
- Sexual needs

Anger, fear, and depression are common. Some surgeries are disfiguring. The person may feel unwhole, unattractive, or unclean. The person and family need support.

Spiritual needs are important. A spiritual leader may provide comfort. To many people, spiritual needs are just as important as physical needs.

Persons dying of cancer often receive hospice care (Chapters 1 and 44). Support is given to the person and family.

See *Focus on Communication: The Person's Needs.*

FOCUS ON **COMMUNICATION**

The Person's Needs

Knowing what to say to a person with cancer can be hard. Talk as you would with any other person. Avoid comments like "I'm sure you will be fine" or "It will be okay."

Often the person needs to talk and have someone listen. Listen and use touch to show you care. Being there when needed is important. You may not have to say anything. Just listen.

MUSCULO-SKELETAL DISORDERS

Musculo-skeletal disorders affect movement. Injury and aging are common causes. Daily living, social activities, and quality of life are affected.

Arthritis

Arthritis means joint (arthr) *inflammation* (itis). Affected joints have swelling, stiffness, and reduced range of motion. The joints are hard to move.

The 2 main types of arthritis are:

- *Osteoarthritis.* Cartilage at the ends of bones is damaged and wears away, causing the bones to rub together. The hands, knees, hips, and spine are often affected (Fig. 40-3).
- *Rheumatoid arthritis (RA).* RA is an autoimmune disorder (p. 524) that attacks the lining of the joints. RA causes inflammation and painful swelling. Many joints are affected at the same time. The wrists, hands, and knees are commonly affected. RA can also affect the neck, shoulders, elbows, hips, ankles, and feet. RA occurs on both sides of the body. For example, both the right and left wrists are affected. RA can cause fever and fatigue and affect other tissues and organs. The lungs, heart, and eyes are examples.

Risk Factors. Arthritis risk factors include:

- *Aging.* The risk increases with age.
- *Being over-weight.* Stress is placed on the weight-bearing joints—knees, hips, and spine.
- *Biological sex.* Arthritis is more common in women.
- *Joint injury.* A previous joint injury or over-use of a joint may develop into osteoarthritis.
- *Family history.* Arthritis tends to run in families.

Treatment. Osteoarthritis and RA have no cure. Treatments are similar.

- *Pain control.* Drugs decrease swelling and inflammation and relieve pain.
- *Heat and cold.* Heat relieves pain, increases blood flow, and reduces stiffness. Sometimes cold is applied after joint use.
- *Exercise.* Exercise helps joint flexibility. It helps with weight control and promotes fitness. The person is taught needed exercises.
- *Rest and joint care.* Good body mechanics, posture, and regular rest protect the joints. Relaxation methods are helpful.
- *Adaptive (assistive) devices.* Canes and walkers provide support. Splints support weak joints and promote alignment. Devices for hands and wrists are useful.

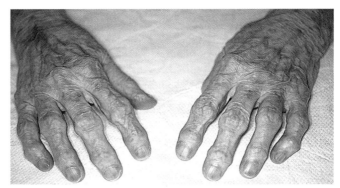

FIGURE 40-3 Osteoarthritis in the finger joints. (From Swartz MH: *Textbook of physical diagnosis: history and examination,* ed 8, Philadelphia, 2021, Elsevier.)

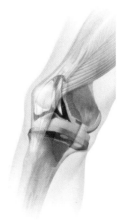

FIGURE 40-4 Knee replacement prosthesis. (Courtesy Zimmer, Inc., A Bristol-Meyers Squibb Company, Warsaw, Ind.)

- *Weight control.* Weight loss reduces stress on weight-bearing joints and prevents further joint injury.
- *Healthy life-style.* The focus is on fitness, exercise, rest, managing stress, and good nutrition.
- *Safety.* Falls are prevented. Help is given with activities of daily living (ADL) as needed. Elevated toilet seats are helpful when hips and knees are affected. So are chairs with higher seats and armrests.
- *Joint replacement surgery. Arthroplasty is the surgical replacement* (plasty) *of a joint* (arthro). The damaged joint is removed and replaced with an artificial joint *(prosthesis).* Hip and knee replacements are common (Fig. 40-4). See Figure 40-5 and Box 40-2 for care measures. Ankle, foot, shoulder, elbow, and finger joints also can be replaced.

Do **Do Not**

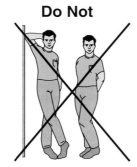

Do not cross your operated leg past the mid-line of the body or turn your kneecap in toward your body.

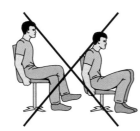

Do not sit in low chairs or cross your legs.

To sit: Use a high chair with arms or add pillows to elevate the seat.

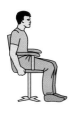

Avoid flexing your hips past 90 degrees.

To bend: Keep the operative leg behind you or as instructed by your therapist.

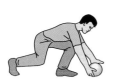

To reach: Use long-handled grabbers or as your therapist advises.

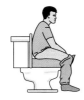

Use an elevated toilet.

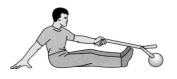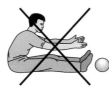

Sleep with a pillow between the legs.

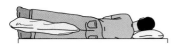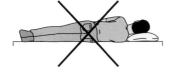

FIGURE 40-5 Measures to protect the hip after hip replacement surgery. (Modified from Monahan FD et al.: *Phipps' medical-surgical nursing: health and illness perspectives,* ed 8, St Louis, 2007, Mosby.)

BOX 40-2 Care After Joint Replacement—Hip or Knee

- Deep-breathing and coughing exercises to prevent respiratory complications.
- Elastic stockings to prevent *thrombi* (blood clots) in the legs.
- Physical therapy and exercises to strengthen the hip or knee.
- Measures to protect the hip as shown in Figure 40-5.
- Food and fluids for tissue healing and to restore strength.
- Safety measures to prevent falls.
- Measures to prevent infection. Wound, urinary tract, and skin infections must be prevented.
- Measures to prevent pressure injuries.
- Assist devices for moving, turning, re-positioning, and transfers.
- Long-handled devices for reaching things.
- Assistance with walking and a walking aid—cane, walker, or crutches.

Osteoporosis

With osteoporosis, the bone *(osteo)* becomes porous and brittle *(porosis).* Bones are fragile and break easily. Fractures (broken bones) can occur during normal daily activities. Spine, hip, and wrist fractures are common. (See "Fractures" on p. 508.)

Risk factors include:
- Aging.
- Biological sex. Women are at higher risk because of the loss of estrogen after menopause.
- Being thin and small.
- A family history of osteoporosis.
- A diet low in calcium and vitamin D.
- Tobacco and alcohol use.
- Eating disorders (Chapter 41).
- Bed rest, immobility, and lack of exercise. Bones must bear weight for strength and to form properly.

A broken bone is often the first sign of osteoporosis. A break in the spine can cause sloped shoulders, curving of the back, loss of height, back pain, and a hunched (bent over) posture.

Prevention is important. Calcium and vitamin supplements may be ordered to prevent bone loss and build new bone. Estrogen is ordered for some women. Other preventive measures include:
- Exercising weight-bearing joints—walking, jogging, stair climbing, weight lifting, dancing, and so on
- Eating foods that contain calcium and vitamin D
- No smoking and limiting alcohol
- Safety measures to prevent falls and accidents
- Good posture and body mechanics
- Safe moving, transfer, turning, and positioning procedures

Fractures

A *fracture is a broken bone.* Fractures are open or closed (Fig. 40-6).

- *Open fracture (compound fracture)*—the broken bone has come through the skin.
- *Closed fracture (simple fracture)*—the bone is broken but the skin is intact.

Falls, accidents, sports injuries, bone tumors, and osteoporosis are some causes. Signs and symptoms of a fracture are:

- Pain
- Swelling and tenderness
- Problems moving the part
- Deformity (the part looks out of place)
- Bruising and skin color changes at the fracture site
- Bleeding (internal or external)
- Numbness and tingling

For healing, bone ends are brought into and held in normal position. This is called *reduction and fixation.*

- Reduction—the bone is moved back into place.
  - Closed reduction—the bone is not exposed.
  - Open reduction—the bone is surgically exposed and moved into alignment.
- Fixation—the bone is held (fixed) in place.
  - External fixation—Pins, screws, or wires are set into the bone outside the skin. The device is removed after healing or when the person is healthy enough for internal fixation of the fracture.
  - Internal fixation—Nails, rods, pins, screws, plates, or wires are surgically placed. The device is under the skin.

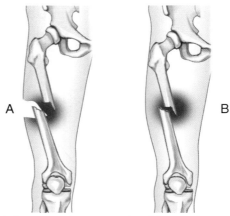

FIGURE 40-6 **A,** Open fracture. **B,** Closed fracture. (From Patton KT, Thibodeau GA: *The human body in health & disease,* ed 7, St Louis, 2018, Elsevier.)

Casts and traction are also used. Devices such as splints and walking boots are common. Healing can take 6 to 8 weeks or longer depending on age, type of fracture, and general health.

Casts. Casts are made of fiberglass or plastic. First, a stockinette and padding are applied to protect the skin. Then, wet plaster or fiberglass strips or rolls are wrapped around the part.

Fiberglass casts dry quickly. A plaster cast dries in 24 to 48 hours. When wet, it is gray and cool and has a musty smell. It is odorless, white, and shiny when dry. The nurse may ask you to assist with care (Box 40-3).

BOX 40-3 Cast Care

The Cast

- Do not cover the cast with blankets, plastic, or other material. A cast gives off heat as it dries. Covers prevent the escape of heat. Burns can occur if heat cannot escape.
- Promote drying of the cast. Turn the person at least every 2 hours or as directed. All cast surfaces need exposure to air.
- Maintain the shape of the cast.
  - Do not place a wet cast on a hard surface. It flattens the cast.
  - Use pillows to support the entire length of the cast (Fig. 40-7).
  - Support the wet cast with your palms to turn and position the person (Fig. 40-8). Fingertips can dent the cast, causing pressure areas and skin breakdown.
  - Report rough cast edges. The nurse may cover the cast edges with tape.
  - Keep the cast dry. A wet cast loses its shape. For casts near the perineal area, the nurse may apply a waterproof material after the cast dries.
- Do not remove stockinette or padding around the cast edges.

Positioning

- Position the person as directed.
- Elevate a casted arm or leg on pillows to reduce swelling.
- Have enough help to turn and re-position the person. Plaster casts are heavy and awkward. Balance is lost easily.

Safety

- Follow the care plan for elimination needs. Some persons use a fracture pan.
- Do not let the person insert things into the cast (pencils, back scratchers, and so on). Itching under the cast causes an intense desire to scratch. Items used to scratch can open the skin, wrinkle the stockinette or padding, or be lost into the cast. Skin breakdown, pressure injury, and infection are risks.
- Do not put powder under the cast.
- Do not let the person wear rings on the fingers or toes. The fingers or toes may swell or be swollen.
- Complete a safety check before leaving the room. (See the inside of the back cover.)

Reporting and Recording

- Report these signs and symptoms at once.
  - *Pain*—pressure injury, poor circulation, nerve damage
  - *Swelling and a tight cast*—reduced blood flow to the part
  - *Pale skin*—reduced blood flow to the part
  - *Cyanosis* (bluish skin color)—reduced blood flow to the part
  - *Odor*—infection
  - *Inability to move the fingers or toes*—pressure on a nerve
  - *Numbness*—pressure on a nerve, reduced blood flow to the part
  - *Temperature changes*—cool skin means poor circulation; hot skin means inflammation
  - *Drainage on or under the cast*—infection or bleeding
  - *Chills, fever, nausea, and vomiting*—infection

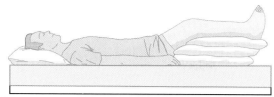

FIGURE 40-7 Pillows support the entire length of the wet cast.

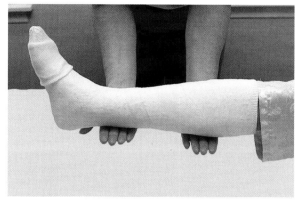

FIGURE 40-8 The cast is supported with the palms.

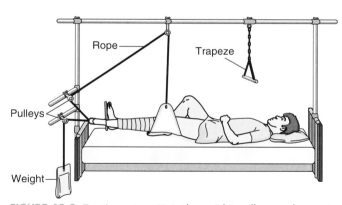

FIGURE 40-9 Traction set-up. Note the weight, pulleys, and rope. A trapeze is used to raise the upper body off of the bed. (Modified from Monahan FD et al.: *Phipps' medical-surgical nursing: health and illness perspectives*, ed 8, St Louis, 2007, Mosby.)

BOX 40-4 Traction Care

- Keep the person in good alignment.
- Do not remove the traction.
- Keep the weights off of the floor. Weights must hang freely from the traction set-up (see Fig. 40-9).
- Do not add or remove weights.
- Check for frayed ropes. Report fraying at once.
- Perform range-of-motion (ROM) exercises for uninvolved joints as directed.
- Position the person as directed. Usually only the supine position is allowed. Slight turning may be allowed.
- Provide the fracture pan for elimination.
- Give skin care as directed.
- Put bottom linens on the bed from the top down. The person uses a trapeze to raise the body off of the bed (see Fig. 40-9).
- Check pin, nail, wire, or tong sites for redness, drainage, and odors. Report observations at once.
- Observe for the signs and symptoms listed under cast care (see Box 40-3). Report them at once.
- Complete a safety check before leaving the room. (See the inside of the back cover.)

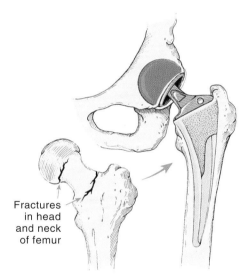

FIGURE 40-10 Hip fracture repaired with a prosthesis. (Modified from Cooper K, Gosnell K: *Adult health nursing*, ed 8, St Louis, 2019, Elsevier.)

Hip Fractures. Common in older persons, hip fractures require surgical repair or a hip replacement (Fig. 40-10). Adduction, internal rotation, external rotation, and severe hip flexion are avoided after surgery. Rehabilitation is usually needed.

Post-operative problems present life-threatening risks. They include pneumonia, urinary tract infections, and *thrombi* (blood clots) in the leg veins or lungs. Pressure injuries, constipation, and confusion are other problems. Box 40-5 (p. 510) describes the required care.

Traction. With traction, a steady pull from 2 directions keeps the bone in place. Weights, ropes, and pulleys are used (Fig. 40-9). Traction is applied to the neck, arms, legs, or pelvis. To assist with the person's care, see Box 40-4.

BOX 40-5 Hip Fracture Care

- Give good skin care. Skin breakdown can be rapid.
- Prevent pressure injuries.
- Prevent wound, skin, and urinary tract infections.
- Encourage deep-breathing and coughing exercises as directed.
- Turn and position the person as directed. Usually the person is not positioned on the operative side.
- Prevent external rotation of the hip. Use trochanter rolls, pillows, or sandbags.
- Keep the leg abducted at all times. Use pillows (Fig. 40-11) or a hip abduction wedge (abductor splint).
- Do not exercise the affected leg. The physical therapist helps the person with rehabilitation exercises.
- Provide a straight-back chair with armrests. The person needs a high, firm seat.
- Place the chair on the unaffected side for transfers.
- Use assist devices to move, turn, re-position, and transfer the person.
- Do not let the person stand on the operated leg unless allowed by the doctor.
- Elevate the leg following the care plan. With an internal fixation device, the leg is not elevated when the person sits in a chair. Elevating the leg puts strain on the device.
- Apply elastic stockings as directed to prevent *thrombi* (blood clots) in the legs.
- Assist with walking according to the care plan. The person may use a walker.
- Follow measures to protect the hip. (The measures from Figure 40-5 apply.) The person:
  - Does not cross the affected leg past the mid-line of the body.
  - Does not turn the kneecap on the affected side in toward the body.
  - Does not sit in low chairs.
  - Does not cross the legs.
  - Does not flex the hips past 90 degrees.
  - Uses long-handled devices for reaching.
  - Uses an elevated toilet seat.
  - Sleeps with a pillow between the legs.
- Practice safety measures to prevent falls.
- Complete a safety check before leaving the room. (See the inside of the back cover.)

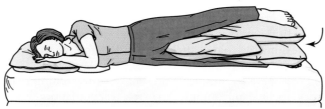

FIGURE 40-11 Pillows are used to keep the hip in abduction. (From Monahan FD et al.: *Phipps' medical-surgical nursing: health and illness perspectives*, ed 8, St Louis, 2007, Mosby.)

Loss of Limb

An *amputation* is the removal of all or part of an extremity. Severe injuries, tumors, severe infection, gangrene, and vascular disorders are common causes. Diabetes can cause vascular changes leading to amputation.

Gangrene is a condition in which there is death of tissue. Causes include poor blood flow from infection, injuries, or vascular disorders. Tissues do not get enough oxygen and nutrients. Tissues become black, cold, shriveled, and die (Fig. 40-12). Surgery is needed to remove dead tissue. Gangrene can cause death.

A *prosthesis* is an artificial replacement for a missing body part (Fig. 40-13). Occupational and physical therapists help the person learn to use the prosthesis.

The person may feel that the limb is still there. Aching, tingling, and itching are common sensations. Or the person complains of pain in the amputated part (*phantom pain*). This is a normal reaction. It may occur for a short time or for many years.

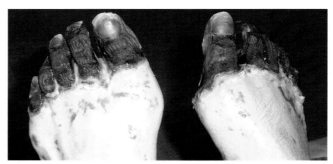

FIGURE 40-12 Gangrene. (From Centers for Disease Control and Prevention/Christina Nelson, MD, MPH, 2012.)

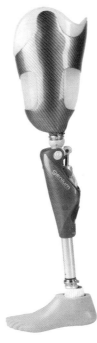

FIGURE 40-13 Above-the-knee prosthesis. (Courtesy Otto Bock Health Care, Minneapolis, Minn.)

NERVOUS SYSTEM DISORDERS

Nervous system disorders can affect mental and physical function. They can affect the ability to speak, understand, feel, see, hear, touch, think, control bowels and bladder, and move.

Stroke

Stroke *(brain attack* or *cerebrovascular accident [CVA])* occurs when 1 of these happens.
* A blood vessel in the brain bursts and bleeds into the brain (cerebral hemorrhage).
* A blood clot blocks a blood vessel in the brain. Blood flow stops.

Brain cells in the affected area do not get enough oxygen and nutrients. Brain damage occurs. Functions controlled by that part of the brain are lost (Fig. 40-14).

Stroke is a leading cause of disability and death in the United States. The person needs emergency care.

Stroke Signs and Symptoms. Stroke occurs suddenly. See Box 40-6 for the major signs and symptoms. Nausea and vomiting, seizures, or loss of consciousness may occur.

When signs and symptoms only last a few minutes, this is called a *transient ischemic attack (TIA). (Transient* means *temporary* or *short term. Ischemic* means *to hold back* [ischein] *blood* [hemic].) During a TIA, blood supply to the brain is interrupted for a short time. A TIA may occur before a stroke.

All stroke-like symptoms signal the need for emergency care. Blood flow to the brain must be restored as soon as possible.

BOX 40-6 Stroke—Signs and Symptoms

* Sudden numbness or weakness of the face, arm, or leg, especially on 1 side of the body
* Sudden confusion, trouble speaking or understanding speech
* Sudden trouble seeing in 1 or both eyes
* Sudden trouble walking, dizziness, loss of balance or coordination
* Sudden, severe headache with no known cause

From National Institute of Neurological Disorders and Stroke: *Know stroke. Know the signs. Act in time.* NIH Publication Number 13-4872, Bethesda, Md, July 2013, National Institutes of Health.

Effects on the Person. If the person survives, some brain damage is likely. Effects of stroke include:
* Loss of face, hand, arm, leg, or body control
* *Hemiplegia—paralysis* (plegia) *on 1 side* (hemi) *of the body*
* Changing emotions—crying easily or mood swings sometimes for no reason
* Difficulty swallowing *(dysphagia)*
* Aphasia or slowed or slurred speech (Chapter 39)
* Changes in sight, touch, movement, and thought
* Impaired memory
* Urinary frequency, urgency, or incontinence
* Loss of bowel control or constipation
* Depression and frustration
* Behavior changes

Rehabilitation starts at once. The person may depend in part or totally on others for care. The goal is to regain the highest possible level of function (Box 40-7, p. 512).

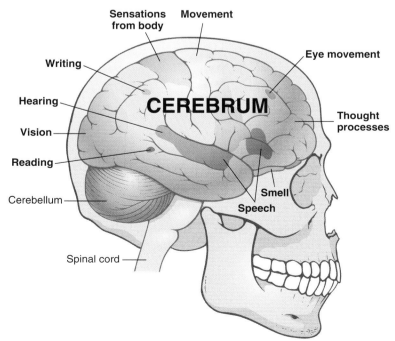

FIGURE 40-14 Functions lost from a stroke depend on the area of brain damage. (From Chabner DE: *The language of medicine,* ed 12, St Louis, 2021, Elsevier.)

BOX 40-7 Stroke Care Measures

- Position the person in the side-lying position to prevent aspiration.
- Keep the bed in semi-Fowler's position.
- Approach the person from the strong (unaffected) side. The person may have loss of vision on the affected side.
- Turn and re-position the person at least every 2 hours.
- Use assist devices to move, turn, re-position, and transfer the person.
- Encourage deep breathing and coughing.
- Prevent contractures. Assist with ROM exercises.
- Prevent pressure injuries.
- Meet food and fluid needs. A dysphagia diet is common (Chapter 29).
- Apply elastic stockings as directed to prevent *thrombi* (blood clots) in the legs.
- Meet elimination needs. Follow the care plan for:
  - Catheter care or bladder training
  - Bowel training
- Practice safety precautions.
  - Keep the call light and other needed items within reach on the strong (unaffected) side.
  - Check the person often. Follow the care plan.
  - Use bed rails according to the care plan.
  - Prevent falls and other injuries.
- Encourage as much self-care as possible. This includes turning, positioning, and transferring. The person uses adaptive (assistive) devices and walking aids as needed.
- Do not rush the person. Movements are slower after a stroke.
- Follow established communication methods.
- Give support, encouragement, and praise.
- Complete a safety check before leaving the room. (See the inside of the back cover.)

Parkinson's Disease

Parkinson's disease is a progressive disorder affecting movement. It occurs when nerve cells in the brain do not produce enough of a chemical called *dopamine*. Dopamine is needed for smooth, purposeful movement. Persons over the age of 60 are at higher risk.

Signs and symptoms are mild at first on 1 side of the body (Fig. 40-15). They worsen over time and affect both sides of the body. The main signs are:

- *Tremors*—often start in the hand. Pill-rolling movements (rubbing the thumb and index finger) may occur. There may be trembling in the hands, arms, legs, jaw, and face. Shaking has a rhythmic back-and-forth motion.
- *Rigid, stiff muscles*—occur in the arms, legs, neck, and trunk. (The trunk [torso] is the chest and abdomen.)
- *Slow movement*—the person develops short, shuffling steps. Simple tasks are hard to do.
- *Stooped posture and impaired balance*—it is hard to walk. Falls are a risk.

Other signs and symptoms develop over time. They include swallowing and chewing problems, constipation, sleep problems, depression, and emotional changes (fear, insecurity). Memory loss and slow thinking can occur. The person may have slow, monotone, and soft speech. A fixed stare and trouble blinking and smiling can occur.

With no cure, drugs are used to control the disease. Exercise and physical therapy help improve strength, posture, balance, and mobility. Therapy is needed for speech and swallowing problems. The person may need help with eating and self-care. Normal elimination is a goal. Safety measures are needed to prevent falls and injuries.

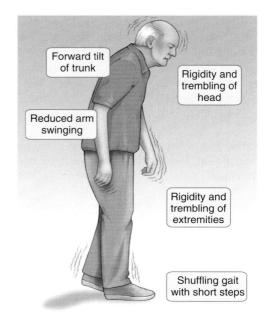

FIGURE 40-15 Signs of Parkinson's disease. (From Patton KT, Thibodeau GA: *The human body in health & disease*, ed 7, St Louis, 2018, Elsevier.)

Multiple Sclerosis

Multiple means *many*. *Sclerosis* means *hardening* or *scarring*. In multiple sclerosis (MS), the myelin (which covers nerve fibers) in the brain and spinal cord is destroyed. Nerve impulses between the body and brain are not sent in a normal way. Functions are impaired or lost.

Symptoms usually start between the ages of 20 and 40. Whites and women are at greater risk than other groups. The risk increases if a family member has MS.

Signs and symptoms of MS vary widely depending on the nerves affected. They may include:

- Blurred or double vision; blindness in 1 eye
- Muscle weakness in the arms and legs
- Balance and coordination problems
- Tingling, prickling, or numb sensations
- Partial or complete paralysis
- Pain
- Speech problems
- Tremors
- Dizziness
- Concentration, attention, memory, and judgment problems
- Depression
- Bladder problems
- Problems with sexual function
- Hearing loss
- Fatigue

MS can present in many ways. For example:

- Symptoms appear for a while then seem to go away. The person is in *remission*. Later, symptoms flare up again *(relapse)*.
- More symptoms appear. The condition worsens.
- There are remissions and relapses at first. Eventually symptoms become worse. More symptoms occur with each flare-up. The person's condition declines.

MS has no cure. Some drugs can slow the disease and help control symptoms. Persons with MS are kept as active and as independent as possible. The care plan reflects changing needs. Skin care, hygiene, and ROM exercises are important. So are turning, positioning, and deep breathing and coughing. Elimination needs are met. Injuries and complications from bed rest are prevented.

Amyotrophic Lateral Sclerosis

Amyotrophic lateral sclerosis (ALS) affects the nerve cells in the brain and spinal cord that control voluntary muscles. Muscles in the arms and legs and those used for chewing and talking are voluntary. Commonly called *Lou Gehrig's disease*, it is rapidly progressive and fatal. (Lou Gehrig was a New York Yankees baseball player who died of the disease.)

ALS usually strikes persons between 55 and 75 years of age. Most die 3 to 5 years after onset.

Affected nerve cells in the brain and spinal cord stop sending messages to the voluntary muscles. Muscles weaken, waste away *(atrophy)*, and twitch. Over time, the brain cannot start or control voluntary movements. The person cannot move the arms, legs, and body. Muscles for speaking, chewing and swallowing, and breathing also are affected. Eventually respiratory muscles fail.

The disease usually does not affect the mind, intelligence, or memory. Sight, smell, taste, hearing, and touch are not affected. Usually bowel and bladder functions remain intact.

ALS has no cure. Some drugs can slow the disease and improve symptoms. However, damage cannot be reversed. The person is kept active and independent to the extent possible. The care plan reflects changing needs.

Spinal Cord Injury

Spinal cord injury usually results from a sudden, traumatic blow to the spine. Common causes are vehicle accidents, falls, violence (knife and gunshot wounds), and sports injuries. Cancer and other diseases can also cause injury.

Serious damage to the nervous system can occur. Problems depend on the amount of damage to the spinal cord and the level of injury. *Paralysis (loss of muscle function)* can result. Sensation and body functions are also affected. The higher the level of injury, the more functions lost (Fig. 40-16).

- Lumbar injuries—occur in the low back. Sensory and muscle function in the legs is lost. The person has paraplegia. *Paraplegia is paralysis in the legs and lower trunk. (Para means beyond; plegia means paralysis).*
- Thoracic injuries—occur in the middle and upper back. Sensory and muscle function below the chest is lost. The person has paraplegia.
- Cervical injuries—occur at the neck. Sensory and muscle function of the arms, legs, and trunk is lost. *Paralysis in the arms, legs, and trunk is called* **quadriplegia** *(tetraplegia). Quad and tetra mean 4. Plegia means paralysis.*

Cervical traction with a special bed may be needed. The spine is kept straight at all times. See Box 40-8 (p. 514) for care measures. Emotional needs are great. Reactions to paralysis and loss of function are often severe. If the person lives, rehabilitation is needed.

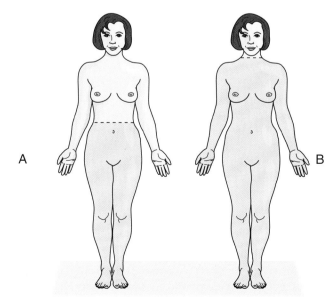

FIGURE 40-16 The *shaded areas* show the area of paralysis. **A,** Paraplegia. **B,** Quadriplegia (tetraplegia).

BOX 40-8 Paralysis—Care Measures

- Practice safety measures to prevent falls. Use bed rails as directed.
- Keep the bed in a low position. Follow the care plan.
- Keep the call light and other needed items within reach. If unable to use the call light, check the person often.
- Prevent burns. Check bath water, heat applications, and food for proper temperature.
- Turn (logroll) and re-position the person at least every 2 hours.
- Prevent pressure injuries. Follow the care plan.
- Use supportive devices for good alignment.
- Follow bowel and bladder training programs.
- Keep intake and output records.
- Maintain muscle function and prevent contractures. Assist with ROM exercises.
- Assist with food and fluid needs. Provide adaptive (assistive) devices as ordered.
- Give emotional and psychological support.
- Follow the person's rehabilitation plan.
- Complete a safety check of the room. (See the inside of the back cover.)

Head Injuries

Head injuries result from trauma to the scalp, skull, or brain. Injuries range from a minor bump to a serious, life-threatening brain injury.

Traumatic brain injury (TBI) occurs from violent injury to the brain. Falls, vehicle accidents, and violence (assaults, gunshots) are common causes. So are sports and combat injuries.

Brain tissue is bruised or torn. Bleeding is in the brain or in nearby tissues. Spinal cord injuries are likely. If the person survives, some permanent damage is likely. Disabilities depend on the severity and site of injury. They include:

- Cognitive problems—thinking, memory, reasoning
- Sensory problems—sight, hearing, touch, taste, smell
- Communication problems—expressing or understanding language
- Emotional problems—depression, anxiety, personality changes, aggressive behavior, acting out, socially inappropriate behavior
- Changes in level of consciousness:
  - Stupor—the person is unresponsive but can be briefly aroused by a strong stimulus (such as pain).
  - Coma—the person is unconscious, does not respond, is unaware, and cannot be aroused.
  - Vegetative state—the person is unconscious and unaware of surroundings. The person has sleep-wake cycles and may open the eyes, make sounds, or move.
  - Brain death—despite complete loss of brain function, the heart continues to beat. Reflex activity, movement, and spontaneous respirations are absent.

Rehabilitation is required. Nursing care depends on the person's needs and abilities.

CARDIOVASCULAR DISORDERS

Cardiovascular disorders are leading causes of death in the United States. Problems occur in the heart or blood vessels.

Hypertension

With every heartbeat, blood is pumped into arteries. Blood pressure is the force of blood pressing against artery walls. Pressure is higher when the heart beats (systole). Pressure is lower when the heart rests (diastole).

Hypertension means high blood pressure. Blood pressure is high when:

- The systolic pressure is 140 mm Hg (millimeters of mercury) or higher.
- The diastolic pressure is 90 mm Hg or higher.

When risk factors are present (Box 40-9), a systolic pressure between 130 and 139 mm Hg or a diastolic pressure between 80 and 89 mm Hg may signal hypertension. Report abnormal blood pressures at once.

Hypertension often does not cause symptoms. Measuring blood pressure regularly is important. Over time, hypertension causes the heart to work harder, leading to other disorders. Heart attack (p. 516), heart failure (p. 516), stroke (p. 511), and kidney failure (p. 522) are examples.

Life-style changes can lower blood pressure. A diet low in fat and salt, a healthy weight, and regular exercise are needed. No smoking is allowed. Alcohol and caffeine are limited. Managing stress and sleeping well also lower blood pressure. Certain drugs lower blood pressure.

BOX 40-9 Cardiovascular Disorders—Risk Factors

Factors You Cannot Control

- Age—45 years or older for men; 55 years or older for women
- Biological sex—risk increases for women after menopause; having diabetes increases the risk more in women than in men
- Race—African Americans are at greater risk
- Family history—tends to run in families; early onset in a close family member increases the risk

Factors You Can Control

- Being over-weight
- Stress
- Smoking and tobacco use
- Poor diet—high in fat, salt, sugar, and cholesterol
- Excessive alcohol use
- Lack of exercise
- Not getting enough sleep
- High blood pressure
- Unhealthy blood cholesterol levels
- Diabetes

Modified from MedlinePlus: *How to prevent heart disease*, Bethesda, Md, updated December 3, 2021, U.S. National Library of Medicine.

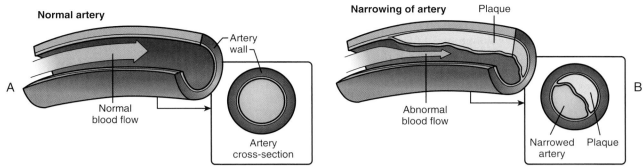

FIGURE 40-17 **A,** Normal artery. **B,** Plaque on the artery wall in atherosclerosis.

Coronary Artery Disease

The *coronary arteries* supply the heart muscle with blood. In coronary artery disease (CAD) (coronary heart disease, heart disease), the coronary arteries become hardened and narrow. One or all are affected. The heart muscle gets less blood and oxygen (O_2).

The most common cause is atherosclerosis (Fig. 40-17). Plaque—made up of cholesterol, fat, and other substances—collects on artery walls. The narrowed arteries block some or all blood flow. Blood clots can form along the plaque and block blood flow.

Major complications of CAD are angina, heart attack, heart failure, irregular heartbeats, and sudden death. The more risk factors present (see Box 40-9), the greater the chance of CAD and its complications.

Treatment goals are to:
* Relieve symptoms (see "Angina")
* Slow or stop atherosclerosis
* Lower the risk of blood clots
* Widen or bypass clogged arteries
* Prevent complications

CAD requires life-style changes (see "Hypertension"). Some drugs decrease the heart's workload and relieve symptoms. Drugs may be used to delay medical and surgical procedures that open or bypass diseased arteries (Fig. 40-18).

Angina

Angina is chest pain from reduced blood flow to part of the heart muscle *(myocardium)*. *(Angina* comes from the Latin word *angor* that means *strangling.)* It occurs when the heart needs more O_2. Normally blood flow to the heart increases when O_2 needs increase. Exertion, a heavy meal, stress, and excitement increase the heart's need for O_2. So does smoking and very hot or cold temperatures. In CAD, narrowed vessels prevent increased blood flow.

Chest pain is described as tightness, pressure, squeezing, or burning in the chest. Pain can occur in the shoulders, arms, neck, jaw, or back (Fig. 40-19). The person may also have nausea, fatigue, dyspnea, sweating, lightheadedness, and weakness.

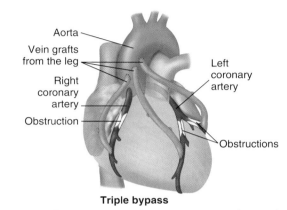

Triple bypass

FIGURE 40-18 Coronary artery bypass surgery. Arteries or veins from other parts of the body are used to bypass (go around) narrowed coronary arteries. (Modified from Patton KT, Thibodeau GA: *The human body in health & disease,* ed 7, St Louis, 2018, Elsevier.)

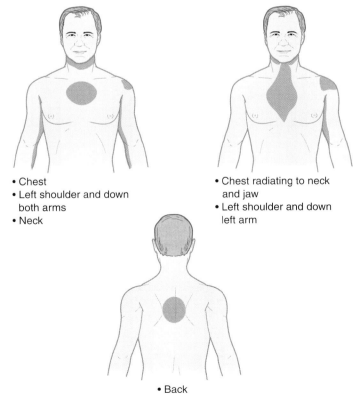

* Chest
* Left shoulder and down both arms
* Neck

* Chest radiating to neck and jaw
* Left shoulder and down left arm

* Back

FIGURE 40-19 *Shaded areas* show common locations and patterns of angina. (Modified from Harding M et al.: *Lewis's Medical-surgical nursing: assessment and management of clinical problems,* ed 11, St Louis, 2020, Elsevier.)

Rest often relieves symptoms in a few minutes. Persons with angina need to know:

- The usual pattern of their symptoms. This includes the causes, usual description and duration of the pain, and if rest or drugs relieve pain.
- What drugs to use and how to use them. *Nitroglycerin* dissolved under the tongue is common.
- How to control angina. Avoiding triggers like physical exertion, stress, and large meals are examples.
- The limits of physical activity. The person should stop activity before symptoms occur.
- When to get emergency care. Pain that is severe, lasts longer than a few minutes, or is not relieved by rest or drugs may signal a heart attack. Emergency care is needed.

See "Coronary Artery Disease" for the treatment of angina. Increased blood flow to the heart lowers the risk of heart attack and death.

Myocardial Infarction

Myocardial refers to the *heart muscle*. *Infarction* means *tissue death*. With myocardial infarction (MI), part of the heart muscle dies from sudden blockage of blood flow in a coronary artery. A thrombus (blood clot) in an artery with atherosclerosis blocks blood flow (Fig. 40-20).

MI also is called:

- Heart attack
- Acute myocardial infarction (AMI)
- Acute coronary syndrome (ACS)

CAD, angina, and previous MI are risk factors. See Box 40-10 for signs and symptoms. MI is an emergency. Efforts are made to:

- Relieve pain.
- Reduce the heart's workload.
- Restore blood flow to the heart.
- Stabilize vital signs.
- Give O_2.
- Calm the person.
- Prevent death and life-threatening problems.

The person may need medical or surgical procedures to open or bypass the diseased artery. Cardiac rehabilitation is needed. The goals are to:

- Recover and resume normal activities.
- Prevent another MI.
- Prevent complications such as heart failure or sudden cardiac arrest (sudden cardiac death) (Chapter 43).

Heart Failure

Heart failure or congestive heart failure (CHF) occurs when the weakened heart cannot pump normally. Blood backs up. Tissue congestion occurs. Heart failure is caused by conditions that damage or over-work the heart muscle. CAD, heart attack, and hypertension are some causes.

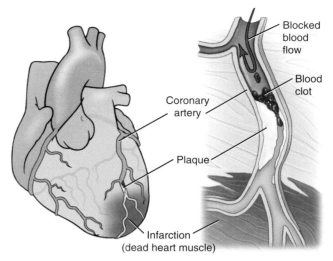

FIGURE 40-20 Myocardial infarction. Blood flow to part of the heart muscle is blocked, causing death of heart tissue.

BOX 40-10 Myocardial Infarction—Signs and Symptoms

- Chest pain or discomfort
  - Usually in the center or on the left side of the chest
  - Lasts more than a few minutes or goes away and comes back
  - Described as pressure, squeezing, fullness, pain, heartburn, or indigestion
  - Mild or severe
  - Different from usual angina pattern or is not relieved by rest or nitroglycerin
- Upper body discomfort—pain in 1 or both arms, the back, shoulders, neck, jaw, or upper stomach
- *Dyspnea* (difficulty breathing)
  - May be the only symptom or may occur before or with chest pain
  - Can occur with rest or during mild physical activity
- Breaking out in a cold sweat
- Unexplained fatigue (especially in women)
- Nausea and vomiting
- Light-headedness or sudden dizziness

Modified from National Heart, Lung, and Blood Institute; National Institutes of Health; U.S. Department of Health and Human Services: *Heart attack*, Bethesda, Md, National Institutes of Health.

Heart failure can affect 1 or both sides of the heart.

- Left side—when the left side of the heart cannot pump normally, blood backs up into the lungs. Respiratory congestion occurs.
- Right side—when the right side of the heart cannot pump normally, blood backs up into the venous system. Swelling occurs (*edema*).
- Both left side and right side—the body does not get enough blood. Signs and symptoms occur from the effects on other organs. See Box 40-11.

Pulmonary edema (fluid in the lungs) can result from heart failure. It is an emergency. The person can die.

Drugs are used to strengthen the heart, decrease strain on the heart, and reduce fluid buildup. A sodium-controlled diet and fluid restriction are often ordered. Oxygen is given. Semi-Fowler's position is preferred for breathing. Rest and activity are balanced. Good skin care and regular position changes are needed due to tissue swelling, poor circulation, and fragile skin. Intake and output (I&O), daily weight, elastic stockings, and ROM exercises are part of the care plan.

RESPIRATORY DISORDERS

The respiratory system brings O_2 into the lungs and removes carbon dioxide (CO_2) from the body. Respiratory disorders interfere with this function and threaten life.

Chronic Obstructive Pulmonary Disease

Chronic obstructive pulmonary disease (COPD) involves 2 disorders—emphysema and chronic bronchitis (Fig. 40-21). These disorders interfere with O_2 and CO_2 exchange in the lungs. They obstruct (block) airflow. Lung function is gradually lost.

Most people with COPD have both emphysema and chronic bronchitis. The severity of each varies for each person.

Cigarette smoking is the greatest risk factor. Pipe, cigar, and other smoking tobaccos are also risk factors. So is exposure to second-hand smoke. Not smoking is the best way to prevent COPD. COPD has no cure.

Emphysema. In emphysema, the alveoli are damaged (see Fig. 40-21). Alveoli lose their shape and become less elastic. They do not expand and shrink normally. As a result, air is trapped and not exhaled. Over time, more alveoli are involved. O_2 and CO_2 exchange cannot occur in affected alveoli.

The person has shortness of breath and a cough. At first, shortness of breath occurs with exertion. Over time, it occurs at rest. Fatigue is common. The body does not get enough O_2. Breathing is easier when sitting upright and slightly forward (Chapter 37).

The person must stop smoking. Respiratory therapy, breathing exercises, oxygen, and drug therapy are ordered.

Chronic Bronchitis. *Bronchitis* means *inflammation* (itis) *of the bronchi* (bronch). With chronic bronchitis, airways are narrowed from inflammation and mucus (see Fig. 40-21).

The main symptom is an on-going cough or a cough that produces a lot of mucus (*smoker's cough*). The person has difficulty breathing and tires easily. The body cannot get enough O_2. Wheezing and chest tightness can occur.

The person must stop smoking. Oxygen therapy and breathing exercises are common. Drugs are given to open airways. Respiratory tract infections are prevented. If one occurs, prompt treatment is needed.

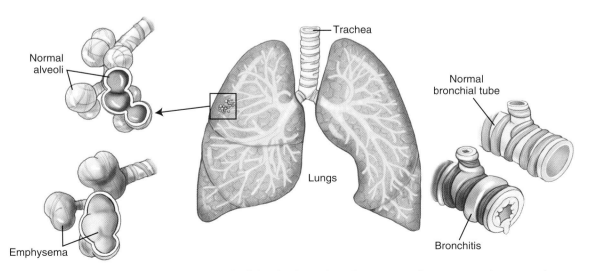

FIGURE 40-21 COPD. Emphysema damages the inner walls of alveoli. Chronic bronchitis causes inflammation and mucus in the airways. (Modified from Brooks ML, Brooks DL: *Exploring medical language: a student-directed approach*, ed 11, St Louis, 2022, Elsevier.)

Asthma

With asthma, the airway becomes inflamed and narrow. Extra mucus is produced. Coughing, wheezing, chest tightness, and shortness of breath can occur.

Asthma usually is triggered by allergies. Other triggers include air pollutants and irritants, smoking and second-hand smoke, respiratory infections, exertion, and cold air.

Asthma is treated with drugs. Episodes of worsening symptoms (asthma attacks) can be life-threatening. Severe attacks require emergency care.

Influenza

Influenza (flu) is a respiratory infection caused by viruses. In the United States, "flu season" occurs in the fall and winter months. During these months—usually ranging from October through March—flu activity is highest. Older persons are at great risk. Pneumonia is a common complication.

Coughing and sneezing spread flu viruses. The virus is also spread when a person touches a contaminated surface or object and then touches the mouth, eyes, or nose.

Signs and symptoms of flu include fever, chills, fatigue, headache, and muscle or body aches. Chest discomfort and cough are common and can be severe. The person may have a runny nose, stuffy nose, or sore throat.

Treatment involves fluids and rest. Drugs are ordered for symptom relief and to shorten the flu episode. Standard Precautions and Droplet Precautions are needed (Chapter 15).

See *Focus on Older Persons: Influenza.*

FOCUS ON OLDER PERSONS

Influenza

Older persons may not have the usual flu signs and symptoms. The following may signal flu in older persons.
- Changes in mental status or behavior
- Worsening of other health problems
- A body temperature below the normal range
- Fatigue
- Decreased appetite and fluid intake

Pneumonia

Pneumonia means inflammation and infection of lung tissue. (Pneumo means lungs.) Affected tissues fill with fluid. O_2 and CO_2 exchange is affected. Bacteria, viruses, and other microbes are causes.

Signs and symptoms of pneumonia include fever, chills, fatigue, productive cough, and shortness of breath. Chest pain with breathing or coughing; nausea, vomiting, or diarrhea; headache; and muscle aches are others.

Drugs are ordered for infection and pain. Fluid intake is increased for fever and to thin secretions. Thin secretions are easier to cough up. Intravenous (IV) therapy and oxygen may be needed. Semi-Fowler's position eases breathing. Rest and mouth care are important. Standard Precautions are followed. Transmission-Based Precautions depend on the cause. Mouth care is important. Frequent linen changes are needed because of fever.

See *Focus on Older Persons: Pneumonia.*

FOCUS ON OLDER PERSONS

Pneumonia

Changes from aging, diseases, and decreased mobility increase the risk of pneumonia in older persons. Decreased mobility after surgery is a risk factor. Aspiration pneumonia is common. For older adults, pneumonia can be life-threatening.

Older persons may not have the usual signs and symptoms. Older persons may have lower than normal body temperature. Confusion or changes in mental awareness can occur.

Tuberculosis

Tuberculosis (TB) is a bacterial infection in the lungs. TB is spread by airborne droplets with coughing, sneezing, speaking, singing, or laughing. Nearby persons can inhale the bacteria. Those with close, frequent contact with an infected person are at risk. TB is more likely to occur in close, crowded areas. Age (very young or very old), poor nutrition, and HIV (human immunodeficiency virus) infection are other risk factors.

TB can be present in the body but not cause signs and symptoms (latent TB). *Latent* means *present but not active.* An active infection may not occur for many years. Only persons with an active infection can spread the disease to others.

Chest x-rays and TB testing can detect the disease. Signs and symptoms are fatigue, loss of appetite, weight loss, fever, chills, and night sweats. The person has a bad cough that lasts 3 weeks or longer. Sputum may contain blood. Chest pain occurs.

Drugs for TB are given. Standard Precautions and Airborne Precautions are needed (Chapter 15). The person must cover the mouth and nose with tissues when sneezing, coughing, or producing sputum. Tissues are discarded in a no-touch waste container. Hand-washing after contact with sputum is essential.

See *Focus on Older Persons: Tuberculosis.*

FOCUS ON OLDER PERSONS

Tuberculosis

With aging, persons infected long ago can develop active TB from declining general health. Other older people with extended contact with those infected can become infected. Nursing center residents are examples.

DIGESTIVE DISORDERS

The digestive system breaks down food into nutrients for the body to absorb. Solid wastes are eliminated. See Chapter 27 for diarrhea, constipation, flatulence, fecal incontinence, and ostomy care.

Vomiting

Vomitus (emesis) is the food and fluids expelled from the stomach through the mouth. Vomiting signals illness or injury. Aspirated vomitus can obstruct the airway. Vomiting large amounts of blood can lead to shock (Chapter 43). Provide for safety and comfort when vomiting occurs.

- Follow Standard Precautions and the Bloodborne Pathogen Standard.
- Turn the person's head well to 1 side if the person is supine. This prevents aspiration.
- Place a kidney basin under the chin.
- Move vomitus away from the person.
- Provide oral hygiene. This helps remove the bitter taste of vomitus.
- Eliminate odors.
- Provide comfort measures. (See the inside of the back cover.)
- Report your observations.
  - Observe vomitus for blood, color, odor, and undigested food. If it looks like coffee grounds, it contains blood.
  - Measure, report, and record the amount of vomitus and your observations.
  - Save a specimen for laboratory study if needed.
  - Dispose of vomitus after the nurse observes it.

Diverticular Disease

Small pouches can develop in the colon. The pouches bulge outward through weak spots in the colon wall (Fig. 40-22). A pouch is called a *diverticulum*. (*Diverticulare* means *to turn inside out*). *Diverticulosis* is the condition of having these pouches. (*Osis* means *condition of.*) The pouches can become infected or inflamed—*diverticulitis*. (*Itis* means *inflammation.*)

Diverticular disease becomes more common with aging. Obesity, smoking, lack of exercise, low-fiber diet, a diet high in animal fat, and some drugs are risk factors.

When feces enter the pouches, they can become inflamed and infected. The person has abdominal pain and tenderness in the lower left abdomen. Fever, nausea and vomiting, bloating, and constipation or diarrhea can occur.

Diet changes are ordered. Sometimes antibiotics and probiotics are ordered. *Probiotics*—found in dietary supplements and some foods—are live bacteria normally found in the colon. Surgery is done for severe disease, obstruction, and ruptured pouches. The diseased part of the bowel is removed. A colostomy may be needed (Chapter 27).

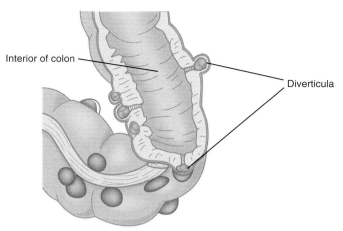

FIGURE 40-22 Diverticulosis. (From Harding M et al.: *Lewis's Medical-surgical nursing: assessment and management of clinical problems*, ed 11, St Louis, 2020, Elsevier.)

Inflammatory Bowel Disease

Inflammatory bowel disease (IBD) involves chronic inflammation of the gastro-intestinal (GI) tract. IBD often occurs before 30 years of age. Risk factors include a family history of IBD and cigarette smoking. Two types of IBD are:

- *Crohn's disease.* Inflammation commonly affects the small intestine and the beginning of the large intestine. However, any part of the GI tract from the mouth to the anus can be affected.
- *Ulcerative colitis.* The lining of the large intestine and rectum is inflamed and has ulcers.

Signs and symptoms include:

- Persistent diarrhea
- Abdominal pain and cramping
- Fever
- Rectal bleeding and bloody stools
- Fatigue
- Weight loss

Complications include bowel obstruction, abnormal passages in the body (fistulas), infected areas (abscesses), tears in the anus (anal fissures), ulcers in the GI tract, poor nutrition, and dehydration. Persons with IBD may be at higher risk for colon cancer.

Treatment involves diet changes and drug therapy for inflammation, infection, diarrhea, pain, and nutrition. Surgery may be needed to remove damaged parts of the small intestine or colon. A colostomy or ileostomy (Chapter 27) may be necessary.

Hepatitis

Hepatitis is inflammation *(itis)* and infection of the liver *(hepat)* caused by a virus. See Box 40-12 for signs and symptoms. Some people have no symptoms. There are 5 major types of hepatitis. See Box 40-12 for the methods of transmission for each type.

- *Hepatitis A* is caused by the hepatitis A virus. It is spread through contact with feces (stools) from an infected person. Handle bedpans, toilets, commodes, incontinence products, and rectal thermometers carefully. The hepatitis A vaccine protects against the disease.
- *Hepatitis B* is caused by the hepatitis B virus (HBV). It is spread through contact with infected blood or body fluids. The hepatitis B vaccine protects against the disease.
- *Hepatitis C* is caused by the hepatitis C virus. It is spread through contact with infected blood. A person may have no symptoms but can spread the disease. Serious liver disease and damage may appear years later. There is no vaccine for hepatitis C.
- *Hepatitis D* is caused by the hepatitis D virus. It is spread through contact with infected blood or body fluids. It only infects persons who have hepatitis B. Vaccination for hepatitis B protects against hepatitis D.
- *Hepatitis E* is caused by the hepatitis E virus. There are different types. This disease is not common in developed countries.

See *Promoting Safety and Comfort: Hepatitis.*

PROMOTING SAFETY AND COMFORT

Hepatitis

Safety

Hepatitis is contagious. Protect yourself and others. Practice hand-washing and follow Standard Precautions and the Bloodborne Pathogen Standard. Transmission-Based Precautions are ordered as necessary (Chapter 15). Assist the person with hygiene and hand-washing after BMs, before preparing or eating food, and as needed. Also, people should avoid sharing personal care items with an infected person—toothbrush, razor, nail clippers, and so on.

Cirrhosis

Cirrhosis is a liver condition caused by chronic liver damage. *(Cirrho* means *yellow-orange. Osis* means *condition.)* Scarred liver tissue blocks blood flow through the liver. Normal liver functions are affected. Chronic alcohol abuse, chronic hepatitis B or C, and extra fat in the liver are common causes.

BOX 40-12 Hepatitis

Signs and Symptoms
- *Jaundice*—yellowish color of the skin or whites of the eyes
- Fatigue
- Pain: abdominal, joint
- Appetite: loss of
- Nausea and vomiting
- Diarrhea
- Bowel movements (BMs): light, clay-colored
- Urine: dark
- Fever
- Itching: severe
- Weight loss

Transmission

Hepatitis A

Spread through contact with an infected person's feces (stools) by:
- Eating food prepared by the infected person with poor hand-washing after a BM
- Drinking untreated water
- Eating food washed in untreated water
- Placing a finger or object that is contaminated with the infected person's feces (stools) into the mouth
- Close personal contact with an infected person—sex, providing care

Hepatitis B

Spread through contact with an infected person's blood, semen, or other body fluids by:
- Being born to an infected mother
- Having unprotected sex with an infected person
- Sharing drug needles or materials with an infected person
- Getting an accidental stick with a needle that was used on an infected person
- Being tattooed or pierced with tools not cleaned properly after use on an infected person
- Having contact with blood or open sores of an infected person
- Using an infected person's razor, toothbrush, or nail clippers

Hepatitis C

Spread through contact with an infected person's blood (see Hepatitis B)

Hepatitis D

Spread through an infected person's blood or body fluids by:
- Sharing drug needles or materials with an infected person
- Having unprotected sex with an infected person
- Getting an accidental stick with a needle that was used on an infected person

Hepatitis E

Different types are spread by:
- Drinking water contaminated with feces (stools) of an infected person
- Eating raw or under-cooked pork, venison, wild boar, or shellfish

Modified from National Institute of Diabetes and Digestive and Kidney Diseases: What is viral hepatitis, May 2017; Hepatitis A, September 2019; Hepatitis B, June 2020; Hepatitis C, March 2020; Hepatitis D, May 2017; Hepatitis E, June 2017.

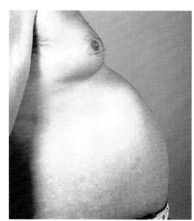

FIGURE 40-23 Fluid in the membrane lining the abdominal cavity *(ascites).* (From Chabner DE: *The language of medicine,* ed 12, St Louis, 2021, Elsevier.)

Signs and symptoms of cirrhosis may occur as the disease progresses.

- Weakness and fatigue
- Loss of appetite and weight loss
- Nausea and vomiting
- Pain or discomfort in the right upper abdomen
- *Ascites*—abdominal bloating from fluid buildup in the abdomen (Fig. 40-23)
- *Edema* (swelling) in the feet and legs
- Itching (severe)
- Dark urine color
- Jaundice

Cirrhosis has many serious complications. Infection, bruising, and bleeding occur. Blood vessels in the esophagus and stomach enlarge and burst. Gallstones may develop. Toxins build up in the brain, causing confusion, personality changes, and memory loss. Liver cancer is a risk.

Treating the underlying cause can prevent cirrhosis from getting worse. Complications are treated. Diuretic drugs (water pills) are ordered to remove fluid. Antibiotics are ordered for infection. The person must avoid alcohol and may need a liver transplant. These measures may be part of the person's care plan.

- Provide good skin care and prevent itching. Follow the care plan for what cleanser to use. Apply lotion to the skin. Discourage the scratching of itchy skin.
- Follow diet and fluid orders. A low-sodium diet and fluid restriction are needed for edema and ascites.
- Provide mouth care before meals and every 2 hours.
- Measure I&O and daily weight.
- Promote comfort and the ability to breathe. Bloating from ascites makes breathing difficult. Semi-Fowler's or Fowler's position, pillows under the arms for support, and coughing and deep-breathing exercises are common.
- Assist with ambulation and ADL as needed.
- Turn the person at least every 2 hours.
- Prevent complications from bed rest—pneumonia, blood clots, pressure injuries.
- Observe vomitus and stools for blood.

URINARY SYSTEM DISORDERS

Disorders can occur in urinary system structures—kidneys, ureters, bladder, and urethra. Men can develop prostate problems.

Urinary Tract Infections

A urinary tract infection (UTI) is an infection in any part of the urinary system. UTIs most often involve the lower urinary tract (bladder and urethra). Microbes can enter the system through the urethra. Urological exams, intercourse, poor perineal hygiene, immobility, and poor fluid intake are common causes. Persons with urinary catheters are at high risk (Chapter 26). UTI is a common healthcare-associated infection (Chapter 14). The infection can spread to other urinary structures.

See Box 40-13 for signs and symptoms and 2 types of UTIs. UTIs are treated with antibiotics. Fluids, especially water, are encouraged to flush bacteria from the urinary tract. Normal elimination is promoted. The person should urinate when the urge is felt. For prevention and treatment, proper perineal care and catheter care are needed.

BOX 40-13 Urinary Tract Infections

Signs and Symptoms
- Urinary frequency
- Urgency
- Burning on urination
- *Oliguria*—scant *(olig)* urine *(uria)*
- *Dysuria*—difficult or painful *(dys)* urination *(uria)*
- *Hematuria*—blood *(hemat)* in the urine *(uria)*
- *Pyuria*—pus *(py)* in the urine *(uria)*
- Cloudy urine
- Urine that appears red, pink, or dark
- Fever
- Fatigue
- Weakness
- Pressure in the lower abdomen
- Urine odor
- Pelvic pain—women
- Rectal pain—men

Types of Urinary Tract Infections
- *Cystitis* (bladder infection)—a bladder *(cyst)* infection *(itis)* caused by bacteria. Specific symptoms:
  - Pelvic pressure
  - Lower abdominal discomfort
  - Frequent, painful urination
  - Hematuria
- *Pyelonephritis* (kidney infection)—inflammation *(itis)* of the kidney *(nephr)*. *(Pyelo* relates to the renal pelvis.) Specific symptoms:
  - Flank pain—pain in the back between the ribs and the hip
  - High fever
  - Nausea and vomiting
  - Shaking and chills

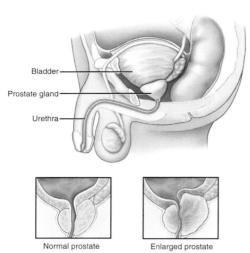

FIGURE 40-24 Enlarged prostate. The prostate presses against the urethra. Urine flow is obstructed.

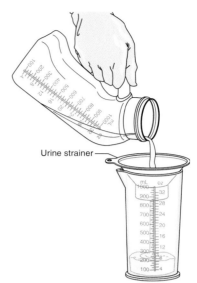

FIGURE 40-25 Urine is poured through a strainer to collect stones.

Prostate Enlargement

The prostate is a walnut-shaped gland in men. It lies just below the bladder (Chapter 9). The prostate surrounds the urethra. The prostate grows larger (enlarges) as the man grows older. This is called benign prostatic hyperplasia (BPH). *Benign* means *non-malignant. Hyper* means *excessive. Plasia* means *formation* or *development.* Benign prostatic hypertrophy is another name for enlarged prostate. *(Trophy* means *growth.)*

BPH is common in older men. The enlarged prostate presses against the urethra, obstructing urine flow (Fig. 40-24). The following are signs and symptoms of BPH.

- Urinary frequency—voiding 8 or more times a day
- Urgency—cannot delay voiding
- Trouble starting a stream
- Weak or "stop and start" urine stream
- Dribbling after voiding
- Frequent voiding during sleep *(nocturia)*
- Urinary retention—the bladder does not empty; urine remains in the bladder
- Urinary incontinence
- Pain during urination *(dysuria)*
- Urine has an unusual color or smell

For mild BPH, drugs can shrink the prostate or stop its growth. Procedures or surgery may be needed to remove tissue or widen the urethra. A transurethral resection of the prostate (TURP) is a common surgical procedure used to treat BPH. The surgery uses a scope inserted through *(trans)* the urethra *(urethral)* to remove prostate tissue. *Resection* involves removing tissue.

Kidney Stones

Kidney stones *(renal calculi)* are hard, pebble-like materials that develop in 1 or both kidneys. They vary in size—from a grain of sand to pea-sized. Larger stones can develop. Stones may be smooth or jagged. They are usually yellow or brown.

Signs and symptoms include:
- Severe, sharp pain in the back, side, lower abdomen, or groin
- *Dysuria*—difficult or painful *(dys)* urination *(uria)*
- Urinary frequency and urgency
- Inability to urinate or can only urinate a small amount
- *Hematuria*—blood *(hemat)* in the urine *(uria)*
- Cloudy urine
- Foul-smelling urine
- Nausea and vomiting
- Fever and chills

Drugs are given for pain relief. The person needs to drink 2000 to 3000 mL (milliliters) a day. Fluids help flush stones out through the urine. All urine is strained (Fig. 40-25). Medical or surgical removal of the stone may be necessary. Diet changes may prevent stones.

Chronic Kidney Disease

In chronic kidney disease (CKD), the kidneys are damaged and do not function normally. Waste products are not removed from the blood. Fluid is retained. Heart failure and hypertension easily result.

CKD can worsen over time and may lead to kidney failure (end-stage renal disease; ESRD). ESRD requires a kidney transplant or dialysis. *Dialysis* is the process of removing waste products from the blood. The measures in Box 40-14 are common when caring for persons with CKD.

BOX 40-14 Kidney Disease—Care Measures

- A diet low in protein, potassium, and sodium
- Fluid restriction
- Measuring blood pressure in the supine, sitting, and standing positions
- Measuring daily weight
- Measuring and recording I&O
- Turning and re-positioning at least every 2 hours
- Measures to prevent pressure injuries
- ROM exercises
- Measures to prevent itching (bath oils, lotions, creams)
- Measures to prevent injury and bleeding
- Frequent oral hygiene
- Measures to prevent infection
- Deep-breathing and coughing exercises
- Measures to prevent diarrhea or constipation
- Measures to meet emotional needs
- Measures to promote rest

REPRODUCTIVE DISORDERS

Aging affects the reproductive system (Chapter 10). Injuries, diseases, and surgeries can affect reproductive structures and functions.

Sexually Transmitted Diseases

Sexually transmitted diseases (STDs) are passed from person to person through sexual contact. They are also known as sexually transmitted infections (STIs). Common infection sites are the genitals, rectum, mouth, and throat.

STDs/STIs can be caused by:

- Bacteria. Gonorrhea, syphilis, and chlamydia are common bacterial STDs/STIs.
- Parasites. Trichomoniasis is an example.
- Viruses. Human papillomavirus (HPV), genital herpes, and HIV/AIDS (p. 525) are caused by viruses. STDs/STIs caused by a virus cannot be cured. Treatment can reduce symptoms and the risk of transmission to others.

Signs and symptoms vary depending on the cause. A person may not have signs and symptoms and still spread infection. Vaginal, anal, and oral sex can transmit STDs/STIs. Needle sharing (injection drug use) can spread HIV and other bloodborne infections.

Correct use of latex condoms reduces the risk of becoming infected or spreading STDs/STIs. Not having vaginal, anal, or oral sex is the best way to avoid infection. In health care settings, Standard Precautions and the Bloodborne Pathogen Standard are followed.

See *Focus on Older Persons: Sexually Transmitted Diseases.*

FOCUS ON OLDER PERSONS

Sexually Transmitted Diseases

Many older people are sexually active. They get and can spread STDs/STIs in the same ways as younger persons. However, many do not think they are at risk. Always practice Standard Precautions and follow the Bloodborne Pathogen Standard. Do not assume that older people are too old to have sex.

ENDOCRINE DISORDERS

The endocrine system is made up of glands. The endocrine glands secrete hormones that affect other organs and glands. Diabetes is the most common endocrine disorder.

Diabetes

In diabetes, the body cannot produce or use insulin properly. Insulin is needed for glucose to move from the blood into the cells. The pancreas secretes insulin. Without any or enough insulin, sugar builds up in the blood. Blood glucose (sugar) is high. Cells do not have enough sugar for energy and cannot function.

Types of Diabetes. A family history of the disease is a common risk factor for the 3 types of diabetes.

- *Type 1 diabetes.* Occurs most often in children and young adults but can develop at any age. The pancreas makes no insulin. Too much glucose stays in the blood. Onset is rapid.
- *Type 2 diabetes.* This is the most common type. It occurs most often in middle and older adulthood. It can develop during childhood. In type 2 diabetes, the body does not make enough insulin or use insulin well. Risk factors include being age 45 or older, having a family history of diabetes, being over-weight or obese, and being physically inactive.
- *Gestational diabetes.* This type develops during pregnancy. (*Gestation* comes from *gestare.* It means *to bear.*) This type usually goes away after the baby is born. However, the mother is at risk for type 2 diabetes later in life.

Signs and Symptoms. Signs and symptoms of diabetes are:

- Being very thirsty
- Frequent urination
- Feeling very hungry or tired
- Weight loss without trying
- Sores that heal slowly
- Tingling or loss of feeling in the feet or hands
- Blurred vision

Complications. Diabetes must be controlled to prevent complications. High blood glucose levels can cause serious health problems. Heart disease, stroke, kidney disease, eye problems, and nerve damage are examples. So are dental disease and foot problems.

Treatment. Type 1 diabetes is treated with daily insulin therapy, healthy eating (Chapter 28), and exercise. Type 2 diabetes is treated with healthy eating, exercise, and weight loss if needed. Type 2 may require oral drugs or insulin. Types 1 and 2 involve controlling blood pressure, cholesterol, and the risk factors for coronary artery disease.

Good foot care is needed. Corns, blisters, calluses, and other foot problems can lead to an infection and amputation. See Chapters 23 and 35.

TABLE 40-1 Hypoglycemia and Hyperglycemia

Hypoglycemia (Low Blood Sugar)		Hyperglycemia (High Blood Sugar)	
Causes	Signs and Symptoms	Causes	Signs and Symptoms
• Too much insulin or diabetic drugs • Increased exercise • Skipping or delaying a meal • Eating too little food • Vomiting • Drinking alcohol	**Mild to Moderate** • Shaky or jittery • Sweaty • Hunger • Headache • Blurred vision • Sleepy or tired • Dizzy or being light-headed • Confused or disoriented • Skin: pale • Uncoordinated movements • Irritable or nervous • Arguing or being combative • Behavior or personality changes • Trouble concentrating • Weakness • Pulse: rapid or irregular **Severe** • Cannot eat or drink • Seizures or convulsions • Unconsciousness	• Not enough insulin or diabetic drugs • Too little exercise • Eating too much food • Emotional stress • Infection or sickness • Undiagnosed diabetes	**Early** • Frequent urination • Increased thirst • Blurred vision • Being tired • Headache **Late** • Breath that smells fruity • Weakness • Dry mouth • Shortness of breath • Nausea and vomiting • Confusion • Abdominal pain • Coma

Blood sugar level can fall too low or go too high:
- *Hypoglycemia means low* (hypo) *sugar* (glyc) *in the blood* (emia).
- *Hyperglycemia means high* (hyper) *sugar* (glyc) *in the blood* (emia).

Blood glucose is monitored as often as ordered (Chapter 34). For example, type 1 testing may be done 4 to 10 times a day. For type 2, testing can range from daily to 4 times a day—before meals and at bedtime.

See Table 40-1 for the causes, signs, and symptoms of hypoglycemia and hyperglycemia. Both can lead to death if not corrected. Call for the nurse at once.

IMMUNE SYSTEM DISORDERS

The immune system protects the body from microbes, cancer cells, and other harmful substances. It defends against threats inside and outside the body. Immune system disorders occur from problems with the immune response. The response may be inappropriate, too strong, or lacking.

Autoimmune Disorders

Autoimmune disorders occur when the immune system attacks the body's own *(auto)* healthy cells, tissues, or organs. Most autoimmune disorders are chronic. The body parts affected depend on the type of disorder.

Common autoimmune disorders include:
- *Celiac disease.* The person cannot tolerate gluten—a substance in wheat, rye, and barley. When gluten is ingested, the immune system responds and damages the small intestines. Over time, the damage prevents nutrient absorption. Diarrhea, fatigue, weight loss, bloating, and anemia occur. Poor nutrition and serious complications can result. A gluten-free diet is needed (Chapter 28).
- *Graves' disease.* The thyroid gland produces too much thyroid hormone *(hyperthyroidism)*. The person has irritability, problems sleeping, rapid heart rate, weight loss, sweating, fatigue or muscle weakness, shaky hands, and bulging eyes. A goiter (enlarged thyroid) may cause the neck to look swollen.
- *Hashimoto's disease.* The thyroid gland does not produce enough thyroid hormone *(hypothyroidism)*. The person has fatigue, weakness, weight gain, sensitivity to cold, muscle aches, stiff joints, facial swelling, and constipation. A goiter (enlarged thyroid) can also occur with Hashimoto's disease.
- *Lupus.* This disease can damage the joints, skin, kidneys, heart, lungs, and other body parts. A rash across the nose and cheeks is common.
- *Rheumatoid arthritis* (p. 506).
- *Multiple sclerosis* (p. 512).
- *Inflammatory bowel disease* (p. 519).
- *Type 1 diabetes* (p. 523).

HIV/AIDS

Acquired immunodeficiency syndrome (AIDS) is caused by the *human immunodeficiency virus (HIV)*. HIV attacks the immune system. Therefore it destroys the body's ability to fight infections and disease.

HIV is spread through certain body fluids—blood, semen, vaginal fluids, rectal fluids, and breast-milk (from mother to baby). HIV is not spread by air, water, saliva, tears, sweat, insects, casual contact (shaking hands, hugging, dancing, sharing dishes), closed mouth or social kissing, or toilet seats.

HIV is transmitted *mainly* by:

- Having sex with someone who has HIV.
  - Anal sex
  - Vaginal sex
  - Multiple sex partners
- Sharing needles, syringes, rinse water, or other equipment used to prepare injection drugs.

If untreated, HIV progresses in stages. AIDS is the most severe stage. The immune system is badly damaged. The person is at risk for infections, illnesses, and cancers. Box 40-15 lists the signs and symptoms of AIDS. Some HIV-infected persons are symptom-free for more than 10 years. However, they carry HIV and can spread it to others.

Drugs are used to treat or reduce HIV symptoms. They also reduce complications and prolong life. AIDS has no vaccine and no cure at present. Without treatment, persons with AIDS live for about 3 years.

You may care for persons who are HIV positive, are HIV carriers, or have AIDS (see Box 40-15). You may have contact with the person's blood or body fluids. Protect yourself and others. Follow Standard Precautions and the Bloodborne Pathogen Standard. A person may have the HIV virus but no symptoms. In some persons, HIV or AIDS is not yet diagnosed.

See *Focus on Older Persons: HIV/AIDS.*

FOCUS ON OLDER PERSONS

HIV/AIDS

According to the Centers for Disease Control and Prevention (CDC), the following factors affect HIV prevention in older persons.

- Older persons are less likely to discuss sexual activity and drug use with their doctors. They may:
  - Not consider themselves at risk.
  - Be embarrassed to discuss sex.
  - Mistake symptoms as normal aging.
- While older persons have many of the same risk factors as younger people, they may be less likely to use prevention measures. Using condoms, reducing the number of sexual partners, avoiding risky sexual behaviors, and taking drugs for prevention (prophylaxis) are examples.
- Older persons are more likely to have late-stage HIV infection when diagnosed. More immune system damage occurs when HIV treatment is started later.
- Older persons may avoid treatment or not disclose their HIV status due to fears of isolation or negative attitudes from others.

Both aging and HIV increase the risk for heart disease, COPD, bone loss, and some cancers. Drug interactions can occur between drugs used to treat HIV and those for other conditions. Hypertension, diabetes, high cholesterol, and obesity are examples.

BOX 40-15 AIDS

Signs and Symptoms

- Rapid weight loss
- Recurring fever
- Night sweats
- Fatigue: extreme and unexplained
- Swollen lymph glands: underarms, groin, neck
- Diarrhea lasting more than 1 week
- Pneumonia
- Sores: mouth, anus, genitals
- Red, brown, pink, or purple blotches: on or under the skin; inside the mouth, nose, or eyelids
- Memory loss
- Depression
- Loss of coordination
- Paralysis

Care Measures

- Follow Standard Precautions and the Bloodborne Pathogen Standard.
- Provide daily hygiene. Avoid irritating soaps.
- Follow the care plan for oral hygiene. A toothbrush with soft bristles is best.
- Provide oral fluids as ordered.
- Measure and record intake and output.
- Measure weight daily.
- Encourage deep-breathing and coughing exercises as ordered.
- Prevent pressure injuries.
- Assist with ROM exercises and ambulating as ordered.
- Encourage self-care. The person may use adaptive (assistive) devices (walker, commode, eating devices).
- Encourage the person to be as active as possible.
- Change linens and garments when damp or wet.
- Listen and provide emotional support.

SKIN DISORDERS

There are many types of skin disorders. Alopecia, hirsutism, dandruff, lice, and scabies are discussed in Chapter 23. Skin tears and pressure injuries are discussed in Chapters 35 and 36. Burns are discussed in Chapter 43.

Shingles

Shingles (herpes zoster) is caused by the same virus that causes chicken pox. The virus lies dormant in nerve tissue. (*Dormant* means *to be inactive.*) The virus can become active years later.

At first there is pain, itching, or tingling of the skin. Then the person has a painful rash of fluid-filled blisters. This usually occurs on 1 side of the face or body (Fig. 40-26).

Persons who have had chicken pox are at risk. So are persons with weakened immune systems from HIV infection, certain cancers and cancer treatments, immuno-suppressive drugs, and stress. The risk of getting shingles increases with age.

Anti-viral drugs and pain-relief drugs are used. For many healthy people, the rash is gone in 2 to 4 weeks. Pain can last for months or years after the rash heals. A vaccine is available to prevent shingles. The CDC recommends that persons age 50 and older be vaccinated against shingles.

Fluid from the blisters can spread the virus to persons who have not had chicken pox or the chicken pox vaccine.

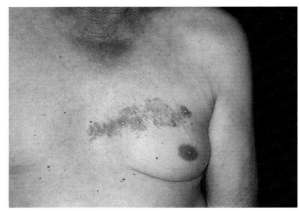

FIGURE 40-26 Shingles. (Courtesy Department of Dermatology, School of Medicine, University of Utah, Salt Lake City, Utah.)

The blisters usually develop a crust (scab) within 7 to 10 days. Shingles lesions are infectious until they crust over. The person needs to cover the rash, avoid touching or scratching the rash, and practice hand hygiene often.

Avoid contact with an infected person if you:
- Have never had chicken pox or the vaccine to prevent chicken pox.
- Are pregnant and have not had chicken pox or the vaccine to prevent chicken pox.
- Have a weakened immune system.

FOCUS ON P R I D E

The Person, Family, and Yourself

P ersonal and Professional Responsibility

Understanding health problems allows you to safely assist with care. You may want to know more about a health problem. Or a person may have a disorder you did not learn about in your training. Ask the nurse for more information. You can also look up the problem in a medical dictionary or on the Internet. Take pride in learning more.

R ights and Respect

The person and family have many reactions to illness—fear, anger, worry, guilt. Families respond in different ways. Family bonds are stronger when the family relies on each other during stress. A helpful, supportive family benefits the person's quality of life.

Promote pride in the family. Show respect. Compliment their efforts. Encourage the family's help and support.

I ndependence and Social Interaction

Some choices are unhealthy. For example, a person with COPD continues to smoke. Or a person with CAD chooses not to exercise or make diet changes. The health team teaches the person the risks and encourages healthy changes. They cannot force changes. However, they must be sure the person understands the risks.

While aware of the risks, some persons choose not to change. You may not agree with the person's decision, but you must continue to treat the person well. Independence and personal choice promote quality of life.

D elegation and Teamwork

A person's condition can change quickly. A person with angina may have an MI. Hypertension may lead to a stroke. A person may have a severe asthma attack.

Sudden condition changes require the nurse's attention. Assist as directed. You may need to help other patients or residents while the nurse gives care. Help willingly. The entire nursing team must give "extra effort" during an emergency.

E thics and Laws

With chronic health problems, staff may care for a person many times. Staff get to know the person's likes, dislikes, and preferences. Staff learn about the person's family, school or work, hobbies, and so on. Interest in the person adds to quality of care.

Maintaining professional boundaries can be hard when caring for persons you see often and get to know well. However, you must protect the person's privacy and rights. Watch your behavior closely to avoid crossing boundaries (Chapter 4).

FOCUS ON PRIDE: *Application*

Choose a disorder in this chapter. What life-style changes are needed? Discuss the impact on the person and family. How does the health team help the person and family adjust?

Circle the BEST answer.

1 Metastasis means that
   a Cancer cells have been killed
   b A benign tumor has grown larger
   c A malignant tumor has spread to other body parts
   d Healthy cells have been damaged by cancer treatments

2 A person receiving chemotherapy becomes sad when talking about fatigue, hair loss, and nausea. You should
   a Change the subject
   b Talk about how other patients respond to treatment
   c Tell the person: "It will be okay"
   d Listen

3 A person has arthritis. Care includes
   a Keeping joints abducted
   b Applying traction to affected areas
   c Wearing a cast to prevent movement
   d Rest balanced with exercise

4 A person had hip replacement surgery. Which should you question?
   a Do not cross the legs.
   b Provide a chair with a low seat.
   c Keep a hip abduction wedge between the legs.
   d Provide a long-handled brush for bathing.

5 A person with osteoporosis is at risk for
   a Fractures
   b An amputation
   c Phantom pain
   d Paralysis

6 A cast needs to dry. Which should you question?
   a Turn the person so the cast dries evenly.
   b Cover the cast with plastic.
   c Elevate the cast on pillows.
   d Support the cast by the palms when lifting.

7 A person is in traction. Care includes
   a Avoiding ROM exercises
   b Keeping the weights on the floor
   c Removing the weights if the person is uncomfortable
   d Using a fracture pan for elimination

8 After hip surgery the operated leg is kept
   a Abducted
   b Adducted
   c Externally rotated
   d Flexed

9 Sudden weakness on 1 side of the body and trouble speaking and walking are signs of
   a Stroke
   b Heart attack
   c Cancer
   d Hyperglycemia

10 A person had a stroke. Which should you question?
   a Leave the bed in semi-Fowler's position.
   b Perform ROM exercises every 2 hours.
   c Turn and re-position the person every 2 hours.
   d Place needed items on the weak (affected) side.

11 Which statement about Parkinson's disease is *true*?
   a There is a cure.
   b Mental function is affected first.
   c Tremors, slow movements, and a shuffling gait occur.
   d Paralysis occurs but mental function is intact.

12 A person with multiple sclerosis is in remission. This means that symptoms
   a Have gone away for a while
   b Are worsening
   c Will not return
   d Are being treated

13 A person has quadriplegia from a spinal cord injury. Care includes
   a Active ROM exercises
   b Pressure injury prevention
   c Removing the call light from the room
   d Using a long-handled device for reaching

14 In hypertension
   a The diastolic pressure is higher than the systolic pressure
   b The systolic pressure is 140 mm Hg or higher
   c The diastolic pressure is 70 mm Hg or higher
   d Chest pain is a common symptom

15 A person with angina has pain that is severe and not relieved by rest or drugs. This
   a Is normal angina pain
   b Signals hypertension
   c Signals heart failure
   d Signals a heart attack

16 A person complains of sudden squeezing chest pain. You should
   a Report the pain if it is not relieved in 15 minutes
   b Report the pain at once
   c Give the person a nitroglycerin tablet
   d Give the person oxygen

17 A person has heart failure. Which should you question?
   a Encourage fluids.
   b Measure intake and output.
   c Measure weight daily.
   d Perform ROM exercises.

18 The most common cause of COPD is
   a Smoking
   b Allergies
   c Being over-weight
   d A high-sodium diet

19 A person has emphysema. Which is *true*?
   a The person has an infection.
   b Breathing is usually easier lying down.
   c The person has dyspnea and a cough.
   d There is swelling in an arm or leg.

20 The flu virus is spread by
   a Coughing and sneezing
   b The fecal-oral route
   c Blood
   d Needle sharing

21 Which position eases breathing in the person with pneumonia?
   a Supine
   b Prone
   c Semi-Fowler's
   d Trendelenburg's

22 A person with TB coughs on your hand. You should
   a Watch for signs of latent TB
   b Get a TB vaccine
   c Ask the nurse about being treated
   d Wash your hands

Continued

23 A person is vomiting. You should
   a Position the person supine
   b Leave to get the nurse
   c Do nothing
   d Turn the person's head to the side

24 A person has diverticular disease. How will you assist with care?
   a Giving antibiotics
   b Promoting normal bowel elimination
   c Dietary teaching and planning
   d Assessing risk factors

25 Crohn's disease and ulcerative colitis can cause
   a Flank pain and dysuria
   b Jaundice and itching
   c Diarrhea and bloody stools
   d Ascites and edema

26 Which is spread by food or water contaminated with feces from an infected person?
   a Hepatitis A
   b Hepatitis B
   c Hepatitis C
   d Hepatitis D

27 A vaccine is available to protect against
   a Chronic kidney disease
   b Benign prostatic hyperplasia (BPH)
   c Hepatitis B
   d Diabetes

28 A person has cirrhosis. Which should you question?
   a Measure I&O.
   b Weigh the person daily.
   c Apply lotion after bathing.
   d Encourage fluids.

29 A person has cystitis. This is a
   a Kidney infection
   b Kidney stone
   c Sexually transmitted disease (infection)
   d Bladder infection

30 BPH causes urinary problems because
   a An enlarged prostate presses against the urethra
   b Stones in the kidneys block urine flow
   c Kidney damage reduces urine output
   d Cancer cells damage the bladder

31 Which statement about STDs/STIs is *true?*
   a Older persons do not get them.
   b They only affect the genital area.
   c Some persons have no signs or symptoms.
   d They can all be cured with antibiotics.

32 A person with diabetes is confused, weak, and shaky after an exercise activity. These are signs of
   a Hypoglycemia
   b Hyperglycemia
   c Jaundice
   d Bleeding

33 HIV is spread through
   a Blood and certain body fluids
   b Coughing and sneezing
   c Using public phones and restrooms
   d Hugging or dancing with an infected person

34 HIV can be prevented by
   a Taking immuno-suppressive drugs
   b Getting an HIV vaccine
   c Using antibiotics
   d Avoiding risky sexual behaviors

35 A person with shingles needs to
   a Avoid contact with persons who have had chicken pox
   b Keep the rash covered until lesions crust over
   c Gently scratch areas of the rash that itch
   d Avoid pain-relief drugs

Answers to Chapter 40 questions are on p. 589.

FOCUS ON **PRACTICE**

Problem Solving

After a stroke a person has hemiplegia, aphasia, and dysphagia. How will you modify the care measures listed below? Apply learning from this and other chapters.
- Transferring from the bed to the wheelchair
- Dressing and undressing
- Assisting with food and fluids
- Explaining a procedure
- Performing a safety check of the room

CHAPTER 41

Mental Health Disorders

OBJECTIVES

- Define the key terms and key abbreviations in this chapter.
- Explain mental health and the effects of mental health disorders.
- Identify the risk factors and warning signs of mental health disorders.
- Describe anxiety disorders and the defense mechanisms used to relieve anxiety.
- Describe schizophrenia.
- Describe mood disorders.
- Describe personality disorders.
- Describe substance use disorder and addiction.
- Describe 3 eating disorders.
- Describe suicide and the persons at risk.
- Describe the care required by persons with mental health disorders.
- Explain how to promote PRIDE in the person, the family, and yourself.

KEY TERMS

addiction A chronic disease involving substance-seeking behaviors and use that is compulsive and hard to control despite the harmful effects

anxiety A feeling of worry, nervousness, or fear about an event or situation

compulsion An over-whelming urge to repeat certain rituals, acts, or behaviors

coping Strategies to manage stress and reduce negative emotions caused by stress

defense mechanism An unconscious reaction that blocks unpleasant or threatening feelings

delusion A false belief

delusion of grandeur An exaggerated belief about one's importance, fame, wealth, power, or talents

delusion of persecution A false belief that one is being mistreated, abused, or harassed

detoxification The process of removing a toxic substance from the body

flashback Reliving a trauma over and over in thoughts during the day and in nightmares during sleep

hallucination Seeing, hearing, smelling, feeling, or tasting something that is not real

mental health Involves a person's emotional, psychological, and social well-being

mental health disorder A serious illness that can affect a person's thinking, mood, behavior, function, and ability to relate to others; psychiatric disorder

obsession A frequent, upsetting, and unwanted thought, idea, or image

panic An intense and sudden feeling of fear, anxiety, or dread

personality The set of attitudes, values, behaviors, and traits of a person

phobia An intense fear of something that has little or no real danger

psychosis A condition that affects the mind and causes a loss of contact with reality

stress The response or change in the body caused by any emotional, psychological, physical, social, or economic factor

stressor The event or factor that causes stress

suicide To end one's life on purpose

suicide contagion Exposure to suicide or suicidal behaviors within one's family, one's peer group, or through media reports of suicide

withdrawal syndrome The physical and mental response after stopping or severely reducing the use of a substance that was used regularly

KEY ABBREVIATIONS

BPD Borderline personality disorder
GAD Generalized anxiety disorder

OCD Obsessive-compulsive disorder
PTSD Post-traumatic stress disorder

Mental health involves a person's emotional, psychological, and social well-being. Important from childhood through old age, mental health affects how a person:
- Thinks.
- Feels.
- Acts when coping with life.
- Handles stress. *Stress is the response or change in the body caused by any emotional, psychological, physical, social, or economic factor.*
- Relates to others.
- Makes choices.

Mental health disorders (psychiatric disorders) are serious illnesses that can affect a person's thinking, mood, behavior, function, and ability to relate to others. Risk factors and early warning signs are listed in Box 41-1. Mental health disorders are common. They may be occasional or long-term. Many persons recover completely.

ANXIETY DISORDERS

Anxiety is a feeling of worry, nervousness, or fear about an event or situation. Some anxiety is normal. It is a normal reaction to stress. Anxiety disorders happen when anxiety cannot be controlled and interferes with every-day activities, work, school, and relationships. The anxiety does not go away and can get worse over time. See Box 41-2 for signs and symptoms.

Anxiety level depends on the stressor. A *stressor is the event or factor that causes stress.* It can be physical, emotional, social, or economic. Past experiences and the number of stressors affect how a person reacts.

Coping and defense mechanisms may help relieve anxiety.
- *Coping involves strategies to manage stress and reduce negative emotions caused by stress.* Unhealthy coping includes over-eating, drinking alcohol, smoking, and fighting. Healthy coping includes discussing the problem, exercising, listening to music, and having time alone or being with others who are helpful.
- *Defense mechanisms are unconscious reactions that block unpleasant or threatening feelings* (Box 41-3). (*Unconscious reactions* are experiences and feelings that cannot be recalled.) Some use of defense mechanisms is normal. In mental health disorders, they are used poorly.

Anxiety disorders often occur with other mental health disorders. Depression (p. 533), eating disorders (p. 536), and substance use disorder (p. 534) are examples. Anxiety may be linked to health problems. Heart disease, diabetes, thyroid problems, and respiratory disorders are examples.

BOX 41-1 Mental Health Disorders

Risk Factors
- Genetics and family history. Mental health disorders tend to run in families.
- Life experiences. Stress or history of abuse are examples.
- Chemical imbalances in the brain.
- Traumatic brain injury.
- Fetal exposure to viruses or toxic chemicals.
- Use of alcohol or recreational drugs.
- Serious health problems.
- Having few friends and feeling lonely or isolated.

Early Warning Signs
- Eating or sleeping too much or too little
- Pulling away from people or usual activities
- Having low or no energy
- Feeling numb or like nothing matters
- Having unexplained aches and pains
- Feeling helpless or hopeless
- Smoking, drinking, or using drugs more than usual
- Feeling unusually confused, forgetful, on edge, angry, upset, worried, or scared
- Yelling or fighting with family and friends
- Having severe mood swings that cause relationship problems
- Having persistent thoughts and memories
- Hearing voices or believing things that are not true
- Thinking of harming oneself or others
- Being unable to perform daily tasks

Modified from MentalHealth.gov: *What is mental health*, Washington, D.C., updated May 28, 2020, U.S. Department of Health & Human Services and MedlinePlus: *Mental disorders*, Washington, D.C., updated December 7, 2021, U.S. Department of Health & Human Services.

BOX 41-2 Anxiety—Signs and Symptoms

- Weakness
- Breathing problems: shortness of breath, smothering or choking sensations
- Rapid heart rate; pounding heartbeat
- Nausea
- Abdominal pain
- Hot flashes (women)
- Dizziness
- Chest pain
- Nightmares
- Restlessness
- Fatigue
- Difficulty concentrating
- Irritability
- Muscle tension
- Sleep problems
- Sweating
- Trembling or shaking
- Tingling or numb hands

BOX 41-3 Defense Mechanisms

Compensation. *Compensate* means *to make up for, replace, or substitute.* A weakness is replaced with a strength.
EXAMPLE: Not good in sports, a child develops another talent.

Conversion. *Convert* means *to change.* An emotion is changed into a physical symptom.
EXAMPLE: Not wanting to read out loud in school, a child complains of a headache.

Denial. *Deny* means *refusing to accept or believe something that is true.* The person refuses to accept unpleasant or threatening things.
EXAMPLE: A person ignores pain and refuses to see a doctor.

Displacement. *Displace* means *to move or take the place of.* Behaviors or emotions are moved from one person, place, or thing to a safe person, place, or thing.
EXAMPLE: Angry at your boss, you yell at a friend.

Identification. *Identify* means *to relate to or associate with.* A person assumes the ideas, behaviors, or traits of another person.
EXAMPLE: Fearing rejection, a person acts differently around peers.

Projection. *Project* means *to blame another.* Unacceptable behaviors, thoughts, or emotions are attributed to someone else.
EXAMPLE: Not understanding a lesson, a student thinks: "The teacher does not understand it enough to teach it well."

Rationalization. *Rational* means *sensible, reasonable, or logical.* An acceptable reason—not the real reason—is given for behaviors or actions.
EXAMPLE: A student did not study and failed a test. The student thinks: "I failed because I wasn't feeling well."

Reaction formation. A person acts in a way opposite to how the person truly feels.
EXAMPLE: A worker does not like the boss. The worker gives the boss a gift.

Regression. *Regress* means *to move back or to retreat.* The person retreats or moves back to an earlier time or condition.
EXAMPLE: A 3-year-old wants a baby bottle when a new baby arrives.

Repression. *Repress* means *to hold down or keep back.* Unpleasant or painful thoughts or experiences are kept from the conscious mind. They cannot be recalled or remembered.
EXAMPLE: A child was sexually abused. Now 33 years old, there is no memory of the event.

Generalized Anxiety Disorder

The person with generalized anxiety disorder (GAD) has extreme anxiety, fear, or worry. GAD occurs on most days for at least 6 months. The person has worry and concern about many things. Health, work, social situations, and every-day life are examples. Serious problems in such areas can result.

Panic Disorder

Panic is an intense and sudden feeling of fear, anxiety, or dread. The person with panic disorder has sudden, recurring periods of panic when there is no real danger. *Panic attacks* can be unexpected or brought on by a trigger—fear of an object or situation. The person cannot function. Signs and symptoms of anxiety are severe (see Box 41-2).

Panic attacks can occur at any time and can last several minutes or longer. The person may try to avoid places or situations where panic attacks have occurred.

Call for the nurse if the person has severe signs and symptoms of anxiety. During a panic attack, these actions can help.
- Help the person to a quiet area.
- Stay with the person and remain calm.
- Speak in short, simple sentences. Give reminders of the person's safety.
- Talk the person through deep-breathing exercises (Chapter 37) or other relaxation methods (Chapter 33). Follow the person's care plan.
See *Focus on Communication: Panic Disorder.*

FOCUS ON COMMUNICATION

Panic Disorder

A calm and focused approach can help reduce stress in a stressful situation. Pay attention to your voice tone, posture, and facial expressions. Help the person focus and relax. This is an example.

You are safe. I am with you. The nurse is coming. Let's focus on taking slow breaths. Breathe in through your nose. (Wait and allow the person to follow the instruction. Do the action with the person. Make eye contact. Give positive feedback.) *Good job. Now breathe out through your mouth.*

Phobias

A phobia is an intense fear of something that has little or no real danger. Common phobias are fear of:
- Being in an open, crowded, or public place (*agoraphobia—agora* means *marketplace*)
- Water (*aquaphobia—aqua* means *water*)
- Being in or trapped in an enclosed or narrow space (*claustrophobia—claustro* means *closing*)
- The slightest uncleanliness (*mysophobia—myso* means *anything that is disgusting*)
- Night or darkness (*nyctophobia—nycto* means *night or darkness*)
The person avoids what is feared. When faced with the fear, the person has high anxiety and cannot function.

Obsessive-Compulsive Disorder

Obsessive-compulsive disorder (OCD) occurs when a person has recurring thoughts, behaviors, or both that cannot be controlled.

- An **obsession** *is a frequent, upsetting, and unwanted thought, idea, or image.* Microbes, dirt, order and neatness, violent thoughts, or sexual acts are common obsessive thoughts.
- A **compulsion** *is the over-whelming urge to repeat certain rituals, acts, or behaviors.* The compulsion is done in response to obsessive thoughts and the resulting anxiety. Hand-washing, counting, checking on things, cleaning, hoarding, and doing things in a certain order are examples.

OCD behaviors can take a long time, are very distressing, and affect daily life.

Post-Traumatic Stress Disorder

Post-traumatic stress disorder (PTSD) occurs in some people after a terrifying, traumatic, scary, or dangerous event. There was harm or threat of harm. PTSD can develop at any age after:

- Being harmed or after a loved one was harmed
- Seeing a harmful event happen to a loved one or stranger
- The sudden, unexpected death of a loved one
- Traumatic events:
  - War, terrorist attack, bombing
  - Abuse, mugging, rape, torture
  - Kidnapping, being held captive
  - Crashes—vehicle, train, plane
  - Natural disaster—flood, tornado, hurricane, earthquake

Signs and symptoms may begin within 3 months or years after the event (Box 41-4). Flashbacks are common. A **flashback** *is reliving a trauma over and over in thoughts during the day and in nightmares during sleep.* Every-day things can trigger them—words, objects, situations, thoughts, or reminders of the event. During a flashback, the trauma seems to be happening all over again. The person has symptoms of PTSD.

Some people recover within 6 months. For others, PTSD is a chronic condition. Depression, substance use disorder, and other anxiety disorders may occur with PTSD.

PSYCHOTIC DISORDERS

Psychosis describes a condition that affects the mind and causes a loss of contact with reality. Psychotic disorders cause abnormal thinking and perceptions. (To *perceive* means *to become aware of something through the mind or the senses—sight, hearing, touch, smell, and taste.*) In a psychotic state, the person has lost touch with what is real.

Two main symptoms of a psychosis are:

- **Delusions**—*false beliefs.*
- **Hallucinations**—*seeing, hearing, smelling, feeling, or tasting something that is not real.* Hearing voices is a common hallucination. "Voices" may comment on the person's behavior or order the person to do things, warn of danger, or talk to other voices.

Schizophrenia is one disorder that causes psychosis. Other causes include sleep deprivation, alcohol and some drugs, brain tumors, brain infections, and stroke.

See *Focus on Communication: Psychotic Disorders.*

FOCUS ON COMMUNICATION

Psychotic Disorders

Delusions and hallucinations can frighten a person. Good communication is important.

- Speak slowly and calmly.
- Do not pretend to experience what the person does. Help the person focus on reality.
- Do not try to convince the person that the experience is not real. To the person, it is real.

For example, a person hears voices. You can say: "I don't hear the voices. But I believe you do. Try to listen to my voice and not the other voices."

Schizophrenia

Schizophrenia is a serious brain illness affecting how a person thinks, feels, and behaves. *Schizophrenia* means split *(schizo)* mind *(phrenia).* Age of onset is usually between 16 and 30. Gradual changes in mood, thinking, and social function begin before the first episode of psychosis. Signs and symptoms (Box 41-5) make it hard to perform daily tasks.

People with schizophrenia do not tend to be violent. However, if a person becomes violent, it is often directed at oneself. Some persons with schizophrenia attempt suicide (p. 536).

BOX 41-4 Post-Traumatic Stress Disorder—Signs and Symptoms

- Flashbacks
- Nightmares or bad dreams
- Frightening thoughts
- Avoiding places, events, or things that are reminders of the trauma
- Avoiding thoughts or feelings related to the trauma
- Being easily startled or frightened
- Feeling tense or "on edge"
- Sleep problems
- Angry outbursts
- Problems remembering key parts of the trauma
- Negative thoughts about oneself or the world
- Feeling guilt or blame
- Loss of interest in enjoyed activities

Modified from National Institute of Mental Health: *Post-traumatic stress disorder,* National Institutes of Health, revised May 2019.

BOX 41-5 Schizophrenia—Signs and Symptoms

- Hallucinations
- Delusions
  - *Delusions of grandeur*—exaggerated beliefs about one's importance, fame, wealth, power, or talents
  - *Delusions of persecution*—false beliefs that one is being mistreated, abused, or harassed
- Abnormal thinking and speech
  - Trouble organizing or logically connecting thoughts
  - Stopping speech in the middle of a thought
  - Making up words that have no meaning
- Abnormal body movements
  - Repeating motions over and over
  - Sitting for long periods without moving, speaking, or responding
- Emotional and behavioral problems
  - Dull voice
  - No facial expression (flat affect)
  - Trouble being happy
  - Trouble planning and staying with an activity
  - Socially withdrawn
- Cognitive problems
  - Trouble paying attention, understanding, or remembering
  - Trouble making decisions

BOX 41-6 Bipolar Disorder—Signs and Symptoms

Manic Episode
- Feeling very up, high, or happy, or very irritable or touchy
- Feeling jumpy, wired, or more active than usual
- Racing thoughts
- Decreased need for sleep
- Talking fast about many different things ("flight of ideas")
- Excessive appetite for food, drinking, sex, or other pleasurable activities
- Thinking one can do many things at once without getting tired
- Feeling unusually important, talented, or powerful

Depressive Episode
- Feeling very down, sad, or anxious
- Feeling slowed down or restless
- Problems concentrating or making decisions
- Trouble falling asleep, waking up too early, or sleeping too much
- Talking very slowly, feeling that one has nothing to say, or forgetting a lot
- Lack of interest in almost all activities
- Unable to do simple things
- Feeling hopeless or worthless
- Thinking about death or suicide

Modified from National Institute of Mental Health: *Bipolar disorder*, U.S. Department of Health and Human Services, October 2018.

MOOD DISORDERS

Mood disorders are also called affective disorders. (*Affect* relates to *feelings, emotions, and mood*.) Feeling sad, irritable, or in a bad mood from time to time is normal. Mood disorders can cause feelings of constant sadness, loss of interest in life, and extremes in feeling happy and sad. Bipolar disorder and depression are 2 types.

Bipolar Disorder

Bipolar means 2 (*bi*) poles or ends (*polar*). The person with bipolar disorder has severe extremes in mood, energy, and function. There are emotional highs or "ups" (*mania*) and emotional lows or "downs" (*depression*). Therefore the disorder is sometimes called manic-depressive disorder.

The disorder runs in families. It usually develops during the late teens or early adulthood. Signs and symptoms range from mild to severe (Box 41-6). Mood changes are called "episodes."

If not treated, bipolar disorder can cause problems with relationships, school, or work. Some persons are suicidal. Life-long management is needed.

Depression

Depression (major depressive disorder; clinical depression) is a mood disorder that affects feeling, thinking, and daily activities. See "Depressive Episode" in Box 41-6 for signs and symptoms. The person has prolonged feelings of sadness, loss, anger, or frustration that affect daily life. Work, study, sleep, eating, and other activities are affected.

Depression is thought to be caused by a combination of factors. Persons with a family history are at higher risk. Major life changes, trauma, and stress are other risk factors. Depression can occur with other illnesses.

Diabetes, cancer, heart disease, stroke, and Parkinson's disease are examples. Depression can make an illness worse. Or an illness can make depression worse. Some drugs have the side effect of depression.

Depression in Older Persons. Depression occurs in older persons. However, it is not a normal part of aging. Older persons have many losses—death of family and friends, loss of body functions, loss of independence. See Box 41-7 for the signs and symptoms of depression in older persons.

Depression in older persons is often overlooked or a wrong diagnosis is made. Instead of depression, the person is thought to have a cognitive disorder (Chapter 42). Therefore the depression goes untreated.

BOX 41-7 Depression in Older Persons—Warning Signs

- Changes in mood, energy level, or appetite
- Feeling "flat" or trouble feeling good emotions
- Problems sleeping or sleeping too much
- Problems concentrating
- Feeling restless, worried, or "on edge"
- Angry, irritable, or aggressive behaviors
- On-going headaches, gastro-intestinal problems, or pain
- Need for alcohol or drugs
- Feeling sad or hopeless
- Suicidal thoughts
- High-risk activities
- Obsessive thinking or compulsive behavior
- Thoughts or behaviors that interfere with work, family, or social activities
- Unusual thinking or behaviors about people

Modified from National Institute of Mental Health: *Older adults and mental health*, revised March 2018.

PERSONALITY DISORDERS

Personality is the set of attitudes, values, behaviors, and traits of a person. Personality development starts at birth. Genes, growth and development, environment, parenting, and social experiences influence personality. Normally, people can form relationships and cope with normal stresses.

Personality disorders involve long-term patterns of thoughts, feelings, and behaviors that can:

- Interfere with daily life.
- Cause problems at school or work.
- Cause problems in relationships.

There are many types of personality disorders. Two examples are described in this chapter.

Antisocial Personality Disorder

A person has a long-term pattern of manipulating, exploiting, or violating the rights and safety of others. Behavior is often criminal. Setting fires and animal cruelty during childhood are often seen. Symptoms include:

- Being witty and charming
- Flattering and manipulating (conning) others for personal gain or pleasure
- Breaking the law repeatedly—lying, stealing, fighting
- Having no regard for the safety of self and others
- Having problems with substance use
- Showing no guilt or remorse (regret, sorrow)
- Being angry
- Feeling superior or more important than others

Borderline Personality Disorder

In borderline personality disorder (BPD), the person has a long-term pattern of unstable moods, behaviors, and emotions. Relationship problems and impulsive actions often result. (To be *impulsive* means *to be reckless or act in haste without considering the consequences.*) Genes and family and social factors may be causes. Childhood abandonment, abuse, and family problems are risk factors.

Signs and symptoms of BPD include:

- Changing interests and values rapidly
- Viewing things in terms of extremes—all good or all bad
- Shifting and changing feelings about other people—liking a person one day but not the next
- Having an intense fear of being abandoned
- Being unable to stand being alone
- Feeling empty and bored
- Inappropriate anger
- Impulsive substance use or sexual relationships
- Self-injury such as wrist cutting or over-dosing
- Suicide attempts or suicide

SUBSTANCE USE DISORDER

Substance use disorder is when the use of alcohol or another substance (a drug) leads to health issues or problems at work, school, or home. Addiction is the most severe form of substance use disorder.

The exact cause is unknown. Influencing factors include genetics, how the substance affects the person, peer pressure, anxiety, depression, and stress. The person with substance use disorder may have other mental health problems.

Legal substances (such as alcohol) and illegal substances (such as heroin) are used. Legal drugs are approved for use in the United States. Illegal drugs are not approved for use. Legal drugs may be bought or obtained illegally. Commonly used substances include:

- *Opiates and other narcotics.* These drugs are strong painkillers that cause drowsiness. Some cause an intense feeling of well-being, happiness, excitement, and joy.
- *Stimulants.* These drugs stimulate the brain and nervous system.
- *Depressants.* These drugs depress the nervous system, causing drowsiness and reduced anxiety. Alcohol is a depressant.
- *Hallucinogens.* These drugs cause sensations and images (hallucinations) that are not real.
- *Marijuana.* This drug affects the brain, causing a "high." Seeing brighter colors and mood changes are common. Legal in some states, medical use includes pain management and nausea from cancer therapy.

Signs and symptoms of substance use disorder are listed in Box 41-8.

See *Focus on Older Persons: Substance Use Disorder.*

FOCUS ON OLDER PERSONS

Substance Use Disorder

Aging can lead to physical and social changes that may increase the risk of substance use. Some older adults use substances to cope with life changes such as retirement, grief and loss, health problems, or a change in living situation. Sometimes the effects of substance use are mistaken for other health problems. When this happens, substance use disorder can be overlooked.

Older adults often have more prescription drugs than other age-groups. This can lead to accidental mis-use of drugs. A person may forget to take a drug, take a drug too often, or take the wrong amount.

Alcohol is the most used substance among older adults. Drinking too much alcohol over a long time can:

- Cause health problems. Certain types of cancer, liver damage, immune system disorders, and brain damage are examples.
- Worsen some health problems. Osteoporosis, diabetes, high blood pressure, stroke, memory loss, and mood disorders are examples.
- Make it hard to diagnose and treat some health problems. For example, body changes from alcohol use can dull the pain that signals a heart attack.
- Cause confusion and forgetfulness. These may be mistaken as signs of Alzheimer's disease (Chapter 42).

Changes from aging can affect how the body handles alcohol. Alcohol use increases the risk for falls, fractures, vehicle crashes, and other injuries. Mixing alcohol with some prescribed drugs is harmful.

BOX 41-8 Substance Use Disorder—Signs and Symptoms

Behavior Changes
- Missing school or work; decreased school or work performance
- Getting into trouble—fights, violence, accidents, car crashes, illegal activities
- Using a substance in hazardous situations—driving, using a machine
- Secretive or suspicious behaviors; hiding substance use
- Appetite: changes in
- Sleep pattern: changes in
- Personality and attitude: changes in
- Mood swings
- Irritability
- Angry outbursts
- Hyperactivity
- Agitation
- Giddiness
- Motivation: lacking
- Fearful, anxious, or paranoid behaviors for no reason

Physical Changes
- Eyes: bloodshot, abnormal pupil size
- Weight: loss or gain
- Appearance: decline in
- Smells: body, breath, clothing
- Tremors
- Speech: slurred
- Coordination: impaired

Social Changes
- Sudden change in friends, hangouts, hobbies
- Legal problems related to substance use
- Unexplained need for money
- Financial problems
- Continued substance use despite harmful effects on health, work, or family

Modified from U.S. Department of Health & Human Services: *Mental health and substance use disorders*, MentalHealth.gov, updated March 22, 2019.

Addiction

Addiction is a chronic disease involving substance-seeking behaviors and use that is compulsive and hard to control despite the harmful effects. See Box 41-9 for behaviors that signal addiction. The person must have the substance.

In *drug addiction*, there is a strong urge or craving to use the substance. The person cannot stop using the drug. Tolerance develops—needing more of the drug for the same effect.

Alcoholism (alcohol dependence) involves:
- *Craving*—a strong need to drink
- *Loss of control*—not being able to stop drinking once started
- *Physical dependence*—withdrawal symptoms
- *Tolerance*—the need for more alcohol for the same effect

BOX 41-9 Signs of Addiction
- The substance is taken in larger amounts. Or it is taken for longer than intended.
- The person tries to cut down or stop using the substance.
- The person craves or has a strong urge for the substance.
- Dangerous activities occur during or after substance use.
- Much time is spent using the substance or recovering from its effects. Or the person spends much time trying to obtain the substance. This interferes with family, work, school, or interests. Substance use continues despite problems.
- The person continues to use the substance even when it causes depression or anxiety or worsens other health problems.
- Substance use causes impaired memory *(blackouts)*.
- The person has tolerance to the substance.
  - The substance has less and less effect on the person.
  - More of the substance is needed for the same effect.
- The person has withdrawal symptoms. *Withdraw* means *to stop, remove, or take away.* **Withdrawal syndrome** *is the physical and mental response after stopping or severely reducing the use of a substance that was used regularly.* The body responds with anxiety, restlessness, insomnia, irritability, poor attention, and physical illness.

Persons with drug or alcohol addiction cannot stop taking the substance without treatment. Treatment for substance use disorder is a long-term process. The person may *relapse*—use the substance again after stopping. Treatment may involve:
- Emergency treatment. An over-dose is life-threatening. Treatment depends on the substance used.
- Detoxification (detox). A *toxin* is a harmful substance that can cause death or serious illness. *Detoxification is the process of removing a toxic substance from the body.*
- Drug therapy. A drug with a similar action on the body is slowly given to reduce withdrawal effects.
- Counseling. See "Care and Treatment" on p. 537.

Complications
Complications of substance use disorder include:
- Sudden death. This can occur from one use of the substance.
- Stroke.
- Lung disease.
- Cancer. Cancers of the mouth and throat, esophagus, larynx, liver, and breast are linked to alcohol.
- Infection. HIV/AIDS and hepatitis B and C are risks from shared needles (Chapter 40).
- Job loss.
- Depression.
- Memory and concentration problems.
- Problems with police and legal issues.
- Relationship problems.
- Unsafe sexual practices. Unwanted pregnancy, sexually transmitted disease (infection), HIV/AIDS, or hepatitis can result.
- Suicide.

EATING DISORDERS

An eating disorder involves a severe disturbance in eating behavior with thoughts and emotions related to eating. Eating disorders often develop during the teen years or in young adulthood. However, they can develop during childhood or later in life. The person may have other mental health disorders.

Eating disorders include:

- *Anorexia nervosa. Anorexia* means no (*a*) appetite (*orexis*). *Nervosa* relates to *nerves* or *emotions.* The person has an intense fear of gaining weight. A fat body image is felt despite being quite thin. Eating very small amounts, exercising excessively, forcing vomiting, and using laxatives (drugs to promote bowel movements) are common. Serious health problems can result. Death is a risk from cardiac arrest or suicide.
- *Bulimia nervosa.* Binge-eating occurs—eating large amounts of food. Over-eating is followed by forced vomiting and intense exercise. Enema and laxative use rid the body of food. Diuretic misuse may occur. (Diuretics cause the kidneys to produce large amounts of urine. Weight loss occurs with the fluid loss.)
- *Binge-eating disorder.* The person often eats large amounts of food. Eating is out of control. Binge-eating is not followed by purging, fasting, or exercise. Often the person is over-weight or obese. High blood pressure, heart disease, diabetes, and joint pain can occur.

SUICIDE

Suicide means to end one's life on purpose. Violence is directed at oneself. The action results in death. If the person survives, it is called a *suicide attempt.*

Risk factors are listed in Box 41-10. Talking about wanting to die or feeling empty, hopeless, or having no reason to live are warning signs. *If a person mentions or talks about suicide, take the person seriously. Call for the nurse at once. Do not leave the person alone.*

Agencies treating persons with mental health disorders must identify persons at risk for suicide. They must:

- Identify specific factors or features that increase or decrease the risk for suicide.
- Meet the person's immediate safety needs.
- Provide the most appropriate setting to treat the person.
- Provide crisis information to the person and family. A crisis "hotline" phone number is an example.
  See *Focus on Communication: Suicide.*
  See *Focus on Older Persons: Suicide.*

BOX 41-10 Suicide Risk Factors

- Prior suicide attempt
- Depression or other mental health disorders
- Substance use disorder
- Chronic pain
- Family history of a mental health disorder, substance use disorder, or suicide
- Family violence (including physical or sexual abuse)
- Guns or other firearms in the home
- Being in prison or jail recently
- Exposure to the suicidal behavior of others (family, peers, media figures)

Modified from National Institute of Mental Health: *Frequently asked questions about suicide*, NIH publication No. 21-MH-6389, Bethesda, Md, revised 2021, National Institutes of Health.

FOCUS ON COMMUNICATION

Suicide

A person thinking about suicide may say:

- "I just don't want to live anymore."
- "I wish I was dead."
- "I wish I had never been born."
- "Everyone would be better off without me."

A person may ask you not to tell anyone about the suicidal thoughts. Protecting personal information is important. But the person's safety is the priority. Never promise that you will not tell anyone. *Call for the nurse at once if a person talks about suicide.*

FOCUS ON OLDER PERSONS

Suicide

Many older persons suffer from depression (p. 533). Depression can severely affect an older person's health. It can worsen conditions such as heart disease, diabetes, and stroke. Especially when untreated, depression can lead to suicide.

Depression in older persons is treatable. Noticing and reporting the warning signs (see Box 41-7) can prevent depression from being overlooked and untreated.

Suicide Contagion

Suicide contagion is exposure to suicide or suicidal behaviors within one's family, one's peer group, or through media reports of suicide. The exposure has led to suicides and suicidal behaviors in persons at risk. Adolescents and young adults are at risk for suicide contagion.

Following suicide exposure, those close to the victim need evaluation by a mental health professional. They include family, friends, peers, and co-workers. Persons at risk for suicide need mental health services.

CARE AND TREATMENT

Treatment of mental health disorders involves therapy, prescription drugs, or both. Counseling and psycho-therapy (talk therapy) help a person identify and change troubling emotions, thoughts, and behaviors. There are different therapy types.

The care plan reflects the needs of the total person. This includes physical, safety and security, and emotional needs.

Communication is important. Be alert to nonverbal communication—the person's and your own. The person may respond to stress with anxiety, panic, anger, or violence. Protect yourself. Once you are safe, the health team can protect the person and others. To protect yourself:

- Call for help. Do not try to handle the situation on your own.
- Keep a safe distance between you and the person.
- Be aware of your setting. Do not let the person block your exit.

See *Focus on Communication: Care and Treatment.*

FOCUS ON **COMMUNICATION**
Care and Treatment

Nonverbal communication involves eye contact, tone of voice, facial expressions, body movements, and posture. Persons with depression often have little eye contact, poor posture, and speak softly. Some do not say much at all. Facial expressions may not change. Some persons cry.

Persons with anxiety may be restless, unable to sit still, and talk fast. Eye contact may be prolonged and intense. Others have poor eye contact. The eyes may dart about. Be alert to nonverbal cues. Report what you observe.

Your nonverbal communication is important. When interacting with persons with mental health disorders:

- Face the person.
- Maintain eye contact.
- Position yourself near the person but not too close. Do not invade the person's space.
- Crouch, sit, or stand at the person's level if safe to do so.
- Show interest and concern through your posture and facial expressions.
- Speak calmly.

FOCUS ON P R I D E
The Person, Family, and Yourself

P ersonal and Professional Responsibility

Just as a person does not choose to have a physical illness, a person does not choose a mental health disorder. How you view the disorder affects how you treat the person. Treat the person with kindness, respect, and compassion. Provide quality care.

R ights and Respect

Agencies have strict rules to protect the person's rights to privacy and confidentiality (Chapter 2). Do not talk about the person with your family or friends. Never give information to someone not involved in the person's care. This includes the person's family. Direct questions to the nurse. Follow agency policies. Take pride in protecting the person's rights.

I ndependence and Social Interaction

Social support is important in treating mental health disorders. Family and friends provide support and a sense of worth and belonging. *Support groups* connect people who share common problems. People can share experiences and coping strategies. Groups may be in-person or on-line.

D elegation and Teamwork

Mental health disorders can be very distressing for the person. Some situations are urgent. If someone calls for help, respond at once. Assist as the nurse directs. Take pride in working as a team.

E thics and Laws

Sometimes a person's speech or behaviors may seem strange or odd to you. You must show professional and ethical conduct. Never laugh at or insult a person. Do not joke with others about a person. Treat the person with dignity and respect.

FOCUS ON **PRIDE:** *Application*

Why are persons with mental health disorders at risk for violations of their rights? How must the health team protect the person's rights?

REVIEW QUESTIONS

Circle the BEST answer.

1 Stress is
   a A way to cope with or adjust to every-day living
   b A response or change in the body caused by some factor
   c A mental health disorder
   d An unwanted thought or idea

2 These statements are about defense mechanisms. Which is *true?*
   a Using them signals a mental health disorder.
   b They can help relieve anxiety.
   c They prevent mental health disorders.
   d Persons with mental health disorders use them well.

3 A phobia is
   a The event that causes stress
   b A false belief
   c An intense fear of something
   d A ritual

4 A person cleans and cleans in response to anxious thoughts. This behavior is
   a A delusion
   b A hallucination
   c A compulsion
   d Panic

5 Flashbacks with PTSD can cause the person to
   a Relive the trauma in thoughts and during sleep
   b Forget the past
   c Regress to an earlier time
   d Be violent toward others

6 A person with schizophrenia has delusions and hallucinations. This means that the person has
   a Enhanced sensation and awareness
   b Anger and aggression
   c Impulsive and violent behavior
   d False beliefs and perceptions

7 Bipolar disorder means that the person
   a Is very suspicious
   b Has anxiety
   c Is very unhappy and feels unwanted
   d Has severe extremes in mood

8 In bipolar disorder, an "emotional high" is called
   a Depression
   b A hallucination
   c Mania
   d An obsession

9 Which is a sign of depression in older persons?
   a Hallucinations
   b Appetite changes
   c Memory loss
   d Slurred speech

10 In antisocial personality disorder, the person
   a Lacks regard for the rights and safety of others
   b Has a sad, anxious, or empty mood
   c Withdraws from people and interests
   d Is paranoid and avoids social situations

11 Which statement about substance use disorder is *true?*
   a Legal substances cannot cause addiction.
   b Substance use causes problems at work, home, or school.
   c Complications of substance use disorder are minor.
   d There is no treatment for substance use disorder.

12 A person has withdrawal syndrome. This means that
   a The person has a physical and mental response when the drug is not taken
   b The person needs higher doses of the drug
   c The effect is reduced with the same amount of drug
   d The person has a relapse after treatment

13 Binge-eating followed by forced vomiting occurs in
   a Anorexia nervosa
   b Binge-eating disorder
   c Bulimia nervosa
   d Borderline personality disorder

14 A person talks about suicide. What should you do?
   a Call for the nurse.
   b Identify factors that increase the risk of suicide.
   c Ask what method the person plans to use.
   d Restrain the person.

15 A patient's family member asks what to say when the person talks about suicide. You should
   a Give advice
   b Direct the question to the nurse
   c Suggest a local support group
   d Call a crisis hotline

Answers to Chapter 41 questions are on p. 589.

FOCUS ON PRACTICE

Problem Solving

A person with panic disorder becomes restless in a group setting. The person feels short of breath and hot and says: "My heart is pounding. I need to leave." What might be the cause? What will you do?

CHAPTER 42

Confusion and Dementia

OBJECTIVES

- Define the key terms and key abbreviations in this chapter.
- Describe confusion and its causes.
- List the measures that help confused persons.
- Explain the difference between delirium and dementia.
- Describe the signs, symptoms, and behavior and function changes that can occur with Alzheimer's disease (AD).

- Explain the care required by persons with AD and other dementias.
- Describe the effects of AD on the family.
- Explain validation therapy.
- Explain how to promote PRIDE in the person, the family, and yourself.

KEY TERMS

cognitive function Involves memory, thinking, reasoning, ability to understand, judgment, and behavior
confusion A state of being disoriented to person, time, place, situation, or identity
delirium A state of sudden, severe confusion and rapid changes in brain function
delusion A false belief
dementia The loss of cognitive function that interferes with daily life and activities

elopement When a patient or resident leaves the agency without staff knowledge
hallucination Seeing, hearing, smelling, feeling, or tasting something that is not real
paranoia A disorder *(para)* of the mind *(noia)*; false beliefs (delusions) and suspicion about a person or situation
sundowning Signs, symptoms, and behaviors of dementia increase during hours of darkness

KEY ABBREVIATIONS

AD   Alzheimer's disease
ADL   Activities of daily living

NIA   National Institute on Aging

Changes in the brain and nervous system occur with certain diseases and with age (Box 42-1). Cognitive function may be affected. *(Cognitive* relates to *knowledge.) Cognitive function involves memory, thinking, reasoning, ability to understand, judgment, and behavior.* Changes in function affect quality of life.

CONFUSION

Confusion is a state of being disoriented to person, time, place, situation, or identity. Disoriented means to be apart from (dis) *one's awareness* (oriented). Memory and the ability to make good judgments are lost. Daily activities may be affected.

BOX 42-1 Nervous System Changes From Aging

- Nerve cells are lost.
- Nerve conduction slows.
- Reflexes, responses, and reaction times are slower.
- Vision, hearing, taste, smell, and touch decrease.
- Sensitivity to pain decreases.
- Blood flow to the brain is reduced.
- Sleep patterns change.
- Memory is shorter; forgetfulness occurs.
- Dizziness can occur.

A person may not know people, the time, or the place. Behavior changes are common—anger, restlessness, depression, irritability.

Disease, brain injury, infections, hearing and vision loss, and drug side effects are some causes. Reduced blood flow to the brain with aging can cause personality and mental changes. Depending on the cause, onset may be fast or slow. Report sudden onset of confusion at once. Confusion may be temporary or permanent.

Treatment is aimed at the cause. Some measures help improve function (Box 42-2). You must meet the person's basic needs.

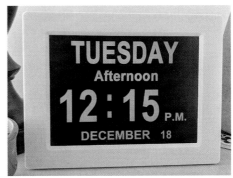

FIGURE 42-1 A large clock can help persons who are confused.

BOX 42-2 Confusion—Care Measures

- Follow the care plan.
- Provide for safety.
- Face the person. Speak clearly.
- Call the person by name each time you have contact.
- State your name. Show your name tag.
- Give the date and time each morning. Repeat as needed during the day or evening.
- Explain what you are going to do and why.
- Give clear, simple directions and answers to questions.
- Break tasks into small steps.
- Ask clear and simple questions. Allow time to respond.
- Make sure the person can see a calendar and clock (Fig. 42-1). Remind the person of holidays, birthdays, and other events.
- Have the person wear needed eyeglasses and hearing aids.
- Use touch to communicate (Chapter 6).
- Place familiar objects and photos within view.
- Provide newspapers, magazines, TV, radio, phone, and any other personal electronic devices. Read to the person if appropriate.
- Discuss current events.
- Maintain the day-night cycle.
  - Open window coverings during the day. Close them at night.
  - Use night-lights in rooms, bathrooms, hallways, and other areas at night.
  - Have the person wear day-time clothes during the day.
- Provide a calm, relaxed, and peaceful setting. Prevent loud noises, rushing, and crowded hallways and dining rooms.
- Follow the person's routine. Meals, bathing, exercise, TV, bedtime, and other activities have a schedule. This promotes a sense of order and what to expect.
- Do not re-arrange furniture or the person's belongings.
- Encourage the person to take part in self-care.

Delirium

Delirium is a state of sudden, severe confusion and rapid changes in brain function. Usually temporary and reversible, it can occur with physical or mental illness. Surgery, drug side effects, severe lack of sleep, electrolyte imbalances, and substance use disorder or withdrawal (Chapter 41) are some causes. Infections such as urinary tract infections and pneumonia can cause delirium (Chapter 40).

Onset is usually fast—within hours or a few days. Signs and symptoms (Box 42-3) may come and go during the day and worsen at night. Delirium often lasts for about 1 week. However, it may take several weeks for normal mental function to return.

Delirium signals illness. It is an emergency. The cause must be found and treated.

See *Focus on Older Persons: Delirium.*

FOCUS ON OLDER PERSONS

Delirium

Older persons in a hospital or long-term care setting are at risk for delirium. Do not assume the nurse knows about a problem. Report the signs and symptoms in Box 42-3 or a change in the person's normal behavior at once.

BOX 42-3 Delirium—Signs and Symptoms

- Alertness: changes in (usually more alert in the morning and less alert at night)
- Sensation and perception: changes in
- Awareness and level of consciousness: changes in
- Movement: very active or slow moving
- Drowsiness, changes in sleep patterns
- Confusion about time or place
- Thinking: disorganized
- Memory: decreased short-term memory and recall (cannot remember events since the delirium began)
- Concentration: problems with
- Speech: does not make sense
- Incontinence
- Emotional or personality changes: agitation, anger, depression, euphoria (overly happy), irritability

Modified from MedlinePlus: *Delirium*, Bethesda, Md, updated January 11, 2022, U.S. National Library of Medicine, National Institutes of Health.

DEMENTIA

Dementia is the loss of cognitive function that interferes with daily life and activities. (De means from. Mentia means mind.) Changes in personality, mood, behavior, and communication are common. Dementia is a group of symptoms, not a specific disease.

Dementia is caused by damage to brain cells. Some conditions cause thinking and memory problems that can be reversed when the cause is treated. Depression, drug side effects, excess alcohol use, thyroid problems, and vitamin deficiencies are examples. Head injury and blood clots, tumors, or infections in the brain are other treatable causes.

Permanent dementias result from changes in the brain (Box 42-4). There is no cure. Function declines over time.

Dementia is not a normal part of aging. The risk increases with age. Persons over 65 and those with a family history of dementia are at higher risk.

Early warning signs include:
- Memory loss (losing things, forgetting names)
- Problems with common tasks (dressing, cooking, driving)
- Problems with language and communication; forgetting simple words
- Getting lost in familiar places
- Misplacing things and putting things in odd places (for example, putting a watch in the oven)
- Personality, mood, and behavior changes
- Poor or decreased judgment (for example, going out in the snow without shoes)
  See *Focus on Older Persons: Dementia.*

BOX 42-4 Types of Permanent Dementia

- Alzheimer's disease—most common type. See "Alzheimer's Disease."
- Vascular dementia—stroke or other blood vessel problems damage vessels that supply blood to the brain.
- Lewy body dementia—abnormal protein deposits in the brain (Lewy bodies) affect chemicals in the brain.
- Fronto-temporal disorders—nerve cells in certain areas of the brain (front and sides) break down.
- Mixed dementia—2 or more types of dementia occur together.

FOCUS ON OLDER PERSONS

Dementia

Depression is a common mental health disorder in older persons. Confusion and attention problems from depression may be mistaken for dementia. Dementia, depression, aging, and some drug side effects have similar signs and symptoms. See "Depression in Older Persons" in Chapter 41.

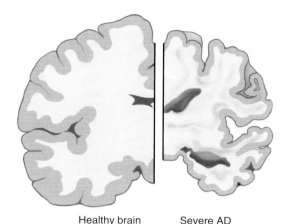

FIGURE 42-2 Nerve cell death and tissue loss shrink the brain in the person with AD. (Redrawn from National Institute on Aging: *Alzheimer's disease fact sheet*, National Institutes of Health, U.S. Department of Health and Human Services, content reviewed July 8, 2021.)

ALZHEIMER'S DISEASE

Alzheimer's disease (AD) is the most common type of permanent dementia. Many brain cells are destroyed and die. Connections between nerve cells are lost. Over time, the brain shrinks from nerve cell death and tissue loss (Fig. 42-2). Two abnormal structures are thought to cause damage.
- *Plaques*—protein pieces that build up in the spaces between nerve cells.
- *Tangles*—twisted protein fibers that build up inside cells.

With aging, most people develop some plaques and tangles. In AD, plaque and tangle development is severe. Memory areas of the brain are often affected before other areas.

AD onset is gradual. Most persons with AD are age 65 and older. However, it can occur in younger persons.

AD is progressive. Symptoms gradually get worse over time. Currently, there is no cure. The goals of treatment are to slow the progression of symptoms and improve quality of life. Persons with AD can live for 4 to 8 years or longer.

Risk Factors

The greatest risk factor for AD is increasing age. The risk increases after age 65. A family history of AD increases the person's risk. More persons with AD are women because women often live longer than men.

The National Institute on Aging (NIA) recommends the following to maintain cognitive health.

- Get regular exercise.
- Eat a healthy diet.
- Maintain a healthy weight.
- Spend time with family and friends.
- Keep the mind active.
- Control type 2 diabetes and maintain healthy blood pressure and cholesterol levels (Chapter 40).
- Do not smoke.
- Get help for depression (Chapter 41).
- Avoid excess alcohol intake.
- Get enough sleep.

Signs of AD

According to the Alzheimer's Association, the most common early symptom of AD is difficulty remembering newly learned information. *The classic sign is a gradual loss of short-term memory.* At first, the only symptom may be forgetfulness.

Box 42-5 lists early signs and symptoms of AD. AD is not a normal part of aging. See Box 42-6 for the differences between AD and normal age-related changes.

Stages of AD

Signs and symptoms become more severe as AD progresses. The disease ends in death. AD is described in 3 stages. See Box 42-7 and Figure 42-3.

BOX 42-5 Alzheimer's Disease—Early Signs and Symptoms

Memory Loss That Disrupts Daily Life
- Forgets newly learned information
- Forgets important dates or events
- Asks the same questions over and over
- Relies more on memory aids—reminder notes, electronic devices
- Relies on family members for things usually handled alone

Problems With Planning or Problem Solving
- Has trouble making a plan or working with numbers
- Has problems following a recipe
- Has trouble keeping track of monthly bills
- Difficulty concentrating
- Takes longer to do things than before

Problems Completing Familiar Tasks
- Has a hard time with tasks in the home, at work, or with recreation
- Has problems driving to familiar places
- Has trouble organizing a grocery list
- Forgets the rules to a favorite game

Confusion With Time or Place
- Loses track of dates, seasons, and passing of time
- Has trouble understanding something that is not happening right away
- Forgets the current location
- Forgets the method of arrival (how the person got to the current location)

Problems With Vision and Spatial Relationships
- Balance problems
- Difficulty reading
- Difficulty judging distance
- Has problems with color or contrast
- Has trouble driving

Problems With Speaking or Writing
- Has trouble following or joining a conversation
- Stops in the middle of a conversation and does not know how to continue
- Repeats things
- Has trouble finding the right word
- Calls things by the wrong name—calling a "watch" a "hand-clock" is an example

Misplacing Items and Being Unable to Find Them
- Puts things in strange places
- Loses things and is unable to retrace steps to find them
- Accuses others of stealing

Decreased or Poor Judgment
- Changes in judgment or decision making
- Poor judgment with money—giving away large amounts is an example
- Pays less attention to hygiene and grooming

Withdrawal From Work or Social Activities
- No longer does hobbies, social activities, work projects, or sports
- Has trouble keeping up with a favorite sports team
- Has trouble remembering how to do a hobby
- Avoids being social

Mood and Personality Changes
- Is confused
- Is depressed
- Is suspicious, afraid, or anxious
- Is easily upset at home, at work, with friends, or outside of the usual setting

Modified from Alzheimer's Association: *10 early signs and symptoms of Alzheimer's,* 2022.

BOX 42-6 Alzheimer's Disease and Normal Aging

Signs of AD	Normal Age-Related Changes
• Poor judgment and decision making.	• Makes a bad decision once in a while.
• Cannot manage a budget.	• Misses a monthly payment.
• Loses track of the date or season.	• Forgets which day it is but remembers later.
• Problems having a conversation.	• Sometimes forgets which word to use.
• Misplaces things. Cannot retrace steps to find them.	• Loses things from time to time.

Modified from Alzheimer's Association: *10 early signs and symptoms of Alzheimer's,* 2022.

BOX 42-7 Alzheimer's Disease—Stages

Mild AD
- Memory loss
- Poor judgment, bad decisions
- Loss of spontaneity and initiative
- Taking longer to do daily tasks
- Repeating questions
- Problems handling money and paying bills
- Wandering and getting lost
- Losing things or misplacing them in odd places
- Mood and personality changes
- Anxiety or aggression

Moderate AD
- Increased memory loss and confusion
- Cannot learn new things
- Problems with language, reading, writing, and working with numbers
- Trouble with thoughts and thinking logically
- Shortened attention span
- Problems coping with new situations
- Problems with tasks having multiple steps—getting dressed is an example
- Problems recognizing family and friends
- Hallucinations, delusions, and paranoia
- Impulsive behavior—undressing at inappropriate times or places and using vulgar language are examples
- Outbursts of anger
- Restlessness, agitation, anxiety, tearfulness
- Wandering—especially in the late afternoon or evening
- Repetitive statements or movements, occasional muscle twitches

Severe AD
- Depends on others for care
- In bed most or all of the time
- Cannot communicate
- Weight loss
- Seizures
- Skin infections
- Difficulty swallowing
- Groaning, moaning, or grunting
- Increased sleeping
- Loss of bowel and bladder control

Modified from National Institute on Aging: *What are the signs of Alzheimer's disease?*, content reviewed May 16, 2017, National Institutes of Health.

Behavior and Function Changes

AD changes how a person behaves and acts. Besides the signs and symptoms in Boxes 42-5 and 42-7, these common behaviors and changes of AD are described in the following pages.
- Wandering and getting lost
- Sundowning
- Hallucinations
- Delusions
- Paranoia
- Catastrophic reactions
- Agitation and aggression
- Communication changes
- Screaming
- Repetitive behaviors
- Rummaging and hiding things
- Changes in intimacy and sexuality
  Besides brain changes, the following can affect behavior.
- Health problems—illness, pain, infection, drugs, lack of sleep, constipation, hunger, thirst, poor vision or hearing, alcohol abuse, too much caffeine
- Emotions—sadness, fear, feeling overwhelmed, stress, anxiety
- Changes in routine
- Problems in the person's setting:
  - A strange setting. The person does not know the setting well.
  - Too much noise (TV, music, people talking at once) can cause confusion and frustration.
  - Not understanding signs. The person may think that a *WET FLOOR* sign means to urinate on the floor.
  - Mirrors. The person may think that a mirror image is another person in the room.

See *Promoting Safety and Comfort: Behavior and Function Changes.*

PROMOTING SAFETY AND COMFORT
Behavior and Function Changes

Safety
Some behaviors are caused by illness, injury, or drugs—not AD. Without treatment, life may be threatened. Always report changes in behavior.

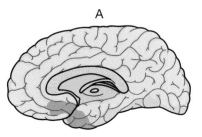
Very Early AD

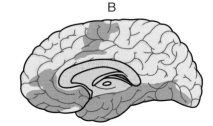
Mild to Moderate AD

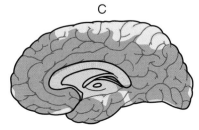
Severe AD

FIGURE 42-3 **A,** Very early AD. **B,** Mild to moderate AD. **C,** Severe AD. (NOTE: Blue shading shows the areas of the brain affected.) (Redrawn from National Institute on Aging: *Alzheimer's disease: unraveling the mystery*, Bethesda, Md, September 2008, National Institutes of Health.)

Wandering and Getting Lost. Persons with AD are often not oriented to person, time, and place. They may wander off and not find their way back. Wandering is by foot, car, bike, or other means. They may be with you one moment and gone the next.

Judgment is poor. They cannot tell what is safe or dangerous. Life-threatening accidents are great risks. They can walk into traffic or a nearby river, lake, ocean, or forest. If not properly dressed, heat or cold exposure is a risk.

Wandering may have no cause. Or the person is looking for something or someone—the bathroom, the bedroom, a child, or a partner. Pain, drug side effects, stress, restlessness, too much stimulation, and anxiety are other causes. A wandering pattern may reflect a life-long routine—leaving work, getting children from school, and so on. Sometimes finding the cause prevents wandering.

See *Promoting Safety and Comfort: Wandering and Getting Lost.*

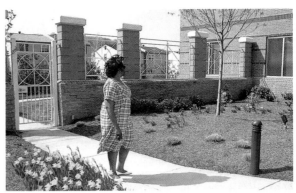

FIGURE 42-4   An enclosed garden allows persons with AD to wander in a safe setting.

PROMOTING SAFETY AND COMFORT

Wandering and Getting Lost

Safety

Patients and residents may try to wander to another nursing unit or out of the agency. *Leaving the agency without staff knowledge is called* **elopement**. Serious injury and death have resulted. State and federal guidelines to prevent elopement are followed.

   All staff must be alert to persons who wander. Wandering is allowed in safe areas (Fig. 42-4). Unsafe areas include kitchens, shower rooms, and utility rooms.

   Tell other staff that a person wanders. You cannot be with the person all the time. All staff can help monitor the person. Help other staff in the same way. If you see a person wandering into an unsafe area, gently guide the person to a safe place (Fig. 42-5). Tell the nurse.

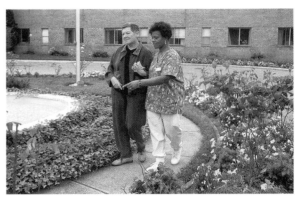

FIGURE 42-5   Guide the person who wanders to a safe area.

Alert Systems. Some states have safety alert systems for older persons who are missing. Called "Silver Alert" or "Code Silver" in some states, such programs involve reporting and alert procedures to help locate older persons with dementia who are lost.

MedicAlert® + Alzheimer's Association Safe Return® is a nationwide 24-hour emergency service for persons who wander or have a medical emergency. The purpose is to find and safely return persons who wander and become lost. A small fee is charged.

A family member provides required information and a photo. The person receives an ID (wallet card and bracelet or necklace). If reported missing, the person's information is sent to the police. When the person is found, someone calls the toll-free number on the ID. *MedicAlert® + Alzheimer's Association Safe Return®* then calls the family member or caregiver. The person is returned home.

Sundowning. With **sundowning**, *signs, symptoms, and behaviors of dementia increase during hours of darkness.* As daylight ends and darkness starts, confusion and restlessness increase. So do anxiety, agitation, and other symptoms. Behavior is worse after sundown. It may continue during the night.

Brain changes affecting the sleep-wake cycle may cause sundowning. Other possible causes include fatigue, hunger or thirst, depression, pain, and boredom. Confusion and fear can occur when poor lighting and shadows cause the person to see things that are not there.

Hallucinations and Delusions. A **hallucination** *is seeing, hearing, smelling, feeling, or tasting something that is not real.* Affected persons see animals, insects, or people that are not present. Some hear voices. They may feel bugs crawling or feel that they are being touched.

Poor vision or hearing may be a cause. The person should wear needed eyeglasses and hearing aids. Other causes include infection, pain, and drugs.

Delusions *are false beliefs.* To the person, the beliefs are real. People with AD may think they are another person. Some believe they are in jail, are being killed, or are being attacked. A person may believe the caregiver is someone else. Many other false beliefs can occur.

Paranoia. *Paranoia is a disorder* (para) *of the mind* (noia). *The person has false beliefs (delusions) and suspicion about a person or situation.* Paranoia is a type of delusion. The person believes others are mean, lying, not fair, or intend harm. The person may be suspicious, fearful, or jealous.

Paranoia may worsen as memory loss gets worse. For example, the person thinks misplaced items have been stolen. Or the person no longer recognizes a caregiver. The person does not trust the caregiver.

The person may express loss through paranoia. Reasons for the loss do not make sense. Therefore the person blames or accuses others.

See *Promoting Safety and Comfort: Paranoia.*

PROMOTING SAFETY AND COMFORT

Paranoia

Safety

Behaviors may not mean paranoia. Fears of harm, strangers, stealing, mistreatment, and so on may be real. Some people abuse vulnerable adults (Chapter 4). This includes sexual and financial abuse.

Abuse may be by phone, mail, e-mail, or in person. The abuser may be a friend or family member. Financial abuse occurs when money or belongings are stolen. Financial abuse can include:

- Forging checks or cashing checks without permission
- Taking retirement and Social Security benefits
- Using the person's credit cards or bank accounts
- Changing names on wills, bank accounts, insurance policies, or titles to homes or cars
- "Scams" such as identity theft, phone prizes, and threats
- Borrowing money and not paying it back
- Giving away or selling the person's property without permission
- Forcing the person to sign over property
  Protect the person from harm, abuse, and mistreatment.

Report the following at once.

- What the person is saying
- The person seems afraid or worried about money
- Missing items
- The person's behaviors
- Signs and symptoms of problems
- Visitors or family members acting strangely

Catastrophic Reactions. These are extreme responses to normal events or things. The person reacts as if there is a disaster or tragedy. The person may scream, cry, or be agitated or combative (ready to fight). These reactions are common from too many stimuli. Eating, music or TV playing, and being asked questions all at once can overwhelm the person.

Agitation and Aggression. When agitated, the person is restless or worried and cannot settle down. The person may pace, move about, or not sleep. Agitation may lead to aggression. The person may yell, scream, swear, hit, pinch, grab, or try to hurt someone. Common causes are:

- Pain or discomfort.
- Anxiety, depression, or stress.
- Loneliness.
- Drug interactions.
- Fatigue.
- Too many stimuli. Too much noise or too many people in the room are examples.
- Hunger or thirst.
- Elimination needs, constipation, or incontinence.
- Feeling lost or abandoned.
- A feeling of loss. Missing driving or caring for children are examples.
- Care measures (bathing, dressing) that upset or frighten the person.
- Feeling pressured to do something that is now hard or impossible. Remembering an event or person are examples.
- Change in routine, caregiver, or setting.
- Caregivers. A caregiver may rush the person or be impatient. Or mixed verbal and nonverbal messages are sent. For example, a caregiver talks too fast or too loud. Consider how your behaviors affect the person.

Communication Changes. Communication skills gradually decline. The person has trouble expressing thoughts and emotions. Communication changes include:

- Struggling to find the right word
- Problems understanding the meaning of words
- Attention problems during conversations
- Losing one's train of thought when talking
- Problems blocking background noises—radio, TV, music, phones, others talking, and so on
- Frustration with communication problems
- Being sensitive to touch, tone, and voice volume

As the person loses the ability to talk clearly, other communication methods may be used. Facial expressions and gestures are examples. In time, the person cannot understand others and communicate verbally.

See *Caring About Culture: Communication Changes.*
See *Focus on Communication: Communication Changes,* p. 546.

 ### CARING ABOUT CULTURE

Communication Changes

For some, English is a second language. For example, the first language learned is Spanish, Italian, French, Russian, Chinese, or Japanese. With AD, the person may forget or no longer understand English. The person uses and understands only the first language learned.

FOCUS ON COMMUNICATION

Communication Changes

To promote communication with the person with AD, see Box 42-8. Avoid:

- *Giving orders.* For example: "Sit down and eat" is bossy. It does not show respect. Instead say: "Let me help you sit down."
- *Wanting the truth.* For example, do not say: "Don't you remember?" or "What day is it?" Instead say: "Today is Friday."
- *Correcting errors.* For example, do not say: "I just told you it's time to get dressed. You already had breakfast." Instead say: "Let me help you get dressed."
- *Pointing out errors.* Instead of saying: "You missed a button," say: "Let's try it this way."
- *Giving many choices.* For example: "What would you like for dinner?" involves many choices. Instead, limit choices. Say: "Do you want potatoes or rice?"
- *Asking open-ended questions.* For example, do not say: "How do you feel?" Instead, ask "yes" or "no" questions. You can say: "Are you tired?"

Screaming. At first, persons with AD have problems finding the right words. As AD progresses, they speak in short sentences or just words. Often speech is not understandable.

Screaming to communicate is common in persons who are very confused and have poor communication skills. They may scream a word or a name. Or they just make screaming sounds.

Possible causes include hearing and vision problems, pain or discomfort, fear, and fatigue. Too much or not enough stimulation is another cause. A person may react to a caregiver or family member by screaming. The following measures and those in Box 42-8 may be helpful.

- Provide a calm, quiet setting.
- Play soft music.
- Have the person wear hearing aids and eyeglasses.
- Have a family member or favorite caregiver comfort and calm the person.
- Use touch to calm the person.

Repetitive Behaviors. *Repetitive* means *to do over and over.* The person repeats the same motions, words, or questions over and over. For example, the same napkin is folded over and over. Or the person says the same words or asks the same question over and over. Such behaviors are not harmful. However, they can annoy caregivers and the family.

Rummaging and Hiding Things. To *rummage* means *to search for things by moving things around, turning things over, or looking through something such as a drawer or closet.* The behavior may have no meaning. Or the person is looking for a certain item but cannot tell you what or why.

The person may hide things, throw things away, or lose things. Eyeglasses, hearing aids, and dentures must stay with the person. Always make sure these items are safe. Money, jewelry, and other important items usually are sent home with the family.

BOX 42-8 Dementia Care—Communication

- Treat the person with dignity and respect.
- Approach the person in a calm, quiet manner.
- Approach the person from the front—not from the side or the back. This avoids startling the person.
- Make eye contact to get the person's attention. Maintain eye contact.
- Have the person's attention before you start speaking.
- Identify yourself and other people by name.
- Call the person by name.
- Avoid pronouns (he, she, them, it, and so on). For example, instead of saying: "They are here," say: "Jon and Stacy are here."
- Follow the rules and measures to promote communication (Chapter 6).
- Do not talk about the person as if the person is not there.
- Control distractions and noise. TV, radio, and music are examples.
- Speak in a calm, gentle voice. Be patient.
- Be aware of your body language. Smile and avoid frowning, grimacing, or other negative actions. Standing with the arms folded tightly signals tension or anger.
- Use gestures or cues. Point to objects.
- Watch the person's facial expressions and gestures. Expressions may show sadness, anger, or frustration. Pulling at under-garments may signal incontinence or elimination needs.

- Comfort the person with touch. Hold the person's hand while you talk.
- Speak slowly. Use simple words and short sentences.
- Do not "baby talk" or use a "baby voice."
- Ask or say 1 thing at a time. Present 1 idea, statement, or question at a time.
- Give simple, step-by-step instructions.
- Explain all procedures and activities.
- Repeat instructions as needed. Allow time to respond or react.
- Ask simple questions with simple answers. Do not ask complex questions.
- Let the person speak. Do not interrupt or rush the person.
- Give the person time to respond.
- Try other words if the person does not seem to understand.
- Provide the word if the person is struggling to communicate a thought.
- Do not criticize, correct, interrupt, argue, or try to reason with the person.
- Give consistent responses.
- Practice the measures in Chapter 39:
  - To promote hearing
  - To communicate with speech-impaired persons
  - For blind and visually impaired persons

Changes in Intimacy and Sexuality. *Intimacy* is a special bond between people who love and respect each other. It includes the way people talk and act toward each other. *Sexuality* involves the way partners physically express feelings for each other. The person with AD may:

- Depend on and cling to a partner.
- Not remember life with a partner.
- Not remember feelings for a partner.
- Express affection for another person.
- Have side effects from drugs that affect sexual interest.
- Have memory loss, brain changes, or depression that affects sexual interest.
- Have abnormal sexual behaviors. Sexual behaviors are labeled abnormal because of how and when they occur—wrong person, wrong place, or wrong time. Persons with AD cannot control the behavior.

Healthy persons do not undress or expose themselves in front of others. They do not masturbate or engage in sexual acts in public. They know their sexual partners. Persons with AD may mistake someone else for a sexual partner. The person kisses and hugs the other person.

Appropriate affection is encouraged. The nurse encourages the person's partner to show affection with the couple's usual practices. Hand-holding, hugging, kissing, touching, and dancing are examples. Distraction and privacy measures may be helpful when actions occur with the wrong person or in public (undressing, masturbating). For example, a resident is distracted with an activity or guided to the resident's room.

Some behaviors are not sexual. Touching, scratching, and rubbing the genitals can signal infection, pain, or discomfort in the urinary or reproductive systems. Poor hygiene and incontinence are other causes. Good hygiene prevents itching. Clean the person promptly and thoroughly after elimination. Do not let the person stay wet or soiled.

CARE OF PERSONS WITH AD AND OTHER DEMENTIAS

The person may be cared for at home until symptoms become severe. Adult day care may help. Often assisted living or nursing center care is required. Other illnesses may require hospital care. The person may need hospice care as death nears (Chapter 44). You may care for persons with AD or other dementias in such settings. The person and family need your support and understanding.

People with dementia do not choose the signs and symptoms of the disease. They cannot control what is happening to them. *The disease is responsible, not the person.* Often, the person's behavior is an attempt to communicate needs. See "Meeting Basic Needs" on p. 549.

You must treat persons with dementia with dignity and respect. They have the same rights as everyone else. The care plan addresses the person's specific needs related to behavior changes. See Box 42-9 for examples. See Box 42-8 for measures to promote communication.

BOX 42-9 Dementia Care—Behavior Changes

Wandering
- Follow agency policy for locking doors and windows. Some doors lock automatically. Staff enter a code into an electronic key pad for entry and exit. Some doors have manual locks in places the person is not likely to look (Fig. 42-6, p. 548).
- Keep door alarms and electronic doors turned on. Respond to alarms at once.
- Follow agency policy for fire exits. Everyone must be able to leave the building for a fire.
- Have the person wear an ID bracelet or *MedicAlert*® + *Alzheimer's Association Safe Return*® ID at all times.
- Know when the person is more likely to wander.
- Follow the care plan for daily routine, activities, and exercise. Meet food, fluid, and elimination needs.
- Involve the person in activities—folding napkins, dusting a table, sorting socks, rolling yarn, sweeping, sanding blocks of wood, or watering plants.
- Do not use restraints. They tend to increase confusion and disorientation. See Chapter 13.
- Do not argue with the person who wants to leave. The person will not understand.
- Go with the person who insists on going outside. Provide proper clothing. Guide the person inside after a few minutes.
- Allow wandering in enclosed and safe areas.

Sundowning
- Complete treatments and activities early in the day.
- Encourage exercise and activity early in the day.

Sundowning—cont'd
- Avoid too many activities in a day.
- Allow for rest during the day if needed. If a nap is needed, it should be short and not late in the day.
- Keep the person on a schedule. Waking up, meal times, and bedtime should involve a set routine.
- Avoid caffeine (coffee, tea, colas, chocolate), sweets, and alcohol late in the day.
- Provide a calm, quiet setting late in the day.
- Do not restrain the person.
- Meet nutrition and elimination needs. Unmet needs can increase restlessness.
- Use night-lights at night.
- Do not try to reason with the person. The person will not understand.
- Do not ask the person to explain the problem. Communication changes impair understanding and speech.
- Promote sleep at night. See p. 549.

Hallucinations and Delusions
- Have the person wear eyeglasses and hearing aids as needed.
- Do not argue with the person. The person will not understand.
- Reassure the person. Say that you will keep the person safe.
- Distract the person with an item or activity. Or take the person to another room or for a walk.
- Turn off TV or movies when violent and disturbing programs are on. The person may believe the story is real.

Continued

BOX 42-9 Dementia Care—Behavior Changes—cont'd

Hallucinations and Delusions—cont'd
- Provide comfort if the person seems afraid. Gentle touch may calm and reassure some persons (Fig. 42-7).
- Eliminate noises that can be misinterpreted. TV, radio, music, furnaces, and air conditioners are examples.
- Check lighting. Eliminate glares, shadows, or reflections.
- Cover or remove mirrors. The person could misinterpret the reflection.
- Remove anything that could be used to hurt the self or others.
- Report behavior changes. They may signal a physical illness.

Paranoia
- Do not react if the person blames you for something.
- Do not argue with the person.
- Give reminders of the person's safety.
- Use touch correctly. Know how the person responds to touch. Touch can comfort some people. Others do not like being touched.
- Search for missing things to distract the person. Talk about what you found. For example, talk about a photo you found.

Catastrophic Reactions
- Approach the person from the front. Do not startle from behind or the side.
- Be calm. Do not appear rushed. Give the person time to calm down.
- Use touch correctly. See "Paranoia."
- Explain in simple terms what you want the person to do. For example: "It's time for bed. I'll help you into bed."
- Do not argue with the person.
- Follow the person's daily routine, including naps and bedtime.
- Distract the person with an item or activity.

Agitation and Aggression
- Look at how your behaviors affect the person.
- Provide a calm, quiet setting.
- Follow the care plan and a set routine for activities of daily living (ADL). Meet basic needs.
- Observe for early signs of agitation and aggression. Try to remove the cause before the agitation or aggression worsens.
- Do not ignore the problem. Try to find the cause.
- Allow personal choice to the extent possible.
- Try to distract the person. A snack or activity may help.
- Reassure the person.
  - Speak calmly.
  - Listen to concerns.
  - Try to show that you understand the person's anger or fears.
- Keep personal items within the person's sight. Photos and treasures are examples.
- Reduce glares, noise, and clutter.

Agitation and Aggression—cont'd
- Limit the number of people in the room.
- Use touch correctly. See "Paranoia."
- Provide soothing music.
- Read to the person with a gentle voice.
- Try taking the person for a walk.
- Provide quiet times.
- Limit the amount of caffeine (coffee, tea, colas, chocolate) and sweets.
- See Chapter 6 for dealing with the angry person.
- See Chapter 11 for workplace violence.

Repetitive Behaviors
- Allow harmless acts. Holding a purse, folding napkins, caring for a doll, and petting a stuffed animal are examples.
- Look for a reason for the repetition. The action may have meaning if it occurs around certain people, in certain places, or at certain times.
- Know when repetitive behaviors are likely. For example, a person constantly calls for a nurse at bedtime.
- Consider how the person may be feeling. Think about the emotion instead of reacting to the behavior.
- Engage the person in a pleasant activity. Boredom may be the cause.
- Take the person for a walk.
- Turn the action into an activity. For example, a person has repetitive hand motions. You provide a pile of washcloths and ask the person to help fold laundry.
- Use a calm voice and gentle touch. Be patient.
- Do not argue with the person.
- Answer questions. You may have to answer the same question many times.
- Follow the care plan for memory aids when the person asks the same questions over and over. Clocks, calendars, and photos are examples.

Rummaging and Hiding Things
- Keep harmful items and products out of sight and reach.
- Remove spoiled items from refrigerators and cabinets. The person may look for food and eat whatever is found.
- Guide the person away from other patient or resident rooms.
- Keep wastebaskets covered or out of sight. The person may rummage through a wastebasket or throw things away.
- Check wastebaskets, linens, and food trays. Look for items thrown away or hidden.
- Keep bathroom doors closed and toilet seats down. The person cannot flush things down the toilet.
- Allow rummaging in a safe place. The agency may have a drawer, closet, bag, box, basket, or chest with safe items.

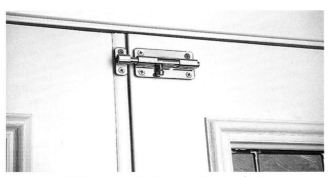

FIGURE 42-6 A slide lock is at the top of a door.

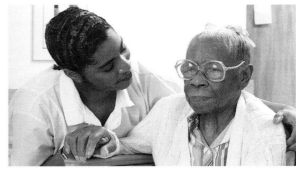

FIGURE 42-7 Gentle touch can be calming for some persons.

Meeting Basic Needs

Over time, the person depends on others more and more for care. Safety, hygiene, food and fluids, elimination, and activity needs must be met. So must comfort and sleep needs. Good skin care and alignment prevent skin breakdown and contractures. The agency's safety plan and the person's care plan will include many of the measures listed in Box 42-10.

The person can have other health problems and injuries. However, the person may not be aware of pain, fever, constipation, incontinence, or other signs and symptoms. Carefully observe the person. Report any change in usual behavior.

Infection is a risk. Infection can occur from poor hygiene. This includes poor skin care, oral hygiene, and perineal care after elimination. Inactivity and immobility can cause pneumonia and pressure injuries.

See *Focus on Surveys: Meeting Basic Needs*, p. 551.

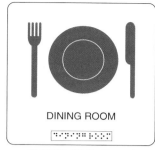
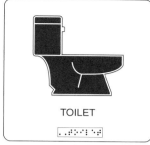

DINING ROOM   TOILET

FIGURE 42-8 Signs give cues to persons with dementia.

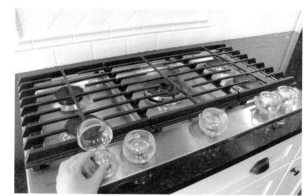

FIGURE 42-9 Safety covers are on stove knobs.

BOX 42-10 Dementia Care—Meeting Basic Needs

Environment
- Follow set routines. Avoid changing roommates or rooms.
- Place picture signs by room doors, bathrooms, dining rooms, and other areas (Fig. 42-8).
- Keep personal items where the person can see and reach them.
- Stay within the person's sight to the extent possible.
- Place memory aids (large clocks and calendars) where the person can see them.
- Keep noise levels low.
- Play music and show movies from the person's past.

Safety
- Reassure the person that you are there to help.
- Remove harmful, sharp, and breakable items from the area. This includes knives, scissors, glasses, dishes, razors, and tools.
- Provide plastic eating and drinking utensils. They help prevent breakage and cuts.
- Practice electrical safety measures (Chapter 11). Also remove electric appliances from the bathroom. Hair dryers, curling irons, make-up mirrors, and electric shavers are examples.
- Provide safe storage for:
  - Personal care items (shampoo, deodorant, lotion, and so on)
  - Cleaners and drugs
  - Dangerous equipment and tools
  - Cigarettes, cigars, pipes, matches, and other smoking materials
  - Car keys
- Keep childproof caps on drug containers and cleaners.
- Remove knobs from stoves or place safety covers on the knobs (Fig. 42-9).

Safety—cont'd
- Remove dangerous appliances, power tools, and firearms and weapons from the home.
- Supervise the person who smokes.
- Practice safety measures to prevent:
  - Falls (Chapter 12)
  - Fires (Chapter 11)
  - Burns (Chapter 11)
  - Poisoning (Chapter 11)
- Lock doors to kitchens, utility rooms, and housekeeping closets. Keep them locked.

Sleep
- Develop a regular bedtime. Bedtime should be the same each evening.
- Perform activities that use more energy early in the day.
- Provide a quiet, peaceful mood in the evening—dimmed lights, low noise level, and soft music.
- Follow bedtime rituals.
- Use night-lights in rooms, hallways, bathrooms, and other areas. They help the person see and prevent accidents and disorientation.
- Limit caffeine.
- Limit naps during the day.
- Follow the person's exercise plan. Play music to the exercise.
- Reduce noises.

Oral Care
- Allow the person to do as much as possible.
- Explain what to do 1 step at a time. For example: "Pick up the toothpaste. Take off the cap. Squeeze the toothpaste on the toothbrush. Put the toothbrush in your mouth. Brush."
- Show the person how to brush the teeth step-by-step.
- Help the person clean dentures.
- Try a long-handled, angled, or electric toothbrush.

Continued

BOX 42-10 Dementia Care—Meeting Basic Needs—cont'd

Bathing
- Follow the care plan for how often to give a bath or shower. Bathing 2 to 3 times a week is enough. A partial bath is done on other days.
- Follow the person's habits and routines.
  - Use the person's preferred bathing method—tub bath, shower. Follow the care plan. Some persons may need complete bed baths.
  - Perform the bath at the same time—in the morning, before bed.
- Practice safety measures. See Chapter 22.
  - Do not leave the person alone in the bath or shower.
  - Check for a comfortable water temperature.
  - Use a hand-held shower head.
  - Use a bath mat and grab (safety) bars.
  - Use a sturdy shower chair.
  - Do not use bath oils. They make the tub slippery and may increase the risk of urinary tract infection.
- Expect that bathing will be a difficult task. Plan ahead to calm the person. Before the bath:
  - Gather supplies—soap, washcloths, towels, shampoo, and so on.
  - Make sure the bathroom is warm and well lit.
  - Play soft music if this relaxes the person.
  - Be matter-of-fact. Say: "It is time for a bath now." Try the bath when the person is calm. Never use force.
  - Provide privacy.
- Promote comfort and independence. During the bath or shower:
  - Be gentle and respectful.
  - Tell the person what you will do step-by-step.
  - Do not rush the person.
  - Allow the person to do as much as possible. This shows dignity and helps the person feel in control.
  - Give the person a washcloth to hold.
  - Put a towel over the shoulders or lap. The person feels less exposed. Clean under the towel with a washcloth.
  - Talk to the person about something else. This may distract the person.
- Dry the skin well after bathing to prevent a rash or infection. Dry well between skin folds.

Hygiene and Grooming
- Provide good skin care.
- Provide incontinence care as needed. Apply a barrier cream or moisturizer (cream, lotion, paste) as directed by the nurse and care plan.
- Help the person apply make-up if this is a routine. Do not apply eye make-up.
- Use an electric razor for shaving. Help the person as needed.
- Keep the nails clean and trimmed without rough edges.

Dressing and Undressing
- Choose clothing that is comfortable and simple to put on. Front-opening garments are easy to put on. Pullover tops are harder. And the person may become frightened when the head is inside a garment.
- Select clothing that closes with Velcro. Such items are easy to put on and take off. Buttons, zippers, snaps, and other closures can frustrate the person.
- Apply slip-on shoes that will not slide off or shoes with Velcro straps.
- Offer simple clothing choices (Fig. 42-10). Let the person choose between 2 shirts or 2 blouses, 2 pants or 2 slacks, and so on.
- Lay clothing out in the order it will be put on. Hand the person 1 item at a time. Tell or show the person what to do. Do not rush.

Meals
- Maintain a routine. Have meals at usual times. Serve food in a familiar place and in a consistent way.
- Serve favorite foods.
- Respect personal, cultural, and religious food preferences.
- Use the meal as a time for social interaction. Use a kind and pleasant tone of voice.
- Play music during the meal.
- Be patient. Give the person time to eat.
- Provide finger foods.
- Avoid coffee, tea, and cola. The caffeine can increase restlessness, confusion, and agitation.
- Cut food and pour liquids as needed.
- Tell the nurse about changes in eating habits and appetite.
- Watch for signs of dysphagia (Chapter 29) and dehydration (Chapter 30).

Other Basic Needs
- Follow a daily routine. This helps the person know when certain things will happen.
- Promote urinary and bowel elimination and prevent incontinence.
- Promote exercise and activity during the day. This helps reduce wandering and sundowning behaviors. The person may also sleep better.
- Provide a quiet, restful setting. Soft music is better than loud TV programs.
- Have equipment ready for any procedure. This lessens the time for care measures.
- Observe for signs and symptoms of health problems (Chapter 7). Common health problems include:
  - Dental problems (Chapter 21)
  - Incontinence (Chapters 25 and 27)
  - Constipation and diarrhea (Chapter 27)
  - Dehydration (Chapter 30)
  - Flu and pneumonia (Chapter 40)
  - Fever—may signal infection, dehydration, heat-related illness, or constipation
- Prevent infection.

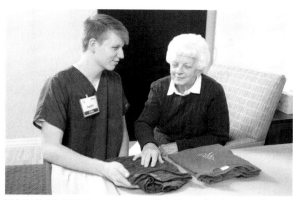

FIGURE 42-10 The person is offered simple clothing choices.

Secured Units

Many nursing centers have secure memory care units (Chapter 1). Entrances and exits are locked. Residents cannot wander away. They have a safe setting to move about. Some persons have aggressive behaviors that disrupt or threaten others. They need a secured unit.

According to the Centers for Medicare & Medicaid Services (CMS), persons on a secured unit must be protected from involuntary seclusion (Chapter 4). The agency must identify the reason for placement on the unit. The reason must not be:

- For staff convenience or discipline.
- Based on a diagnosis alone. Placement is made on an individual basis.
- By request of the family or the person's representative without a medical reason.

The person's medical record must include:

- The reason for placement on the unit.
- How the resident or resident's representative was involved in the decision.
- If the secured unit is the least restrictive approach to protect the person.
- The person's reaction to placement on the unit.
- On-going review and revision of the care plan as needed. For example, are interventions meeting the resident's needs? Is a secured unit still needed?

At some point, the secured unit is no longer needed. For example, a person's condition progresses to severe AD (see Box 42-7). The person cannot sit or walk. Wandering is not a concern. The person is transferred to another unit.

Activities

Persons with dementia need to feel useful, worthwhile, and active. This promotes self-esteem. Therapies and activities focus on strengths and past successes. For example:

- A person who used to cook helps clean fruit.
- Once a good dancer, activities are planned so the person can dance.
- A person who likes to clean helps with dusting.

Supervised activities meet the person's needs and cognitive abilities. Activities are based on what the person enjoys and can do. Some people like crafts, exercise, gardening, and listening and moving to music. Others like sing-alongs, board games, and reminiscing. (*Reminiscence* or *to reminisce* means *to talk about or recall past events.*) Some like to string beads, fold towels, or roll dough.

Massage, soothing touch, music, and aromatherapy are comforting and relaxing.

The Family

The person may live at home or with a partner, children, or other family members. Or someone stays with the person. Home care may help for a while. Adult day care and assisted living are options (Chapter 1). Nursing center care is needed when:

- The family cannot meet the person's needs.
- The person no longer knows the caregiver.
- Family members have health problems.
- The person's behavior presents dangers to self and others.

Doctor's visits, drugs, home care, and assisted living are costly. So is nursing center care. The person's medical care can drain finances.

Home care and nursing center care are stressful. The family has physical, emotional, social, and financial stresses. Adult children are in the *sandwich generation.* Their own children need attention while an ill parent needs care. Caring for 2 families is stressful. Often adult children have jobs too.

Caregivers can suffer from anger, anxiety, guilt, depression, and sleep problems. Some cannot concentrate or are irritable. Health problems can develop. They need to focus on their own health. They need a healthy diet, exercise, and plenty of rest. Asking family and friends for help is hard for some people.

Caregivers need support and encouragement. The NIA suggests how family members can take care of themselves. See Box 42-11. AD support groups are sponsored by hospitals, nursing centers, and the Alzheimer's Association. The Alzheimer's Association has chapters across the country. Support groups offer encouragement and advice. Members share feelings, anger, frustration, guilt, and other emotions. They also share coping and caregiving ideas.

BOX 42-11 Family Caregivers—Taking Care of Yourself

- Ask for help when you need it. Asking for something specific may be useful. For example:
  - "Can you make Mom's dinner Sunday night?"
  - "Can you stay with Dad from 2 to 4 Monday afternoon?"
  - "Can Mom stay at your house Saturday afternoon?"
- Join a support group.
- Take breaks every day.
- Spend time with friends.
- Maintain hobbies and interests.
- Eat healthy foods and exercise often.
- See a doctor regularly.
- Keep health, legal, and financial information current.
- Remember that these feelings are normal—being sad, lonely, frustrated, confused, angry. Say to yourself:
  - "I'm doing the best I can."
  - "What I'm doing would be hard for anyone."
  - "I'm not perfect and that's okay."
  - "I can't control some things."
  - "I need to do what works for right now."
  - "Even when I do everything I can, there will still be problems. This is caused by the illness, not by what I do."
  - "I will enjoy our peaceful times together."
  - "I will get counseling if caregiving becomes too much."
- Meet spiritual needs—attending religious services, believing that larger forces or a higher power is at work.
- Understand that you may feel powerless and hopeless about what is happening.
- Understand that you may feel a sense of loss and sadness.
- Understand why you are caring for a person with AD. Was the choice made out of love, loyalty, duty, religious obligation, money concerns, fear, habit, or self-punishment?
- Let yourself feel "uplifts." Examples include good feelings about the person, support from caring people, and time for your interests.

Modified from National Institute on Aging: *Alzheimer's caregiving: caring for yourself*, Bethesda, Md, content reviewed May 17, 2017, National Institutes of Health.

The family often feels hopeless. No matter what is done, dementia gets worse. Much time, money, energy, and emotion are needed to care for the person. Anger and resentment may result. Guilt feelings are common. The family knows that the person did not choose the disease and its signs, symptoms, and behaviors. Sometimes behaviors are embarrassing. The family may be upset and angry that the loved one cannot show love or affection.

The family is an important part of the health team. They help plan care when possible. The nurse and support group help the family learn how to provide a safe home setting and give needed care. They learn how to bathe, feed, dress, and give oral care.

In nursing centers, some family members take part in unit activities. For many persons, family members provide comfort. They also need support and understanding from the health team.

Validation Therapy

Validation therapy is a way to communicate with persons with dementia. *Validate* means *to show that a person's feelings and needs are fair and have meaning*. Behaviors signal the need to express feelings and needs—safety, security, comfort, love and belonging, feeling useful, and so on. Caregivers help the person express feelings and needs verbally or nonverbally. With validation, the person's reality (what the person thinks is real and true) is accepted. The person is treated with dignity and self-worth.

Validation therapy is based on these principles.

- All behavior has meaning.
- A person may have unresolved issues and emotions from the past.
- A person's mind may return to the past to resolve issues and emotions.
- Caregivers need to listen and provide empathy.
- Attempts are not made to correct thoughts or bring the person back to reality (reality orientation). For example:
  - A person talks about waiting for the bus to go to work. The caregiver does not say: "You don't work anymore." Instead, the caregiver says: "Tell me about your work."
  - A resident says she is at the train station waiting for her husband. Killed in a war, her husband never came home. The caregiver does not remind the resident of what happened. Instead, the caregiver asks the resident about her husband.
  - A patient was 3 years old when his father died. He holds a ball constantly. He calls for his father and repeats "play ball, play ball." The caregiver does not remind the patient that his father is not alive. Instead, the caregiver says: "Tell me about playing ball."

Validation therapy is useful for some persons. If used in your agency, you will be trained to use validation therapy correctly.

FOCUS ON P R I D E

The Person, Family, and Yourself

P ersonal and Professional Responsibility

Everyone has different talents, abilities, and interests. Persons with dementia are no different. Understanding the person's past, hobbies, talents, family, and work helps you give better care.

Learn about the person. Engage the person in activities once enjoyed. Treat each person as unique with a history, interests, strengths, and needs.

R ights and Respect

The person has the right to privacy and confidentiality. Protect the person from exposure. Only those involved in the person's care are present during care. The person is allowed to visit in private. Do not share information about the person with others.

The person has the right to keep and use personal items. A pillow, blanket, or sweater may have meaning. The person may not know why or recognize the item. Still, it is important and provides comfort. Keep personal items safe. Protect property from loss or damage.

I ndependence and Social Interaction

Maintaining routines can help persons with dementia remain independent longer. For example, a person uses the bathroom, washes hands, brushes teeth, brushes hair, and dresses in the morning. The person is more independent when ADL are done in this order. Changing the order causes confusion.

Break down tasks into simple steps. Patiently tell the person each step. Repeat directions as needed. Allow extra time for each task. Resist the urge to take over. Let the person do what is safely possible.

D elegation and Teamwork

Persons with dementia may respond better to certain staff or caregivers. This can vary by day or time of day. Do not be offended if someone else provides care. The team works together to meet the person's needs.

Sometimes the person resists care from everyone. Convincing the person to allow care is often useless. Use a calm and caring approach. Try giving care at a different time. Never use force.

E thics and Laws

Patience and kindness are very important qualities when caring for persons with dementia. If you find yourself feeling impatient or frustrated, tell the nurse. You may need an assignment change. Never act out against the person. You cannot yell at the person or be rough. The person must be protected from verbal and physical abuse and mistreatment.

FOCUS ON PRIDE: *Application*

Caregivers affect the person's quality of life. Describe care that values the person. What qualities must the caregiver have? How must the caregiver treat the person?

REVIEW QUESTIONS

Circle the BEST answer.

1 A person is confused. Which should you question?
 a Restrain in bed at night.
 b Give clear, simple directions.
 c Use touch to communicate.
 d Open drapes during the day.

2 A person has AD. Which is *true*?
 a AD is a normal part of aging.
 b Diet and drugs can cure the disease.
 c AD and delirium are the same.
 d AD ends in death.

3 During the final stage of AD, the person is likely to
 a Wander and become lost
 b Follow simple commands
 c Need total assistance with ADL
 d Repeat questions over and over

4 Which is common in persons with AD?
 a Paralysis
 b Dyspnea
 c Vision loss
 d Sleep disturbances

Continued

5 A person has AD. To communicate, you should
   a Give orders
   b Limit choices
   c Correct mistakes
   d Ask open-ended questions

6 A person with AD is screaming. You know that this is
   a A way to communicate
   b An agitated reaction
   c Caused by a delusion
   d A repetitive behavior

7 Which statement about sundowning is *true*?
   a AD behaviors improve at night.
   b Encouraging activity late in the day can help.
   c Being tired or hungry can increase restlessness.
   d Dim lighting or darkness is calming.

8 A person with AD has delusions. Which should you question?
   a Distract the person with an activity.
   b Tell the person you will provide protection.
   c Tell the person the beliefs are not real.
   d Use touch to calm the person.

9 Which can cause delusions in persons with AD?
   a Mirrors
   b Eyeglasses
   c Hearing aids
   d Night-lights

10 A person with AD keeps telling you that someone is stealing things. What should you do?
   a Nothing. The person has paranoia.
   b Tell the nurse. Someone could be abusing the person.
   c Tell the person not to worry.
   d Send other items home with the family.

11 A person with AD is at risk for elopement. Which should you question?
   a Make sure door alarms are turned on.
   b Make sure an ID bracelet is worn.
   c Assist with exercise as ordered.
   d Remind the person not to wander.

12 Which can help with rummaging?
   a Keep the person's room locked.
   b Provide safe places to rummage.
   c Ask the person to explain the behavior.
   d Hide items the person looks for.

13 A person with AD is upset. Which is a *correct* response?
   a Try to reason with the person.
   b Ask what is bothering the person.
   c Ignore the problem.
   d Provide reassurance and try to find the cause.

14 Which is *unsafe* for persons with AD?
   a Utility rooms are locked.
   b Cleaners and drugs are locked up.
   c The person keeps smoking materials.
   d Sharp objects are removed from the setting.

15 You are preparing to give oral care to a person with moderate AD. Which will you do?
   a Give step-by-step directions.
   b Brush the teeth yourself if the person resists.
   c Help the person to the bathroom before gathering supplies.
   d Play loud music to distract the person.

16 You need to help a person with AD change clothes. You should
   a Ask the person to get clothes from the closet and signal for you when ready.
   b Dress the person quickly to prevent agitation.
   c Avoid showing the person what to do.
   d Offer 2 clothing options that are comfortable and easy to put on.

17 You are caring for a person with AD. You should avoid
   a Trying to bring the person back to reality
   b Offering support to the family
   c Following a set routine
   d Providing a quiet setting

18 Validation therapy involves
   a Support groups and counseling for persons with severe AD
   b Drugs to treat AD
   c Helping the person with AD express needs and feelings
   d Orienting the person with AD to reality

Answers to Chapter 42 questions are on p. 589.

FOCUS ON **PRACTICE**

Problem Solving

A person has moderate AD. While preparing for a bath, the person becomes upset and repeats: "Go away" over and over. How will you respond? How might you meet hygiene needs?

Emergency Care

OBJECTIVES

- Define the key terms and key abbreviations in this chapter.
- Describe the rules of emergency care.
- Identify the signs of cardiac arrest and the emergency care required.
- Describe the emergency care for respiratory arrest.
- Describe the emergency care for poisoning.
- Describe the emergency care for heart attack.

- Describe the emergency care for hemorrhage, fainting, and shock.
- Describe the emergency care for stroke.
- Explain how to care for a person during a seizure.
- Describe the emergency care for concussions.
- Describe the emergency care for burns.
- Explain how to promote PRIDE in the person, the family, and yourself.

KEY TERMS

anaphylaxis A life-threatening sensitivity to an antigen

cardiac arrest See "sudden cardiac arrest"

cardiopulmonary resuscitation (CPR) An emergency procedure performed when the heart and breathing stop

convulsion See "seizure"

fainting The sudden loss of consciousness from an inadequate blood supply to the brain; syncope

first aid The emergency care given to an ill or injured person before medical help arrives

hemorrhage The excessive loss *(rrhage)* of blood *(hemo)* in a short time

respiratory arrest Breathing stops but heart action continues for several minutes

resuscitate To revive from apparent death or unconsciousness using emergency measures

seizure Violent and sudden contractions or tremors of muscle groups caused by abnormal electrical activity in the brain; convulsion

shock Results when tissues and organs do not get enough blood

sudden cardiac arrest (SCA) The heart stops suddenly and without warning; cardiac arrest

KEY ABBREVIATIONS

AED	Automated external defibrillator
CPR	Cardiopulmonary resuscitation
EMS	Emergency Medical Services

RRS	Rapid Response System
SCA	Sudden cardiac arrest
VF; V-fib	Ventricular fibrillation

Emergencies can occur anywhere. Sometimes you can save a life if you know what to do.

The information in this chapter is basic. First aid and cardiopulmonary resuscitation (CPR) courses provide more training and practice. Most agencies require nursing assistants to be CPR certified. *You need a CPR course for health care providers.* Ask your instructor about courses in your area or on-line.

CPR guidelines are updated as new information becomes available. You are responsible for following current guidelines. Updates can be found on-line at the American Heart Association's website.

EMERGENCY CARE

First aid is the emergency care given to an ill or injured person before medical help arrives. The goals of first aid are to:
- Prevent death.
- Prevent injuries from becoming worse.

In an emergency, the Emergency Medical Services (EMS) system is activated. Emergency personnel (paramedics, emergency medical technicians) give advanced emergency care. They treat, stabilize, and transport persons with life-threatening problems. They have guidelines for care and communicate with doctors in hospital emergency rooms. EMS ambulances have emergency drugs, equipment, and supplies.

To activate the EMS system, do 1 of the following.
- Dial 911.
- Call the local fire or police department.

Each emergency is different. The rules in Box 43-1 apply to any emergency. Hospitals and other agencies have procedures for advanced emergency care. In hospitals, a Rapid Response System (RRS) is activated when a person shows signs of a life-threatening condition. An RRS team may include a doctor, a nurse, and a respiratory therapist. The RRS team brings emergency drugs, supplies, and equipment to the bedside. The goal is to prevent death.

See *Focus on Communication: Emergency Care.*
See *Promoting Safety and Comfort: Emergency Care.*

FOCUS ON COMMUNICATION

Emergency Care

Some illnesses and injuries are life-threatening. You may need to ask questions to find out what happened and the person's condition. For example:
- "Are you okay?"
- "Are you choking?"
- "Tell me what's wrong."
- "Where does it hurt?"
- "Can you point to where it hurts?"
- "Can you move your arms and legs?"

PROMOTING SAFETY AND COMFORT

Emergency Care

Safety
Contact with blood and body fluids is likely. Follow Standard Precautions and the Bloodborne Pathogen Standard to the extent possible.

For an emergency in an agency, call for the nurse at once. You may need to activate the EMS system or the RRS. Or you take the person's vital signs (Chapter 31). Assist as the nurse instructs.

Comfort
Mental comfort is important. Help the person feel safe and secure. Give reassurance. Explain the care you provide. Use a calm approach.

BOX 43-1 Emergency Care Rules

- Call for help. Or have someone activate the EMS system. *Do not hang up until the operator (dispatcher) has hung up.* Give the following information.
  - Your location—street address and city, cross streets or roads, and landmarks
  - Phone number you are calling from
  - What seems to have happened (for example: heart attack, crash, fire)—police, fire equipment, and ambulances may be needed
  - How many people need help
  - Conditions of victims, obvious injuries, and life-threatening situations
  - What aid is being given
- Wait for help if the scene is not safe enough to approach.
- Know your limits. Do not do more than you are able. Do not perform an unfamiliar procedure. Do what you can under the circumstances.
- Stay calm. This helps the person feel more secure.
- Know where to find emergency supplies.
- Follow Standard Precautions and the Bloodborne Pathogen Standard to the extent possible.
- Check for life-threatening problems. Check for breathing, a pulse, and bleeding.
- Keep the person lying down or as the person was found (unless emergency measures require re-positioning). Moving the person could make an injury worse.
- Move the person only if the setting is unsafe. Examples include:
  - A burning car or building
  - A building that might collapse
  - Stormy conditions with lightning
  - In water
  - Near electrical wires
- Perform necessary emergency measures.
- Do not remove clothes unless you have to. To remove clothing, tear or cut garments along the seams. (For CPR, remove clothing or move it out of the way. See p. 558.)
- Keep the person warm. Cover the person with a blanket, coats, or sweaters.
- Reassure the person. Explain what is happening and that help was called.
- Do not give the person fluids.
- Keep on-lookers away. They invade privacy and tend to stare, give advice, and comment about the person's condition. This can worry the person.

SUDDEN CARDIAC ARREST

Sudden cardiac arrest (SCA) or *cardiac arrest* *is when the heart stops suddenly and without warning.* Within seconds, breathing stops too. Blood and oxygen are not supplied to the body. Brain and other organ damage occurs within minutes.

SCA is a sudden, unexpected, and dramatic event. It can occur anywhere and at any time—while driving, shoveling snow, playing golf or tennis, watching TV, eating, or sleeping. Common causes include cardiovascular disorders (Chapter 40) and dysrhythmias (arrhythmias). Electrical shock, chest trauma, and substance use (Chapter 41) are other causes. The person is at risk for an abnormal heart rhythm called ventricular fibrillation (p. 561). The heart cannot pump blood. A normal rhythm must be restored or the person will die.

Signs of Sudden Cardiac Arrest

There are 3 major signs of SCA.

- *No response.*
- *No breathing or no normal breathing.* The person may have *agonal gasps (agonal respirations)* early during SCA. (*Agonal* means *to struggle.* Agonal relates to death and dying.) Agonal gasps do not bring enough oxygen into the lungs. Agonal gasps are not normal breathing.
- *No pulse.*

The skin is cool, pale, and gray. The person is not coughing or moving.

To check for SCA:

1 *Check for a response.* In an adult, tap or gently shake the person. Call the person by name, if known. Shout: "Are you okay?" Get help and emergency equipment if there is no response.
2 *Check for breathing and a pulse at the same time.* Do so for 5 to 10 seconds.
   - Look for no breathing or only gasping.
   - In an adult, check the carotid pulse (Fig. 43-1).

CPR

Cardiopulmonary resuscitation (CPR) is an emergency procedure performed when the heart and breathing stop. Cardio relates to the heart. *Pulmonary* relates to the lungs. To *resuscitate means to revive from apparent death or unconsciousness using emergency measures.* CPR must be started at once when a person has SCA. CPR provides blood and oxygen to the heart, brain, and other organs until advanced emergency care is given.

CPR involves:

- Giving chest compressions
- Opening the airway and giving breaths
- Defibrillation

See *Focus on Communication: CPR.*
See *Promoting Safety and Comfort: CPR.*

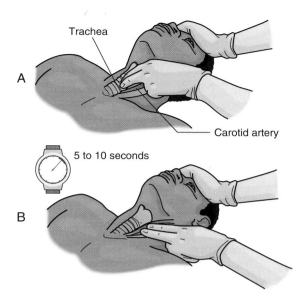

FIGURE 43-1 Checking the carotid pulse. **A,** Place 2 fingers on the trachea. **B,** Move the fingertips down into the groove of the neck to the carotid artery. Feel for a pulse for at least 5 seconds but no more than 10 seconds.

FOCUS ON **COMMUNICATION**

CPR

Getting help is a critical part of CPR. Advanced emergency care is needed at once. Follow the agency's procedure for activating the RRS or EMS. Outside the work setting, use a phone to call 911. For an adult:

- *If you are alone and have a phone*—call while giving care.
- *If you are alone without a phone*—leave the person to call 911 before starting CPR.
- *If you are not alone*—have someone call 911.

PROMOTING SAFETY AND COMFORT

CPR

Safety

Rescuer safety: The area must be safe for you to approach. If unsafe, wait for help to arrive. Do not approach the person. Only move the person if needed for safety and if it is safe enough to do so.

Trauma: If the person has injuries, special measures are used to position the person for CPR and open the airway for breathing (p. 559). Such measures are learned during a CPR certification course.

Nursing centers: In nursing centers, a nurse decides when to activate the EMS system. The nurse tells you how to help. For SCA, the nurse may start CPR. Some agencies allow nursing assistants to start CPR. Others do not. Know your agency's policy.

Infants and children: CPR guidelines for infants and children differ from those for adults. The content in this chapter applies to adults. You will learn CPR for infants and children in a CPR certification course.

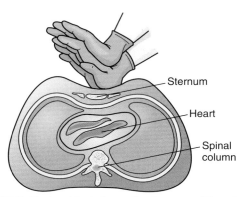

FIGURE 43-2 The heart lies between the sternum and the spinal column. The heart is compressed when pressure is applied to the sternum.

Chest Compressions

Chest compressions force blood through the circulatory system. When pressure is applied to the chest, the sternum compresses the heart (Fig. 43-2). For effective compressions, the person must be supine on a hard, flat surface.

To position the hands for compressions on an adult:

- Expose the chest. Remove clothing or move it out of the way.
- Place the heel of 1 hand (usually the dominant hand) in the center of the bare chest (Fig. 43-3, A). The hand is between the nipples on the lower half of the sternum.
- Place the heel of the other hand on top of the heel of the first hand (Fig. 43-3, B).

When giving compressions, the arms are straight. The shoulders are directly over the hands. Fingers are interlocked. See Figure 43-4. Press down and release pressure without removing the hands. Releasing pressure allows the chest to recoil—to return to its normal position. Recoil lets the heart fill with blood. Do not lean on the chest.

Compressions are given fast—at a rate of 100 to 120 per minute. The chest is pressed down at least 2 inches for an adult. Compressions are stopped only when necessary and for a short time—less than 10 seconds. Without compressions, blood does not flow to the heart, brain, and other organs.

See *Promoting Safety and Comfort: Chest Compressions.*

PROMOTING SAFETY AND COMFORT
Chest Compressions

Safety

The person must be on a hard, flat surface—floor or backboard. For the person in bed, place a board under the person. Logroll the person so there is no twisting of the spine. Place the arms alongside the body.

In a hospital, the RRS team brings a back-board. The headboard can be removed in some hospital beds for use as a backboard. Other hospital beds have a CPR button that lowers and deflates the mattress for a hard surface.

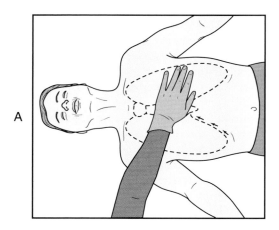

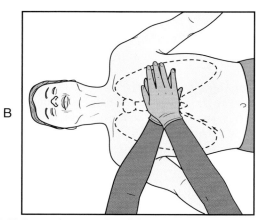

FIGURE 43-3 Hand position for adult CPR. **A,** The heel of the dominant hand is in the center of the chest. It is between the nipples and on the lower half of the sternum. **B,** The heel of the non-dominant hand is on top of the dominant hand.

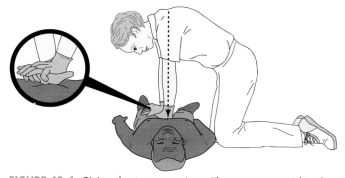

FIGURE 43-4 Giving chest compressions. The arms are straight. The shoulders are over the hands. The fingers are interlocked.

Airway and Breathing

The airway is often obstructed (blocked) during SCA. The tongue falls to the back of the throat and blocks the airway. The airway must be open to give breaths. The head tilt–chin lift method is used to open the airway. See Figure 43-5.

The rescuer breathes air into the person's mouth. To give mouth-to-mouth breaths to an adult (Fig. 43-6):

1 Keep the airway open with the head tilt–chin lift method.
2 Pinch the nostrils shut to keep air from coming out of the nose. Use the fingers on the hand on the person's forehead.
3 Take a normal breath.
4 Place your mouth tightly over the person's mouth. Seal the mouth with your lips.
5 Blow air into the person's mouth. The breath is given over 1 second. *The chest should rise as the lungs fill with air.*
6 Repeat the head tilt–chin lift if the chest did not rise.
7 Remove your mouth from the person's mouth. Take in another breath.
8 Give another breath. Watch for the chest to rise.

Masks. A mask or other barrier device is used to give breaths when possible (Fig. 43-7). The device prevents contact with the person's mouth and blood and body fluids. Place the mask over the person's mouth and nose (see Fig. 43-7). Make a tight seal. Open the airway and blow through the mouth-piece to give breaths.

EMS and hospital staff often use a bag valve mask (Fig. 43-8) to give breaths. The device consists of a hand-held bag attached to a mask. The mask is held securely to the face. The bag is squeezed to give breaths. The bag can be connected to an oxygen source.

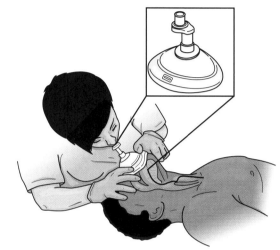

FIGURE 43-7 A mask is used to give breaths.

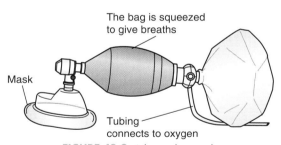

FIGURE 43-8 A bag valve mask.

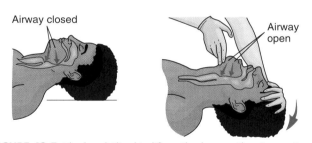

FIGURE 43-5 The head tilt–chin lift method opens the airway. One hand is on the forehead. Pressure is applied to tilt the head back. The chin is lifted with the fingers of the other hand.

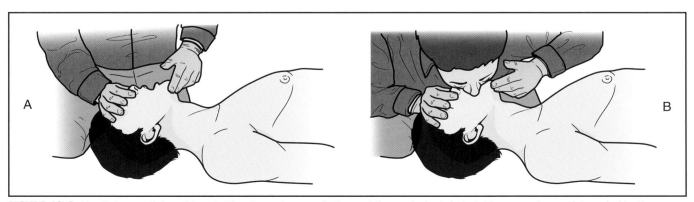

FIGURE 43-6 Mouth-to-mouth breathing. A, The airway is opened. The nostrils are pinched shut. B, The person's mouth is sealed by the rescuer's mouth.

Adult CPR Cycle

For an adult, a cycle of CPR involves 30 chest compressions and 2 breaths. Continue cycles of 30 compressions followed by 2 breaths until the person responds or help takes over. CPR is paused briefly to use a defibrillator. See "Defibrillation." Then CPR continues with compressions first. See Figure 43-9 for the sequence of CPR for an adult.

CPR is done by 1, 2, or more rescuers (Fig. 43-10). With more rescuers, a team approach promotes effective CPR. For example, with 2 rescuers:

- Rescuer 1 checks for a response. If no response, rescuer 1 tells rescuer 2 to call 911 and get an automated external defibrillator (AED).
- Rescuer 2 leaves to call for help and get an AED.
- Rescuer 1 gives CPR alone until rescuer 2 returns.
- Rescuer 2 returns and uses the AED.
- Rescuer 2 resumes compressions after AED use. (Rescuer 1 needs a break from compressions.)
- Rescuer 1 gives 2 breaths after every 30 compressions.
- Both rescuers continue CPR. They switch roles about every 2 minutes to avoid fatigue and inadequate compressions. They follow the AED's prompts to repeat AED use.

See *Focus on Communication: Adult CPR Cycle.*

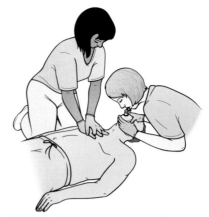

FIGURE 43-10 Two people perform CPR.

FOCUS ON COMMUNICATION

Adult CPR Cycle

Good communication is needed when 2 rescuers give CPR. The rescuer giving compressions counts out loud so the other rescuer is ready to give breaths. Clear communication prevents delays and lessens interruptions in chest compressions.

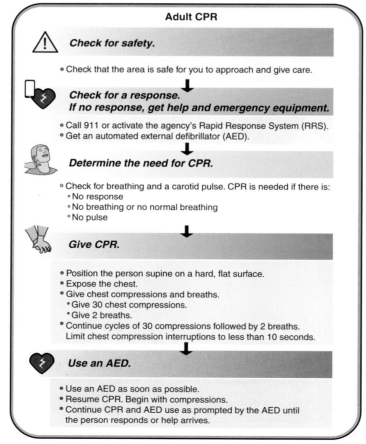

Adult CPR

⚠ **Check for safety.**

- Check that the area is safe for you to approach and give care.

Check for a response.
If no response, get help and emergency equipment.

- Call 911 or activate the agency's Rapid Response System (RRS).
- Get an automated external defibrillator (AED).

Determine the need for CPR.

- Check for breathing and a carotid pulse. CPR is needed if there is:
  - No response
  - No breathing or no normal breathing
  - No pulse

Give CPR.

- Position the person supine on a hard, flat surface.
- Expose the chest.
- Give chest compressions and breaths.
  - Give 30 chest compressions.
  - Give 2 breaths.
- Continue cycles of 30 compressions followed by 2 breaths. Limit chest compression interruptions to less than 10 seconds.

Use an AED.

- Use an AED as soon as possible.
- Resume CPR. Begin with compressions.
- Continue CPR and AED use as prompted by the AED until the person responds or help arrives.

FIGURE 43-9 Sequence of adult CPR. (Note: Follow Standard Precautions and the Bloodborne Pathogen Standard to the extent possible. This includes the use of gloves and a mask or other barrier device.)

Defibrillation

Ventricular fibrillation (VF, V-fib) is an abnormal heart rhythm (Fig. 43-11). It causes SCA. Rather than beating in a regular rhythm, the heart quivers and does not pump blood.

A *defibrillator* delivers a shock to the heart. The shock stops the VF (V-fib). This may allow a regular rhythm to return. Defibrillation as soon as possible after the onset of VF (V-fib) increases the chance of survival.

AEDs are found in health care agencies and in many public places (Fig. 43-12). Some persons have them at home.

See Box 43-2 for how to use an AED on an adult. Use an AED as soon as possible. You will learn more about AEDs in a CPR certification course.

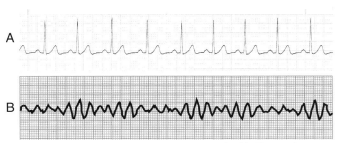

FIGURE 43-11 A, Normal rhythm. **B,** Ventricular fibrillation. (From Ignatavicius DD, Workman ML: *Medical-surgical nursing: concepts for interprofessional collaborative care,* ed 10, St Louis, 2021, Elsevier.)

BOX 43-2 Using an AED

Follow these steps to use an AED on an adult.
1 Open the AED case.
2 Turn on the AED (Fig. 43-13, *A*).
3 Apply adult electrode pads to the chest (Fig. 43-13, *B*). Follow the AED's instructions and diagram.
4 Attach the connecting cables to the AED (Fig. 43-13, *C*).
5 Clear away from the person. Make sure no one is touching the person (Fig. 43-13, *D*).
6 Let the AED check the heart rhythm.
7 Make sure everyone is clear of the person if the AED advises a "shock" (see Fig. 43-13, *D*). Loudly tell others not to touch the person. Say: "Everyone, clear!" Look to make sure no one is touching the person.
8 Press the *SHOCK* button if the AED advises a "shock" (Fig. 43-13, *E*).
9 Resume CPR beginning with compressions. Continue cycles of CPR.
10 Repeat steps 5 through 8 when prompted by the AED—after about 2 minutes of CPR. (NOTE: With 2 rescuers, rescuers switch roles at this step to avoid fatigue and inadequate compressions.)
11 Continue CPR and use of the AED until help takes over or the person responds.

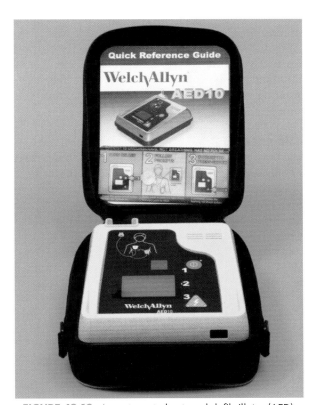

FIGURE 43-12 An automated external defibrillator (AED).

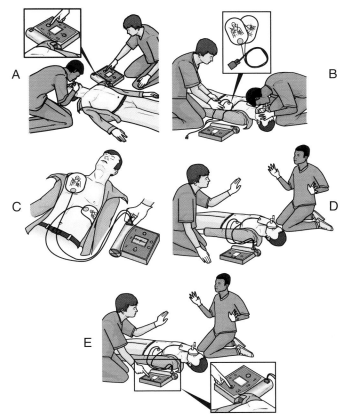

FIGURE 43-13 Using an AED. **A,** The rescuer turns on the AED. **B,** Electrode pads are placed on the chest. **C,** The cables are connected to the AED. **D,** The rescuers "clear" the person. The rescuers make sure no one is touching the person. **E,** The *SHOCK* button is pressed to deliver a shock.

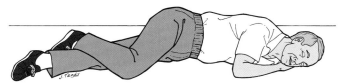

FIGURE 43-14 Recovery position.

Recovery Position

The recovery position is used after CPR when the person is breathing and has a pulse (Fig. 43-14). The person may not be responding. The position helps keep the airway open and prevents aspiration.

Logroll the person into the recovery position. Keep the head, neck, and spine straight. A hand supports the head. *Do not use this position if the person might have neck injuries or other trauma.*

Hands-Only CPR

With SCA, survival depends on others nearby. In public, bystanders may worry that they will not do CPR correctly or may cause injury. The "hands-only" method of CPR involves only chest compressions. Breaths are not given.

Hands-only CPR is intended for adults and adolescents with SCA. There are only 2 steps.

1 Call 911.
2 Push hard and fast in the center of the chest.

This method is for persons in public who are not trained in CPR. With training and practice, you will learn all of the steps of CPR. As a health care provider, you will use the CPR method learned in your CPR certification course.

CPR Skills Testing

CPR certification courses involve:
- Training
- Skills practice
- A multiple-choice test
- A skills test

The American Heart Association's CPR training may be done in a classroom or on-line. For on-line training, a skills test with an evaluator is completed after the on-line portion.

A current training manual (print or electronic) is required. The manual includes the steps you must perform to pass the skills test.

You are tested on providing CPR and using an AED. An evaluator watches you perform the skills on a mannequin. To receive certification, you must pass the multiple-choice test and the skills test.

CHOKING

Foreign bodies can obstruct (block) the airway. This is called *choking* or *foreign-body airway obstruction (FBAO)*. Air cannot pass into the lungs. The body does not get enough oxygen. It can lead to cardiac arrest.

Airway obstruction can be mild or severe. With severe airway obstruction, air does not move in and out of the lungs. If the obstruction is not removed, the person will die. Abdominal thrusts are used to relieve severe airway obstruction. See Chapter 11 for emergency care of the choking person.

RESPIRATORY ARREST

Respiratory arrest is when breathing stops but heart action continues for several minutes. If breathing is not restored, cardiac arrest occurs. Respiratory arrest can occur from:
- Blocked airflow—choking (Chapter 11), drowning, suffocation
- Problems affecting nerves, muscles, or areas of the brain that control breathing—amyotrophic lateral sclerosis (ALS), spinal cord injuries, stroke (Chapter 40); drug or alcohol over-dose; drug side effects
- Lung disorders and problems—pneumonia, chronic obstructive pulmonary disease (Chapter 40), pulmonary embolism (Chapter 35), chest injuries
- Inhaling harmful substances—smoke, chemicals, fumes

Rescue Breathing

Rescue breaths are given when there is a pulse but no breathing or only agonal gasping. To give rescue breaths for an adult:
- Open the airway (p. 559).
- Give 1 breath every 6 seconds.
- Give each breath over 1 second. The chest should rise when breaths are given.

Follow the rules in Box 43-1. This includes activating the EMS system. Check the pulse every 2 minutes. If there is no pulse, begin CPR.

POISONING

A *poison* is any substance harmful to the body when ingested (swallowed), inhaled, injected, or absorbed through the skin. See Chapter 11 for measures to prevent poisoning.

Some common signs and symptoms of poisoning are:

* Burns or redness around the mouth and lips
* A chemical odor to the breath
* Burns, stains, or odors on the person, on clothing, or around the person
* Empty drug bottles or spilled drugs
* Vomiting
* *Dyspnea*—difficulty (*dys*) breathing (*pnea*)
* Drowsiness
* Confusion
* Seizures (p. 565)

If you think a person has had contact with a poison, call the Poison Control Center (1-800-222-1222) or 911. Follow the rules in Box 43-1 for basic emergency care. Also follow the directions given by the Poison Control Center. Such directions may include:

* *Poison in the eyes*—rinse the eyes with running water.
* *Poison on the skin*—remove clothing in contact with the poison. Rinse the skin with running water.
* *Inhaled poison*—leave the area. Get the person to fresh air at once.
* *Swallowed poison*—do not have the person try to vomit or give the person anything to cause vomiting. Do not give the person anything to eat or drink unless told to do so by the Poison Control Center.

Call 911 to activate the EMS system if the person stops responding, stops breathing, or has a seizure. Follow the guidelines for CPR and rescue breathing. See p. 565 for emergency care for seizures.

HEART ATTACK

Heart attack (myocardial infarction) occurs when part of the heart muscle dies from the sudden blockage of blood flow in a coronary artery (Chapter 40). Signs and symptoms include:

* Chest pain (not relieved by rest)
* Pain or discomfort in 1 or both arms, the back, neck, jaw, or stomach
* Shortness of breath
* Perspiration (sweating) and cold, clammy skin
* Feeling light-headed
* Nausea and vomiting

If you suspect a heart attack, activate the EMS system at once. Prompt treatment can reduce the amount of heart muscle damage. Have the person sit and rest. Loosen tight clothing. Follow the rules in Box 43-1. Start CPR for cardiac arrest.

HEMORRHAGE

Life and body functions need an adequate blood supply. If a blood vessel is cut or torn, bleeding occurs. The larger the blood vessel, the greater the bleeding and blood loss. **Hemorrhage** *is the excessive loss* (rrhage) *of blood* (hemo) *in a short time.* If bleeding is not stopped, the person will die.

Hemorrhage is internal or external. You cannot see internal hemorrhage. The bleeding is inside body tissues and body cavities. Pain, shock (p. 564), vomiting blood, coughing up blood, cold and moist skin, and loss of consciousness signal internal hemorrhage. There is little you can do for internal bleeding.

* Follow the rules in Box 43-1. This includes activating the EMS system.
* Keep the person warm, flat, and quiet until help arrives.
* Do not give fluids.

If not hidden by clothing, external bleeding is usually seen. Bleeding from an artery occurs in spurts. There is a steady flow of blood from a vein. To control bleeding:

* Follow the rules in Box 43-1. This includes activating the EMS system.
* Do not remove any objects that have pierced or stabbed the person.
* Place a sterile dressing directly over the wound. Or use any clean material (handkerchief, towel, cloth, or sanitary napkin).
* Apply firm pressure directly over the bleeding site (Fig. 43-15). Do not release pressure until the bleeding stops. If needed, wrap an elastic bandage firmly over the dressing or material.
* Do not remove the dressing or material. If bleeding continues, apply more dressings on top and apply more pressure.
* Bind the wound when bleeding stops. Tape or tie the dressing in place. You can tie the dressing with such things as clothing, a scarf, or a necktie.

See *Promoting Safety and Comfort: Hemorrhage*, p. 564.

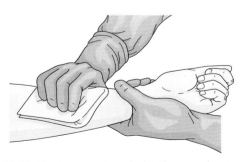

FIGURE 43-15 Direct pressure is applied to the wound to stop bleeding.

> ### PROMOTING SAFETY AND COMFORT
> *Hemorrhage*
>
> **Safety**
> Contact with blood is likely with hemorrhage. Follow Standard Precautions and the Bloodborne Pathogen Standard to the extent possible. Wear gloves if possible. Practice hand hygiene as soon as you can.

FAINTING

Fainting (syncope) is the sudden loss of consciousness from an inadequate blood supply to the brain. Hunger, fatigue, fear, and pain are common causes. Some people faint at the sight of blood or injury. Standing in 1 position too long and being in a warm, crowded room are other causes. Hemorrhage and other serious problems can cause fainting.

Dizziness, perspiration (sweating), weakness, and vision changes are warning signs. The person looks pale. The pulse is weak. Respirations are shallow if consciousness is lost.

If a person has warning signs of fainting:
- Have the person sit or lie down to prevent fainting.
  - If sitting, the person bends forward and places the head between the knees (Fig. 43-16).
  - If lying down, raise the person's legs.
- Loosen tight clothing (belts, ties, scarves, collars, and so on).

If fainting occurs:
- Activate the EMS system.
- Keep the person lying down. Raise the feet about 12 inches.
- Start CPR for cardiac arrest. Give rescue breathing for respiratory arrest.
- Help the person to a sitting position after recovery from fainting. Do not let the person get up quickly. Observe for warning signs of fainting as the person recovers.

SHOCK

Shock results when tissues and organs do not get enough blood. Blood loss, allergic reaction, poisoning, heart attack, burns, and severe infection are causes. Signs and symptoms include:
- Low or falling blood pressure
- Rapid and weak pulse
- Rapid respirations
- Cold, moist, and pale skin
- Thirst
- Nausea and vomiting
- Restlessness
- Confusion and loss of consciousness as shock worsens

Shock is possible in any acutely ill or severely injured person. Follow the rules in Box 43-1. Keep the person lying down. If there are no injuries from trauma, raise the feet about 6 to 12 inches. Lower the feet if the position causes pain. Maintain an open airway and control bleeding. Start CPR for cardiac arrest.

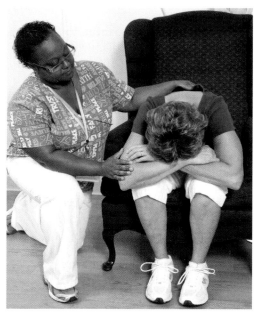

FIGURE 43-16 The person bends forward and lowers the head to prevent fainting.

Anaphylactic Shock

Some people are allergic or sensitive to foods, insects, chemicals, and drugs. For example, allergies to *penicillin* are common. An *antigen* is a substance that the body reacts to. The body releases chemicals to fight or attack the antigen. The person may react with an area of redness, swelling, or itching. Or the reaction may involve the entire body.

Anaphylaxis is a life-threatening sensitivity to an antigen. (*Ana* means *without. Phylaxis* means *protection.*) The reaction can occur within seconds. Signs and symptoms include:
- An itchy rash
- Swelling of the face, eyes, or lips
- Flushed or pale skin
- Feeling warm
- Dyspnea or wheezing from airway narrowing or a swollen tongue or throat
- Feeling that there is a "lump" in the throat
- A fast and weak pulse
- Nausea, vomiting, or diarrhea
- A feeling of dread or doom
- Dizziness or fainting
- Signs and symptoms of shock

Anaphylactic shock is an emergency. The EMS system must be activated. Drugs are needed to reverse the allergic reaction. Keep the person lying down and the airway open. Start CPR for cardiac arrest. Give rescue breathing for respiratory arrest.

Some persons carry *epinephrine*—a drug used to treat life-threatening allergic reactions. The person injects the drug into the outer thigh. One dose is given for anaphylaxis. The person may give a second dose if:
- There is no response to the first dose.
- EMS arrival will take longer than 5 to 10 minutes.

STROKE

Stroke (cerebrovascular accident) occurs when the brain is suddenly deprived of its blood supply (Chapter 40). Usually only part of the brain is affected. A stroke may be caused by a thrombus, an embolus, or hemorrhage if a blood vessel in the brain ruptures.

Signs of stroke vary (Chapter 40). They depend on the size and location of brain injury. The National Institute of Neurological Disorders and Stroke lists these major signs.

- Sudden numbness or weakness of the face, arm, or leg, especially on 1 side of the body
- Sudden confusion or trouble speaking or understanding speech
- Sudden trouble seeing in 1 or both eyes
- Sudden trouble walking, dizziness, or loss of balance or coordination
- Sudden, severe headache with no known cause

With stroke, getting treatment quickly can lessen brain damage. The acronym FAST is used as a reminder to check for signs of stroke and act immediately if you suspect stroke. See Box 43-3. The most effective stroke treatments must be given within 3 hours of symptom onset. Activate the EMS system at once. Find out when symptoms began. Tell the EMS staff the time.

While waiting for EMS to arrive, follow the rules in Box 43-1. Keep the person comfortable, warm, and quiet. Give emergency care for seizures if necessary. Start CPR for cardiac arrest. Give rescue breathing for respiratory arrest.

BOX 43-3 Stroke Emergency Care—FAST

F—Face: Ask the person to smile. Does 1 side of the face droop (hang down)?

A—Arms: Ask the person to raise both arms. Does 1 arm drift downward?

S—Speech: Ask the person to repeat a simple phrase. Is speech slurred or strange?

T—Time: If any of these signs are present, call 911 right away.

Modified from National Center for Chronic Disease Prevention and Health Promotion, Division for Heart Disease and Stroke Prevention, Centers for Disease Control and Prevention: *Stroke signs and symptoms*, page reviewed August 28, 2020.

SEIZURES

Seizures (convulsions) are violent and sudden contractions or tremors of muscle groups caused by abnormal electrical activity in the brain. Movements are uncontrolled. The person may lose consciousness. Causes include head injury during birth or from trauma, high fever, brain tumors, poisoning, and nervous system disorders or infections. Lack of blood flow to the brain can also cause seizures.

Seizures are generalized or focal.

- *Generalized seizures*—affect both sides of the brain. There are 2 types.
  - *Absence (petit mal) seizures*—cause staring and rapid blinking. The seizure lasts a few seconds.
  - *Tonic-clonic (grand mal) seizures*—have 2 phases. In the *tonic* phase, muscles become stiff. The person loses consciousness and falls to the floor. The *clonic* phase follows. Muscles contract and relax. Jerking and shaking movements occur. The person may be incontinent. After the seizure, the person is often tired.
- *Focal (partial) seizures*—affect 1 area of the brain. A body part may twitch or have sensation changes. A strange taste or smell is an example. The person may be confused or unable to respond for a few minutes.

You cannot stop a seizure. However, you can protect the person from injury.

- Follow the rules in Box 43-1.
- Do not leave the person alone.
- Lower the person to the floor. This protects the person from falling.
- Note the time the seizure started.
- Place something soft under the head (Fig. 43-17). It prevents the head from striking the floor. You can use a pillow, a cushion, or a folded blanket, towel, or jacket. Or cradle the person's head in your lap.
- Remove eyeglasses and loosen tight jewelry and clothing around the neck. Ties, scarves, collars, and necklaces are examples.
- Turn the person onto the side. Make sure the head is turned to the side. See Figure 43-17.
- Do not put any object or your fingers between the teeth. Your fingers or the person's teeth or jaw can be injured.
- Do not try to stop the seizure or control movements.
- Move furniture, equipment, and sharp objects out of the way. The person may strike these objects during the seizure.

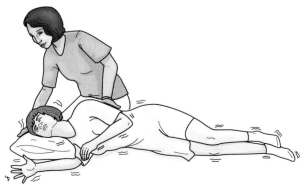

FIGURE 43-17 A pillow protects the person's head during a seizure. The person is turned onto the side.

Monitor the person's breathing during and after a seizure. Gasping or pauses may occur when chest muscles tighten during a seizure. Rescue breathing and CPR usually are not needed. Breathing should return to normal after the seizure.

Note the time the seizure ends. Make sure the mouth is clear of food, fluids, and saliva after the seizure. Do not give food or fluids until the person is fully alert. Also, do not let the person drive after a seizure. See Box 43-4 for when to activate the EMS system.

BOX 43-4 Seizures—Activating EMS

Activate the EMS system for any of the following.
- This is the person's first seizure.
- The person has trouble breathing after the seizure.
- The person has difficulty awakening after the seizure.
- The seizure lasts longer than 5 minutes.
- The person has another seizure soon after the first seizure.
- The person is or may be injured.
- The seizure happened in water.
- The person has diabetes or heart disease.
- The person is pregnant.

Modified from National Center for Chronic Disease Prevention and Health Promotion, Centers for Disease Control and Prevention: *Seizure first aid*, page reviewed January 2, 2022.

CONCUSSIONS

Head injuries can be minor or serious and life-threatening. Concussion is the most common brain injury. A concussion results from a bump or blow to the head or jolt to the head or body. The head and brain move quickly back and forth.

The following danger signs in adults signal the need for emergency care.
- Headache—gets worse or does not go away
- Stiff neck
- Weakness
- Numbness
- Decreased coordination
- Nausea or vomiting more than once
- Slurred speech
- Very sleepy; drowsy; cannot be awakened
- One eye pupil is larger than the other
- Convulsions or seizures
- Cannot recognize people, places, or things
- Confusion
- Restlessness
- Agitation
- Unusual behavior
- Loss of consciousness

Emergency care for a concussion includes the following.
- Follow the rules in Box 43-1. This includes activating the EMS system.
- Start CPR for cardiac arrest. Give rescue breathing for respiratory arrest.
- Place your hands on both sides of the head to keep the head aligned with the spine. Prevent movement.
- Apply firm pressure with a clean cloth to a bleeding area. See "Hemorrhage" on p. 563. Be careful not to move the person's head.
- Do not apply direct pressure to the skull if the skull may be fractured. Cover the wound with sterile gauze dressing.
- Do not remove any object from a wound.
- Logroll the person as a unit onto the side if vomiting occurs.
- Apply ice packs to swollen areas.

BURNS

Burns can severely disable a person. They can also cause death. Most burns occur in the home. Infants, children, and older persons are at risk. Common causes of burns and fires are:
- Scalds from steam or hot liquids
- Playing with matches or lighters
- Electrical injuries
- Cooking accidents (barbecues, microwave ovens, stoves, ovens)
- Falling asleep while smoking
- Fireplaces
- Space heaters
- No smoke alarms or non-functioning smoke alarms
- Sunburns
- Fireworks
- Chemicals

Some burns are severe (Fig. 43-18). Severity depends on burn size and depth, the body part involved, and age. Burns to the face, hands, feet, groin, buttocks, or over a joint are more serious than burns to an arm or leg. Infants, young children, and older persons are at high risk for complications and death.

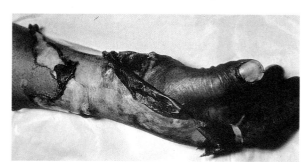

FIGURE 43-18 A severe burn. (From Ignatavicius DD, Workman ML: *Medical-surgical nursing: patient-centered collaborative care*, ed 10, St Louis, 2021, Elsevier.)

Emergency care for severe burns includes the following.

- Follow the rules in Box 43-1. This includes activating the EMS system.
- Do not touch the person if the person is in contact with an electrical source. Have the power source turned off. Do not approach the person or try to remove the electrical source with any object until the power source is turned off.
- Remove the person from the fire or burn source.
- Stop the burning process. Put out flames with water or roll the person in a blanket. Or smother flames with a coat, sheet, or towel.
- Apply cold or cool water for 10 to 15 minutes. Water temperature is between 59°F and 77°F (Fahrenheit) (15°C and 25°C [centigrade]). Do not put ice directly on the burn.
- Remove hot clothing that is not sticking to the skin. If you cannot remove hot clothing, cool the clothing with water.
- Remove jewelry and any tight clothing that is not sticking to the skin.
- Provide rescue breathing and CPR as needed.
- Cover burns with sterile, dry dressings. Or use a sheet or any other clean cloth.
- Do not put oil, butter, salve, or ointments on burns.
- Keep blisters intact. Do not break blisters.
- Elevate the burned area above heart level if possible.
- Cover the person with a blanket or coat to prevent heat loss.

FOCUS ON P R I D E

The Person, Family, and Yourself

P ersonal and Professional Responsibility

Practicing CPR skills improves confidence. Never practice CPR on another person. Serious damage can be done. Practice on a mannequin. Take pride in learning CPR. Your training can save a life.

R ights and Respect

Protect the right to privacy. Do not expose the person unnecessarily. The person may be in a lounge, dining area, or public place. Do what you can to provide privacy. As always, treat the person with dignity and respect.

I ndependence and Social Interaction

Quality of life and independence are important. In an emergency, choices may be few. However, they are given when possible. For example, the person has the right to choose a hospital.

The EMS staff has guidelines if a person refuses care. For example, the person must be competent and able to legally make medical decisions. The person must also be informed of the risks, benefits, and alternatives to recommended care.

D elegation and Teamwork

On-lookers can threaten privacy and confidentiality. Your main concern is the person's illness or injuries. You cannot give care and manage on-lookers. Ask someone else to deal with on-lookers. If someone else is giving care, keep on-lookers away from the person. Work together to protect the person's privacy.

E thics and Laws

People are curious. They want to know what happened, the extent of injuries or illness, and if the person will be okay. Do not discuss the situation. Do not offer ideas of what is wrong. Information about care, treatment, and condition is confidential. Keep the person's information private. It is the right thing to do.

FOCUS ON PRIDE: *Application*

Emergencies are stressful. A calm, professional approach helps the person and family feel more secure. Describe professional conduct in an emergency. Explain how you will prepare yourself to respond.

Circle the BEST answer.

1 When giving first aid, you should
   a Know your own limits
   b Move the person
   c Give the person fluids
   d Keep the person cool

2 The signs of sudden cardiac arrest are
   a Restlessness, rapid breathing, and a weak pulse
   b Confusion, hemiplegia, and slurred speech
   c No response, no normal breathing, and no pulse
   d Dizziness, pale skin, and slow breathing

3 A person is not responsive. To check for breathing
   a Use the head tilt–chin lift method to open the airway
   b Look for no breathing or agonal gasping
   c Look, listen, and feel for air moving in and out of the lungs
   d Take 10 to 15 seconds to listen for breathing

4 Which pulse is checked for an unresponsive adult?
   a The carotid pulse
   b The apical pulse
   c The brachial pulse
   d The femoral pulse

5 Which hand placement is correct for adult chest compressions?
   a 1 hand in the center of the chest
   b 2 hands below the sternum
   c 2 hands on the lower half of the sternum
   d 2 fingers on the lower half of the sternum

6 Which compression rate is used for CPR?
   a 30 compressions per minute
   b 100 to 120 compressions per minute
   c 15 compressions per minute
   d 60 to 100 compressions per minute

7 For adult CPR
   a Give 2 breaths after every 15 compressions
   b Give 2 breaths after every 30 compressions
   c Give 1 breath after every 5 compressions
   d Give 2 breaths when you are tired from giving compressions

8 Two rescuers are giving adult CPR. When should the AED be used?
   a After 5 cycles of CPR
   b After 2 minutes of CPR
   c As soon as the AED arrives
   d When EMS staff arrives

9 Rescue breathing for an adult involves
   a Giving each breath over 2 seconds
   b Watching the abdomen rise with each breath
   c Giving a breath every 3 seconds
   d Giving a breath every 6 seconds

10 A person swallowed a chemical. You should
   a Have the person drink a glass of water
   b Have the person try to vomit
   c Call the Poison Control Center
   d Contact the chemical's manufacturer

11 Which statement about heart attack is *true*?
   a It is the same as cardiac arrest.
   b It can cause cardiac arrest.
   c Symptoms resolve with rest.
   d It is a severe response to an antigen.

12 A person is hemorrhaging from the forearm. Your *first* action is to
   a Lower the arm
   b Apply pressure to the brachial artery
   c Tape a dressing in place
   d Apply direct pressure to the wound

13 A person is about to faint. What should you do?
   a Have the person sit or lie down.
   b Take the person outside for fresh air.
   c Have the person stand very still.
   d Raise the head if the person is lying down.

14 Which signals shock?
   a High blood pressure
   b Slow pulse
   c Slow and deep respirations
   d Cold, moist, and pale skin

15 Emergency care for stroke involves
   a Asking when the person's symptoms began
   b Giving the person sips of water
   c Controlling bleeding
   d Positioning the person bent forward with the head lowered

16 A person is having a tonic-clonic (grand mal) seizure. You should
   a Place an object between the person's teeth
   b Loosen tight jewelry and clothing around the neck
   c Try to stop the person's movements
   d Place the person's head on a firm surface

17 After falling down stairs, a person is confused and has a headache. You should
   a Place the person in the recovery position
   b Give the person a pain-relief drug
   c Prevent movement of the head and neck
   d Help the person to bed to lie down

18 While waiting for help to arrive, cover a severe burn with
   a A sterile, dry dressing or clean cloth
   b Butter or oil
   c Salve or an ointment
   d Nothing

Answers to Chapter 43 questions are on p. 589.

FOCUS ON **PRACTICE**

Problem Solving

A resident has a tonic-clonic (grand mal) seizure during an activity. What emergency care will you provide? How will you and the nursing team provide for the person's privacy?

44

End-of-Life Care

OBJECTIVES

- Define the key terms and key abbreviations in this chapter.
- Describe palliative care and hospice care.
- Describe the factors affecting attitudes about death.
- Describe the 5 stages of dying.
- Explain how to meet the needs of the dying person and family.
- Explain the purposes of the *Patient Self-Determination Act.*

- Describe 3 advance directives.
- Identify the signs of approaching death and the signs of death.
- Explain how to assist with post-mortem care.
- Perform the procedure in this chapter.
- Explain how to promote PRIDE in the person, the family, and yourself.

KEY TERMS

advance directive A document stating a person's wishes about health care when that person is unable to make decisions
autopsy The examination of the body after death
end-of-life care The support and care given during the time surrounding death
palliative care Care that relieves or reduces the intensity of uncomfortable symptoms without producing a cure

post-mortem care Care of the body after *(post)* death *(mortem)*
rigor mortis The stiffness or rigidity *(rigor)* of skeletal muscles that occurs after death *(mortis)*
terminal illness An illness or injury from which the person will not likely recover

KEY ABBREVIATIONS

CPR	Cardiopulmonary resuscitation	ID	Identification
DNR	Do Not Resuscitate	OBRA	Omnibus Budget Reconciliation Act of 1987

*E*nd-of-life care *describes the support and care given during the time surrounding death.* For some, death is sudden. For others, the process is gradual and death is expected. End-of-life care may involve days, weeks, or months.

Your feelings about death affect the care you give. You will help meet the dying person's physical, psychological, social, and spiritual needs. Therefore you must understand the dying process. Then you can approach the dying person with caring, kindness, and respect.

TERMINAL ILLNESS

Many illnesses and diseases have no cure. The body cannot function after some injuries. Recovery is not expected. The disease or injury ends in death. *An illness or injury from which the person will not likely recover is a* **terminal illness.**

Types of Care

Terminally ill persons may need palliative care or hospice care. The person may opt for palliative care and then change to hospice care.

- *Palliative care. Palliate* means *to soothe or relieve.* **Palliative care** *relieves or reduces the intensity of uncomfortable symptoms without producing a cure.* The focus is on comfort. The intent is to improve quality of life and provide family support. Palliative care can be given along with disease treatment.
- *Hospice care.* The focus is on the physical, emotional, social, and spiritual needs of dying persons and their families (Chapter 1). Often the person has less than 6 months to live. Cure or life-saving measures are not concerns. Pain relief and comfort are stressed. The goal is to improve quality of life. Follow-up care and support groups for survivors are hospice services. Hospice also supports the health team in dealing with a person's death.

ATTITUDES ABOUT DEATH

Experiences, culture, religion, and age influence attitudes about death. Many people fear death. Others do not believe they will die. Some look forward to and accept death. Attitudes about death often change as a person grows older and with changing needs.

Cultural and Spiritual Needs

Practices and attitudes about death differ among cultures. In some cultures, dying people are cared for at home by the family. Some families prepare the body for burial.

Spiritual needs relate to the human spirit and to religion and religious beliefs. Many people strengthen religious beliefs when dying. Religion can comfort the dying person and the family.

Attitudes about death are often closely related to religion. Some believe life after death is free of suffering and hardship. They also believe in reunion with loved ones. Many believe sins and misdeeds are punished in the afterlife. Others do not believe in the afterlife. To them, death is the end of life.

There are also religious beliefs about the body's form after death. Some believe the body keeps its physical form. Others believe that only the spirit or soul is present in the afterlife. *Reincarnation* is the belief that the spirit or soul is reborn in another human body or in another form of life.

Many religions have rites and rituals during the dying process and at the time of death and after. Prayers, blessings, scripture readings, and religious music are common sources of comfort. So are visits from a cleric.

See *Caring About Culture: Cultural and Spiritual Needs.*

See *Focus on Communication: Cultural and Spiritual Needs.*

CARING ABOUT CULTURE
Cultural and Spiritual Needs

In *Vietnam*, dying persons may be helped to recall past good deeds and to achieve a fitting mental state. Death at home may be preferred. In some areas, a coin or jewels (a wealthy family) or rice (a poor family) is put in the dead person's mouth. The belief is that they will help the soul go through encounters with gods and devils and the soul will be born rich in the next life.

In *India*, Hindu persons are often accepting of God's will. The person's desire to be clear-headed as death nears must be assessed in planning treatment. The family and person need a time and place for prayer. The Hindu priest reads from holy Sanskrit books. Some priests tie strings (meaning a blessing) around the neck or wrist. Cremation is usually preferred.

NOTE: *Each person is unique. A person may not follow all of the beliefs and practices of his or her culture. Follow the care plan.*

Modified from D'Avanzo CE: *Pocket guide to cultural health assessment*, ed 4, St Louis, 2008, Mosby.

FOCUS ON COMMUNICATION
Cultural and Spiritual Needs

Your cultural or religious practices and beliefs may differ from those of patients and residents. Do not judge the person by your standards. Do not make negative comments or insult the person's beliefs. Respect the person as a whole. This includes the person's beliefs and customs.

Age

Infants and toddlers do not understand death. They know or sense that something has changed. They sense a caregiver's absence or a different caregiver. They also sense changes in when and how their needs are met. They may feel a sense of loss.

Between about 3 and 6 years old, children understand more. They know when family members or pets die. They notice dead birds or bugs. Some children think death is temporary. (The person will come back to life.) Such ideas come from fairy tales, cartoons, movies, video games, and TV. Children this age often blame themselves when someone or something dies. Answers to questions about death often cause fear and confusion. Children who are told the person is "sleeping" may be afraid to go to sleep.

School-age children learn that death is final. They do not think they will die. Death happens to others, especially adults. It can be avoided. Children relate death to punishment and body mutilation. It also involves witches, ghosts, goblins, and monsters. Understanding increases as children grow older and have more experiences with death.

Adults may fear pain and suffering, dying alone, and the invasion of privacy. They also may fear loneliness and separation from loved ones. Worries about the care and support of those left behind are common. Adults often resent death because it affects plans, hopes, dreams, and ambitions.

Older persons know death will occur. Many have lost family and friends. Some welcome death as freedom from pain, suffering, and disability. Like younger adults, many fear dying alone.

THE STAGES OF DYING

Dr. Elisabeth Kübler-Ross described 5 stages of dying. They also are called the "stages of grief." *Grief* is the person's response to loss.

- *Stage 1: Denial.* The person refuses to believe that death will occur soon. "No, not me" is a common response. The person believes a mistake was made.
- *Stage 2: Anger.* The person thinks "Why me?" There is anger and rage. Dying persons may envy and resent those with life and health. Family, friends, and the health team are often targets of anger.
- *Stage 3: Bargaining.* Anger has passed. The person now says: "Yes, me but…" The person may bargain with God or a higher power for more time. Promises are made in exchange for more time. Bargaining is usually private and spiritual.
- *Stage 4: Depression.* The person thinks "Yes, me" and is very sad. The person mourns lost things and the future loss of life. The person may cry or say little. Sometimes the person talks about people and things that will be left behind.
- *Stage 5: Acceptance.* The person is calm, at peace, and accepts death. The person has said what needs to be said. Unfinished business is complete. This stage may last for many months or years. Reaching the acceptance stage does not mean death is near.

Dying persons do not always pass through each stage. A person may stay in one stage. Some move back and forth between stages. For example, a person moves from acceptance back to bargaining and then moves forward to acceptance.

COMFORT NEEDS

End-of-life care involves physical, mental and emotional, and spiritual comfort. See "Cultural and Spiritual Needs." Comfort goals are to:

- Prevent or relieve suffering to the extent possible.
- Respect and follow end-of-life wishes.

Dying persons may want family and friends present. They may want to talk about fears, worries, and anxieties. Some want to be alone. Often they need to talk during the night. Things are quiet, distractions are few, and there is more time to think.

You need to listen and use touch.

- *Listening.* The person may need to talk and share worries and concerns. Let the person express feelings and emotions. Do not worry about saying the wrong thing or finding comforting words. You do not need to say anything. Being there is what counts.
- *Touch.* Touch shows care and concern when words cannot. Sometimes the person does not want to talk but needs you nearby. Do not feel that you must talk. Silence, along with touch, is a powerful and meaningful way to communicate.

Some people want to see a spiritual leader. Or they want to take part in religious practices. Provide privacy during prayer and spiritual times. Be courteous to the spiritual leader. The person has the right to have religious items nearby—medals, pictures, statues, writings, and so on. Handle them with care and respect.

See *Focus on Communication: Comfort Needs.*
See *Focus on Older Persons: Comfort Needs.*

FOCUS ON **COMMUNICATION**
Comfort Needs

Knowing what to say to the dying person is hard for many health team members. Unless you have been near death yourself, do not say: "I understand what you are going through." The statement is a communication barrier. Instead, you can say:

- "Would you like to talk? I have time to listen."
- "You seem sad. Can I help?"
- "Can I quietly sit with you for a while?"

FOCUS ON **OLDER PERSONS**
Comfort Needs

Persons with advanced Alzheimer's disease cannot share their concerns, discomforts, or problems. It can be hard to provide emotional and spiritual comfort. Focus on the person's senses—hearing, touch, sight—to promote comfort. Comforting touch or massage can be soothing. So can soft music or sounds from nature—birds chirping, gentle breezes, ocean waves, and so on.

Physical Needs

Dying may take a few minutes, hours, days, or weeks. Body processes slow. The person is weak. Levels of consciousness change. The person is independent to the extent possible. As the person weakens, basic needs are met by others. Every effort is made to promote physical and psychological comfort. The person is allowed to die in peace and with dignity.

Pain. Pain can range from none to severe. Report signs and symptoms of pain at once (Chapter 33). Some persons cannot tell you about pain. Watch for signs of pain or discomfort.

* Restlessness
* Agitation
* Frowning, grimacing
* Sighing
* Moaning
* Whimpering, crying
* Tense muscles
* Rapid pulse

Skin care, personal and oral hygiene, back massages, and good alignment promote comfort. So do frequent position changes and supportive devices. Turn the person slowly and gently. Follow the care plan to prevent and control pain. The nurse can give pain-relief drugs.

Breathing Problems. Shortness of breath and difficulty breathing *(dyspnea)* are common end-of-life problems. Semi-Fowler's position and oxygen (Chapter 37) are helpful. An open window for fresh air may be helpful. So might a fan circulating air.

Noisy breathing—the *death rattle*—is common as death nears. This is from mucus collecting in the airway. These measures may help.

* The side-lying position.
* Suctioning by the nurse. *Suctioning* removes secretions.
* Drugs to reduce the amount of mucus.

Vision, Hearing, and Speech. Vision blurs and gradually fails. The person turns toward light. A darkened room may frighten the person. The eyes may be half-open. Secretions may collect in the eye corners.

Because of failing vision, explain who you are and what you are doing to the person or in the room. The room should be lit to meet the person's needs. Avoid bright lights and glares.

Good eye care is needed (Chapter 22). If the eyes stay open, a nurse may apply a protective ointment. Then the eyes are covered with moist pads to prevent injury.

Hearing is one of the last functions lost. Many people hear until the moment of death. Even unconscious persons may hear. Always assume that the person can hear. Speak in a normal voice. Give reassurance and explain care. Offer words of comfort. Avoid upsetting topics. Do not talk about the person.

Speech becomes harder. It may be hard to understand the person. Sometimes the person cannot speak. Anticipate needs. Do not ask questions with long answers. Ask a few "yes" or "no" questions. Despite speech problems, you must talk to the person.

Mouth, Nose, and Skin. Oral hygiene promotes comfort. Give routine mouth care if the person can eat and drink. Give frequent oral hygiene as death nears and when taking oral fluids is difficult. Oral hygiene is needed if mucus collects in the mouth and the person cannot swallow. A lip balm may be used for dry lips.

Crusting and irritation of the nostrils can occur. Nasal secretions, an oxygen cannula, and a naso-gastric tube are common causes. Carefully clean the nose. Apply lubricant as directed by the nurse and the care plan.

Circulation fails. Body temperature changes as death nears. The skin is cool, pale, and mottled (blotchy). Sweating increases. Skin care, bathing, and preventing pressure injuries are necessary. Linens and gowns are changed as needed. Although the skin feels cool, only light bed coverings are needed. Blankets may cause warmth and restlessness. However, observe for signs of cold—shivering, hunching shoulders, and pulling covers. Prevent drafts and provide more blankets.

Nutrition. Nausea, vomiting, and loss of appetite are common at the end of life. Drugs for nausea and vomiting are ordered.

You may need to feed the person. Favorite foods may help loss of appetite. So may small, frequent meals.

As death nears, loss of appetite is common. The person may choose not to eat or drink. Do not force the person to eat or drink. Tell the nurse.

Elimination. Urinary and fecal incontinence may occur. Use incontinence products or waterproof under-pads as directed. Give perineal care as needed. Constipation and urinary retention are common. A catheter may be needed. Follow the care plan for catheter care and bowel elimination.

The Person's Room. Provide a comfortable and pleasant room. Remove unnecessary equipment. Some equipment is upsetting to see (suction machines, drainage containers). If possible, keep such items out of the person's sight.

Mementos, pictures, cards, flowers, and religious items provide comfort. The person and family arrange the room as they wish. This helps meet love, belonging, and esteem needs. The room should reflect the person's choices.

Mental and Emotional Needs

Mental and emotional needs are very personal. Some persons are calm and at peace. Others are anxious or depressed or have specific fears and concerns. Examples include:

* Severe pain
* When and how death will occur
* What will happen to loved ones
* Dying alone

Simple measures may be soothing—touch, holding hands, back massage, soft lighting, music at a low volume.

THE FAMILY

The family usually gathers at the bedside to comfort the person and each other. This is a hard time for the family. It may be hard to find comforting words. To show you care, use touch and be available, courteous, and considerate.

Sometimes the family keeps a *vigil*. That is, someone is always with the person even at night. They watch over or pray for the person. Provide for the family's comfort.

Respect the right to privacy. The person and family need time together. However, do not neglect care because the family is present. Most agencies let family members help give care. Or you can suggest that they take a beverage or meal break.

The family may be very tired, sad, and tearful. Watching a loved one die is very painful. So is dealing with the eventual loss of that person. The family goes through stages like the dying person. They need support, understanding, courtesy, and respect. A spiritual leader may provide comfort. Communicate this request to the nurse at once.

LEGAL ISSUES

Much attention is given to the right to die. Many people do not want machines or other measures keeping them alive. Consent is needed for any treatment. When able, the person makes care decisions. Some people make end-of-life wishes known.

Advance Directives

The *Patient Self-Determination Act* and the *Omnibus Budget Reconciliation Act of 1987 (OBRA)* give persons the right to accept or refuse treatment. They also give the right to make advance directives. An ***advance directive*** *is a document stating a person's wishes about health care when that person is unable to make decisions.* Advance directives usually forbid certain care if there is no hope of recovery. Quality of care cannot be less because of the person's advance directives.

Agencies must inform all persons of the right to advance directives on admission. The medical record documents whether or not the person has made them.

See *Focus on Surveys: Advance Directives.*

FOCUS ON SURVEYS

Advance Directives

Advance directives are a focus of surveys. Nursing staff must know the person's current wishes. Surveyors review medical records and perform interviews to check that advance directives are current. The health team must regularly review the advance directive with the person or the person's representative to be sure that it reflects the person's current wishes.

Living Wills. A living will is about measures that support or maintain life when death is likely. Tube feedings, ventilators, and resuscitation are examples. A living will may instruct doctors:

- Not to start measures that prolong dying
- To remove measures that prolong dying

Durable Power of Attorney for Health Care. This advance directive gives the power to make health care decisions to another person. That person is often called a *health care proxy.* Usually this is a family member, friend, or lawyer. When a person cannot make health care decisions, the health care proxy can do so. This advance directive does not cover property or financial matters.

"Do Not Resuscitate" Orders. "Do Not Resuscitate" (DNR) or "No Code" orders mean that the person will not be resuscitated. Cardiopulmonary resuscitation (CPR) is not done (Chapter 43). The person is allowed to die with peace and dignity. The orders are written after consulting with the person and family. The family and doctor make the decision if the person is not mentally able to do so.

SIGNS OF DEATH

As death nears, these signs may occur fast or slowly.

- Movement, muscle tone, and sensation are lost. This usually starts in the feet and legs. Mouth muscles relax, the jaw drops. The mouth may stay open. The facial expression is often peaceful.
- Gastro-intestinal functions slow down. Abdominal distention, fecal incontinence, nausea, and vomiting are common.
- Body temperature changes. The person feels cool or cold, looks pale, and perspires heavily.
- Circulation fails. The pulse is fast or slow, weak, and irregular. Blood pressure starts to fall.
- The respiratory system fails. Slow or rapid and shallow respirations are observed. Mucus collects in the airway. Breathing sounds are noisy and gurgling *(death rattle)*.
- Pain decreases as the person loses consciousness. However, some people are conscious until the moment of death.

The signs of death include *no pulse, no respirations,* and *no blood pressure.* A doctor determines that death has occurred and pronounces the person dead. If a doctor is not present in a nursing center, a nurse calls the doctor to report the signs of death. The time and place are noted for the death certificate.

CARE OF THE BODY AFTER DEATH

Care of the body after (post) *death* (mortem) *is called **post-mortem care***. You may be asked to assist the nurse. Post-mortem care begins when the person is pronounced dead.

Post-mortem care is done to maintain a good appearance of the body. Discoloration and skin damage are prevented. Valuables and personal items are gathered for the family.

Within 2 to 4 hours after death, rigor mortis develops. *Rigor mortis is the stiffness or rigidity* (rigor) *of skeletal muscles that occurs after death* (mortis). The body is positioned in normal alignment before rigor mortis sets in. The body should appear in a comfortable and natural position when the family sees the body.

In some agencies, the body is prepared only for viewing by the family. The funeral director completes post-mortem care.

Sometimes an autopsy is done. An *autopsy is the examination of the body after death. (Autos* means *self. Opsis* means *view.)* It is done to determine the cause of death. Post-mortem care is not done. Doing so could remove or destroy evidence.

Post-mortem care involves bathing soiled areas and positioning the body in good alignment. When moving the body, air in the lungs, stomach, and intestines can be expelled. When air is expelled, sounds are produced. Do not let those sounds alarm or frighten you. They are normal and expected.

See *Delegation Guidelines: Care of the Body After Death.*

See *Promoting Safety and Comfort: Care of the Body After Death.*

See procedure: *Assisting With Post-Mortem Care.*

DELEGATION GUIDELINES
Care of the Body After Death

To assist with post-mortem care, you need this information from the nurse.
- If dentures are inserted or placed in a denture cup
- If tubes and dressings are removed or left in place
- If rings are removed or left in place
- If the family wants to view the body
- Special agency policies and procedures

PROMOTING SAFETY AND COMFORT
Care of the Body After Death

Safety

Standard Precautions and the Bloodborne Pathogen Standard are followed. You may have contact with blood or body fluids.

   NOTE: *A task may require more than 1 pair of gloves. Change gloves as needed. Use careful judgment. Remember to practice hand hygiene after removing gloves.*

Comfort

Respect and dignity must be maintained during post-mortem care. Provide privacy. Keep the body covered as much as possible. Move the body gently. Handle the person's valuables with care. Consider the family and the dignity they would want shown to the person.

Assisting With Post-Mortem Care

Pre-Procedure

1 Follow *Delegation Guidelines: Care of the Body After Death.* See *Promoting Safety and Comfort: Care of the Body After Death.*
2 Practice hand hygiene and get the following supplies.
   - Post-mortem kit (shroud or body bag, gown, identification [ID] tags, gauze squares, safety pins)
   - Disposable bed protectors
   - Wash basin
   - Bath towel and washcloths
   - Denture cup
   - Items for shaving facial hair (Chapter 23)
   - Tape
   - Dressings
   - Cotton balls
   - Valuables envelope
   - Gloves
   - Laundry bag
3 Arrange items in the room.
4 Provide for privacy.
5 Raise the bed for body mechanics.
6 Make sure the bed is flat.

Assisting With Post-Mortem Care—cont'd

Procedure

7 Put on the gloves.
8 Position the body supine. Arms and legs are straight. A pillow is under the head and shoulders. Or raise the head of the bed 15 to 20 degrees if this is agency policy.
9 Close the eyes. Gently pull the eyelids over the eyes. Apply moist cotton balls gently over the eyelids if the eyes do not stay closed.
10 Insert dentures or put them in a labeled denture cup. Follow agency policy.
11 Close the mouth. If necessary, place a rolled towel under the chin to keep the mouth closed.
12 Follow agency policy for jewelry. In some agencies, jewelry is removed except for a wedding ring. List any jewelry that is removed. Place the jewelry and the list in a valuables envelope.
13 Place a cotton ball over rings. Tape them in place as the nurse directs.
14 Remove drainage containers.
15 Remove tubes and catheters with gauze squares as the nurse directs.
16 Remove soiled dressings. Replace them with clean ones.
17 Shave facial hair if agency policy or if desired by the family. Some men normally grow facial hair (beard, mustache). If so, do not shave facial hair.
18 Bathe soiled areas with plain water. Dry thoroughly.
19 Place a disposable bed protector under the buttocks.

20 Remove and discard the gloves. Practice hand hygiene. Put on clean gloves.
21 Put a clean gown on the body. Position the body as in step 8.
22 Brush and comb the hair if necessary.
23 Cover the body to the shoulders with a sheet if the family will view the body.
24 Gather belongings. Put them in a bag labeled with the person's name. Be sure to include eyeglasses, hearing aids, and other valuables.
25 Remove supplies, equipment, and linens. Straighten the room. Provide soft lighting.
26 Remove and discard the gloves. Practice hand hygiene.
27 Let the family view the body. Provide for privacy. Return to the room after they leave.
28 Practice hand hygiene. Put on gloves.
29 Fill out the ID tags. Tie 1 to the ankle or to the right big toe.
30 Place the body in the body bag or cover it with a sheet. Or apply a shroud (Fig. 44-1).
  a Position the shroud under the body.
  b Bring the top down over the head.
  c Fold the bottom up over the feet.
  d Fold the sides over the body.
  e Pin or tape the shroud in place.
31 Attach the second ID tag to the shroud, sheet, or body bag.
32 Leave the denture cup with the body.
33 Remove and discard the gloves. Practice hand hygiene.

Post-Procedure

34 Maintain privacy measures. Leaving the privacy curtain, window coverings, and door closed are examples. Follow the nurse's instructions.
35 Clean the unit after the body has been removed. Wear gloves for this step.

36 Remove and discard the gloves. Practice hand hygiene.
37 Report the following.
   • The time the body was taken by the funeral director
   • What was done with jewelry, other valuables, and personal items
   • What was done with dentures

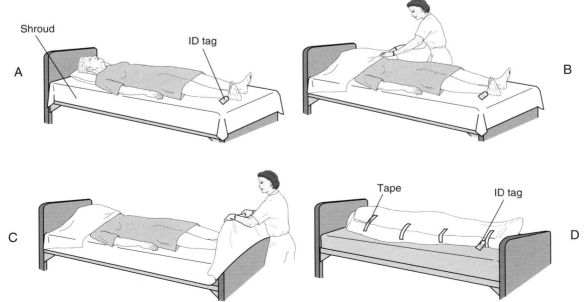

FIGURE 44-1 Applying a shroud. **A,** Position the shroud under the body. **B,** Bring the top down over the head. **C,** Fold the bottom up over the feet. **D,** Fold the sides over the body. Tape or pin the sides together. Attach an ID tag to the outside of the shroud.

FOCUS ON   P R I D E

The Person, Family, and Yourself

P ersonal and Professional Responsibility

To give quality care to the dying person and family:
- Promote comfort. Report signs of pain at once. Follow the comfort measures in the care plan. Ask about the family's comfort. Offering a drink or a blanket shows concern.
- Provide support to the person and family. Be kind. Show compassion and respect.
- Give the family time alone with the person.

Take pride in supporting the person and family during a difficult time. The family has many emotions during the dying process and after a loved one's death (Fig. 44-2).

R ights and Respect

Understanding the person's needs and desires allows you to give better care. The desire to die in peace and with dignity is respected. The right to privacy and the right to be treated with dignity and respect apply after death.

I ndependence and Social Interaction

Some days the person can do more and interact more than other days. Consider the person's physical and mental limits. Do not force more. Allow rest. Tell the nurse if you suspect that the family or visitors are tiring the person.

D elegation and Teamwork

Over time, the health team often bonds with the person. This is common in hospice and long-term care. The person's death is difficult for the staff. Sadness and grief may occur.

Tell the nurse if you have trouble coping with a person's death. Support others who need help. A kind word, a hug, or taking time to listen show concern. Take pride in being a part of a caring and supportive team.

E thics and Laws

The dying person has rights under OBRA.
- *The right to privacy before and after death.* Proper draping and screening are important.
- *The right to visit others in private.* Moving the dying person to a private room provides privacy. Family can usually stay with the person.
- *The right to confidentiality before and after death.* The final moments and cause of death are confidential. So are statements, conversations, and family reactions.
- *The right to be free from abuse, mistreatment, and neglect.* The person has the right to kind and respectful care before and after death. Report signs of abuse, mistreatment, or neglect at once.
- *Freedom from restraint.* Restraints are used only if ordered by the doctor. Dying persons are often too weak to be dangerous to themselves or others.
- *The right to personal possessions.* The person may want photos and religious items nearby. Protect the person's property from loss or damage before and after death. Such items are often family treasures or mementos.
- *The right to a safe and home-like setting.* Everyone must keep the setting safe and home-like. Try to keep equipment and supplies out of view. The room should be free from unpleasant odors and noises. Do your best to keep the room neat and clean.
- *The right to personal choice.* The dying person may refuse treatment. Advance directives are common. The health team must respect choices to refuse treatment or not prolong life.

FOCUS ON PRIDE: *Application*

Genuine concern for the dying person is shown in the care you give. How can you show respect at the end of life and with post-mortem care? How can you show care and concern for the grieving family?

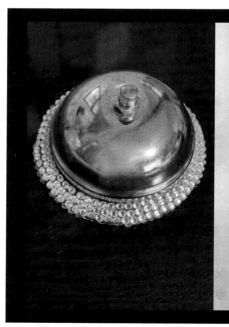

ROGER'S BELL

Mom neared the end of her travail,
she suffered much...so thin, so frail.
I worried a lot; "What if she fell?"
Then I remembered "Roger's Bell!"
I put the bell beside her bed.
"Just ring it anytime," I said,
"and I'll be there to help you stand,
or rub your back, or hold your hand."
I'd tell Mom most every night
to ring that bell if things weren't right.
And once or twice she rang the bell,
she did it for me, I could tell.
The final weeks were Carol's hell...
yet she ignored the nightstand bell.

The bell was quiet the day she died,
when friends she barely knew had cried.
I went to the nightstand...said a prayer,
picked up the bell...Do I dare?
"Why have it there beside your bed,
when now I need your help instead?"
She answered, "If you're sad and lonely too,
ring the bell and I'll be there with you!"
– Now Mom doesn't need my steady hand,
– she marches on...leading the band.
Her ordeal is over, her task complete,
and she watches over me, till again we meet.

–Bob Pinkerton

FIGURE 44-2   When he was dying of cancer, Linda Pinkerton Davis gave her husband, Roger, a nightstand bell. Several years later, "Roger's bell" was decorated and passed on to Linda's mom, Carol, who had cancer. Carol's husband wrote this poem for his four daughters after their mother died. (Bell photo courtesy Becky MacMillan; "Roger's Bell" poem printed with permission from Robert Pinkerton, July 2017.)

Circle the BEST answer.

1 Which is *true*?
   a Death from terminal illness is sudden.
   b Doctors know when death will occur.
   c An illness is terminal when recovery is not likely.
   d All severe injuries end in death.

2 Reincarnation is the belief that
   a There is no afterlife
   b The spirit or soul is reborn into another human body or form of life
   c The body keeps its physical form in the afterlife
   d Only the spirit or soul is present in the afterlife

3 Adults and older persons usually fear
   a Reincarnation
   b The 5 stages of dying
   c Advance directives
   d Dying alone

4 Persons in the stage of denial
   a Are angry
   b Are calm and at peace
   c Refuse to believe they are dying
   d Are sad and quiet

5 A person tries to gain more time during the stage of
   a Anger
   b Bargaining
   c Depression
   d Acceptance

6 When caring for the dying person, you should
   a Use touch and listen
   b Do most of the talking
   c Ask questions with long answers
   d Speak in a loud voice

7 As death nears, the last sense lost is
   a Sight
   b Taste
   c Smell
   d Hearing

8 The dying person's care includes the following. Which should you question?
   a Eye care
   b Mouth care
   c Active range-of-motion exercises
   d Position changes

9 The dying person is positioned in
   a The supine position
   b The Fowler's position
   c Good body alignment
   d The dorsal recumbent position

10 A "DNR" order means that
   a CPR will not be done
   b A representative will make decisions for the person
   c Life-prolonging measures will be carried out
   d Comfort measures will not be given

11 The signs of death are
   a Convulsions and incontinence
   b No pulse, respirations, or blood pressure
   c Loss of consciousness and no muscle movements
   d A rigid body and pale skin

12 Post-mortem care is done
   a After rigor mortis sets in
   b When the funeral director arrives for the body
   c After the family has viewed the body
   d After the doctor pronounces the person dead

Answers to Chapter 44 questions are on p. 589.

FOCUS ON **PRACTICE**

Problem Solving

A person is nearing the end of life. You want to provide mouth care. The family arrives. Is this a good time to give care? What will you say to the family?

CHAPTER 45

Getting a Job

OBJECTIVES

- Define the key terms and key abbreviations in this chapter.
- Identify the sources for jobs and places to work.
- Describe what employers look for when hiring staff.
- Describe how to prove completion of a nursing assistant training and competency evaluation program (NATCEP).
- Explain how to complete a job application.
- Describe in-person, phone, and video interviews.
- Explain how to prepare and dress for an interview.
- Identify common interview questions.
- Explain how to conduct yourself during an interview.
- Describe the questions you cannot be asked during an interview or on a job application.
- Explain what to do after an interview.
- Explain how to accept or decline a job offer.
- Explain how to promote PRIDE in the person, the family, and yourself.

KEY TERMS

discrimination Unjust treatment based on personal qualities

job application An agency's official form listing questions that require factual answers from the person seeking employment; employment form

job interview When an employer asks a job applicant questions about the applicant's education and career

reasonable accommodation To assist or change a position or workplace to allow an employee to do a job despite having a disability

KEY ABBREVIATIONS

EEOC	Equal Employment Opportunity Commission
NATCEP	Nursing assistant training and competency evaluation program
OBRA	Omnibus Budget Reconciliation Act of 1987

Successfully completing a nursing assistant training and competency evaluation program (NATCEP) is a step toward employment. This chapter will help you find a job in a professional and efficient manner.

SOURCES OF JOBS

There are easy ways to learn about jobs and places to work.
- The Internet—job sites and social media sites
- Newspaper ads
- Local and state employment services
- Agencies you would like to work at
- People you know—instructor, family, and friends
- Your school's or college's job placement counselors
- Job fairs
- Your clinical experience site

Your clinical experience site is an important source. The staff observe students as future employees. They look for good work ethics. They watch how students treat patients or residents, their instructor, other students, and staff. They look for the qualities and traits of a nursing assistant described in Chapter 5. If your clinical agency is not hiring, the staff may suggest other places to apply.

WHAT EMPLOYERS LOOK FOR

If you owned a business, who would you hire? Your answer helps you better understand the agency's point of view. Agencies want staff who:

- Are dependable
- Have needed job skills and training
- Have values and attitudes that fit with the agency
- Have a professional appearance

To function well, you need good work ethics. Review Chapter 5 and the *Focus on PRIDE* boxes at the end of each chapter to help you develop positive attitudes and work practices.

You must be at work on time and when scheduled. Undependable people cause everyone problems. Other staff have extra work. Fewer staff give care. Quality of care suffers. You want co-workers to work when scheduled. Otherwise, you have extra work. You have less time to spend with patients or residents. Likewise, co-workers expect you to work when scheduled.

Job Skills and Training

The agency checks the nursing assistant registry and requests proof of successful NATCEP completion. An agency will accept 1 or more of the following.

- A certificate of course completion from your training program
- A high school, college, or technical school transcript
- An official grade report (report card)

Give the agency a *copy* of your certificate, transcript, or grade report. Never give the original to anyone. Keep originals in a safe place for future use. Some agencies want a transcript sent directly from the school or college.

See *Promoting Safety and Comfort: Job Skills and Training.*

PROMOTING SAFETY AND COMFORT

Job Skills and Training

Safety

To work in long-term care, you must complete a state-approved NATCEP. This is a requirement of the *Omnibus Budget Reconciliation Act of 1987 (OBRA)*. The agency requests proof of training. The nursing assistant registry is checked. Nursing centers cannot hire persons convicted of abuse, neglect, or mistreatment. This also is an OBRA requirement.

JOB APPLICATIONS

A *job application (employment form) is an agency's official form listing questions that require factual answers from the person seeking employment* (Fig. 45-1, pp. 580–581). Personal information (legal name, address, phone number), work history, education, qualifications, and references are examples. The same information is required of all applicants.

You get a job application from the *personnel office (human resources office)* or on-line through an agency's website. For a paper application, use a pen with black ink to complete the form. You can complete the application at the agency or take it home to return by mail or in person. You must be well groomed and behave pleasantly when seeking or returning a job application. It may be your first chance to make a good impression.

On-line job applications require an electronic device—computer, tablet, phone. Follow the agency's website instructions for completing an on-line application.

Completing a Job Application

To complete a job application, see Box 45-1, p. 582. The application may be your first chance to impress the agency. A neat, readable, and complete application gives a good image. A sloppy or incomplete one does not.

A job application is easier to complete if you keep a file of your education and work history. The file should contain:

- A copy of your high school diploma or general equivalency diploma (GED).
- A copy of any grade reports, college degrees, certificates, or military training.
- A copy of your nursing assistant training program certificate of completion.
- NATCEP test results.
- Nursing assistant registry information for each state in which you are certified (licensed, registered).
- Copies of communications with your state's nursing assistant registry agency.
- Copies of court records for criminal convictions.
- A copy of your Social Security card.
- Names, addresses, and phone numbers of references.
- Names, addresses, and phone numbers of current and past employers. Include:
  - Your job title
  - Dates employment started and ended
  - Your supervisor's name
  - Hourly salary
- Proof of in-services attended and continuing education units (CEUs).

When requesting a job application, also ask for the agency's nursing assistant job description (Chapter 3).

EMPLOYMENT APPLICATION

All information listed on this application will be considered and handled as personal and confidential. Please print or write legibly.

AN EQUAL OPPORTUNITY EMPLOYER

This employer provides equal opportunity to all persons without regard to disability, race, color, religion, gender, age, or national origin.

Name

Date of Application

Address   City   State   Zip

Home Phone   Cell Phone   Social Security Number

GENERAL INFORMATION

Position applied for:

Available to work: ☐ Full-time   ☐ Part-time   ☐ Temporary   Date available to start work:

Will transportation be a problem for you? _____ ☐ No ☐ Yes

Do you have the legal right to work in the United States? _____ ☐ No ☐ Yes

Were you given a job description? _____ ☐ No ☐ Yes

Do you understand the functions of the job? _____ ☐ No ☐ Yes

Can you perform the functions of the job with or without reasonable accommodation? ____ ☐ No ☐ Yes

Have you ever been convicted of a felony? _____ ☐ No ☐ Yes

If yes, explain:

EDUCATION

	Name and Address of School	Major/Degree(s)	Number of Years Completed	Did You Graduate?
High School				
Community College				
4-Year Institution				
Vocational				
Other (specify)				

Describe specialized training, skills, seminars, courses, in-services, continuing education, or extra-curricular activities:

FIGURE 45-1 A sample job application.

EMPLOYMENT RECORD

Beginning with your current employer, please list your work experience over the last ten years. You may include pertinent volunteer activities.

Name and Address of Employer

Start Date   End Date

Phone

Job Title   Supervisor   Phone

Start Salary   End Salary

Duties

Reason for Leaving

Name and Address of Employer

Start Date   End Date

Phone

Job Title   Supervisor   Phone

Start Salary   End Salary

Duties

Reason for Leaving

Name and Address of Employer

Start Date   End Date

Phone

Job Title   Supervisor   Phone

Start Salary   End Salary

Duties

Reason for Leaving

REFERENCES

Only include persons familiar with your work ability. Do not include family.

Name and Title   Address   Phone

Name and Title   Address   Phone

Name and Title   Address   Phone

Name and Title   Address   Phone

SIGNATURE

I certify that the information provided on this application is true and complete. I understand that any false information or omissions may result in rejection of my application or job loss at any time during employment. I authorize verification of my education and past employment. I release all persons, schools, and past employers from liability for supplying such information.

I understand that the employer will conduct a criminal background check.

I understand that the use of illegal drugs is prohibited during employment. I am willing to submit to drug testing before and during employment.

Signature   Date

FIGURE 45-1, cont'd

BOX 45-1 Guidelines for Completing a Job Application

- Read and follow the directions. They may ask you to print using black ink. Following directions on the job application gives insight about your ability to follow directions on the job.
- Write neatly. Writing must be readable. A messy application gives a bad image. Readable writing gives the correct information. The agency cannot contact you if unable to read your phone number. You may miss getting the job.
- Complete the entire form. If an item does not apply to you, write "N/A" for non-applicable. Or draw a line through the space. This shows that you read the section. It also shows that you did not skip the item on purpose.
- Give information about employment gaps. If you did not work for a time, the agency wonders why. Providing this information shows you are honest. Some reasons are an illness, school, raising children, or caring for a family member.
- Tell why you left a job, if asked. Be brief but honest. People leave jobs for one that pays better. Some leave for career advancement. Others leave for reasons given for employment gaps. If fired from a job, give an honest but positive answer. Do not talk badly about the former agency.
- Give references. List the names, titles, addresses, and phone numbers of at least 4 non-family references. Have this information with you before completing an application. (Always ask references if an agency can contact them.) You may get the job faster if the agency can check references quickly. The agency should not have to wait for missing or incomplete information. This wastes your time and the agency's time. Also, the agency wonders if you are hiding something with incomplete reference information.
- Be prepared to provide the following.
  - Social Security number
  - Proof of the legal right to work in the United States
  - Proof of successful NATCEP completion
  - Identification—driver's license or government-issued ID card
- Report any felony convictions as directed. Write "no" or "none" as appropriate. Criminal background and fingerprint checks are common requirements (Chapter 3).
- Give honest answers. Lying on an application is fraud. It is grounds for being fired.
- Complete a final review of your application. Make sure you have provided all required information.

THE JOB INTERVIEW

A *job interview* is when an employer asks a job applicant questions about the applicant's education and career. The agency gets to know and evaluate you. You learn about the agency.

The interview may be when you complete the job application. Some agencies review applications before scheduling interviews. An interview may be conducted by 1 person or 2 or more people.

When an interview is scheduled, write down the interviewer's name and the interview date and time. If you need directions to the agency, ask for them when the interview is scheduled.

When expecting a call from the agency, answer your phone. Do not let your phone go to voice mail. If the caller has to leave a message, you need an appropriate and professional greeting. Sometimes an agency will contact you through a text or e-mail message. Return messages within 24 hours.

Types of Interviews

Interviews may be in-person, by phone, or by video. You need good communication skills. (See Chapters 6 and 7.)
- *In-person interview.* You and the interviewer meet in the same room face-to-face. Appropriate dress and body language are needed.
- *Phone interview.* A phone interview may be used to decide if an in-person interview will follow. If distance is a factor, a phone interview may work for the agency and you.
- *Video interview.* You use a computer or other electronic device at home or another site. Appropriate dress and body language are needed.

For phone and video interviews:
- Use a quiet room. Turn off phones, music, TV, and other devices. Do not use a room where phones ring, people are talking, or pets are present.
- Be ready to answer the phone or turn on the electronic device at the scheduled time.
- Have your electronic device charged. Consider plugging into a power source to prevent the device from turning off.
- Speak clearly and slowly. Do not shout.
- Listen carefully. Let the interviewer finish speaking before you answer.
- Smile. Smile even for a phone interview. Attitude and facial expression affect your voice tone.

Preparing for the Interview

Box 45-2 lists common interview questions. Prepare your answers ahead of time. Also prepare a list of your skills for the interviewer.

You must present a good image. You need to be neat, clean, and well groomed. How you dress is important. Follow the guidelines in Box 45-3.

Show that you are dependable. No matter the type of interview, be on time. For an in-person interview, do a practice run (dry run). Go to the agency some day before the interview. Note how long it takes to get there and where to park. Also find the personnel office. A practice run gives an idea of the time needed from your home to the personnel office.

BOX 45-2 Common Interview Questions

What the Interviewer May Ask
- Tell me about yourself.
- Tell me about your career goals.
- What are you doing to reach these goals?
- Describe what *professional* behavior means to you.
- Tell me about your last job. Why did you leave?
- What did you like the most about your last job? The least?
- What would your supervisor and co-workers tell me about you? Your dependability? Your skills? Your flexibility?
- Which functions are hard for you? How do you handle this difficulty?
- How do you set priorities?
- How have your experiences prepared you for this job?
- What would you like to change about your last job?
- How do you handle problems with patients, residents, families, and co-workers?
- Why do you want to work here?
- Why should this agency hire you?

What to Ask the Interviewer
- Which job functions are the most important?
- What employee qualities and traits are important to you?
- What nursing care pattern is used here (Chapter 1)?
- Who will I work with?
- When are performance evaluations done? Who does them? How are they done?

What to Ask the Interviewer—cont'd
- What performance factors are evaluated?
- How does the supervisor handle problems?
- What are the most common reasons that nursing assistants lose their jobs here? What are common reasons for resigning? (To *resign* means *to leave a job.*)
- How do you see this job in the next year? In the next 5 years?
- What is the greatest reward from this job? The greatest challenge?
- What do you like the most about nursing assistants who work here? The least?
- Why should I work here rather than in another agency?
- How much will I make an hour?
- What hours will I work?
- What uniforms are required?
- What benefits do you offer?
  - Health and dental insurance?
  - Continuing education?
  - Vacation time?
- Do you have a new employee orientation program? How long is it?
- May I have a tour of the agency and the unit I will work on? Can I meet the nurse manager and unit staff?
- Can I have a few minutes to talk to the nurse manager?

BOX 45-3 Grooming and Dressing for an Interview

- Bathe and brush your teeth. Wash your hair. Men should shave facial hair or groom beards and mustaches.
- Use deodorant or antiperspirant.
- Make sure your hands and fingernails are clean.
- Apply make-up in a simple, attractive manner (if worn).
- Style your hair in a neat and attractive way.
- Do not wear jeans, shorts, yoga pants, tank tops, halter tops, or other casual clothing. Also do not wear distracting colors or prints. Do not wear lacy, sheer, tight, or low-cut garments.
- Iron clothing. Sew on loose buttons and mend garments.
- Wear clothing that covers tattoos (body art).
- Wear clothing that looks professional. Slacks and a shirt or blouse are common (Fig. 45-2). A long-sleeved shirt with a simple pattern or single color (white, light blue, black) is best. A jacket or tie is optional. A simple dress or skirt of an appropriate length may be worn.
- Wear socks, hose, or tights. Hose should be free of runs and snags.
- Make sure shoes are clean and in good repair.
- Avoid heavy perfumes, colognes, and after-shave lotions. A light fragrance is okay.
- Wear only simple jewelry that complements your clothes. Avoid adornments in body piercings. For multiple ear piercings, wear only 1 set of earrings.
- Brush your teeth again before leaving for the interview. Do not smoke or chew gum before the interview. You must have fresh breath.
- Stop in the restroom when you arrive at the agency. Check your hair, make-up, clothes, and hands.

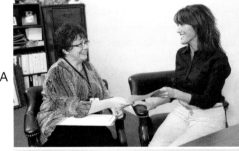
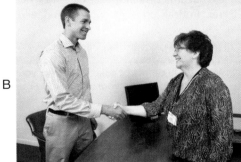

FIGURE 45-2 Dress for an interview. **A,** This applicant wears a simple blouse and slacks. **B,** This applicant wears a simple shirt and slacks.

Arriving at the Agency. When you arrive at the agency, turn off your phone and other devices. Tell the receptionist your name, why you are there, and the interviewer's name. Then sit quietly in the waiting area. Do not smoke, chew gum, or use your phone or other devices for calls, e-mails, text messages, or other reasons.

While waiting, review your answers to the common interview questions. Waiting may be part of the interview. The interviewer may ask staff about how you acted while waiting. Smile and be polite and friendly.

During the Interview

Politely greet and address the interviewer as Miss, Mrs., Ms., Mr., or Doctor. For an in-person interview, give a firm hand-shake. Stand until asked to sit. Sit with good posture and in a professional way. If offered a beverage, you may accept. Be sure to thank the person.

Good eye contact is needed for in-person and video interviews. Look directly at the interviewer to answer or ask questions. Poor eye contact sends negative information—shy, insecure, dishonest, or lacking interest.

Watch your body language (Chapter 6)—facial expressions, gestures, posture, and body movements. What you say is important. However, your body tells a great deal. Avoid distracting habits—slumping; biting nails; playing with jewelry, clothing, or your hair; crossing your arms; and crossing and swinging legs back and forth. Focus on the interview. Do not touch or read things on the person's desk.

Give complete and honest answers. Speak clearly and with confidence. Avoid short and long answers. "Yes" and "no" answers give little information. Briefly explain "yes" and "no" responses.

The interviewer will ask about your skills. Share your skills list. An agency-required skill may not be on your list. Explain that you are willing to learn if your state allows nursing assistants to perform the skill.

Review the job description with the interviewer. Ask questions. Advise the interviewer of functions you cannot perform because of training, legal, ethical, or religious reasons. Honesty now prevents problems later.

Find the right job for you. An employer wants to hire staff who will be happy in the job and the agency. Box 45-2 lists some questions for you to ask at the end of the interview. The interviewer's answers will help you decide if the job is right for you.

The interview usually lasts 15 to 20 minutes. You may be offered a job at this time. Or you are told when to expect a call or letter. Follow-up is acceptable. Ask when you can check on your application. Always thank the interviewer. Say: "I look forward to hearing from you." Shake the person's hand after an in-person interview.

Questions You Cannot Be Asked. The U.S. Equal Employment Opportunity Commission (EEOC) is a government agency. To guard against discrimination in hiring, the EEOC has guidelines for questions that cannot be asked during an interview or on a job application. *Discrimination involves unjust treatment based on personal qualities.* Age, race, biological sex, gender identity, sexuality, pregnancy, religion, and disability are examples. See Box 45-4.

See *Focus on Communication: Questions You Cannot Be Asked.*

FOCUS ON COMMUNICATION

Questions You Cannot Be Asked

If asked a question listed in Box 45-4, you have the right to decline to answer. Decline politely. You can say: "I'm sorry, but the EEOC does not allow that question during an interview. What else can I answer for you?"

After the Interview

A thank-you letter or note is advised within 24 hours after the interview (Fig. 45-3). Write neatly and clearly. Use a computer, another electronic device, or a typewriter if your writing is hard to read. The thank-you note should include:

- The date
- The interviewer's formal name with Miss, Ms., Mrs., Mr., or Dr.
- A statement thanking the person for the interview
- Comments about the interview, the agency, and your eagerness to hear about the job
- Your signature, using your first and last names

BOX 45-4 Interview Questions Not Allowed by the EEOC

- *Age.* Generally, you cannot be asked your age, your birth date, or any question that refers to your age. However, under OBRA, you must be at least 16 years old. Some states have limits on the tasks allowed for persons under 18 years of age.
- *Color, race, or national origin.* This includes questions related to your place of birth or that of your parents; language spoken; or how you learned to read, write, or speak a language.
- *Religion or spiritual beliefs.* You cannot be asked about your religion, religious practices, church, priest or pastor, or religious holidays observed.
- *Gender or sexuality.* No questions are allowed about gender identity (Chapter 6) or your sexuality.
- *Pregnancy or plans for pregnancy.* You cannot be asked if you are pregnant or planning to get pregnant or about your pregnancy history.
- *Marital status.* You cannot be asked if you are married, single, divorced, separated, engaged, or widowed.
- *Children.* You cannot be asked if you have children, how many children or their ages, or who will care for children while you are at work.
- *Arrest record.* You cannot be asked about arrests. However, you can be asked about criminal convictions.
- *Finances.* You cannot be asked about credit cards or bank accounts or if you own your home or car.
- *Disabilities.* You cannot be asked if you have disabilities or what they are. This includes treatment for alcoholism. However, you can be asked if you can perform the job with reasonable accommodation. *Reasonable accommodation means to assist or change a position or workplace to allow an employee to do a job despite having a disability.*
- *Number of sick days used in the last year.* You cannot be asked about your medical history. However, you may have to take a medical exam or have some tests done after a job offer is made.
- *Citizenship.* You cannot be asked if you are a United States citizen. You cannot be asked to provide proof of citizenship. However, if hired, you can be asked to provide proof of the legal right to work in the United States.

December 12

Dear [Interviewer's name],

Thank you for the interview yesterday. I enjoyed meeting you and learning more about the nursing center. I was impressed by the friendliness of the staff and would enjoy working in that environment.

Again, thank you. I look forward to hearing from you soon.

Sincerely,
[Your full name]

FIGURE 45-3 Sample thank-you note written after a job interview.

ACCEPTING OR DECLINING A JOB OFFER

You can apply to many places and have many interviews. Think about all offers before accepting one. You might have more questions about an agency. Ask them before accepting a job. To help you decide, discuss the offer with a family member, friend, co-worker, or your instructor.

When you accept a job, agree on a starting date, pay rate, and work hours. Ask where to report on your first day. Ask for all information in writing. That way you and the agency have the same understanding of the job offer. Use the written offer later if questions arise. Also ask for the employee handbook and other agency information. Read everything before you start working.

Accept the best job for you. To decline a job offer, thank the person for offering you a job. If asked why you are refusing, give a positive response. For example: "Thank you for offering me a job. I'm going to accept a job closer to my home."

Sometimes a job is not offered. You may not hear from the agency. Or the agency calls, writes, or e-mails saying that you will not be offered the job. If this happens, thank the person for letting you know. Ask that the agency keep your application active. For example: "Thank you for letting me know. Please keep me in mind for other openings."

DRUG TESTING

State laws vary about drug testing. Drug testing may be part of the application process. If so, review the job application before signing it. The application usually states 1 of the following (see Fig. 45-1).
- Drug testing is part of the application screening process for new staff.
- A job offer depends on passing a drug test.

FOCUS ON PRIDE
The Person, Family, and Yourself

P ersonal and Professional Responsibility

Agencies invest much time and money in new staff. Frequently changing jobs can reflect poorly on you. Before applying, find out about the agency. This helps you decide if the agency is a good fit for you. Also, your interest in the agency can make a good impression during an interview.

R ights and Respect

You have the right to protection from discrimination. Application and interview questions must relate to your ability to do the job. See Box 45-4 for questions that are not allowed.

Job-related questions are allowed if asked to all applicants. These questions are allowed.
- What languages do you read, write, and speak fluently?
- Can you perform the duties of this job? Do you need any special accommodations to perform the job?
- Have you ever been convicted of a crime?
Know your rights. Plan how to respond if you suspect a question violates your rights.

I ndependence and Social Interaction

Some agencies perform social media background checks. State laws vary about what information can be accessed—public or private. Employers must focus only on information related to the job. Show good judgment when using social media (Chapter 5). Be professional. Agencies may view postings on social media sites.

D elegation and Teamwork

Non–health care work experiences, education, and training are important. They give employers information about your dependability, teamwork, and work quality. Draw from your experiences. Give examples of your positive work ethics.

E thics and Laws

Agencies watch for safe and ethical conduct. They must act when conduct is unsafe or unethical. Background checks, drug testing, and interview questions help agencies decide if an applicant will meet safety and ethical standards.

Poor conduct outside of work can affect your job. Take pride in making good choices inside and outside the workplace.

FOCUS ON PRIDE: *Application*

Being prepared for an interview is helpful. You may be nervous about what questions will be asked, how you will answer, and if you will make a good impression. Describe how you will prepare yourself for a job interview.

REVIEW QUESTIONS

Circle the BEST answer.

1. When should you ask questions about your job description?
   a. After completing the job application
   b. Before completing the job application
   c. When your interview is scheduled
   d. During the interview

2. Lying on a job application is
   a. Negligence
   b. Fraud
   c. Libel
   d. Defamation

3. When completing a job application
   a. Use pencil
   b. Leave spaces blank that do not apply to you
   c. Give information about employment gaps
   d. List family members as references

4. For an interview, you show you are dependable when you
   a. Are on time
   b. Smile
   c. Are well groomed
   d. Shake the interviewer's hand

5. What should you wear to a job interview?
   a. A uniform
   b. Party clothes
   c. Slacks and a shirt or blouse
   d. Whatever is most comfortable

6. For a phone interview you should
   a. Shout answers so they are heard
   b. Take another call during the interview
   c. Have the interviewer leave a message
   d. Use a quiet room

7. Which is poor behavior during a job interview?
   a. Crossing your arms and legs
   b. Good eye contact with the interviewer
   c. Shaking hands with the interviewer
   d. Asking the interviewer questions

8. Which is the *best* response to an interview question?
   a. Brief explanations
   b. "Yes" or "no"
   c. Long answers
   d. A written response

9. An interviewer asks the following. Which should you decline to answer?
   a. Tell me about yourself.
   b. Are you married?
   c. Have you ever been convicted of a crime?
   d. What are your career goals?

10. After an interview
    a. Ask if the agency plans to hire you
    b. Ask to be paid for your time at the interview
    c. Write a thank-you note
    d. Do not apply to any other agencies

11. When accepting a job offer, avoid discussing
    a. Starting date
    b. Personal finances
    c. Pay rate
    d. Work hours

12. Drug testing may be required before an agency hires you.
    a. True
    b. False

Answers to Chapter 45 questions are on p. 589.

FOCUS ON **PRACTICE**

Problem Solving

You are asked the following questions at a job interview. How will you respond to each?

- Why did you decide to become a nursing assistant?
- What are your strengths and weaknesses?
- Describe a problem in your clinical training. How did you resolve it?
- Give an example of when you had to prioritize. How did you decide what to do first, second, and so on?

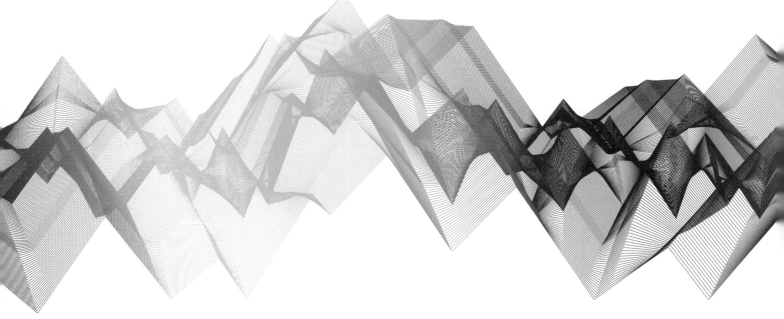

Review Question Answers

CHAPTER 1
1. c
2. d
3. b
4. c
5. a
6. b
7. b
8. a
9. d
10. c
11. a
12. b
13. a
14. d
15. c
16. c
17. b
18. d

CHAPTER 2
1. a
2. b
3. b
4. c
5. d
6. c
7. d
8. b
9. a
10. a
11. c
12. d
13. c
14. b
15. d
16. a
17. c
18. d
19. b
20. d
21. a
22. b

CHAPTER 3
1. d
2. c
3. d
4. c
5. a
6. b
7. c
8. a
9. c
10. b
11. d
12. d
13. a
14. d
15. a

CHAPTER 4
1. c
2. d
3. a
4. b
5. d
6. c
7. b
8. b
9. d
10. a
11. c
12. a
13. b
14. d
15. c
16. a
17. d
18. b
19. c
20. a

CHAPTER 5
1. b
2. d
3. c
4. a
5. d
6. b
7. a
8. d
9. d
10. a
11. c
12. b
13. c
14. a
15. b
16. d
17. a
18. c
19. d
20. b

CHAPTER 6
1. c
2. d
3. b
4. c
5. a
6. a
7. d
8. c
9. b
10. a
11. b
12. d
13. c
14. c
15. a
16. b
17. d
18. b

CHAPTER 7
1. d
2. c
3. b
4. a
5. a
6. d
7. c
8. a
9. b
10. c
11. a
12. d
13. a
14. b
15. b
16. d
17. a
18. c

CHAPTER 8
1. c
2. b
3. a
4. c
5. b
6. c
7. d
8. d
9. b
10. d
11. b
12. a
13. c
14. a
15. a
16. c
17. d
18. b
19. d
20. b
21. a
22. c

CHAPTER 9
1. a
2. b
3. a
4. c
5. c
6. a
7. d
8. b
9. c
10. d
11. d
12. c
13. b
14. a
15. b
16. b
17. b
18. c
19. d
20. b
21. a
22. a

CHAPTER 10
1. b
2. a
3. b
4. d
5. a
6. d
7. b
8. c
9. c
10. d
11. b
12. a
13. a
14. d
15. c
16. d

CHAPTER 11
1. a
2. d
3. c
4. b
5. c
6. d
7. b
8. d
9. a
10. c
11. b
12. a
13. b
14. a
15. b
16. d
17. a
18. c
19. a
20. c
21. b
22. d

CHAPTER 12
1. a
2. c
3. c
4. a
5. b
6. c
7. d
8. b
9. c
10. b
11. a
12. c
13. c
14. d
15. d

CHAPTER 13
1. b
2. c
3. d
4. b
5. c
6. a
7. a
8. b
9. d
10. c
11. a
12. b
13. a
14. c
15. d

CHAPTER 14
1. b
2. a
3. c
4. b
5. d
6. a
7. c
8. b
9. a
10. b
11. d
12. a
13. b
14. d
15. d
16. c
17. a
18. c
19. a
20. b
21. d
22. c

CHAPTER 15
1. a
2. b
3. a
4. c
5. c
6. d
7. b
8. d
9. c
10. d
11. a
12. b
13. b
14. d
15. a

CHAPTER 16
1. a
2. b
3. c
4. a
5. a
6. c
7. b
8. a
9. d
10. a
11. c
12. d
13. b
14. b
15. c
16. a

CHAPTER 17
1. c
2. d
3. b
4. a
5. b
6. c
7. c
8. a
9. d
10. b
11. a
12. c
13. b
14. d
15. c

CHAPTER 18
1. b
2. d
3. c
4. b
5. a
6. c
7. a
8. d
9. c
10. a
11. c
12. b
13. c
14. d

CHAPTER 19
1. d
2. b
3. d
4. d
5. c
6. c
7. a
8. a
9. b
10. b
11. a
12. c
13. a
14. d
15. c

CHAPTER 20
1. c
2. d
3. b
4. a
5. d
6. a
7. b
8. d
9. a
10. c
11. c
12. b

CHAPTER 21
1. c
2. d
3. b
4. d
5. a
6. d
7. a
8. c
9. c
10. a
11. b
12. c

CHAPTER 22
1. c
2. b
3. a
4. b
5. b
6. d
7. c
8. a
9. d
10. c
11. d
12. a
13. d
14. a
15. b
16. c
17. b
18. a

CHAPTER 23
1. d
2. b
3. b
4. c
5. a
6. d
7. d
8. a
9. c
10. c
11. b
12. d
13. a
14. c
15. a

CHAPTER 24
1. d
2. d
3. b
4. a
5. c
6. d
7. a
8. c

CHAPTER 25
1. c
2. d
3. a
4. a
5. b
6. b
7. a
8. d
9. c
10. b
11. c
12. d
13. a
14. c

CHAPTER 26
1. c
2. d
3. a
4. a
5. c
6. b
7. d
8. c
9. a
10. d

CHAPTER 27
1. b
2. a
3. d
4. b
5. c
6. d
7. c
8. a
9. b
10. d
11. a
12. b

CHAPTER 28
1. b
2. b
3. a
4. c
5. d
6. a
7. c
8. b
9. a
10. a
11. b
12. a
13. d
14. c
15. c

CHAPTER 29
1. b
2. c
3. d
4. d
5. a
6. a
7. b
8. c
9. d
10. b
11. a
12. c
13. a
14. c
15. d

CHAPTER 30
1. c
2. d
3. a
4. b
5. a
6. d
7. b
8. c
9. d
10. b
11. a
12. c
13. b
14. b
15. a

CHAPTER 31
1. b
2. a
3. c
4. a
5. d
6. c
7. d
8. c
9. c
10. a
11. d
12. c
13. d
14. b
15. b
16. a
17. c
18. c

CHAPTER 32
1. b
2. d
3. a
4. b
5. c
6. c
7. a
8. d
9. c
10. a
11. b
12. a
13. c
14. d
15. d
16. b
17. c
18. a

CHAPTER 33
1. a
2. d
3. b
4. c
5. d
6. a
7. b
8. c
9. d
10. d
11. b
12. a

CHAPTER 34
1. c
2. d
3. b
4. a
5. a
6. c
7. d
8. c
9. b
10. a
11. b
12. a

CHAPTER 35
1. c
2. b
3. a
4. d
5. b
6. d
7. a
8. a
9. c
10. b
11. c
12. b
13. a
14. c
15. b
16. a

CHAPTER 36
1. b
2. d
3. d
4. a
5. d
6. c
7. b
8. c
9. a
10. b
11. d
12. a
13. b
14. a
15. b
16. c
17. d
18. c

CHAPTER 37
1. c
2. c
3. b
4. b
5. d
6. c
7. d
8. a
9. b
10. a
11. c
12. d
13. a
14. c
15. a

CHAPTER 38
1. d
2. c
3. b
4. b
5. a
6. c
7. d
8. a
9. c
10. c

CHAPTER 39
1. b
2. d
3. b
4. a
5. d
6. c
7. a
8. d
9. a
10. b
11. a
12. b
13. c
14. d
15. d
16. c

CHAPTER 40
1 c
2 d
3 d
4 b
5 a
6 b
7 d
8 a
9 a
10 d
11 c
12 a
13 b
14 b
15 d
16 b
17 a
18 a
19 c
20 a
21 c
22 d
23 d
24 b
25 c
26 a
27 c
28 d
29 d
30 a
31 c
32 a
33 a
34 d
35 b

CHAPTER 41
1 b
2 b
3 c
4 c
5 a
6 d
7 d
8 c
9 b
10 a
11 b
12 a
13 c
14 a
15 b

CHAPTER 42
1 a
2 d
3 c
4 d
5 b
6 a
7 c
8 c
9 a
10 b
11 d
12 b
13 d
14 c
15 a
16 d
17 a
18 c

CHAPTER 43
1 a
2 c
3 b
4 a
5 c
6 b
7 b
8 c
9 d
10 c
11 b
12 d
13 a
14 d
15 a
16 b
17 c
18 a

CHAPTER 44
1 c
2 b
3 d
4 c
5 b
6 a
7 d
8 c
9 c
10 a
11 b
12 d

CHAPTER 45
1 d
2 b
3 c
4 a
5 c
6 d
7 a
8 a
9 b
10 c
11 b
12 a

Appendix A

The Patient Care Partnership—Understanding Expectations, Rights, and Responsibilities (A Summary)

High-Quality Care

- The hospital provides needed care with skill, compassion, and respect.
- The patient has the right to know the identities of those involved in care.
  - Doctors, nurses, and other staff
  - Students and other trainees

Clean and Safe Setting

- There are policies and procedures to:
  - Avoid mistakes.
  - Prevent abuse and neglect.
- The patient is told of unexpected or significant events.
  - What happened
  - Needed changes in care

Involvement in Care

- The patient has the right to make informed decisions about treatment choices.
  - What are the benefits and risks of each treatment?
  - Is the treatment experimental or part of a research study?
  - What can be expected from treatment?
  - How might long-term effects of treatment affect quality of life?
  - What will the patient and family need to do after discharge?
  - What are the costs for uncovered services or providers?
- The patient has the right to consent to or refuse treatment. The person is told of the effects of refusing treatment.
- The patient is expected to give information about:
  - Past illnesses, surgeries, or hospital stays
  - Allergic reactions
  - Drugs or dietary supplements that are taken
  - Health insurance plan admission requirements
- The patient's health care goals, values, and spiritual beliefs are respected. The patient is responsible for sharing his or her wishes with the doctor, family, and health team.
- The patient is expected to communicate about who makes decisions when the patient is unable.
  - *Power of attorney*, *living will*, or *advance directive* documents are shared with the doctor, family, and health team (Chapter 44).
  - Help is provided with making difficult decisions. Counselors or chaplains are available.

Protection of Privacy

- The hospital protects the confidentiality of:
  - The patient's relationships with the doctor and health team
  - Information about the patient's health and care
- A "Notice of Privacy Practices" is provided describing:
  - How patient information is used, disclosed, and protected
  - How to obtain a copy of hospital records about patient care

Preparing to Leave the Hospital

- Sources for follow-up care are identified. The hospital's financial interest in any referrals is disclosed.
- Hospital activities are coordinated with community caregivers. The hospital requests permission to share information.
- Information and training are given about self-care at home.

Help With Bills and Insurance Claims

- The hospital files insurance, Medicare, or Medicaid claims.
- Patients can contact the business office for questions about insurance coverage.
- The hospital tries to find financial help or make other arrangements if the person is without health coverage. The patient provides needed information to obtain coverage or assistance.

Modified from American Hospital Association: *The patient care partnership: understanding expectations, rights, and responsibilities*, Chicago, 2003.

Appendix B

National Nurse Aide Assessment Program (NNAAP®) Written Examination Content Outline

The NNAAP® written examination is comprised of 70 multiple-choice items; 10 of these items are pretest (non-scored) items on which statistical information will be collected.

I Physical Care Skills

A Activities of Daily Living   9 questions
  1 Hygiene
  2 Dressing and Grooming
  3 Nutrition and Hydration
  4 Elimination
  5 Rest/Sleep/Comfort

B Basic Nursing Skills   23 questions
  1 Infection Control
  2 Safety/Emergency
  3 Therapeutic and Technical Procedures
  4 Data Collection and Reporting

C Restorative Skills   5 questions
  1 Prevention
  2 Self Care/Independence

II Psychosocial Care Skills

A Emotional and Mental Health Needs   6 questions

B Spiritual and Cultural Needs   2 questions

III Role of the Nurse Aide

A Communication   4 questions
B Client Rights   4 questions
C Legal and Ethical Behavior   2 questions
D Member of the Health Care Team   5 questions

National Nurse Aide Assessment Program (NNAAP®) Skills Evaluation

List of Skills

1 Hand hygiene (hand washing)
2 Applies one knee-high elastic stocking
3 Assists to ambulate using transfer belt
4 Assists with use of bedpan
5 Cleans upper or lower denture
6 Counts and records radial pulse
7 Counts and records respirations
8 Donning and removing PPE (gown and gloves)
9 Dresses client with affected (weak) right arm
10 Feeds client who cannot feed self
11 Gives modified bed bath (face and one arm, hand, and underarm)
12 Measures and records electronic blood pressure (state specific)
13 Measures and records urinary output
14 Measures and records weight of ambulatory client
15 Performs modified passive range of motion (PROM) for one knee and one ankle
16 Performs modified passive range of motion (PROM) for one shoulder
17 Positions on side
18 Provides catheter care for female
19 Provides foot care on one foot
20 Provides mouth care
21 Provides perineal care (peri-care) for female
22 Transfers from bed to wheelchair using transfer belt
23 Measures and records manual blood pressure (state specific)

Appendix C

Minimum Data Set: Selected Pages

Resident _____ Identifier _____ Date _____

Section G	Functional Status

G0110. Activities of Daily Living (ADL) Assistance
Refer to the ADL flow chart in the RAI manual to facilitate accurate coding

Instructions for Rule of 3
- When an activity occurs three times at any one given level, code that level.
- When an activity occurs three times at multiple levels, code the most dependent, exceptions are total dependence (4), activity must require full assist every time, and activity did not occur (8), activity must not have occurred at all. Example, three times extensive assistance (3) and three times limited assistance (2), code extensive assistance (3).
- When an activity occurs at various levels, but not three times at any given level, apply the following:
  ○ When there is a combination of full staff performance, and extensive assistance, code extensive assistance.
  ○ When there is a combination of full staff performance, weight bearing assistance and/or non-weight bearing assistance code limited assistance (2).

If none of the above are met, code supervision.

1. ADL Self-Performance
Code for **resident's performance** over all shifts - not including setup. If the ADL activity occurred 3 or more times at various levels of assistance, code the most dependent - except for total dependence, which requires full staff performance every time

Coding:
Activity Occurred 3 or More Times
0. **Independent** - no help or staff oversight at any time
1. **Supervision** - oversight, encouragement or cueing
2. **Limited assistance** - resident highly involved in activity; staff provide guided maneuvering of limbs or other non-weight-bearing assistance
3. **Extensive assistance** - resident involved in activity, staff provide weight-bearing support
4. **Total dependence** - full staff performance every time during entire 7-day period

Activity Occurred 2 or Fewer Times
7. **Activity occurred only once or twice** - activity did occur but only once or twice
8. **Activity did not occur** - activity did not occur or family and/or non-facility staff provided care 100% of the time for that activity over the entire 7-day period

2. ADL Support Provided
Code for **most support provided** over all shifts; code regardless of resident's self-performance classification

Coding:
0. **No** setup or physical help from staff
1. **Setup** help only
2. **One** person physical assist
3. **Two+** persons physical assist
8. ADL activity itself **did not occur** or family and/or non-facility staff provided care 100% of the time for that activity over the entire 7-day period

	1. Self-Performance	2. Support
	↓ Enter Codes in Boxes ↓	
A. Bed mobility - how resident moves to and from lying position, turns side to side, and positions body while in bed or alternate sleep furniture	☐	☐
B. Transfer - how resident moves between surfaces including to or from: bed, chair, wheelchair, standing position (**excludes** to/from bath/toilet)	☐	☐
C. Walk in room - how resident walks between locations in his/her room	☐	☐
D. Walk in corridor - how resident walks in corridor on unit	☐	☐
E. Locomotion on unit - how resident moves between locations in his/her room and adjacent corridor on same floor. If in wheelchair, self-sufficiency once in chair	☐	☐
F. Locomotion off unit - how resident moves to and returns from off-unit locations (e.g., areas set aside for dining, activities or treatments). **If facility has only one floor**, how resident moves to and from distant areas on the floor. If in wheelchair, self-sufficiency once in chair	☐	☐
G. Dressing - how resident puts on, fastens and takes off all items of clothing, including donning/removing a prosthesis or TED hose. Dressing includes putting on and changing pajamas and housedresses	☐	☐
H. Eating - how resident eats and drinks, regardless of skill. Do not include eating/drinking during medication pass. Includes intake of nourishment by other means (e.g., tube feeding, total parenteral nutrition, IV fluids administered for nutrition or hydration)	☐	☐
I. Toilet use - how resident uses the toilet room, commode, bedpan, or urinal; transfers on/off toilet; cleanses self after elimination; changes pad; manages ostomy or catheter; and adjusts clothes. Do not include emptying of bedpan, urinal, bedside commode, catheter bag or ostomy bag	☐	☐
J. Personal hygiene - how resident maintains personal hygiene, including combing hair, brushing teeth, shaving, applying makeup, washing/drying face and hands (**excludes** baths and showers)	☐	☐

Resident _____ Identifier _____ Date _____

Section G	**Functional Status**

G0120. Bathing

How resident takes full-body bath/shower, sponge bath, and transfers in/out of tub/shower (**excludes** washing of back and hair). Code for **most dependent** in self-performance and support

Enter Code [ ]
A. Self-performance
0. **Independent** - no help provided
1. **Supervision** - oversight help only
2. **Physical help limited to transfer only**
3. **Physical help in part of bathing activity**
4. **Total dependence**
8. **Activity itself did not occur** or family and/or non-facility staff provided care 100% of the time for that activity over the entire 7-day period

Enter Code [ ]
B. Support provided
(Bathing support codes are as defined in item **G0110 column 2, ADL Support Provided**, above)

G0300. Balance During Transitions and Walking

After observing the resident, **code the following walking and transition items for most dependent**

Coding:
0. **Steady at all times**
1. **Not steady, but able to stabilize without staff assistance**
2. **Not steady, only able to stabilize with staff assistance**
8. **Activity did not occur**

↓ **Enter Codes in Boxes**

[ ] **A. Moving from seated to standing position**
[ ] **B. Walking** (with assistive device if used)
[ ] **C. Turning around** and facing the opposite direction while walking
[ ] **D. Moving on and off toilet**
[ ] **E. Surface-to-surface transfer** (transfer between bed and chair or wheelchair)

G0400. Functional Limitation in Range of Motion

Code for limitation that interfered with daily functions or placed resident at risk of injury

Coding:
0. **No impairment**
1. **Impairment on one side**
2. **Impairment on both sides**

↓ **Enter Codes in Boxes**

[ ] **A. Upper extremity** (shoulder, elbow, wrist, hand)
[ ] **B. Lower extremity** (hip, knee, ankle, foot)

G0600. Mobility Devices

↓ **Check all that were normally used**

[ ] **A. Cane/crutch**
[ ] **B. Walker**
[ ] **C. Wheelchair** (manual or electric)
[ ] **D. Limb prosthesis**
[ ] **Z. None of the above** were used

G0900. Functional Rehabilitation Potential
Complete only if A0310A = 01

Enter Code [ ]
A. Resident believes he or she is capable of increased independence in at least some ADLs
0. **No**
1. **Yes**
9. **Unable to determine**

Enter Code [ ]
B. Direct care staff believe resident is capable of increased independence in at least some ADLs
0. **No**
1. **Yes**

From Centers for Medicare & Medicaid Services: MDS 3.0, http://www.cms.gov/Medicare/Quality-Initiatives-Patient-Assessment-Instruments/NursingHomeQualityInits/MDS30RAIManual.html.

Glossary

A

abbreviation A shortened form of a word or phrase

abduction Moving a body part away from the mid-line of the body

abuse
- The willful infliction of injury, unreasonable confinement, intimidation, or punishment that results in physical harm, pain, or mental anguish
- Depriving the person (or the person's caregiver) of the goods or services needed to attain or maintain well-being

accountable To answer to one's self and others about one's choices, decisions, and actions

acetone See "ketone"

activities of daily living (ADL) The activities usually done during a normal day in a person's life

acute illness An illness of rapid onset and short duration; the person is expected to recover

acute pain Pain that is sharp or severe; felt suddenly from injury, disease, trauma, or surgery

addiction A chronic disease involving substance-seeking behaviors and use that is compulsive and hard to control despite the harmful effects

adduction Moving a body part toward the mid-line of the body

admission The official entry of a person into a health care setting

advance directive A document stating a person's wishes about health care when that person is unable to make decisions

advocate Someone who acts or speaks on behalf of another person

afebrile Without (*a*) a fever (*febrile*)

affected side The side of the body with weakness from illness or injury; weak side

alopecia Hair loss

ambulation The act of walking

anaphylaxis A life-threatening sensitivity to an antigen

anorexia The loss of appetite

antibiotic A drug that kills bacteria

anxiety A feeling of worry, nervousness, or fear about an event or situation

aphasia The total or partial loss (*a*) of the ability to use or understand language (*phasia*)

apnea The lack or absence (*a*) of breathing (*pnea*)

artery A blood vessel that carries blood away from the heart

arthritis Joint (*arthr*) inflammation (*itis*)

arthroplasty The surgical replacement (*plasty*) of a joint (*arthro*)

asepsis The absence (*a*) of disease-producing microbes (*sepsis* means *infection*)

aspiration Breathing fluid, food, vomitus, or an object into the lungs

assault Intentionally attempting or threatening to touch a person's body without the person's consent

assessment Collecting information about the person; see "nursing process"

assisted living residence (ALR) Provides housing, personal care, support services, health care, and social activities in a home-like setting to persons needing some help with daily activities

atrophy The decrease in size or wasting away of tissue

autopsy The examination of the body after death

B

base of support The area on which an object rests

bath blanket A covering used for privacy and warmth during bathing, hygiene, and other care measures

battery Touching a person's body without consent

bed mobility How a person moves to and from a lying position, turns from side to side, and re-positions in a bed or other sleeping furniture

bed rail A device that serves as a guard or barrier along the side of the bed; side rail

bed rest Restricting a person to bed and limiting activity for health reasons

benign tumor A tumor that does not spread to other body parts

biohazardous waste Items contaminated with blood or other potentially infectious materials (OPIM); regulated medical waste, infectious waste

blindness The absence of sight

bloodborne pathogens Microbes that are present in blood and can cause infection

blood pressure (BP) The amount of force exerted against the walls of an artery by the blood

body alignment The way the head, trunk, arms, and legs align with one another; posture

body language Messages sent through facial expressions, gestures, posture, hand and body movements, gait, eye contact, and appearance

body mechanics Using the body in an efficient and careful way

body temperature The amount of heat in the body that is a balance between the amount of heat produced and the amount lost by the body

bony prominence An area where the bone sticks out or projects from the flat surface of the body; pressure point

boundary crossing
- A brief act or behavior of being over-involved with the person
- The intent of the act or behavior is to meet the person's needs

boundary sign An act, behavior, or thought that warns of a boundary crossing or boundary violation

boundary violation An act or behavior that meets your needs, not the person's

bradycardia A slow (*brady*) heart rate (*cardia*); less than 60 beats per minute

bradypnea Slow (*brady*) breathing (*pnea*); respirations are fewer than 12 per minute

braille A touch reading and writing system that uses raised dots for each letter of the alphabet; the first 10 letters also represent the numbers 0 through 9

bullying Repeated attacks or threats of fear, distress, or harm by a bully toward a target

burnout A job stress resulting in being physically or mentally exhausted, having doubts about your abilities, and having doubts about the value of your work

C

calorie The fuel or energy value of food

cancer See "malignant tumor"

capillary A very tiny blood vessel; nutrients, oxygen, and other substances pass from capillaries into the cells

cardiac arrest See "sudden cardiac arrest"

cardiopulmonary resuscitation (CPR) An emergency procedure performed when the heart and breathing stop

carrier A human or animal that is a reservoir for microbes but does not develop the infection

catheter A tube used to drain or inject fluid through a body opening

catheterization The process of inserting a catheter

cell The basic unit of body structure

certification Official recognition by a state that standards or requirements have been met

chart See "medical record"

chemical restraint Any drug used for discipline or convenience and not required to treat medical symptoms

Cheyne-Stokes respirations Respirations gradually increase in rate and depth and then become shallow and slow; breathing may stop (*apnea*) for 10 to 20 seconds

child abuse and neglect The intentional harm or mistreatment of a child under 18 years old that:
- Involves any recent act or failure to act on the part of a parent or caregiver
- Results in death, serious physical or emotional harm, sexual abuse, or exploitation
- Presents a likely or immediate risk for harm

cholesterol A soft, waxy substance found in the bloodstream and all body cells

chronic illness A long-term health condition that may not have a cure; it can be controlled and complications prevented with proper treatment

chronic pain Pain that continues for a long time (longer than 12 weeks, occurs off and on, or is persistent [constant])

circumcised The fold of skin (foreskin) covering the glans of the penis was surgically removed

civil law Laws concerned with relationships between people

clean technique See "medical asepsis"

cognitive function Involves memory, thinking, reasoning, ability to understand, judgment, and behavior

colostomy A surgically created opening (*stomy*) between the colon (*colo*) and the body's surface

coma A prolonged state of unconsciousness

comatose Being unable to respond to stimuli; unconscious

comfort A state of well-being; the person has no physical or emotional pain and is calm and at ease

communicable disease A disease caused by a pathogen that can spread to others; contagious disease

communication The exchange of information—a message sent is received and correctly interpreted by the intended person

compulsion An over-whelming urge to repeat certain rituals, acts, or behaviors

condom catheter A soft sheath that slides over the penis and is used to drain urine

confidentiality Trusting others with personal and private information

confusion A state of being disoriented to person, time, place, situation, or identity

constipation The passage of a hard, dry stool

constrict To narrow

contagious disease See "communicable disease"

contamination The process of becoming unclean

contracture Decreased motion and stiffness of a joint caused by shortening (*contracting*) of a muscle

convulsion See "seizure"

coping Strategies to manage stress and reduce negative emotions caused by stress

crime An act that violates a criminal law

criminal law Laws concerned with offenses against the public and society in general

cross-contamination Passing microbes from 1 person to another by contaminated hands, equipment, or supplies

culture The characteristics of a group of people—language, values, beliefs, habits, likes, dislikes, customs—passed from 1 generation to the next

cyanosis Bluish color (*cyano*) to the skin, lips, mucous membranes, and nail beds

D

dandruff Excessive amounts of dry, white flakes from the scalp

deafness Hearing loss in which it is impossible for the person to understand speech through hearing alone

deconditioning The loss of muscle strength from inactivity

defamation Injuring a person's name and reputation by making false statements to a third person

defecation The process of excreting feces from the rectum through the anus; bowel movement

defense mechanism An unconscious reaction that blocks unpleasant or threatening feelings

dehydration A decrease in the amount of water in the body

delegate To authorize or direct a nursing assistant to perform a nursing task

delegation The process a nurse uses to direct a nursing assistant to perform a nursing task; allowing a nursing assistant to perform a nursing task that is beyond the nursing assistant's usual role and not routinely done by the nursing assistant

delirium A state of sudden, severe confusion and rapid changes in brain function

delusion A false belief

delusion of grandeur An exaggerated belief about one's importance, fame, wealth, power, or talents

delusion of persecution A false belief that one is being mistreated, abused, or harassed

dementia The loss of cognitive and social function caused by changes in the brain; the loss of cognitive function that interferes with daily life and activities

denture A removable replacement for missing teeth

detoxification The process of removing a toxic substance from the body

development Changes in mental, emotional, and social function

developmental task A skill that must be completed during a stage of development for development to continue

diarrhea The frequent passage of liquid stools

diastolic pressure The pressure in the arteries when the heart is at rest

digestion The process that breaks down food physically and chemically so it can be absorbed for use by the cells

dilate To expand or open wider

disability Any lost, absent, or impaired physical or mental function

disaster A harmful event that can affect the agency, patient or resident population, community, or larger geographic area

discharge The official departure of a person from a health care setting

discomfort See "pain"

discrimination Unjust treatment based on personal qualities

disinfection The process of killing pathogens

dorsal recumbent position The back-lying or supine position

dorsiflexion Bending the toes and foot up at the ankle

drawsheet A small sheet placed over the middle of the bottom sheet to keep the mattress and bottom linens clean

dysphagia Difficulty (*dys*) swallowing (*phagia*)

dyspnea Difficult, labored, or painful (*dys*) breathing (*pnea*)

dysuria Painful or difficult (*dys*) urination (*uria*); burning on urination

E

edema The swelling of body tissues with water

elder abuse Any knowing, intentional, or negligent act by a caregiver or any other person to an older adult that causes harm or serious risk of harm

electronic health record (EHR) An electronic version of a person's medical record; electronic medical record

electronic medical record (EMR) See "electronic health record"

elopement When a patient or resident leaves the agency without staff knowledge

emesis See "vomitus"

enabler A device that limits freedom of movement but is used to promote independence, comfort, or safety

end-of-life care The support and care given during the time surrounding death

end-of-shift report A report that the nurse gives at the end of the shift to the on-coming shift; change-of-shift report

endorsement A state recognizes the certificate, license, or registration issued by another state; reciprocity or equivalency

enema The introduction of fluid into the rectum and lower colon

enteral nutrition Giving nutrients into the gastro-intestinal (GI) tract (*enteral*) through a feeding tube

entrapment Getting caught, trapped, or entangled in spaces created by the bed rails, the mattress, the bed frame, the head-board, or the foot-board

equivalency See "endorsement"

ergonomics The science of designing a job to fit the worker; *ergo* means *work*, *nomos* means *law*

esteem The worth, value, or opinion one has of a person

ethics Knowledge of what is right conduct and wrong conduct

evaluation To measure if goals in the planning step were met; see "nursing process"

extension Straightening a body part

external rotation Turning the joint outward

F

fainting The sudden loss of consciousness from an inadequate blood supply to the brain; syncope

false imprisonment Unlawful restraint or restriction of a person's freedom of movement

febrile With a fever

fecal impaction The prolonged retention and buildup of feces in the rectum

fecal incontinence The inability to control the passage of feces and flatus through the anus

feces The semi-solid mass of waste products in the colon that is expelled through the anus; stool or stools

fever Elevated body temperature

first aid The emergency care given to an ill or injured person before medical help arrives

flashback Reliving a trauma over and over in thoughts during the day and in nightmares during sleep

flatulence The excessive formation of gas or air in the stomach and intestines

flatus Gas or air passed through the anus

flexion Bending a body part

flow rate The number of drops per minute (gtt/min) or milliliters per hour (mL/hr)

footdrop The foot falls down at the ankle; permanent plantar flexion

Fowler's position A semi-sitting position; the head of the bed is raised between 45 and 60 degrees

fracture A broken bone

fraud Saying or doing something to trick, fool, or deceive a person

friction The rubbing of 1 surface against another

full visual privacy Having the means to be completely free from public view while in bed

functional incontinence The person has bladder control but cannot use the toilet in time

G

gait belt See "transfer belt"

garment An item of clothing

gavage The process of giving a tube feeding

gender identity A person's sense or feelings of being male, female, a combination of male and female, or neither male nor female

geriatrics The care of aging people

gerontology The study of the aging process

glucometer A device for measuring (*meter*) blood glucose (*gluco*); glucose meter

glucosuria Sugar (*glucose*) in the urine (*uria*)

gossip To spread rumors or talk about the private matters of others

graduate A measuring container for fluid

growth The physical changes that are measured and that occur in a steady, orderly manner

H

hallucination Seeing, hearing, smelling, feeling, or tasting something that is not real

harassment To trouble, torment, offend, or worry a person by one's behavior or comments

hazard Anything in the person's setting that could cause injury or illness

hazardous chemical Any chemical that is a physical hazard or a health hazard

healthcare-associated infection (HAI) An infection that develops in a person cared for in any setting where health care is given; the infection is related to receiving health care

health team The many health care workers whose skills and knowledge focus on the person's total care; interdisciplinary health care team

hearing loss Not being able to hear the range of sounds associated with normal hearing

hematuria Blood (*hemat*) in the urine (*uria*)

hemiplegia Paralysis (*plegia*) on 1 side (*hemi*) of the body

hemoglobin The substance in red blood cells that carries oxygen and gives blood its red color

hemoptysis Bloody (*hemo*) sputum (*ptysis* means *to spit*)

hemorrhage The excessive loss (*rrhage*) of blood (*hemo*) in a short time

high-Fowler's position A variation of Fowler's position; the head of the bed is raised 60 to 90 degrees

hirsutism Excessive body hair

holism A concept that considers the whole person; the whole person has physical, psychological, social, and spiritual parts that are woven together and cannot be separated

hormone A chemical substance secreted by the endocrine glands into the bloodstream

hospice A health care agency or program that promotes comfort and quality of life for the dying person and the person's family

hygiene The cleanliness practices that promote health and prevent disease

hyperextension Excessive straightening of a body part

hyperglycemia High (*hyper*) sugar (*glyc*) in the blood (*emia*)

hypertension High blood pressure

hyperventilation Breathing (*ventilation*) is rapid (*hyper*) and deeper than normal

hypoglycemia Low (*hypo*) sugar (*glyc*) in the blood (*emia*)

hypotension Low blood pressure

hypoventilation Breathing (*ventilation*) is slow (*hypo*), shallow, and sometimes irregular

hypoxia Cells do not have enough (*hypo*) oxygen (*oxia*)

I

ileostomy A surgically created opening (*stomy*) between the ileum (small intestine [*ileo*]) and the body's surface

immobility The inability to move

immunity Protection against a disease or condition; the person will not get or be affected by the disease

implementation To perform or carry out nursing interventions (nursing measures, nursing actions, nursing tasks) in the care plan; see "nursing process"

incident Any event that has harmed or could harm a patient, resident, visitor, or staff member

indwelling catheter A catheter left in the bladder so urine drains constantly into a drainage bag; retention or Foley catheter

infection A disease state resulting from the invasion and growth of microbes in the body

infection control Practices and procedures that prevent the spread of infection

informed consent The process by which a person receives and understands information about a treatment or procedure and is able to decide to receive or refuse the treatment or procedure

insomnia A chronic condition in which the person cannot sleep or stay asleep all night

intact skin Normal skin and skin layers without damage or breaks

intake The amount of fluid taken in; input

internal rotation Turning the joint inward

intimate partner violence (IPV) Physical violence, sexual violence, stalking, or psychological aggression by a current or former partner

intravenous (IV) therapy Giving fluids through a tube inserted into a vein; IV and IV infusion

invasion of privacy Violating a person's right not to have his or her name, photo, or private affairs exposed or made public without giving consent

involuntary seclusion Separating a person from others against the person's will, keeping the person to a certain area, or keeping the person away from his or her room without consent

J

job application An agency's official form listing questions that require factual answers from the person seeking employment; employment form

job description A document that describes what the agency expects you to do

job interview When an employer asks a job applicant questions about the applicant's education and career

joint The point at which 2 or more bones meet to allow movement

K

ketone A substance appearing in urine from the rapid breakdown of fat for energy; acetone, ketone body

ketone body See "ketone"

Kussmaul respirations Very deep and rapid respirations

L

lateral position The person lies on 1 side or the other; side-lying position

lateral transfer When a person moves between 2 horizontal surfaces

law A rule of conduct made by a government body

left semi-prone position The person lies on the left side of the abdomen; the upper leg (right leg) is sharply flexed (bent) so it is not on the lower leg (left leg); the lower arm (left arm) is behind the person

libel Making false statements in print, in writing (including e-mail and text messages), through pictures or drawings, through broadcast (radio, TV, or video), posted on-line on websites, or through video sites and social media sites

lice See "pediculosis"

licensed practical nurse (LPN) A nurse who has completed a practical nursing program and has passed a licensing test; called *licensed vocational nurse (LVN)* in California and Texas

licensed vocational nurse (LVN) See "licensed practical nurse (LPN)"

logrolling Turning the person as a unit, in alignment, with 1 motion

low vision Vision loss that cannot be corrected with eyeglasses, contact lenses, drugs, or surgery; vision loss interferes with every-day activities

M

malignant tumor A tumor that invades and destroys nearby tissues and can spread to other body parts; cancer

malpractice Negligence by a professional person

medical asepsis Practices used to reduce the number of microbes and prevent their spread from 1 person or place to another person or place; clean technique

medical record The legal account of a person's condition and response to treatment and care; chart

melena A black, tarry stool

menopause The time when menstruation stops and menstrual cycles end; there has been at least 1 year without a menstrual period

menstruation The process in which the lining of the uterus (endometrium) breaks up and is discharged from the body through the vagina

mental health Involves a person's emotional, psychological, and social well-being

mental health disorder A serious illness that can affect a person's thinking, mood, behavior, function, and ability to relate to others; psychiatric disorder

metabolism How the body uses nutrients to provide energy and maintain body functions

metastasis The spread of cancer to other body parts

microbe See "microorganism"

microorganism A small (*micro*) living thing (*organism*) seen only with a microscope; microbe

mixed incontinence The combination of stress incontinence and urge incontinence

mobility A person's ability to move

musculo-skeletal disorders (MSDs) Injuries and disorders of the muscles, tendons, ligaments, joints, and cartilage

N

need Something necessary or desired for maintaining life and mental well-being

neglect When a caregiver or responsible person fails to:
- Protect a vulnerable person from harm
- Provide food, water, clothing, shelter, health care, or basic activities of daily living to a vulnerable person

negligence An unintentional wrong in which a person did not act in a reasonable and careful manner and a person or the person's property was harmed

nocturia Frequent urination (*uria*) at night (*noc*)

non-pathogen A microbe that does not usually cause an infection

nonverbal communication Communication that does not use words

normal flora Microbes that live and grow in a certain area

nursing assistant A person who has passed a nursing assistant training and competency evaluation program (NATCEP); performs delegated nursing tasks under the supervision of a licensed nurse

nursing care plan A written guide about the person's nursing care; care plan

nursing diagnosis A health problem that can be treated by nursing measures; see "nursing process"

nursing intervention An action or measure taken by the nursing team to help the person reach a goal; nursing action, nursing measure, nursing task

nursing process The method nurses use to plan and deliver nursing care; its 5 steps are assessment, nursing diagnosis, planning, implementation, and evaluation

nursing task Nursing care or a nursing function, procedure, skill, or activity

nursing team Those who provide nursing care—RNs, LPNs/LVNs, and nursing assistants

nutrient A substance that is ingested, digested, absorbed, and used by the body

nutrition The processes involved in the ingestion, digestion, absorption, and use of food and fluids by the body

O

objective data Information that is seen, heard, felt, or smelled by an observer; signs

observation Using the senses of sight, hearing, touch, and smell to collect information

obsession A frequent, upsetting, and unwanted thought, idea, or image

occupied In use

oliguria Scant amount (*olig*) of urine (*uria*); less than 500 mL in 24 hours

ombudsman Someone who supports or promotes the needs and interests of another person

opposition Touching an opposite finger with the thumb

oral hygiene The practices that promote healthy tissues and structures of the mouth; mouth care

organ Groups of tissue that function together

orthopnea Breathing (*pnea*) deeply and comfortably only when sitting (*ortho*)

orthopneic position Sitting up (*ortho*) and leaning over a table to breathe (*pneic*)

orthotic A device used to support a muscle, promote a certain motion, or correct a deformity; *ortho* means *to straighten*

ostomy A surgically created opening that connects an internal organ to the body's surface; see "colostomy" and "ileostomy"

output The amount of fluid lost

over-flow incontinence Small amounts of urine leak from a full bladder

oxygen concentration The amount (percent [%]) of hemoglobin containing oxygen

P

pain To ache, hurt, or be sore; discomfort

palliative care Care that relieves or reduces the intensity of uncomfortable symptoms without producing a cure

panic An intense and sudden feeling of fear, anxiety, or dread

paralysis Loss of muscle function

paranoia A disorder (*para*) of the mind (*noia*); false beliefs (delusions) and suspicion about a person or situation

paraphrasing Re-stating the person's message in your own words

paraplegia Paralysis in the legs and lower trunk

pathogen A microbe that is harmful and can cause an infection

pediculosis Infestation with wingless insects that feed on blood; lice

pericare See "perineal care"

perineal care Cleaning the genital and anal areas; pericare

peristalsis Involuntary muscle contractions in the digestive system that move food down the esophagus through the alimentary canal

personality The set of attitudes, values, behaviors, and traits of a person

personal protective equipment (PPE) The clothing or equipment worn by staff for protection against a hazard

person's unit The space, furniture, and equipment used by the person in the agency

phobia An intense fear of something that has little or no real danger

physical restraint Any manual method or physical or mechanical device, material, or equipment that:
- Is attached to or near the person's body
- Cannot be removed easily by the person
- Restricts freedom of movement or normal access to the body

pivot To turn one's body from a set standing position

planning Setting priorities and goals; see "nursing process"

plantar flexion Bending the foot down at the ankle

pneumonia Inflammation and infection of lung tissue

poison Any substance harmful to the body when ingested, inhaled, injected, or absorbed through the skin

polyuria Abnormally large amounts (*poly*) of urine (*uria*)

position change alarm Any physical or electronic device that monitors a person's movement and alerts staff of movement

post-mortem care Care of the body after (*post*) death (*mortem*)

postural hypotension Abnormally low (*hypo*) blood pressure when the person suddenly stands up (*postural*); orthostatic hypotension

posture See "body alignment"

prefix A word element at the beginning of a word; it changes the meaning of the word

pressure injury Localized damage to the skin and underlying soft tissue; the injury is usually over a bony prominence or related to a medical or other device and results from pressure or pressure in combination with shear

pressure point See "bony prominence"

priority The most important thing at the time

professional boundary That which separates helpful actions and behaviors from those that are not helpful

professionalism Following laws, being ethical, having good work ethics, and having the skills to do your work

professional sexual misconduct A violation of professional interactions with an act, behavior, or comment that is sexual in nature

pronation Turning the joint downward

prone position The person lies on the abdomen with the head turned to 1 side

prosthesis An artificial replacement for a missing body part

protected health information Identifying information and information about the person's health care that is maintained or sent in any form (paper, electronic, oral)

psychosis A condition that affects the mind and causes a loss of contact with reality

pulse The beat of the heart felt at an artery as a wave of blood passes through the artery

pulse oximetry Measures *(metry)* the oxygen *(oxi)* concentration in arterial blood

pulse rate The number of heartbeats or pulses in 1 minute

Q

quadriplegia Paralysis in the arms, legs, and trunk; tetraplegia

R

range of motion (ROM) The movement of a joint to the extent possible without causing pain

reasonable accommodation To assist or change a position or workplace to allow an employee to do a job despite having a disability

reciprocity See "endorsement"

recording The written account of care and observations; charting, documentation

reflex The body's response (function or movement) to a stimulus

reflex incontinence Urine is lost at predictable intervals when a specific amount of urine is in the bladder

registered nurse (RN) A nurse who has completed a 2-, 3-, or 4-year nursing program and has passed a licensing test

regulations Rules made by government agencies

regurgitation The backward flow of stomach contents into the mouth

rehabilitation The process of restoring a person's highest possible level of physical, psychological, social, and economic function

religion Spiritual beliefs, needs, and practices

reporting The oral account of care and observations

representative Someone with the legal right to act on the patient's or resident's behalf when the person cannot do so alone

respiration The process of supplying cells with oxygen and removing carbon dioxide from them; breathing air into (inhalation) and out of (exhalation) the lungs

respiratory arrest Breathing stops but heart action continues for several minutes

rest To be calm, at ease, and relaxed with no anxiety or stress

restorative aide A nursing assistant with special training in restorative nursing and rehabilitation skills

restorative nursing care Care that helps persons regain health and strength for safe and independent living

resuscitate To revive from apparent death or unconsciousness using emergency measures

rigor mortis The stiffness or rigidity *(rigor)* of skeletal muscles that occurs after death *(mortis)*

risk factor Something that increases the chance of illness or injury

root A word element that contains the basic meaning of the word

rotation Turning the joint

S

scabies A skin disorder caused by a female mite

seizure Violent and sudden contractions or tremors of muscle groups caused by abnormal electrical activity in the brain; convulsion

self-esteem Thinking well of oneself and seeing oneself as useful and having value

self-neglect A person's behaviors and way of living that threaten the person's own health, safety, and well-being

semi-Fowler's position A variation of Fowler's position; the head of the bed is raised 30 degrees

sexuality The physical, emotional, social, cultural, and spiritual factors that affect a person's feelings, attitudes, and behaviors about one's gender identity and sexual behavior

shear When layers of the skin rub against each other; when the skin remains in place and underlying tissues move and stretch, tearing underlying capillaries and blood vessels and causing tissue damage

shearing When the skin sticks to a surface while muscles slide in the direction the body is moving

shock Results when tissues and organs do not get enough blood

side-lying position See "lateral position"

signs See "objective data"

skin tear A break or rip in the outer layers of the skin; the epidermis (top skin layer) separates from the underlying tissues

slander Making false statements through the spoken word, sounds, sign language, or gestures

sleep apnea Pauses *(a)* in breathing *(pnea)* that occur during sleep

sleep deprivation The amount and quality of sleep are not adequate, causing reduced function and alertness

sleepwalking When the person leaves the bed and walks about while sleeping

sputum Mucus from the respiratory system that is expectorated (expelled) through the mouth

standard of care The skills, care, and judgments required by a health team member under similar conditions

sterile The absence of *all* microbes

sterile technique See "surgical asepsis"

sterilization The process of destroying *all* microbes

stethoscope An instrument used to listen to the sounds produced by the heart, lungs, and other body organs

stimulus Anything that excites or causes a body part to function, become active, or respond

stoma A surgically created opening seen on the body's surface; see "colostomy" and "ileostomy"

stool Excreted feces; stools

straight catheter A catheter that drains the bladder and then is removed

stress The response or change in the body caused by any emotional, psychological, physical, social, or economic factor

stress incontinence When urine leaks during exercise and certain movements that cause pressure on the bladder

stressor The event or factor that causes stress

subjective data Things a person tells you about that you cannot observe through your senses; symptoms

sudden cardiac arrest (SCA) The heart stops suddenly and without warning; cardiac arrest

suffix A word element at the end of a word; it changes the meaning of the word

suffocation When breathing stops from the lack of oxygen; asphyxia

suicide To end one's life on purpose

suicide contagion Exposure to suicide or suicidal behaviors within one's family, one's peer group, or through media reports of suicide

sundowning Signs, symptoms, and behaviors of dementia increase during hours of darkness

supination Turning the joint upward

supine position The back-lying or dorsal recumbent position

suppository A cone-shaped, solid drug that is inserted into a body opening; it melts at body temperature

surgical asepsis Practices used to remove *all* microbes; sterile technique

survey The formal review of an agency through the collection of facts and observations

surveyor A person who collects information by observing and asking questions

symptoms See "subjective data"

system Organs that work together to perform special functions

systolic pressure The pressure in the arteries when the heart contracts

T

tachycardia A rapid *(tachy)* heart rate *(cardia)*; more than 100 beats per minute

tachypnea Rapid *(tachy)* breathing *(pnea)*; respirations are more than 20 per minute

teamwork Staff members work together as a group; everyone does their part to give safe and effective care

terminal illness An illness or injury from which the person will not likely recover

thermometer A device used to measure *(meter)* temperature *(thermo)*

tinnitus A ringing, roaring, hissing, or buzzing sound in the ears or head

tissue A group of cells with similar functions

transfer How a person moves to and from a surface

transfer belt A device applied around the waist and used to support a person who is unsteady or disabled; gait belt

transient incontinence Temporary or occasional incontinence that is reversed when the cause is treated

treatment The care provided to maintain or restore health, improve function, or relieve symptoms

tumor A new growth of abnormal cells that is benign or malignant

U

ulcer A shallow or deep crater-like sore of the skin or mucous membrane

unaffected side The side of the body opposite the affected side; strong side

uncircumcised Foreskin covers the head of the penis

unconscious Being unaware of one's setting and being unable to react or respond to people, places, or things

under-garment An item of clothing worn next to the skin under clothing

urge incontinence The loss of urine in response to a sudden, urgent need to void; the person cannot get to a toilet in time

urinary frequency Voiding at frequent intervals

urinary incontinence (UI) The involuntary loss or leakage of urine

urinary retention Not being able to completely empty the bladder

urinary urgency The need to void at once

urination The process of emptying urine from the bladder; voiding

V

vein A blood vessel that returns blood to the heart

verbal communication Communication that uses written or spoken words

vertigo Dizziness

vital signs Temperature, pulse, respirations, and blood pressure; pulse oximetry and pain are included in some agencies

voiding See "urination"

vomitus The food and fluids expelled from the stomach through the mouth; emesis

vulnerable adult A person 18 years old or older who has a disability or condition that causes the person to be at risk for harm

W

waterproof under-pad An absorbent pad with a quilted top layer and a waterproof bottom layer

withdrawal syndrome The physical and mental response after stopping or severely reducing the use of a substance that was used regularly

word element A part of a word

work ethics Behavior in the workplace

workplace violence Violent acts (including assault or threat of assault) directed toward persons at work or while on duty

wound A break in the skin or mucous membrane

Key Abbreviations

AD	Alzheimer's disease
ADA	American Dental Association
ADL	Activities of daily living
AE	Anti-embolism; anti-embolic
AED	Automated external defibrillator
AFO	Ankle-foot orthosis
AIDS	Acquired immunodeficiency syndrome
ALR	Assisted living residence
ALS	Amyotrophic lateral sclerosis
AMD	Age-related macular degeneration
ANA	American Nurses Association
APRN	Advanced practice registered nurse
ASL	American Sign Language
BM	Bowel movement
BON	Board of nursing
BP	Blood pressure
BPD	Borderline personality disorder
BPH	Benign prostatic hyperplasia
C	Centigrade
CAD	Coronary artery disease
CAUTI	Catheter-associated urinary tract infection
CDC	Centers for Disease Control and Prevention
C. diff	*Clostridioides difficile; Clostridium difficile*
CKD	Chronic kidney disease
CMS	Centers for Medicare & Medicaid Services
CNS	Central nervous system
CO_2	Carbon dioxide
COPD	Chronic obstructive pulmonary disease
CPAP	Continuous positive airway pressure
CPR	Cardiopulmonary resuscitation
CVA	Cerebrovascular accident
DNR	Do Not Resuscitate
DON	Director of nursing
E. coli	*Escherichia coli*
EEOC	Equal Employment Opportunity Commission
EHR	Electronic health record
EMR	Electronic medical record
EMS	Emergency Medical Services
EPHI; ePHI	Electronic protected health information
ESRD	End-stage renal disease
F	Fahrenheit
FBAO	Foreign-body airway obstruction
FDA	Food and Drug Administration

GAD	Generalized anxiety disorder
GI	Gastro-intestinal
gtt	Drops
gtt/min	Drops per minute
HAI	Healthcare-associated infection
HBV	Hepatitis B virus
Hg	Mercury
HHS	U.S. Department of Health & Human Services
HIPAA	Health Insurance Portability and Accountability Act of 1996
HIV	Human immunodeficiency virus
IBD	Inflammatory bowel disease
ID	Identification
I&O	Intake and output
IPV	Intimate partner violence
IV	Intravenous
L/min	Liters per minute
LPN	Licensed practical nurse
LVN	Licensed vocational nurse
MDRO	Multidrug-resistant organism
MDS	Minimum Data Set
mg	Milligram
MI	Myocardial infarction
mL	Milliliter
mL/hr	Milliliters per hour
mm	Millimeter
mm Hg	Millimeters of mercury
MRSA	Methicillin-resistant *Staphylococcus aureus*
MS	Multiple sclerosis
MSD	Musculo-skeletal disorder
NATCEP	Nursing assistant training and competency evaluation program
NCSBN	National Council of State Boards of Nursing
NG	Naso-gastric
NIA	National Institute on Aging
NPIAP	National Pressure Injury Advisory Panel
NPO	Nothing by mouth
O_2	Oxygen
OBRA	Omnibus Budget Reconciliation Act of 1987
OCD	Obsessive-compulsive disorder
OPIM	Other potentially infectious materials
OSHA	Occupational Safety and Health Administration
oz	Ounce

PASS	*Pull* the safety pin, *aim* low, *squeeze* the lever, *sweep* back and forth	**TB**	Tuberculosis
PHI	Protected health information	**TIA**	Transient ischemic attack
PNS	Peripheral nervous system	**TJC**	The Joint Commission
PPE	Personal protective equipment	**TPR**	Temperature, pulse, and respirations
PROM	Passive range of motion		
PTSD	Post-traumatic stress disorder	**U/A; UA**	Urinalysis
		UI	Urinary incontinence
RA	Rheumatoid arthritis	**USDA**	United States Department of Agriculture
RACE	Rescue, alarm, confine, extinguish	**UTI**	Urinary tract infection
RBC	Red blood cell		
RN	Registered nurse	**VF; V-fib**	Ventricular fibrillation
ROM	Range of motion; range-of-motion	**VRE**	Vancomycin-resistant *Enterococci*
RRS	Rapid Response System		
		WBC	White blood cell
SCA	Sudden cardiac arrest	**WHO**	World Health Organization
SDS	Safety data sheet		
SNF	Skilled nursing facility		
SpO$_2$	Saturation of peripheral oxygen (oxygen concentration)		
STD	Sexually transmitted disease		
STI	Sexually transmitted infection		

Index

A

Abandonment, 36
Abbreviations, 78, 84, 85t
Abdominal binder, 456, 456f
Abdominal quadrants, 83–84, 83f
Abdominal thrusts, for choking, 121, 122b, 123f
Abduction, 412, 414b
Abuse, 30–31
  child, 37, 38t
  elder, 36–37
  freedom from, 13
  physical, 36, 37b
  reporting, 35–39, 35b–36b
  sexual, 115
  vulnerable adult, 31, 36, 36b
Accidents
  choking, 121–122, 121f–123f, 121b–122b
  equipment, 124–125, 124f, 124b
  reporting of, 130
  risk factors for, 118
Accountable, definition of, 18
Acetone. See Ketone
Acoustic nerve, 97, 97f
Acquired immunodeficiency syndrome
  (AIDS), 525–526, 525b
ACTH. See Adrenocorticotropic hormone
Activities director, 4t
Activities of daily living (ADL), 486–487
Activity needs, 412–424, 412b, 423b–424b
Acute care agencies, 2
Acute illness, 1–2
Acute pain, 425, 427
Acute problem, 486
AD. See Alzheimer's disease
Adaptive (assistive) devices, for hygiene, 272f
Addiction, 535, 535b
  definition of, 529
Adduction, 412, 414b
ADEAR. See Alzheimer's Disease Education
  and Referral Center
Adenoids, 100
ADH. See Antidiuretic hormone
ADL. See Activities of daily living
Administrator, 3
Admission, 1, 232
  information, 65
Adrenal gland, 105f, 105t
Adrenocorticotropic hormone (ACTH), 105t
Advance directives, 12, 573, 573b
  definition of, 569
Advocate, 10
AE. See Anti-embolism
Afebrile, 388
Affected side, definition of, 304–305
AFO. See Ankle-foot orthosis
Age
  accidents and, 118
  as factors affecting eating and nutrition,
    366
  sleep and, 431
Age-related macular degeneration (AMD),
  497, 497f
Agencies, types of, 2–3
Aggressive behavior, 60, 118, 547b–548b
Aging
  Alzheimer's disease and, 542b
  nervous system changes from, 539b
  physical changes caused by, 110, 111t–113t
  social changes caused by, 110, 110f, 110b

Agitated behavior, 118
Agitation, 148, 545, 547b–548b
Agonal gasps, 562
AIDS. See Acquired immunodeficiency
  syndrome
AIIR. See Airborne infection isolation room
Air flotation bed, 472, 472f
Airborne infection isolation room (AIIR), 178b
Airborne precautions, 178b
Airway management, 559, 559f
Airway obstruction, 121
Alcohol, 43
Alcohol-based hand rub, 167f, 167b
Alcoholism, 535
Alimentary canal, 101
Alopecia, 291–292
ALR. See Assisted living residence
ALS. See Amyotrophic lateral sclerosis
Alveoli, 100
Alzheimer's disease (AD), 541–547, 541f,
  548f–549f, 551f, 551b
  aggression, 545
  aging and, 542b
  agitation, 545
  behavior and function changes with,
    543–547, 543b
  care of persons with, 547–553, 547b–550b
  catastrophic reactions, 545, 547b–548b
  communication changes, 545–546,
    545b–546b
  delusions, 544, 547b–548b
  family caregivers, 551–552, 552b
  getting lost, 544, 544f, 544b
  hallucinations, 544
  hygiene and grooming, 549b–550b
  intimacy, 547
  onset, 541
  paranoia, 545, 545b, 547b–548b
  repetitive behaviors, 546, 547b–548b
  rummaging, 546, 547b–548b
  screaming, 546, 546b
  sexuality, 547
  signs of, 542, 542b
  stages of, 542, 543f, 543b
  sundowning, 544, 547b–548b
  validation therapy for, 552–553
  wandering, 544, 544f, 544b, 547b–548b
Alzheimer's Disease Education and Referral
  Center (ADEAR), 56b
Ambulation, 421–424, 421f, 421b–423b
  definition of, 412, 421
  helping with, 422b
AMD. See Age-related macular degeneration
American Sign Language, 494f
Amputation, 510
Amputee sling, 225
Amyotrophic lateral sclerosis (ALS), 513
Anal sphincter, 94
Anaphylactic shock, 564
Anaphylaxis, 564
  definition of, 555
Aneroid manometer, 402, 402f
Anger, 60
Angina, 515–516, 515f
Ankle, exercise for, 415b–416b, 417f
Ankle-foot orthosis (AFO), 418t–419t
Anorexia, 365–366
Anorexia nervosa, 536
Anterior, term, 84
Anti-embolism (AE), 450
Antibiotics, 159–160
Antibodies, 104
Anticoagulant, 297

Antidiuretic hormone (ADH), 105t
Antigens, 104
Antiseptics, 169
Antisocial personality disorder, 534
Anxiety, 530, 530b
  definition of, 529
  disorders, 530–532
Aorta, 99, 99f
Aortic valve, 99f
Aphasia, 489, 493, 496
Apical pulse, 397, 398f, 399b–400b
Apnea, 475–476, 476f
Appearance, 44, 44f–45f, 44b
Appetite, as factors affecting eating and
  nutrition, 366
Apraxia of speech, 496
Aquathermia pad, 458t–459t
Aqueous chamber, 97
Aqueous humor, 97
Arachnoid, 96
Arachnoid space, 96
Arterial ulcers, 448, 449f
Arteriole, 99
Artery, 89, 99, 99f
Arthritis, 506–507, 506f–507f
  definition of, 503
  joint replacement surgery for, 506, 506f, 507b
  osteoarthritis, 506
  rheumatoid, 506
Arthroplasty, 506
  definition of, 503
Asepsis
  definition of, 159, 162
  medical, 162–169
  practices, 162, 163f, 163b, 170f, 170b
  surgical, 162
Aspiration, 261, 265, 365
  definition of, 367
  precautions for, 367b
  prevention of, 374
Assault, 30, 33
Assessment, 68, 68b–69b
Assignment sheets, 70, 70b, 71f
Assisted living residence (ALR), 1, 3
Assistive devices, for eating, 366f
Asthma, 518
Atherosclerosis, 515, 515f
Athlete's foot, 449f, 449b
Atria, 98
Atrophy, 412–413, 413f
Attendance, 45, 46b
Attention (focus), 47
Attitude, 46
Audiologist, 4t
Auditory canal, 97, 97f
Auricle, 97
Autoclave, 169f
Autoimmune disorders, 524
Automated external defibrillator, 561f
Autonomic nervous system, 97
Autopsy, 574
  definition of, 569, 574
Axillary temperature, 393b, 394f

B

B lymphocytes (B cells), 104
Back injuries, 191, 191b
Back massage, 429–430, 429b–430b, 430f
Ball-and-socket joint, 93, 93f
Bariatric bed, 239, 239f, 239b
Bariatric needs, 62
Bariatric sling, 225
Barriers, to prevent wandering, 136f

Page numbers followed by "f" indicate figures,
"b" indicate boxes, and "t" indicate tables.

604

Base of support, 189–190, 190f
Basic needs, 179, 179b
Bath blanket, 244, 271
Bathing, 272–284, 274b–275b
　　complete bed bath, 272, 275–279,
　　　　276b–277b, 278f–279f
　　frequency of, 272
　　partial, 279–280, 279f, 279b–280b
　　partial bed bath, 272
　　rules for, 273b, 274f
　　tub baths and showers and, 280–284, 281f,
　　　　282b–284b
Bathing sling, 225
Bathroom, 241, 241f
Battery, 30, 33
Beans, 356t–357t
Beard, care for, 300
Bed, 235–239, 236b
　　air flotation, 472, 472f
　　bariatric, 239, 239f, 239b
　　closed, 244, 245f, 249–254, 249b–250b,
　　　　251f–253f
　　electric, 235, 235f–236f
　　manual, 235, 235f–236f
　　moving persons in, 202–206, 202b
　　　　to side of bed, 204b–206b, 205–206, 205f
　　　　up in, 203–205, 203f–204f, 203b–204b
　　occupied, 244, 245f, 254–258, 254b–255b,
　　　　256f–257f
　　open, 244, 245f, 254
　　positions in, 236, 237t
　　safety in, 238, 238f
　　shampooing in, 295
　　surgical, 244, 245f, 258–260, 258b, 259f
　　transferring of person
　　　　to bed, from chair or wheelchairs,
　　　　　　221–222, 221f, 221b–222b
　　　　to chair or wheelchair, 218–221,
　　　　　　218b–219b, 220f
　　types of, 244, 245f
Bed cradle, 418t–419t, 472
Bed frame, restraint in, 151f
Bed mobility, 199
Bed rail protector, 152f
Bed rails, 133, 137, 137f, 138b, 146, 147f, 239
Bed rest, 412
Bedmaking, 244–260, 248b–249b, 259b–260b
　　drawsheet in, 245, 246f, 252f
　　linens and, 245–246, 246f–247f, 248b
　　types of beds and, 244, 245f
Bedpans, 318–321, 318f, 319f–320b, 320f–321f
Bedrest, 413
　　complications of, 413, 413f, 414b
　　positioning during, 418, 418t–419t
Bedside stand, 239, 239f
Behavior issues, 60, 61b
Behavioral problems, 533b
Belonging, 54
Belt restraints, 150f, 152, 153f, 154b
Benign prostatic hyperplasia (BPH), 522
Benign tumor, 504, 504f
　　definition of, 503
Between-meal snacks, 362
Bilevel positive airway pressure (BiPAP), 483
Binders, 456–457, 456f, 457b
Binge-eating disorder, 536
BIOHAZARD symbol, 171, 171f
Biohazardous waste, 159, 172
BiPAP. *See* Bilevel positive airway pressure
Bipolar disorder, 533, 533b
Bladder, 102
Blanchable skin, 467, 467f
Bland diet, 359t–360t
Blindness, 493, 496, 498, 499b
Blisters, 449f, 449b
Bloating, 348

Blood, 98
Blood glucose testing, 444–445, 444f
　　equipment, 444–445
Blood pressure (BP), 388, 401–406
　　abnormal, 401–402, 401b
　　definition of, 401
　　measuring, 403–406, 403b–406b, 404f–405f
　　　　equipment for, 402–403, 402f, 402b
　　normal, 401–402, 401b
Blood vessels, 99, 99f
Bloodborne Pathogen Standard, 170–173
Bloodborne pathogens, 159
Board of directors, 3
Board of trustees, 3
Body, structure and function of, 89–107,
　　106b–107b
Body alignment, 189
Body language, 53, 58, 582
Body mechanics, 43, 189–198, 198b
　　definition of, 189
　　principles of, 189–190, 190f, 190b
Body reactions, as factors affecting eating and
　　nutrition, 366
Body temperature, 92
　　definition of, 388–394
　　normal, 390t
　　procedure for taking, 392–394, 392b
　　sites for, 389–390, 390b
Bomb threats, 126
Bone marrow, 92
Bones, 92, 93f
Bony prominence, 464, 465f
Borderline personality disorder (BPD), 534
Boundary, 31
　　crossing, 30, 32
　　signs, 30, 32, 32b
　　violation, 30, 32
Bowel elimination
　　comfort during, 346–347, 346b–347b
　　common problems in, 347–348
　　normal, 345–346, 345b–346b
　　safety during, 346–347, 346b–347b
Bowel movement, 346–347, 346b
Bowel needs, 344–354, 345b, 353b–354b
Bowel training, 348, 349f
BP. *See* Blood pressure
BPD. *See* Borderline personality disorder
BPH. *See* Benign prostatic hyperplasia
Braces, 418t–419t
Bradycardia, 388
Bradypnea, 475–476, 476f
Braille, 493, 498, 498f
Brain, 95, 96f
Brainstem, 95, 96f
Breaks, 48
Breast binder, 456, 456f
Breasts, 104
Breathing, end-of-life care, 572
Broca's aphasia, 496
Bronchioles, 100
Bronchitis, 517
Brushing
　　of hair, 293–295, 293b–294b, 294f
　　of teeth, 262–267, 263b, 264f
Bulimia nervosa, 536
Bullying, 42, 50
Bunions, 449f, 449b
Burnout, 48, 49b
Burns, 566–568, 566f
　　prevention of, 120, 120b

C
CAD. *See* Coronary artery disease
Call lights, 240, 240f–241f, 241b
Call system, 240–241, 240f–241f, 241b
　　safety in, 241

Calluses, 449b
Calorie, 355
　　counts, 362, 363f, 363b
Calorie-controlled diet, 359t–360t
Cancer, 504–506
　　chemotherapy for, 505
　　definition of, 503
　　person's needs, 505–506, 505b
　　radiation therapy for, 505
　　risk factors for, 504
　　signs and symptoms of, 505b
　　treatment of, 505
Canes, 420, 420f, 420b
Capillary, 89, 99
Carbohydrates, 358
Cardiac muscle, 94
Cardiopulmonary resuscitation (CPR), 555,
　　557–568, 557b
　　adult, 560–561, 560f, 560b
　　airway, 559, 559f
　　breathing, 559, 559f
　　chest compressions, 558–559, 558f, 558b
　　defibrillation, 561, 561f, 561b
　　hands-only, 562
　　recovery position after, 562, 562f
Cardiovascular disorders, 514–517, 514b
　　angina, 515–516, 515f
　　coronary artery disease, 515, 515f
　　heart failure, 516–517, 517b
　　hypertension, 514
　　myocardial infarction, 516, 516f, 516b
Care conferences, 70, 70b
Caregivers, children as, 110
Carpooling, 45
Carrier, 159, 161
Cartilage, 93
Case management, 6
Case manager, 6
Casts, 508, 508b, 509f
Cataracts, 496, 497f, 497b
Catheter-associated urinary tract infection
　　(CAUTI), 335
Catheterization, 333
Catheters, 333
　　urinary, 333–343, 333b–334b, 342b–343b
　　　　care for, 335–338, 335f, 336b–337b,
　　　　　　338f
　　　　condom, 333, 340–343, 340f, 340b–342b
　　　　indwelling, 333–334, 334f, 335b, 336f
　　　　purpose of, 334
　　　　securing, 336f
　　　　straight, 333–334
　　　　types of, 334
CAUTI. *See* Catheter-associated urinary tract
　　infection
Celiac disease, 524
Cell, 89–90, 90f–91f
Cell membrane, 90, 90f
Centers for Medicare & Medicaid Services
　　(CMS), in restraints, 144
Central nervous system, 95–96, 95f
Central vision, 497
Cerebellum, 95, 96f
Cerebral cortex, 96, 96f
Cerebrospinal fluid, 96
Cerebrum, 95, 96f
Certification, 18, 20, 20b–21b
Cerumen, 97
Cervical traction, 513
Cervix, 103
Chain of infection, 161–162, 161f
Chair position, 196–198, 196f
Chairs, 240
　　re-positioning in, 211–213, 211f–212f
　　transferring from bed to, 218–221,
　　　　218b–219b, 220f

Chart, 64
Chemical restraints, 144, 146–147, 146b
Chemotherapy, 505
Chest compressions, 558–559, 558f, 558b
Chest pain, 476b
Chest thrusts, for choking, 122, 122f
Chewing problems, as factors affecting eating and nutrition, 367
Cheyne-Stokes respirations, 475–476, 476f
Child abuse and neglect, 30, 37, 38t
Childcare, 45
Children, as caregivers, 110
Choking, 121–122, 121f–123f, 121b–122b, 562
Cholesterol, 355, 358
Choroid, 97
Chromosomes, 90
Chronic bronchitis, 517
Chronic illness, 1–2
Chronic kidney disease, 522, 523b
Chronic obstructive pulmonary disease (COPD), 517
Chronic pain, 425, 427
Chronic problem, 486
Chyme, 101
Cigarette smoking, 517
Ciliary muscle, 97
Circulatory system, 98–99, 98f–99f, 111t–113t
Circulatory ulcers, 448–453
    elastic bandages for, 452–453, 452b, 454f
    elastic stockings for, 450–452, 450b–451b, 451f–452f
    prevention of, 448–453, 448b
    treatment of, 448–453
Circumcised, definition of, 271, 284, 284f
Civil law, 30, 33
Clarifying, 59
Cleansing enema, 349
Clear-liquid diet, 359t–360t
Cleric, 4t
Clinical laboratory technician, 4t
Clinical nurse specialist, 4t, 5
Clitoris, 104
Closed bed, 244, 245f, 249–254, 249b–250b, 251f–253f
Closed fracture, 508, 508f
Closed reduction, 508
Cochlea, 97, 97f
Cognitive function, 539
    definition of, 539
Cognitive problems, 533b
Cold applications, for wound care, 458, 458t–459t, 460–463, 460b–462b
Cold compress, 458t–459t
Cold packs, 458t–459t
Cold temperature, ranges of, 460t
Color-coded wristbands, 129–130, 129f
Colostomy, 344, 352, 352f
Coma, 117–118
Comatose, 53, 61
Comfort, 233b–234b, 234–235, 425–429, 426b
    end-of-life care, 571–572, 571b
    enteral nutrition, 374–375, 374f
    lighting, 235, 235b
    measures, 428, 428b
    needs in, 425–433, 432b–433b
    noise and, 234–235, 234b
    odors and, 235
    temperature and ventilation and, 234, 234b
Commodes, 323–325, 323f, 323b–324b
Common health problems, 503–528, 526b, 528b
Communicable disease, 159, 161

Communication, 56–60, 56b, 65, 65b
    barriers to, 60, 60b
    body language, 53, 58
    changes, Alzheimer's disease and, 545–546, 545b–546b
    clarifying, 59
    in delegation, 26, 27b
    with dementia patients, 56b
    direct questions, 59
    eye contact during, 58b, 59f
    focusing, 59
    hearing loss, 494, 494b
    listening, 59
    methods, 59–60
    nonverbal, 53, 58
    open-ended questions, 59
    paraphrasing, 59
    with persons from other cultures, 59b
    rehabilitation of, 489, 489b
    rules for, 56
    silence, 59–60, 60b
    with speech-impaired persons, 496b
    verbal, 53, 56–57, 57f, 57b
Competency
    evaluation of, 19–20
    maintaining, 21, 21b
Complete bed bath, 272, 275–279, 276b–277b, 278f–279f
Complete (full) dentures, 267
Comprehensive care plan, 70
Compression garments, 456–457, 457f, 457b
Compression stockings, 446–450
Compulsion, 532
    definition of, 529
Concussions, 566
Condom catheters, 333, 340–343, 340f, 340b–342b
Confidentiality, 12, 42, 46, 46b
Conflict, 49
    resolving, 49, 50b
Confusion, 3b, 539–554, 540f, 540b, 553b
    definition of, 539
Connective tissue, 91
Constipation, 344, 347
Constrict, definition of, 446, 457
Contact lenses, 500
Contact precautions, 178b
Contamination, 159, 162
Continuous positive airway pressure (CPAP), 483, 484f
Contracture, 193, 412–413, 413f
COPD. See Chronic obstructive pulmonary disease
Coping, 529
Cornea, 97
Corns, 449f, 449b
Coronary artery disease (CAD), 515, 515f
Corpus callosum, 96f
Corpus cavernosum, 103f
Corpus spongiosum, 103f
Corrective lenses, 500, 500b
Cough, 476b
    etiquette, 176b
Coughing, 178b, 479–481, 479b–480b, 480f
Courtesies, 47
Cowper's glands, 103
CPAP. See Continuous positive airway pressure
CPR. See Cardiopulmonary resuscitation
Cracked skin, 449f, 449b
Cranial nerves, 96
Crime, 30
Criminal law, 30, 33
Crohn's disease, 519
Cross-contamination, 159, 162, 163f
Crutches, 421

Culture, 55, 56b
    definition of, 53
    eye contact based on, 58b
    facial expressions based on, 58b
    as factors affecting eating and nutrition, 366, 366b
    health care beliefs and, 55b
    sick care practices and, 55b
    spiritual needs and, 570
    touch practices based on, 58b
Cushions, 472, 472f
Cyanosis, 475, 476b
Cytoplasm, 90, 90f

D
Dairy products, 356t–357t
Dandruff, 291–292
Dangling, 209–211, 209b–211b, 211f
Dark green vegetables, 356t–357t
Deafness, 493–494
Death, 110
    age, 570–571
    attitudes about, 570–571, 570b
    care of body after, 574–577, 574b
    cultural attitudes, 570, 570b
    post-mortem care, 574
        definition of, 569
    rattle, 572
    signs of, 573
    spiritual needs, 570, 570b
Deconditioning, 412–413
Deep, term, 84
Deep breathing, 479–481, 479b, 480f
Defamation, 30, 33, 33b
Defecation, 344–345
Defense mechanisms, 530, 531b
    definition of, 529
Defibrillation, 561, 561f, 561b
Dehydration, 344, 347, 377–378, 378b
Delegate, 18
Delegation, 8b, 18, 25–28, 28b, 40b, 51b, 62b
    accepting task in, 28
    assessment in, 26
    body mechanics and, 197b
    five rights of, 27b
    infection and, 173b
    isolation precautions and, 187b
    in moving of person, 212b
    nursing assistant's role in, 27–28
    persons allowed to delegate, 25, 25b
    process, 26–27, 26f
    refusing task in, 28, 28b
    restraints and, 157b
Delirium, 540–541, 540b
    definition of, 539
Delusions, 532, 544
    definition of, 529, 539
Delusions of grandeur, 533b
    definition of, 529
Delusions of persecution, 533b
    definition of, 529
Demanding behavior, 60
Dementia, 539–554, 541b, 553b
    care of persons with, 547–553, 547b–551b, 548f–549f, 551f
    definition of, 117, 118b, 539
    patients, communication with, 56b
Denture, 261, 267–269, 267f
    care for, 267–269, 267f, 267b–269b, 269f
Depression, 533, 533b, 541b
Dermis, 92, 92f
Detoxification, 535
    definition of, 529
Development, 108
Developmental task, 108, 109f, 109b

Diabetes, 105t, 523–524
  foot care, 449b
  meal plan, 359t–360t, 362
Diabetic foot ulcers, 448
Diabetic retinopathy, 497f, 498
Diaphragm, 101
Diarrhea, 344, 347–348, 347b–348b
Diastole, 98
Diastolic pressure, 388, 401
Diet
  diabetes meal plan, 362
  dysphagia, 362
  general, 359
  liquid, 359t–360t
  regular, 359
  sodium-controlled, 361
  special, 359–362, 359t–360t
Dietitian, 4t
Digestion, 89
Digestive disorders, 519–521
  cirrhosis, 520–521, 521f
  diverticular disease, 519, 519f
  hepatitis, 520, 520b
  inflammatory bowel disease, 519
  vomiting, 519
Digestive system, 101, 101f, 111t–113t
Digit, 72b
Digital thermometer, 391t
Dignity, 14b
Dilate, definition of, 446, 457
Dining programs, 368
Direct questions, 59
Directional terms, 84, 84f
Director of nursing (DON), 5
Disability, 486
  definition of, 53, 61
  etiquette considerations for, 61b
  as factors affecting eating and nutrition,
    366
Disasters, 117, 126–128, 126b
Discharge, 1
Discipline, 145b
Discrimination, 578, 584
Disinfection, 159, 169, 169b
Disorientation, 3b
Distal, term, 84
Diverticular disease, 519, 519f
Diverticulosis, 519, 519f
"Do Not Resuscitate" orders, 573
DON. *See* Director of nursing
Dorsal recumbent position, 189, 195
Dorsiflexion, 412, 414b
Double-bagging, 186
Drainage systems, for indwelling catheters,
    338–343, 338b–339b, 339f
Drawsheets, 244–245, 246f, 252f
Dressing, 304–315, 305f, 305b, 309b–310b,
    310f–312f, 315b, 453–456
  applying, 454–456, 454b–455b
  dry, non-sterile, 455b–456b
  functions of, 453
  for interview, 583f, 583b
  securing, 453–454
Drinking water, 383–384, 383f–384f,
    383b–384b
Droplet precautions, 178b
Drug addiction, 535
Drug testing, 51, 585–586
Drugs, 43
  as factors affecting eating and nutrition,
    366
  sleep and, 431
Dry applications, 458
Dry cold applications, 458
Dry heat applications, 458
Dry skin, 449f, 449b

Dura mater, 96
Durable power of attorney for health care,
    573
Dying
  comfort needs during, 571, 571b, 576b
  stages of, 571
Dysarthria, 496
Dysphagia, 355, 362, 365, 367, 367f, 367b,
    488
  diet for, 362
Dyspnea, 475–476, 572
Dysuria, 316–317

E
Ear, 97, 97f
Eardrum, 97, 97f
Eating
  assistive devices for, 366f
  device, 487f
  disorders, 536
  factors affecting, 366–367
Edema, 377–378
EHR. *See* Electronic health record
Ejaculatory duct, 103, 103f
Elastic bandages, 452–453, 452b
  applying, 453b, 454f
Elastic stockings, 450–452, 450b, 451f
  applying, 451b, 452f
Elbow, exercise for, 415b–416b, 416f
Elbow protectors, 472, 472f
Elder abuse, 36–37
  definition of, 30
  reporting, 36
  signs of, 37f, 37b
Electric bed, 235, 235f–236f
Electrical equipment, 124, 125f
Electrical shock, 124
Electrolytes, 102
Electronic communications, wrongful use of,
    34, 34b–35b
Electronic devices, 75, 75b
Electronic health record (EHR), 64–65
Electronic manometer, 402, 402f
Electronic recording, 74, 74f
Elimination, 487
  comfort during, 346–347, 346b–347b
  end-of-life care and, 572
  normal, 345–346, 345b–346b
  safety during, 346–347, 346b–347b
Elopement, 117, 128, 544b
  definition of, 539
Embolus, 450
Emergency care, 555–568, 567b–568b
  for burns, 566–568, 566f
  for choking, 562
  for concussions, 566
  description of, 556–557, 556b
  for fainting, 564, 564f
  for heart attack, 563
  for hemorrhage, 563–564, 563f
  for poisoning, 563
  Rapid Response System, 556
  rules of, 556b
  for seizures, 565–566, 565f, 566b
  for shock, 564
  for stroke, 565, 565b
Emotional abuse, 36
Emotional problems, 533b
  sleep and, 431
Emphysema, 517, 517f
Enablers, 147
Encourage fluids, 379t
End-of-life care, 569–577, 576b–577b
  breathing problems, 572
  comfort needs in, 571–572, 571b
  definition of, 569

End-of-life care *(Continued)*
  dying, stages of, 571
  elimination, 572
  emotional needs, 572
  family considerations, 573
  hearing, 572
  legal issues, 573
  mental needs, 572
  mouth, 572
  nose, 572
  nutrition, 572
  oral hygiene, 572
  pain management, 572
  person's room, 572
  physical needs, 571–572
  skin, 572
  speech, 572
  vision, 572
End-of-shift report, 64, 73, 73b
Endocardium, 98, 99f
Endocrine disorders, 523–524
Endocrine glands, 105
Endocrine system, 105, 105f
Endometrium, 103
Endorsement, 18, 21
Enema
  cleansing, 349
  definition of, 344, 349–351
  delegation of, 349b
  oil-retention, 351, 351b
  safety of, 349b
  small-volume, 349–351, 349b–350b,
    351f
Engineering controls, 171, 171f
Enteral nutrition, 365, 373–375
  observations in, 374
Entrapment, 232, 238
  zones for, 238f
Environment, of microbes, 160
Epidemic, 128
Epidermis, 92, 92f
Epididymis, 103, 103f
Epiglottis, 100
Epinephrine, 105t
Epithelial tissue, 91
Equipment
  accidents, prevention of, 124–125, 124f,
    124b
  in Bloodborne Pathogen Standard, 172
  for teeth, 262
    denture care, 267
Equivalency, 18
Ergonomics, 189, 191, 192b
Erythrocytes, 98
Eschar, 467, 468f–469f
Esophagus, 101
Esteem, 53
Estrogen, 103
Ethical aspects, 67
Ethics, 8b, 28b, 30–41, 40b–41b, 51b, 62b
  body mechanics and, 197b
  codes of, 31, 31b
  definition of, 30
  infection and, 173b
  isolation precautions and, 187b
  in moving of person, 212b
  restraints and, 157b
Eustachian tube, 97, 97f
Evaluation, 70
  in delegation, 27b
Exercises, 43, 412–424, 412b, 423b–424b
  range-of-motion, 414–418, 414b–416b,
    416f
  sleep and, 431
Exposure incidents, 172–173
Expressive aphasia, 496

Extension, 412, 414b
External ear, 97
External female genitalia, 104, 104f
External rotation, 412, 414b
Eye, 97, 97f
Eye contact, during communication, 58b, 59f
Eye disorders, 496–500, 501b–502b
Eyeglasses
    caring for, 500b
    removing, 501f

F
Face shields, 180, 180b, 182f
Facial expressions, 58b
Fainting, 564, 564f
    definition of, 555
Fall prevention, 133–143, 133b, 142b–143b
    bed rails for, 133, 137, 137f, 138b, 146, 147f
    communication for, 134b
    grab bars for, 138, 138f
    hand rails for, 138, 138f
    programs, 134–138, 136b
    safety measures for, 135b
    transfer belts for, 133, 139–141, 139f–140f, 139b–140b
    wheel locks for, 138, 138f
Fallopian tube, 103, 103f
Falls
    causes of, 134, 134b
    help during, 141–143, 141f, 141b
    risk factors for, 134, 134b
False imprisonment, 30, 33, 148
Family, 62
    of Alzheimer's disease patient, 551–552, 552b
    of dying patient, 573
Fat-controlled diet, 359t–360t
Fats, 358
FBAO. *See* Foreign-body airway obstruction
Febrile, 388
Fecal impaction, 344
Fecal incontinence, 344, 348, 348b
Feces, 101, 344–345
Feedback, 27
Feeding the person, 371–373, 371f, 371b–373b
Feeding tubes, 373, 373f
Female perineal care, 285f, 286b–287b, 287f
Female reproductive system, 103–104, 103f–104f
Fertilization, 104
Fever, 388–389
Fiber-restricted diet, 359t–360t
Finances, as factors affecting eating and nutrition, 366
Financial exploitation, 36
Finger cushion, 418t–419t
Fingers, exercise for, 415b–416b, 417f
Fire extinguisher, 127, 127f, 127b
Fire safety, 126–127, 126b–127b, 127f
First aid, 556
    definition of, 555
Flashback, 532
    definition of, 529
Flat bones, 92
Flatulence, 344, 348
Flatus, 344, 348
Flexion, 412, 414b
Floor cushion, 136f
Flora, normal, 159
Flossing, of teeth, 262, 264f
Flow rate, 377, 385, 385f, 385b
    oxygen, 483
Flow sheets, 67f

Fluid
    needs, 377–387, 386b–387b
    orders, special, 378
    requirements, normal, 378
Fluid balance, 378, 378f, 378b
Fluid-filled pads, 472
Focal (partial) seizure, 565
Focusing, 59
Food labels, 358–359, 358f, 359b
Foods
    groups of, 356, 356t–357t
    high-sodium, 361b
    intake of, 362–364, 363f, 363b
        percent of, 362, 362f
Foot, exercise for, 415b–416b, 417f
Foot-board, 418t–419t
Foot care, 44, 300–303, 300b–302b, 301f
Foot ulcers, diabetic, 448
Footdrop, 412, 418t–419t
Forearm, exercise for, 415b–416b, 416f
Foreign-body airway obstruction (FBAO), 121, 562
Fowler's position, 189, 194–195, 194f, 194b, 237t, 465f
Fracture pans, 318, 318f
Fractures, 508–509
    closed, 508
    definition of, 503
    hip, 509, 509f–510f, 510b
    open, 508
Fraud, 30, 33
Freedom of movement, 145b
Friction, 199, 201
Friction-reducing devices, 201–202, 201f–202f, 201b
Friends, 62
Fruits, 356t–357t
Full denture, 267f
Full visual privacy, 232, 240
Functional incontinence, 316, 325
Functional nursing, 6
Fungal infection, 449f, 449b

G
GAD. *See* Generalized anxiety disorder
Gait belt, 133, 139–141, 139f–140f, 139b–140b
Gangrene, 448, 510, 510f
Garment, 304–312, 305b–306b
Gastrostomy tube, 373, 374f
Gavage, 365, 373, 374f
Gel-filled pads, 472
Gender identity, 53–54
Generalized anxiety disorder (GAD), 531
Geriatrics, 108
Gerontology, 108
Gestational diabetes, 523
GH. *See* Growth hormone
Glaucoma, 498
Global aphasia, 496
Gloves, 178b, 180, 181f–184f, 181b, 186f
Glucocorticoids, 105t
Glucometer, 434
Glucosuria, 434, 439
Gluten-free diet, 359t–360t
Goggles, 180, 180b, 182f
Gonads, 105t
Gossip, 42, 46
Gowns
    changing of, 312–315, 312f–313f, 313b–314b
    description of, 176b, 178b, 180, 182f
Grab bars, 138, 138f, 241
Graduate, 377, 379, 380f
Grains, 356t–357t
Graves' disease, 524

Grievances, right to, 13
Grieving, 110
Grooming, 291–303, 291f, 291b, 302b–303b
    in Alzheimer's disease, 549b–550b
    changing garments for, 304–312, 305f, 305b–306b
    changing patient gowns in, 312–315, 312f–313f, 313b–314b
    dressing for, 304–315, 305f, 305b, 309b–310b, 310f–312f
    foot care in, 300–303, 300b–302b, 301f
    hair care in, 292–295
    for interview, 583f, 583b
    nail care in, 300–303, 300b–302b, 301f
    shaving in, 297–300, 297f–298f, 298b–299b
    undressing in, 304–315, 305b, 307b, 308f
Group insurance, 6
Growth, 108
Growth hormone (GH), 105t

H
HAI. *See* Healthcare-associated infection
Hair
    anatomy of, 92
    brushing of, 293–295, 293b–294b, 294f
    care of, 292–295
    combing of, 293–295, 293b–294b, 294f
    shampooing of, 295, 295f, 295b–297b
    skin and scalp conditions, 292–293, 292b
Hallucinations, 532, 544
    definition of, 529, 539
Hammer toes, 449f, 449b
Hand grip, 418t–419t
Hand hygiene, 163–168, 164b, 165f–166f, 166b
Hand rails, 138, 138f
Hand roll, 418t–419t
Hand-washing, 165f–166f, 166b, 176b
Harassment, 42, 50, 50b
Hashimoto's disease, 524
Hazard, 117
Hazardous chemical, 117, 125, 125f
Head injuries, 514
Head tilt-chin lift method, 122b, 123f, 559, 559f
Health, 43
Health care, 1–9, 8b–9b
    beliefs, 55, 56b
    paying for, 6–7, 7b
    practices, 55
    purposes of, 2
Health history, 65
Health Insurance Portability and Accountability Act of 1996 (HIPAA), 34b
Health team, 1, 4, 4t, 4b
    communications, 64–77, 76b–77b
Healthcare-associated infection (HAI), 159, 162
Hearing, 493–502
    end-of-life care considerations in, 572
    loss of, accident risks and, 118
    measures to promote, 495b
Hearing aids, 495, 495f, 495b
Hearing disorders, 493–495, 501b–502b
Hearing dogs, 494
Hearing loss, 493–495, 494b
Heart, 98, 98f–99f
Heart attack, 563
Heart failure, 516–517, 517b
Heat applications, for wound care, 457, 457f, 458t–459t, 460b–462b
Heat temperature, ranges of, 460t
Heel elevators, 472f
Heel protectors, 472, 472f
Height measurements, 406–411, 407f–408f, 407b–409b, 410f

Heimlich maneuver, 121
Hematuria, 316–317, 434, 439
Hemiplegia, 511
  definition of, 503
Hemoglobin, 89, 98
Hemoptysis, 434, 442b
Hemorrhage, 563–564, 563f, 564b
  definition of, 555
Hepatitis A, 520
Hepatitis B, 520
  vaccination, 171
Hepatitis C, 520
Hepatitis D, 520
Hepatitis E, 520
High-calorie diet, 359t–360t
High-fiber diet, 359t–360t
High-fiber foods, 346
High-Fowler's position, 189, 237t
High-iron diet, 359t–360t
High-protein diet, 359t–360t
High-sodium foods, 361b
Hinge joint, 93, 93f
Hip, exercise for, 415b–416b, 417f
Hip abduction wedge, 418t–419t
Hip fractures, 509, 509f–510f, 510b
HIPAA. *See* Health Insurance Portability and
  Accountability Act of 1996
Hirsutism, 291–292
HIV. *See* Human immunodeficiency virus
Holism, 53
Home care agencies, 3
Hormone, 89, 105
Hospice care, 570
Hospices, 1, 3
Hospitals, 2, 2f
Host, 160, 161f
  susceptible, 162, 170b
Hot-cold balance, 56b
Hot compress, 461b–462b
Hot pack, 458t–459t
Hot soak, 458t–459t, 461b–462b
Human immunodeficiency virus (HIV),
  525–526, 525b
Humidifier, 483f
Hydration, 378
Hygiene, 43–44, 261–262
  adaptive (assistive) devices for, 272f
  in Alzheimer's disease, 549b–550b
  bathing and, 272–284
  daily, 271–290, 289b–290b
  daily care and, 272, 272b–273b
  hand, 163–168, 164b, 165f–166f, 166b,
    168f, 168b, 176b
  perineal care and, 284–289, 284b–288b,
    285f, 287f–288f
  reporting and recording, 289–290, 289b
Hymen, 103
Hyperextension, 412, 414b
Hyperglycemia, 503, 524, 524t
Hypertension, 388, 401, 503, 514
Hyperventilation, 475–476, 476f
Hypoglycemia, 503, 524, 524t
Hypotension, 388, 401
Hypothalamus, 96f
Hypoventilation, 475–476, 476f
Hypoxemia, 481
Hypoxia, 475–476, 476b

I
Ice bags, 458t–459t
Identification, of person, 119, 119f, 119b
Identification bracelet, 119, 119f
Ileostomy, 344, 351, 351f
Illness
  as factors affecting eating and nutrition, 366
  sleep and, 431

Immobility, 412–414
Immune system
  description of, 104–105, 111t–113t
  disorders, 524–526
Immunity, 89, 104, 171
Impaired vision, 498, 499b
Implementation, 70
In-patient care, 2
In-person interview, 582
Incident, 117
Incident reports/reporting, 130
Incontinence brief, 328b–329b, 330f
Incus, 97, 97f
Independence, 8b, 28b, 40b, 51b, 62b
  body mechanics and, 197b
  infection and, 173b
  isolation precautions and, 187b
  in moving of person, 212b
  restraints and, 157b
Indwelling catheter, 333–334, 334f, 335b,
  336f
  care of, 335f, 336b
  drainage systems for, 338–343, 338b–339b,
    339f
Infection, 160–162, 161b
  chain of, 161–162, 161f
  control, 159, 175
  definition of, 159–160
  healthcare-associated, 159, 162
  preventing, 159–174, 174b
  signs and symptoms of, 160b
Inferior, term, 84
Inferior vena cava, 99, 99f
Inflammatory bowel disease, 519
Influenza, 518, 518b
Information, right to, 12, 12b
Informed consent, 30, 35, 35b, 148
Ingrown toenails, 449f, 449b
Inner ear, 97
Insomnia, 425, 431
Insulin, 105t, 362
Intact skin, 464–465, 465f
Intake, 377, 379–383
  measuring, 379–383, 379b, 381f,
    381b–382b
Intake and output record, 379, 380f
Integumentary system, 92, 92f, 111t–113t
Intentional torts, 33–34, 33b–34b
Intercom systems, 46
Interdisciplinary health care team, 4
Internal rotation, 412, 414b
International time, 71
Interview
  during, 584
  job, 582–584, 585f
  preparing for, 582–583
  questions, 583b
    cannot asked for, 584, 584b
  thank-you letter or note after, 584
  types of, 582
Intimacy, changes in, 547
Intimate partner violence (IPV), 30, 39, 39b
Intravenous (IV) therapy, 377, 384–387,
  384f
  assisting, 385–387, 385b–386b
Invasion of privacy, 30, 33–34, 34f, 34b
Involuntary muscles, 94
Involuntary seclusion, 10, 13, 35
IPV. *See* Intimate partner violence
Iris, 97
Irregular bones, 92
Isolation precautions, 175–188, 188b
  rules for, 179b
  standard precautions in, 175, 176b
  transmission-based precautions, 177–179,
    177f, 178b–179b

J
Jacket restraints, 152–154, 153f, 154b–156b
Job, 585b–586b
  losing, 51, 51b
  offer, accepting or declining, 585
  resigning from, 50
  skills and trainings, 579, 579b
  sources of, 578
Job application, 579, 582b
  completing, 579
  definition of, 578
  sample, 580f–581f
Job description, 18, 22, 22b, 23f–24f
Job interview, 582–584, 585f
  definition of, 578
Job safety, 47
Joint, 89, 93, 93f

K
Ketone, 434, 439
Ketone body. *See* Ketone
Kidney stones, 522, 522f
Kidneys, description of, 102
Knee, exercise for, 415b–416b, 417f
Kübler-Ross, Elisabeth, 571
Kussmaul respirations, 475–476, 476f

L
Labeling, of hazardous substances, 125,
  125f
Labia majora, 103f, 104
Labia minora, 103f, 104
Lactose-free diet, 359t–360t
Language, 46
Large intestine, 101
Lateral, term, 84
Lateral position, 189, 196, 196f, 465f, 470
Lateral transfer, 214, 223, 224f, 224b
Laundry, contaminated, 172, 172b
Laws, 8b, 28b, 30–41, 41b, 51b, 62b
  body mechanics and, 197b
  civil, 30, 33
  criminal, 30, 33
  definition of, 30, 33, 40b
  ethics and, 33–35
  infection and, 173b
  isolation precautions and, 187b
  medical records and, 67
  in moving of person, 212b
  restraints and, 148, 148b, 157b
Left atrium, 98, 99f
Left lower quadrant (LLQ), 83
Left semi-prone position, 189, 196, 196f
Left upper quadrant (LUQ), 83
Left ventricle, 98, 99f
Legs, shaving of, 300
Leukocytes, 98
Libel, 30, 33
Lice, 292, 292f. *See also* Pediculosis
Licensed practical nurse (LPN), 1, 4t, 5
Licensed vocational nurse (LVN), 1, 4t, 5
Life-long residents, 3b
Ligaments, 93
Lighting, comfort and, 235, 235b
Linens, 245–246, 246f–247f, 248b
Liquid diet, 359t–360t
Liquid oxygen system, 481, 482f
Listening, 59
Living wills, 573
LLQ. *See* Left lower quadrant
Local infection, 160
Logrolling, 199, 208–209, 208b–209b,
  209f
Long bones, 92
Long-term care centers, 2–3
Loss of limb, 510

Lotion, for back massage, 429
Love, 54
Low-stimulation dining, 368
Low vision, 493, 498
Lower esophageal sphincter, 94
LPN. *See* Licensed practical nurse
Lupus, 524
LUQ. *See* Left upper quadrant
LVN. *See* Licensed vocational nurse
Lymph, 100
Lymph nodes, 100
Lymphatic system, 100, 100f
Lymphatic vessels, 100
Lymphocytes, 100, 104

M
MA-C. *See* Medication assistant-certified
Male perineal care, 288f, 288b
Male reproductive system, 103, 103f
Malignant tumor, 504, 504f
    definition of, 503
Malleus, 97, 97f
Malpractice, 31, 33
Mammary glands, 104
Mania, 533
Manometer, 402, 405f
Masks, 176b, 180, 182f–184f, 186f
Maslow, Abraham, 54, 54f
Masturbation, 114
Material safety data sheet (MSDS), 125
MDROs. *See* Multidrug-resistant organisms
MDS. *See* Minimum Data Set
Meals
    breaks, 48
    dining program for, 368
    preparing for, 368–369, 368b–369b
    serving of, 369, 370b
Measurements, 388–411, 410b–411b
Mechanical lifts
    slings as, 225
    transferring person with, 224–231,
        224f–225f, 226b–228b, 227f, 229f
Mechanical soft diet, 359t–360t
Medial, term, 84
Medicaid, 6
Medical asepsis
    cleaning in, 169
    definition of, 159, 162–169
    disinfection in, 159, 169, 169b
    hand hygiene in, 163–168, 164b, 165f–166f,
        166b, 168b
    supplies and equipment for, 169
Medical device-related pressure injuries,
    467
Medical devices, in pressure injuries, 471b
Medical diagnosis, 68
Medical record, 64–67, 65f, 66t
Medical symptom, 145b
Medical terminology, 78–88, 87b–88b
Medical terms, 78–83
    common terms and phrases, 86, 86t
    defining, 78, 83, 83t
MedicAlert® + Alzheimer's Association Safe
    Return®, 544
Medicare, 6
Medication assistant-certified (MA-C), 4t
Medulla, 96, 96f
Melena, 344, 434
Membrane, 91
Memory care units, 3
Meniere's disease, 493–494
Menopause, 108
Menstruation, 89, 104
Mental abuse, 36
Mental health, 530
    definition of, 529

Mental health disorders, 529–538, 530b,
    537b–538b
    anxiety, 530–532
    bipolar, 533, 533b
    care and treatment for, 537–538, 537b
    definition of, 529
    depression, 533, 533b
    personality, 534
    schizophrenia, 532–533, 533b
    substance use, 534–535, 534b–535b
Mercury manometer, 403f
Metabolism, 89, 105t
Metastasis, 504
    definition of, 503
Methicillin-resistant *Staphylococcus aureus*
    (MRSA), 160
Mexican Americans, 56b
Microorganisms, 159–160
Midbrain, 96, 96f
Middle ear, 97
Midstream urine specimen, 437–438, 437f,
    437b–438b
Military time, 71
Mineralocorticoids, 105t
Minerals, 358
Minimum Data Set (MDS), 68
Mistreatment, freedom from, 13
Mitered corner, 251f
Mitosis, 90, 91f
Mitral valve (bicuspid valve), 98, 99f
Mitt restraints, 152, 153f, 154b–156b
Mixed aphasia, 496
Mixed incontinence, 316, 325
mm Hg, 401
Mobility, 412–414, 488, 489f, 498
    accident risks and, 118
    bed, 199
Moist applications, 458
Moist cold applications, 458
Moist heat applications, 458
Mons pubis, 103f, 104
Montgomery straps, 454, 454f
Mood disorders, 533
Mouth, end-of-life care considerations to, 572
Mouth-to-mouth breathing, 559, 559f
Moving, of person, 199–213, 199b–200b,
    213b
    in bed, 202b–204b, 203–205, 203f–204f
    dangling, 209–211, 209b–211b, 211f
    from floor, 142, 142f
    re-positioning, in chair or wheelchair,
        211–213, 211f–212f
    to side of bed, 204b–206b, 205–206, 205f
    skin in, protection of, 201–202, 201f, 201b
    work-related injuries in, prevention of,
        202b–203b
MRSA. *See* Methicillin-resistant *Staphylococcus
    aureus*
MSDS. *See* Material safety data sheet
MSDs. *See* Musculo-skeletal disorders
Mucosal membrane pressure injuries, 467
Multidrug-resistant organisms (MDROs), 160
Multiple sclerosis (MS), 512–513
Muscle tissue, 91
Muscles, 94, 94f
Musculo-skeletal disorders (MSDs), 189, 191,
    191b–192b, 506–510
    arthritis. *See* Arthritis
    loss of limb, 510
    osteoporosis, 507
Musculo-skeletal system, 92–94, 111t–113t
Mustaches, care for, 300
Myelin sheath, 95
Myocardial infarction, 516, 516f, 516b
Myocardium, 98, 99f
MyPlate, 356, 356f

N
Nails
    anatomy of, 92
    care of, 300–303, 300b–302b, 301f
Nasal cannula, 482t
Naso-gastric tube, 373, 373f
NATCEP. *See* Nursing assistant training and
    competency evaluation program
National Council of State Boards of Nursing,
    25
National Pressure Injury Advisory Panel
    (NPIAP), 464
Neck, exercise for, 415b–416b, 416f
Needs, 53–54, 54f, 179, 179b
Neglect
    child, 30, 37, 38t
    elder, 31, 36
    freedom from, 13
Negligence, 31, 33
Nephron, 102, 102f
Nerve tissue, 91
Nervous system, 95–97, 95f, 111t–113t
    central, 95–96, 95f
    peripheral, 96–97, 96f
Nervous system disorders, 511–514
    amyotrophic lateral sclerosis, 513
    head injuries, 514
    multiple sclerosis, 512–513
    Parkinson's disease, 512, 512f
    spinal cord injury, 513, 513f, 514b
    stroke, 511, 511f, 511b–512b
Nitroglycerin, 516
Nocturia, 316–317
Noise, comfort and, 234–235, 234b
Non-blanchable skin, 467, 467f
Non-pathogen, 159–160
Non-rebreather mask, 482t
Non-specific immunity, 104
Nonverbal communication, 53, 58, 537b
Norepinephrine, 105t
Nose, 100
    end-of-life care considerations in, 572
Nothing by mouth, 379t, 383
Nourishment, of microbes, 160
NPIAP. *See* National Pressure Injury
    Advisory Panel
Nucleus, 90, 90f
Nurse managers, 5
Nurse practice acts, 19
Nurse practitioner, 4t
Nursing assistant, 1, 4t, 5, 18–29, 28b–29b
    roles and responsibilities of, 21–22,
        21b–22b
    standards for, 22, 22b
Nursing assistant registry, 20
Nursing assistant training and competency
    evaluation program (NATCEP), 45, 578
Nursing care patterns, 6, 6f
Nursing care plan, 64, 70
Nursing center care, 113, 113f
Nursing center residents, identification of,
    119, 119f
Nursing centers, 3
    personal belongings in, 130
Nursing diagnosis, 64, 68–70
Nursing education, 5
Nursing interventions, 70
Nursing process, 64, 67–71, 68f
    assessment in, 68, 68b–69b
    evaluation in, 70
    implementation in, 70
    nursing diagnosis in, 68–70
    planning in, 70, 70b
Nursing service, 5
Nursing supervisors, 5
Nursing task, 18, 21

Nursing team, 1, 5
Nutrients
 definition of, 355
 types of, 358
Nutrition, 355–364, 363b–364b, 488
 definition of, 355
 end-of-life care, 572
 enteral, 365, 373–375
 factors affecting, 366–367
 MyPlate, 356, 356f
 needs
  meeting, 365–376, 365b, 375b–376b
  special, assisting, 373–375, 373b
 sleep and, 431
Nutritionist, 4t

O

Obesity
 chest thrusts for choking in patients with, 122b
 definition of, 62
Objective data, 64, 68
OBRA. *See* Omnibus Budget Reconciliation Act of 1987
Observation, 64, 67, 68b
Obsession, 532
 definition of, 529
Obsessive-compulsive disorder (OCD), 532
Occupational Safety and Health Administration (OSHA)
 in moving the person, 199
 work-related injuries, 191
 workplace violence prevention programs, 128, 128b–129b
Occupational therapist registered (OTR), 4t
Occupied, definition of, 244
Occupied bed, 244, 245f, 254–258, 254b–255b, 256f–257f
OCD. *See* Obsessive-compulsive disorder
Odors, comfort and, 235
Oil glands, 92
Oil-retention enema, 351, 351b
Oils, 358
Older person, 108–116, 115b–116b
 depression in, 533, 533b
Oliguria, 316–317
Ombudsman, 10, 15
Omnibus Budget Reconciliation Act of 1987 (OBRA), 10, 19–21, 37
 dignity and privacy promotion, 14b
Open bed, 244, 245f, 254
Open dining, 368
Open-ended questions, 59
Open fracture, 508, 508f
Open reduction, 508
OPIM. *See* Other potentially infectious materials
Opposition, 412, 414b
Optic nerve, 97
Oral hygiene, 261–270, 269b–270b
 brushing and flossing teeth in, 262–267, 263b, 264f
 denture care in, 267–269, 267f, 267b–269b, 269f
 end-of-life care of, 572
 purpose of, 262, 262b
 reporting and recording of, 269–270
 for the unconscious person, 265–267, 265f, 265b–266b
Oral temperature, 390b, 393b
Organ, 89, 91
Organization, 3–5, 5f
Orthopnea, 475–476
Orthopneic position, 475, 479, 479f
Orthostatic hypotension, 413
Orthotic devices, 412

OSHA. *See* Occupational Safety and Health Administration
Ossicles, 97
Osteoarthritis, 506
Osteomyelitis, 473
Osteoporosis, 507
Ostomy
 colostomy, 344, 352, 352f
 definition of, 344, 351–354
 ileostomy, 344, 351, 351f
 pouches, 352–354, 353f
Other potentially infectious materials (OPIM), 170
OTR. *See* Occupational therapist registered
Out-patient (ambulatory) care, 2
Output, 377, 379–383
 measuring, 379–383, 379b, 381f, 381b–382b
Ovaries, 103, 103f, 105f
Over-bed table, 239, 239f
Over-flow incontinence, 316, 325
Ovulation, 103
Oxygen, 475
 coughing, 479–481, 479b–480b, 480f
 deep breathing, 479–481, 479b, 480f
 devices, 482, 482t
 fire and, 126, 127b
 flow rates, 483
 needs, 475–485, 484b–485b
  meeting, 478–481, 478b
 positioning for, 479, 479f
 safety, 483, 483f, 483b
 sources of, 481–482, 481f–482f, 481b
Oxygen concentration, 475, 477
Oxygen concentrator, 481, 482f
Oxygen tank, 481, 481f
Oxygen therapy, assisting with, 481–483
Oxytocin, 105t

P

Padded waterproof drawsheet, 246f
Pain, 406, 425–428, 426b
 acute, 425, 427
 back massage for, 429–430, 429b–430b, 430f
 chronic, 425, 427
 definition of, 426
 description of, 4295
 factors affecting, 427, 426b
 intensity of, 427
 location of, 427
 management of, in end-of-life care, 572
 onset and duration of, 427
 phantom, 427, 510
 precipitating factors of, 427
 in pressure injuries, 473
 radiating, 427, 427f
 signs and symptoms of, 427–428, 428b
 types of, 427
 vital signs, 427
Pain rating scale, 427, 427f
Palliative care, definition of, 569–570
Pancreas, 105f, 105t
Pandemics, 128
Panic, 531
 definition of, 529
Panic disorder, 531, 531b
Paralysis, 117–118, 511, 513, 513f, 514b
 definition of, 503
Paranoia, 545, 545b, 547b–548b
 definition of, 539
Paraphrasing, 53, 59
Paraplegia, 513, 513f
 definition of, 503
Parasympathetic nervous system, 97
Parathormone, 105t

Parathyroid gland, 105f, 105t
Parenteral, 172
Parkinson's disease, 512, 512f
Partial bed bath, 272, 279–280, 279f, 279b–280b
Partial denture, 267, 267f
Pathogen, 159–160
Patient Care Partnership: Understanding Expectations, Rights, and Responsibilities, 10
Patient-focused care, 6
Patient Protection and Affordable Care Act of 2010, 6
Patient rights, 10
Patients, definitions of, 2
Peas, 356t–357t
Pediculosis, 291–292, 292f
Penis, 103
Pericardium, 98
Pericare, 271
Perineal care, 271, 284–289, 284b–288b, 285f, 287f–288f
 female, 285f, 286b–287b, 287f
 male, 288f, 288b
Periosteum, 92
Peripheral nervous system, 96–97, 96f
Peristalsis, 89, 101
Person, 61b
 addressing, 54
 communicating with, 53–63, 63b
 whole, 53–54, 54f
Personal belongings, 130, 242–243
Personal care items, 240, 240f
Personal choice
 as factors affecting eating and nutrition, 366
 right to, 12, 13f
Personal items, right to, 13, 14f
Personal matters, 47
Personal protective equipment, 169, 172, 176b, 180–182, 182f, 182b, 185b
Personal responsibility, 8b, 28b, 40b, 51b, 62b
 body mechanics and, 197b
 infection and, 173b
 isolation precautions and, 187b
 in moving of person, 212b
 restraints and, 157b
Personality, 529
Personality disorders, 534
Person's unit, 232–243, 233f, 233b, 242b–243b
Petit mal seizure, 565
Phagocytes, 104, 105f
Phantom pain, 427, 510
Pharmacist, 4t
Pharynx, 100
Phobias, 531
 definition of, 529
Phone communications, 75, 76b
Phone interview, 582
Physical abuse, 36, 37b
Physical activity, 356, 356b
Physical changes, 110, 111t–113t
Physical needs, 54
Physical restraints, 144, 146–147, 146b
Physical therapist, 4t
Physical violence, 39
Physician, 4t
Pia mater, 96
Pillowcases, 252f–253f
Pineal gland, 96f, 105f
Pinna, 97
Pituitary gland, 96f, 105f, 105t
Pivot, 214
Pivot joint, 93, 93f

Planning, 64, 70, 70b
    in delegation, 26–27
Plantar flexion, 412, 414b
Plantar warts, 449f, 449b
Plaque, 262
Plasma, 98
Platelets (thrombocytes), 98
Pleura, 101
Pneumonia, 518, 518b
    definition of, 503
Podiatrist, 4t
Poison, 117, 120
Poisoning, 563
    prevention of, 120, 120b
Policies, 7
Polyuria, 316–317
Pons, 96, 96f
Position change alarm, 133, 136–137, 136f
    promoting safety and comfort, 137
Positional terms, 84
Positioning, 193–198, 193b–194b
    during bedrest, 418, 418t–419t
    chair position, 196–198, 196f
    Fowler's position, 194–195, 194f, 194b
    lateral position, 189, 196, 196f
    prone position, 189, 195, 195f
    supine position, 189, 195, 195f
Post-mortem care, 574
    assisting with, 574b–575b
    definition of, 569
Post-traumatic stress disorder (PTSD), 532,
    532b
Posterior, term, 84
Postural hypotension, 412–413
Postural supports, 197, 197f
Prefixes, 78–79, 78f, 79t, 80f
Pregnancy, chest thrusts for choking during,
    122b
Pressure injuries, 464–474, 464f, 473b–474b
    complications of, 473–474
    definition of, 464
    observations of, 469, 470b
    persons at risk in, 466, 466b
    prevention of, 470–472, 470b–471b
    protective devices for, 472, 472f
    risk factors for, 466, 466f, 466b
    sites of, 467–469
    stages of, 467, 467f–469f
    30-degree lateral position, 470
    treatment of, 470–472, 470b
Pressure point, 464, 465f
Primary nursing, 6
Priority, 42, 48
Privacy
    curtains, 240
    invasion of, 30, 33, 34f, 34b
    promotion of, 14b
    as resident rights, 12, 12f
Private insurance, 6
Procedures, 7
Professional appearance, 44f–45f, 44b
Professional boundary, 31–32, 32f, 32b
Professional responsibility, 8b, 28b, 40b, 51b,
    62b
    body mechanics and, 197b
    infection and, 173b
    isolation precautions and, 187b
    in moving of person, 212b
    restraints and, 157b
Professional sexual misconduct, 31–32
Professionalism, 42
Progesterone, 103
Progress notes, 67f
Pronation, 412, 414b
Prone position, 189, 195, 195f, 465f
Prospective payment systems, 7

Prostate enlargement, 522, 522f
Prostate gland, 103f
Prosthesis, 486, 488, 510
    above-the-knee, 510f
Protected health information, 31, 34b
Protecting rights, 15
Protective devices, for pressure injuries, 472,
    472f
Protein, 358
    foods, 356t–357t
Proximal, term, 84
Psychological aggression, 39
Psychological changes, 110, 110b
Psychosis, 532
    definition of, 529
Psychotic disorders, 532–533, 532b
Pulmonary artery, 99f
Pulmonary edema, 517
Pulmonary embolism, 450
Pulmonary veins, 99f
Pulse, 396–400
    definition of, 388, 396
    rhythm and force, 396, 396f
    sites for, 396f
    stethoscope for, 388, 396–397, 396f–397f,
        396b–397b
    taking of, 397–400, 397f–398f, 398b
Pulse oximetry, 406, 475, 477–478, 477f,
    477b–478b
Pulse rate, 388, 396
Pupil, 97
Pyloric sphincter, 94, 95f

Q
Quadriplegia, 513, 513f
    definition of, 503
Quality of life, 491–492
    restraints and, 148
    right to, 14–15, 14b
        activities and, 15, 15f, 15b
        environment and, 14
Questions, 59

R
Radial pulse, 397, 399b
Radiating pain, 427, 427f
Radiographer/radiologic technologist, 4t
Random urine specimen, 435–437, 436b
Range of functions, 21
Range of motion (ROM), 412
Range-of-motion exercises, 414–418, 414b
    for ankle, 417f
    for elbow, 416f
    for fingers, 417f
    for foot, 417f
    for forearm, 416f
    for hip, 417f
    for knee, 417f
    for neck, 416f
    performing, 415b–416b
    for shoulder, 416f
    for thumb, 417f
    for toes, 417f
    for wrist, 417f
Rapid Response System (RRS), 556
Razors, safety, 297, 298b
RBCs. See Red blood cells
Re-positioning, in chair or wheelchair,
    211–213, 211f–212f
Reasonable accommodation, definition of, 578
Receptive aphasia, 496
Reciprocity, 18
Recording, 72b–73b, 73–74, 74f
    definition of, 64, 71–74
    in restraints, 156, 157f
    of time, 71–72, 72b

Recreational therapist, 4t
Rectal temperature, 390b, 392b–393b
Red and orange vegetables, 356t–357t
Red blood cells (RBCs), 98
Refined grains, 356t–357t
Reflex, 95
Reflex incontinence, 316, 325
Registered nurse (RN), 1, 4t, 5
Registration, 20b
Regulations, 1
Regurgitation, 365, 374
    prevention of, 374
Rehabilitation, 2, 486
    assisting with, 490b
    communication in, 489, 489b
    definition of, 486
    economic aspects in, 489
    elimination, 487
    mobility in, 488, 489f
    needs, 486–492, 487b, 491b–492b
    nutrition in, 488
    person's setting, 490
    physical aspects of, 487–488
    programs, 490
    psychological aspects in, 489, 489b
    quality of life in, 491–492
    self-care, 487, 487f–488f, 488b
    social aspects in, 489, 489b
    whole person, 487–489, 487b
Rehabilitation team, 490
    role in, 490, 490b
Religion, 53, 55, 55b
    as factors affecting eating and nutrition,
        366
Reporting, 72–73, 72f, 72b
    definition of, 64, 71–74
    of incidents, 130
    in restraints, 156, 157f
    of time, 71–72, 72b
Representative, 10
Reproductive disorders, 523
Reproductive system, 523
    description of, 102–104, 103f–104f,
        111t–113t
Rescue breathing, 562
Reservoir, of microbes, 160
Resident groups, 13
Resident rights, 10–15, 11b
    to confidentiality, 12
    to freedom from abuse, mistreatment, and
        neglect, 13
    to freedom from restraint, 13
    to grievances, 13
    to information, 12, 12b
    to personal choice, 12, 13f
    to personal items, 13, 14f
    to privacy, 12, 12f
    to quality of life, 14–15, 14b
    to refuse treatment, 12
    to resident groups, 13
    to work, 13
Residents, definition of, 2
Residue-restricted diet, 359t–360t
Respect, 8b, 28b, 40b, 51b, 62b
    body mechanics and, 197b
    infection and, 173b
    isolation precautions and, 187b
    in moving of person, 212b
    restraints and, 157b
Respirations, 89, 100, 388, 400–401, 400b
    abnormal, 476, 476f
    counting, 401b
    function, altered, 476, 476b
Respirator, 180, 180f
Respiratory arrest, 562
    definition of, 555

Respiratory disorders, 517–519
  asthma, 518
  chronic bronchitis, 517
  chronic obstructive pulmonary disease, 517
  emphysema, 517, 517f
  influenza, 518, 518b
  pneumonia, 518, 518b
  tuberculosis, 518–519, 518b
Respiratory hygiene, 176b
Respiratory system, 100–101, 101f, 111t–113t
Respiratory tests, 477–478
Respiratory therapist, 4t
Respite care, 3b
Rest, 425, 430
  needs in, 425–433, 432b–433b
Restaurant-style menus, 368
Restorative aides, 486–487
Restorative nursing care, 486–487
Restraints, 144–158, 157b–158b
  alternatives to, 145, 145b, 146f
  application of, 154, 154b–156b, 156f
  belt, 150f, 152, 153f, 154b–156b
  chemical, 144, 146–147, 146b
  freedom from, 13
  hand and, 152f
  history of, 145
  informed consent for, 148
  jacket, 152–154, 153f, 154b–156b
  law, rules, and guidelines in, 148, 148b
  least restrictive method, 148
  mitt, 152, 153f, 154b–156b
  physical, 144, 146–147, 146b
  quick-release buckles for, 150f
  quick release knot for, 151f
  reporting and recording in, 156, 157f
  risks from, 147, 147b
  safety guidelines in, 148, 149b–150b, 154b
  strangulation caused by, 147, 147f
  vest, 150f, 152–154, 154b–156b
  wrist, 152, 153f, 155b–156b
Restrict fluids, 379t
Resuscitate, definition of, 555
Retina, 97
Retirement, 110
Reverse Trendelenburg's position, 237t
Rheumatoid arthritis, 506
Right atrium, 98, 99f
Right lower quadrant (RLQ), 83
Right lymphatic duct, 100
Right upper quadrant (RUQ), 83
Right ventricle, 98, 99f
Rights, 8b, 10–17, 16b–17b, 28b, 40b, 51b, 62b
  body mechanics and, 197b
  infection and, 173b
  isolation precautions and, 187b
  in moving of person, 212b
  patient, 10
  resident, 10–15, 11b
  restraints and, 157b
Rigor mortis, 574
  definition of, 569
Risk factor, 53
Risk management, 129–130
RLQ. See Right lower quadrant
RN. See Registered nurse
Roles and responsibilities, 21–22, 21b–22b
ROM. See Range of motion
Room furniture and equipment, 235–243
  bathroom and, 241, 241f
  bed as, 236b
  bedside stand as, 239, 239f
  call system as, 240–241, 240f–241f, 241b
  chairs as, 240
  closet and drawer space in, 241–242, 241b
  over-bed table as, 239, 239f
  privacy curtains as, 240

Roots, 78–79, 78f, 80f, 81t
Rotation, 412, 414b
Rummaging, 546, 547b–548b
RUQ. See Right upper quadrant

S
Saccule, 97f
Safe handling programs, 193, 193b
Safe move, planning of, 200–201, 200b
Safety, 117–132, 118b, 131b–132b
  accident risk factors in, 118
  burn prevention, 120, 120b
  choking and, 121–122, 121f–123f, 121b–122b
  disasters and, 117, 126–128, 126b
  electrical, 124, 125f
  equipment accident prevention, 124–125, 124f, 124b
  fall prevention and, 135b. See also Fall prevention
  fire, 126–127, 126b–127b, 127f
  hazardous chemical, 117, 125, 125f
  identification of person, 119, 119f, 119b
  job, 47
  poisoning prevention, 120, 120b
  promotion of, 118b
  quality and, 7–8, 7b
  risk management in, 129–130
  stretcher, 125
  suffocation prevention, 121–122, 121b
  wheelchair, 125
Safety bars, 241
Safety data sheets, 125
Safety needs, 54
Safety razors, 297, 298b
Salivary glands, 101
SCA. See Sudden cardiac arrest
Scabies, 291–292, 292f
Schizophrenia, 532–533, 533b
School, preparing for, 45
Sclera, 97
Scope of practice, 21
Scrotum, 103, 103f
Security needs, 54
Seizures, 565–566
  definition of, 555
  emergency care for, 565f, 566b
Self-actualization, 54
Self-care, 487, 487f–488f, 488b
Self-centered behavior, 60
Self-esteem, 53–54
Self-neglect, 31
Semen, 103
Semi-Fowler's position, 189, 237t
Semicircular canals, 97, 97f
Seminal vesicle, 103, 103f
Sense organs, 97
Sexual abuse, 36, 115
Sexual behavior, inappropriate, 60
Sexual harassment, 50
Sexual misconduct, professional, 31–32
Sexual needs, 114, 114b
Sexual violence, 39
Sexuality, 108, 114–115, 114f, 114b, 547
Sexually aggressive behaviors, 115, 115b
Sexually transmitted diseases (STDs), 523, 523b
Shampoo caps, 295
Shampooing, of hair, 295, 295f, 295b–297b
Shaving, 297–300, 297f–298f, 298b–299b
Shear, 464–465
Shearing, 199, 201, 201f
Shingles, 526–527, 526f
Shock, 564
  definition of, 555
Short bones, 92

Short-term residents, 3b
Shoulder, exercise for, 415b–416b, 416f
Shower benches, 280, 281f
Shower chairs, 280, 281f
Shower trolleys, 280, 281f
Showers, 280–284, 282b–284b
  safety in, 281–284, 282b
Shroud, 575f
Silence, 59–60, 60b
Simple face mask, 482t
Sitting position, 465f
Sitz bath, 458t–459t, 461b–462b
Skilled nursing facilities, 3
Skin
  anatomy of, 92, 92f
  disorders, 526–527, 526f
  end-of-life care considerations in, 572
  functions of, 92
  protection of, in moving, of person, 201–202, 201f, 201b
Skin care, in pressure injuries, 471b
Skin tears, 446–448, 447f, 447b
  preventing, 447b
Skull, 96f
Slander, 31, 33
Sleep, 430–433
  deprivation, 425, 431
  disorders in, 431
  factors affecting, 431, 431b
  promoting, 431–433, 432b
Sleep apnea, 425, 431
  devices for, 483–485
Sleepwalking, 425, 431
Slings, 225, 225f
Slough, 467, 468f–469f
Small intestine, 101
Small-volume enema, 349–351, 349b–350b, 351f
Smell, impaired, accident risks and, 118
Smoke, odors from, 235
Smoking, 43, 517
Social changes, 110, 110f, 110b
Social dining, 368, 368f
Social distancing (physical distancing), 128
Social interaction, 8b, 28b, 40b, 51b, 62b
  body mechanics and, 197b
  infection and, 173b
  isolation precautions and, 187b
  in moving of person, 212b
  restraints and, 157b
Social relationships, 110, 110f
Social worker, 4t
Sodium-controlled diet, 359t–360t, 361
Solid fats, 358
Source individual, 172
Special beds, 472, 472f
Special needs, persons with, 61–62
Specific immunity, 104
Specimen collection, 186–187, 434–445, 435b, 444b–445b
  sputum, 442–444, 442b–443b, 443f
  stool, 440–442, 440b–442b, 442f
  urine, 435–440, 435b
Speech, 46, 493–502, 572
Speech disorders, 496, 501b–502b
Speech-language pathologist/speech therapist, 4t
Sperm, 103
Sphincters, 94
Sphygmomanometer, 402, 402f
Spinal cord, 96, 96f
Spinal cord injury, 513, 513f, 514b
Spinal nerves, 96
Spiritual needs, 570, 570b
Spleen, 100
Splints, 418t–419t

Sputum, 476b
    collection of, 442–444, 442b–443b, 443f
    definition of, 434, 442
Staffing, 5
Stand and pivot transfers, 217–223, 217f, 217b
Standard electronic thermometer, 391t
Standard full-sling, 225
Standard precautions, 171, 175, 176b
Standards, 7
Stapes, 97, 97f
Starchy vegetables, 356t–357t
Stasis ulcers, 448
STDs. *See* Sexually transmitted diseases
Sterile, 159, 162
Sterilization, 159, 169, 169f
Stethoscope, 388, 396–397, 396f–397f, 396b–397b
Stimulus, 95
Stoma, 344, 351f
Stomach, 101
Stool specimens, 440–442, 440b–442b, 442f
Stools, 344–345, 345f–346f
Straight catheter, 333–334
Strangulation, 147, 147f
Stress, 42, 48–49, 530
    definition of, 529
    managing, 49
Stress incontinence, 316, 325
Stressor, 529
Stretcher safety, 125, 215, 216f–217f, 216b
Stroke, 511, 511f, 511b–512b, 565, 565b
Sub-acute care, 2
Subcutaneous tissue, 92, 92f
Subjective data, 64, 68
Substance use disorder, 534–535, 534b–535b
Sudden cardiac arrest (SCA), 557, 557f
    definition of, 555
Suffixes, 78–79, 78f, 82f, 82t
Suffocation, 117, 121
    prevention of, 121–122, 121b
Suicide, 536, 536b
    definition of, 529
Suicide contagion, 536
    definition of, 529
Sundowning, 544, 547b–548b
    definition of, 539
Superficial, term, 84
Superior, term, 84
Superior vena cava, 99, 99f
Supervision, in delegation, 25
Supination, 412, 414b
Supine position, 189, 195, 195f, 465f
Support devices, 197–198, 197f
Suppository, 344, 348
Surgical asepsis, 159
Surgical bed, 244, 245f, 258–260, 258b, 259f
Survey, 1, 7, 8b
Surveyor, 1, 8b
Susceptible hosts, 162
Swallowing, 101
    problems, as factors affecting eating and
        nutrition, 367
Sweat, 92
Sweat glands, 92, 92f
Sympathetic nervous system, 97
Synovial fluid, 93
Synovial membrane, 93
System, 90f
    circulatory, 98–99, 98f–99f, 111t–113t
    definition of, 89–90
    digestive, 101, 101f, 111t–113t
    endocrine, 105, 105f
    immune, 104–105
    integumentary, 92, 92f, 111t–113t
    lymphatic, 100, 100f

System *(Continued)*
    musculo-skeletal, 92–94, 111t–113t
    nervous, 95–97, 111t–113t
    reproductive, 102–104, 103f–104f, 111t–113t
    respiratory, 100–101, 101f, 111t–113t
    urinary, 102, 102f, 111t–113t
Systemic infection, 160
Systole, 98, 401
Systolic pressure, 388, 401

T
T lymphocytes (T cells), 104
Tachycardia, 388
Tachypnea, 475–476, 476f
Tape, 453–454, 454f, 454b
Tartar, 262
Taste buds, 97, 101
TB. *See* Tuberculosis
TBI. *See* Traumatic brain injury
Team nursing, 6
Teamwork, 8b, 28b, 40b, 42, 45–48, 51b, 62b
    body mechanics and, 197b
    infection and, 173b
    isolation precautions and, 187b
    in moving of person, 212b
    restraints and, 157b
TED. *See* Thrombo-embolic disease
Teeth
    brushing and flossing of, 262–267, 263b, 264f
    structure and function of, 261, 261f
Temperature, comfort and, 234, 234b
Temporal artery temperature, 390b
Temporal artery thermometer, 391t
Temporal bone, 97f
Tendons, 94
Terminal illness, 1–2, 569–570
    definition of, 569
Testes, 103, 103f, 105f
Testosterone, 103
Tetany, 105t
Thalamus, 96f
The Joint Commission, restraint guidelines
    and, 145
Thermometers
    definition of, 388–389
    electronic, 391t, 392f, 393b, 394f
    glass, 394–396, 395f, 395b
    types of, 390, 390b, 391t
Thickened liquids, 379t
Thoracic duct (left lymphatic duct), 100
Threats, 39
    bomb, 126
Thrombo-embolic disease (TED), 450
Thrombus, 450
Thumb, exercise for, 415b–416b, 417f
Thymosin, 105t
Thymus gland, 100, 105f, 105t
Thyroid gland, 105f, 105t
Thyroid hormone, 105t
Thyroid-stimulating hormone (TSH), 105t
TIA. *See* Transient ischemic attack
Time, 71f, 72b
Tinnitus, 493
Tissue, 89, 91
Toes, exercise for, 415b–416b, 417f
Toilet, transferring the person to and from,
    222–223, 222b–223b, 223f
Toileting sling, 225
Tonic-clonic (grand mal) seizures, 565
Tonsils, 100
Torts, 33
Touch, 58
    impaired, accident risks and, 118
    sexuality and, 114

Trachea, 100
Traction, 509, 509f, 509b
    cervical, 513
Training program, 19, 19f, 19b
Transfer, 214
    wheelchair to tub, 489f
Transfer belts, 133, 139–141, 139f–140f, 139b–140b, 211f, 217
Transferring the person, 214–231, 214b, 216f–217f, 230b–231b
    from bed, to chair or wheelchair, 218–221, 218b–219b, 220f
    to bed, from chair or wheelchairs, 221–222, 221f, 221b–222b
    delegation guidelines for, 215b
    lateral transfer for, 223, 224f, 224b
    mechanical lift for, 224–231, 224f–225f, 226b–228b, 227f, 229f
    promoting safety and comfort, 215b
    slings for, 225
    stand and pivot, 217–223, 217f, 217b
    to and from the toilet, 222–223, 222b–223b, 223f
Transient incontinence, 316, 325
Transient ischemic attack (TIA), 511
Translators, 60b
Transmission-based precautions, 177–179, 177f, 178b–179b
    face shields, 180, 180b, 182f
    gloves, 178b, 180, 181f–184f, 181b
    goggles, 180, 180b, 182f
    gowns, 176b, 178b, 180, 182f
    masks, 176b, 180, 182f–184f, 186f
    specimens, collection of, 186–187
    transporting persons, 187–188
Transplant, 162
Transportation, 45
Transporting persons, 187–188
Traumatic brain injury (TBI), 514
Treatment
    definition of, 10
    refusing, 12
Tremors, 512
Trendelenburg's position, 237t
    reverse, 237t
Tricuspid valve, 98, 99f
Trimming, of nails, 300, 301f
Trochanter roll, 418t–419t
TSH. *See* Thyroid-stimulating hormone
Tub baths, 280, 281f, 282b–284b
    safety in, 281–284, 282b
Tub transfer, wheelchair to, 489f
Tube feeding, 373f
Tuberculosis (TB), 518–519, 518b
Tumor, 504, 504f
    in breast, 504f
    definition of, 503
Turn clock, 470
Turning pad, 201f
Turning persons, 206–209, 206b–208b, 207f
    logrolling in, 199, 208–209, 208b–209b, 209f
24-hour urine specimen, 439
Tympanic membrane temperature, 393b, 394f
Tympanic membrane thermometer, 391t
Type 1 diabetes, 523
Type 2 diabetes, 523

U
Ulcer, 446, 464–465
Ulcerative colitis, 519
Unaffected side, definition of, 304–305
Uncircumcised, definition of, 271, 284, 284f
Unconscious, definition of, 117
Unconscious person, oral hygiene for,
    265–267, 265f, 265b–266b

Under-garment, definition of, 304
Underarms, shaving of, 300
Undressing, 304–315, 305b, 307b, 308f, 315b
Unethical student behavior, 51
Unintentional torts, 33
Ureter, 102
Urethral sphincters, 94
Urge incontinence, 316, 325
Urinals, 321–323, 321b–322b, 322f
Urinary elimination, safety of, 317b
Urinary frequency, 316–317
Urinary incontinence, 325–331
    bladder training for, 331–332
    definition of, 316–317
    functional incontinence, 316, 325
    managing, 325–326, 325b–326b
    mixed incontinence, 316, 325
    over-flow incontinence, 316, 325
    products for, 327–331, 327f, 327b–329b,
        330f
    reflex incontinence, 316, 325
    stress incontinence, 316, 325
    transient incontinence, 316
    types of, 325
    urge incontinence, 316
Urinary needs, 316–332, 317b, 331b–332b
Urinary retention, 316–317
Urinary system
    description of, 102, 102f, 111t–113t
    disorders, 521–522, 521b
Urinary tract infection, 521, 521b
Urinary urgency, 316–317
Urination
    bedpans for, 318–321, 318f, 319b–320b,
        320f–321f
    commodes for, 323–325, 323f, 323b–324b
    definition of, 316
    normal, 317–325, 317b, 318f
    rules for, 317b
    urinals for, 321–323, 321b–322b, 322f
Urine
    color chart for, 318f
    description of, 102
    observation of, 317
Urine specimens, 435–440, 435b
    catheter, 438, 438f
    midstream, 437–438, 437f, 437b–438b
    pan for collecting, 436f
    random, 435–437, 436b
    24-hour, 439
Urine testing, 439–440, 439b
    using reagent strips, 439f, 440b
Uterus, 103, 103f

V
Vaccination, 171
Vaccine, 171
Vagina, 103, 103f
Validation therapy, 552–553
Valves, 98
Vancomycin-resistant *Enterococci* (VRE), 160
Vas deferens, 103, 103f
Vascular ulcers, 448
Vegetables, 356t–357t
Vein, 89, 99, 99f
Venous ulcers, 448, 448f
Ventilation, comfort and, 234, 234b
Ventricles, 98
Ventricular fibrillation (VF, V-fib), 561, 561f
Verbal abuse, 36
Verbal communication, 53, 56–57, 57f, 57b
Vertigo, 493
Vest restraints, 150f, 152–154, 153f,
    154b–156b
Video interview, 582
Vietnamese Americans, 56b
Vision
    central, 497
    end-of-life care considerations of, 572
    impaired, 498, 499b
    loss of, accident risks and, 118
    low, 493, 498
Vision problems, 493–502
Visually impaired persons, 371, 371f
Vital signs
    body temperature. *See* Body temperature
    definition of, 388
    description of, 389–406, 389b
    factors affecting, 389b
    pulse. *See* Pulse
    respirations, 388, 400–401, 400b
Vitamins, 358
Vitreous humor, 97
Voiding equipment, 318, 318b
Voluntary muscles, 94
Vomiting, 519
Vomitus, 519
    definition of, 503
VRE. *See* Vancomycin-resistant *Enterococci*
Vulnerable adult, 31, 36, 36b
Vulva, 104

W
Walkers, 420, 420f–421f, 421b
Walking aids, 420–421
Wall outlet, 481, 481f
Wandering, 544f, 547b–548b

Water, 358, 383–384, 383f–384f, 383b–384b
    of microbes, 160
Waterproof under-pad, 244–245, 246f
WBCs. *See* White blood cells
Weight measurements, 406–411, 407f–408f,
    407b–409b, 410f
Wernicke's aphasia, 496
Wheel locks, 138, 138f
Wheelchair
    parts of, 216f
    re-positioning in, 211–213, 211f–212f
    restraint straps, 151f
    safety in, 215, 216f–217f, 216b
        considerations for, 125
    transferring from bed to, 218–221,
        218b–219b, 220f
    to tub transfer, 489f
White blood cells (WBCs), 98
Whole grains, 356t–357t
Withdrawal, 60
Withdrawal syndrome, 535b
    definition of, 529
Wong-Baker FACES® Pain Rating Scale,
    427, 427f
Word element, 78
    learning, 79
Work
    in another state, 21
    planning, 48, 48b
    preparing for, 45
    right to, 13
Work ethics, 42–52, 43f, 44b, 45f, 52b
Work practice controls, 171, 171f
Work-related injuries, 191–193, 192b
    prevention of, in moving, of person,
        202b–203b
Workplace violence, 117, 128, 128b–129b
Wound
    cleaning, 454f
    definition of, 446
Wound care, 446–463, 447b, 462b–463b
    circulatory ulcers, 448–453, 448f, 448b
    skin tears, 447–448, 447f, 447b
Wound dressings, 453–456
    applying, 454–456, 454b–455b
    dry, non-sterile, 454f, 455b–456b
    functions of, 453
    securing, 453–454
Wrist
    exercise for, 415b–416b, 417f
    restraints, 152, 153f, 155b–156b